呼吸与危重症医学 2019—2020

Respiratory & Critical Care Medicine 2019—2020

顾　　问	罗慰慈	朱元珏	钟南山	刘又宁		
名誉主编	王　辰	陈荣昌				
主　　编	瞿介明					
副 主 编	曹　彬	陈良安	李为民	李时悦	沈华浩	
学术秘书	代华平	刘亚君				

编　　委（以姓氏汉语拼音为序）

蔡后荣	曹　彬	曹　洁	陈　虹	陈良安	陈荣昌	代华平
高占成	葛慧青	韩　芳	贺　蓓	胡成平	季颖群	赖国祥
赖克方	黎毅敏	李惠萍	李　琦	李　强	李庆云	李时悦
李为民	梁宗安	林江涛	刘辉国	刘晓菊	刘亚君	马　壮
宁　文	潘频华	冉丕鑫	瞿介明	单广良	申昆玲	沈华浩
施举红	施　毅	时国朝	宋元林	孙德俊	孙加源	孙永昌
王长征	王　辰	王广发	王　健	王　玮	文富强	肖　丹
肖　伟	肖　毅	解立新	熊维宁	徐金富	徐作军	应颂敏
曾奕明	瞿振国	詹庆元	张　艰	张　杰	张湘燕	郑劲平
郑则广	周建英	周　新				

中华医学电子音像出版社
CHINESE MEDICAL MULTIMEDIA PRESS
北　京

图书在版编目(CIP)数据

呼吸与危重症医学. 2019—2020 / 瞿介明主编. —北京:中华医学电子音像出版社,2020.12
ISBN 978 - 7 - 83005 - 333 - 8

Ⅰ. ①呼… Ⅱ. ①瞿… Ⅲ. ①呼吸系统疾病-险症-诊疗 Ⅳ. ①R56

中国版本图书馆 CIP 数据核字(2020)第 231186 号

网址:www.cma-cmc.com.cn(出版物查询、网上书店)

呼吸与危重症医学 2019—2020

HUXI YU WEIZHONGZHENG YIXUE 2019—2020

主　　编:	瞿介明
策划编辑:	史仲静　崔竹青青
责任编辑:	崔竹青青
校　　对:	张　娟
责任印刷:	李振坤
出版发行:	中华医学电子音像出版社
通信地址:	北京市西城区东河沿街 69 号中华医学会 610 室
邮　　编:	100052
E-mail:	cma - cmc@cma.org.cn
购书热线:	010 - 51322677
经　　销:	新华书店
印　　刷:	北京云浩印刷有限责任公司
开　　本:	889mm×1194mm　1/16
印　　张:	38.75
字　　数:	1570 千字
版　　次:	2020 年 12 月第 1 版　2020 年 12 月第 1 次印刷
定　　价:	98.00 元

版权所有　侵权必究

购买本社图书,凡有缺、倒、脱页者,本社负责调换

内容提要

本书为"呼吸与危重症年度进展"系列丛书之一，体现呼吸与危重症医学新进展、新观点，是每年中华医学会呼吸病学分会年会学术交流的重要资料。2020年新型冠状病毒肺炎疫情突发，疫情之下出版的此书仍然秉持最前沿、最客观、最实用的理念，旨在为呼吸与危重症医学同道系统地了解呼吸与危重症医学前沿讯息提供简便、客观的途径。本书内容涵盖了烟草病学、慢性阻塞性肺疾病、支气管哮喘、呼吸系统感染、间质性肺疾病、肺癌、睡眠呼吸障碍、危重症医学、肺功能检查、纵隔与胸膜疾病及介入呼吸病学11个领域年度关注的重点问题，具有学术引领性和规范性的特点。本书囊括了近1年来世界范围内呼吸与危重症医学最前沿的学术动向，紧密围绕呼吸与危重症医学临床及基础研究的焦点、难点问题，具有权威性、学术性、先进性和实用性。本书可作为呼吸与危重症医学医疗、护理从业者，实习医师，研究生的案头工具书和参考用书。

编者名单（以姓氏汉语拼音为序）

白　冲	海军军医大学附属长海医院呼吸与危重症医学科
白　莉	陆军军医大学第二附属医院呼吸与危重症医学科
蔡柏蔷	中国医学科学院北京协和医院呼吸与危重症医学科
蔡绍曦	南方医科大学南方医院呼吸与危重症医学科
蔡湘龙	武警特色医学中心呼吸和重症医学科
曹　洁	天津医科大学总医院呼吸与危重症医学科
陈成水	温州医科大学附属第一医院呼吸与危重症医学科
陈恩国	浙江大学医学院附属邵逸夫医院呼吸与危重症医学科
陈　昉	南方医科大学中西医结合医院呼吸与危重症医学科
陈　宏	哈尔滨医科大学附属第二医院呼吸与危重症医学科
陈　虹	重庆医科大学附属第一医院呼吸与危重症医学科
陈丽嫦	南方医科大学珠江医院呼吸与危重症医学科
陈良安	解放军总医院第一医学中心呼吸与危重症医学科
陈　平	中南大学呼吸疾病研究所　中南大学湘雅二医院呼吸与危重症科　湖南省呼吸疾病诊治中心
陈　茜	浙江大学医学院附属第一医院呼吸与危重症医学科
陈荣昌	深圳市人民医院呼吸与危重症医学科　深圳市呼吸疾病研究所　广州医科大学附属第一医院国家呼吸系统疾病临床医学研究中心
陈　锐	苏州大学附属第二医院呼吸科
陈　夕	重庆医科大学附属第二医院呼吸与危重症医学科
陈小蓉	厦门大学附属中山医院呼吸与危重症医学科
陈亚红	北京大学第三医院呼吸与危重症医学科
陈延斌	苏州大学附属第一医院呼吸与危重症医学科
陈　燕	中南大学湘雅二医院呼吸与危重症医学科
陈玥晗	广州医科大学附属第一医院呼吸与危重症医学科　国家呼吸医学临床研究中心　呼吸疾病国家重点实验室　广州呼吸健康研究院
陈志华	浙江省呼吸疾病诊治及研究重点实验室　浙江大学医学院附属第二医院呼吸与危重症医学科
褚淑媛	桂林医学院附属医院呼吸与危重症医学科
崔节伟	解放军总医院第一医学中心呼吸内科
崔景华	广东省人民医院（广东省医学科学院）呼吸与危重症医学科
崔亚楠	中南大学湘雅二医院呼吸与危重症医学科
崔　烨	首都医科大学基础医学院免疫学系
崔越亭	山西医科大学第二医院呼吸与危重症医学科
代华平	中日友好医院国际呼吸医学中心呼吸与危重症医学科
戴然然	上海交通大学医学院附属瑞金医院呼吸与危重症医学科
戴　威	温州医科大学附属第二医院呼吸与危重症医学科
戴　钰	解放军总医院第一医学中心呼吸与危重症医学科
戴元荣	温州医科大学附属第二医院呼吸与危重症医学科
邓海怡	广州医科大学附属第一医院呼吸与危重症医学科　国家呼吸系统疾病临床研究中心　呼吸疾病

	国家重点实验室　广州呼吸健康研究院
邓　琳	广州医科大学附属第一医院呼吸与危重症医学科　国家呼吸系统疾病临床医学研究中心　呼吸疾病国家重点实验室　广州呼吸健康研究院
邓　旺	重庆医科大学附属第二医院呼吸与危重症医学科
董　亮	山东大学齐鲁医院呼吸与危重症医学科
杜旭菲	浙江大学医学院附属第二医院呼吸与危重症医学科
段玉香	上海交通大学医学院附属同仁医院呼吸与危重症医学科
范　红	四川大学华西医院呼吸与危重症医学科
范亚丽	首都医科大学附属北京朝阳医院职业病与中毒医学科　间质性肺疾病临床诊疗与研究中心　北京呼吸疾病研究所
范雨辰	重庆医科大学附属第一医院呼吸与危重症医学科
方媛媛	华中科技大学同济医学院附属同济医院呼吸与危重症医学科
费广鹤	安徽医科大学第一附属医院呼吸与危重症医学科
冯　缤	暨南大学第一附属医院呼吸与危重症医学科
冯起校	南方医科大学中西医结合医院呼吸与危重症医学科
高兴林	广东省人民医院呼吸与危重症医学科
高　怡	广州医科大学附属第一医院呼吸与危重症医学科　国家呼吸系统疾病临床医学研究中心　呼吸疾病国家重点实验室　广州呼吸健康研究院
高占成	北京大学人民医院呼吸与危重症医学科
耿　菁	中日友好医院国际呼吸医学中心呼吸与危重症医学科
郭　建	中国医学科学院北京协和医院呼吸与危重症医学科
郭　健	上海市肺科医院呼吸与危重症医学科
郭述良	重庆医科大学附属第一医院呼吸与危重症医学科
郭佑民	西安交通大学第一附属医院呼吸与危重症医学科
何婉媚	中山大学附属第一医院呼吸与危重症医学科
何　炜	复旦大学附属上海市第五人民医院呼吸与危重症医学科
何玉坤	北京大学人民医院呼吸与危重症医学科
贺斌峰	陆军军医大学第二附属医院（重庆新桥医院）呼吸与危重医学科
洪　谊	广州医科大学附属第一医院呼吸与危重症医学科　国家呼吸系统疾病临床医学研究中心　呼吸疾病国家重点实验室　广州呼吸健康研究院
胡　斌	复旦大学附属中山医院徐汇医院呼吸与危重症医学科
胡　克	武汉大学人民医院呼吸与危重症医学二科
胡雪君	中国医科大学附属第一医院呼吸与危重症医学科
黄丹辉	南方医科大学南方医院呼吸与危重症医学科
黄凤祥	郑州大学第一附属医院呼吸与危重症医学科
黄　红	中国医科大学附属第一医院呼吸与危重症医学科
黄　怡	海军军医大学第一附属医院呼吸与危重症医学科
季婷芬	浙江大学医学院附属第一医院呼吸与危重症医学科
简文华	广州医科大学附属第一医院呼吸与危重症医学科　国家呼吸系统疾病临床医学研究中心　呼吸疾病国家重点实验室　广州呼吸健康研究院
姜淑娟	山东省立医院呼吸与危重症医学科
蒋军红	苏州大学附属第一医院呼吸与危重症医学科
蒋紫玉	广州医科大学附属第一医院呼吸与危重症医学科　国家呼吸系统疾病临床医学研究中心　呼吸疾病国家重点实验室　广州呼吸健康研究院
解立新	解放军总医院呼吸与危重症医学部
金旭如	温州医科大学附属第一医院呼吸与危重症医学科

柯明耀	厦门医学院附属第二医院呼吸病医院呼吸与危重症医学科
赖克方	广州医科大学附属第一医院呼吸与危重症医学科　国家呼吸医学临床研究中心　呼吸疾病国家重点实验室　广州呼吸健康研究院
李　丹	吉林大学第一医院呼吸与危重症医学科
李风森	新疆医科大学第四附属医院(新疆维吾尔自治区中医医院)呼吸与危重症医学科
李国强	武警特色医学中心呼吸和重症医学科
李和权	浙江大学医学院附属第一医院呼吸与危重症医学科
李　静	广东省人民医院(广东省医学科学院)呼吸与危重症医学科
李　俊	中日友好医院国际呼吸医学中心呼吸与危重症医学科
李　明	同济大学附属第十人民医院呼吸与危重症医学科
李　强	同济大学附属东方医院呼吸与危重症医学科
李庆云	上海交通大学医学院附属瑞金医院呼吸与危重症医学科　上海交通大学医学院呼吸病研究所
李善群	复旦大学附属中山医院呼吸内科
李时悦	广州医科大学附属第一医院呼吸与危重症医学科　广州呼吸健康研究院　国家呼吸系统疾病临床医学研究中心
李诗琪	上海交通大学医学院附属瑞金医院呼吸与危重症医学科　上海交通大学医学院呼吸病研究所
李雯邹	浙江大学医学院附属第二医院呼吸与危重症医学科
李亚清	中国科学院大学附属肿瘤医院/浙江省肿瘤医院呼吸与危重症医学科
李鋆璐	郑州大学第一附属医院呼吸与危重症医学科
梁红阁	北京协和医院呼吸与危重症科
梁晓林	广州医科大学附属第一医院呼吸与危重症医学科　国家呼吸系统疾病临床医学研究中心　呼吸疾病国家重点实验室　广州呼吸健康研究院
梁振宇	深圳市人民医院呼吸与危重症医学科　深圳市呼吸疾病研究所　国家呼吸系统疾病临床医学研究中心
梁志欣	解放军总医院第一医学中心呼吸内科
林　山	中山大学附属第一医院呼吸与危重症医学科
刘国梁	中日医院呼吸中心呼吸与危重症医学科
刘宏炜	上海市奉贤区中心医院呼吸与危重症医学科
刘辉国	华中科技大学同济医学院附属同济医院呼吸与危重症医学科
刘锦铭	上海市肺科医院呼吸与危重症医学科
刘瑞麟	同济大学附属同济医院呼吸与危重症医学科
刘远灵	广东省人民医院呼吸与危重症医学科
刘耘充	北京大学第三医院呼吸与危重症医学科
刘正媛	浙江大学医学院附属第二医院呼吸与危重症医学科　浙江省呼吸疾病诊治及研究重点实验室
逯　勇	首都医科大学附属北京朝阳医院北京呼吸疾病研究所
罗　娅	中国医学科学院基础医学研究所　北京协和医学院基础学院
马金铃	湖南省人民医院呼吸与危重症医学科
马千里	陆军军医大学第二附属医院(重庆新桥医院)呼吸与危重症医学科
马　青	重庆医科大学附属第二医院呼吸与危重症医学科
马昕茜	北京大学人民医院呼吸与危重症医学科
麦仲伦	南方医科大学中西医结合医院呼吸与危重症医学科
茅　靖	上海市松江区方塔中医医院呼吸与危重症医学科
苗丽君	郑州大学第一附属医院呼吸与危重症医学科
莫碧文	桂林医学院附属医院呼吸与危重症医学科
欧　琼	广东省人民医院(广东省医学科学院)呼吸与危重症医学科睡眠中心
欧阳若芸	中南大学湘雅二医院呼吸与危重症医学科

潘瑞丽	北京协和医院呼吸与危重症科
彭丽萍	吉林大学第一医院呼吸与危重症医学科
齐　咏	河南省人民医院呼吸与危重症医学科
祁亚楠	河南省人民医院呼吸与危重症医学科
任　玺	南方医科大学中西医结合医院呼吸与危重症医学科
任雁宏	中日友好医院国际呼吸医学中心呼吸与危重症医学科
邵喆婳	浙江大学呼吸疾病研究所
佘丹阳	解放军总医院第一医学中心呼吸科
申永春	四川大学华西医院呼吸与危重症医学科　生物治疗国家重点实验室呼吸病学研究室
沈华浩	浙江大学医学院附属第二医院呼吸与危重症医学科
沈　凌	浙江大学医学院附属杭州市第一人民医院呼吸内科
沈　宁	北京大学第三医院呼吸与危重症医学科
施　毅	南京大学医学院附属金陵医院呼吸与危重症医学科
史文佳	解放军总医院呼吸与危重症学部
时国朝	上海交通大学医学院附属瑞金医院呼吸与危重症医学科
史兆雯	上海中医药大学附属普陀医院呼吸与危重症医学科
宋新宇	广州医科大学附属第一医院呼吸与危重症医学科　广州呼吸健康研究院　国家呼吸医学中心
孙　兵	首都医科大学附属北京朝阳医院呼吸与危重症医学科　北京呼吸疾病研究所
孙德俊	内蒙古自治区人民医院呼吸与危重症医学科
孙加源	上海交通大学附属胸科医院呼吸与危重症医学科
孙永昌	北京大学第三医院呼吸与危重症医学科
汤　楠	北京生命科学研究所
汤　葳	上海交通大学医学院附属瑞金医院呼吸与危重医学科
唐学义	河南省人民医院呼吸与危重症医学科
童　瑾	重庆医科大学附属第二医院呼吸与危重症医学科
童　翔	四川大学华西医院呼吸与危重症医学科
汪金林	广州医科大学附属第一医院呼吸与危重症学科　广州呼吸健康研究院
汪　蜀	上海同济大学附属东方医院呼吸与危重症医学科
王　蓓	山西医科大学第二医院呼吸与危重症医学科
王昌惠	上海市第十人民医院呼吸与危重症医学科
王导新	重庆医科大学附属第二医院呼吸与危重症医学科
王　飞	广州医科大学附属第一医院呼吸与危重症医学科　国家呼吸系统疾病临床医学研究中心　呼吸疾病国家重点实验室　广州呼吸健康研究院
王凤燕	深圳市人民医院呼吸与危重症医学科　深圳市呼吸疾病研究所　国家呼吸系统疾病临床医学研究中心
王关嵩	陆军军医大学第二附属医院(重庆新桥医院)呼吸与危重医学科
王广发	北京大学第一医院呼吸和危重症医学科
王华南	解放军总医院第一医学中心呼吸内科
王　瑾	上海市静安区市北医院呼吸与危重症医学科
王　婧	苏州大学附属第二医院呼吸科
王　婧	中国医学科学院基础医学研究所　北京协和医学院基础学院
王　娟	解放军总医院第一医学中心呼吸内科
王李强	广州医科大学附属第一医院呼吸与危重症医学科　国家呼吸系统疾病临床研究中心　呼吸疾病国家重点实验室　广州呼吸健康研究院
王拢拢	广东省人民医院(广东省医学科学院)呼吸与危重症医学科睡眠中心
王　平	解放军总医院呼吸与危重症学部

王　强	青岛大学附属医院呼吸与危重症医学科
王　冉	中南大学呼吸疾病研究所　中南大学湘雅二医院呼吸与危重症科　湖南省呼吸疾病诊治中心
王　睿	首都医科大学附属北京朝阳医院呼吸与危重症医学科　北京呼吸疾病研究所
王　玮	中国医科大学附属第一医院呼吸与危重症医学科
王晓丹	复旦大学附属中山医院呼吸与危重症医学科
王晓斐	上海交通大学医学院附属瑞金医院呼吸与危重症医学科
王晓娜	北京协和医院呼吸与危重症医学科
王雄彪	上海中医药大学附属普陀医院呼吸与危重症医学科
王　彦	天津医科大学总医院呼吸与危重症医学科
王一喆	中国医科大学附属第一医院呼吸与危重症医学科
王译民	广州医科大学附属第一医院呼吸与危重症医学科　国家呼吸系统疾病临床医学研究中心　呼吸疾病国家重点实验室　广州呼吸健康研究院
王悦虹	浙江大学医学院附属第一医院呼吸与危重症医学科
卫　平	同济大学附属上海市肺科医院呼吸与危重症医学科
文富强	四川大学华西医院呼吸与危重症医学科　生物治疗国家重点实验室呼吸病学研究室
吴琳颖	浙江大学医学院附属第一医院呼吸与危重症医学科
吴　珍	解放军总医院第一医学中心呼吸与危重症医学科
夏敬文	复旦大学附属华山医院呼吸与危重症医学科
肖　毅	北京协和医院呼吸与危重症医学科
谢俊刚	华中科技大学同济医学院附属同济医院呼吸与危重症医学科
邢丽华	郑州大学第一附属医院呼吸与危重症医学科
熊维宁	上海交通大学医学院附属第九人民医院呼吸与危重症医学科
徐金富	同济大学附属上海市肺科医院呼吸与危重症医学科
徐　瑜	陆军军医大学第二附属医院呼吸与危重症医学科
徐作军	北京协和医院呼吸与危重症医学科
许婷婷	广州医科大学附属第一医院呼吸与危重症医学科　国家呼吸医学临床研究中心　呼吸疾病国家重点实验室　广州呼吸健康研究院
杨文兰	上海市肺科医院肺功能科
杨新艳	广州医科大学附属第一医院呼吸与危重症医学科
杨　震	中国人民解放军总医院呼吸与危重症医学部
叶　枫	广州医科大学附属第一医院呼吸与危重症医学科　广州呼吸健康研究院
叶　俏	首都医科大学附属北京朝阳医院职业病与中毒医学科　间质性肺疾病临床诊疗与研究中心　北京呼吸疾病研究所
义　敏	浙江大学医学院附属第二医院呼吸与危重症医学科
应颂敏	浙江大学医学院附属第二医院呼吸与危重症医学科
于化鹏	南方医科大学珠江医院呼吸与危重症医学科
于　楠	陕西中医药大学附属医院呼吸与危重症医学科
袁海波	吉林大学第一医院呼吸与危重症医学科
云春梅	内蒙古自治区人民医院呼吸与危重症医学科
云俊杰	上海交通大学医学院附属第九人民医院呼吸与危重症医学科
曾惠清	厦门大学附属中山医院呼吸与危重症医学科
曾　勉	中山大学附属第一医院呼吸与危重症医学科
曾运祥	广州医科大学附属第一医院呼吸与危重症学科　广州呼吸健康研究院
詹　晨	广州医科大学附属第一医院呼吸与危重症医学科　国家呼吸系统疾病临床医学研究中心　呼吸疾病国家重点实验室　广州呼吸健康研究院
詹文志	广州医科大学附属第一医院呼吸与危重症医学科　国家呼吸系统疾病临床医学研究中心　呼吸

	疾病国家重点实验室　广州呼吸健康研究院
张　超	浙江大学呼吸疾病研究所
张冀松	浙江大学医学院附属邵逸夫医院呼吸与危重症医学科
张　艰	空军军医大学第一附属医院呼吸与危重症医学科
张剑青	昆明医科大学第一附属医院呼吸与危重症医学科
张锦涛	山东大学齐鲁医院呼吸与危重症医学科
张　静	北京大学第三医院呼吸与危重症医学科
张立强	北京大学第三医院呼吸与危重医学科
张　旻	上海交通大学附属第一人民医院呼吸与危重症医学科
张　娜	河南省人民医院呼吸与危重症医学科
张挪富	广州医科大学附属第一医院呼吸与危重症医学科　广州呼吸健康研究院
张清玲	广州医科大学附属第一医院呼吸与危重症医学科　国家呼吸系统疾病临床医学研究中心　呼吸疾病国家重点实验室　广州呼吸健康研究院
张韶泽	湖南省人民医院呼吸与危重症医学科
张　笋	广州医科大学附属第一医院呼吸与危重症医学科　广州呼吸健康研究院
张　伟	上海交通大学附属胸科医院呼吸与危重症医学科
张文静	陆军军医大学第二附属医院呼吸与危重症医学科
张晓雷	中日友好医院呼吸与危重症医学科
张　新	复旦大学附属中山医院呼吸与危重医学科
张旭华	宁夏医科大学总医院呼吸与危重医学科
张　岩	浙江大学呼吸与危重医学科
赵桂华	河南省人民医院呼吸与危重医学科
赵洪文	中国医科大学附属一院呼吸与危重症医学科
赵　立	中国医科大学附属盛京医院呼吸与危重症医学科
赵丽敏	河南省人民医院呼吸与危重症医学科
赵　帅	哈尔滨医科大学附属第二医院呼吸与危重症医学科
赵　微	解放军总医院第一医学中心呼吸与危重症医学科
赵亚滨	中国医科大学附属第一医院呼吸与危重症医学科
郑劲平	广州医科大学附属第一医院呼吸与危重症医学科　国家呼吸系统疾病临床医学研究中心　呼吸疾病国家重点实验室　广州呼吸健康研究院
郑青松	温州医科大学附属第二医院呼吸与危重症医学科
钟志成	深圳大学总医院呼吸内科
周承志	广州医科大学附属第一医院呼吸与危重症医学科　国家呼吸系统疾病临床研究中心　呼吸疾病国家重点实验室　广州呼吸健康研究院
周国武	中日友好医院国际呼吸医学中心呼吸与危重症医学科
周　佳	重庆医科大学附属第一医院呼吸与危重症医学科
周建英	浙江大学医学院附属第一医院呼吸与危重症医学科
周　敏	上海交通大学医学院附属瑞金医院呼吸与危重症医学科
周明娟	广东省中医院肺功能科
周　玮	宁夏医科大学总医院呼吸与危重症医学科
周　新	上海交通大学附属第一人民医院呼吸与危重症医学科
周　英	空军军医大学第一附属医院呼吸与危重症医学科
朱惠莉	复旦大学附属华东医院呼吸与危重症科
朱黎明	湖南省人民医院呼吸与危重症医学科

前 言

2020年注定是不平凡的一年。这一年,全球遭遇新型冠状病毒肺炎(以下简称"新冠肺炎")疫情,截至目前全球感染新冠病毒者近3600多万人,由此造成死亡人数超过100万人。在应对这场突发新冠肺炎疫情的阻击战中,呼吸学科和呼吸人以其训练有素的专业水准、职业精神和责任担当,义不容辞地成为这次抗击新冠肺炎疫情的中流砥柱。近年来呼吸学科推行的"三架马车"——呼吸与危重症医学(PCCM)专培、专修与单修,PCCM科室规范化建设,PCCM专科联合体,驱动了全国呼吸学科的蓬勃发展和学科队伍的不断发展壮大,使得呼吸学科和呼吸人在面对突如其来的新冠肺炎疫情中经受住了考验。

看不见的新冠肺炎病毒改变了世界,也催生了新的学术交流形式。2020年的中华医学会呼吸病学分会年会(CTS2020)也推迟到10月,并以现场会议和网络视频会议相结合的形式召开。为配合呼吸病学年会而编的《呼吸与危重症医学2019—2020》也将到时与广大读者见面。该书主要是根据各个学组提出的本年度关注的重点问题,配合年会上安排的讲者和内容,形成本书的框架和目录。各个学组的组长对该学组的书稿把关,最后汇编成书。因此,该书体现的是呼吸与危重症医学的年度进步与近年来关注的热点问题,以及临床上常见和困惑的问题。编写中众多学者参与的各章节内容和风格将展示出"百花齐放、各展所长"的特点,同时,也可以让读者能够博取众长,读后有所收获。

CTS2020已经成为呼吸与危重症医学的年度盛会。每年凝练主题,指出呼吸学科发展方向:2011年——呼吸病学与危重症医学实行捆绑式发展战略;2012年——呼吸学科应当在多学科交融的呼吸疾病防治中发挥主导作用;2013年——在我国建立呼吸与危重症医学(PCCM)专科医师规范化培训制度;2014年——加强临床医学研究的体系与能力建设;2015年——携手基层医生,推动呼吸疾病防治;2016年——构建多学科立体交融的现代呼吸学科体系;2017年——推动结核病防治与呼吸学科的历史性回归;2018年——加强合作研究,共推学科发展;2019年——把握精准医学内涵推动呼吸疾病诊治;2020年——持续推进PCCM学科建设,引领呼吸道传染病防治,与今年的新冠肺炎疫情防控相呼应。纵观这些主题,均体现了呼吸与危重症医学学科发展的核心理念与关键环节,成为学科发展的指引。

感谢为本书撰写付出辛勤工作和做出贡献的所有专家、学者。我们相约于2020年10月23日至10月25日在深圳或在云端相见,共同迎接2020年呼吸盛会和本书的正式出版。

瞿介明
CTS2020年会主席
中华医学会呼吸病学分会主任委员
2020年10月

目　录

第一部分　烟草病学

1. 电子烟相关性肺损伤 …………………………………………………………………………（3）
2. 烟草控制与中国经济之关系 ………………………………………………………………（11）
3. 中国烟草病学发展现状与展望 ……………………………………………………………（14）
4. 根据发生机制和临床表现甄别烟草戒断症状与药物不良反应 …………………………（17）
5. 呼吸疾病患者的戒烟现状与研究进展 ……………………………………………………（22）
6. 戒烟门诊就诊人群的吸烟行为与吸烟网络初步分析 ……………………………………（25）
7. 戒烟在呼吸康复中的作用 …………………………………………………………………（29）
8. 电子烟上海专家共识简洁版 ………………………………………………………………（33）
9. 烟草、巨噬细胞与肺部疾病 …………………………………………………………………（34）
10. 烟草暴露与慢性阻塞性肺疾病预防进展 …………………………………………………（40）
11. 吸烟增加COVID-19感染风险的机制 ……………………………………………………（43）
12. 阻塞性睡眠呼吸暂停相关的恶性心律失常 ………………………………………………（47）
13. 吸烟相关疾病与DNA甲基化关系的研究进展 …………………………………………（53）
14. 新型冠状病毒肺炎与吸烟的关系 …………………………………………………………（57）

第二部分　慢性阻塞性肺疾病

1. 慢性阻塞性肺疾病年度研究进展（2019—2020）…………………………………………（63）
2. 从GOLD2020更新看慢性阻塞性肺疾病个体化治疗 ……………………………………（68）
3. 慢性阻塞性肺疾病及其主要合并症的机制关联研究进展 ………………………………（72）
4. 肺纤维化合并肺气肿综合征的最新认识 …………………………………………………（76）
5. 慢性阻塞性肺疾病频繁急性加重的对因治疗 ……………………………………………（80）
6. 基于气道炎症的COPD精准化治疗探讨 …………………………………………………（83）
7. 经典与旁路炎症通路与COPD ……………………………………………………………（88）
8. 气道黏液高分泌是慢性阻塞性肺疾病一个新表型吗？……………………………………（93）
9. 嗜酸性粒细胞在慢性阻塞性肺疾病不同时期的意义 ……………………………………（97）
10. 靶向诱导粒细胞死亡：慢性气道疾病防治的新靶点？……………………………………（102）
11. 慢性阻塞性肺疾病合并症与肺康复结局探讨 ……………………………………………（106）
12. 慢性阻塞性肺疾病合并焦虑抑郁的病因及诊断进展 ……………………………………（108）
13. 肺结核与慢性阻塞性肺疾病关系研究进展 ………………………………………………（114）
14. 慢性阻塞性肺疾病的中枢损害与认知功能障碍最新认识 ………………………………（118）
15. 慢性阻塞性肺疾病与肺曲霉菌病病管理的挑战和思路转变 ……………………………（125）
16. 免疫治疗在慢性阻塞性肺疾病合并肺癌治疗中的进展 …………………………………（130）
17. 低风险慢性阻塞性肺疾病的早期干预 ……………………………………………………（134）
18. 慢性阻塞性肺疾病表观遗传研究进展 ……………………………………………………（137）
19. 肌肉评估在慢性阻塞性肺疾病治疗中的重要性 …………………………………………（141）
20. 从队列研究认识慢性阻塞性肺疾病诊断标准的争议 ……………………………………（145）
21. HFNC及NPPV在慢性阻塞性肺疾病急性加重期治疗中的地位与选择 ………………（148）

第三部分　支气管哮喘

1. 《成人和青少年咳嗽型哮喘和嗜酸性粒细胞性支气管炎（NAEB）》—ACCP 指南解读 ……… (155)
2. 重度激素抵抗型哮喘新型治疗方法探索及机制 ……………………………………………… (160)
3. EGPA 的肺部表现带来的临床挑战 …………………………………………………………… (166)
4. ABPA 激素、抗真菌、靶向药物之争 …………………………………………………………… (170)
5. 非 Th2 相关性支气管哮喘的研究进展 ………………………………………………………… (174)
6. 酷似哮喘的 VCD 研究进展 …………………………………………………………………… (178)
7. 趋化因子与哮喘 ………………………………………………………………………………… (184)
8. 上皮因子与过敏性哮喘 ………………………………………………………………………… (187)
9. 哮喘气道重塑的免疫标志物和个体化治疗前景 ……………………………………………… (190)
10. 《支气管哮喘防治指南（2020 年更新版）》解读 ……………………………………………… (196)
11. 哮喘合并胃食管反流性疾病的诊疗 …………………………………………………………… (200)

第四部分　呼吸系统感染

1. 糖尿病合并肺炎诊治路径中国专家共识 ……………………………………………………… (207)
2. 新型冠状病毒肺炎特异性免疫治疗的现状与展望 …………………………………………… (215)
3. 新型冠状病毒肺炎继发感染的诊断与治疗 …………………………………………………… (221)
4. 当前支原体肺炎诊治中面临的困难和挑战 …………………………………………………… (226)
5. 支气管镜技术在肺部感染的应用进展 ………………………………………………………… (228)
6. 重症甲流的肺外损伤机制 ……………………………………………………………………… (230)
7. 脑卒中相关性肺炎诊治中国专家共识解读 …………………………………………………… (234)
8. 肺炎影像学复查的争议与探讨 ………………………………………………………………… (236)
9. 新型冠状病毒的实验室检测 …………………………………………………………………… (239)
10. 糖皮质激素在 COVID-19 及其他病毒性肺炎的应用及潜在机制 …………………………… (244)

第五部分　间质性肺疾病

1. 间质性肺疾病的影像学新进展：多模态成像定量影像学研究进展与临床应用 …………… (251)
2. 间质性肺疾病药物治疗进展 …………………………………………………………………… (264)
3. 尘肺中的免疫防御机制研究进展：2019—2020 年 …………………………………………… (268)
4. 肺纤维化诊断与预测的生物标志物 …………………………………………………………… (273)
5. 经支气管冷冻肺活检术诊断间质性肺疾病的临床应用进展 ………………………………… (280)
6. 特发性肺纤维化的随访和管理 ………………………………………………………………… (284)
7. 特异性肺纤维化的全新发病机制 ……………………………………………………………… (291)
8. 肺纤维化动物模型的制备与评价 ……………………………………………………………… (295)

第六部分　肺　癌

1. ALK 阳性非小细胞肺癌的治疗进展 …………………………………………………………… (301)
2. 晚期非小细胞肺癌分子靶向治疗现状与进展 ………………………………………………… (305)
3. 肺癌免疫治疗现在与展望 ……………………………………………………………………… (309)
4. 液体活检在肺癌诊治中的应用和挑战 ………………………………………………………… (312)
5. 肿瘤新抗原预测程序 …………………………………………………………………………… (318)
6. 中国肿瘤专科护士在免疫治疗中的角色功能及作用 ………………………………………… (324)
7. 人工智能病理诊断系统在肺癌诊断及预后判断中的应用 …………………………………… (328)
8. 雾霾与肺癌 ……………………………………………………………………………………… (332)
9. 导航支气管镜新技术在肺癌诊断的应用进展 ………………………………………………… (334)

10	生物标志物在肺癌免疫治疗中的预测价值	(339)
11	肺癌免疫治疗相关生物标记物的应用现状	(343)
12	真实世界肺癌免疫治疗的有关问题和思考	(350)

第七部分　睡眠呼吸障碍

1	阻塞性睡眠呼吸暂停2019年年度进展	(359)
2	阻塞性睡眠呼吸暂停与免疫功能	(363)
3	抗击新冠肺炎疫情对医务人员睡眠心理状态的影响	(366)
4	阻塞性睡眠呼吸暂停与视神经病变的关系	(369)
5	从睡眠呼吸调控辨析呼吸衰竭——临床病例评析	(374)
6	新型冠状病毒肺炎患者的睡眠呼吸障碍	(377)
7	PSG数据后处理及其临床应用	(382)
8	阻塞性睡眠呼吸暂停低通气综合征与肿瘤免疫	(387)
9	阻塞性睡眠呼吸暂停致靶器官损伤的免疫学机制	(392)
10	评估量表在OSA患者中的应用	(396)
11	阻塞性睡眠呼吸暂停与肠道菌群	(400)
12	阻塞性睡眠呼吸暂停患者的炎症损伤与认知功能障碍	(404)
13	ICU获得性衰弱与睡眠障碍的相关性研究	(409)
14	阻塞性睡眠呼吸暂停相关的恶性心律失常	(413)
15	减重在睡眠呼吸疾病治疗中的价值	(419)
16	基于标准PSG数据的OSA临床表型分析	(423)

第八部分　危重症医学

1	新型冠状病毒肺炎呼吸支持介入时机	(429)
2	从COVID-19重症病例救治谈俯卧位在ARDS患者中的应用	(431)
3	$ECCO_2R$促进ARDS超保护性通气是否可行？	(434)
4	脓毒症与免疫失衡：个体化诊疗的希望	(439)
5	重症患者血液净化和抗生素剂量调整——慎思笃行	(444)
6	跨肺压指导的机械通气策略在ECMO支持的ARDS患者中的应用	(450)
7	肥胖ARDS患者的机械通气	(453)
8	大环内酯类药物的免疫调节作用：在重症患者中的治疗潜力	(457)
9	感染性疾病与炎症风暴	(462)

第九部分　肺功能检查

1	膈肌功能评价与训练方法研究进展	(473)
2	2019 ATS/ERS肺量计检测标准变迁	(476)
3	呼出气一氧化氮检测技术的现状与指南变迁	(487)
4	肺龄指标适用于推广普及肺功能检查及呼吸慢病防控	(496)
5	新冠肺炎患者的呼吸功能评估和康复	(498)
6	不同肺功能检测在小气道阻塞中优劣敏感性的对比及小气道的靶向药物治疗	(502)
7	支气管激发试验可疑阳性患者的长期跟踪随访研究	(509)
8	人工智能结合肺量计检查在慢性呼吸疾病中的应用	(511)
9	侵入性心肺运动试验在不明原因呼吸困难鉴别诊断中的应用	(515)
10	围术期气道反应测定与手术安全性管理	(518)
11	医院血气分析POCT管理	(522)
12	肺功能检查临床应用研究进展（2019—2020年）	(526)

第十部分　纵隔与胸膜疾病：诊断技术

1　生物学标志物在渗出性胸腔积液诊断的研究进展 …………………………………………………………（533）
2　结节病的诊治进展 ……………………………………………………………………………………………（538）
3　恶性胸膜病变光动力治疗现状与探索 ………………………………………………………………………（543）
4　恶性胸腔积液的免疫微环境与免疫治疗新思路 ……………………………………………………………（546）

第十一部分　介入呼吸病学

1　关于介入呼吸病学与转化医学的几点思考 …………………………………………………………………（551）
2　支气管镜新技术在肺小结节诊断中的应用策略 ……………………………………………………………（554）
3　TTS气道支架的基础与临床研究 ……………………………………………………………………………（558）
4　硅酮支架的现场加工技巧与应用 ……………………………………………………………………………（561）
5　呼吸介入转化医学研究 ………………………………………………………………………………………（564）
6　2020早期肺癌微创介入治疗年度回顾 ………………………………………………………………………（568）
7　慢性血栓栓塞性肺动脉高压的介入诊疗 ……………………………………………………………………（572）
8　经支气管肺活检和消融治疗进展 ……………………………………………………………………………（573）
9　从呼吸介入发展谈临床创新 …………………………………………………………………………………（576）
10　人工智能-快速现场评估场景的研发及应用 ………………………………………………………………（583）
11　肺结节工作室建设与运行 ……………………………………………………………………………………（584）
12　活瓣肺减容的患者选择和并发症的处理 ……………………………………………………………………（588）
13　再生医学在气道疾病中的应用 ………………………………………………………………………………（594）
14　致知力行　继往开来　相聚2020世界支气管和介入呼吸病学大会 ……………………………………（600）

第一部分

烟草病学

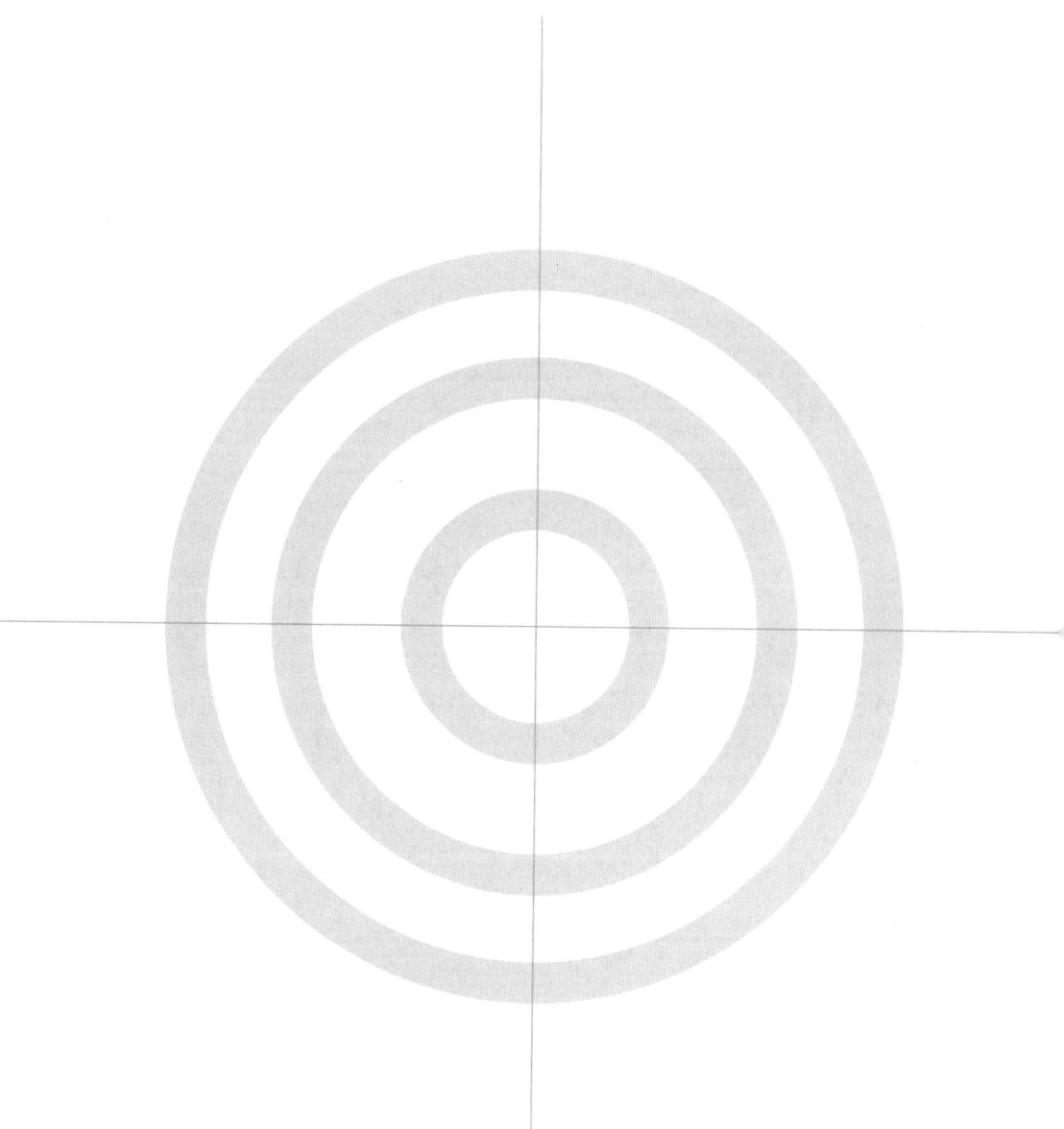

1 电子烟相关性肺损伤

陈延斌

电子烟(electronic cigarettes,e-cigarettes),在英文文献中常被称为 vapes,e-hookahs,vape pens,tank systems,mods,electronic nicotine delivery systems(ENDS,电子尼古丁传输系统);使用或吸入电子烟的过程通常称作 vaping。第一代电子烟是采用电池加热电子烟液产生烟雾(气溶胶)供使用者吸入的电子尼古丁传输系统,主要由三部分组成:电池、加热元件和烟液容器。同第一代电子烟不同,第二、三、四代产品采用可充电的锂电池;第三、四代产品还增加了对工作电压及其温度的可调节功能,从而增加了对电子烟设备的可操控性。与电子烟设备更新相伴行的是电子烟液的成分及所谓"口味"持续不断的更新。

第一个电子烟的专利可以追溯到1927年,不过当时并没有尝试进行商业化生产。第一款商业化的电子烟于2003年在中国制造,并很快成功进入欧美市场,2007年电子烟开始在美国销售。此后,电子烟的生产制造和消费规模呈迅速上升趋势。在美国,电子烟生产企业的注册资金高达25亿美元。2014年,美国电子烟生产企业每年用于市场营销的投入高达12 500万美元,且逐年递增。其营销策略包括鼓吹电子烟更健康、价格更便宜、品种繁多、"口味"各异、更符合当代的社交和消费时尚、能规避控烟政策限制等。电子烟产品问世之初,被标榜为具有辅助戒烟功效的"灵丹妙药",一度出现了大量传统纸烟使用者纷纷改吸电子烟的局面,但正如《Smoking Cessation: A Report of the Surgeon General 2020》所述,目前仍缺乏足够的证据支持电子烟可以提高戒烟成功率。

常用的电子烟液有尼古丁、四氢大麻醇(tetrahydrocannabinol,THC)、大麻二醇(cannabidiol,CBD)、丁烷杂油等。一般而言,电子烟液还含有保湿剂,如丙二醇和植物甘油等基本成分,其他成分包括化学调味剂和增香剂、矿物油和中链甘油、丙酮、甲醛、亚硝基去甲烟碱、亚硝胺等。

起初,使用电子烟设备吸入尼古丁或大麻制品导致的肺损伤只有零星报道。2019夏季,因吸电子烟导致肺损伤的病例数激增,短短数月内,美国出现了数以千计的病例,病死病例数也迅速攀升,且以年轻人为主,吸电子烟引发的肺损伤成为一个突出的公共健康问题,引起广泛关注。因此,美国疾病控制与预防中心(Centers for Disease Control and Prevention,CDC)正式将这一急性或亚急性综合症候群命名为电子烟产品使用相关性肺损伤(E-cigarette or vaping product use-associated lung injury,EVALI),本文简称为电子烟相关性肺损伤,也有文献称之为电子烟相关性肺病(vaping associated pulmonary illness,VAPI)。

一、EVALI 的流行病学

据统计,2017年,约有210万(2.8%)美国成人吸电子烟;2018年增至360万人;目前至少有810万美国成人吸电子烟。据世界卫生组织(WHO)估算,2011年,全球有700万人吸电子烟,2018年猛增至4100万人。

2016年,澳大利亚12~17岁和18~19岁年龄人群中,吸电子烟者占比分别为7.1%和16%。2017—2018年,9%的英国年轻人吸电子烟。2017年,加拿大15~24岁年龄人群中,既往30d内吸电子烟的人数多达27.2万人。

再以美国学生群体为例,2011—2018年,美国高中生的电子烟吸烟率由1.5%飙升至20.8%,初中生的电子烟吸烟率由0.6%升至4.9%;相当于每5名高中生和每20名初中生中就有1人吸电子烟。美国国立卫生研究院的数据表明:2017年,27.8%的美国12年级学生在既往1年中曾吸过电子烟,2018年增至37.3%;2019年,12岁中学生中,14%的学生报道既往30d内都吸过含有大麻的电子烟。根据美国2019年青少年烟草消费报告的统计数据,高中生吸电子烟的比列为27.5%,初中生为10.5%,是2017年的2倍多,上升态势一目了然。

EVALI 的报道最早可以追溯到2012年。2019年8月,伊利诺伊州报道了全美第一例因 EVALI 致死的病例。随后,Marlière 等报道了欧洲第一例 EVALI 病死病例。EVALI 主要发生于年轻人群,由于各研究样本均较小,中位患病年龄有所不同:来自费城的研究显示,EVALI 的中位患病年龄只有16岁;伊利诺伊州和威斯康星州的中位患病年龄只有19岁;宾夕法尼亚州36例 EVALI 的中位患病年龄为21岁,男性占78%,19%需气管插管机械通气,6%需体外膜肺氧合(extracorporeal membrane oxygenation,ECMO),平均住院天数为8d,出院后再住院率为8%,多集中在3d内;犹他州的报道表明 EVALI 的中位发病年龄为27岁,男性居多,占80%。

研究表明,1个月内吸入含 THC 电子烟气溶胶而患 EVALI 的概率为76.9%,吸入含尼古丁电子烟气溶胶而患 EVALI 的概率为56.8%,单纯吸入 THC 患 EVALI 的概率为36%,单纯吸入尼古丁而患EVALI的概率为16%。

截至2020年2月18日,美国CDC共收到因EVALI住院的病例报告2807例,其中病死68例,病死率约为2%。CDC对2668例EVALI患者(病例时间截至2020年1月14日)的综合统计分析显示:66%的EVALI患者为男性;中位患病年龄为24岁(13~85岁),18岁以下者占15%,18~24岁者占37%,25~34岁者占24%,35岁以上者占24%;82%的EVALI患者吸含有THC的电子烟,57%的EVALI患者吸含有尼古丁的电子烟;德克萨斯州和伊利诺伊州EVALI病例数最多,均超过200例;纽约州和加利福尼亚州紧随其后,均超过150例。这是目前关于EVALI的最大数据综合分析报告。

二、EVALI的发病机制

电子烟的电池电压通常为3~6V,可将金属圈加热至1000℃,使电子烟液气化,形成气溶胶,便于使用者吸入。电子烟液及加热后形成的气溶胶中含有多种有害成分,如维生素E醋酸酯(vitamin E acetate,VEA)和中链脂肪酸三酰甘油(medium-chain triglycerides,MCT);还包含溶媒类(丙二醇、植物甘油)、调味剂类(香草香精、肉桂、大马烯酮、薄荷醇、萜烯、苯甲醇、甲醛、吡嗪类)、羰基化合物、甲苯、苯和重金属(镍、铅、铬、锌、镁、钴)、其他类(多环芳烃化合物、亚硝胺、热分解产物、丙烯醛、杂质类(矿物质、植物油、杂油)等。有报道称,气溶胶中还含有微生物毒素,包括内毒素。有的还含有杀虫剂成分,如乙基毒死蜱(chlorpyrifos ethyl)和三福林(trifluralin)。研究表明,MCT和VEA可诱导产生活性氧簇及细胞毒反应。吸入电子烟气溶胶后,气道上皮屏障功能减弱、氧化应激和炎症反应增强、细胞因子如IL-6和IL-8分泌增多,诱发EVALI,出现诸如机化性肺炎、弥漫性肺泡损伤、纤维素性渗出、黏液栓和透明膜形成、Ⅱ型肺泡上皮增生等改变;肺泡结构破坏和黏液清除能力降低,还可使肺功能进一步受损。EVALI发生的可能机制还包括支气管上皮细胞蛋白表达改变、气道重构、巨噬细胞活化等。二乙酰、2,3-戊二酮、乙偶姻等化合物等破坏纤毛的功能,导致闭塞性细支气管炎和"爆米花肺(popcorn lung)"。电子烟液气溶胶还可引起气道上皮细胞凋亡、坏死直至病死;也可引起巨噬细胞焦亡,表现为细胞渗漏、细胞质外溢、加剧局部炎症反应;同时,还可使巨噬细胞的吞饮功能减弱,对功能异常受损细胞的清除能力受损。如前所述,美国CDC的数据表明82%的住院EVALI患者使用含THC的电子烟,而VEA是含THC电子烟液的稀释剂,多数EVALI患者的支气管肺泡灌洗液(bronchoalveolar-lavage fluid,BALF)中可以发现VEA,说明VEA可能是EVALI发生的主要原因。反复吸入丙二醇、甘油、挥发性有机物、直径低于100 nm的超细颗粒、自由基等物质,会对机体造成进一步危害。电子烟液加热时还可产生有毒的烯酮气体,与EVALI的暴发流行密切相关。也有报道发现,吸入不含尼古丁及THC的电子烟液同样可导致重症EVALI。Krishnan等的一例病例报告显示:一例38岁女性,吸电子烟4年,其电子烟液既不含尼古丁,也不含THC,为"西瓜味",因咳嗽、眩晕、呼吸困难4d入院,病情迅速恶化,先后经历气管插管、大剂量糖皮质激素冲击、俯卧位通气、ECMO、气管切开等治疗,住院46d病情方获改善。有报道认为植物甘油与脂质性肺炎(类质性肺炎,lipoid pneumonia)密切相关,且也有EVALI表现为脂质性肺炎的报道,这些患者的BALF中也确实发现了油红O染色阳性的富含脂质的巨噬细胞。然而,脂质性肺炎是否与EVALI有关,仍存争议,需进一步研究。据不完全统计,美国2014年有450多种品牌的电子烟产品,包含了近8000种不同"口味"的电子烟,此后几乎每月要新增250多种"口味"的电子烟,目前有超过15 500种"口味"的电子烟液。在英国,约有41 000种不同"口味"的电子烟。不同品种的电子烟,其烟液的成分不同,加热后所产生的气溶胶成分也不同,吸入后产生EVALI的原因和表现也必然不同,值得深入研究。

三、EVALI的临床表现

基于目前的病例资料,EVALI患者以年轻男性居多。

全身非特异性症状的发生率高达88%~100%,主要包括发热(78%~83%)、乏力不适(48%~75%)、寒战(25%~58%)、多汗(42%)、头痛(28%)、消瘦(12%~26%)、肌肉酸痛(17%)、心动过速(64%),有的还可表现为盗汗和眩晕等。

几乎所有的EVALI患者都有呼吸道症状,占比高达92%~98%,其中85%~91%的患者呼吸困难、78%~83%的患者咳嗽、35%~55%的患者胸膜炎性胸痛、43%~55%的患者非胸膜炎性胸痛、33%的患者咳痰、77%的患者低氧血症、9%~12%的患者咯血。若EVALI患者合并有哮喘或COPD等基础疾病,发生EVALI时,可诱发哮喘或COPD的急性发作。

81%~92%的EVALI患者有消化道症状,恶心和呕吐最常见,发生率分别为64%~75%和66%~91%;此外,腹痛者达27%~47%,腹泻者占27%~40%。值得注意的是,有的EVALI患者仅表现为消化道症状;如Matta等报道了一名16岁男性EVALI患者,每天吸含尼古丁的电子烟多次,持续2年,发病前数月夜间开始吸含THC的电子烟,入院前近3个月,患者仅表现为消瘦、餐后恶心、食欲缺乏、间或呕吐,而无任何呼吸道症状。

吸电子烟时,电池加热的温度可高达1000℃,还可能发生烧伤和爆炸伤,也可能引发癫痫。

四、EVALI的影像学表现

EVALI影像学的异常表现与电子烟的吸入频率、剂量、烟液的化学组分、甚至所用的设备有关。常见影像学改变包括急性肺损伤、过敏性肺炎、急性嗜酸性粒细胞性肺炎、弥漫性肺泡损伤、机化性肺炎、脂质性肺炎、巨细胞性间质性肺炎等。

一个含14例EVALI患者的小样本数据显示：胸部X线片异常率达100%,多显示为双肺弥漫浸润性磨玻璃影（ground glass opacities,GGO），提示存在弥漫性肺损伤、闭塞性支气管炎及机化性肺炎;GGO的发生率为100%,实变率为57%，呈双肺分布;93%的病灶呈双肺对称分布;下叶分布为主的有50%;病变范围超过肺容积75%的有29%,50%~75%的有36%,25%~50%的有29%,不足25%的有7%;气胸或纵隔气肿和双侧少量胸腔积液的各占7%;由于小叶间隔增厚，通常可见Kerley B线;胸部X线片的敏感性远不及CT;CT显示100%的患者都有GGO,实变发生率为64%,14%的有小叶间隔增厚,14%的表现为小叶中心性分布的磨玻璃结节，所有患者的病变均呈双肺分布，对称分布的达93%,下叶为主的占50%，胸膜下及支气管血管束周围鲜有累及是其突出特点,79%的患者胸膜下没有累及,36%的可见反晕征或环礁征，病变范围超过肺容积75%的有71%,50%~75%的有14%，不足25%的有14%,纵隔气肿的有14%,双侧少量胸腔积液的占7%。GGO多表现为双肺弥漫性分布的斑片状或融合性并呈重力依赖性分布，可与实变、小叶间隔增厚、铺路石征并存;牵拉性支扩或蜂窝肺发生率则高达35%;可有肺门和（或）纵隔淋巴结肿大。急性嗜酸性粒细胞性肺炎、弥漫性肺泡损伤、弥漫性肺泡出血、机化性肺炎和脂质性肺炎多呈弥漫性分布的GGO和实变，以下叶为主，胸膜下鲜有累及;过敏性肺炎则以中上叶GGO和机化性肺炎为主，多见于肺的外周。

（一）急性肺损伤（ALI）/急性呼吸窘迫综合征（ARDS）

多数EVALI患者在其发病的过程中都会出现ALI/ARDS,CT可表现为双肺弥漫性分布的GGO、斑片影，甚至是实变影，与其他原因所致的肺损伤不易区别，但EVALI鲜有胸膜下受累，为其重要特点。Sakla等报道了一例25岁女性EVALI患者，在过去一年间，每周吸3次电子烟，每次吸2~3h,因干咳、胸痛、呼吸困难2d急诊入院，迅速进展为ARDS,气管插管机械通气后病情仍不能改善，最终借助于ECMO技术，治疗方获成功。

（二）机化性肺炎

主要表现为双肺弥漫性分布GGO、实变影，以外周及小叶周分布为主;也可表现为局灶性结节和急性纤维素性肺炎伴机化;胸膜下及心脏周围通常不受累及，实变通常较轻;可见反晕征或环礁征及铺路石征。上述征象可在糖皮质激素治疗后快速缓解。

（三）弥漫性肺泡损伤

提示急性肺损伤的程度更为严重、病情更重、更有可能需要机械通气，甚至是ECMO才能维持氧合;在弥漫性肺泡损伤的急性渗出期、肺容积通常减小，并可见下叶为主的非均一性实变和GGO,也可见小叶间隔增厚及铺路石征;随着病变进展到机化期，肺容积更小，并可见牵拉性支气管扩张改变;弥漫性肺泡损伤可与机化性肺炎重叠存在。

（四）急性嗜酸性粒细胞性肺炎

小样本资料显示，97%的患者表现为双肺弥漫性分布的GGO,88%的患者合并少量胸腔积液，68%的患者同时存在小叶间隔增厚,52%的患者表现为小叶中心性分布的磨玻璃结节,37%的患者表现为实变影,18%的患者有支气管血管束增厚,8.3%的患者可出现树芽征。而气腔实变后，由于改变了通气/血流比值，在发生呼吸衰竭的EVALI患者中出现的频率更高，可作为病情严重性的标志。有文献报道了一例16岁女性患者，吸含THC电子烟1年，咳嗽、气急3个月，腹部不适、腹泻、发热、胸痛1周入院,CT提示双肺节段性分布的GGO伴纵隔淋巴结肿大，尿液中检出THC,BALF中嗜酸性粒细胞占比62%,并可见Charcot-Leyden结晶体，符合嗜酸性粒细胞性肺炎病理改变。糖皮质激素治疗24h后迅速缓解,4周内逐步减量至停药。

（五）过敏性肺炎

可呈急性或亚急性,CT多表现为中上肺为主的GGO,边界不清的小叶中心性磨玻璃结节，小叶间隔增厚，可有胸腔积液。

（六）细支气管炎

CT可表现为气体陷闭征象。弥漫性分布的小叶中心性结节提示细支气管炎改变，并与过敏性肺炎相关，通常以上叶多见。

（七）弥漫性肺泡出血

多见于吸食可卡因和大麻者。一例33岁男性患者，吸电子烟2个月，以咯血和呼吸困难为主要表现,CT表现为双肺弥漫分布的GGO及斑片状实变影,BALF及肺楔形切除活检证实为弥漫性肺泡出血，经无创通气及激素治疗后完全缓解。另一例22岁男性，吸含THC的电子烟，出现咯血和急性呼吸衰竭，经气管插管机械通气,BALF证实为弥漫性肺泡出血，尿中检出THC代谢产物，给予糖皮质激素治疗，逐步缓解，康复出院。

（八）呼吸性细支气管炎伴间质性肺病

相对少见,Flower等报道了一例33岁男性患者，由吸传统纸烟改为吸电子烟3个月后,CT表现为双肺新发多发的边界不清的磨玻璃结节影，沿支气管血管束分布，经胸腔镜活检病理证实，为呼吸性细支气管炎伴间质性肺病。

（九）巨细胞性间质性肺炎

与电子烟气溶胶中的重金属在肺内沉积有关,CT表现为双肺GGO,支气管扩张，沿支气管周围分布的线样磨玻璃改变。

（十）急性脂质性肺炎

CT表现为GGO、实变影、铺路石征,BALF中可见油红O染色阳性的泡沫样巨噬细胞或富含脂质的巨噬细胞。有报道发现,67%的EVALI患者BALF中有油红O染色阳性的富含脂质的巨噬细胞，比例高达50%~75%。有文献报道了一例27岁男性患者，因干咳、发热、呼吸困难5d入院，吸含THC和尼古丁的电子烟2年,CT扫描可见双肺弥漫性分布的GGO和实变，胸膜下没有累及。BALF可见油红O染色阳性的肺泡巨噬细胞，经支气管镜肺活检病理符合急性肺损伤之机化性肺炎改变，并可见特征性巨噬细胞呈空泡改变，支持脂质性肺炎的诊断。另一例46岁男性患者，因气急、乏力、寒战、发热、咳嗽等流感样症状入院,近4~6个月开始吸含大麻的电子烟,右下叶支气管镜肺活检可见肺泡内泡沫样巨噬细胞及活化的Ⅱ型肺泡上皮细胞等炎症反应细胞,与机化性肺炎表现一致;BALF中可见油红O染色阳性的富含脂质的巨噬细胞,肺泡巨噬细胞内可见棕黑色色素沉着,与脂质性肺炎表现一致。然而,有学者认为,BALF或肺活检标本的脂肪染色并不能区分EVALI及其他原因导致的急性肺损伤,对此仍需进一步研究。

(十一)纵隔气肿或气胸

多见于年轻男性,发生率高达16%,若合并有基础疾病或需正压通气,则更易发生。

有的EVALI可以表现为双肺弥漫性分布的树芽征及结节影,酷似转移瘤。长期吸电子烟者还可引起气管、支气管软化等严重并发症。

五、EVALI的组织病理学表现

EVALI在组织病理学上以急性肺损伤为主要表现,但缺乏特异性改变。

肺活检的病理结果具有异质性,可能与使用糖皮质激素干预有关。主要包括非特异性急性炎症反应、泡沫样巨噬细胞、急性弥漫性肺泡损伤、间质性/支气管周围性肉芽肿性炎、透明膜形成、肺泡细胞空泡化、Ⅱ型肺泡上皮细胞增生、肺泡腔内可见局灶性纤维蛋白沉积、局灶性毛细血管增生及机化性肺炎等。活检及尸检病理表明,在渗出期和机化期均可见弥漫性肺泡损伤,并可见泡沫样巨噬细胞散在分布。

有限的肺活检资料显示,弥漫性肺泡损伤、急性纤维素性肺炎和机化性肺炎最为常见,三者共占约96%。这些急性肺损伤改变由吸入电子烟液气溶胶导致的化学性炎症及高温气雾导致的热损伤共同作用引起。

小样本的病理资料显示,76%的EVALI患者有机化性肺炎,48%表现为急性纤维素性肺炎伴机化,24%有弥漫性肺泡损伤,84%有泡沫样或空泡状巨噬细胞,100%可见泡沫样或空泡状肺泡细胞,88%可见肺泡腔内纤维蛋白,78%有细支气管炎,67%有支气管黏膜溃疡,65%有间质水肿,40%可见中性粒细胞性炎症,56%有慢性间质性炎症,41%可见巨噬细胞有色素沉着,28%可见嗜酸性粒细胞。极少数患者可表现为类上皮样细胞及多核巨细胞性肉芽肿。镜下亦可见富含含铁血黄素的巨噬细胞,与弥漫性肺泡出血密切相关。

一个包含8例EVALI患者的小样本研究显示,肺活检标本中均可发现急性肺损伤征象,具体表现为机化性肺炎、弥漫性肺泡损伤、未分类的机化性急性肺损伤。机化性肺炎以肺泡腔内成纤维细胞的匍行性生长或息肉样成纤维细胞栓为特点,可伴有间质性炎症改变。弥漫性肺泡损伤可与机化性肺炎共存,以透明膜形成和肺泡间隔增厚为特点。也有的表现为机化性急性肺损伤,但无法进一步分类。肺泡腔内可有纤维素性渗出伴不同程度的机化,多呈局灶性分布。间质的慢性炎症则以淋巴细胞浸润为主,免疫组织化学染色证实,以$CD3^+$ T淋巴细胞为主,$CD20^+$的B淋巴细胞极少。肺泡腔内还有数量不等的巨噬细胞浸润。

六、EVALI的诊断与鉴别诊断

由于EVALI缺乏特征性的临床、实验室、影像和病理学改变,诊断标准为排他性。

EVALI多表现为急性炎症反应,81%的患者WBC计数$>11.0×10^9$/L,超过94%的患者中性粒细胞比例>80%,97%的EVALI患者ESR>30mm/h。少数患者可有肝功能异常,41%的患者AST或ALT>35U/L,10%的患者>105U/L。31%的患者有低钠血症(<135mmol/L)、35%的患者有低钾血症(<3.5mmol/L),多数EVALI患者尿液中可检出THC。来自EVALI发病中位年龄为17.1岁的小样本研究显示,部分患者康复出院后短期内(中位随访时间4.5周)可出现阻塞性或限制性通气功能障碍及一氧化碳弥散功能降低。BALF中可以看到巨噬细胞和中性粒细胞为主的炎症反应,如不合并呼吸道感染,一般检测不到病原体。

美国CDC于2019年8月30日提出了EVALI的诊断标准:①症状发作前90d内有电子烟吸入史;②胸部X线片或CT扫描提示双肺弥漫性浸润影或磨玻璃影;③排除肺部感染(定义为呼吸道病毒检测阴性、流感病毒PCR阴性、痰培养及尿肺炎球菌抗原阴性、军团菌检测阴性、BALF培养阴性);④排除心脏疾病或肿瘤性疾病。

随着病例的积累及对EVALI诊治能力的提高,2019年11月19日,CDC对上述标准进行了修订,内容包括:①对于新出现呼吸道、消化道及全身症状的患者,应询问其电子烟的使用情况;②临床疑诊EVALI时,及时进行氧合情况及胸部影像学评估;③对临床情况稳定的EVALI患者,给予门诊治疗;④检测是否存在流感病毒感染,特别是在流感流行季节,并据检测结果,给予抗感染治疗;⑤鉴于目前的证据尚不足,对于门诊治疗的EVALI患者,糖皮质激素的使用应持谨慎态度;⑥劝戒电子烟;⑦强调每年接种流感疫苗的重要性。

同EVALI一样,新型冠状病毒肺炎(COVID-19)也可引起急性呼吸衰竭,也有相似的主诉,影像学上也可表现为GGO。在新型冠状病毒肺炎流行的大背景下,所有的EVALI患者均需进行新型冠状病毒肺炎核酸检测,排除COVID-19感染。首先,COVID-19患者外周血WBC计数通常正常或降低,淋巴细胞计数则明显减少;而多数EVALI患者WBC计数明显升高,小样本研究发现,92%的EVALI患者WBC升高达$15.3×10^9$/L。其次,"典型"的EVALI,特别是重症EVALI患者的发病年龄更小,而COVID-19,特别是重症COVID-19患者普遍以高龄为主。最后,多数EVALI患者对激素治疗反应良好,一般1~3d即可起效;而对于COVID-19,激素的作用依然存在争议。

由于多数EVALI患者合并有恶心、呕吐、腹痛、腹泻等消化道症状,因此还需与具有类似症状的消化道疾病相鉴别。EVALI还需与流感、社区获得性肺炎、肺血栓栓塞症、糖尿病酮症酸中毒、ANCA相关性血管炎、肺孢子菌肺炎、心功能不全等相鉴别。EVALI与流感合并存在时,往往提示病情危重、预后不良。Akkanti等报道了一例27岁男性EVALI合并甲型流感的患者,病情快速恶化,经气管插管机械通气、VV-ECMO、VA-ECMO、主动脉内球囊反搏等治疗,最终依然抢救失败。

有学者建议,根据EVALI患者对氧的需求程度将其进行严重程度分级,以便更好地对患者进行分级治疗:若无须氧疗,则为轻度,门诊治疗并密切随访即可;若需1～5L/min鼻导管供氧,则为中度,需要住院治疗;若需6L/min及以上的鼻导管供氧或需无创甚至有创通气支持,则为重度EVALI,一般需要入住到ICU进一步治疗。

七、EVALI的治疗

若呼吸空气的条件下,$SaO_2>95\%$,没有呼吸窘迫,不合并可能会导致呼吸功能恶化的基础疾病,不再吸电子烟,则可门诊治疗。由于本病可快速进展,CDC建议门诊治疗的患者需在24～48h复诊。

90%的EVALI患者需住院治疗,54%需入住重症监护病房(ICU)。

对于EVALI的治疗,CDC提出了3条总的原则:①经验性使用广谱抗生素覆盖可能的病原体;②使用糖皮质激素(最佳剂量及疗程尚未明确);③氧疗、最佳支持治疗并密切监护。

由于最初EVALI患者的表现与肺部感染难以区分,因此CDC建议经验性使用广谱抗生素,但随着EVALI病例数的增加及诊治经验的积累,若非合并肺部感染,一般不再推荐抗感染治疗。

使用糖皮质激素是EVALI患者的主要治疗措施。关于其使用剂量和疗程,目前尚无统一的推荐。有学者建议,甲泼尼龙琥珀酸钠40mg,1次/8h,2周内逐步减量至停药;也有学者建议静脉使用甲泼尼龙琥珀酸钠125mg/d(120～240mg),平均2d,然后逐步减量,平均使用11d;少数重症患者糖皮质激素的使用量可达1g/d。84%的EVALI患者经糖皮质激素治疗后可缓解。目前多推荐中等剂量的糖皮质激素,如泼尼松40～60mg/d,疗程为5～10d。也有研究发现,对EVALI患者,单纯停吸电子烟后,临床情况即可获得改善,并无须使用糖皮质激素,因此,对于糖皮质激素的使用指征,还需进一步探讨。

82%的EVALI患者需要氧疗,包括鼻导管高流量氧疗(47%)、无创正压通气(30%)、气管插管机械通气(22%)。有的患者虽然接受了大剂量糖皮质激素治疗,仍出现呼吸衰竭的快速进展并需接受ECMO治疗。有报道一例16岁女孩,住院期间经2次VV-ECMO,分别持续应用16d和30d,最终获得康复。病情极为严重者还需要肺移植治疗。

50岁以下者中位住院时间为5～6d,50岁以上者则需住院12d;24%的患者出院时仍需氧疗。近10%的患者短期内仍需再次住院,再住院的中位时间为4d(其中有一半是因复吸所致),再住院患者的中位年龄是57岁,需要再次住院的EVALI患者多数(70.6%)合并基础疾病,病死的EVALI患者合并基础疾病的比例更是高达83.3%,而无须住院也未病死的EVALI患者,其合并基础疾病的比例则比较低,为25.6%。

美国CDC发布了EVALI住院患者出院标准:出院前24～48h临床情况稳定,包括实验室数据正常,生命体征、体格检查、氧合及运动耐力稳定;门诊可提供理想的治疗、心理健康保健及成瘾物质滥用监测。对于出院的EVALI患者,建议密切随访2～4周,并建议1～2个月后复查影像学及肺功能。

有限的数据表明,糖皮质激素治疗前后,EVALI患者的1s用力呼气量(FEV_1)、用力肺活量(FVC)、肺总量、肺一氧化碳弥散功能均得到明显改善。对一例18岁男性患者的随访表明,康复出院后8个月,仍存在肺功能的明显异常,使用支气管舒张剂后,FEV_1仅为预计值的53%,FEV_1/FVC为55%,磁共振肺功能显像提示双肺上叶仍存在通气功能异常,说明EVALI可对患者的肺功能造成较长时间的负面影响。

八、EVALI的预后

需特别关注的情况是:目前已知的有关EVALI信息均来自住院患者,而更多的症状轻微者或无症状者可能因不曾就诊致使统计到的EVALI发病率远低于真实情况。

尽管有危重病例,EVALI总体预后较好,病死率为2%左右,病死的中位年龄是27岁。

所有出院后病死的EVALI患者都曾入住ICU,都曾经历呼吸衰竭和气管插管、机械通气。因此,CDC推荐,对于所有出院的EVALI患者,48h内都要进行密切随访,特别是具有慢性基础疾病的老年人、入住ICU并行气管插管和机械通气的EVALI患者。

犹他州的报道显示,EVALI患者出院2周内再次入院者,有一半因复吸电子烟所致。因此,建议所有人,特别是青少年、孕妇不要吸电子烟;吸电子烟者,需尽早戒除并避免复吸;如出现相应症状,及早就医。

关于EVALI,还有许多问题值得进一步探讨。例如,电子烟在美国销售已有12年之久,为何只在2019年出现EVALI的暴发流行?难道仅仅与2019年大规模使用含THC的电子烟液有关?是否还有其他未知的原因?又如,英国吸电子烟的现象同样非常普遍,为何没有像美国一样出现EVALI的暴发流行?这与英国只允许销售含尼古丁的电子烟液是否有关?如前文所述,有的EVALI患者所吸的电子烟液既不含THC,也不含尼古丁,其发病原因又是什么?再比如,EVALI为何会表现出消化道症状?这仅仅只与电子烟液中含有的大麻成分有关吗?这些关于EVALI的诸多问题,都值得关注并进行深入研究。

参 考 文 献

[1] Norris MR. Vaping-associated pulmonary injury. Ann Intern Med,2020,172(12):841.

[2] Cobb NK,Solanki JN. E-cigarettes,vaping devices,and acute lung injury. Respir Care,2020,65(5):713-718.

[3] Jonas AM,Raj R. Vaping-related acute parenchymal lung injury:a systematic review. Chest,2020,158(4):1555-1565.

[4] Winnicka L,Shenoy MA. EVALI and the pulmonary toxicity of electronic cigarettes:a review. J Gen Intern Med,2020,35(7):2130-2135.

[5] Mazer-Amirshahi M,Garlich FM,Calello DP,et al. ACMT position statement:limiting harms of vaping and e-cigarette use. J Med Toxicol,2020.

[6] Hage R,Fretz V,Schuurmans MM. Electronic cigarettes and vaping associated pulmonary illness(VAPI):a narrative review. Pulmonology,2020,26(5):291-303.

[7] Muthumalage T,Lucas JH,Wang Q,et al. Pulmonary toxicity and inflammatory response of E-cigarette vape cartridges containing medium-chain triglycerides oil and vitamin E acetate:implications in the pathogenesis of EVALI. Toxics,2020,8(3):E46.

[8] King BA,Jones CM,Baldwin GT,et al. The EVALI and youth vaping epidemics—implications for public health. N Engl J Med,2020,382(8):689-691.

[9] Gilley M,Beno S. Vaping implications for children and youth. Curr Opin Pediatr,2020,32(3):343-348.

[10] Cai H,Garcia JGN,Wang C. More to add to E-cigarette regulations:unified approaches. Chest,2020,157(4):771-773.

[11] Fonseca Fuentes X,Kashyap R,Hays JT,et al. VpALI-vaping-related acute lung injury:a new killer around the block. Mayo Clin Proc,2019,94(12):2534-2545.

[12] Besaratinia A,Tommasi S. Vaping epidemic:challenges and opportunities. Cancer Causes Control,2020,31(7):663-667.

[13] Carroll BJ,Kim M,Hemyari A,et al. Impaired lung function following e-cigarette or vaping product use associated lung injury in the first cohort of hospitalized adolescents. Pediatr Pulmonol,2020,55(7):1712-1718.

[14] Essa A,Macaraeg J,Jagan N,et al. Review of cases of E-cigarette or vaping product use-associated lung injury(EVALI) and brief review of the literature. Case Rep Pulmonol,2020,2020:1090629.

[15] Salzman GA,Alqawasma M,Asad H. Vaping associated lung injury(EVALI):an explosive United States Epidemic. Mo Med,2019,116(6):492-496.

[16] Landman ST,Dhaliwal I,Mackenzie CA,et al. Life-threatening bronchiolitis related to electronic cigarette use in a Canadian youth. CMAJ,2019,191(48):E1321-E1331.

[17] McCauley L,Markin C,Hosmer D. An unexpected consequence of electronic cigarette use. Chest,2012,141(4):1110-1113.

[18] Munsif M,Hew M,Dabscheck E,et al. E-cigarette or vaping product use-associated lung injury(EVALI):a cautionary tale. Med J Aust,2020,213(3):109-110.

[19] Layden JE,Ghinai I,Pray I,et al. Pulmonary illness related to E-cigarette use in Illinois and Wisconsin—final report. N Engl J Med,2020,382(10):903-916.

[20] Lozier MJ,Wallace B,Anderson K,et al. Update:demographic,product,and substance-use characteristics of hospitalized patients in a nationwide outbreak of E-cigarette,or vaping,product use-associated lung injuries-United States,December 2019. MMWR Morb Mortal Wkly Rep,2019,68(49):1142-1148.

[21] Marlière C,De Greef J,Gohy S,et al. Fatal e-cigarette or vaping associated lung injury(EVALI):a first case report in Europe. Eur Respir J,2020,56(1):2000077.

[22] Chidambaram AG,Dennis RA,Biko DM,et al. Clinical and radiological characteristics of e-cigarette or vaping product use associated lung injury. Emerg Radiol,2020,27(5):495-501.

[23] Zou RH,Tiberio PJ,Triantafyllou GA,et al. Clinical characterization of E-cigarette,or vaping,product use associated lung injury in 36 patients in Pittsburgh,PA. Am J Respir Crit Care Med,2020,201(10):1303-1306.

[24] Blagev DP,Harris D,Dunn AC,et al. Clinical presentation,treatment,and short-term outcomes of lung injury associated with e-cigarettes or vaping:a prospective observational cohort study. Lancet,2019,394(10214):2073-2083.

[25] Wang KY,Jadhav SP,Yenduri NJS,et al. E-cigarette or vaping product use-associated lung injury in the pediatric population:imaging features at presentation and short-term follow-up. Pediatr Radiol,2020,50(9):1231-1239.

[26] Ind PW. E-cigarette or vaping product use-associated lung injury. Br J Hosp Med(Lond),2020,81(4):1-9.

[27] Callahan SJ,Harris D,Collingridge DS,et al. Diagnosing EVALI in the Time of COVID-19. Chest,2020,2020,158(5):2034-2037.

[28] Werner AK,Koumans EH,Chatham-Stephens K,et al. Hospitalizations and deaths associated with EVALI. N Engl J Med,2020,382(17):1589-1598.

[29] Ali M,Khan K,Buch M,et al. A Case Series of Vaping-Induced Lung Injury in a Community Hospital Setting. Case Rep Pulmonol,2020,2020:9631916.

[30] Aberegg SK,Maddock SD,Blagev DP,et al. Diagnosis of EVALI:General Approach and the Role of Bronchoscopy. Chest. 2020,158(2)820-827.

[31] Xantus GZ,Gyarmathy AV,Johnson CA,et al. Smouldering ashes:burning questions after the outbreak of electronic cigarette or vaping-associated lung injury(EVALI). Postgrad Med J,2020,96(1141):686-692.

[32] Jiang H,Ahmed CMS,Martin TJ,et al. Chemical and toxicological characterization of vaping emission products from commonly used vape juice diluents. Chem Res Toxicol,2020,33(8):2157-2163.

[33] Attfield KR,Chen W,Cummings KJ,et al. Potential of Ethenone(ketene)to Contribute to E-cigarette,or Vaping,Product

Use-Associated Lung Injury. Am J RespirCrit Care Med, 2020,202(8):1187-1189.

[34] Hamberger ES, Halpern-Felsher B. Vaping in adolescents: epidemiology and respiratory harm. CurrOpinPediatr, 2020, 32(3):378-383.

[35] Muthumalage T, Lucas JH, Wang Q, et al. Pulmonary toxicity and inflammatory response of e-cigarettes containing medium-chain triglyceride oil and vitamin E acetate: Implications in the pathogenesis of EVALI but independent of SARS-COV-2 COVID-19 related proteins. BioRxiv, 2020, 8(3):46.

[36] Knapp S. Knapp S. Vaping: Cell Damage at the Receiving ENDS. Am J Respir Cell Mol Biol,2020,63(3):271-272.

[37] Blount BC, Karwowski MP, Shields PG, et al. Vitamin E Acetate in Bronchoalveolar-Lavage Fluid Associated with EVALI. N Engl J Med,2020,382(8):697-705.

[38] Kligerman S, Raptis C, Larsen B, et al. Radiologic, Pathologic, Clinical, and Physiologic Findings of Electronic Cigarette or Vaping Product Use-associated Lung Injury (EVALI): Evolving Knowledge and Remaining Questions. Radiology, 2020,294(3):491-505.

[39] Strongin RM. Toxic ketene gas forms on vaping vitamin E acetate prompting interest in its possible role in the EVALI outbreak. Proc Natl AcadSci U S A, 2020, 117 (14): 7553-7554.

[40] Krishnan S, Thind GS, Soliman M, et al. A case of vaping-induced acute respiratory distress syndrome requiring extracorporeal life support. Perfusion,2020.

[41] Fedt A, Bhattarai S, Oelstrom MJ. Vaping-Associated Lung Injury: A New Cause of Acute Respiratory Failure. J Adolesc Health,2020,66(6):754-757.

[42] De Jesús VR, Silva LK, Newman C, et al. Novel Methods for the Analysis of Toxicants in Bronchoalveolar Lavage Fluid Samples from E-cigarette, or Vaping, Product Use-Associated Lung Injury(EVALI)Cases: Terpenes. Rapid Commun Mass Spectrom,2020:e8898.

[43] Matta P, Hamati JN, Unno HL, et al. E-cigarette or Vaping Product Use-Associated Lung Injury (EVALI) Without Respiratory Symptoms. Pediatrics,2020,145(5):e20193408.

[44] Cao DJ, Aldy K, Hsu S, et al. Review of Health Consequences of Electronic Cigarettes and the Outbreak of Electronic Cigarette, or Vaping, Product Use-Associated Lung Injury. J Med Toxicol,2020,16(3):295-310.

[45] Carlos WG, Crotty Alexander LE, Gross JE, et al. ATS Health Alert-Vaping-associated Pulmonary Illness (VAPI). Am J RespirCrit Care Med,2019,200(7):15-16.

[46] Daffolyn Rachael Fels Elliott, Rupal Shah, Catherine Ann Hess, et al. Giant cell interstitial pneumonia secondary to cobalt exposure from e-cigarette use. EurRespir J,2019,54(6): 1901922.

[47] Casanova GS, Amaro R, Soler N, et al. An imported case of e-cigarette or vaping associated lung injury in Barcelona. EurRespir J,2020,55(2):1902076.

[48] Sharma M, Anjum H, Bulathsinghala CP, et al. A Case Report of Secondary Spontaneous Pneumothorax Induced by Vape. Cureus,2019,11(11):e6067.

[49] Bonilla A, Blair AJ, Alamro SM, et al. Recurrent spontaneous pneumothoraces and vaping in an 18-year-old man: a case report and review of the literature. J Med Case Rep, 2019, 13 (1):283.

[50] Cedano J, Sah A, Cedeno-Mendoza R, et al. Confirmed E-cigarette or vaping product use associated lung injury (EVALI) with lung biopsy: A case report and literature review. Respir Med Case Rep,2020,30:101122.

[51] Artunduaga M, Rao D, Friedman J, et al. Pediatric Chest Radiographic and CT Findings of Electronic Cigarette or Vaping Product Use-associated Lung Injury (EVALI). Radiology, 2020,295(2):430-438.

[52] Freathy S, Kondapalli N, Patlolla S, et al. Acute lung injury secondary to e-cigarettes or vaping. Proc (BaylUniv Med Cent),2019,33(2):227-228.

[53] MacMurdo M, Lin C, Saeedan MB, et al. e-Cigarette or Vaping Product Use-Associated Lung Injury: Clinical, Radiologic, and Pathologic Findings of 15 Cases. Chest,2020,157(6): e181-e187.

[54] Mull ES, Erdem G, Nicol K, et al. Eosinophilic Pneumonia and Lymphadenopathy Associated With Vaping and Tetrahydrocannabinol Use. Pediatrics,2020,145(4):e20193007.

[55] ChaabanT. Chaaban T. Acute eosinophilic pneumonia associated with non-cigarette smoking products: a systematic review. AdvRespir Med,2020,88(2):142-146.

[56] Sakla NM, Gattu R, Singh G, et al. Vaping-associated acute respiratory distress syndrome. EmergRadiol, 2020, 27 (1): 103-106.

[57] Wilhite R, Patel T, Karle E, et al. Diffuse Alveolar Hemorrhage: An Uncommon Manifestation of Vaping-associated Lung Injury. Cureus,2019,11(12):e6519.

[58] Shehata M, Kocher T. Vaping-associated diffuse alveolar hemorrhage-A case report. Respir Med Case Rep, 2020, 30:101038.

[59] Flower M, Nandakumar L, Singh M, et al. Respiratory bronchiolitis-associated interstitial lung disease secondary to electronic nicotine delivery system use confirmed with open lung biopsy. Respirol Case Rep,2017,5(3):e00230.

[60] Henry TS, Kligerman SJ, Raptis CA, et al. Imaging Findings of Vaping-Associated Lung Injury. AJR Am J Roentgenol, 2020,214(3):498-505.

[61] Davidson K, Brancato A, Heetderks P, et al. Outbreak of Electronic-Cigarette-Associated Acute Lipoid Pneumonia-North Carolina, July-August 2019. MMWR Morb Mortal Wkly Rep,2019,68(36):784-786.

[62] O'Carroll O, Sharma K, Fabre A, et al. Vaping-associated lung injury. Thorax,2020,11(11):e6216.

[63] Alzghoul BN, Innabi A, Mukhtar F, et al. Rapid Resolution of Severe Vaping Induced Acute Lipoid Pneumonia Following Corticosteroid Treatment. Am J RespirCrit Care Med, 2020, 202(2):32-33.

[64] Gay B, Field Z, Patel S, et al. Vaping-Induced Lung Injury: A Case of Lipoid Pneumonia Associated with E-Cigarettes Containing Cannabis. Case Rep Pulmonol,2020,2020:7151834.

[65] Carlos WG, Crotty Alexander LE, Gross JE, et al. Vaping-associated Pulmonary Illness (VAPI). Am J RespirCrit Care Med, 2019, 200(7):13-14.

[66] Mittal A, Baig A, Zulfikar R, et al. Chronic Vaping Related Tracheomalacia (TM): A Case of Vaping Induced Altered Innate Immunity that Culminated in Severe TM. Cureus, 2020, 12(4):e7571.

[67] Cecchini MJ, Mukhopadhyay S, Arrossi AV, et al. E-Cigarette or Vaping Product Use-Associated Lung Injury: A Review for Pathologists. Arch Pathol Lab Med, 2020, 144(12):1490-1500.

[68] Priemer DS, Gravenmier C, Batouli A, et al. Overview of Pathologic Findings of Vaping in the Context of an Autopsy Patient With Chronic Injury. Arch Pathol Lab Med, 2020, 144(11):1408-1413.

[69] Butt YM, Smith ML, Tazelaar HD, et al. Pathology of Vaping-Associated Lung Injury. N Engl J Med, 2019, 381(18):1780-1781.

[70] Khan MS, Khateeb F, Akhtar J, et al. Organizing pneumonia related to electronic cigarette use: A case report and review of literature. Clin Respir J, 2018, 12(3):1295-1299.

[71] Fryman C, Lou B, Weber AG, et al. Acute Respiratory Failure Associated With Vaping. Chest, 2020, 157(3):e63-e68.

[72] Villeneuve T, Prevot G, Le Borgne A, et al. Diffuse alveolar haemorrhage secondary to e-cigarette "vaping" associated lung injury (EVALI) in a young European consumer. Eur Respir J, 2020, 2000143.

[73] Mukhopadhyay S, Mehrad M, Dammert P, et al. Lung Biopsy Findings in Severe Pulmonary Illness Associated With E-Cigarette Use (Vaping). Am J Clin Pathol, 2020, 153(1):30-39.

[74] Siegel DA, Jatlaoui TC, Koumans EH, et al. Update: Interim Guidance for Health Care Providers Evaluating and Caring for Patients with Suspected E-cigarette, or Vaping, Product Use Associated Lung Injury-United States, October 2019. MMWR Morb Mortal Wkly Rep, 2019, 68(41):919-927.

[75] Schier JG, Meiman JG, Layden J, et al. Severe Pulmonary Disease Associated with Electronic-Cigarette-Product Use-Interim Guidance. MMWR Morb Mortal Wkly Rep, 2019, 68(36):787-790.

[76] Jatlaoui TC, Wiltz JL, Kabbani S, et al. Update: Interim Guidance for Health Care Providers for Managing Patients with Suspected E-cigarette, or Vaping, Product Use-Associated Lung Injury-United States, November 2019. MMWR Morb Mortal Wkly Rep, 2019, 68(46):1081-1086.

[77] Armatas C, Heinzerling A, Wilken JA. Notes from the Field: E-cigarette, or Vaping, Product Use-Associated Lung Injury Cases During the COVID-19 Response-California, 2020. MMWR Morb Mortal Wkly Rep, 2020, 69(25):801-802.

[78] Ahmad M, Aftab G, Rehman S, et al. Long-term Impact of E-cigarette and Vaping Product Use-associated Lung Injury on Diffusing Capacity for Carbon Monoxide Values: A Case Series. Cureus, 2020, 12(2):e7002.

[79] Foust AM, Winant AJ, Chu WC, et al. Pediatric SARS, H1N1, MERS, EVALI, and Now Coronavirus Disease (COVID-19) Pneumonia: What Radiologists Need to Know. AJR Am J Roentgenol, 2020, 215(3):736-744.

[80] Cerepani MJ, Lynch M, Ramponi DR. Vaping: What Every Emergency Nurse Practitioner Should Know! Adv Emerg Nurs J, 2020, 42(2):90-95.

[81] Aftab G, Ahmad M, Frenia D. Vaping-associated Lung Injury. Cureus, 2019, 11(11):e6216.

[82] Akkanti BH, Hussain R, Patel MK, et al. Deadly combination of Vaping-Induced lung injury and Influenza: case report. DiagnPathol, 2020, 15(1):83.

[83] Crotty Alexander LE, Ware LB, Calfee CS, et al. NIH Workshop Report: E-cigarette or Vaping Product Use Associated Lung Injury (EVALI): Developing a Research Agenda. Am J RespirCrit Care Med, 2020, 202(6):795-802.

[84] Kalininskiy A, Bach CT, Nacca NE, et al. E-cigarette, or vaping, product use associated lung injury (EVALI): case series and diagnostic approach. Lancet Respir Med, 2019, 7(12):1017-1026.

[85] Aldy K, Cao DJ, McGetrick M, et al. Severe E-Cigarette, or Vaping, Product Use Associated Lung Injury Requiring Venovenous Extracorporeal Membrane Oxygenation. PediatrCrit Care Med, 2020, 21(4):385-388.

[86] Patterson CM, Valchanov K, Barker A, et al. Severe acute respiratory distress syndrome requiring extracorporeal membrane oxygenation support: a consequence of vaping. ERJ Open Res, 2020, 6(2):00013-2020.

[87] Huey S, Granitto M. Discharge guidelines for patients with EVALI. Nursing, 2020, 50(6):18.

[88] Rao DR, Maple KL, Dettori A, et al. Clinical Features of E-cigarette, or Vaping, Product-Associated Lung Injury in Teenagers. Pediatrics, 2020, 146(1):e20194104.

[89] Eddy RL, Serajeddini H, Knipping D, et al. Pulmonary Functional MRI and CT in a Survivor of Bronchiolitis and Respiratory Failure Due to E-cigarette Use. Chest, 2020, 158(4):147-151.

[90] Deliwala S, Sundus S, Haykal T, et al. E-cigarette, or Vaping, Product Use-associated Lung Injury (EVALI): Acute Lung Illness within Hours of Switching from Traditional to E-cigarettes. Cureus, 2020, 12(4):e7513.

[91] Odish MF, Bellinghausen A, Golts E, et al. E-cigarette, or vaping, product use associated lung injury (EVALI) treated with veno-venous extracorporeal membrane oxygenation (VV-ECMO) and ultra-protective ventilator settings. BMJ Case Rep, 2020, 13(7):e234771.

2 烟草控制与中国经济之关系

赵 帅 陈 宏

烟草危害是严重的公共卫生问题,全世界每年因为吸烟导致死亡人数达到600万。世界卫生组织已经将烟草依赖列入国际疾病分类,确认了烟草对健康有严重的危害。中国是世界上最大烟草消费国和生产国,根据中国烟草局统计,2018年中国烟草种植总面积约为1057.86千公顷,全年烟草产量224.1万吨,2019年中国卷烟总产量呈上升趋势,总产量为23642.5亿支,同比2018年增加286.3亿支。2020年1～2月,全国卷烟产量为5187.4亿支,较2019年同比增长4.4%。中国现吸烟总人数达3.01亿,15岁以上吸烟率达到28.1%。中国目前至少有7.4亿人正在被动吸烟,72.4%的非吸烟者不得不暴露于二手烟环境中。中国每年吸烟导致死亡人数多于100万,占死亡总人数的12%。吸烟所导致的经济损失已经超过烟草行业所带来的社会财富。

烟草行业是一个完整的产业链条,包括烟草种植、烟草加工、包装生产、烟草生产线制造、卷烟销售、烟叶贸易等。烟草行业属于中国经济的重要组成部分,故而烟草控制与经济有着密切的联系。

一、个人吸烟的经济学成因

经济学家Becker和Murphy提出了理性成瘾理论,认为吸烟者是寻找经济效用最大化的理性人。吸烟者会尝试计算吸烟的成本和效益,比如购买卷烟的花费、健康损失和当前享乐之间的关系。如果吸烟者觉得效益大于成本,就会选择吸烟。这一理论认为,吸烟是烟民理性选择。也有经济学家对此提出质疑,Gruber提出烟民具有偏好不稳定性,他发现吸烟者被迫戒烟后,不会不开心,反而变得很高兴。他认为,吸烟者具有"双重自我","今天的自我"希望立刻享受吸烟的乐趣,而"明天的自我"考虑到健康和经济问题,希望戒烟。当明天变为今天时,吸烟者便会每天推迟戒烟行动。他认为吸烟者缺乏自我约束能力是吸烟的重要原因。提高烟草税,可以迫使一部分吸烟者开始戒烟行动,解决自制力缺乏的问题。

根据以上理论,我们可以分析吸烟的主观期望效用:①吸烟能带来明显的及时的效用:吸烟者点燃一支烟,经过广泛的肺泡的吸收,尼古丁能够迅速的进入血液,快速地给吸烟者带来愉悦。这种效用是吸烟者易于体会到的。在经济学中,期望效用越靠近现在,那么决策权重越大,时间越远,决策权重越小。②吸烟的短期和长期成本都不明显:吸烟者承担的短期成本不明显,随着经济水平的提高,卷烟的开销在烟民经济收入的占比越来越小。另外,吸烟者产生的环境污染、对他人的二手烟吸入并不需要负明确的责任。长期成本来看,由于时间较远,故而对当前吸烟决策的影响权重就偏小。由于吸烟带来的损失不明显,吸烟者往往会推迟戒烟,虽然吸烟有害健康的结论已经证实,但是吸烟者基于生活经验,往往低估这种损害,当下一支烟的享乐比远期的的危害要更加真实。

二、烟草工业在国家经济中的地位

1991年,中国出台了《烟草专卖法》,确定了中国的烟草专卖制度。在专卖制度的保护下,中国烟草行业一直稳步增长。根据国家烟草专卖局数据,中国烟草种植区分为5个一级和26个二级烟草种植区。中国共有烟农130余万户,500余万户零售商。2018年,烟草行业卷烟销量达到3557.54万箱,同比2017年增长2.34%,烟草行业工业总产值同比2017年增长9.04%。烟草相关劳动人数达到2000余万。中国烟草行业有17家省级烟草专卖公司、30家烟草生产企业和上千家烟草销售企业。烟草具有成瘾性,再加上烟草专卖制度的控制,所以烟草销量受到经济影响很小。中国长期卷烟产销比接近1:1,无库存积压,仓储成本低,市场销量稳中有涨。中国50%以上的烟草生产基地位于经济不发达地区,局部地区的经济水平高度依赖烟草业,在这些地区,烟草行业对人口就业及社会保障,经济发展有着密切的关系。我们不能脱离经济因素,孤立的探讨控烟问题。巨大的经济问题,导致控烟困难重重。在改革开放的发展过程中,烟草提供了可观的财政收入。20世纪80年代开始,烟草行业成为中国最大的财税来源。从2011年到2015年,烟草行业贡献税利占全国一般公共预算收入的7%以上(表1-2-1)。对于云南、贵州这样的烟草

表 1-2-1 2013－2017 年中国烟草行业工商税利情况

年份	烟草行业工商税利(亿元)	全国一般公共预算收入(亿元)	烟草税利占全国一般公共预算收入百分比(%)
2013	9559.86	129 210	7.4
2014	10 517.60	140 370	7.49
2015	11 436.00	152 269	7.51
2016	10 759.00	159 605	6.77
2017	11 145.10	172 593	6.46

种植省份来说,烟草提供的财政收入尤为显著。烟草利税占云南省财政收入多年超过40%,个别年份甚至超过60%。

三、烟草外部性成本造成的经济负担巨大

烟草除了危害人体健康,对经济发展也造成相当的危害,这往往是我们医学工作者容易忽略的。

经济学概念:外部性成本包括正外部性和负外部性。正外部性是指行为人实施的行为对他人或者公共环境的利益有溢出效应,即是有益的行为;负外部性是指行为人实施的行为对他人或者公共环境造成减损,即有害的行为。吸烟造成的人体疾病、环境污染、灾害发生等均属于烟草的外部性成本。外部性成本对经济造成损害,我们不能忽视,也不能孤立的评价人体疾病与控烟的关系,而忽略经济因素。

随着中国国民整体素质逐步提高,医疗卫生知识通过媒体获得了广泛的普及,吸烟有害健康被人民群众广泛认可。但是,由于中国经济的飞速发展,人们消费能力大幅度提高。烟草产品作为价格相对低廉,人们随处可得的享受类产品,获得了越来越广泛的消费群体,尤其是年轻消费者比例有升高的趋势。因为烟草对人体的损害有滞后性,在使用和消费烟草产品的时候,使用者往往容易忽略烟草的危害。这部分负面成本会被转移到将来,对计算烟草外部性成本造成一定困难。以下从烟草外部成本的三个方面进行讨论。

(一)吸烟导致医疗成本

中国是世界上吸烟人口数最大的国家,原卫生部发布的《中国吸烟危害健康报告》中提到,中国吸烟人群超过3亿,二手烟危害人群达到7.4亿,中国每年因吸烟相关疾病死亡人数达到100万人,因二手烟导致的死亡人数达到10万人。有证据表明,吸烟可以导致呼吸系统疾病、肿瘤、心血管疾病等。二手烟也可以导致以上疾病的发生,二手烟对孕妇及儿童也会带来长期潜在的危害。吸烟的医疗外部成本包括:吸烟导致的早逝、直接医疗损失、间接陪护造成的损失等。医疗成本呈现逐年增加趋势,2014年医疗外部成本为4577.02亿元,2015年为5167.986亿元。2017年,主动吸烟造成的医疗外部成本为6007.16亿元,被动吸烟造成的医疗外部成本为270.63亿元,总的医疗外部成本为6277.79亿元。

(二)烟草导致的环境成本

烟草导致的环境外部成本包括:烟草产品生产制造的环境成本,烟蒂、烟灰垃圾清理成本。

中国烟草生产以烤烟为主,制作烤烟需要大量的煤炭。煤炭燃烧产生一氧化碳、二氧化碳、二氧化硫等有害气体,这些有害气体会导致温室效应和酸雨等自然环境灾害。另外生产卷烟需要消耗大量的纸张,生产纸张带来的环境污染(以水体富营养化为主)是极其严重的。烟蒂、烟灰是烟草消费带来的垃圾,这类垃圾体积小,易藏匿,不容易清理。室内的烟蒂会破坏居住和工作环境,室外的烟蒂则影响市容、市貌。所以,这部分成本涉及每个家庭、每家公司,更影响大型公共场所。每年清理烟蒂、烟灰垃圾,也会造成客观的外部成本。中国烟草导致温室效应造成的经济损失为18.038亿~34.239亿元。而烟草导致的酸雨造成的经济损失为0.168亿元。温室效应导致的环境成本也呈现逐渐增加的趋势。烟蒂等固体废弃物造成的经济损失为51.9亿~103.8亿元。

(三)烟草相关灾害导致的成本

未熄灭的烟蒂、打火机和火柴的不正确使用,是导致火灾发生的重要原因之一。其中,随意丢弃的烟蒂非常容易导致火灾发生。全世界每年有约20%的火灾由吸烟导致。火灾所造成的经济损失包括火灾中直接烧毁的财务、火灾伤残导致的劳动力损失、火灾造成的医疗成本。根据中国应急管理部每年公布数据,吸烟导致的普通火灾造成经济损失2.52亿~3.6亿元。2003—2017年平均每年吸烟引发的火灾占火灾总数的6.71%。吸烟引起森林火灾所造成的经济损失也不能忽略,2017年该类损失为0.349亿~0.524亿元。

综上,2017年,中国烟草引起的医疗外部成本为6277.789亿元,温室效应导致的外部成本为18.038亿~34.239亿元,酸雨造成的经济损失为0.168亿元,普通火灾造成的经济损失为2.52亿~3.6亿元,森林火灾经济损失为0.349亿~0.524亿元,其中医疗外部成本为烟草外部成本的最主要组成部分。2017年,中国烟草税费收入为5293.569亿元,尚不足以抵消医疗外部成本。因此,烟草行业对于中国经济发展总体来说是负作用。

四、中国烟草税费对控烟影响

赋税是一种常用的经济手段。烟草税在国际上是公认的效果明显、方便操作的控烟政策。在《烟草控制框架公约》中,通过提高烟草税来减少烟草消费是缔约国的义务。与国际社会对比,中国烟草税一直处在较低水平。

上文的计算表明烟草行业对中国经济发展带来了不利的影响,如果不控制烟草,将会阻碍中国经济的健康发展。提高烟草税是控烟手段中最基本的也是效果最明显的手段。提高烟草税会导致烟草产品零售价格提高,间接减少烟草的消费。提高烟草税还可以解决烟草外部成本带来的经济损害,使得吸烟者自行承担部分烟草外部成本。由于烟草产品的成瘾性,烟草价格变化导致的消费弹性较低,所以提高烟草税可以带来增量的财政收入。2008年以来,中国卫生医疗支出增长率接近20%,超过了同期GDP增长,为了进一步推动中国的医疗改革,公共财政也需要新的资金增长点,此时,提高烟草税的作用就得以发挥。

中国于1994年建立消费税制度,针对包括烟草在内的消费品征税。之后,中国多次调整烟草税率。其中2015年的烟草消费税调整作用尤为显著,卷烟批发环节从价税提高到11%,并增加了每支0.005元的从量税。政策推行后,烟草消费税额保持稳定,烟草消费数量首次出现减少趋势。

同时,我们也不能忽略提高烟草税可能带来的副作用:第一,提高烟草税可能促进非法交易。提高烟草税的

政策,很大程度地限制和减少了烟草商的合法经营利润;客观上,非法经营的利润空间增加,非法经营者可能增加交易量。所以在增加烟草税的同时,还需要加强针对非法烟草经营行为的执法力度,严格处罚,有效抑制烟草的非法经营行为。第二,提高烟草税可能导致吸烟者的补偿行为。在提高烟草税后,吸烟者每天吸烟数减少,但因烟草的成瘾性客观存在,吸烟者为了缓解烟草的戒断症状,会尝试补偿行为。这种补偿行为包括使用价格低廉同时含有更多烟碱和烟焦油的烟草产品,甚至直接使用未经深加工的烤烟叶。这样虽然每日吸烟支数减少,但客观上摄入的烟碱和焦油量并未下降,甚至可能上升。这些副作用也是税务部门需要慎重考虑的。

五、综合经济因素,综合手段推进控烟工作

疾病治疗的花费和劳动力减少的损失,对经济造成了巨大的影响,远远超过了当年烟草行业上缴的税额。尽管如此,我们发现,一些部门的控烟工作依旧进展缓慢。从经济角度分析,这其中有经济负担转移的功利因素:①医疗花费主要在个人,对财政消耗不大。虽然现在全民医保覆盖越来越完善,但是在几年前,中国公民医疗过程中大量的开销由个人负担。所以,疾病所导致的经济负担更多表现在家庭经济上,对地方财政影响较小。地方财政的烟草税利成为一些部门的净收益。②医疗负担由现在转向未来。烟草依赖性疾病是一种慢性疾病,从开始吸烟到发病过程,一般需要几年到几十年。由烟草疾病所导致的劳动力损失,也需要几十年后才能体现出来,而政府部门收到的烟草税利在当年就立竿见影。面对眼前的快速的显而易见的收益和未来的漫长的不显著的疾病负担,在部门决策中的优先级就有较大落差。

综上,在控烟工作中,对经济因素的重视尤为重要。目前总的财政对烟草税利仍有依赖,同时一部分地区的经济支柱是烟草行业,所以必须考虑经济因素,才能开拓控烟的康庄大道。①烟草管理部门与烟草企业分离:中国烟草企业与烟草管理部门没有明显的界限,在具体控烟工作中,难以要求烟草行业自己限制自己,自己缩减自己的经济利益。这也是在目前控烟形势轰轰烈烈的背景下,烟草行业仍能够获得一定发展空间的主要原因之一。所以让烟草企业归于市场,烟草管理部门一心服务于行政,让两者划清界限,才是高效的控烟策略。②减少地方经济对烟草行业的依赖:中国烟草种植区共划分为31个种植区。其中云南、四川、贵州、湖南和河南是最主要的烟草种植区。而且这些地区多为经济欠发达地区,当地经济高度依赖烟草生产。所以解决当地的经济问题,成为解决控制烟草生产的重要途径。发展替代产业,将烟草行业劳动力转移到其他产业,保持当地经济继续繁荣,是需要当地政府重点解决的问题。③提高烟草税,减少烟草消费量:控制烟草消费的重要手段是提高烟草税。提高烟草税率,导致烟草价格上涨,可以有效减少烟草的消费。尤其是提高价格低廉的卷烟的售价,对于控烟尤其有效。低价格卷烟的主要消费群体属于价格敏感群体;高价卷烟的消费人群对卷烟价格变化并不敏感。当卷烟价格提高后,消费能力低的人群就会减少烟草的消费。通过时间的积累,卷烟销量逐渐减少,烟草生产销售,乃至整个烟草行业就会逐渐萎缩。根据《2015年中国成人烟草调查报告》资料分析:吸烟者自吸的购买卷烟平均价格为9.9元/盒,而接受馈赠的卷烟价格平均为17元/盒。自己吸用的属于三类卷烟,而作为馈赠礼品的卷烟属于一类卷烟,甚至部分属于名贵卷烟范畴。针对高价卷烟,政府也在着手进行限制,包括限制生产制造和限制销售流通。这样既可以减少卷烟的高消费,同时一定程度上减少腐败滋生的土壤。提高烟草税,还能抵消一部分烟草销量减少导致的财政收入减少。与其他国家横向比较,中国烟草税率水平低于国际平均水平,仍然有很大的税率提高空间。

参 考 文 献

[1] 中华人民共和国卫生部.中国吸烟危害健康报告.北京:人民卫生出版社,2012.
[2] Eriksen M,Mackay J,Ross H. The tobacco Atlas. (4th edition). World Lung Foundation and American Cancer Society,2013.
[3] 国家烟草专卖局.《2019年1-1月卷烟统计信息》. http://www.tobacco.gov.cn/html/56/9015347_n.html(2020-06-23).
[4] 中国疾病预防控制中心.2010年全球成人烟草调查-中国报告.北京:中国三峡出版社,2011.
[5] 杨功焕,胡鞍钢.控烟与中国未来:中外专家中国烟草使用与烟草控制联合评估报告.北京:经济日报出版社,2011.
[6] 黄馨缘,郑频频.2006—2015年中国控烟干预实践文献分析.环境与职业医学,2016,33(5):461-465.
[7] 国家烟草专卖局.《2018年1—9月卷烟产销统计信息》. http://www.tobacco.goc.cn/html/56/87400267_n.html (2018-10-23).
[8] 国家烟草专卖局.《中国烟草控制规划(2012—2015年)发布 http://www.tobacco.goc.cn/html/49/425349_n.html (2012-12-21).
[9] 张森荣,张海芳.从社会与经济视角论我国控烟政策.健康教育促进,2012,7(2):119-123.
[10] Markowitz S. The effecticeess of cigarette regulations in reducing cases of sudden infant death syndrome. Journal of Health Economics,2008,27(1):106-133.
[11] 赵世鑫.烟草消费税与烟草消费的外部成本.上海海关学院,2019.
[12] da Costae Silva VL,Fishburn B. Tobacco use and control:determinants of consumption, intervention strategies, and the role of the tobacco industry. Toxicology,2004,198(1-3):9-18.
[13] 清水.揭开《2015年中国成人烟草调查报告》面纱 http://www.tobaccochina.com/revision/takematter/wu/20161/20161616343_707174.shtml.(2016-01-11)[2016-01-22].

3 中国烟草病学发展现状与展望

孙德俊

烟草病学是研究烟草对健康影响的医学学科,其学科框架包括吸烟行为和烟草依赖,吸烟及二手烟的流行状况、主要危害,戒烟的健康益处,烟草依赖的治疗。

近年来,烟草病学学科体系在中国逐步走向成熟。在几代呼吸病学研究人员的不断努力下,中国于2011年成立了以推广烟草病学相关学术研究为目标的"中华医学会呼吸病学分会烟草病学学组"及"中国医师协会呼吸医师分会疾病预防工作委员会烟草控制工作组"。世界卫生组织戒烟与呼吸疾病预防合作中心落户北京,同时成立了中国戒烟联盟及各地多层级的戒烟机构,有力地推动了中国各地的控烟工作。中国也在烟草控制、烟草与呼吸疾病发病的关系、戒烟技术等多方面开展了一系列较为深入的研究,取得了一系列的成绩。

一、中国烟草流行情况

自20世纪以来,各种各样的烟草制品在全球广泛流行。连续多年的烟草流行状况调查显示中国烟草流行状况依然严峻。

2015年中国成人烟草调查的结果显示:15岁及以上人群现吸烟率为27.7%,2015年吸烟者总数为3.16亿;男性吸烟率为52.1%,女性为2.7%。2018年中国成人烟草调查的结果显示:中国15岁及以上人群吸烟率为26.6%,男性为50.5%,女性为2.1%,农村为28.9%,城市为25.1%。与既往调查结果相比,吸烟率呈现下降趋势,但与实现《"健康中国2030"规划纲要》的控烟目标——"2030年15岁及以上人群吸烟率下降至20%"仍有较大差距。

2015年对二手烟流行情况调查显示,与2010年相比,在工作场所看到有人吸烟的比例由60.6%降至54.3%。在政府大楼看到有人吸烟的比例从54.9%降至38.1%;在医疗机构看到有人吸烟的比例从36.8%降至26.9%;在中小学(室内和室外)看到有人吸烟的比例从34.6%降至17.2%;在餐馆看到有人吸烟的比例从87.6%降至76.3%;在公共交通工具看到有人吸烟的比例从29.0%降至16.4%;在家中看到有人吸烟的比例由64.3%降至57.1%。2018年的调查显示,二手烟的总体暴露率为68.1%。50.9%的室内工作者在工作场所看到有人吸烟。44.9%的调查对象报告有人在自己家中吸烟。二手烟暴露最严重的室内公共场所为:网吧(89.3%)、酒吧和夜总会(87.5%)、餐馆(73.3%)。与2015年调查结果相比,二手烟暴露情况整体有所改善。

从2015年开始,公众对室内公共场所和工作场所全面禁烟的支持度逐步增高。即使是吸烟者,对各类公共场所室内全面禁烟也有很高的支持度。人群在电视或报纸/杂志上看到控烟信息的比例为61.1%。然而与2010年相比,人群看见烟草广告和促销信息的比例均有所增加,其中在销售卷烟的商店里看到烟草广告的比例增幅仍然最大。与既往调查结果相比,2018年的调查中发现,公众支持在室内公共场所、工作场所和公共交通工具场所全面禁烟的比例进一步上升。公众支持工作场所全面禁烟的比例为90.9%。超过九成的公众支持在医院(97.1%)、中小学校(96.7%)、公共交通工具(96.1%)、出租车(92.9%)和大学(92.7%)全面禁烟。支持餐馆室内全面禁烟的比例为79.9%。

在戒烟方面,2015年调查显示,医务人员向吸烟者提供戒烟建议的比例由2010年的33.2%上升至58.2%。戒烟比(每日吸烟者中戒烟者在所有曾经和现在每日吸烟者中的比例)为14.4%,现在吸烟者考虑在未来12个月内戒烟(包括计划在1个月内)的比例为17.6%,与2010年相比无明显差异。2018年的调查显示,中国成年吸烟人群戒烟意愿普遍较低,戒烟率未呈现明显变化。中国15岁及以上人群戒烟率为20.1%;每日吸烟者戒烟率为15.6%。16.1%的吸烟者打算在未来12个月内戒烟,计划在1个月内戒烟的比例仅为5.6%。在过去12个月吸烟的人中,19.8%尝试过戒烟。尝试戒烟的前三位原因分别是担心继续吸烟影响今后健康(38.7%)、已经患病(26.6%)和家人反对吸烟(14.9%)。

调查显示,2015年到2018年烟草制品的可负担性情况为:吸烟者购买20支机制卷烟的费用中位数为9.9元,无明显变化。购买100盒卷烟的花费占同年人均国内生产总值的比例由2015年的2.0%降至1.5%,这也是导致青少年吸烟率持续升高的重要原因之一。烟草广告、促销和赞助仍是青少年尝试吸烟的重要影响因素。在接受调查前30d内,调查对象看到过烟草广告、促销或赞助的比例为18.1%,其中在15～24岁年龄组中,该比例为28.5%。看过烟草广告的人中,在销售卷烟的商店和互联网看到烟草广告的比例相对较高,分别为43.3%和42.3%。另外,影视作品中的吸烟镜头对青少年尝试吸烟有非常重要的诱导作用。此次调查发现在调查前30d内,61.1%的人在电视、录像、视频或者电影中看到吸烟镜头,在15～24岁年龄组中,该比例高达68.3%。

中国学者发表在《柳叶刀－呼吸》的研究报道了

2003—2013年中国吸烟流行趋势及其对慢性病的影响。此后，全国范围内的系列横断面调查也就相关问题进行了研究。

研究表明，中国吸烟率从15～24岁急剧上升，在40～50岁的人群中达到高峰，50岁后下降。曾经吸烟的总人数中戒烟的比例较低，但在50岁或50岁以上人群中戒烟的比例高于50岁以下人群。同时研究显示了青少年吸烟率大幅度增加。

青少年性别标准化吸烟率从8.3%上升到12.5%，在男性青少年中，吸烟率从16.0%上升到23.5%，在女性青少年中，从0.4%上升到1.1%；非学生青少年的吸烟率是学生青少年的10倍以上。2003年学生青少年吸烟率为0.5%，2013年为1.9%，非学生青少年吸烟率2003年为13.1%，2013年为19.9%。调查显示77.9%的吸烟者在青春期开始吸烟。2013年，15～19岁人群吸烟率增幅最高（60.2%），其次为19～24岁人群（18.1%）。

新型烟草制品的出现，无疑对青少年吸烟者具有更强的吸引力和更便捷的可得性。2018年的调查发现，使用电子烟的人群主要以年轻人为主，15～24岁年龄组人群电子烟使用率为1.5%。获得电子烟最主要的途径是互联网（45.4%）。值得关注的是，与2015年相比，听说过电子烟、曾经使用过电子烟，以及现在使用的比例均有所提高。新型烟草制品带来的问题也是烟草病学面临的新的挑战。

二、烟草流行对中国呼吸系统疾病的影响

与慢性非传染性疾病（NCDs）发生的主要吸烟相关危险因素是开始吸烟年龄和吸烟时间。

已经有明确的证据表明，吸烟和二手烟暴露与全身各个部位的肿瘤和慢性疾病的发生有明确的相关关系。尤其在中国，吸烟和二手烟暴露对常见慢性呼吸系统疾病发病造成明显的影响。基于2010年全球成人烟草调查报告、全球青少年烟草调查报告、中国慢性病前瞻性研究、开滦煤矿队列研究和广州生物样本库队列研究等经典研究结果，《中国慢性呼吸疾病流行状况与防治策略》白皮书阐述了吸烟和二手烟暴露对中国常见慢性呼吸疾病发病的影响。

随着时间的推移，NCDs患病率在男性和女性人群中都急剧上升，女性从2003年的8.3%上升到2013年的13.6%，男性从7.3%上升到12.7%；所有受调查的年份中，男性和女性的非传染性疾病患病率均随年龄稳步上升；经常吸烟的人比不吸烟的人患NCD的风险更高，与过早开始吸烟相关的风险增加。吸烟者中消化性溃疡发病率最高，其次是支气管肺癌或肺癌、慢性阻塞性肺疾病（以下简称慢阻肺）和口腔疾病。男性NCDs顺位为：消化性溃疡、支气管肺癌或肺癌、慢阻肺、口腔疾病和类风湿关节炎；女性NCDs顺位为：消化性溃疡、慢性阻塞性肺疾病、缺血性心脏病和脑血管疾病。

（一）肺癌

吸烟是肺癌的首要危险因素。中国前瞻性吸烟研究和中国慢性病前瞻性研究结果显示，开始吸烟年龄越早、吸烟量越大，肺癌的死亡风险越高。例如，城市男性开始吸烟年龄小于20岁者的肺癌死亡风险为不吸烟者的3.78倍，开始吸烟年龄25岁及以上者肺癌死亡风险为不吸烟者的2.23倍；城市男性每日吸烟量小于15支者，肺癌死亡风险为非吸烟者的2.28倍，而每日吸烟量超过25支者肺癌死亡风险为不吸烟者的4.12倍。在中国二手烟暴露导致非吸烟肺癌患者中超过22 000例死亡。

（二）慢阻肺

吸烟是导致慢阻肺最主要的危险因素，开始吸烟年龄越小、吸烟量越大，慢阻肺死亡风险越高。CPHS研究显示，与慢阻肺关系最密切的因素是吸烟和空气污染。

（三）哮喘

中国学者的研究显示，吸烟可以显著增加哮喘急性发作风险及急诊就诊。母亲妊娠期吸烟可增加儿童哮喘的发病率。存在二手烟暴露风险的儿童哮喘风险显著升高。

（四）小气道病变

中国CPHS研究结果显示，经标准肺功能检查发现小气道病变普遍存在于人群中，研究发现中国小气道病变（SAD）发病率为43.5%，推测SAD患者数4.26亿。而吸烟与小气道病变发生关系最密切。

三、烟草依赖治疗研究进展

近年来，越来越多的研究集中在烟草依赖治疗的相关药物研究，包括尼古丁替代类药物、伐尼克兰、安非他酮等的戒烟效果、药物相关不良反应等，同时开展了药物戒烟后时包括心血管系统、呼吸系统、消化系统等各个系统的影响的研究。

现存的戒烟药物主要是以nAChR为靶点，以nAChR介导的尼古丁诱导多巴胺和去甲肾上腺素释放作为药物开发方向，存在疗效有限且高复发率的问题。而nAChR亚型选择性激动剂和拮抗剂均可被开发为新一代治疗药物，都具有潜在的优势和局限性。nAChR受体拮抗剂（部分或全部）可以代替使用烟草时产生的快感，通常具有良好的耐受性及患者依从性；nAChR激动剂（部分或完全）可以缓解戒断症状的发生。尽管尼古丁的替代疗法是戒烟的主要方法，但同样存在一些新的、潜在的以nAChR部分激动剂作为治疗药物的治疗方法。nAChR部分激动剂代替尼古丁作为治疗方法，可缓解戒断症状的产生和减少对烟草的渴求，同时还可以减少尼古丁的强化和由nAChR介导的尼古丁重复给药引起的药物的释放。目前，靶向nAChR的戒烟药物分为三类：①尼古丁替代品；②nAChR部分激动剂；③nAChR拮抗剂。

nAChR部分激动剂除伐尼克兰外，还有金雀花碱及类似物，以及法国赛诺菲-安万特公司开发的用于治疗尼古丁成瘾的部分激动剂Dianicline，Abbott公司开发的神经型α4β2 nAChR全激动剂ABT-418和nAChR部分激动剂ABT-089。用作戒烟试剂的nAChR拮抗剂主要有安非他酮、bPiDDB、r-bPiDDB、18-MC和美卡拉明。

在中国，传统中医学在戒烟中的作用也是临床研究的

热点,其中包括穴位(埋线)治疗、针灸治疗辅助戒烟等。

四、展望

(一)新型烟草带来的挑战

新型烟草制品的出现无疑给烟草病学带来新的挑战。一方面,新型烟草制品如电子烟带来了新的社会、经济问题;另一方面,也带来了新型烟草依赖和危害,给临床戒烟和控烟工作提出了新的问题和要求。

(二)控烟问题给烟草病学带来的挑战

近年来青少年的吸烟率大幅度增加,除了青少年对烟草危害的知识缺乏,对烟草的无知、猎奇心理、模仿、耍酷行为等之外,也伴随着青春期心理和行为的变化。因此烟草病学仍需要从社会学、心理学、行为学、药物学等多个方面对吸烟行为和烟草依赖,以及相关综合干预开展更为深入的研究工作,用科学的态度、观点和实证有力推动控烟工作。

4 根据发生机制和临床表现甄别烟草戒断症状与药物不良反应

童 瑾 陈 夕

《2015中国成人烟草调查报告》中显示中国成人吸烟率为27.7%,吸烟人数3.16亿,但戒烟率仅18.7%。2003年国家卫生服务调查的39 904名现在吸烟者中,15.8%(城市17.3%、农村15.3%)为戒烟后复吸,而复吸原因之一是混淆戒断反应与戒烟药物(安非他酮和伐尼克兰)不良反应而致戒烟者依从性降低,擅自停药。因两者引起的症状极为相似,国内外也鲜少有其区别的研究报道,很多医务人员和戒烟者难以准确鉴别,导致提前停药,增加复吸可能,故对两者鉴别的需求极为迫切。此外,对于药物不良反应的早期处理也有利于规避药物引起的严重后果。

本文从戒断反应和安非他酮、伐尼克兰药物不良反应的不同时间进程、常见和少见但需警惕的症状进行甄别。

一、时间进程特点

目前戒断反应的确切时间进程尚不清楚。有研究表明,经历戒断症状和吸烟渴求的受试者比例在第1天最高,第2天开始下降,第1周又反跳(除外易怒和渴求),1年内逐渐降至基线水平。Hughes等则认为戒断症状多在第1~2天开始,第1周达到高峰,持续2~4周。除吸烟渴求和饥饿外,很少长期持续存在(即6个月或以上)。也有研究发现另外的时间规律,即初期戒断反应由高到低,3周后反跳。上述不同的结论可能与回顾性报告中的偏倚或描述时间进程所使用的方法不同有关。

安非他酮戒烟时,1/3~2/3的患者于用药后数小时至数天内出现不良反应,随时间延长而减弱,多为轻、中度,但有7%~12%不良事件导致停药。

伐尼克兰的不良反应多在几周内可消退,轻度多见,但其停药率仍可达7.9%。对伐尼克兰不良反应时间演变的研究显示,失眠、头痛、便秘和口干仅为一过性症状,恶心和梦境异常从第6周减少,仅肠胃胀气可持续于整个治疗过程。

对于服药(安非他酮或伐尼克兰)的第1周,即戒烟日前1周,此时因未完全戒烟,如出现明显不适感需考虑药物不良反应。

二、常见难区分的症状

戒断反应中,烦躁易怒、焦虑、睡眠障碍、口干、恶心及头痛常易与安非他酮或伐尼克兰的不良反应相混淆。

戒烟后体内尼古丁水平降低,多巴胺(dopamine,DA)被重摄取而减少,引起戒断反应。其机制可能包括:①与脑内N型乙酰胆碱受体(nicotinic acetylcholinesterase receptors,nAChRs)上调和脱敏有关。其中躯体方面的戒断反应主要由中枢和外周nAChRs介导,α_7、α_3、α_5、β_4、α_2 nAChRs亚基和$\alpha_3\beta_4$ nAChRs亚型参与其中,其分布于内侧缰核到脚间核通路;心理方面则通过中枢nAChRs介导,主要由β_2和α6nAChRs亚基参与,其分布多在大脑中的伏隔核、内侧缰核到脚间核通路、杏仁核和海马等区域。此外,也有研究表明,戒断反应的快感缺失由位于中脑腹侧被盖区的α_4和β_2 nAChRs亚型介导,认知障碍由海马区内$\alpha_4\beta_2$ nAChRs介导。②钙依赖机制参与了躯体方面的戒断反应,可能与额下回中的钙离子/钙调素依赖性蛋白激酶Ⅱ总蛋白和磷酸化蛋白水平,以及神经递质释放所必需的囊泡相关蛋白的总蛋白和磷酸化蛋白水平降低有关。③γ-氨基丁酸、谷氨酸、多巴胺和5-羟色胺3(5-hydroxytryptamine,5-HT_3)神经递质参与了躯体和心理方面的戒断反应。nAChRs的激活促进脑中上述神经递质的释放,戒烟时则可因为这些神经递质改变产生戒断反应。④肽能传递物质(甘丙肽、促肾上腺素皮质激素释放因子、src激酶、G蛋白偶联受体激酶5、降钙素、神经激肽、脑源性神经营养因子)、内源性阿片样物质和大麻素也或多或少与躯体和心理方面的戒断反应有关。⑤有假说还认为,戒断症状可能是对失去强化物的一种简单行为反应。

(一) 心理症状

1. 情绪异常 主要表现为烦躁易怒和焦虑。对戒断反应而言,前者在戒烟第1周内达高峰,可持续2周或以上;后者开始于第1~3天,约持续2周。安非他酮的上述症状多在服药后数天内出现,且随时间而减弱。而伐尼克兰的上述症状则多发生在戒烟1~2周。此外,安非他酮引起的烦躁易怒机制与增加去甲肾上腺素(norepinephrine,NE)能和DA能,激活NE和D_2受体有关;焦虑则由激动α_1和D_1受体,增加警醒度引起。但焦虑与安非他酮剂量成反比,剂量越低,焦虑更重,可见安非他酮有一定的抗焦虑作用。有研究证实,因尼古丁戒断导致颅内自身刺激(ntracranialself-stimulation,ICSS)阈值升高,脑奖赏功能减低,促进烦躁易怒和焦虑发生。而伐尼克兰则可减少戒断引起的ICSS阈值升高,减轻这些症状。结合上述机制和研究考虑,情绪异常更多见于戒断反应,少见于安非他酮和伐尼克兰。如服药2周(戒烟日1周)后出现较重的情绪异常,考虑戒断反应可能性大。

处理方式:症状较轻者,无须处理,多数随时间而改善;较重者,若使用安非他酮,则可换为伐尼克兰,也可换用或加用尼古丁替代治疗(nicotine replacement therapy, NRT)。经过上述处理未好转者,在医务工作者监督下可使用药物抗焦虑(如地西泮、甲丙氨酯和丁螺环酮)。

2. 睡眠障碍　戒断症状的睡眠障碍可表现为睡眠持续时间和效率降低、入睡困难、睡眠分裂(包括夜间觉醒、睡眠阶段转换、入睡后的清醒时间等)和梦境异常。安非他酮所致睡眠障碍可表现为降低快速眼动潜伏期,增加快速眼动时间,引起频繁觉醒,导致睡眠障碍。伐尼克兰的睡眠障碍则表现为失眠、梦境异常及难以入睡。有研究提出,频繁的夜间觉醒可能多见于尼古丁戒断,而难以入睡可能多是由于药物引起,其中梦境异常多见于伐尼克兰,安非他酮更易失眠。戒断的睡眠障碍多在戒烟后的第1周内出现,3~12个月后改善。安非他酮所致睡眠障碍时间及机制均与焦虑类似。伐尼克兰的睡眠障碍不良作用可能与胆碱能增强和(或)DA能减弱有关。可在治疗第1周达峰值,然后逐渐下降,第2~12周达到治疗前水平。其与安非他酮对产生此不良作用均有剂量依赖性。故睡眠障碍在服药1周内出现,需考虑药物引起;若2周(戒烟日1周)后出现或加重,则戒断反应可能性大。

处理方式:如果持续性失眠,可先改变或减少药物剂量,或取消安非他酮夜间用药。若效果不佳,可通过非药物和药物干预。非药物干预包括:睡眠卫生宣教和各种行为矫正(如认知疗法、放松和睡眠限制等)。药物干预包括:苯二氮䓬类(艾司唑仑、氯西泮、地西泮、替马西泮和三唑仑)和非苯二氮䓬类(曲唑酮和唑吡坦)。对于入睡困难可使用喹硫平或奥氮平诱导睡眠。

(二)躯体症状

主要有恶心、头痛和口干。戒烟后恶心会短暂增加,口干无明显增加。安非他酮致口干和恶心的机制可能为:阻断尼古丁受体,引起唾液分泌减少和增加NE能产生拟交感神经效应。其口干舌燥具有剂量依赖性,还可能与其唾液中浓度是血浆浓度的5倍有关。伐尼克兰的恶心机制为:①肠神经系统中的神经元调节神经元间胆碱传递的树突状和突触前nAChRs,后者表达的大量nAChRs亚单位(包括α_3、α_5、α_7、β_2和β_4)构成了引起其恶心的nAChRs。②通过激动纹状体DA释放调节的突触前α_4、α_6和$5-HT_3$受体引发恶心。有研究表明,恶心最多见于伐尼克兰,高峰在用药后第2周出现,具有剂量依赖性。口干则多见于安非他酮。上述两种症状戒断反应均少见。

研究发现,对于戒断反应的头痛与安慰剂组相比无明显增加。安非他酮引起头痛的机制是阻断NE和DA再摄取而增加其在突触间隙的浓度,二者均可激动α_1受体,引起脑血管收缩,发生缺血缺氧性头痛,可停药后2~3d基本缓解。伐尼克兰头痛机制是因其为部分nAChRs激动剂,作用于中枢烟碱受体而影响脑血管调节,引起可逆性节段性脑血管收缩;还可因$5-HT_3$受体

的激动引起,发生率为12%~24%。头痛在药物不良反应中较常见,停药后有好转。多为暂时性且轻、中度,随服药时间延长而减轻。

处理方式:头痛明显,可减少药物剂量和(或)换为NRT;若仍持续,可停药,使用尼莫地平或非甾体抗炎药对症镇痛。恶心、呕吐则可通过饭时服药和(或)缓慢增加剂量,或使用抗恶心或止吐药物来缓解。口干通常是短暂的,多迅速消退。

三、少见但需警惕的症状

(一)癫痫发作

戒断反应与癫痫发作无明显相关性。而安非他酮较伐尼克兰更易诱发癫痫,其机制尚不清,可能与抑制性γ-氨基丁酸能和兴奋性谷氨酸能之间的不平衡,以及抑制突触前DA和NE再摄取转运蛋白致NE能增加有关。安非他酮可降低癫痫发作阈值,其发生率可达0.1%~0.4%。常在服药后0.5~24h发作,多自限性,但严重时也可危及生命。安非他酮过量可引发癫痫发作,剂量低于300mg/d时,其风险约0.1%;450mg/d时,增至0.4%;超过450mg/d则风险可增加10倍。

伐尼克兰与癫痫发作虽罕见,但也有报道,其可能机制:伐尼克兰作用的$\alpha_4\beta_2$ AChRs和α_7 nAChRs在大脑各处表达,尤其是皮质和皮质下区域,具有较高的Ca^{2+}通透性。所以伐尼克兰可激活这些受体而诱导细胞内Ca^{2+}水平升高,这是神经元兴奋和癫痫发作的常见机制。另外可能的原因:由于大脑皮质的兴奋性控制依赖于兴奋性和抑制性传递之间的良好平衡,伐尼克兰通过激活nAChRs,调节轴突终末神经递质的释放,使谷氨酸能和氨基丁酸能系统失衡,致癫痫发作,并多发生在初始治疗的第1个月内。

所以用药期间诱发的癫痫发作需考虑药物因素。在下述情况,戒烟药物应警惕使用:①有任何癫痫发作病史(包括儿童发热或酒精戒断引起的癫痫发作);②服用降低癫痫发作阈值的药物(如抗精神病药、抗抑郁药、茶碱类和全身皮质类固醇激素等);③酗酒;④既往有严重闭合性脑外伤、大脑结构异常(如脑卒中或肿瘤);⑤癫痫发作家族史;⑥因糖尿病使用降糖药或胰岛素;⑦因兴奋剂和药物引起的厌食症。

处理方式:若为药物引起,必须停药。癫痫发作时或发作前出现震颤、幻觉、心动过速及激动等症状,均可使用苯二氮䓬类药物。此外,还可采用包括胃肠净化(包括活性炭、全肠灌洗等)、碱化、气管插管及机械通气等对症处理。

(二)严重心血管不良反应

戒烟对心血管疾病有明显益处。而安非他酮和伐尼克兰目前有报道的其心血管不良事件(adverse events, AE)包括:心血管相关死亡、非致死性心肌梗死、不稳定型心绞痛、冠状动脉疾病、接受冠状动脉血运重建手术、心律失常、充血性心力衰竭、短暂性脑缺血发作和卒中等。

安非他酮因增加NE能,激动心脏β_1受体和血管α_1

受体，引起心率增加和冠状动脉及外周血管收缩，致心肌耗氧量增大和血压升高，增加急性心血管病风险，故冠心病患者慎用。法国的一项研究发现，安非他酮引起缺血性心脏病和2周内猝死的发生率分别达10.1%和2.3%，不过此研究未排除有冠状动脉疾病高风险的吸烟群体。为解释此问题，两项荟萃分析也表明，较安慰剂组，安非他酮对心血管疾病高危人群的戒烟有显著益处。最近一项荟萃分析也显示，安非他酮组人群其主要心血管AE未见增加，反而因其可减少心血管应激，具有心脏保护作用。总之，安非他酮戒烟人群的心血管AE并不常见，也未发现其相关性。

伐尼克兰因对外周神经节$\alpha_3\beta_4$ nAChRs作用引起乙酰胆碱和儿茶酚胺释放，及对$\alpha_4\beta_2$ AChRs和α_7 nAChRs的作用影响血压而增加心血管风险，尤其是对非神经内皮细胞α_7 nAChRs的作用，可使内皮功能和(或)血管生成产生不良影响。美国食品药品监督管理局（Food and Drug Administration，FDA）发布了对15项临床试验的荟萃分析结果：较安慰剂组，伐尼克兰戒烟的心血管AE有所增加，这提醒患者和医务人员权衡其风险和益处，在发生新的或恶化的心血管症状时保持警惕。Singh等的荟萃分析提出，伐尼克兰组较安慰剂组的心血管严重不良事件（serious adverse event，SAE）发生率增加。但由Prochaska和Hilton进行的后续荟萃分析中发现其较安慰剂组的心血管SAE发生率无显著差异。澳大利亚食品和药物管理局发布的荟萃分析也发现其心血管AE未见增加。吸烟本身与心血管疾病有关，戒烟可以显著改善长期预后。所以伐尼克兰对心血管的益处远超过任何潜在增加的风险。

处理方法：现有研究未明确表明上述药物与心血管不良反应存在因果关系，所以仍作为戒烟的一线药物推荐给心血管疾病患者。但因考虑到研究的局限性，用药时需警惕急性心血管症状发生，如出现则立即停药就诊。

（三）严重神经精神不良反应

戒烟与严重神经精神不良反应发生无直接因果关系。而安非他酮可通过以下机制引起神经精神不良反应：①引起血清素水平过高和破坏黑质纹状体及结节漏斗通路中的多巴胺能神经元导致锥体外系反应（静坐不能、肌张力障碍、帕金森症运动和迟发性运动障碍）。②增加DA能和NE能，激动D_2受体引起精神病。③阻断尼古丁受体，抑制伏膈核DA释放，引起快感缺失和心绪不宁，导致抑郁表现。④增加DA能，使冲动性增加，当抑郁加冲动时，则可促发自杀行为。2009年，FDA报告了用于戒烟的安非他酮与59起（30起自杀意念及29起自杀行为）神经精神症状之间的联系。并增加安非他酮"黑框"警告，建议对此保持警惕。但在英国的一些大型研究则表明，没有证据证明用于戒烟的安非他酮与神经精神症状之间存在必然联系。同样在一项荟萃分析中，两者也尚未建立因果关系。随后，FDA也基于EAGLES研究的结果移除了安非他酮的"黑框"警告。

伐尼克兰的神经精神症状可能因刺激中脑边缘多巴胺系统致多巴胺释放而引发，但也可能是因吸烟者戒烟前已存在。2008年FDA提出伐尼克兰与行为改变、情绪激动和低落、自杀意念和行为风险的增加可能存在关联，并随后更改其警告和药物指南。Tonstad等指出伐尼克兰引起的神经精神症状与戒断反应存在复杂的相关性，需区分混杂因素后，两者的因果关系才能明确。EAGLES试验对伐尼克兰、安非他酮、NRT和安慰剂进行了比较：与安慰剂相比，不论是否存在有精神病病史，伐尼克兰和安非他酮均未与中重度神经精神AE的增加存在相关性。因此，2016年，FDA也取消了伐尼克兰的"黑框"警告。

处理方式：虽未发现上述药物与神经精神不良反应有明显关联。但因吸烟者对其可能联系的担忧，故临床医师应告知其潜在风险，并予以监督。在已有精神病史（如抑郁症、焦虑症或精神分裂症等）的患者更应警惕。如发生上述严重情况则需立即停药就诊。

对上述常见及少见症状在戒断反应和药物不良反应的发生情况综合对比见表1-4-1。

表1-4-1 常见及少见症状在戒断反应和药物不良反应的发生情况对比

		戒断反应	安非他酮不良反应	伐尼克兰不良反应
心理症状	烦躁易怒	最多见	少见	少见
	焦虑	最多见	少见	少见
	睡眠障碍	频繁的夜间觉醒多见	难以入睡、失眠多见	难以入睡、梦境异常多见
躯体症状	恶心	少见	少见	最多见
	口干	少见	最多见	较戒断反应多见
	头痛	少见	多见	多见
少见但需警惕的症状	癫痫	无明显关联	较伐尼克兰多见	有罕见报道
	严重心血管症状	无明显关联	无明显因果关系，但有报道	无明显因果关系，但有报道
	严重神经精神症状	无明显关联	无明显因果关系，但有报道	无明显因果关系，但有报道

四、总　结

因戒断反应与药物不良反应极为相似,易混淆,导致药物使用欠规范,戒烟失败。故本文针对这些误区进行区分,并给出其处理方法,使临床医师更好的优化戒烟方案,使吸烟者得到科学的戒烟指导,最终成功戒烟。

参 考 文 献

[1] 杨焱,南奕,屠梦昊,等.2015中国成人烟草调查报告概要.中华健康管理学杂志,2016,10(2):85-87.

[2] 卫生部统计信息中心.第三次国家卫生服务调查分析报告.北京:中国协和医科大学出版社,2004:1-8.

[3] Seung-Hyun Yu, Myeong-Jun Kim, Jin Jeon, et al. Short-Term Success Rates of Smoking Cessation Support Programs and Factors Predicting Smoking Relapse: Using Data From a Smoking Cessation Clinic in a Hospital. Korean J Fam Med, 2019, 40(6):373-379.

[4] E R Gritz, C R Carr, A C Marcus. The Tobacco Withdrawal Syndrome in Unaided Quitters. Br J Addict,1991,86(1):57-69.

[5] Hughes JR, Gust SW, Keenan RM, et al. Effect of dose on nicotine's reinforcing, withdrawal-suppression and self-reported effects. J Pharmacol Exp Ther, 1990, 252(3):1175-1183.

[6] Piasecki, Jorenby, Smith, et al. Smoking withdrawal dynamics: I. Abstinence distress in lapsers and abstainers. J Abnorm Psychol,2003,112(1):3-13.

[7] Cahill K, Stevens S, Perera R, et al. Pharmacological interventions for smoking cessation: an overview and network meta-analysis. Cochrane Database Syst Rev, 2013, 31(5):CD009329.

[8] Halperin AC, McAfee TA, Jack LM, et al. Impact of symptoms experienced by varenicline users on tobacco treatment in a real world setting. J Subst Abuse Treat, 2009, 36(4):428-434.

[9] Raich A, Ballbè M, Nieva G, et al. Safety of Varenicline for Smoking Cessation in Psychiatric and Addicts Patients. Subst Use Misuse,2016,51(5):649-657.

[10] McLaughlin I1, Dani JA, De Biasi M. Nicotine Withdrawal. Curr Top Behav Neurosci,2015,24:99-123.

[11] K. J. Jackson, P. P. Muldoon, M. De Biasi, et al. New mechanisms and perspectives in nicotine withdrawal. Neuropharmacology,2015,96:223-234.

[12] Falk JL. The origins and functions of adjunctive behavior. Anim Learn Behav,1977,5:325-335.

[13] Gilbert DG, McClernon FJ, Rabinovich NE, et al. Mood disturbance fails to resolve across 31 days of cigarette abstinence in women. J Consult Clin Psychol,2002,70(1):142-152.

[14] Ward MM, Swan GE, Jack LM. Self-reported abstinence effects in the first month after smoking cessation. Addict Behav,2001,26(3):311-327.

[15] Foulds J, Russ C, Yu CR, et al. Effect of Varenicline on Individual Nicotine Withdrawal Symptoms: A Combined Analysis of Eight Randomized, Placebo-Controlled Trials. Nicotine Tob Res,2013,15(11):1849-1857.

[16] 喻东山.安非他酮的不良反应.临床精神医学杂志,2016,26(6):427-428.

[17] Johnston JA, Fiedler-Kelly J, Glover ED, et al. Relationship between drug exposure and the efficacy and safety of bupropion sustained release for smoking cessation. Nicotine Tob Res,2001,3:131-140.

[18] Igari M, Alexander JC, Ji Y, et al. Varenicline and cytisine diminish the dysphoric-like state associated with spontaneous nicotine withdrawal in rats. Neuropsychopharmacology, 2014,39(2):455-465.

[19] Robert West, Christine L. Baker, Joseph C. Cappelleri, et al. Effect of varenicline and bupropion SR on craving, nicotine withdrawal symptoms, and rewarding effects of smoking during a quit attempt. Psychopharmacology, 2008, 197:371-377.

[20] Cahill K, Stevens S, Perera R, et al. Pharmacological interventions for smoking cessation: an overview and nework meta-analysis. Cochrane Database Syst Rev, 2013, (5):CD009329.

[21] Paul M. Cinciripini, Jason D. Robinson, Maher Karam-Hage, et al. Effects of Varenicline and Bupropion Sustained-Release Use Plus Intensive Smoking Cessation Counseling on Prolonged Abstinence From Smoking and on Depression, Negative Affect, and Other Symptoms of Nicotine Withdrawal. JAMA Psychiatry,2013,70(5):522-533.

[22] Ashare RL, Lerman C, Tyndale RF, et al. Sleep Disturbance During Smoking Cessation: Withdrawal or Side Effect of Treatment? J Smok Cessat,2017,12(2):63-70.

[23] Hajek P, Belcher M. Dream of absent-minded transgression: an empirical study of a cognitive withdrawal symptom. J Abnorm Psychol,1991,100(4):487-491.

[24] Polini F, Principe R, Scarpelli S, et al. Use of varenicline in smokeless tobacco cessation influences sleep quality and dream recall frequency but not dream affect. Sleep Med, 2017,30:1-6.

[25] Foley KF, DeSanty KP, Kast RE. Bupropion: pharmacology and therapeutic applications. Expert Rev Neurother, 2006, 6(9):1249-1265.

[26] Patterson F, Grandner MA, Malone SK, et al, Sleep as a Target for Optimized Response to Smoking Cessation Treatment. Nicotine Tob Res,2019,21(2):139-148.

[27] Hajek P, Gillison F, McRobbie H. Stopping smoking can cause constipation. Addiction,2003,98(11):1563-1567.

[28] Ross S, Williams D. Bupropion: risks and benefits. Expert Opin Drug Saf,2005,4(6):995-1003.

[29] Swan GE, Javitz HS, Jack LM, et al. Varenicline for smoking cessation: nausea severity and variation in nicotinic receptor

genes. Pharmacogenomics J,2012,12(4):349-358.
[30] Nakamura M,Oshima A,Fujimoto Y,et al. Efficacy and tolerability of varenicline,an alpha4beta2 nicotinic acetylcholine receptor partial agonist, in a 12-week, randomized, placebo-controlled, dose-response study with 40-week follow-up for smoking cessation in Japanese smokers. Clin Ther,2007,29(6):1040-1056.
[31] De la Torre-Colmenero JD,Arjona-Padillo A,Fernandez-Perez J. Reversible cerebral vasoconstriction syndrome following smoking cessation and treatment with bupropion. Rev Neurol,2018,66(9):322-323.
[32] Valença MM. Bath-related headache induced by varenicline. Arq Neuropsiquiatr. 2012,70(11):908.
[33] Johannessen Landmark C,Henning O,Johannessen SI. Proconvulsant effects of antidepressants-What is the current evidence? Epilepsy Behav,2016,61:287-291.
[34] Noda AH,Schu U,Maier T,et al. Epileptic seizures,coma and EEG burst-suppression from suicidal bupropion intoxication. Epileptic Disord,2017 1,19(1):109-113.
[35] Haydar Ali Erken,Gülten Erken,Hasan Simşek,et al. Single Dose Varenicline May Trigger Epileptic Activity. Neurol Sci,2014, 35(11):1807-1812.
[36] U. S. Food and Drug Administration. FDA Drug Safety Communication:FDA updates label for stop smoking drug Chantix(varenicline) to include potential alcohol interaction, rare risk of seizures, and studies of side effects on moodbehavioror thinking[EB/OL](2015-03-09)[2015-04-05]. http://www. fda. Gov/Drugs/DrugSafety/ ucm436494. htm.
[37] Horst WD,Preskorn SH. Mechanisms of action and clinical characteristics of three atypical antidepressants:venlafaxine, nefazodone, bupropion. J Affect Disord, 1998, 51 (3): 237-254.
[38] Foley KF,DeSanty KP,Kast RE. Bupropion:pharmacology and therapeutic applications. Expert Rev Neurother,2006,6(9):1249-1265.
[39] Shepherd G,Velez LI,Keyes DC. Intentional bupropion overdoses. J Emerg Med,2004,27(2):147-151.
[40] Beyens MN,Guy C,Mounier G,et al. Serious adverse reactions of bupropion for smoking cessation:analysis of the French Pharmacovigilance Database from 2001 to 2004. Drug Saf,2008,31:1017-1026.
[41] Suissa K,Larivière J,Eisenberg MJ,et al. Efficacy and safety of smoking cessation interventions in patients with cardiovascular disease: a network meta - analysis of randomized controlled trials. Circ Cardiovasc Qual Outcomes,2017,10:e002458.
[42] Grandi SM,Shimony A,Eisenberg MJ. Bupropion for smoking cessation in patients hospitalized with cardiovascular disease: a systematic review and meta-analysis of randomized controlled trials. Can J Cardiol,2013,29:1704-1711.
[43] Mills EJ,Thorlund K,Eapen S,et al. Cardiovascular events associated with smoking cessation pharmacotherapies: a network meta-analysis. Circulation,2014,129(1):28-41.
[44] Sterling LH,Windle SB,Filion KB,et al. Varenicline and Adverse Cardiovascular Events: A Systematic Review and Meta - Analysis of Randomized Controlled Trials. J Am Heart Assoc,2016,22;5(2).
[45] Prochaska JJ,Hilton JF,et al. Risk of cardiovascular serious adverse events associated with varenicline use for tobacco cessation: systematic review and meta-analysis. BMJ, 2012, 344:e2856.
[46] Yeh JS,Sarpatwari A,Kesselheim AS. Food and Drug Administration. Ethical and Practical Considerations in Removing Black Box Warnings from Drug Labels. Drug Saf, 2016,39(8):709-714.
[47] Singh S,Loke YK,Spangler JG,et al. Risk of serious adverse cardiovascular events associated with varenicline:a systematic review and meta-analysis. CMAJ,2011,183:1359-1366.
[48] Prochaska JJ,Hilton JF. Risk of cardiovascular serious adverse events associated with varenicline use for tobacco cessation: systematic review and meta - analysis. BMJ, 2012, 344:e2856.
[49] Mills EJ,Thorlund K,Eapen S,et al. Cardiovascular events associated with smoking cessation pharmacotherapies: a network meta - analysis. Circulation,2014,129:28-41.
[50] US Food and Drug Administration. The smoking cessation aids varenicline(marketed as Chantix)and bupropion(marketed as Zyban and generics): suicidal ideation and behavior. FDA Safety Newsletter,2009,2(1):1-4.
[51] Boshier A,Wilton LV,Shakir SAW. Evaluation of the safety of bupropion(Zyban) for smoking cessation from experience gained in general practice use in England in 2000. Eur J Clin Pharmacol,2003,59:767-773.
[52] Hubbard R,Lewis S,West J,et al. Bupropion and the risk of sudden death: a self-controlled case-series analysis using The Health Improvement Network. Thorax,2005,60:848-850.
[53] Hughes JR, Stead LF, Lancaster T. Antidepressants for smoking cessation. Cochrane Database Syst Rev, 2007, (1):CD000031.
[54] Taha Can Tuman. Psychosis Induced by Varenicline in a Patient With No Psychiatric History. Prim Care Companion CNS Disord,2017,19(4):15101918.
[55] Xi ZX. Preclinical Pharmacology, Efficacy and Safety of Varenicline in Smoking Cessation and Clinical Utility in High Risk Patients. Drug Healthc Patient Saf,2010,(2):39-48.
[56] Anthenelli RM,Benowitz NL,West R,et al. Neuropsychiatric safety and efficacy of varenicline, bupropion, and nicotine patch in smokers with and without psychiatric disorders(EAGLES):a double-blind, randomised, placebo-controlled clinical trial. Lancet,2016,387(10037):2507-2520.

5 呼吸疾病患者的戒烟现状与研究进展

周 佳 范雨辰 陈 虹

烟草危害是当今世界最严重的公共卫生问题之一,全球每年因吸烟导致的死亡人数高达600万,中国每年约100万人死于烟草相关的疾病。吸烟是慢性阻塞性肺疾病(chronic obstructive pulmonary disease,COPD)、肺结核等呼吸系统慢性疾病的独立危险因素,并可导致多系统的恶性肿瘤,尤其是肺癌。肺癌、肺结核及COPD是呼吸系统常见的疾病,对人民健康及生命财产安全构成了极大的威胁。

被动和主动暴露于烟草烟雾已被证明与肺结核的发病有关,同时吸烟的肺结核患者预后更差。Thomas等调查了印度南部结核病患者复发的预测因素,发现吸烟与肺结核复发独立相关。研究显示,若每年减少1%的吸烟率,预计到2050年,可以预防2 700 000万人的吸烟合并结核相关的死亡。研究表明,确诊肺癌后继续吸烟可缩短患者的生存期、降低生活质量、增加肺癌复发率,以及增加第二原发肿瘤的发生率。肺癌行根治性切除后,继续吸烟的患者与戒烟的患者相比,复发率高1.9倍,再发第二肿瘤的发生率高2.3倍,总病死率高2.9倍。

烟草相关疾病是可以有效预防的。研究显示戒烟可以提高肺癌患者放、化疗的疗效,并降低肺癌复发的风险。同时,戒烟还可以降低放疗期间放射性肺炎和感染的发生率,并延长小细胞肺癌放化疗的中位生存期。对于许多接受姑息治疗的肺癌患者而言,戒烟具有改善肺功能,增加体重和改善整体生活质量的优势。对于COPD患者而言,戒烟是疾病干预最为重要及有效的方法,也是减少肺功能下降并改善COPD患者预后的最有效干预措施。已有研究证实,戒烟可有效降低肺结核患者的病死率。

全球成人烟草调查(global adult tobacco survey,GATS)报道,46.6%的吸烟者有戒烟的意愿。但多项研究发现,部分罹患肺癌、COPD和肺结核的患者在确诊后仍继续吸烟,少数患者尝试戒烟一段时间后复吸的比例高,戒烟成功率低。目前我国呼吸系统疾病患者的戒烟及复吸情况、戒烟的影响因素及复吸的原因不十分清楚,不同呼吸系统疾病之间的戒烟率是否存在差异也存在争议。掌握呼吸系统慢病患者的戒烟情况和影响因素,对我国控烟工作的开展具有非常重要的指导意义。

一、呼吸疾病患者的戒烟情况

2010年GATS-中国报告显示,目前中国吸烟人群中的戒烟成功率非常低(16.9%),其中只有11.7%的人戒烟两年或更长时间,而33.1%的人曾经戒烟,但是又复吸,中国人群的戒烟现状很不乐观。

一项研究显示,中国结核患者中吸烟的比例为54.6%,显著高于健康对照组的45.1%。尽管54.9%的吸烟者在被诊断出结核病后停止吸烟,但在随访期间复吸率超过18%。其中,戒烟后的6~9个月和12~15个月复吸的比例更高。

研究表明,大部分吸烟肺癌患者初期戒烟意愿强烈,这被认为是戒烟劝解成功的重要时机,这种现象在其他疾病中也存在。有研究报道,在给予针对性的戒烟干预及治疗后,肺癌患者6个月后的戒烟率为22%。另外两项研究中,在戒烟6个月后随访,约有50%的肺癌患者仍不吸烟。

调查显示,约40%的COPD患者在诊断COPD后继续吸烟,而肺癌患者的持续戒断率更是高达71%。也有研究表明,超过50%的吸烟者在诊断结核病后成功戒烟。不同研究之间的结果存在差异,且不同病种之间的戒烟情况也有所不同,但总体戒烟情况不容乐观。因疾病特点的关系,肺癌的戒烟率较COPD等其他呼吸系统慢性疾病高。任何时候戒烟对吸烟者均是有益的,如果吸烟者在诊断呼吸道疾病之前戒烟,呼吸系统疾病的发病率和病死率均可能会降低。因此,早期干预对于吸烟者在诊断之前甚至在呼吸道症状出现之前戒烟具有非常重要的意义。

二、呼吸疾病患者戒烟是否成功的影响因素

(一)尼古丁依赖、个人及社会因素对戒烟的影响

是否成功戒烟受遗传、个人因素及社会环境之间交互作用的共同影响,其中个人因素包括吸烟动机、自我效能、焦虑、年龄、教育水平、吸烟量与年限、吸烟危害认知程度等。上述各个因素构成了一个复杂的交互网络系统,决定戒烟是否成功。其中,尼古丁依赖程度是影响戒烟成功与否最主要的因素之一。

年龄可影响戒烟成功率。一般情况下,年龄大的吸烟者因为患病或担心患病,选择戒烟,并且当他们身体健康状况很差时,戒烟的动力会更大,也更容易戒烟成功。研究表明,在吸烟的肺癌患者中,年轻、早期以及伴侣也吸烟的患者戒烟意愿更强烈。

戒烟受个人、社会、尼古丁依赖等综合因素影响,戒烟

干预需要综合上述多种因素制定有效措施。

（二）疾病诊断对呼吸疾病患者戒烟情况的影响

研究显示，不管戒烟成功与否，大部分人戒烟的原因是他们担心患病或者已经患病。许多患者被诊断出患有呼吸系统疾病后由于持续的呼吸道症状导致生活质量下降，进而尝试戒烟。而老年人的因罹患肺结核、COPD等慢性呼吸系统疾病，导致健康状况更差，所以他们可能更希望通过戒烟来减少吸烟的危害。此外，随着年龄的增长，老年人对尼古丁及其代谢物可替宁的代谢功能降低，他们体内尼古丁含量降低的速度更慢，维持体内一定浓度的尼古丁水平所需要的吸烟量较少，因此其吸烟严重程度相对较低。本课题组研究发现，健康对照组的戒烟成功率仅为10.2%，而NSCLC、COPD和肺结核患者在疾病诊断2年后的戒烟率分别高达76.8%、62.8%和63.7%（相关资料待发表），进一步证实疾病的诊断对于戒烟具有正向驱动作用。

三、呼吸疾病患者复吸情况及原因

大多数肺癌、COPD及肺结核患者在疾病诊断时均有强烈的戒烟意愿。然而，对于许多吸烟者而言，戒烟后的情感障碍、强烈的吸烟者身份感、烦躁、烟草的渴望、饥饿和体重增加等，可增加患者的复吸率。这主要源于尼古丁依赖所致的戒断症状，单纯的行为干预或者戒烟建议可能导致戒烟失败，因此往往需要药物治疗的辅助。

本课题组前期研究发现，肺癌、COPD和肺结核患者疾病诊断后的戒烟率分别为76.8%、62.8%和63.7%，复吸率分别为5.5%、24.8%和25.4%。肺癌组戒烟率最高（$P<0.01$），复发率最低（$P<0.01$），而COPD和肺结核患者之间的戒烟和复吸率没有显著差异（相关资料待发表）。肺癌、COPD和肺结核患者复吸率不仅与疾病本身有关，也与年龄、受教育程度等有关。研究显示，接受教育时间＜6年的肺结核患者，其复吸率显著高于受教育时间≥6年的患者，提示肺结核患者复吸可能与受教育程度有关。研究还发现，新近诊断的肺结核患者复吸率低于以往诊断的肺结核患者。在确诊肺结核患者人群中，年龄＞65岁为戒烟后复吸的高危因素，提示高龄肺结核患者需要进行强化督导戒烟。研究显示，以胸部CT作为肺癌筛查方式，可促进戒烟。其中筛查小结节每3个月随访复查胸部CT为成功戒烟的预测因素，而连续复查阴性与复吸明确相关。

综上所述，复吸受疾病本身、年龄、受教育程度、疾病诊断时间、尼古丁依赖等多种因素的影响，规范、全面、有效的戒烟干预措施有助于降低复吸率。

四、降低复吸的措施

目前已有多种用于结核病患者戒烟的行为方法，例如，简短的戒烟建议，已被证明可大大提高这些受试者的戒烟率。国际抗结核和肺病联盟提出了实施简短戒烟建议的不同方法，也是一种简洁易行的方法。但对于重度烟草依赖的患者，大量研究表明简短的戒烟建议联合药物治疗可有效降低复吸率。对于COPD患者而言，高强度行为干预和药物治疗（尼古丁替代疗法，伐尼克兰，安非他酮）的联合是吸烟COPD患者最有效的治疗策略。没有药物治疗的行为干预措施并不比简单的戒烟建议更有效，而强烈的戒烟动机可帮助戒烟成功，降低复吸率。

通常医生都建议患者戒烟，但目前我国戒烟门诊的普及率比较低，大多数医生只是简单地向患者提及戒烟的好处，并未给予科学的戒烟建议。研究证实，经过规范、系统的联合干预，患者6个月结束时的戒烟为71.7%，显著高于简短咨询组和对照组，复吸率也较低。因此，强烈建议设置专门的戒烟门诊，提高呼吸系统慢性疾病患者的戒烟成功率。

参 考 文 献

[1] Chen Z, Peto R, Zhou M, et al. China Kadoorie Biobank collaborative, g. Contrasting male and female trends in tobacco-attributed mortality in China: evidence from successive nationwide prospective cohort studies. Lancet, 2015, 386: 1447-1456.

[2] Thomas A, Gopi PG, Santha T, et al. Predictors of relapse among pulmonary tuberculosis patients treated in a DOTS programme in South India. Int J Tuberc Lung Dis, 2005, 9: 556-561.

[3] Basu S, Stuckler D, Bitton A, et al. Projected effects of tobacco smoking on worldwide tuberculosis control: mathematical modelling analysis. BMJ, 2011, 343: d5506.

[4] Garces YI, Yang P, Parkinson J, et al. The relationship between cigarette smoking and quality of life after lung cancer diagnosis. Chest, 2004, 126: 1733-1741.

[5] Fox JL, Rosenzweig KE, Ostroff JS. The effect of smoking status on survival following radiation therapy for non-small cell lung cancer. Lung Cancer, 2004, 44: 287-293.

[6] Jimenez-Ruiz CA, Andreas S, Lewis KE, et al. Statement on smoking cessation in COPD and other pulmonary diseases and in smokers with comorbidities who find it difficult to quit. Eur Respir J, 2015, 46: 61-79.

[7] Andreas S, Rittmeyer A, Hinterthaner M, et al. Smoking cessation in lung cancer-achievable and effective. Dtsch Arztebl Int, 2013, 110: 719-724.

[8] Park ER, Japuntich SJ, Rigotti NA, et al. A snapshot of smokers after lung and colorectal cancer diagnosis. Cancer, 2012, 118: 3153-3164.

[9] Wang J, Shen H. Review of cigarette smoking and tuberculosis in China: intervention is needed for smoking cessation among tuberculosis patients. BMC Public Health, 2009, 9: 292.

[10] van der Aalst CM, van den Bergh KA, Willemsen MC, et al. Lung cancer screening and smoking abstinence: 2 year follow-

up data from the Dutch-Belgian randomised controlled lung cancer screening trial. Thorax,2010,65:600-605.
[11] Sanderson Cox L,Patten CA,Ebbert JO,et al. Tobacco use outcomes among patients with lung cancer treated for nicotine dependence. J Clin Oncol,2002,20:3461-3469.
[12] Cooley ME,Wang Q,Johnson,BE,et al. Factors associated with smoking abstinence among smokers and recent-quitters with lung and head and neck cancer. Lung Cancer,2012,76:144-149.
[13] Vogelmeier C,Hederer B,Glaab T,et al. Tiotropium versus salmeterol for the prevention of exacerbations of COPD. N Engl J Med,2011,364:1093-1103.
[14] Cooley ME,Emmons KM,Haddad R,et al. Patient-reported receipt of and interest in smoking-cessation interventions after a diagnosis of cancer. Cancer,2011,117:2961-2969.
[15] Kim SS,Son H,Nam KA. Personal factors influencing Korean American men's smoking behavior:addiction,health,and age. Arch Psychiatr Nurs,2005,19:35-41.
[16] Vuong K,Hermiz O,Razee H,et al. The experiences of smoking cessation among patients with chronic obstructive pulmonary disease in Australian general practice:a qualitative descriptive study. Fam Pract,2016,33:715-720.
[17] Santoro A,Tomino C,Prinzi G,et al. Tobacco Smoking:Risk to Develop Addiction,Chronic Obstructive Pulmonary Disease,and Lung Cancer. Recent Pat Anticancer Drug Discov,2019,14:39-52.
[18] Taylor KL,Cox LS,Zincke N,et al. Lung cancer screening as a teachable moment for smoking cessation. Lung Cancer,2007,56:125-134.
[19] Anderson CM,Yip R,Henschke CI,et al. Smoking cessation and relapse during a lung cancer screening program. Cancer Epidemiol Biomarkers Prev,2009,18:3476-3483.
[20] Gomez MM,LoBiondo-Wood G. Lung Cancer Screening With Low-Dose CT:Its Effect on Smoking Behavior. J Adv Pract Oncol,2013,4:405-414.
[21] Ashraf H,Tonnesen P,Holst Pedersen J,et al. Effect of CT screening on smoking habits at 1-year follow-up in the Danish Lung Cancer Screening Trial(DLCST). Thorax,2009,64:388-392.
[22] Underner M,Perriot J,Peiffer G. Smoking cessation in smokers with chronic obstructive pulmonary disease. Rev Mal Respir,2014,31:937-960.
[23] Aryanpur M,Hosseini M,Masjedi MR,et al. A randomized controlled trial of smoking cessation methods in patients newly-diagnosed with pulmonary tuberculosis. BMC Infect Dis,2016,16:369.

6 戒烟门诊就诊人群的吸烟行为与吸烟网络初步分析

张剑青 沈 凌

吸烟作为人类的一种行为,具有一定的社会性,在社交中具有一定的社会功能,但同时又可能诱发多种疾病。1998年世界卫生组织正式将烟草依赖作为一种慢性高复发性疾病列入国际疾病分类(ICD-10)(F17.2),烟草依赖对身体健康危害极大。据世界卫生组织调查,在工业发达的国家中,吸烟所致疾病致死比例分别为:死于肺癌:90%;死于支气管炎:75%;死于心肌梗死:25%。吸烟不但给本人带来危害,而且还殃及子女。对5200个孕妇调查分析发现父亲每天吸烟的数量与胎儿产前的死亡率和先天畸形儿的出生率成正比。父亲不吸烟的,子女先天畸形比为0.8%;父亲每天吸烟1~10支的其比为1.4%;每天吸10支以上的其比为2.1%。孕妇本人吸烟数量的多少,也直接影响到婴儿出生前后的死亡率。例如,每天吸烟不足一包的,婴儿死亡危险率为20%;每天吸烟一包以上的,婴儿死亡危险率为35%以上。

在中国,吸烟行为不容乐观。中国疾病预防控制中心发布的《2018年中国成人烟草调查报告》显示,在全国31个省(自治区、直辖市)的200个监测县(区)中,2018年我国15岁及以上人群吸烟率为26.6%,其中,男性为50.5%,女性为2.1%,农村为28.9%,城市为25.1%。与既往调查结果相比,吸烟率虽呈现下降趋势,但与实现《"健康中国2030"规划纲要》的控烟目标——"2030年15岁以上人群吸烟率下降至20%"仍有较大差距。非吸烟者的二手烟暴露率为68.1%。50.9%的室内工作者在工作场所看到有人吸烟。44.9%的调查对象报告有人在自己家中吸烟。二手烟暴露最严重的室内公共场所为:网吧(89.3%)、酒吧和夜总会(87.5%)和餐馆(73.3%)。与既往调查结果相比,二手烟暴露情况整体有所改善。

调查还显示,我国成年吸烟人群戒烟意愿普遍较低,戒烟率未呈现明显变化。我国15岁及以上人群戒烟率为20.1%;每日吸烟者戒烟率为15.6%。16.1%的现在吸烟者打算在未来12个月内戒烟,计划在1个月内戒烟的比例仅有5.6%。在过去12个月吸烟的人群中,19.8%尝试过戒烟。尝试戒烟的前三位原因分别是担心继续吸烟影响今后健康(38.7%)、已经患病(26.6%)和家人反对吸烟(14.9%)。

总体说来,我国15岁及以上人群吸烟率与既往调查结果相比呈下降趋势,二手烟暴露情况有所改善,但是戒烟形式依然严峻。

针对戒烟者成功率较低,复吸率居高不下的情况,相关戒烟团队使用了简短戒烟干预、戒烟热线和戒烟门诊,戒烟模式包括基于心理社会学模式、基于医学模式、联合戒烟干预模式、干戒法等,戒烟效果都达不到预期。鉴于以上戒烟方法都是以个体为中心,很多学者开始考虑应用社会网络理论(social network theory,SNT)于戒烟的活动中。

我们生活的世界由各种各样的系统组成,或简单、或复杂。系统科学认为,系统是由元素组成的,元素之间相互联系、相互作用,组成一个整体。如果用节点表示元素,用边表示元素之间的相互联系与作用,系统就构成了一个网络。网络既是实际系统的一种模型,又是系统存在的普遍形式。整个自然界或人类社会,或两者的综合即整个世界,都是多层次、多结构、多姿态的复杂网络。

社会网络被定义为人、组织、政治实体(国家或民族)之间的联系。社会网络理论起源于社会学,为研究个体与个体之间、组织与组织之间的关系与互动提供了新的视角。社会网络分析是一种理论视角,也是一套用于理解这些关系,以及理解关系如何影响相关者行为的技术方法。社会网络分析对网络关系如何影响吸烟行为提供了很好的方法,例如,在吸烟者受到与他们有重要联系的人向他们施加戒烟压力时他们就会戒烟。

根据SNA理论,在社会活动中,每一个人都会存在于一个大的社会网络中,这个网络由很多个小的网络构成,每个小的网络中包括一定数量性质接近的成员,如:社会支持网络,吸烟网络,性伴网络,同学网络等。每个人拥有的小的网络数量、大小、成员、功用等不同,这些不同都与个体的背景、行为、交往等特征有关。就一个特定的吸烟网络来说,吸烟网络的特征,包括人员构成、机构大小、关系情况、交往频率等都会影响吸烟行为的变化。为了测定这些网络的特征,SNA定义了一系列指标来测量网络参数,包括:节点、连线、中心性、体积等。SNA有一套特殊的工具来收集网络数据,使用R软件、UCINET、NETMINNER等专用软件,可以对网络数据进行整理分析,探讨网络特征与相关行为之间的关系和转归,进而对行为的干预和改变提出意见和建议。

本研究依托昆明市多家医院的戒烟门诊,使用自制的吸烟网络调查问卷,对来戒烟门诊就诊的患者进行调查,重点关注吸烟网络特征与吸烟行为之间的关系,以下内容为本次调查数据的初步分析结果。

一、对象和方法

(一)对象

2019年1—6月,在选定的云南省昆明市8家三甲医院的戒烟门诊中对前来就诊患者进行随即问卷调查,共发放问卷360份,剔除废卷,回收351份,回收率为97.5%。

(二)方法

采用本课题组编制的"戒烟门诊就诊人员吸烟网络与吸烟行为调查问卷"对戒烟门诊患者进行问卷调查。调查问卷主要由四大部分组成:①戒烟者的人口学特征;②吸烟的具体情况;③社会支持网络;④吸烟网络。每个部分又由若干具体的小问题组成,由经过培训的戒烟门诊医师指导并协助患者填写问卷,涉及的社会人口学特征则通过调查员面对面询问调查对象获得。

(三)统计分析

运用R统计软件进行数据分析,包括描述性统计方法、卡方检验、t检验。描述性统计方法用于描述戒烟门诊吸烟者的基本信息和吸烟网络特征,卡方分析与t检验用于分析社会人口学特征、吸烟状况、吸烟史、戒烟史等的差异。

二、结　果

(一)一般情况

2019年1—6月,共调查到昆明市8家三甲医院戒烟门诊就诊的人员351人,最多一家医院调查182人,平均每家医院44人。

在调查的351人中,男性占97.4%,汉族占71%,60%以上患者不信教,文化程度为大专及以上的人员占66%以上;医保方面,使用新型农村合作医疗的患者和职工医疗保险的患者基本一致,各占1/3;职业方面,公司员工占20%,农民、技术人员和其他人员均超过10%,政府公务员最少,只占到3%左右。

本次调查对象年龄跨度比较大,最小19岁,最大70岁,平均33.53岁;个人收入差距比较大,最高25 000元/月,平均5000元/月;家庭收入差距很大,平均8000元/月;同屋居住人数差距同样很大,最多10人一起居住,平均2人一起居住,超过35%的患者和小孩一起居住,接近40%的患者与配偶一起居住。

(二)吸烟情况

在调查的患者中,上个月吸烟天数差别较大,从0 d到30 d都存在,平均22 d;上个月吸烟花费最高8000元,平均550元;每天吸烟数量最多3包,平均半包;吸烟的支出超过60%来自工资;在香烟的价位方面,5元左右的最受欢迎,占比接近40%,5~10元的香烟接近1/4,10~20元的香烟占1/5;超过50%的患者经常在家吸烟,在社交中吸烟的人员占1/7(表1-6-1);超过70%的患者有戒烟的打算;接近50%的患者是由于家里人劝阻,才来进行戒烟活动;接近70%的患者认为吸烟一定对健康有危害地点。

表1-6-1　吸烟地点情况表

吸烟地点	百分比(%)	有效百分比(%)	累计百分比(%)
家	53.6	53.6	53.6
办公室	10.5	10.5	64.1
餐厅	4.0	4.0	68.1
朋友家	5.7	5.7	73.8
社交场所	14.0	14.0	87.7
公共场所	7.7	7.7	95.4
其他	4.5	4.5	100.0
总计	100.0	100.0	

(三)吸烟网络情况

在调查患者的吸烟网络中(表1-6-2),吸烟网络尺寸大小为4人左右;接近1/3的患者喜欢5人规模一起吸烟,喜欢10人以上规模一起吸烟的有7%左右,喜欢2人吸烟的只占1%;网络中,同性别吸烟占比超过90%;超过40%的吸烟网络成员喜欢经常在一起吸烟;网络成员吸烟的价格明显高于平时吸烟的水平,20元以上的香烟占50%以上;吸烟网络中,35%为朋友,17%为同事,15%为酒友,7%为同学;一起吸烟的人群中,非常亲近的人员占比超过40%,一点也不亲近的只有2%;在网络中,接近30%的成员影响力很大,可以改变调查对象的决定和选择;接近40%的网络成员,通过经常谈话交流的方式,影响其他成员的思想和决定,只有1%左右的成员通过非物质的作用影响其他成员的行为;70%的成员用工资购买香烟;网络成员中购买20元以上香烟占比超过40%;吸烟地点频率从大到小,依次是:家,社交场所,公共场所;过去一年中,有40%的网络成员尝试戒烟;超过60%的网络成员认为吸烟一定有害;吸烟网络中,超过15%的成员承认有与吸烟有关的疾病。

表1-6-2　吸烟网络成员关系情况

	吸烟网络成员	百分比(%)	有效百分比(%)	累计百分比(%)
有效	配偶	0.2	0.2	0.2
	兄弟姐妹	4.2	4.4	4.6
	父母	2.8	3.0	7.6
	祖父母	0.3	0.3	7.9
	孩子	0.3	0.3	8.2
	酒友	15.7	16.7	24.9
	领导	2.5	2.6	27.5
	朋友	34.9	37.2	64.6
	同事	17.8	19.0	83.6
	同学	7.6	8.1	91.7
	医生	0.2	0.2	91.9
	护士	3.0	3.2	95.1
	其他	10.5	10.8	100.0
总计		100.0	100.0	

三、讨 论

（一）戒烟门诊就诊患者的人口学特征

本次调查结果表明，自愿到戒烟门诊接受戒烟干预的吸烟者主要是男性，平均年龄33.53岁，大专及以上的学历，职业公司员工，新型农村合作医疗或者城镇职工医保，和配偶一起居住。和文献相比，本次调查的戒烟患者年龄明显偏小、学历层次较高、公司职员较多，提示戒烟人群的组成逐渐发生改变。戒烟患者出于对自己健康的关注，逐步了解烟草对健康的损害，再加上周围戒烟宣传环境对自身影响等因素，开始尝试戒烟，这也体现了戒烟宣传的效果和间接作用。但是戒烟的患者人数依然不多，推动戒烟进程，到达"健康中国2030"的目标，还需要有关部门通力合作，继续努力。

（二）调查对象吸烟特征情况

本次调查中，戒烟患者每个月吸烟平均花费550元，每天平均消费半包香烟，5元左右的卷烟吸得最多，喜欢在家中吸烟，多数人认识到吸烟有害健康并有戒烟的打算，多数人是在家人的劝阻下才来医院就诊。与文献相比，患者前往戒烟门诊尝试戒烟的比例是上升的，对戒烟的意愿也是呈上升状态。应以此为契机，加大宣传力度、创新宣传方式，吸引更多的吸烟人员到戒烟门诊，持续推进戒烟活动，不断改善吸烟人群的健康水平。

（三）调查对象吸烟网络情况

本次调查的戒烟患者的吸烟网络尺寸为4人，中等规模（5人）的网络在吸烟群体中受到欢迎，网络中吸烟的卷烟价格明显高于个体的水平，吸烟网络中，以朋友、酒友、同事和同学等社会背景相似的人员为主；多数网络成员通过经常谈话交流的方式影响其他成员，网络成员的影响力较大，可以改变其他成员的决定和选择。

吸烟网络作为个体社会网络中的组成部分，同样体现社会网络的基本特征和性质，吸烟网络中的成员都吸烟，多具有相同的社会背景和经济地位等特征。同社会网络一样，一部分吸烟网络中的成员具有相当的影响力，能够改变其他成员的决定和选择；这些成员在网络中处于信息流通和传播的关键位置和地位，利用这些成员的特性，我们可以把健康知识、戒烟知识等信息流导入到吸烟网络中，提高网络成员的对健康、戒烟等概念的认识，进而推动其态度、行为的改变。

总之，把社会网络分析方法应用于吸烟干预中，利用吸烟网络的特征进行戒烟干预活动，是戒烟领域的一个新尝试和发展，我们期待有更多的调查研究使用这种方法和思路，不断推动戒烟活动的开展，早日实现"健康中国2030"的目标。

参 考 文 献

[1] Anwar K, Sherouk F, Ali M, et al. Cigarette smoking blocks the benefit from reduced weight gain for insulin action by shifting lipids deposition to muscle. Clinical Science(Lond), 2020, 134(13):1659-1673.

[2] 中国疾病预防控制中心. 2015年中国成人烟草调查报告. 北京：人民卫生出版社, 2016.

[3] 翁心植. 我国戒烟情况和促进戒烟的建议. 心肺血管病杂志, 2001, 20(2):118-119.

[4] 孙月, 姬忠飞, 吴小领. 中国吸烟者戒烟意愿Meta分析. 中国健康教育, 2018, 34(10):879-881, 897.

[5] 张婷婷, 南奕, 姜垣. 戒烟服务现状概述. 中国健康教育, 2015, 31(8):779-781, 794.

[6] 刘疆东, 张建国. 戒烟的干预模式及实施方式. 中华全科医师杂志, 2017, 16(4):324-327.

[7] 李建, 杨廷忠, 李鲁. 几种吸烟干预方法的比较和戒烟心理健康效益评价. 中国校医, 2000, 14(4):259-260.

[8] 马丽娜, 黄希骥, 李玲, 等. 湖北省6家戒烟门诊戒烟服务现状分析. 实用预防医学, 2017, 24(8):938-940.

[9] Nazzal Z, Odeh D, Fatima Azahraa Haddad FA, et al. Effects of waterpipe tobacco smoking on the spirometric profile of university students in Palestine:a cross-sectional study. Canadian Respiratory Journal, 2020(3):1-6.

[10] 季莉莉, 郭海健, 曲晨, 等. 不同戒烟方式戒烟效果Meta分析. 江苏预防医学, 2015, 26(6):131-133.

[11] 中华人民共和国卫生部. 中国吸烟危害健康报告. 北京：人民卫生出版社, 2012.

[12] Kang SH, Joo JH, Jang SI, et al. Association of exposure to secondhand smoke at home with early age at menarche in South Korea. Public Health, 2020, 185:144-149.

[13] 刘路, 冯国忠. 我国戒烟药市场现状及成因分析. 中南药学, 2012, 10(4):318-320.

[14] Higuchi Y, Fujiwara M, Nakaya N, et al. Trends in smoking rates among individuals with serious psychological distress: Analysis of data from a Japanese national survey, 2007—2016. Psychiatry Research, 2020, 291:113225.

[15] Senyurek VY, Imtiaz MH, Prajakta B, et al. A CNN-LSTM neural network for recognition of puffing in smoking episodes using wearable sensorsBiomedical Engineering Letters, 2020, 10(2):195-203.

[16] Alves RF, Precioso J, Becoña E. Smoking behavior and secondhand smoke exposure among university students in northern Portugal: Relations with knowledge on tobacco use and attitudes toward smoking. Pulmonology, 2020, 10(1):1-10.

[17] Manosij G, Lisa J, Dries S M, et al. Increased telomere length and mtDNA copy number induced by multi-walled carbon nanotube exposure in the workplace. Journal of Hazardous Materials, 2020, 394:122569.

[18] Shuryo F, Nerea M. Evaluation of a smoke-and tobacco-free campus policy: The issue of displacement. Journal of American College Health: J of ACH, 2020:1-9.

[19] Courtney K, Wendy M, Yao TT, et al. Smoking behavior in low-and high-income adults immediately following California proposition 56 tobacco tax increase. American Journal of Public Health, 2020, 110(6):1-8.

[20] 孙铭繁,倪文庆,袁雪丽,等.深圳市福田区慢性病高风险人群吸烟、饮酒和运动行为干预效果评价.中国慢性病预防与控制,2020,28(5):358-362.

[21] Chung WS,Kung PT,Chang HY,et al. Demographics and medical disorders associated with smoking: a population-based study. BMC Public Health,2020,20(702):1-8.

[22] Vicki M,Eimi L,Nurit G,et al. "I can't stand it…but I do it sometimes" parental smoking around children: practices, beliefs, and conflicts-a qualitative study. BMC Public Health,2020,20(693):1-10.

[23] 林镇涛.中距离户外施工人员吸烟行为检测方法研究.成都：电子科技大学,2020.

[24] Tiili EM,Mitiushkina NV,Sukhovskaya OA,et al. The effect of SLC6A3 variable number of tandem repeats and methylation levels on individual susceptibility to start tobacco smoking and on the ability of smokers to quit smoking. Pharmacogenetics and Genomics,2020,30(6):117-123.

[25] Chu WC,Chen CH. Smoking behavior and survival outcomes in bladder cancer patients. Urological Science,2020,31(3):1-8.

[26] Yip D,Gubner N,Le T,et al. Association of medicaid expansion and health insurance with receipt of smoking cessation services and smoking behaviors in substance use disorder treatment. The Journal of Behavioral Health Services & Research: Official Publication of the National Council for Behavioral Health,2020,47(2):264-274.

[27] James L,Steve A,Glantz SA. Predictive validation and forecasts of short-term changes in healthcare expenditure associated with changes in smoking behavior in the United States. PLoS One,2020,15(1):e0227493.

[28] Wang XF,Xue T,Dong F,et al. The changes of brain functional networks in young adult smokers based on independent component analysis. Brain Imaging and Behavior,2020,4:1-10.

[29] Brailovskaia J,Ströse F,Schillack H,et al. Less Facebook use-more well-being and a healthier lifestyle? An experimental intervention study. Computers in Human Behavior,2020,108:106332.

7 戒烟在呼吸康复中的作用

张韶泽　马金铃　朱黎明

呼吸康复是基于患者全面评估，为患者量身定制的一个综合性干预治疗方案，能改善慢性呼吸系统疾病患者的身体和心理状况。吸烟是慢性阻塞性肺疾病、支气管肺癌和哮喘的高危因素，也是世界上导致过早死亡和残疾的主要原因之一，而戒烟是世界上唯一一个可避免过早死亡的最重要因素。戒烟教育作为呼吸康复的重要组成部分，对改善疾病预后、提高患者生活质量起着至关重要的作用。

一、吸烟对呼吸系统的危害

吸烟是可预防的第一大死亡原因，全球每年因吸烟造成的死亡人数达 700 多万，终身吸烟者在 1/2～2/3 的情况下死于与吸烟直接相关的疾病，因此吸烟成为世界重大的公共卫生问题。

吸烟是导致慢性阻塞性肺疾病、支气管哮喘和原发性支气管肺癌的重要危险因素。烟草中的焦油、尼古丁和氢氰酸等化学物质可以使支气管上皮纤毛变短、不规则，纤毛运动功能发生障碍，导致气道炎症和重塑的加重，通过引起气道壁及肺实质的慢性炎症和结构的改变，导致局部抵抗力下降，降低灭菌作用，通过副交感神经亢进作用，引起支气管平滑肌的痉挛收缩，气道阻力增加，气流受限。有 10%～15% 的长期吸烟者，1s 用力呼气容积（FEV_1）下降速度提前并增快，甚至早期即出现临床症状，停止吸烟后受损的肺功能无法恢复。一氧化碳是烟草烟雾的主要成分之一，与血红蛋白的亲和力比氧气高 200 倍，它可以降低血液对氧气的结合力，并减少氧气向肌肉线粒体的转运。焦油、氰化物及香烟烟雾中存在的自由基，可以损害线粒体呼吸链功能，影响细胞的新陈代谢。慢性吸烟者的碳氧血红蛋白水平增加 9%，这与低氧血症一样导致缺氧。

有学者认为 87% 的肺癌死亡可直接归因于吸烟。吸烟并接受非小细胞肺癌手术的患者出现心脏和肺部合并症的风险增加，同时也增加了术后感染及伤口延迟愈合的风险。肺癌诊断后继续吸烟者将导致预后不良、生存率降低、罹患第二原发癌及复发的风险增加、患者生活质量下降、化疗药物的不良反应发生率增加。烟草烟雾中的尼古丁可以诱导细胞增生和血管生成，抑制顺铂药物诱导癌细胞凋亡的潜能。

二、吸烟对骨骼肌的影响

肌纤维分红肌纤维与白肌纤维，红肌纤维也称Ⅰ型纤维，白肌纤维又称Ⅱ型纤维，Ⅰ型纤维依靠氧化磷酸化产生能量引起肌肉收缩，与耐力相关，而Ⅱ型纤维依靠糖酵解途径产生能量，耗氧量要小得多。长时间吸烟后人和动物运动肌纤维类型发生潜在糖酵解转变，Ⅱ型肌肉纤维向Ⅰ型或Ⅰ/ⅡA型纤维的转变，会降低肌肉耐力。急性吸烟也可能直接触发骨骼肌糖酵解的转变，可能会导致运动能力下降。即使在无明显肺部疾病发生前，吸烟者的运动能力水平可能也要低于不吸烟者。慢性吸烟可能会降低骨骼肌的收缩功能，增加炎症因子和肌肉蛋白降解因子的表达，导致肌肉萎缩。暴露于香烟烟雾 14 周的雄性大鼠戒烟 2 周后可以逆转吸烟引起的线粒体功能障碍、肢体肌肉质量下降和膈肌萎缩的情况。卫星细胞是赋予骨骼肌可塑性以适应不断变化需求的肌肉干细胞，烟雾的长期暴露会阻止这些干细胞活化，同时吸烟也使促炎因子的表达增强，放大骨骼肌损伤部位的局部炎症反应，进一步阻止卫星细胞的活化，导致肌肉损伤和收缩功能恶化。人体研究表明，吸烟会损害肌肉蛋白质合成过程，增加与受损的肌肉维持能力相关的基因表达，表明吸烟可能提高患肌肉减少症的风险，并且肌肉功能障碍可能会在慢性阻塞性肺疾病（简称慢阻肺）发生之前发生，同时吸烟也可能会对膈肌产生负面影响。

三、吸烟的成瘾性

吸烟是一种成瘾行为，其中烟草中生物碱尼古丁起主要作用。尼古丁以游离碱的形式穿过肺泡-毛细血管屏障，与大脑中的特定烟碱型乙酰胆碱受体迅速结合，刺激突触前的乙酰胆碱受体，从而增强 ACh 的释放和代谢，同时诱导多巴胺的释放，多巴胺所引起的愉悦、放松、注意力集中、疲劳减轻是出现满足感的主要原因，这导致吸烟者对烟草的心理需求增加，增强他们继续吸烟的欲望。血清素系统、γ-氨基丁酸（GABA）系统和去甲肾上腺素能系统等也可能参与了尼古丁成瘾的分子机制。

烟草依赖的能力，与所输送尼古丁的量和到达大脑的速度有关。在没有尼古丁摄入的情况下，依赖性吸烟者会出现"渴望"戒断症候群。戒断综合征在戒烟的第1周达到顶峰，但是"渴望"有时会在戒烟消失后的几个月持续存在，如果有信号触发吸烟，则吸烟可延迟恢复。尼古丁戒断会对人的内分泌系统产生严重影响，尼古丁在人体内的半衰期短，只有2h，戒烟症状可能在吸最后一支香烟后2h开始出现，除了食欲增加外，这些症状可能需要4周才能消失。体重也可能在戒烟后的第一年增加5kg左右。脑部暴露于烟草会引起神经系统可塑性的改变，并经常与焦虑症或抑郁症有关。患有精神疾病和社会经济劣势的吸烟者更容易上瘾，戒烟的可能性更小，对健康的不利影响更大。焦虑、抑郁患者比无焦虑、抑郁的吸烟者感觉到更严重的呼吸道症状。

四、戒烟的益处

戒烟是对慢阻肺自然病程影响最大的措施，65岁时戒烟伴随着男性预期寿命从1.4岁增加到2岁，女性从2.7岁增加到3.7岁，早期戒烟行为是预防慢阻肺患者早期死亡的重要原因，并且能减少癌症、心血管、呼吸道疾病的发生。戒烟是唯一能减缓慢阻肺患者肺功能下降的干预措施，对慢阻肺患者的预后、生活质量、生存期起关键作用。通过微观模拟，从1998年到2017年美国实施烟草控制措施后，明尼苏达州癌症患者减少12 298例，因心血管疾病和糖尿病住院的患者减少72 208例，因呼吸系统疾病的住院患者减少31 913例，归因于吸烟的死亡减少140 063例，归因于吸烟的医疗支出减少102亿美元。戒烟显著改善夜间血氧饱和度降低的戒烟者的CAT评分、6min的步行距离及FEV_1。

五、戒烟在呼吸康复中的作用

呼吸康复是在全面系统评估后给予患者的个体化综合干预的治疗措施，旨在改善呼吸系统疾病患者的病理生理和心理状态，减轻呼吸困难症状，提高运动耐量，减少住院次数及致残率，提高患者生存率及社会参与能力。呼吸康复包括药物教育、戒烟教育、疾病自我管理教育、力量训练、柔韧性训练、耐力训练等。

吸烟有成瘾性，通常需要教育和药理援助才能戒除，呼吸康复治疗中包括戒烟干预。医生在鼓励患者戒烟、开具戒烟药物及使患者接受呼吸康复的过程中起非常重要的作用，医生可以通过修改和控制患者的诊疗计划来监督其参与呼吸康复治疗。由于尼古丁具有成瘾性，因此患者在戒烟时常需要同时接受非药物治疗和药物治疗，以增加戒烟的成功率，呼吸康复教育就属于非药物治疗。目前能有效增加长期戒烟效果的一线临床戒烟用药包括：尼古丁替代疗法（nicotine replacement therapy，NRT）药物、盐酸安非他酮和酒石酸伐尼克兰，主要是以nAChR亚型为靶点的选择性激动剂和拮抗剂，能缓解戒断症状的产生和减少对烟草的渴求。

吸烟者是否能成功戒烟受到社会心理因素、家人和朋友支持的强烈影响，这在老年人与年轻人通常不同。老年吸烟者因吸烟更容易出现健康问题，这可能是其戒烟的动力；年轻吸烟者因不愿被树立成"坏榜样"可能是他们戒烟的动机。心理和行为戒烟干预广泛应用于不同阶段的吸烟者，通过"5A＋5R干预法"贯穿到患者的整个戒烟过程指导其戒烟，能全面掌握患者的吸烟情况，消除紧张、焦虑情绪，鼓励患者坚持戒烟。5A询问模型包括询问（ask）、建议（advice）、评估（access）、帮助（assist）和随访（arrange）；5R建议模型包括强调健康相关性（relevance）、告知吸烟的危害（risk）、告知戒烟的好处（rewards）、告知可能遇到的困难和障碍（roadblocks）、在每次接触中反复重申建议（repetition）。

呼吸康复能改善慢阻肺吸烟者的生活质量，CAT评分优于未进行康复的慢性阻塞性肺疾病吸烟者，更好的康复依从性，并与较高的自控力呈正相关，我们前期研究发现四肢联动训练、下肢运动训练均能减轻慢阻肺稳定期患者的呼吸困难症状，提高运动耐力及改善生活质量；戒烟组慢阻肺患者运动耐力（6min步行试验）、mMRC评分、CAT评分较未戒烟组显著改善；戒烟组慢阻肺康复患者经呼吸康复治疗后1年再入院次数较未戒烟组增加；戒烟组生存时间明显延长；但对患者的肺功能无明显改善。运动训练可能调控慢性阻塞性肺疾病患者的抗氧化物质TRX1、TRXR蛋白及mRNA的表达，增强机体抗氧化能力，提高运动耐力。

吸烟患者可能降低呼吸康复的依从性，而呼吸康复对患者6min步行距离及生活质量提高有着积极影响，对吸烟者的每日香烟消费量和尼古丁依赖性程度有显著降低。GALERA等发现通过组织集体戒烟教育性研讨会，患者戒烟率显著增加，焦虑抑郁评分显著降低，且戒烟后体重没有显著增加。疾病的自我管理干预重点是识别需求，建立健康信念，增强内在动机；达成个性化目标，制定适当的策略以实现这些目标，评估和重新调整策略。这些行为改变可增强患者对运动锻炼及戒烟动机的信心和能力，通过行为改变增强健康。呼吸康复可以通过戒烟教育及运动锻炼加强对疾病的早期管理，可能阻止疾病进展。

呼吸康复中的治疗教育是控制慢病的重要组成部分，治疗教育计划的目标是促进行为和生活方式的改变，以改善健康状况，同时减少接触风险和增加对治疗的依从性。而我国慢病的管理现状让人担忧，患有吸烟相关性疾病患者很难理解呼吸康复治疗中戒烟教育计划的意义，大多数患者认为接受治疗性教育课程后，就能充分了解他们所患的疾病，但实际上，其知识水平仍然很低。患有呼吸道疾病的吸烟者比没有疾病的吸烟者更可能从医疗保健活动中得到戒烟指导，但仍有许多吸烟者在就诊期间并未得到任何建议或支持。戒烟的成功受到社会心理因素及家人和朋友支持的强烈影响，所以戒烟教育要对患者进行个性化评估后，再个性化干预，比如制订针对患者家属及朋友的个性化处方。呼吸康复具有很强的教育意义，因此无论患者是否吸烟，在需要的情况下，建议广泛纳入呼吸康复治疗计划之中。

参 考 文 献

[1] Leading cause of death, illness and impoverishment. https://www.who.int/en/news-room/fact-sheets/detail/tobacco(accessed 9 March 2018).

[2] Wirth N, Bohadana A, Spinosa A, et al. Evidence based pneumology: 3rd update workshop to the SPLF. Smoking: from prevention to weaning. Rev Mal Respir, 2004, 21(6 Pt 1): 1197-1201.

[3] Fletcher C, Peto R. The natural history of chronic airflow obstruction. Br Med J, 1977, 1(6077): 1645-1648.

[4] Degens H, Gayan-Ramirez G, van Hees HW. Smoking-induced skeletal muscle dysfunction: from evidence to mechanisms. American Journal of Respiratory and Critical Care Medicine, 2015, 191(6): 620-625.

[5] Zevin S, Saunders S, Gourlay SG, et al. Cardiovascular effects of carbon monoxide and cigarette smoking. Journal of the American College of Cardiology, 2001, 38(6): 1633-1638.

[6] National Center for Chronic Disease Prevention and Health Promotion(US) Offifice on Smoking and Health. The health consequences of smoking-50 years of progress: a report of the surgeon general. Atlanta, GA: National Center for Chronic Disease Prevention and Health Promotion, Offifice on Smoking and Health, 2014.

[7] Lugg ST, Tikka T, Agostini PJ, et al. Smoking and timing of cessation on postoperative pulmonary complications after curative-intent lung cancer surgery. J Cardiothorac Surg, 2017, 12(1): 52.

[8] Perlik F. Impact of smoking on metabolic changes and effectiveness of drugs used for lung cancer. Cent Eur J Public Health, 2020, 28(1): 53-58.

[9] Dasgupta P, Kinkade R, & Joshi B, et al. Nicotine inhibits apoptosis induced by chemotherapeutic drugs by up-regulating XIAP and survivin. PNAS, 2006, 103(16): 6332-6337.

[10] Zeng F, Li Y, Chen G, et al. Nicotine inhibits cisplatin induced apoptosis in NCI-H446 cells. Med Oncol, 2012, 29(1): 364-373.

[11] Zhang Y, Gao J, Luo Y. The effect of various durations of cigarette smoke exposure on muscle fibre remodeling in rat diaphragms. Biomed Pharmacother, 2019, 117: 109053.

[12] Kruger K, Dischereit G, Seimetz M, et al. Time course of cigarette smoke-induced changes of systemic inflammation and muscle structure. American Journal of Physiology Lung Cellular and Molecular Physiology, 2015, 309(2): L119-L128.

[13] Cheung KK, Fung TK, Mak JCW, et al. The acute effects of cigarette smoke exposure on muscle fiber type dynamics in rats. PLoS One, 2020, 15(5): e0233523.

[14] Corwin EJ, Klein LC, Rickelman K. Predictors of fatigue in healthy young adults: moderating effects of cigarette smoking and gender. Biological Research for Nursing, 2002, 3(4): 222-233.

[15] Su J, Li J, Lu Y, et al. The rat model of COPD skeletal muscle dysfunction induced by progressive cigarette smoke exposure: a pilot study. BMC PulmMed, 2020, 20(1): 74.

[16] Ajime TT, Serré J, Wüst RCI, et al. Two weeks smoking cessation reverses cigarette smoke-induced skeletal muscle atrophy and mitochondrial dysfunction in mice. Nicotine Tob, 2020.

[17] Chan SMH, Cerni C, Passey S, et al. Cigarette smoking exacerbates skeletal muscle injury without compromising its regenerative capacity. Am J Respir Cell Mol Biol, 2020, 62(2): 217-230.

[18] Petersen AM, Magkos F, Atherton P, et al. Smoking impairs muscle protein synthesis and increases the expression of myostatin and MAFbx in muscle. American Journal of Physiology Endocrinology and Metabolism, 2007, 293: E843-E848.

[19] Nucci RAB, de Souza RR, Suemoto CK, et al. Cigarette smoking impairs the diaphragm muscle structure of patients without respiratory pathologies: an autopsy study. Cell Physiol Biochem, 2019, 53: 648-655.

[20] Tiwari RK, Sharma V, Pandey RK, et al. Nicotine addiction: neurobiology and mechanism. J Pharmacopuncture, 2020, 23(1): 1-7.

[21] Brooks D, Lacasse Y, Goldstein RS. Pulmonary rehabilitation programs in Canada: national survey. Can Respir J, 1999, 6: 55-63.

[22] Perriot J, Underner M, Peiffer G, et al. Helping smoking cessation in COPD, asthma, lung cancer, operated smokers. Rev Pneumol Clin, 2018, 74(3): 170-180.

[23] Higgins ST, Heil SH, Sigmon SC, et al. Addiction potential of cigarettes with reduced nicotine content in populations with psychiatric disorders and other vulnerabilities to tobacco addiction JAMA Psychiatry, 2017, 74(10): 1056-1064.

[24] Ho CSH, Tan ELY, Ho RCM, et al. Relationship of anxiety and depression with respiratory symptoms: comparison between depressed and non-depressed smokers in Singapore. Int J Environ Res Public Health, 2019, 16(1): 163.

[25] Printz C. Stronger nicotine addiction associated with higher risk of lung cancer. Cancer, 2014, 120(23): 3591.

[26] Maciosek MV, St Claire AW, Keller PA, et al. Projecting the future impact of past accomplishments in tobacco control. Tob Control, 2020.

[27] Pezzuto A, Carico E. Effectiveness of smoking cessation in smokers with COPD and nocturnal oxygen desaturation: Functional analysis. Clin Respir J, 2020, 14(1): 29-34.

[28] Garvey C, Fullwood M D, Rigler J. Pulmonary rehabilitation exercise prescription in chronicobstructive lung disease: US survey and review of guidelines and clinical practices. J Cardiopulm Rehabil Prev, 2013, 33(5): 314-322.

[29] Hale AG, Collins KP. Students' attitudes towards patient smoking status during enrollment in a pulmonary rehabilitation program. J Allied Health, 2019, 48(1): 67-71.

[30] Corriea A, Wise LA Review of nonpharmacologic and pharmacologic therapies for smoking cessation. Formulary, 2007, 43: 44-64.

[31] 刘朝, 肖丹, 王辰. 戒烟是慢性阻塞性肺疾病防治的最有效措

施.中华结核和呼吸杂志,2017,40(12):894-897.
[32] Guilleminault L,Rolland Y,Didier A. Characteristics of non-pharmacological interventions in the elderly with COPD. Smoking cessation, pulmonary rehabilitation, nutritional management and patient education. Rev Mal Respir,2018,35(6):626-641.
[33] 徐鸣丽,金媛. 5A+5R干预联合伐尼克兰对COPD患者戒烟效果及肺功能的影响. 临床肺科杂志,2020,25(6):843-846.
[34] Postolache P,Nemeș RM,Petrescu O,et al. Smoking cessation,pulmonary rehabilitation and quality of life at smokers with COPD. Rev Med Chir Soc Med Nat Iasi,2015,119(1):77-80.
[35] 周蔚. 四肢联动训练对慢性阻塞性肺疾病稳定期患者肺康复的影响. 南华大学,2018.
[36] 段文滔. 生脉注射液穴位注射联合运动训练对慢阻肺的康复疗效及对TRXS的作用. 南华大学,2017.
[37] Santana VT,Squassoni SD,Neder JA,et al. Influence of current smoking on adherence and responses to pulmonary rehabilitation in patients with COPD. Rev Bras Fisioter,2010,14(1):16-23.
[38] Galera O,Bajon D,Maoz Z,et al. Effectiveness of therapeutic education against "nicotinophobia" in smokers hospitalized for cardiovas-cular and pulmonary rehabilitation. Rev Pneumol Clin,2018,74(4):221-225.
[39] Blackstock FC,Evans RA. Rehabilitation in lung diseases: 'Education' component of pulmonary rehabilitation. Respirology,2019,24(9):863-870.
[40] Lewis A,Dullaghan D,Townes H,et al. An observational cohort study of exercise and education for people with chronic obstructive pulmonary disease not meeting criteria for formal pulmonary rehabilitation programmes. Chron Respir Dis,2019,16.

8 电子烟上海专家共识简洁版

上海医学会呼吸病学分会烟草病学组

一、专家共识形成背景

电子烟正在逐渐成为新时尚，立法仍处于灰色地带，公众对电子烟的认识不足。为更好地了解电子烟，上海医学会呼吸病学分会烟草病学组特制定《电子烟上海专家共识》(以下简称"共识")。

二、共识组成

共识包括以下部分：概述，电子烟的有害物质和对健康的危害，电子烟的成瘾性，电子烟作为辅助戒烟工具，立法现状，上海共识建议。

三、具体内容

(一) 概述

电子烟指由电池供能，将含有尼古丁和其他成分的混合物转化成气雾，由使用者吸入的一种电子装置。

(二) 电子烟的有害物质和对健康的危害

1. 电子烟的有害物质　电子烟烟油含尼古丁、有机溶剂、调味成分等。经加热后形成的电子烟烟雾，其构成及浓度发生变化，含有多环芳香烃、尼古丁、挥发性有机化合物、超细颗粒、金属及硅酸盐等有害物质。

2. 电子烟对健康的危害　电子烟对健康的影响可分为急性损伤和慢性损伤。急性损伤：电子烟器具可在手掌、口腔内爆炸。慢性损伤：可损伤全身各脏器，某些成分具有致癌性。随着禁烟令实施，公共场所吸烟变得越来越困难，但大部分控烟条例未明确禁止吸食电子烟，因而电子烟成为部分吸烟者在公共场所吸食的替代品。

电子烟对青少年和胎儿的影响：由于青少年好奇心强，且不易建立起对慢性、长期的健康危害的认知，导致青少年使用电子烟越来越多，电子烟成为传统卷烟的入门产品。孕妇吸食电子烟，烟雾毒性物质可进入胎儿循环，对胎儿造成不良影响，孕妇应禁止吸食任何烟草产品，包括电子烟。

(三) 电子烟的成瘾性

与传统卷烟相比，电子烟缺乏生产标准和行业监管。电子烟可提供传统卷烟相当或更高数量的尼古丁，过高的尼古丁水平可能会引起大脑烟碱型乙酰胆碱受体的生理变化，这种受体可以导致电子烟成瘾。

(四) 电子烟作为辅助戒烟工具

电子烟作为戒烟工具尚缺乏循证医学证据，目前并无足够证据表明电子烟可以帮助使用者提高彻底戒烟的意愿，而且会阻碍吸烟者使用安全有效的戒烟药物。

(五) 立法现状

2017年世卫组织关于全球烟草流行报告显示全球195个世卫组织成员国中，30个国家禁止电子烟，65个国家对其实施管制。中国疾控中心发布的《2018年中国成人烟草调查结果》显示，虽然我国电子烟使用率处于较低水平，但较前有显著增加。2018年国家市场监督管理总局、国家烟草专卖局发布了《关于禁止向未成年人出售电子烟的通告》。

(六) 上海共识建议

明确电子烟属性和定位，制定电子烟行业标准，对电子烟制造销售全程监管，杜绝向未成年人兜售电子烟。鼓励开展电子烟相关动物和人群研究，进一步明确电子烟的安全性和对戒烟的有效性。

9 烟草、巨噬细胞与肺部疾病

季婷芬　李和权

烟草严重威胁人类健康,吸烟与多种肺部疾病(如慢性阻塞性肺疾病和肺癌等)密切相关。无论机体处于稳态还是遭受感染和炎症等损伤时,巨噬细胞在清除病原体及坏死组织的过程中都起到至关重要的作用。近几年,随着研究的深入,学界对巨噬细胞的起源、作用及分型都有了新的认识。本文综述了巨噬细胞的起源和分型及其与一些肺部疾病的关系,以及烟草在其中的作用和机制。

一、烟　草

吸烟严重威胁人类的健康,2019年世界卫生组织(WHO)发布的《全球烟草流行报告》指出,2018年全球约有1/3的成年人吸烟,因烟草致死人数高达600万。我国每年死于吸烟相关疾病者近100万,占死亡人数的12%。烟草是呼吸、心血管、感染和癌症等多种疾病的独立危险因素,特别是慢性阻塞性肺疾病、哮喘和肺癌等肺部疾病。近年来,电子烟的使用逐渐普及,电子烟作为传统烟草的一种替代品也并非绝对安全,同样会引起组织损伤,诱导肺部疾病。烟草燃烧的烟雾中含有大量的有害物质,包括烟碱、一氧化碳(CO)、氮氧化物和镉等。然而,市面上烟草、电子烟的成分各不相同,其致病机制十分复杂,有待进一步探索。

(一)传统烟草中的致病物质

1. **生物碱类**　烟草中含有50多种生物碱,其中烟碱(俗称尼古丁)约占生物碱的95%。烟碱是烟草主要的神经活性物质,也是烟草上瘾的主要成分。吸烟者通过吸烟维持大脑烟碱的稳定水平,一旦低于这个水平就会出现烦躁、恶心等症状。烟碱可能导致巨噬细胞免疫功能失调。一方面,烟碱诱导巨噬细胞产生大量的活性氧(ROS)和亚硝酸盐(NO),ROS和NO都是炎症反应中重要的信号分子,可以直接损伤肺组织,也可以通过调节炎症反应损伤肺组织。另一方面,巨噬细胞实现吞噬功能需经过识别、黏附、趋化、吞噬等步骤,但在烟碱暴露下,巨噬细胞黏附时间延长、趋化指数下降、吞噬能力减弱,可能与烟碱引起巨噬细胞形状改变及溶酶体损伤有关。

2. **活性氧**　活性氧是机体细胞内或外界环境中由氧组成的含氧量高且化学性质活泼的一类物质的总称,包括过氧化物、超氧阴离子和氧自由基等。烟草烟雾中含有较高浓度的自由基氧化物,在进入呼吸道后,能够诱导肺泡巨噬细胞聚集并产生大量的氧自由基,促进促炎细胞因子的产生,引起肺组织氧化损伤。

3. **化学致癌物质**　烟草烟雾中含有多种化学致癌物质,包括多环芳香烃(PAH)、亚硝胺和丁二烯等,可以诱导肺部肿瘤。巨噬细胞具有识别并吞噬肿瘤细胞、防止肿瘤细胞转移的作用,烟草烟雾中各种化学致癌物质可能通过抑制巨噬细胞功能诱导肺部肿瘤。

4. **其他**　除了化学致癌物质以外,烟草烟雾中还含有无机化合物,如砷、镉、铬和镍,这些都对巨噬细胞有着明显的毒性作用,诱导巨噬细胞凋亡;烟草烟雾中还含有放射性元素,包括铀和钍核素及其衰变产物,它们通过土壤和肥料进入烟草之中,并通过吸烟被肺组织吸收,可能与肺部肿瘤发生有关。

(二)电子烟中的致病物质

目前,市面上的电子烟的烟液通常由甘油、丙二醇、烟碱及调味剂组成。研究表明电子烟烟嘴产生的气雾中含有大部分与传统烟草相同的有害物质,包括烟碱、活性氧和亚硝胺等。除此之外,电子烟气雾中还有部分传统烟草没有的有害物质,如甘油、丙二醇等,都对呼吸道有强烈刺激作用。Aaron等对不含烟碱的电子烟蒸汽冷凝液的研究表明,肺泡巨噬细胞在冷凝液的暴露下极易发生凋亡坏死且吞噬功能下降。与正常肺泡巨噬细胞相比,暴露于冷凝液的肺泡巨噬细胞对大肠埃希菌和金黄色葡萄球菌的吞噬作用大大减弱。同时冷凝液会促进肺泡巨噬细胞释放ROS、炎性细胞因子、趋化因子和金属蛋白酶,导致氧化应激和炎症反应,损伤肺组织。由此可见,电子烟作为传统烟草的替代产品并不意味着绝对安全,也不能起到戒烟作用,更有研究表明青少年早期吸电子烟,将来吸烟草的可能性增加(约为不吸电子烟青少年的3.6倍)。

二、巨噬细胞

(一)巨噬细胞的起源

巨噬细胞广泛存在于哺乳类动物的各种组织,1893年Elie Metchnikoff首次发现以来,人们认为组织中的巨噬细胞由循环中的单核细胞分化而来,并由其补充维持数量,近年来,随着研究的深入,这一观点得以更新。Epelman等研究发现组织中的巨噬细胞群体在胚胎发育时期就已经从卵黄囊中产生,并具有独立的自我更新能力,但是当机体受到刺激时,循环中的单核细胞可以帮助补充维持肺泡巨噬细胞数目。Hashimoto等报道单核细胞减少症的患者,大部分组织巨噬细胞的数目不发生改变也间接证实了这一点。肺组织的巨噬细胞主要分为两种:大部分是存在于肺泡内较大的肺泡巨噬细胞（AM）及小部分异质性较大的间质巨噬细胞（IM）。近年来，研究人员还根据特殊的表面标志和基因表达谱，在小鼠肺组织发现 IM 的 3 种亚型。肺内的巨噬细胞主要有胚胎卵黄囊中发育的原始巨噬细胞和肝发育的胚胎单核细胞前体两种来源。现已证明 IM 可以转化为 AM，但 IM 能否独立的自我更新，IM 是否来源于 AM 的前体细胞等都还不清楚。

（二）巨噬细胞的分型和功能

1. 巨噬细胞的分型　巨噬细胞极化是巨噬细胞应对不同微环境表达不同表型功能的动态过程。1992 年，Stein 等在研究小鼠模型时提出巨噬细胞暴露于干扰素-γ（IFN-γ）或白介素-4（IL-4）可呈现出抗炎或促炎表型，随后这两种表型被称为 M1/M2。M1 巨噬细胞也称为经典活化巨噬细胞（与 Th1 免疫反应相关），在 Th1 相关细胞因子如 IFN-γ、脂多糖（LPS）及粒细胞-巨噬细胞集落刺激因子（GM-CSF）等刺激下活化。M1 能产生一氧化氮（NO）和多种促炎因子（如 IL-1、TNF-α、IL-12 和 IL-18），抵抗病原体及吞噬病原微生物。M2 巨噬细胞被称为交替活化巨噬细胞（与 Th1 免疫反应相关），Th2 相关细胞因子如集落刺激因子-1（CSF-1）、IL-4、IL-13 等都会促进其极化。M2 巨噬细胞在寄生虫感染、组织重塑、过敏性疾病中都起到重要作用。然而，这种分类并无法准确表达巨噬细胞的生理功能特性，例如，部分属 M1 亚群的巨噬细胞，其功能更接近于 M2 类，目前进一步将其分为 M1、M2a、M2b、M2c 等。近年来，对巨噬细胞进行深入研究后，发现除了 M1、M2 表型外，还有其他单核细胞源性的巨噬细胞，可能在特定情况下发挥作用：①肿瘤相关巨噬细胞（TAM）：与癌症相关的巨噬细胞亚群；②CD169$^+$ 巨噬细胞：在淋巴器官中发现，与免疫耐受和抗原提呈相关；③T 细胞受体阳性巨噬细胞（TCR$^+$）；未受刺激时，肺组织保持轻度抗炎状态，以维持对吸入的粉尘、颗粒的耐受性，表现为 M1、M2 混合表型。当肺组织受到刺激时，更易倾向于转变为 M1 表型，释放相关的细胞因子，促进炎症，但持续的急性炎症反应会损伤肺组织。因此为了维持体内平衡，巨噬细胞向 M2 极化并分泌大量的细胞因子抑制炎症，促进组织修复、重塑、血管生成，但过度的 M2 巨噬细胞会促进细胞增生，导致免疫失调。

2. 巨噬细胞的功能　巨噬细胞是一种单核吞噬细胞，在肺组织内被比喻为"哨兵"，无论是在稳定或遭受感染和炎症等损伤时，其在清除病原体及坏死组织中起着重要作用。巨噬细胞主要有以下作用：①识别、吞噬作用。巨噬细胞具有多种模式识别受体，其中最重要的是 Toll 样受体（TLR），其识别外来病原体，是启动免疫应答的关键。随后，巨噬细胞通过形成酸性环境、溶酶体作用、产生毒性物质等手段对病原微生物进行吞噬。②分泌作用。巨噬细胞具有强大的分泌功能，可以分泌脂质介质、趋化因子、细胞因子、生长因子和活性氧等物质调节免疫反应。巨噬细胞的趋化因子能够招募多种细胞，应对外界刺激。巨噬细胞还能分泌基质金属弹性蛋白酶（MMP-12），这与 COPD 患者的肺气肿病变有关。③抗原提呈作用。除了吞噬杀伤病原体外，近年来，研究发现巨噬细胞同样具有抗原提呈功能，但相对较弱。巨噬细胞能够提呈抗原，激活周围的巨噬细胞及诱导 T 细胞活化，启动机体免疫应答。

三、肺部疾病

呼吸系统疾病是我国最主要的疾病，慢性呼吸系统疾病是 WHO 定义的四大慢病之一，大多数呼吸系统疾病与烟草暴露相关。大部分与烟草相关的肺部疾病最初都以炎症反应起病，而巨噬细胞作为炎症反应的重要组成部分在多数呼吸系统疾病（如 COPD、哮喘、肺癌及弥漫性肺部疾病）的发生发展过程中都起到重要作用。烟草烟雾在其中的作用可能包括以下几个方面：①巨噬细胞数量增加：研究表明吸烟者 BAL 巨噬细胞数目高于健康者，在烟草烟雾暴露下，循环中表达 CXCR2 的单核细胞可以转化为巨噬细胞并聚集，引起巨噬细胞数目增加。②巨噬细胞凋亡、坏死：烟草烟雾中的多种物质都对巨噬细胞有毒性作用，也可能通过氧化应激诱导巨噬细胞发生凋亡、坏死。③巨噬细胞吞噬功能受抑制：巨噬细胞通过形成酸性环境、溶酶体作用、产生毒性物质等手段对病原微生物进行吞噬，但在烟草烟雾暴露下，巨噬细胞形状改变、溶酶体损伤，吞噬杀菌功能下降。④M1/M2 巨噬细胞失衡：正常的肺组织 M1、M2 巨噬细胞处于相对动态平衡状态，烟草烟雾暴露引起 M1/M2 巨噬细胞失衡，影响巨噬细胞分泌功能导致趋化因子、炎症因子、活性氧和蛋白酶数量异常，同时激活其他免疫细胞，可能参与多种肺部疾病的发病机制。

（一）呼吸系统感染性疾病

1. 流行性感冒　流行性感冒是流感病毒引起的急性呼吸道传染病，而甲型流感病毒是最常见的病原体。大量的流行病学研究表明，吸烟与呼吸道感染（如流行性感冒）的发病率增加有关，临床观察也表明，流感症状在吸烟者中更为严重。肺泡巨噬细胞被认为是感染过程中炎症反应的重要启动因子，是抵御呼吸道感染的第一道防线。在首次感染病原体 3~7d 后，单核细胞进入肺组织补充消耗的肺泡巨噬细胞，对抗病原体、修复受损组织。s-IgA 是呼吸道黏膜免疫反应中主要的效应因子，在流感病毒感染的体液免疫中起到重要作用。s-IgA 的分泌主要依靠 B 细胞活化因子（BAFF）的表达，而巨噬细胞是表达 BAFF 的重要细胞之一。虽然短期烟草烟雾暴露对 BAFF 表达无明显影响，但较长期（3~6 个月）的烟草烟雾暴露会显著抑制巨噬细胞表达 BAFF，从而影响 s-IgA 分泌，影响机体对流感病毒的清除。同时，Aegerter 等研究表明肺泡巨噬细胞可以在流感病毒再次入侵时，分泌较高水平的 IL-6 起到较长期的抗菌保护作用。而在长期烟草烟雾暴露下，肺泡巨噬细胞 IL-6 分泌可能减少，机体对流感病毒的反应能力减弱。

2. 结核病　肺结核是一种结核分枝杆菌引起的慢性感染性肺部疾病，但并非所有人吸入结核杆菌后都会感染肺结核，这与肺泡巨噬细胞固有的杀菌吞噬能力有关。多项研究表明，吸烟者和二手烟暴露者更易患肺结核，儿童早期接触二手烟烟雾更易患原发性肺结核。当人体受到结核杆菌感染时,巨噬细胞处于第一防线率先做出反应,并在之后的结核性肉芽肿的形成过程中起关键作用。调节性 T 细胞(Treg)是一群负调节机体免疫反应的淋巴细胞,通常能避免免疫反应过度损伤机体,参与慢性炎症的发展。Bai 等研究表明,在烟草烟雾的暴露下,烟碱通过与烟碱乙酰胆碱受体(nAChR)结合,增强 Treg 功能,抑制巨噬细胞对结核杆菌的吞噬功能,表现为 IL-6、IL-12、TNF-α 水平降低,而 IL-10 升高。Huang 等在肺结核患者肺组织中发现,在坏死性或非坏死性肉芽肿中,巨噬细胞均表达 CD206,而 iNOS 表达较低,表明结核性肉芽肿内 M1 和 M2 巨噬细胞共存,以 M2 巨噬细胞为主,这与上述观点一致,进一步证实了烟草烟雾暴露主要通过增强 Treg 功能,诱导巨噬细胞向 M2 极化,使肺部清除入侵分枝杆菌的防御机制失效。同时,在烟草烟雾的暴露下,NF-κB 信号通路激活导致受结核杆菌感染的巨噬细胞自噬功能抑制,促进了结核杆菌在体内生存和迁移。

(二)慢性气道炎症性疾病

1. **慢性阻塞性肺疾病** 慢性阻塞性肺疾病(COPD)是一种慢性炎性疾病,炎症细胞在气道聚集并激活,分泌大量细胞因子和蛋白酶,引起肺组织损伤,导致肺气肿病变和小气道病变。研究表明与未吸烟正常人群相比,吸烟者小气道、管腔、支气管肺泡灌洗液中巨噬细胞数目均增加;COPD 患者肺泡巨噬细胞数目增加更加明显,且与病情严重程度相关,同时吸烟者肺组织可见 M2 巨噬细胞极化增强,而 COPD 患者 M2 巨噬细胞极化水平更高,提示 M2 巨噬细胞在 COPD 病理变化中具有重要的作用。COPD 患者处于反复多次烟雾暴露中,为了维持机体平衡与稳定,巨噬细胞向 M2 极化。He 等研究表明烟草烟雾的暴露使 M2 巨噬细胞极化,并激活 TGF-β/Smad 通路,促进 M2 巨噬细胞分泌 MMP-9、MMP-12,直接损伤肺实质,引起肺气肿病变。此外,小气道病变主要是气道周围组织的重塑和纤维化及小气道附着肺泡的破坏,此过程均与 TGF-β/Smad 通路相关。这也意味着阻断 M2 巨噬细胞的活化或者抑制 TGF-β/Smad 通路的激活可能可以早期防治 COPD,为 COPD 的治疗提供一个新方向。

2. **哮喘** 哮喘是由多种细胞(包括嗜酸性粒细胞、肥大细胞、辅助性 T 细胞及中性粒细胞等)和细胞组分参与的气道慢性炎症性异质性疾病,巨噬细胞作为气道主要的免疫细胞,参与并调控哮喘的发生和发展。Girodec 及其同事发现随着 MRC1 和 MHC-II 在哮喘患者 BALFs 中表达升高,M2 巨噬细胞显著增加(约为健康对照组的 2.9 倍),这直接支持了 M2 巨噬细胞与过敏性哮喘的关系。妊娠期接触烟草和新生儿早期接触烟草都可能导致哮喘发生。烟草烟雾可直接刺激巨噬细胞和气道上皮细胞分泌细胞因子和趋化因子,在 CCL-17 和 MRC1 的介导下,M2a 巨噬细胞分泌 IL-13、CCL-17、CCL-18、CCL-22 和 CCL-24,激活 Th2 细胞,促进嗜酸性粒细胞浸润,诱发并加剧哮喘。未来研制以 M2 巨噬细胞发育及激活为靶点的药物,可能是治疗过敏性哮喘的新方向。同时,Robbe 等通过研究发现,虽然 M2 巨噬细胞在过敏性哮喘中占主导地位,但 M1 巨噬细胞可能是非过敏性哮喘的主要效应细胞,在非过敏性哮喘中,M1 巨噬细胞极化,Th1 和 Th17 表达增加。此外,M1 巨噬细胞还可能和重症哮喘相关,尤其是对于全身皮质类固醇反应不良的患者。

(三)肺癌

肺癌是全球发病率最高的恶性肿瘤,近年来肺癌的发病率和病死率还在不断增加。浸润于肿瘤间质的巨噬细胞被称为肿瘤相关巨噬细胞(TAM),是肿瘤微环境中含量最丰富的炎性细胞,与肿瘤的发生发展息息相关。吸烟是肺癌最主要的诱因,吸烟者肺组织可见 M2 巨噬细胞极化增强,Yuan 等研究表明在烟草烟雾暴露下,巨噬细胞 TGF-β 分泌量增加,而 TNF-α、IL-12 分泌量减少,提示烟草烟雾可以诱导单核细胞转变为巨噬细胞并向 M2 巨噬细胞极化,并且烟草烟雾可能是通过 STAT6 通路激活诱导 M2 巨噬细胞极化的。当 TAM 呈现 M2 极化表型时,M2 巨噬细胞能分泌血管内皮生长因子(VEGF)、血管生成素(ANG)-Ⅰ 和 ANG-Ⅱ 等促血管生成介质促进血管生成,并通过分泌生长因子和 MMP 介导肿瘤细胞侵袭和转移。由此可见,烟草烟雾不仅可以将肿瘤微环境中的单核细胞活化为 TAM,影响巨噬细胞正常功能,还能促进其向 M2 极化,促进肿瘤细胞的侵袭和转移。

(四)肺部弥漫性疾病

1. **朗格汉斯细胞组织细胞增生症** 朗格汉斯细胞组织细胞增生症(LCH)涉及多个系统,包括肝、脾、肺及造血系统等脏器损害,部分病例存在肺部的单独损害,称为原发性肺朗格汉斯细胞组织细胞增生症(PLCH)。朗格汉斯细胞主要来源于卵黄囊巨噬细胞,通过胚胎组织迁移进入机体组织,随后原位增生产生长期存活的朗格汉斯细胞、小胶质细胞和巨噬细胞。

PLCH 主要与有丝分裂原活化蛋白激酶(MAPK)通路信号突变有关,尤其是 BARF^{v600E} 的突变。并非所有的朗格汉斯细胞都会变为 PLCH 的肿瘤细胞,只有当其遇到特殊刺激,才会出现 PLCH 中的异常增生和破坏。近年来研究发现,绝大多数 PLCH 与吸烟关系密切,认为 PLCH 是一种与吸烟相关的肺组织的过度免疫反应形式,由慢性炎性病变引起,最终导致朗格汉斯细胞沉积到小气道的间质区域。烟草烟雾暴露引起小气道炎症,诱导多种细胞因子和趋化因子(主要是 TNF、GM-CSF、TGF 和 CCL20)释放,引起巨噬细胞、树突状细胞和 T 细胞为主的炎症细胞聚集形成炎性组织肉芽肿。TNF 主要由巨噬细胞和上皮细胞产生,可以促进朗格汉斯细胞激活和分化。GM-CSF 是朗格汉斯细胞的强有丝分裂因子。TGF 除了对朗格汉斯细胞有增生活性,还能参与肺实质的重构和纤维化。此外,烟草烟雾还能促进抗凋亡蛋白的表达,抑制朗格汉斯细胞凋亡。因此,同时满足通路信号突变和刺激引起的异常炎症是 PLCH 发生的必备条件。

2. **结节病** 结节病是一种原因不明的多系统累及的肉芽肿性疾病,主要侵犯肺和淋巴系统。结节病发病机制目前尚不明确,可能是环境刺激触发主要由肺泡巨噬细胞介导的适应性免疫失调,导致肉芽肿的形成。对于烟草烟雾暴露与结节病的关系,不同研究持不同观点。有些认为烟草与结节病的发病无关,是否吸烟或是否处于二手烟的暴露对结节病的临床行为或疾病严重程度没有任何影响；而有些认为 CS 暴露与结节病呈负相关,吸烟者不易患结节病。

一般情况下,遗传易感者受到特定环境刺激后,抗原提呈细胞处理吞噬抗原,巨噬细胞分泌促炎因子介导 Th1 型免疫反应,导致细胞聚集、增生、分化和肉芽肿的形成。大多数患者,肉芽肿会随时间的推移而消失,但少数患者会进展演变为进行性纤维化。多项研究发现,巨噬细胞向 M2 极化可能与结节病的发展、肺纤维化、蜂窝肺等有关。Prasse 等研究报道,在肌样变相关的肺纤维化中,M2 巨噬细胞释放促纤维化趋化因子 CCL18。因此,烟草烟雾通过增强 Treg 细胞功能,促进巨噬细胞交替活化,活化的 M2 巨噬细胞可分泌 TGF-β、CCL18,促进结节病的进展。

3.过敏性肺炎　过敏性肺炎(HP)是一种肺部炎症反应性疾病。HP 通常与职业、粉尘暴露有关,Th1 细胞介导的免疫反应在发病过程中占主导地位。肺泡巨噬细胞是肺泡腔内最早摄取抗原的细胞,肺泡巨噬细胞的初始活化是驱动后续免疫反应的关键因素,激活的肺泡巨噬细胞释放一系列的细胞因子,导致肺泡的炎症,引起炎症细胞聚集并参与炎症反应,最终导致过敏性肉芽肿的形成。

虽然具体的机制不明确,但临床上发现吸烟者很少发生 HP,在相同暴露风险下,非吸烟者更易出现 HP,这可能与烟草烟雾暴露诱发肺部局部免疫功能失调有关。在环境刺激因素作用下,活化的 M1 巨噬细胞提呈抗原并分泌 TNF-α、IL-1β,促进 CD4⁺T 细胞分化为 Th1 细胞,Th1 细胞产生并释放 TNF、IL-12、IL-18 和 INF-γ 发挥作用。然而烟草中的烟碱可以影响巨噬细胞的活化及抑制肺泡巨噬细胞分泌 TNF-α、IL-1 和 INF-γ 等细胞因子,减少肺淋巴细胞数量,导致局部免疫失调。此外,烟碱还能够消耗淋巴细胞中的钙,使淋巴细胞生存周期缩短。

四、讨　论

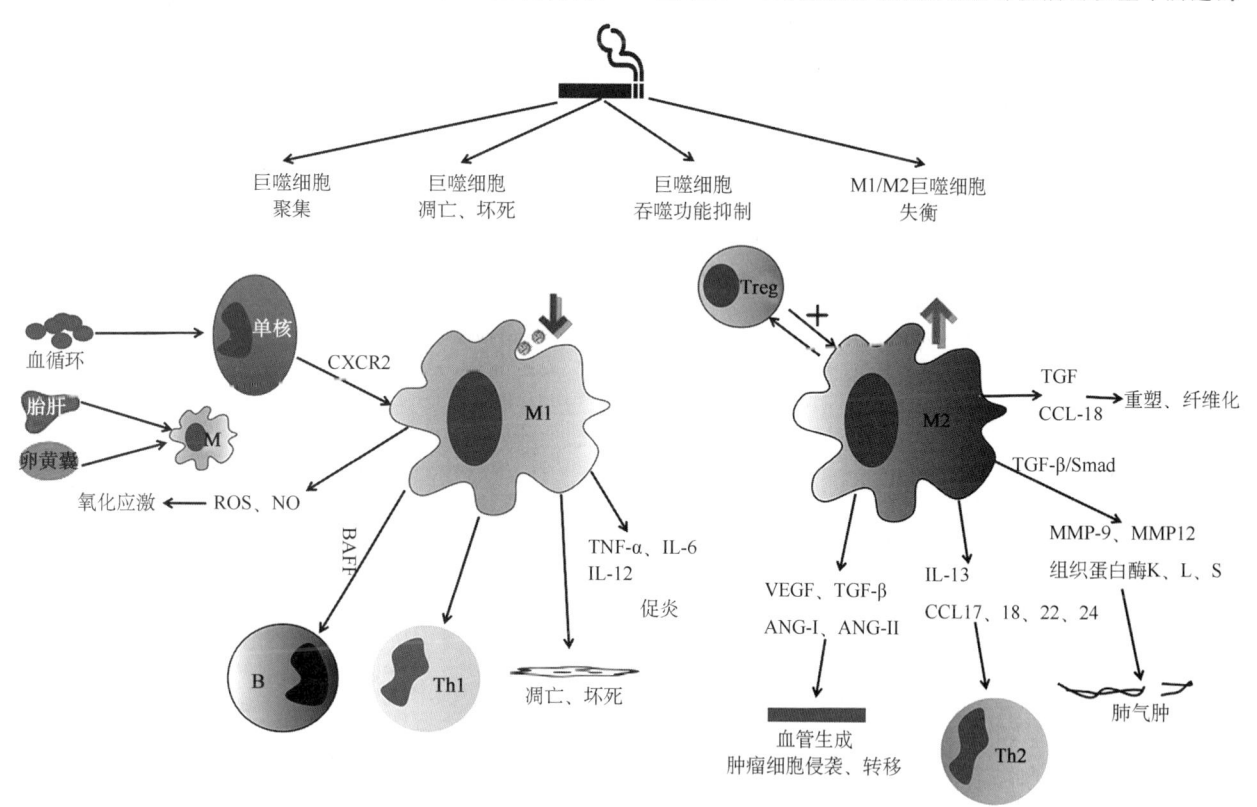

烟草与多种肺部疾病有关,烟草(包括电子烟)中含有多种有害物质,它们可以直接或间接作用于肺泡巨噬细胞,引起肺泡巨噬细胞数量增加、吞噬功能减弱及巨噬细胞相关细胞因子分泌异常等导致肺组织损伤,从而引起肺部疾病。烟草是肺部疾病的多米诺骨牌起点,遗传易感者在此环境暴露下,随后的一系列致病过程才得以发生。巨噬细胞作为炎症反应的重要细胞,几乎每种肺部疾病(包括 COPD、哮喘及肺癌等)都有巨噬细胞的参与。肺组织的巨噬细胞在稳定状态下表现为 M1 和 M2 的混合表型,处于一种动态平衡状态。M1 和 M2 型巨噬细胞像是各种肺部疾病的开关,当气道、肺组织受到烟草烟雾刺激时,这种平衡会遭受破坏,巨噬细胞发生聚集、坏死、凋亡并向不同极型极化,不同极型的巨噬细胞释放相应的细胞因子和蛋白酶,激活其他免疫细胞,可能导致不同肺部疾病的发生(图 1-9-1)。探索巨噬细胞在肺部疾病的发生中所起的

图 1-9-1　烟草烟雾中含有多种有害物质

注:长期烟草烟雾的暴露招募肺泡巨噬细胞,损害巨噬细胞吞噬功能,使巨噬细胞坏死、凋亡并发生极化,导致 M1/M2 巨噬细胞失衡。同时,巨噬细胞分泌细胞因子和蛋白酶并招募其他免疫细胞,导致免疫紊乱。这些过程在各类肺部疾病的发生发展中起到重要作用。M. 巨噬细胞;Treg. 调节性 T 细胞;VEGF. 内皮生长因子;ANG. 血管生成素;TGF. 转化生长因子;CXCR. 趋化因子受体;TNF. 肿瘤坏死因子;IL. 白介素;CCL. 趋化因子;MMP. 基质金属蛋白酶

作用,可能对疾病的发病机制有一个新的认识。同时,巨噬细胞作为一个治疗的方向,可以通过增强或抑制巨噬细胞的功能,来影响疾病的发生与进展。但目前,我们对巨噬细胞的了解还远远不足,有待进一步探索。

参 考 文 献

[1] 姜垣,李强,肖琳,等.中国烟草流行与控制.中华流行病学杂志,2011,32(12):1181-1187.

[2] Ghosh A,Coakley R,Ghio A,et al. Chronic E-cigarette use increases neutrophil elastase and matrix metalloprotease levels in the lung. Am J Respir Crit Care Med,2019,200(11):1392-1401.

[3] Giotopoulou GA,Stathopoulos GT. Effects of inhaled tobacco smoke on the pulmonary tumor microenvironment. Adv Exp Med Biol,2020,1225:53-69.

[4] Mehta H,Nazzal K,Sadikot RT. Cigarette smoking and innate immunity. Inflamm Res,2008,57(11):497-503.

[5] Rong JF,Tao YU,Xu Shu. Research progress of ROS in regulating macrophage polarization. Basic Clin Med,2019,39(1):93-95.

[6] Ween MP,Whittall JJ,Hamon R,et al. Phagocytosis and Inflflammation:Exploring the effects of the components of E-cigarette vapor on macrophages. Physiol Rep,2017,5(16):e13370.

[7] Jenssena BP,Wilson KM. What is new in electronic-cigarettes research?. Curr Opin Pediatr,2019,31(2):262-266.

[8] McGovern N,Schlitzer A,Gunawan M,et al. Human dermal CD14+ cells are a transient population of monocyte-derived macrophages. Immunity,2014,41(3):465-477.

[9] Saradna A,Do DC,Kumar S,et al. Macrophage polarization and allergic asthma. Transl Res,2018,191:1-14.

[10] Epelman S,Lavine KJ,Randolph GJ. Origin and functions of tissue macrophages. Immunity,2014,41(1):21-35.

[11] Hoppstädter J,Diesel B,Zarbock R,et al. Differential cell reaction upon Toll-like receptor 4 and 9 activation in human alveolar and lung interstitial macrophages. Respir Res,2010,11:124.

[12] Cai Y,Sugimoto C,Arainga M,et al. In vivo characterization of alveolar and interstitial lung macrophages in rhesus macaques:implications for understanding lung disease in humans. J Immunol,2014,192:2821-2829.

[13] Stein M,Keshav S,Harris N,et al. Interleukin 4 potently enhances murine macrophage mannose receptor activity:a marker of alternative immunologic macrophage activation. J Exp Med,1992,176(1):287-292.

[14] Moghaddam AS,Mohammadian S,Vazini H,et al. Macrophage plasticity,polarization and function in health and disease. J Cell Physiol,2018,233(9):6425-6440.

[15] Epelman S,Lavine KJ. Randolph GJ. Origin and functions of tissue macrophages. Immunity,2014,41(1):21-35.

[16] Mayer AK,Bartz H,Fey F,et al. Airway epithelial cells modify immune responses by inducing an anti-inflammatory microenvironment. Eur J Immunol,2008,38(6):1689-1699.

[17] Patela VI,Metcalfb JP. Airway macrophage and dendritic cell subsets in the resting human lung. Immunology,2018,38(4):303-331.

[18] Crotty Alexander LE,Shin S,Hwang JH. Inflammatory diseases of the lung induced by conventional cigarette smoke. Chest,2015,148(5):1307-1322.

[19] Wang JM,Li QH,Xie JG,et al. Cigarette smoke inhibits BAFF expression and mucosal immunoglobulin A responses in the lung during influenza virus infection. Respir Res,2015,16(1):37.

[20] Aegerter H,Kulikauskaite J,Crotta S,et al. Influenza-induced monocyte-derived alveolar macrophages confer prolonged antibacterial protection. Nat Immunol,2020,21(2):145-157.

[21] Jafta N,Jeena PM,Barregard P,et al. Association of childhood pulmonary tuberculosis with exposure to indoor air pollution:a case control study. BMC Public Health,2019,19(1):275.

[22] Bai XY,Stitzel JA,Bai A,et al. Nicotine impairs macrophage control of Mycobacterium tuberculosis. Am J Respir Cell Mol Biol,2017,57(3):324-333.

[23] Huang Z,Luo Q,Guo Y,et al. Mycobacterium tuberculosis-induced polarization of human macrophage orchestrates the formation and development of tuberculous granulomas in vitro. PLoS One,2015,10(6):el29744.

[24] He SY,Lu JJ,Sun SH,et al. Characteristics and potential role of M2 macrophages in COPD. Int J Chron Obstruct Pulmon Dis,2017,12:3029-3039.

[25] Peter BJ. Alveolar macrophages as orchestrators of COPD. COPD,2004,1(1):59-70.

[26] Saradna A,Do DC,Kumar S,et al. Macrophage polarization and allergic asthma. Transl Res,2018,191:1-14.

[27] Jie J,Conlon TM,Ballester Lopez C,et al. Cigarette smoke causes acute airway disease and exacerbates chronic obstructive lung disease in neonatal mice. Am J Physiol Lung Cell Mol Physiol,2016,311:L602-L610.

[28] Melgert BN,Oriss TB,Qi Z,et al. Macrophages:regulators of sex differences in asthma?. Am J Respir Cell Mol Biol,2010,42:595-603.

[29] Yuan F,Fu X,Shi H,et al. Induction of murine macrophage M2 polarization by cigarette smoke extract via the JAK2/STAT3 pathway. PLoS One,2014,9(9):e107063.

[30] Shi M,Wang XH,Deng YF,et al. The effects of CSE-induced M2 polarized macrophages on lung carcinoma invasion and migration. Chin J Cell Biol,2019,41(6):1107-1113.

[31] Collin M,Milne P. Langerhans cell origin and regulation. Curr Opin Hematol,2016,23:28-35.

[32] Radzikowska E. Pulmonary Langerhans' cell histiocytosis in adults. Adv Respir Med,2017,85(5):277-289.

[33] Gupta D,Singh AD,Agarwal R,et al. Is Tobacco smoking protective for sarcoidosis? A case-control study from north India. Sarcoidosis Vasc Diffuse Lung Dis,2010,27(1):19-26.

[34] Gomes JP,Watad A,Shoenfeld Y. Nicotine and autoimmuni-

ty:the Lotus' flower in tobacco. Pharmacol Res,2018,128: 101-109.

[35] Fraser SD, Hart SP. Monocytes and macrophages in chronic sarcoidosis pathology. Eur Respir J,2019,54(5):1901626.

[36] Bonifazi M, Gasparini S, Alfieri V, et al. Pulmonary sarcoidosis. Semin Respir Crit Care Med,2017,38(4):437-449.

[37] Selman M, Buendia-Roldán I. Immunopathology, diagnosis, and managementof hypersensitivity pneumonitis. Semin Respir Crit Care Med,2012,33:543-554.

[38] Nizri E, Irony-Tur-Sinai M, Lory O, et al. Activation of the cholinergic anti-inflammatory system by nicotine attenuates neuroinflammation via suppression of Th1 and Th17 responses. J Immunol,2009,183(10):6681-6688.

[39] Sopori ML, Kozak W, Savage SM, et al. Nicotine-induced modulation of T Cell function. Implications for inflammation and infection. Adv Exp Med Biol,1998,437:279-289.

10 烟草暴露与慢性阻塞性肺疾病预防进展

王一喆 胡雪君

慢性阻塞性肺疾病(简称慢阻肺)是目前造成全球人类死亡的第四大疾病,全球每年约有300万人死于慢阻肺。随着吸烟率的持续升高及老龄化加剧,预计慢阻肺的发病率在未来十年仍会继续上升。因此,慢阻肺是全球重要的公共卫生问题。由于慢阻肺是常见的可预防且可治疗的慢性疾病,因此早期干预控制其发病率以及积极治疗避免其致死性合并症的发生对于减轻公共卫生负担具有非常重要的意义。

慢阻肺主要的危险因素是吸烟。90%的慢阻肺患者伴有吸烟史,但并非所有吸烟患者出现呼吸困难、慢性咳嗽、咳痰等呼吸道症状就被诊断为慢阻肺并积极采取戒烟措施。主要原因在于慢阻肺具有严格的诊断标准,即支气管扩张剂使用后肺功能检测$FEV_1/FVC<0.70$证实存在持续的气流受限。然而,在大部分长期吸烟人群中已经更为普遍地出现了小气道功能障碍等慢性肺部疾病的早期病理改变。积极采取戒烟措施对于改善未确诊但具有慢阻肺症状患者的生活质量及预后十分重要。本文综述了烟草暴露导致的慢阻肺病理生理和影像学产生的影响及预防慢阻肺的措施,以期对临床上无论是否合并持续气流受限但已出现慢阻肺病理改变的烟草暴露人群给予重视。

一、烟草暴露与慢阻肺发生发展的关系

吸入香烟烟雾或其他有害颗粒会引起肺部炎症。肺部炎症是正常的生理反应,但长期慢性炎症反应可能导致肺实质组织破坏,并破坏正常的修复和防御机制。这些病理变化将逐渐导致气体滞留及气流受限。既往观点认为慢阻肺是40岁以上人群的成人疾病,现在已认识到围生期、儿童期及早年生活对早期慢阻肺都有影响,比如孕妇吸烟、慢阻肺家族史、遗传因素、接触污染、出生时肺功能低下和(或)出生时ARDS、二手烟暴露等,都是早期慢阻肺的危险因素。

有害颗粒进入下呼吸道时会引起多种炎性细胞、炎性因子向气道及肺间质中聚集,并通过多种细胞通路抑制中性粒细胞凋亡,使得中性粒细胞产生大量蛋白酶和其他细胞因子从而诱导炎症反应。其中,蛋白酶如丝氨酸蛋白酶可以减少细胞外基质蛋白如弹性蛋白的产生,基质金属蛋白酶可降解胶原蛋白和膜基底蛋白,导致肺气肿的产生,加重肺功能的损伤。使用胸部多探头CT扫描检测早期慢阻肺患者的肺部病变,除了显著肺气肿外,也可以观察到终末细支气管的破坏。另外一项研究显示,在未观察到肺气肿病变及肺功能下降的情况下,终末细支气管及细支气管其实已经发生了毁坏或缺失,幸存的支气管管腔变得狭窄且管壁增厚,而此时肺实质其实已经发生了不可逆损伤。早诊断、早治疗是慢阻肺可预防和可治疗的前提,否则一旦形成大面积实质性的肺损伤,肺组织失去其本身应对炎症反应的代偿机制,将会导致肺功能迅速下降,严重影响烟草暴露者的治疗效果及预后。

气道基底细胞的表观遗传重编程也是烟草暴露对早期慢阻肺的重要影响之一。烟草烟雾刺激早期,炎症细胞还没有发生浸润,呼吸系统宿主防御的核心气道基底细胞及纤毛细胞和分泌细胞的干/祖细胞发生表观遗传学改变,不断重塑并增生。合并慢阻肺的吸烟者及部分不合并慢阻肺的吸烟者的小气道上皮细胞的干/祖细胞分化成熟气道上皮的能力受限。除此之外,烟草暴露还可以改变气道上皮细胞中线粒体的结构和功能,导致端粒长度缩短及DNA损伤等促衰老反应,影响肺组织细胞自我更新和修复能力,导致肺功能下降。气道基底干/祖细胞数量减少,自我更新和多向分化潜能衰退与吸烟者肺气肿的发生及慢阻肺的形成过程密切相关,可能成为预测吸烟者对慢阻肺易感性的潜在标志物。

二、烟草暴露与早期慢阻肺影像诊断

轻度(GOLD1级)和中度(GOLD2级)(GOLD: global initiative for obstructive lung disease,慢性阻塞性肺疾病全球倡议)慢阻肺患者在发生肺气肿病变之前,终末细支气管数量显著减少,因此,使用非侵入性技术评估小气道疾病的能力将有可能成为识别吸烟者可能发展为肺气肿患者的潜在手段。随着高分辨率CT在临床上的推广应用,通过影像学特征辅助诊断慢阻肺及定义肺气肿程度成为可能。Galbán等确立了一种新的影像分析方法(parametric response mapping, PRM)用于肺密度的精确体素分类。该技术使用动态图像匹配识别吸气和呼气之间体素密度的变化,将肺区域识别为正常(PRM^{Norm}),气肿(PRM^{Emph})和非气肿性气体滞留(PRM^{fSAD})。这种非气肿性气体滞留由小气道功能性改变引起,反映各种病理变化,因此被称为"小气道功能性疾病"(fSAD)。Dragos等进一步通过离

体肺的超高分辨率CT分析量化小气道和实质结构,并将这些测量结果与肺组织离体前获得的体内胸部CT结果联系起来,从而比较符合PRM^fSAD但分别被诊断为慢阻肺与正常人的肺组织中小气道损伤的实际情况。结果显示,PRM^fSAD可以准确识别出肺组织中的终末细支气管缺失,管腔狭窄和阻塞的区域,证明这种成像生物标志物可以非侵入性地标志终末支气管病理变化,为识别慢阻肺中的小气道损伤提供新方法。

最新研究显示,中国20岁及以上人群中,43.5%的人有小气道功能障碍,总人数约为4.26亿。研究指出,吸烟是小气道功能障碍的主要风险因素之一,与从未吸烟的人群相比,吸烟者更容易发生小气道功能障碍($P<0.0001$)。亚组分析显示,烟草暴露时间越长,平均每日吸烟支数越多,吸烟起始年龄越早,烟龄越长都更容易导致小气道功能障碍($P<0.0001$)。这些结果提示小气道功能障碍是吸烟者普遍存在的肺组织损伤类型,其损伤程度或许与吸烟者慢阻肺易感性及肺功能降低程度密切相关,无气流受限但已出现肺病理改变(如小气道功能障碍、肺气肿等)的研究具有重要临床意义。

三、戒烟与早期慢阻肺治疗与预防

戒烟是预防慢阻肺发展的主要干预措施,可以有效减少呼吸道疾病和慢阻肺发生率。在轻度和中度慢阻肺患者中,强化戒烟并随访5年后肺功能可明显获得改善($FEV_1>50\%$)。尼古丁替代疗法和药物治疗可以增加长期吸烟的戒烟率,然而近期发生急性冠状动脉综合征或卒中患者是尼古丁替代治疗的禁忌证。电子烟作为早期尼古丁替代疗法之一用以辅助戒烟,但其辅助戒烟的功效仍存在争议。有研究发现电子烟中添加的四氢大麻酚(THC)、大麻素(CBD)油、维生素E和其他调味物质与使用者发生严重的急性肺损伤、嗜酸性粒细胞性肺炎、肺泡出血、呼吸道细支气管炎和其他形式的肺部异常有关。

立法禁止吸烟以及医疗专业人员提供的咨询均可以提高人群,尤其低收入群体的戒烟率。无烟政策的实施与戒烟相关行为的积极性和二手烟暴露减少相关。中国关于无烟场所的临床试验显示,虽然对戒烟积极性没有明显提高,但无烟政策可以有效减少烟草暴露的可能($OR=0.56;95\%CI\ 0.51\sim0.60$)。使用电子设备协助戒烟也是大数据时代应运而生的戒烟方式之一,并且取得了良好的戒烟效果,其形式包括手机即时消息通知,手机应用软件管理等。这些方法均可以通过人们常用的通讯设备实时进行戒烟监督和提醒,方便吸烟者寻求戒烟帮助,为希望戒烟的吸烟者提供更多实现戒烟的渠道。然而在这种方法实现推广之前仍有许多问题需要解决,如个体化戒烟方案的定制,管理人员的专业程度与戒烟所付出的时间和经济成本等。

四、展望

随着对慢阻肺及其他肺部疾病的病理生理过程认识的深入,肺功能不再是评估慢阻肺程度的唯一依据。对于肺功能正常但伴随呼吸道症状的人群同样存在预后不良的可能。虽然目前持续气流受限仍然是慢阻肺诊断的金标准,但对于吸烟者来说,发展为慢阻肺的潜在病变可能早就出现。

作为慢阻肺的明确致病因素,烟草暴露对慢阻肺患者的疾病进程、治疗用药等有不同程度的影响。烟草暴露对肺组织的损伤在不断烟雾刺激中已经形成,因此对于轻度慢阻肺患者及尚未诊断为慢阻肺的吸烟者应给予足够的重视。此外,由于烟草依赖及疾病尚未对生活质量造成严重影响,导致这部分人群的依从性较差。除了对症药物治疗,人文关怀和医学教育有助于减少烟草暴露导致的公共卫生问题,对减轻社会疾病负担也具有一定意义。

参考文献

[1] Mortality GBD, Causes of Death C. Global, regional, and national age-sex specific all-cause and cause-specific mortality for 240 causes of death, 1990-2013: a systematic analysis for the Global Burden of Disease Study 2013. Lancet, 2015, 385(9963): 117-171.

[2] Mathers CD, Loncar D. Projections of global mortality and burden of disease from 2002 to 2030. PLoS Med, 2006, 3(11): e442.

[3] Xiao D, Chen Z, Wu S, et al. Prevalence and risk factors of small airway dysfunction, and association with smoking, in China: findings from a national cross-sectional study. Lancet Respir Med, 2020, 8(11): 1081-1093.

[4] Miravitlles M, Soriano JB, Garcia-Rio F, et al. Prevalence of COPD in Spain: impact of undiagnosed COPD on quality of life and daily life activities. Thorax, 2009, 64(10): 863-868.

[5] Postma DS, Bush A, Van Den Berge M. Risk factors and early origins of chronic obstructive pulmonary disease. Lancet, 2015, 385(9971): 899-909.

[6] Xu Y, Li H, Bajrami B, et al. Cigarette smoke(CS) and nicotine delay neutrophil spontaneous death via suppressing production of diphosphoinositol pentakisphosphate. Proc Natl Acad Sci U S A, 2013, 110(19): 7726-7731.

[7] Owen CA. Roles for proteinases in the pathogenesis of chronic obstructive pulmonary disease. Int J Chron Obstruct Pulmon Dis, 2008, 3(2): 253-268.

[8] Mcdonough JE, Yuan R, Suzuki M, et al. Small-airway obstruction and emphysema in chronic obstructivepulmonary disease. N Engl J Med, 2011, 365(17): 1567-1575.

[9] Koo HK, Vasilescu DM, Booth S, et al. Small airways disease in mild and moderate chronic obstructive pulmonary disease: a cross-sectional study. Lancet Respir Med, 2018, 6(8): 591-602.

[10] Sundar IK, Rahman I. Gene expression profiling of epigenetic chromatin modification enzymes and histone marks by ciga-

[11] Crystal RG. Airway basal cells. The "smoking gun" of chronic obstructive pulmonary disease. Am J Respir Crit Care Med,2014,190(12):1355-1362.

[12] Staudt MR,Buro-Auriemma LJ,Walters M S,et al. Airway Basal stem/progenitor cells have diminished capacity to regenerate airway epithelium in chronic obstructive pulmonary disease. Am J Respir Crit Care Med,2014,190(8):955-958.

[13] Shaykhiev R,Crystal RG. Early events in the pathogenesis of chronic obstructive pulmonary disease. Smoking-induced reprogramming of airway epithelial basal progenitor cells. Ann Am Thorac Soc,2014,11 Suppl 5:S252-S258.

[14] Morla M,Busquets X,Pons J,et al. Telomere shortening in smokers with and without COPD. Eur Respir J,2006,27(3):525-528.

[15] Ballweg K,Mutze K,Konigshoff M,et al. Cigarette smoke extract affects mitochondrial function in alveolar epithelial cells. Am J Physiol Lung Cell Mol Physiol,2014,307(11):L895-L907.

[16] Bernstein KE,Ong FS,Blackwell W L,et al. A modern understanding of the traditional and nontraditional biological functions of angiotensin-converting enzyme. Pharmacol Rev,2013,65(1):1-46.

[17] Galban CJ,Han MK,Boes JL,et al. Computed tomography-based biomarker provides unique signature for diagnosis of COPD phenotypes and disease progression. Nat Med,2012,18(11):1711-1715.

[18] Bhatt SP,Soler X,Wang X,et al. Association between Functional Small Airway Disease and FEV1 Decline in Chronic Obstructive Pulmonary Disease. Am J Respir Crit Care Med,2016,194(2):178-184.

[19] Vasilescu DM,Martinez FJ,Marchetti N,et al. Noninvasive Imaging Biomarker Identifies Small Airway Damage in Severe Chronic Obstructive Pulmonary Disease. Am J Respir Crit Care Med,2019,200(5):575-581.

[20] Samet JM. The 1990 Report of the Surgeon General:The Health Benefits of Smoking Cessation. Am Rev Respir Dis,1990,142(5):993-994.

[21] Anthonisen NR,Connett JE,Kiley JP,et al. Effects of smoking intervention and the use of an inhaled anticholinergic bronchodilator on the rate of decline ofFEV1. The Lung Health Study. JAMA,1994,272(19):1497-1505.

[22] Bullen C,Howe C,Laugesen M,et al. Electronic cigarettes for smoking cessation:a randomised controlled trial. Lancet,2013,382(9905):1629-1637.

[23] Hajek P,Phillips-Waller A,Przulj D,et al. E-cigarettes compared with nicotine replacement therapy within the UK Stop Smoking Services:the TEC RCT. Health Technol Assess,2019,23(43):1-82.

[24] Henry TS,Kanne JP,Kligerman SJ. Imaging of Vaping-Associated Lung Disease. N Engl J Med,2019,381(15):1486-1487.

[25] Layden JE,Ghinai I,Pray I,et al. Pulmonary Illness Related to E-Cigarette Use in Illinois and Wisconsin-Final Report. N Engl J Med,2020,382(10):903-916.

[26] Pizacani BA,Maher JE,Rohde K,et al. Implementation of a smoke-free policy in subsidized multiunit housing:effects on smoking cessation and secondhand smoke exposure. Nicotine Tob Res,2012,14(9):1027-1034.

[27] Lin HX,Chang C,Liu Z. The effects of smoke-free workplace policies on individual smoking behaviours in China. Nicotine Tob Res,2020.

[28] Abroms LC,Boal AL,Simmens SJ,et al. A randomized trial of Text2Quit:a text messaging program for smoking cessation. Am J Prev Med,2014,47(3):242-250.

[29] Free C,Knight R,Robertson S,et al. Smoking cessation support delivered via mobile phone text messaging(txt2stop):a single-blind, randomised trial. Lancet,2011,378(9785):49-55.

[30] Colak Y,Nordestgaard BG,Vestbo J,et al. Prognostic significance of chronic respiratory symptoms in individuals with normal spirometry. Eur Respir J,2019,55(1):1902226.

11 吸烟增加COVID-19感染风险的机制

王 强

自2019年年底,新型冠状病毒肺炎(COVID-19)在世界范围内迅速蔓延,截至目前,在某些国家仍然未得到有效控制,至2020年7月20日,世界范围内已有1440多万人感染,死亡人数超过60多万人。

COVID-19是由一种新型致病性冠状病毒——严重急性呼吸综合征冠状病毒2(SARS-CoV-2)引起的肺部疾病,它在系统发育上与SARS-CoV相似,基因组之间约有80%的一致性。SARS-CoV-2主要通过呼吸系统进入人体,临床症状以发热、干咳、乏力为主要表现,少数患者伴有鼻塞、流涕、咽痛、肌痛和腹泻等症状。绝大多数病例为轻症、普通型患者,部分病例病情严重,肺炎进展迅速,短期内发展为重型、危重型患者,出现呼吸衰竭,需要呼吸机辅助通气,甚至发生休克,导致死亡。

已知与COVID-19进展为危重症、甚至导致死亡有关的危险因素包括:65岁以上;反复住院;慢性阻塞性肺疾病;中度至重度哮喘;严重或失代偿性心功能不全;重度高血压;应用免疫抑制药物;尿毒症;高危妊娠;严重肥胖(BMI>40kg/m^2);慢性肝病等。COVID-19还可引起血管内皮功能障碍,导致严重的凝血异常和血栓形成。然而,到目前为止,在控制COVID-19流行的全球指南中,还尚未将吸烟列为重要的危险因素之一。究其原因是自COVID-19爆发以来,吸烟与COVID-19的关系似乎存在很大的争议。争议的起因是有多个研究的临床数据提示COVID-19住院患者中吸烟者的比例明显低于普通人群的吸烟比例。最初是源于中国的数据,此后来自意大利、西班牙、美国等多个国家的数据均提示COVID-19住院患者的吸烟率明显低于普通人群。这似乎说明吸烟可以减少COVID-19感染,对呼吸道具有保护作用。Lippi等对源于中国的5项临床数据的Meta分析,报道了吸烟者与非吸烟者COVID-19进展的合并优势比(OR)为1.69(95% CI 0.41~6.92),得出"吸烟与COVID-19的严重程度无关"的结论,并认为吸烟对COVID-19是一把双刃剑,在吸烟者对COVID-19易感的同时,吸烟还可能对呼吸道具有保护作用。这项研究在科学文献、非主流媒体和各种在线社交网络中被广泛传播,尤其是被烟草行业资助的研究人员或受试者引用、发布,不仅在普通人群中产生吸烟可以预防COVID-19的误解,也误导研究者,导致研究的偏差,如在随后的两项关于吸烟对COVID-19影响的Meta分析中,就引用了Lippi等的研究结论作为否定的依据。甚至有研究者提出尼古丁可能作为治疗COVID-19的新疗法,并开始研究其作用机制。

众所周知,吸烟是呼吸道感染、导致疾病进展的主要危险因素,吸烟者比不吸烟者更容易感染流行性感冒,尤其容易感染重症流行性感冒。吸烟者患流行性感冒/细菌性肺炎和肺结核的比例比不吸烟者增加了1倍。针对中东呼吸综合征冠状病毒(MERS)的研究报道,吸烟是MERS-CoV感染的重要危险因素,并与MERS的高病死率相关。因此,长期吸烟破坏呼吸系统的防御机制,容易导致呼吸道感染,这已经是所有人的共识。COVID-19对呼吸道表现出明显的侵袭性,它竟然成为一个例外,是唯一的不受吸烟影响的呼吸道感染性疾病,这确实有悖于常理,令人费解。

首先是如何解释住院COVID-19患者吸烟人数的比例明显低于普通人群的问题。有研究者对已发表的28项研究的Meta分析发现,其中有25项研究没有记录患者的吸烟史,不能确定纳入研究的非吸烟者是否从未吸过烟。此外,在一些研究中,吸烟状态被分为"吸烟者""前吸烟者"和"不吸烟及吸烟信息缺失者"。把不吸烟者及吸烟信息缺失者归为一类是一个"误导性的类别",会导致作者得到错误的结论。此外,这28项研究都是回顾性分析,数据都是在流行病学的背景下获得的,并没有重点记录吸烟史。所以,大多数研究记录吸烟者状态的一致性和准确性是不统一的。由于疫情紧急,有可能患者的吸烟情况不能被准确记录,有些患者在住院时可能已经处于危重状态,无法报告自己的吸烟情况,这会导致吸烟者的数量被低估,既往吸烟的人可能被认定为从不吸烟者。此外,有严重COVID-19症状的吸烟者可能在住院前已戒烟,未被记录为吸烟者,而WHO对"前吸烟者"的定义是指戒烟至少6个月。所以,对COVID-19住院患者吸烟史的信息记录不全或错误,可能是住院患者中吸烟者比例低的主要原因。

随后有多位研究者对Lippi的研究结论提出质疑,Guo指出Lippi等使用的五项临床数据中,有四项在数据收集上存在缺陷,病例数是错误的,导致Meta分析结果不正确。Ernest等则认为Lippi等使用的统计学方法存在错误,使用零假设显著性检验的方法得出无相关性的结论是不恰当的。并且,Lippi等在结论中犯了一个常见的统计学错误,吸烟与COVID-19严重程度在统计学上没有明显的显著相关性,不等于在临床上吸烟与COVID-19严重程度无关。所以,Lippi和Henry的Meta分析存在大量的错误，得出了误导性的结论。这是迄今为止唯一一篇证明吸烟和COVID-19严重性之间没有关系的研究。此后，至少有17项后续Meta分析对此做了进一步研究，为吸烟与COVID-19的严重程度和进展之间的直接关系提供了明确的证据。与不吸烟的人相比，感染COVID-19的吸烟者发生重症和危重症的概率高3.25倍。WHO已经明确吸烟与COVID-19严重程度明显相关，是COVID-19病情恶化、预后不良的重要的危险因素之一。

吸烟者容易感染COVID-19且病情易恶化的机制包括如下几个方面。

1. 吸烟增加病毒进入人体的机会　吸烟者反复用手接触面部的动作，增加了手口接触的次数，也就增加了病毒侵入人体的机会。当吸烟或运动量增加时，呼吸速度增快，呼吸流量明显增加，导致从鼻到口腔的呼吸状态发生改变，呼吸道黏膜逐渐冷却和干燥，纤毛细胞运动减少、黏膜黏度增加，影响上呼吸道对微生物的过滤，使病毒更容易绕过口腔和上呼吸道的自然防御屏障，促进病毒渗透到下呼吸道和肺泡。

2. 吸烟影响肺的黏膜上皮屏障，导致上皮细胞通透性增加　吸烟引起肺结构的变化包括：黏膜通透性增加，黏膜纤毛间隙增宽，支气管周围炎症和纤维化（气道重塑），这些病理变化使吸烟者对病毒侵入的抵抗力显著减低。吸烟能够引起肺内的氧化应激和炎症反应，导致上皮屏障功能失调，使上皮细胞的通透性明显增加，对吸烟者呼吸道产生严重影响。氧化应激产生的ROS可直接影响血管紧张素转化酶2（ACE2）-血管紧张素-肾上腺素轴，增加呼吸道对病毒（细菌）感染的敏感性，使吸烟者更容易受到细菌（病毒）的感染。

3. 上皮细胞的作用和炎症反应　ACE2和TMPSSR2、SARS-CoV2属于冠状病毒家族，因其冠状外观而得名。这一特征归因于两个功能域——S1和S2的糖基化细胞表面的刺突蛋白。ACE2被证明是SARS-CoV-2病毒进入宿主细胞的受体。病毒刺突包膜的S2结构域与肺上皮的ACE2受体有很高的亲和性。已经发现吸烟者和服用ACE拮抗药物的患者（高血压和糖尿病患者）中ACE2的表达增高，因此更易患COVID-19。此外，ACE2可能在生殖细胞中高表达，即男性比女性表达更多。男性的循环ACE2多于女性，这可能为COVID-19在严重程度上的性别差异提供了证据。ACE2受体大量分布于肺上皮细胞，特别是Ⅱ型肺上皮细胞、杯状细胞、鼻上皮/纤毛细胞和口腔黏膜细胞。最近有研究表明，干扰素刺激的SARS-CoV-2应答通过ACE2和TMPSSR2蛋白酶进入细胞。在吸烟者以及COPD、IPF等烟草相关疾病患者的小气道上皮中ACE2表达上调。因此吸烟者更有可能感染COVID-19。尽管病毒主要通过ACE2进入宿主细胞，但病毒颗粒需要细胞蛋白酶的激活，从而促进病毒的吞噬作用。研究表明在鼻纤毛细胞和杯状细胞中均高表达的TMPSSR2蛋白酶在SARS-CoV-2侵入宿主细胞发挥重要作用，ACE2利用细胞丝氨酸蛋白酶TMPRSS2作用于S蛋白而侵入宿主细胞。此外，通过对多个组织的单细胞RNA测序分析，发现只有少部分ACE2+细胞表达TMPRSS2，这表明可能还存在其他蛋白酶发挥类似的作用。有研究表明，组织蛋白酶B/L在病毒入侵细胞时发挥同样重要的作用。吸烟可以引起组织蛋白酶B表达增加，这可能也是吸烟者容易感染COVID-19的原因之一。另一种细胞蛋白酶是Furin，它能裂解SARS-CoV-2刺突蛋白的S1/S2位点，这对病毒在细胞之间传播至关重要。有证据显示Furin缺乏，增加了小鼠对病毒（甲型流行性感冒病毒）的易感性。丝氨酸蛋白酶抑制剂（Serpin）能调节、控制Furin蛋白酶的活性。而吸烟者Serpin的活性降低，从而影响Furin的活性，使宿主更容易感染COVID-19。

4. 吸烟抑制机体免疫系统　吸烟对免疫系统的影响包括以下方面：首先，吸烟能减少CD4+T细胞（辅助性T细胞）的数量，而辅助性T细胞能促进B细胞产生抗体，并激活杀伤T细胞来攻击病原体。其次，烟草产品中的主要成分尼古丁，能促进儿茶酚胺和皮质类固醇的分泌，这会降低免疫系统的功能，抑制机体抵抗细菌/病毒感染的能力。再次，尼古丁能抑制白介素-22的产生，而白介素-22有助于抑制肺部炎症和修复受损细胞。

5. 吸烟与细胞因子风暴　急性呼吸窘迫综合征（ARDS）是SARS-CoV-2感染最常见的严重合并症之一，是免疫细胞释放促炎细胞因子（趋化因子）导致的"细胞因子风暴"的结果。免疫细胞释放的促炎介质包括IP-10、MCP-3、HGF、MIG、MIP-1α、IL-6、TNF-α、IFN-γ、IL-2、IL-7和GM-CSF等。长期吸烟者体内IL-6、TNF-α和其他促炎因子的表达上调，而自然杀伤（NK）细胞和CD8+T淋巴细胞的两种主要效应蛋白：穿孔素和颗粒酶B的表达水平降低。此外，在COVID-19患者的尸检报告显示肺毛细血管中性粒细胞浸润，伴有纤维蛋白沉积，中性粒细胞外渗进入肺泡腔，提示中性粒细胞胞外杀菌网络（NETs）的形成可能是导致COVID-19患者器官损伤、肺结构重塑的原因。有证据表明，吸烟能影响嗜中性粒细胞的转运、NETs的形成，抑制体液和细胞介导的免疫反应，使疾病更易进展为ARDS，导致疾病恶化。

综上所述，众多的研究证实了吸烟增加COVID-19感染的可能，并且导致病情容易进展、恶化。即使有研究能说明尼古丁可能有抑制SARS-CoV-2生长的药理作用，但是易感COVID-19常见的基础疾病：高血压、心血管疾病、糖尿病、COPD、肿瘤和慢性肾病均是烟草相关疾病，用吸烟预防COVID-19无异于"饮鸩止渴"。当前COVID-19仍在世界范围内蔓延，如何做到有效防控是亟待解决的问题。吸烟可能是最重要的、最可避免的危险因素，戒烟除了可以预防烟草相关疾病外，也能减少戒烟者感染SARS-CoV-2的机会。

参 考 文 献

[1] Walls AC, Park YJ, Tortorici MA, et al. Structure, Function, and Antigenicity of the SARS-CoV-2 Spike Glycoprotein. Cell, 2020, 181(2): 281-292.

[2] World Health Organization. Coronavirus disease(COVID-19) pandemic. https://www.who.int/emergencies/diseases/novel-coronavirus-2019.

[3] Wu C, Chen X, Cai Y, et al. Risk factors associated with acute respiratory distress syndrome and death in patients with coronavirus disease 2019 pneumonia in Wuhan, China. JAMA Intern Med 2020, 180(7): 934-943.

[4] Sardu C, Gambardella J, Morelli MB, et al. Is COVID-19 an endothelial disease? Clinical and basic evidence. J Clin Med, 2020, 9(5): 1417.

[5] Guan WJ, Ni ZY, Hu Y, et al. Clinical Characteristicsof Coronavirus Disease 2019 in China. N Engl J Med, 2020.

[6] Guan WJ, Liang WH, Zhao Y, et al. Comorbidity and its impact on 1590 patients with Covid-19 in China: A Nationwide Analysis. Eur Respir J. 2020.

[7] Farsalinos, K, Barbouni, A, Niaura, R. Smoking, vaping and hospitalization for COVID-19. 2020.

[8] Centers for Disease Control and Prevention. Preliminary Estimates of the Prevalence of Selected Underlying Health Conditions among Patients with Coronavirus Disease 2019; Centers for Disease Control and Prevention: Antlanta, GA, USA, 2020: 382-386.

[9] Creamer, MR, Wang, TW, Babb, S. Tobacco Product Use and CessationIndicators among Adults; Centers for Disease Control and Prevention: Antlanta, GA, USA, 2019: 1013-1019.

[10] Lippi G, Henry BM. Active smoking is not associated with severity of coronavirus disease 2019(COVID-19). Eur J Intern Med, 2020, 3: 14.

[11] Lippi G, Sanchis-Gomar F, Henry BM. Active smoking and COVID-19: a double-edged sword. Eur J Intern Med, 2020, 1(20): 30182-30185.

[12] Patanavanich R, Glantz SA. Smoking is Associated with COVID-19 Progression: A Meta-Analysis. Public and Global Health, 2020, 22(9): 1653-1656.

[13] Zhao Q, Meng M, Kumar R, et al. Theimpact of COPD and smoking history on the severity of Covid-19: A systemic review and meta-analysis. J Med Virol, 2020.

[14] Farsalinos K, Barbouni A, Niaura R. Systematic review of the prevalence of current smokingamong hospitalized COVID-19 patients in China: could nicotine be a therapeutic option? Intern Emerg Med, 2020, 15(5): 845-852.

[15] Groskreutz DJ, Monick MM, Babor EC, et al. Cigarette smoke alters respiratory syncytial virus-induced apoptosis and replication. Am J Respir Cell Mol Biol, 2009, 41: 189-198.

[16] Arcavi L, Benowitz NL. Cigarette smoking and infection. Arch Intern Med, 2004, 164: 2206-2216.

[17] Eapen MS, Sharma P, Moodley YP, et al. Dysfunctional Immunity and Microbial Adhesion Molecules in Smoking-Induced Pneumonia. Am. J. Respir Crit Care Med, 2019, 199: 250-251.

[18] Park JE, Jung S, Kim A, Park JE. MERS transmission and risk factors: a systematic review. BMC Public Health, 2018, 18: 574.

[19] Maria S C, Vincenzo Z, Silvano G, et al. Tobacco smoking and COVID-19 pandemic: old and new issues. A summary of the evidence from the scientific literature. Acta Biomed, 2020, 91(2): 106-112.

[20] Guo FR. Active smoking is associated with severity of coronavirus disease 2019(COVID-19): an update of a meta-analysis. Tob Induc Dis, 2020, 18(6): 37.

[21] Ernest Lo, Benoit Lasnier. Active smoking and severity of coronavirus disease 2019(COVID-19): the use of significance testing leads to an erroneous conclusion, European Journal of Internal Medicine, 2020, 77: 125-126.

[22] Alberto CB, Paula JF, Alvaro SA, et al. Does active smoking worsen Covid-19? European Journal of Internal Medicine, 2020, 77: 129-131.

[23] Silvano Gallus, Alessandra Lugo and Giuseppe Gorini, European Journal of Internal Medicine, 2020, 6: 14.

[24] Patanavanich R, Glantz SA. Smoking is Associated with COVID-19 progression: a meta-analysis. Nicotine Tob Res 2020: ntaa082.

[25] Simons D, Shahab L, Brown J, Perski O. The association of smoking status with SARS-CoV-2 infection, hospitalization and mortality from COVID-19: a living rapid evidence review. (version 7). Addiction, 2020, 10.1111.

[26] WHO. Q&A on smoking and COVID-19. WHO: Geneva. 2020.

[27] Matricardi PM, Dal Negro RW, Nisini R. The First, Comprehensive Immunological Model of COVID-19. Implications for Prevention, Diagnosis, and Public Health Measures. Pediatr Allergy Immunol, 2020, 31(5): 454-470.

[28] Bauer CMT, Morissette MC, Stämpfli MR. The influence of cigarette smoking on viral infections: translating bench science to impact COPD pathogenesis and acuteexacerbations of COPD clinically. Chest, 2013, 143(1): 196-206.

[29] Aghapour M, Raee P, Moghaddam SJ, et al. Airway epithelial barrier dysfunction in chronic obstructive pulmonary disease: role of cigarette smoke exposure. Am J Respir Cell Mol Biol, 2018, 58(2): 157-169.

[30] Hoffmann M, Kleine-Weber H, Schroeder S, et al. SARS-CoV-2 cell entry depends on ACE2 and TMPRSS2 and is blocked by a clinically proven protease inhibitor. Cell, 2020, 181(2): 271-280.

[31] Brake SJ, Barnsley K, Lu W, et al. Smoking upregulates angiotensin-converting Enzyme-2 receptor: a potential adhesion site for novel coronavirus SARS-CoV-2(Covid-19). J Clin Med, 2020, 9(3): 841.

[32] Sungnak W, Huang N, Becavin C, et al. SARS-CoV-2 entry factors are highly expressed in nasal epithelial cells together

with innate immune genes. Nat Med,2020,26(5):681-687.

[33] Leung JM,Yang CX,Tam A,et al. ACE-2 expression in the small airway epithelia of smokers and COPD patients:implications for COVID-19. Eur Respir J,2020,55(5):2000688.

[34] Smith JC,Sheltzer JM. Cigarette smoke triggers the expansion of a subpopulation of respiratory epithelial cells that express the SARS-CoV-2 receptor ACE2. bioRxiv,2020.

[35] Dittmann M,Hoffmann HH,Scull MA,et al. A serpin shapes the extracellular environment to preventinfluenza a virus maturation. Cell,2015,160(4):631-643.

[36] Jean F,Stella K,Thomas L,et al. Alpha1-antitrypsin Portland,a bioengineered serpin highly selective for furin:application as an antipathogenic agent. Proc Natl Acad Sci USA,1998,95(13):7293-7298.

[37] Nouri-Shirazi M,Guinet E. Evidence for the immunosuppressive role of nicotine on human dendritic cell functions. Immunology,2003,109:365-373.

[38] Nguyen HM,Torres JA,Agrawal S,et al. Nicotine impairs the response on lung epithelial cells to IL-22. Mediator Inflamm,2020.

[39] Li X,Geng M,Peng Y,et al. Molecular immune pathogenesis and diagnosis of COVID-19. J Pharm Anal,2020,10(2):102-108.

[40] Barnes BJ,Adrover JM,Baxter-Stoltzfus A,et al. Targeting potential drivers of COVID-19:Neutrophil extracellular traps. J Exp Med,2020,217(6):e20200652.

12 阻塞性睡眠呼吸暂停相关的恶性心律失常

王 彦

越来越多的研究表明阻塞性睡眠呼吸暂停(obstructive sleep apnea,OSA)是多种心血管疾病发病和死亡的独立危险因素,同时也严重影响心脏的电活动,发生心律失常,其中恶性心律失常可在短时间内引起血流动力障碍,导致患者晕厥甚至猝死,从而造成严重后果。

一、恶性心律失常定义

恶性心律失常一般指短时间内引起血流动力障碍,导致患者晕厥甚至猝死的心律失常,是一类根据心律失常的程度及性质分类的严重心律失常,也是一类需要紧急处理的心律失常。OSA患者中较多见的恶性心律失常主要包括室性心动过速(VT)、心室扑动、心室颤动(VF)、高度或三度房室传导阻滞(AVB)等。恶性心律失常的恶性程度高,可在短期内导致严重后果,是心源性猝死(SCD)的首位原因,临床应加强重视,早期识别和积极治疗。

二、OSA基于证据的恶性心律失常

1970年,MacGregor等首先报道Pickwickian综合征患者SCD的相对风险增加23%。1983年,Guilleminault等首次对大型OSA人群(400例)进行24h动态心电图同步多导睡眠监测(PSG),结果发现48%的患者夜间发生心律失常,其中8例持续性室性心动过速,43例窦性停搏(2.5~13s),31例二度AVB。75例频发室性期前收缩(PVC)(>2次/分)。50例因严重心律失常进行了气管切开术。1997年,黄席珍团队首先报道OSA发作时,57%~74%的患者出现室性逸搏,9%~11%的患者出现窦性停搏,4%~8%的患者为二度AVB;并指出窦性停搏>3s应引起临床高度重视。当动脉血氧饱和度(SaO_2)<60%时可出现频繁的室性逸搏或异位性心动过速。在频发OSA周期中,交感神经-副交感神经兴奋性不断变化,恢复呼吸一瞬间,副交感神经兴奋为主转为交感神经兴奋为主的过程中,可使心肌异位兴奋点阈值降低,这种心律失常是引起OSA患者猝死的主要原因。2000年丁殿勋等报道一例OSA患者在急性心肌梗死过程中引起高度窦房、房室传导阻滞和心脏停搏;另一例OSA患者在急性心肌梗死基础上每有OSA发作便激发出VT和(或)VF,抗心律失常药和电复律效果欠佳。因此OSA可能不仅是冠心病的重要危险因子,也是诱发心肌梗死和激发恶性心律失常的直接因素。

(一)快速性恶性心律失常

非持续性室性心动过速(NSVT)定义为连续3个或3个以上PVC,持续时间少于30s。Mehra等发现OSA患者发生NSVT和复杂性室性逸搏(CVE)概率分别为无OSA者的3倍和2倍,即使调整了潜在的混杂因素后,重度OSA患者夜间发生复杂性心律失常的风险为无OSA者的2~4倍。Wang等发现肥厚型梗阻性心肌病患者NSVT患病率随OSA的严重程度而增加(无、轻、中、重度OSA分别为12%、16%、33%和54%)。肥厚型梗阻性心肌病患者OSA的存在及其严重程度与NSVT独立相关,NSVT是该人群SCD和心血管死亡的危险因素。Selim等发现中重度睡眠呼吸障碍(SDB)患者CVE(包括NSVT、二联律、三联律或四联律)和快速性心律失常(包括VT和室上性心动过速)的发生概率是无SDB者的2倍。Mehra等在2911例老年人群中发现SDB严重程度与CVE的风险有关。SDB亚型分析发现CVE与OSA和低氧密切相关。Monahan等调查了2816例SDB患者,其中2%的患者出现心律失常(其中76%为NSVT),且NSVT与先前的呼吸事件存在直接的时间关联。尽管心律失常绝对发生率较低(1次心律失常/4万次呼吸事件),但呼吸事件后90s危险期内NSVT的相对风险显著增加,是正常呼吸后的17.4倍。Koehler等的研究发现有SDB的慢性心力衰竭(CHF)患者NSVT发生率明显高于无SDB者(50%:19%),夜间NSVT的发生率约为白天的2倍,且呼吸暂停低通气指数(AHI)与NSVT相关,因此CHF和SDB的结合易诱发夜间恶性室性心律失常。但Abe等的研究结果发现OSA患者发生NSVT(无、轻、中、重度OSA分别为0、1.0%、1.5%、1.3%)、三度AVB(无、轻、中、重度OSA分别为0、0、0、0.1%)的概率不高($P>0.05$),可能与恶性心律失常发生次数太少有关。Javaheri发现持续性VT与OSA无相关性(对照组和OSA组中持续性VT患者的百分比相似)。Salama等回顾分析了美国三年住院患者18 013 878例,结果发现OSA组VT患病率(2.24%)显著高于无OSA组(1.16%),OSA是VT的独立预测因子($OR=1.22$)。OSA组VF患病率(0.3%)显著高于无OSA组(0.2%),但多变量回归分析后OSA组VF并未显著升高。

动物实验也支持OSA模式间歇低氧(IH)与恶性心律失常的关系。Morand等调查了IH对心肌缺血相关性室性心律失常的发展和严重程度的影响。在体内,暴露于 IH 的大鼠缺血诱导的致死性心律失常的发生率是常氧状态下大鼠的 2 倍。暴露于 IH 的大鼠 VF 总体发生率 66.7% 明显高于常氧状态下大鼠(33.3%)。在体外,暴露于 IH 的大鼠离体心脏在心肌缺血期间 VF 发生率为 34.5%,明显高于常氧状态下大鼠(4.2%)。IH 延长校正后的 QT 间期(QTc)和 T 波顶点到 T 波终末末之间的时间(TpTe 间期),增加心室单相动作电位持续时间(APD)梯度并上调心内膜 L 型钙(LTCC)、瞬时受体电位通道(TRPC)1 和 TRPC6 的表达。因此慢性 IH 通过交感神经激活和心室复极改变,透壁 APD 梯度和心内膜钙通道表达改变,促进心肌缺血相关的致死性室性心律失常。

(二)缓慢性恶性心律失常

有关 OSA 导致缓慢性恶性心律失常的研究很少。Maeno 等报道了一例 54 岁男性 OSA 患者,PSG 同时进行的 24h 动态心电图监测显示高度 AVB,心搏停止长达 6.4s。《2015 年欧洲心脏协会指南》建议心动过缓鉴别诊断时应考虑 OSA。睡眠呼吸暂停和 SaO_2 降低可能是 SDB 患者发生 SCD 的危险因素。

(三)植入型心律转复除颤器治疗

植入型心律转复除颤器(ICD)已经广泛应用于临床治疗恶性心律失常,能有效防止院外 SCD 的发生。Bitter 等发现合并 OSA 的 CHF 患者午夜 0 时至早晨 6 时发生 ICD 除颤电击事件增多,与恶性心动过速事件风险增加相关。Tomaello 等的研究纳入 22 例行 ICD 治疗的 CHF 患者,其中 17 例有 SDB。控制左心室射血分数(LVEF)和心功能分级(NYHA)后,ICD 放电次数与 AHI 正相关($r=0.718$),与夜间最低 SaO_2 负相关($r=-0.619$)。AHI 和睡眠中低氧严重程度是恶性心律失常风险的预测指标。Kwon 等对 9 项前瞻性队列研究进行系统回顾和 Meta 分析,评估 SDB 对 CHF 患者 ICD 治疗的影响,结果发现 SDB 与 ICD 治疗风险增加有关($R^2=1.55$),推断 SDB 与 CHF 患者的心血管病死率增加有关,其中恶性室性心律失常可能起重要作用。Bitter 等随访 255 例植入心脏再同步装置 6 个月后的 CHF 患者 4 年,发现中重度 SDB 患者首次监测到室性心律失常和首次心脏复律除颤治疗的时间明显缩短,发生恶性室性心律失常及需要适当心脏复律除纤颤治疗的风险增加,而且等待首次心脏复律除颤治疗的无事件生存期缩短。Raghuram 等的系统回顾纳入 20 项研究,包括 10 项观察性研究,8 项病例对照研究,1 个病例报告和 1 项 CPAP 干预性研究,发现 OSA 导致室性心律失常的心电图预测因子(如 PVC、QTc 延长、QTcd、T 波改变和心率变异)和 SCD 的风险明显增加,OSA 与 SCD 和适当 ICD 治疗的持续性 VT 独立相关。

(四)心源性猝死

一般人群中 SCD 风险从早上 6 时至中午达到高峰,从午夜至早晨 6 时达到低谷。而 OSA 由于神经激素和电生理异常,可能增加 SCD 的风险,尤其在睡眠期间。Gami 等 2005 年的一项研究首次提示 OSA 和 SCD 之间存在关联:从午夜 0 时至早晨 6 时,46% 的 OSA 患者发生 SCD,明显高于无 OSA 者(21%)和总人群(16%),且 OSA 越严重,夜间 SCD 相对风险越高。Young 等对 1522 例 Wisconsin 睡眠队列进行 18 年的病死率随访,发现随着 SDB 严重程度增加,心血管病死率呈明显增加的趋势。未经治疗的重度 SDB 患者死亡风险最高($HR=5.2$),且不受年龄、性别和体重指数(BMI)的影响。Lee 等发现韩国人 OSA 严重程度与心血管疾病病死率增加有关。重度 OSA 组心血管疾病病死率高于非 OSA 组($HR=4.66$),调整是否接受治疗后仍高于非 OSA 组($HR=4.19$)。Gami 等在接受 PSG 检查的 10 701 名成年人长达 15 年随访中发现,OSA 的存在可预测 SCD 发作,且 SCD 风险程度可通过 OSA 严重性的多个参数预测,包括 AHI>20($HR=1.60$)、夜间平均 $SaO_2<93\%$($HR=2.93$)、最低 $SaO_2<78\%$($HR=2.60$),这些发现提示 OSA 是 SCD 新的危险因素。Shamsuzzaman 等发现先天性长 QT 综合征(LQTS)患者的 OSA 的存在和严重程度与经心率校正的 QT 延长的程度有关,这是 SCD 的重要生物标志。治疗 LQTS 患者的 OSA 可降低 QT 延长,从而降低长 QT 触发 SCD 的风险。Kerns 等前瞻性调查了 558 名血液透析患者中 OSA 与心血管病死率和 SCD 的相关性,结果发现 OSA 的血液透析患者心血管病死率和 SCD 的风险增加。在调整了人口统计学和 BMI 后,OSA 与心血管病死率的高风险相关。调整人口统计学和多种心血管危险因素后,OSA 与 SCD 高风险相关。因此未来的研究应筛查 OSA 并评估以 OSA 为目标的干预措施对终末期肾病死率的影响。Koo 等发现冠状动脉旁路移植术患者睡眠呼吸暂停与主要心脑血管不良事件(包括心血管疾病病死率、SCD 或心搏骤停复苏等)增加独立相关。

三、OSA 诱导恶性心律失常的机制

OSA 通过多种机制导致复杂性心肌损伤。关键因素包括 OSA 相关的自主神经系统波动,其典型特征是呼吸事件时副交感神经活动增强,以及呼吸事件后交感神经活动突然增加,导致心律失常倾向增加。OSA 诱导心律失常的更直接的病理生理影响包括 IH 和高碳酸血症、睡眠片段和胸内压力波动导致心肌紧张。OSA 可能引发心律失常的中间途径包括全身炎症反应、氧化应激、促血栓形成通路上调和血管内皮功能障碍。这些机制导致心室肥大和功能障碍,在组织和细胞水平上表现为多灶性梗死、心肌细胞肥大、细胞凋亡和炎性浸润。长期 OSA 可引起心脏结构和电重构,导致高血压、心室肥大、纤维化和冠状动脉疾病也导致室性心律失常。

(一)自主神经功能失衡

OSA 患者连续的自主神经改变可导致恶性心律失常易感性增强。呼吸暂停事件中迷走神经活动增强导致心动过缓,副交感神经系统的激活还可导致 QTc 延长和心室复极异质性增加,表现为 QTc 离散度增加,增加室性心律失常和心脏猝死的风险。随后呼吸暂停结束上气道张力恢复后,继发于呼吸中枢交感神经耦合、低氧血症、高碳酸血症和正常肺反射启动交感抑制作用缺乏,引发强烈的交感神经系统反应,导致心动过速和左心室后负荷激增。重

度OSA患者不仅夜间交感神经活动增加，而且白天的交感神经活动也增加。交感神经张力增加导致心率和血压升高，常发生室性异位搏动，副交感神经兴奋转为交感神经兴奋时，迷走神经抑制恶性心律失常的保护作用减弱，室颤阈值降低，易发生恶性心律失常，导致猝死。此外，局部心脏舒张反射和压力反射也可能起作用。

(二)间歇低氧

低氧血症直接刺激颈动脉体的化学感受器，促进通气和交感神经放电。此外，低氧会导致周围血管收缩，从而增加前负荷和后负荷，改变心室复极化并增加左心室心内膜钙通道的表达，促进心肌缺血时SCD的发生和发展。此外，上气道阻塞终止后再氧合可能导致活性氧簇（ROS）形成。由于钙通道活性改变和微血管缺血，ROS的产生与心律失常有关。

(三)胸内压力变化

正常人吸气时胸内压通常为$-8cmH_2O$，而OSA患者上气道阻塞产生的胸内负压$<-30cmH_2O$。OSA由于反复上呼吸道阻塞，导致胸内压力剧烈波动，增加右心室静脉回流和左心室后负荷，降低左心室顺应性并增加心脏跨壁压力，这足以引起心室重构。在动物实验中，OSA期间胸腔内压力波动会导致心室复极变化，而中枢性睡眠呼吸暂停（CSA）则未观察到这种变化，并且主要由交感神经激活引起。

(四)心脏结构和电变化

胸腔内负压增大、IH和长期OSA引起的全身性炎症反应和氧化应激上调可导致心脏结构和电重构。心室重构可能导致左、右心室肥大，进而导致心脏收缩和舒张功能障碍。反复缺血性损伤可能会促进心室纤维化。Jiang等的研究表明，OSA可以通过改变钾离子通道的正常功能，导致心肌细胞电位不稳定，从而改变心肌细胞复极，增加QT间期延长和心律失常事件，直至发生恶性心室事件。Sökmen等报道在呼吸暂停阶段，TpTe间期、QT间期、TpTe/QT、TpTe/QTc呈增加趋势，在过度通气阶段呈下降趋势，提示心室复极参数的延长可能导致致死性室性心律失常，其研究结果揭示OSA患者睡眠期间可能存在心室复极参数的改变，从而增加SCD的风险。

(五)心肌缺血

低氧血症、心率和血压升高以及左心室后负荷增加（由于交感神经活性增强和胸内压力增加）的结合，导致心肌耗氧量增加和供氧量减少之间不平衡。此外，OSA还可引起酸中毒、血管内皮功能障碍、全身炎症反应和氧化应激，这些都可能导致心肌缺血，从而增加室性心律失常和SCD的风险。

四、OSA相关恶性心律失常的心电图预测

QT间期可用于评估心室复极，体表心电图TpTe间期可评估QTc，QT离散度（QTd）和复极的透壁离散度。TpTe/QT和TpTe/QTc是代表心律失常的其他心电图指标。OSA患者不仅复极受损，碎片状QRS波（fQRS）是除极异常的标志物。研究已经证实这些参数与室性心律失常和SCD有关。

QT间期代表心室除极和复极的关系，包括折返性心动过速的易感期，它被认为是心室电不稳定的标志，是发生恶性心律失常和SCD的危险因素。QTd是心电图上最大QT间期和最小QT间期之间的差，反映了心室复极化和心肌电不稳定的不均匀性。校正后的QT离散度（QTcd）增加>60ms是心脏死亡的一个独立的重要危险因素。TpTe间期测量心脏复极跨壁离散度，可通过从心内膜（最长）到心外膜细胞（最短）动作电位持续时间的梯度来解释。TpTe间期延长导致早期后除极的易感性增加，并与VT和SCD风险增加有关。未经校正的TpTe间期>100ms的患者发生SCD的风险增加。fQRS是结构性心脏病患者心血管死亡的预测指标，通过不均匀的底物和（或）局部心肌内/室内传导阻滞反映心室的电活动异常。异常的冲动传导通过折返机制为室性心律失常创造了环境。心脏结构中的细胞凋亡和间质纤维化是导致fQRS的机制之一，这可能是继发于慢性缺氧、代谢异常和氧化应激的结果。

Voigt等发现与健康人群相比，患有OSA且无结构性心脏病的患者有更高的QTd或QTcd，这可能是SCD风险增加的标志。Panikkath等发现SCD患者平均TpTe间期明显高于冠心病对照组；QTc正常者TpTe与SCD仍明显相关。因此得出结论：TpTe间期延长与SCD独立相关，是SCD的重要预测因子。Kilicaslan等也发现中重度OSA患者TpTe间期、TpTe/QT和TpTe/QTc延长；AHI与TpTe间期、TpTe/QT和TpTe/QTc呈正相关。Sökmen等的研究发现在呼吸暂停期间TpTe间期、QT间期、TpTe/QT和TpTe/QTc显著增加，而在呼吸暂停后过度通气期间显著下降；QTc间期在呼吸暂停期间增加，在呼吸暂停后过度通气期间仍持续增加。OSA患者这些心室复极参数的变化可能有助于解释SCD的潜在机制。Schmidleitner等回顾性评估100例准备接受冠状动脉旁路移植术（CABG）的患者，发现其中有SDB的患者TpTe、QTc间期、TpTe/QT延长。独立于已知的心律失常危险因素，SDB与CABG术前的心脏复极异常相关，提示SDB可能导致CABG术后发生恶性室性心律失常的风险增加。Morand等在麻醉大鼠中记录II导联心电图，结果发现IH诱导大鼠QTc、TpTe间期明显延长，心内膜APD50明显增加。Adar等研究发现OSA患者（独立于肥胖）中的fQRS，提示心肌电重构。fQRS是OSA患者亚临床左心室功能障碍的独立预测因子，这表明它可以识别出可能存在明显心脏功能障碍风险的OSA患者。有fQRS的OSA患者中较高的C反应蛋白水平提示炎症可能在QRS形态改变中起作用。

五、持续气道正压通气治疗

持续气道正压通气（CPAP）治疗缓解与呼吸暂停相关的低氧血症和睡眠结构紊乱，并消除胸内压力波动过大。CPAP在室性心律失常中可能的作用机制包括改善心肌氧

输送，降低交感活动、左心室透壁压和后负荷。通过减少需氧量和增加供氧量，CPAP可预防缺血性心脏病患者的局部缺血或改善心室复极，并减少心脏交感神经通路。在CPAP治疗组中发现夜尿中去甲肾上腺素水平降低支持此机制。另一种机制可能涉及心室负荷，消除其短暂的机械性扩张，从而减轻电机械分离。已经证明CPAP治疗能改善OSA患者的心脏参数，如心率、QTd、动脉压及每搏输出量。此外通过CPAP治疗，不良心室重塑和异位减少以及心电图标志物得以改善。

Simantirakis等招募了23例中重度OSA患者，所有患者植入能监测心律的可插入式循环记录器持续16个月。CPAP治疗前47%的患者夜间频繁发作心脏停搏＞3s和严重心动过缓＜40次/分。CPAP治疗8周后发作次数明显减少，此后随访6个月中未记录到发作，提示CPAP可显著降低严重缓慢性心律失常发作。Bilal等发现重度OSA患者的QTcd明显高于对照组，且QTcd与AHI、氧减指数正相关。CPAP治疗3个月后QTcd显著降低（从平均62.48ms降至41.42ms）。CPAP治疗可缩短重度OSA患者的QTcd，因此可降低心律失常和心血管疾病的风险。Dursunoglu等发现CPAP治疗可显著降低无高血压的中重度OSA患者QTcd，改善复极的不均匀性，从而降低心血管疾病发病率。而停止CPAP治疗2周时QTc、TpTec间期长度明显增加，且停止CPAP治疗与QTc、TpTec间期延长有关，这可能为OSA和心律失常乃至SCD提供可能的机制联系。Yajima等发现CPAP治疗后RR间期接近正态分布，表明自主神经系统保持平衡。

Javaheri随访29例稳定期心力衰竭患者发现CPAP治疗无效者各种室性心律失常（VT、PVC、成对）每小时发生次数无显著变化。CPAP治疗有效者各种室性心律失常减少，VT从每小时1.1降到0.05，PVC从每小时66降到18，但无统计学差异。Abe等发现CPAP治疗可显著减少心房颤动、PVC、窦性心动过缓和窦性停搏的发生，但CPAP治疗前后NSVT和二度（三度）AVB无统计学差异，可能与例数太少有关。Craig等未发现4周CPAP治疗恶性心律失常的发生率显著降低。Raghuram等的系统回顾提示没有足够的证据表明CPAP治疗显著降低VT或VF，但间接证据表明CPAP治疗可预防SDB患者（特别是AHI≥20）的室性心律失常。总体而言，CPAP治疗的持续时间、治疗依从性、OSA的严重程度和心脏病理学是影响CPAP治疗效果的重要混杂因素。

六、小 结

OSA与恶性心律失常密切相关，OSA的长期心血管损害及存在器质性心脏病是其发生的基础。OSA相关的恶性心律失常诱发机制复杂，且引起特殊的心电图变化，一旦突然发作抢救成功率低，严重威胁生命安全和健康，必须加强重视、早期识别、早期干预。重度OSA患者应在积极治疗原发病的基础上早期应用CPAP治疗，避免发展为恶性心律失常，甚至SCD的风险。

参 考 文 献

[1] MacGregor MI, Block AJ, Ball WC Jr. Topics in clinical medicine: serious complications and sudden death in the Pickwickian syndrome. Johns Hopkins Med J, 1970, 126(5): 279-295.

[2] Guilleminault C, Connolly SJ, Winkle RA. Cardiac arrhythmia and conduction disturbances during sleep in 400 patients with sleep apnea syndrome. Am J Cardiol, 1983, 52(5): 490-494.

[3] 牛楠, 戴玉华, 黄席珍. 阻塞性睡眠呼吸暂停综合征与心律失常. 中华心血管病杂志, 1997, 25(5): 330-333.

[4] 黄席珍, 韩芳, 慈书平, 等. 睡眠呼吸障碍. 中国实用内科杂志, 1998, 18: 195.

[5] 丁殿勋, 杨晔, 康建利, 等. 阻塞性睡眠呼吸暂停综合征引起冠心病急性发作并激发恶性心律失常三例报道. 天津医药, 2000(3): 140-142.

[6] Mehra R, Benjamin EJ, Shahar E, et al. Association of nocturnal arrhythmias with sleep-disordered breathing: The Sleep Heart Health Study. Am J Respir Crit Care Med, 2006, 173(8): 910-916.

[7] Wang S, Cui H, Song C, et al. Obstructive sleep apnea is associated with nonsustained ventricular tachycardia in patients with hypertrophic obstructive cardiomyopathy. Heart Rhythm, 2019, 16(5): 694-701.

[8] Selim BJ, Koo BB, Qin L, et al. The association between nocturnal cardiac arrhythmias and sleep-disordered breathing: the DREAM study. J Clin Sleep Med, 2016, 12(6): 829-837.

[9] Mehra R, Stone KL, Varosy PD, et al. Nocturnal arrhythmias across a spectrum of obstructive and central sleep-disordered breathing in older men: outcomes of sleep disorders in older men(MrOS sleep) study. Arch Intern Med, 2009, 169(12): 1147-1155.

[10] Monahan K, Storfer-Isser A, Mehra R, et al. Triggering of nocturnal arrhythmias by sleep-disordered breathing events. J Am Coll Cardiol, 2009, 54(19): 1797-1804.

[11] Koehler U, Apelt S, Cassel W, et al. Sleep disordered breathing and nonsustained ventricular tachycardia in patients with chronic heart failure. Wien Klin Wochenschr, 2012, 124(3-4): 63-68.

[12] Abe H, Takahashi M, Yaegashi H, et al. Efficacy of continuous positive airway pressure on arrhythmias in obstructive sleep apnea patients. Heart Vessels, 2010, 25(1): 63-69.

[13] Javaheri S. Effects of continuous positive airway pressure on sleep apnea and ventricular irritability in patients with heart failure. Circulation, 2000, 101(4): 392-397.

[14] Salama A, Abdullah A, Wahab A, et al. Is obstructive sleep apnea associated with ventricular tachycardia? A retrospective study from the national inpatient sample and a literature review on the pathogenesis of obstructive sleep apnea. Clin Cardiol, 2018, 41(12): 1543-1547.

[15] Morand J, Arnaud C, Pepin JL, et al. Chronic intermittent hypoxia promotes myocardial ischemia-related ventricular arrhythmias and sudden cardiac death. Sci Rep, 2018, 8(1):2997.

[16] Maeno K, Kasai A, Setsuda M, et al. Advanced atrioventricular block induced by obstructive sleep apnea before oxygen desaturation. Heart Vessels, 2009, 24(3):236-240.

[17] Priori SG, Blomström-Lundqvist C, Mazzanti A, et al. 2015 ESC Guidelines for the management of patients with ventricular arrhythmias and the prevention of sudden cardiac death: The Task Force for the Management of Patients with Ventricular Arrhythmias and the Prevention of Sudden Cardiac Death of the European Society of Cardiology(ESC). Endorsed by: Association for European Paediatric and Congenital Cardiology(AEPC). Eur Heart J, 2015, 36(41):2793-2867.

[18] Bitter T, Fox H, Dimitriadis Z, et al. Circadian variation of defibrillator shocks in patients with chronic heart failure: the impact of Cheyne-Stokes respiration and obstructive sleep apnea. Int J Cardiol, 2014, 176(3):1033-1035.

[19] Tomaello L, Zanolla L, Vassanelli C, et al. Sleep disordered breathing is associated with appropriate implantable cardioverter defibrillator therapy in congestive heart failure patients. Clin Cardiol, 2010, 33(2):E27-E30.

[20] Kwon Y, Koene RJ, Kwon O, et al. Effect of sleep-disordered breathing on appropriate implantable cardioverter-defibrillator therapy in patients with heart failure: a systematic review and Meta-analysis. Circ Arrhythm Electrophysiol, 2017, 10(2):e004609.

[21] Bitter T, Westerheide N, Prinz C, et al. Cheyne-stokes respiration and obstructive sleep apnoea are independent risk factors for malignant ventricular arrhythmias requiring appropriate cardioverter-defibrillator therapies in patients with congestive heart failure. Eur Heart J, 2011, 32(1):61-74.

[22] Raghuram A, Clay R, Kumbam A, et al. A systematic review of the association between obstructive sleep apnea and ventricular arrhythmias. J Clin Sleep Med, 2014, 10(10):1155-1160.

[23] Gami AS, Howard DE, Olson EJ, et al. Day-night pattern of sudden death in obstructive sleep apnea. N Engl J Med, 2005, 352(12):1206-1214.

[24] Young T, Finn L, Peppard PE, et al. Sleep disordered breathing and mortality: eighteen-year follow-up of the Wisconsin sleep cohort. Sleep, 2008, 31(8):1071-1078.

[25] Lee JE, Lee CH, Lee SJ, et al. Mortality of patients with obstructive sleep apnea in Korea. J Clin Sleep Med, 2013, 9(10):997-1002.

[26] Gami AS, Olson EJ, Shen WK, et al. Obstructive sleep apnea and the risk of sudden cardiac death: a longitudinal study of 10,701 adults. J Am Coll Cardiol, 2013, 62(7):610-616.

[27] Shamsuzzaman AS, Somers VK, Knilans TK, et al. Obstructive sleep apnea in patients with congenital long QT syndrome: implications for increased risk of sudden cardiac death. Sleep, 2015, 38(7):1113-1119.

[28] Kerns ES, Kim ED, Meoni LA, et al. Obstructive sleep apnea increases sudden cardiac death in incident hemodialysis patients. Am J Nephrol, 2018, 48(2):147-156.

[29] Koo CY, Aung AT, Chen Z, et al. Sleep apnoea and cadiovascular outcomes after coronary artery bypass grafting. Heart, 2020, 106(19):1495-1502.

[30] Marinheiro R, Parreira L, Amador P, et al. Ventricular arrhythmias in patients with obstructive sleep apnea. Curr Cardiol Revs, 2019, 15(1):64-74.

[31] May AM, VanWagoner DR, Mehra R. Obstructive sleep apnea and cardiac arrhythmogenesis: mechanistic insights. Chest, 2017, 151(1):225-241.

[32] Farré R, Montserrat JM, Navajas D. Morbidity due to obstructive sleep apnea: Insights from animal models. Curr Opin Pulm Med, 2008, 14(6):530-536.

[33] Linz D, Denner A, Illing S, et al. Impact of obstructive and central apneas on ventricular repolarisation: lessons learned from studies in man and pigs. Clin Res Cardiol, 2016, 105(8):639-647.

[34] Sökmen E, Özbek SC, Çelik M, et al. Changes in the parameters of ventricular repolarization during preapnea, apnea, and postapnea periods in patients with obstructive sleep apnea. Pacing Clin Electrophysiol, 2018, 41(7):762-766.

[35] Hayashi T, Fukamizu S, Hojo R, et al. Fragmented QRS predicts cardiovascular death of patients with structural heart disease and inducible ventricular tachyarrhythmia. Circ J, 2013, 77(12):2889-2897.

[36] Voigt L, Haq SA, Mitre CA, et al. Effect of obstructive sleep apnea on QT dispersion: a potential mechanism of sudden cardiac death. Cardiology, 2011, 118(1):68-73.

[37] Panikkath R, Reinier K, Evanado AU, et al. Prolonged Tpeak-to-tend interval on the resting ECG is associated with increased risk of sudden cardiac death. Circ Arrhythm Electrophysiol, 2011, 4(4):441-447.

[38] Kilicaslan F, Tokatli A, Ozdag F, et al. Tp-e interval, Tp-e/QT ratio, and Tp-e/QTc ratio are prolonged in patients with moderate and severe obstructive sleep apnea. Pacing Clin Electrophysiol, 2012, 35(8):966-972.

[39] Schmidleitner C, Arzt M, Tafelmeier M, et al. Sleep-disordered breathing is associated with disturbed cardiac repolarization in patients with a coronary artery bypass graft surgery. Sleep Med, 2018, 42:13-20.

[40] Adar A, Kırış A, Bülbül Y, et al. Association of fragmented QRS with subclinical left ventricular dysfunction in patients with obstructive sleep apnea. Med Princ Pract, 2015, 24(4):376-381.

[41] Simantirakis EN, Schiza SI, Marketou ME, et al. Severe bradyarrhythmias in patients with sleep apnoea: the effect of continuous positive airway pressure treatment: a long-term evaluation using an insertable loop recorder. Eur Heart J, 2004, 25(12):1070-1076.

[42] Bilal N, Dikmen N, Bozkus F, et al. Obstructive sleep apnea is associated with increased QT corrected interval dispersion: the effects of continuous positive airway pressure. Braz J Otorhinolaryngol, 2018, 84(3):298-304.

[43] Dursunoglu D, Dursunoglu N. Effect of CPAP on QT interval dispersion in obstructive sleep apnea patients without hyper-

tension. Sleep Med,2007,8(5):478-483.
[44] Rossi VA,Stoewhas AC,Camen G,et al. The effects of continuous positive airway pressure therapy withdrawal on cardiac repolarization:data from a randomized controlled trial. Eur Heart J,2012,33(17):2206-2212.
[45] Yajima Y,Koyama T,Kobayashi M,et al. Continuous positive airway pressure therapy improves heterogeneity of R-R intervals in a patient with obstructive sleep apnea syndrome. Intern Med,2019,58(9):1279-1282.
[46] Javaheri S. Effects of continuous positive airway pressure on sleep apnea and ventricular irritability in patients with heart failure. Circulation,2000,101(4):392-397.
[47] Craig S,Pepperell JC,Kohler M,et al. Continuous positive airway pressure treatment for obstructive sleep apnoea reduces resting heart rate but does not affect dysrhythmias:a randomised controlled trial. J Sleep Res, 2009, 18(3): 329-336.

13 吸烟相关疾病与DNA甲基化关系的研究进展

祁亚楠 齐 咏

吸烟是许多慢性疾病的坏境风险因素。研究发现吸烟可以通过DNA甲基化介导基因的表达及调控，参与多种系统疾病的发生发展。DNA甲基化是一种表观遗传修饰，遗传因素和环境因素均可调节DNA甲基化水平，进而调节基因表达。DNA甲基化改变可能是烟草暴露的一个生物标志物，研究与吸烟相关疾病的DNA甲基化变化，可能为吸烟相关疾病提供预防、诊断、治疗的靶点。本文对吸烟与呼吸、循环、生殖、消化、内分泌等系统疾病DNA甲基化关系的研究进展进行综述。

一、DNA甲基化概述

DNA甲基化是指在DNA甲基转移酶的催化下，在胞嘧啶残基的5'端位置添加一个甲基来对DNA结构进行可逆修饰的一个过程，不改变DNA序列直接影响DNA片段的活性，进而调节基因表达。DNA甲基化是一个可逆的过程，甲基的供体为甲基硫氨酸，参与的催化酶为DNA甲基转移酶(DNMTs)。DNA序列中富含GC的CpG二核苷酸簇被称为CpG岛，通常基因启动子区域中CpG岛的DNA甲基化会导致基因沉默，而甲基化不足会触发转录激活调控基因表达。

二、吸烟与疾病相关DNA甲基化

(一) 口腔系统疾病

研究发现非吸烟者和吸烟者之间口腔上皮细胞DNA甲基化状态之间存在差异。De等发现慢性牙周炎患者吸烟者唾液的细胞因子信号转导1(SOCS1)基因的启动子甲基化是非吸烟者的7.08倍。通过对口腔角质形成细胞的研究，发现香烟烟雾冷凝物(cigarette smoke condensate, CSC)与 UCHL1、GPX3、LXN 和 LDOC1 基因的甲基化和表达有关，其中 LDOC1 基因启动子甲基化对CSC最敏感，可导致 LDOC1 下调，可能促进早期口腔癌的发生。

(二) 呼吸系统疾病

已知吸烟与呼吸系统的关系最为密切。妊娠期间接触二手烟可降低后代肺单位体积的表面积，使肺泡发育过程受到干扰，进而导致疾病。父亲产前烟草暴露可增加 LMO2 和 IL-10 等免疫基因的甲基化含量，这些基因甲基化状态可从新生儿阶段维持到6岁，并与儿童哮喘的发生发展有关；妊娠期间暴露于烟草烟雾，后代总体DNA甲基化显著低于对照组，哮喘相关基因的甲基化发生改变，从而导致哮喘易感性增加。

吸烟可通过DNA甲基化的介导参与慢性阻塞性肺疾病(chronic obstructive pulmonary disease, COPD)的发病机制如氧化应激、细胞凋亡等。Zeng等发现CSC通过调控Bcl-2启动子甲基化诱导细胞凋亡，在CSC注射小鼠中观察到Bcl-2启动子高甲基化、Bcl-2低表达。吸烟诱导的线粒体转录因子A(mtTFA)启动子高甲基化也通过细胞凋亡参与COPD的发生发展，且CSC暴露以剂量和时间依赖性方式诱导细胞凋亡。同时研究表明通过DNA甲基化酶抑制剂可消除吸烟的毒性作用，减轻吸烟引起的肺细胞凋亡和功能衰竭。

肺中的主要抗氧化剂为谷胱甘肽(GSH)，谷氨酸半胱氨酸连接酶催化亚基(GCLC)对GSH具有调控作用。Cheng等发现吸烟可引起肺组织GCLC启动子的高甲基化，降低了GCLC mRNA的表达及血浆GSH水平，而DNA甲基化酶抑制剂处理后GCLC的表达增高。

Molina-Pinelo等发现DLK1-DIO3簇中的miRNAs靶点含有肿瘤抑制因子，DLK1-DIO3簇的去甲基化可能在当前和曾经吸烟者的肺癌发病机制中发挥作用，其中DNA甲基化与表达水平呈负相关。非小细胞肺癌患者不同的吸烟状态表现出不同的表观遗传特征，一项荟萃分析中显示，7个基因(包括 CDKN2A、RASSF1、MGMT、RARB、DAPK、WIF1 和 FHIT)的高甲基化与非小细胞肺癌患者的吸烟行为显著相关。Zhu等发现非小细胞肺癌患者吸烟可能导致CCGG位点的DNA甲基化水平降低，H3K27me3表达水平降低和细胞凋亡指数降低。吸烟与致癌物BPDE水平升高及p16、DAPK基因启动子高甲基化显著相关，致癌物BPDE和肿瘤抑制基因 TSGs 甲基化在非小细胞肺癌中有独立危险因素。

肺腺癌和肺鳞癌是非小细胞肺癌。王进等发现肺腺癌吸烟患者 SLIT3 和 SPARCL1 基因启动子高甲基化、表达下降，而两个基因的高表达与肺腺癌患者更好地预后有关。SIPA 1L3 基因不同甲基化水平的患者，戒烟对早期肺腺癌生存的影响不同，戒烟干预有利于 SIPA 1L3 低甲基化水平的 LUAD 患者的生存。Freeman等发现吸烟与 WWTR1、NFIX、PLA2G6、NHP2L1、SMUG1 基因的甲基化水平呈正相关，同时发现在肺鳞癌中，基因甲基化与吸烟的相关性比肺腺癌更强。因此不同的肺部肿瘤类型的不同吸烟状态引起的基因甲基化不同,吸烟引起的 DNA 甲基化的标志物的改变,未来可能对肺部肿瘤的诊断、治疗及预后提供帮助。

(三)循环系统疾病

吸烟是心血管疾病的危险因素,吸烟可通过改变醛固酮合成酶的甲基化状态引起原发性高血压风险增加,醛固酮合成酶 CpG1 位点甲基化与年龄呈正相关,CpG3、CpG4 位点甲基化与吸烟呈负相关。烟草烟雾中含有许多芳基烃受体(AhR)通路的激动剂,而 AhR 通路的激活能促进小鼠动脉粥样硬化。AhR 抑制因子(AHRR)的 DNA 甲基化与吸烟量呈负相关。Sabogal 等发现左心室质量与 13 个 CpG 位点甲基化之间存在显著关联,利用这些 CpG 位点构建 DNA 甲基化评分,该评分与 LVM 之间存在显著的相关性。

吸烟与许多在心血管疾病发病机制中起关键作用的基因的差异甲基化相关,尤其是凝血酶信号,包括血小板 F2R、PAR1、GP5、HMOX1、BCL2L1,且女性对烟草诱发的心血管疾病具有更高的易感性。G 蛋白偶联受体 15 参与血管生成和炎症反应,吸烟可通过影响 DNA 甲基化而参与调节 G 蛋白偶联受体 15,随着戒烟时间的增加 GPR15 的表达降低。

孕妇妊娠期间吸烟,后代 GFI1 基因的甲基化水平与青少年心血管危险因素之间存在显著关联。GFI1 基因的 3 个位点甲基化水平较低,与孕产前吸烟有关,8 个位点与成人自身吸烟有关,其中的 cg14179389 位点的 DNA 甲基化水平较低,是孕妇产前吸烟相关最强的位点。GFI1 基因所有位点中 DNA 甲基化水平越低,TG 水平越高。

(四)消化系统疾病

香烟烟雾通过 N 6-甲基腺苷(m6A)修饰引起的 miR-25-3p 过度成熟会促进胰腺癌的发展和进展,吸烟者甲基转移酶样蛋白 3 的甲基化状态在此过程中发挥重要作用。同时尼古丁暴露与正常胰腺上皮细胞抑癌基因高甲基化有关。尼古丁可通过尼古丁乙酰胆碱受体和 MAPK 信号通路介导的胰腺上皮细胞 DNMTs 的上调,导致抑癌基因异常高甲基化,去甲基化药物、尼古丁乙酰胆碱受体的拮抗剂和 p38 MAPK 的抑制剂可减弱尼古丁的毒副作用。

同时研究发现吸烟与结肠直肠癌发病率升高有关,通过对患者肿瘤组织和邻近黏膜的分析,发现抑癌基因 APC 启动子 1A 的甲基化与吸烟及吸烟的持续时间正相关,但高甲基化局限于肿瘤部位,在相邻的黏膜组织中未观察到高甲基化,同时研究发现孕妇吸烟能通过 DNA 甲基化增加后代发生炎症性肠病的可能。

(五)泌尿系统疾病

小鼠产前香烟烟雾暴露,改变了子代肾发育标志物胶质细胞源性神经营养因子和成纤维细胞生长因子 2 的表达,这与出生时肾总体 DNA 甲基化和 DNA 甲基转移酶 1 mRNA 表达增加有关,而通过母体左旋肉碱给药有可能逆转这一结果。

膀胱癌吸烟患者的甲基化代谢物、DNA 甲基转移酶 1 表达明显高于膀胱癌非吸烟患者,甲基化抑制剂可协同治疗,因此甲基化代谢物可作为非侵入性预测生物标志物、分层膀胱癌的风险,在膀胱癌吸烟患者可以帮助早期发现和治疗膀胱癌。吸烟与闭经后妇女膀胱癌的发生有关,具体机制尚不清楚,Jordahl 等发现血液中 AhRR、F2RL3 和 GPR15 基因的甲基化与吸烟之间存在很强的相关性,F2RL3 和 GPR15 基因的甲基化可能介导了吸烟对膀胱癌的影响。

(六)生殖系统与乳腺疾病

吸烟可通过 DNA 甲基化,对精液产生不利影响,增加男性不育的风险,因此 DNA 甲基化可被认为是男性生育能力的一个标志。吸烟会引起精子 H19 基因的低甲基化和 SNRPN 基因的高甲基化,同时 MAPK8IP 和 TKR 基因的甲基化也发生了改变。Zhang 等的进一步研究发现吸烟会改变吸烟者精细胞 MEST、P16、LINE-1 和 GNAS 基因的甲基化,这些基因与精子浓度、FSH 和黄体生成素水平显著相关。妊娠期暴露香烟烟雾,可导致子代卵母细胞染色质结构和 DNA 甲基化水平异常,降低后代卵巢功能的相关指标。

Mitsui 等研究发现吸烟与前列腺肿瘤 DNA 甲基化及前列腺癌的不良预后有关。细胞色素 P450(CYP)1A1 是一种 I 期酶,所有癌细胞株中 CYP1A1 的甲基化水平显著降低,表达高于正常细胞,且甲基抑制剂处理后 CYP1A1 表达进一步增强。在免疫组织中显示 CYP1A1 在前列腺癌中的免疫染色高于正常和良性前列腺增生,吸烟能引起 CYP1A1 启动子低甲基化,并能通过 BCL2 的失调促进前列腺癌的增生和存活。

研究表明吸烟与乳腺癌的发生有关,特定年龄的主动吸烟与 GSTP1、FHIT 和 CDKN2A 的甲基化水平升高以及 SCGB3A1 和 BRCA1 的甲基化水平降低有关。

(七)内分泌系统和营养代谢性疾病

吸烟是糖尿病的一个危险因素,吸烟会加重糖尿病病情。比较目前吸烟者和从未吸烟者,Ligthart 等发现吸烟与糖尿病危险基因 ANPEP、KCNQ1 和 ZMIZ1 的甲基化水平有关,其中 ANPEP 基因 cg23161492 位点甲基化水平升高、表达降低,KCNQ1 基因的低甲基化与较低的空腹胰岛素水平相关。

Chemerin 是一种与肥胖有关的脂肪因子,在肥胖和吸烟个体中升高,妊娠期吸烟母亲所生婴儿 Chemerin mRNA 表达升高,Chemerin DNA 甲基化降低。通过对脂肪组织活检,TSAI 等发现 5 个基因(AHRR、CYP1A1、CYP1B1、CYTL1、F2RL3)在当前吸烟者中甲基化水平降低和表达上调,BHLHE40 和 AHRR 的 DNA 甲基化和基因表达水平是预测未来戒烟后内脏脂肪增加的指标。

(八)神经精神系统疾病

下丘脑-垂体-肾上腺(HPA)轴受烟草和酒精的影响,会引起 HPA 轴外周血 NR3C1 和 FKBP5 基因低甲基化,且与烟酒剂量相关。妊娠期间持续暴露于烟草烟雾可导致子代明显的神经功能缺陷,Chatterton 等研究发现孕妇吸烟会改变胎儿 DNA 甲基化和基因表达的发育模式,并与成熟神经元含量减少有关。比较暴露于烟草和未暴露烟草的胎儿的背外侧前额叶皮质的甲基化谱,在烟草暴露的胎儿中,GNA15 和 SDHAP3 启动子区域低甲基化,同时SDHAP3 mRNA的发育上调被延迟。

通过研究孕妇产前吸烟与后代血液DNA甲基化的关系,发现了69个不同的甲基化位点,其中孕妇烟草暴露的后代的精神疾病发病率增加,cg25189904(GNG12)位点的甲基化水平与精神分裂症有关。

(九)产前吸烟与胎儿生长发育

面裂是发育异常中最常见的一种,第一鳃弓衍生细胞(1-BA细胞)有助于嘴唇和上腭的形成。Mukhopadhyay等通过对1-BA细胞的研究,发现孕妇在妊娠期间吸烟可能通过降低DNA甲基化导致面裂。

孕妇在妊娠期间吸烟会干扰子宫-胎盘的交换,对子代的影响可通过胎盘甲基化来调节,从而增加胎儿低体重出生的风险,孕期吸烟可导致胎盘组织的71个位点甲基化发生变化,其中有7个位点介导了产前吸烟与出生体重之间的关联(*MDS2*、*PBX1*、*CYP1A2*、*VPRBP*、*WBP1L*、*CD28*和*CDK6*基因),关联增强的位点cg22638236,其基因注释于*PBX1*,该基因参与骨骼的发育。胰岛素样生长因子-1在损伤后的生长、分化和修复过程中起重要作用,烟草暴露改变了*Igf1*启动子发育阶段的甲基化,且具有器官和性别特异性,*Igf1*启动子甲基化与mRNA表达呈负相关。

三、结 语

吸烟对全身多系统进行性损害导致各种系统疾病的发生,具体作用机制尚不清楚,DNA甲基化是其研究的热点。DNA甲基化可作为吸烟相关疾病的表观遗传生物标志。迄今为止,大多数研究为横断面研究且药物等干扰因素较多,未来需要进行相关的前瞻性研究,以了解吸烟与疾病及DNA甲基化模式的关联,为疾病的机制、预防、诊断及后期的治疗提供有力的理论依据。

参 考 文 献

[1] De JHMC, Villafuerte KRV, LuchiariHR, et al. Effect of smoking on the DNA methylation pattern of the SOCS1 promoter in epithelial cells from the saliva of patients with chronic periodontitis. J Periodontol,2019,90(11):1279-1286.

[2] Lee CH,Pan KL,Tang YC,et al. LDOC1 silenced by cigarette exposure and involved in oral neoplastic transformation. Oncotarget,2015,6(28):25188-25201.

[3] Wu CC,Hsu TY,Chang JC,et al. Paternaltobacco smoke correlated to offspring asthma and prenatal epigenetic programming. Front Genet,2019,10:471.

[4] Christensen S,Jaffar Z,Cole E,et al. Prenatal environmental tobacco smoke exposure increases allergic asthma risk with methylation changes in mice. Environ Mol Mutagen,2017,58(6):423-433.

[5] Zeng H,Shi Z,Kong X,et al. Involvement of B-cell CLL/lymphoma 2 promoter methylation in cigarette smoke extract-induced emphysema. Exp Biol Med(Maywood),2016,241(8):808-816.

[6] Peng H,Guo T,Chen Z,et al. Hypermethylation of mitochondrial transcription factor A induced by cigarette smoke is associated with chronic obstructive pulmonary disease. Exp Lung Res,2019,45(3-4):101-111.

[7] Cheng L,Liu J,Li B,et al. Cigarettesmoke-induced hypermethylation of the GCLC gene is associated with COPD. Chest,2016,149(2):474-482.

[8] Molina-Pinelo S,Salinas A,Moreno-Mata N,et al. Impact of DLK1-DIO3 imprinted cluster hypomethylation in smoker patients with lung cancer. Oncotarget,2018,9(4):4395-4410.

[9] Huang T,Chen X,Hong Q,et al. Meta-analyses of gene methylation and smoking behavior in non-small cell lung cancer patients. Sci Rep,2015,5:8897.

[10] Zhu K,Deng Y,Weng G,et al. Analysis of H3K27me3 expression and DNA methylation at CCGG sites in smoking and non-smoking patients with non-small cell lung cancer and their clinical significance. Oncol Lett,2018,15(5):6179-6188.

[11] Jin Y,Xu P,Liu X,et al. Cigarettesmoking,BPDE-DNA adducts, and aberrant promoter methylations of tumor suppressor genes(TSGs)in NSCLC from Chinese population. Cancer Invest,2016,34(4):173-180.

[12] 王进,余晓凡,欧阳楠,等. 甲基化调控SLIT3和SPARCL1基因在吸烟致肺腺癌中的表达及其对患者预后的影响. 中华医学杂志,2019,99(20):1553-1557.

[13] Zhang R,Lai L,Dong X,et al. SIPA1L3 methylation modifies the benefit of smoking cessation on lung adenocarcinoma survival:an epigenomic-smoking interaction analysis. Mol Oncol,2019,13(5):1235-1248.

[14] Freeman JR,Chu S,Hsu T,et al. Epigenome-wide association study of smoking and DNA methylation in non-small cell lung neoplasms. Oncotarget,2016,7(43):69579-69591.

[15] Gu T,Mao S,Fan R,et al. Interactions between CYP11B2 promoter methylation and smoking increase risk of essential hypertension. Biomed Res Int,2016,2016:1454186.

[16] Sabogal C,Su S,Tingen M,et al. Cigarette smoking related DNA methylation in peripheral leukocytes and cardiovascular risk in young adults. Int J Cardiol,2020,306:203-205.

[17] Chatziioannou A,Georgiadis P,Hebels D G,et al. Blood-based omic profiling supports female susceptibility to tobacco smoke-induced cardiovascular diseases. Sci Rep,2017,7:42870.

[18] Haase T,Müller C,Krause J,et al. Novel DNA methylation sites influence GPR15 expression in relation to smoking. Biomolecules,2018,8(3).

[19] Parmar P,Lowry E,Cugliari G,et al. Association of maternal prenatal smoking GFI1-locus and cardio-metabolic phenotypes in 18,212 adults. EBio Medicine,2018,38:206-216.

[20] Zhang J,Bai R,Li M,et al. Excessive miR-25-3p maturation via N(6)-methyladenosine stimulated by cigarette smoke promotes pancreatic cancer progression. Nat Commun,2019,

10(1):1858.

[21] Jin T, Hao J, Fan D. Nicotine induces aberrant hypermethylation of tumor suppressor genes in pancreatic epithelial ductal cells. Biochem Biophys Res Commun, 2018, 499(4):934-940.

[22] Barrow TM, Klett H, Toth R, et al. Smoking is associated with hypermethylation of the APC 1A promoter in colorectal cancer: the ColoCare study. J Pathol, 2017, 243(3):366-375.

[23] Wiklund P, Karhunen V, Richmond R C, et al. DNA methylation links prenatal smoking exposure to later life health outcomes in offspring. ClinEpigenetics, 2019, 11(1):97.

[24] Stangenberg S, Nguyen LT, Chan Y L, et al. Maternal L-carnitine supplementation ameliorates renal underdevelopment and epigenetic changes in male mice offspring due to maternal smoking. Clin Exp Pharmacol Physiol, 2019, 46(2):183-193.

[25] Jin F, Thaiparambil J, Donepudi SR, et al. Tobacco-specific carcinogens induce hypermethylation, DNA adducts, and DNA damage in bladder cancer. Cancer Prev Res(Phila), 2017, 10(10):588-597.

[26] Jordahl KM, Phipps AI, Randolph TW, et al. Differential DNA methylation in blood as a mediator of the association between cigarette smoking and bladder cancer risk among postmenopausal women. Epigenetics, 2019, 14(11):1065-1073.

[27] Dong H, Wang Y, Zou Z, et al. Abnormalmethylation of imprinted genes and cigarette smoking: assessment of their association with the risk of male infertility. Reprod Sci, 2017, 24(1):114-123.

[28] Zhang W, Li M, Sun F, et al. Association ofsperm methylation at LINE-1, four candidate genes, and nicotine/alcohol exposure with the risk of infertility. Front Genet, 2019, 10:1001.

[29] Gao J G, Gong L, Wu Z H, et al. Effect of cigarette smoke exposure during pregnancy on offspring of ovarian development and oocyte DNA methylation in female mice Chin J Industr Hygiene Occupat Dis, 2017, 35(6):455-459.

[30] Mitsui Y, Chang I, Kato T, et al. Functional role and tobacco smoking effects on methylation of CYP1A1 gene in prostate cancer. Oncotarget, 2016, 7(31):49107-49121.

[31] Callahan CL, Bonner MR, Nie J, et al. Active and secondhand smoke exposure throughout life and DNA methylation in breast tumors. Cancer Causes Control, 2019, 30(1):53-62.

[32] Ligthart S, Steenaard RV, Peters MJ, et al. Tobacco smoking is associated with DNA methylation of diabetes susceptibility genes. Diabetologia, 2016, 59(5):998-1006.

[33] Reynolds LJ, Chavan NR, Dehoff LB, et al. Smoking during pregnancy increases chemerin expression in neonatal tissue. Exper Physiol, 2019, 104(1):93-99.

[34] Tsai PC, Glastonbury CA, Eliot MN, et al. Smoking induces coordinated DNA methylation and gene expression changes in adipose tissue with consequences for metabolic health. Clin Epigenetics, 2018, 10(1):126.

[35] Dogan MV, Lei MK, Beach SR, et al. Alcohol and tobacco consumption alter hypothalamic pituitary adrenal axis DNA methylation. Psychoneuroendocrinology, 2016, 66:176-184.

[36] Chatterton Z, Hartley BJ, Seok MH, et al. In utero exposure to maternal smoking is associated with DNA methylation alterations and reduced neuronal content in the developing fetal brain. Epigenetics Chromatin, 2017, 10:4.

[37] Mukhopadhyay P, Greene R M, Pisano MM. Cigarette smoke induces proteasomal-mediated degradation of DNA methyltransferases and methyl CpG-/CpG domain-binding proteins in embryonic orofacial cells. Reprod Toxicol, 2015, 58:140-148.

[38] Cardenas A, Lutz SM, Everson TM, et al. Mediation byplacental DNA methylation of the association of prenatal maternal smoking and birth weight. Am J Epidemiol, 2019, 188(11):1878-1886.

[39] Zeng Z, Meyer KF, Lkhagvadorj K, et al. Prenatal smoke effect on mouse offspring Igf1 promoter methylation from fetal stage to adulthood is organ and sex specific. Am J Physiol Lung Cell Mol Physiol, 2020, 318(3):L549-L561.

14 新型冠状病毒肺炎与吸烟的关系

云俊杰　熊维宁

2019年12月,新型冠状病毒肺炎疫情暴发,2020年2月12日WHO将这一疾病正式命名为"Coronavirus Disease 2019(COVID-19)",其病原体命名为"严重急性呼吸综合征冠状病毒-2(severe acute respiratory syndrome coronavirus 2,SARS-Cov-2)"。2020年3月11日,WHO正式宣布新型冠状病毒(以下简称新冠)进入全球大流行状态。吸烟是否增加新冠感染的机会？吸烟是否会导致新冠患者感染更重？随着对疾病的认识不断增加,本文就COVID-19与吸烟关系做一阐述。

一、COVID-19患者吸烟情况的流行病学

Farsalinos等荟萃分析了13项发生在中国,共计5960名COVID-19住院患者的临床研究,并统计了其中合并有关吸烟状况的数据,发现当前的吸烟率从1.4%(95%CI 0.0～3.4%)到12.6%(95%CI 10.6～14.6%)不等。与中国的人群吸烟率相比,荟萃分析发现当前吸烟率异常低(6.5%,95%CI 4.9～8.2%)。将曾经有吸烟史的患者归类为当前吸烟者,发现汇总估计值为7.3%(95%CI 5.7～8.9%)。这项研究首次计算了中国住院COVID-19患者的当前吸烟率。当前吸烟的估计流行率出乎意料的低,约是中国最近估计的吸烟率的1/4。同时发现与女性相比,男性更容易罹患COVID-19。排除数据准确性因素外,Farsalinos等认为这一结论可能与以下因素有关:①COVID-19患者合并吸烟的人群与非吸烟人群因经济、地位等原因,入院机会可能不同;②所记录的吸烟状态的一致性和准确性,例如在这13项研究中,有一项研究中某些患者入院时情况危重,影响了沟通能力从而无法准确报告吸烟情况;另一项研究中将吸烟情况未知归类于未吸烟者但未报告吸烟情况未知者数量等;某些患者可能在发病后不久和入院前就已经戒烟了,有些研究把这些患者归类为曾有吸烟史患者中,从而对结果造成影响。除了这些原因之外,疫情初期的几项研究都在武汉,而当时的情况是大量患者短时间涌入医院,医生争分夺秒救治患者,忽略了相对不重要的吸烟史的确认而被系统默认为不吸烟从而导致后来的统计偏差。另外,有很多患者出于自身原因隐瞒吸烟史。因此,如果想得到准确的流行病学资料,理论上应该是给每位患者进行尼古丁代谢物的血检和尿检。

而在一项针对欧洲38个国家进行的调查研究中显示,吸烟率与COVID-19的患病率之间存在统计学上的显着负相关($P=0.001$)。这项研究存在许多局限性,导致这种关联可能并不意味着存在真实或因果关系,究其原因可能研究中对混杂因素的测量不佳,并且可能存在残留混杂现象。例如:①当地的经济规模,政府政策和COVID-19测试的速度;②忽略了包括空气污染水平,合并症水平,一国之内的COVID-19聚类以及国际旅客的入境率等因素;③当地的严格的抗疫政策;④研究截止日期后每个国家随后COVID-19流行病的进展可能会影响分析结果。

总之,目前没有一项研究支持以下观点:吸烟可作为治疗干预措施或预防措施,以减少COVID-19的影响或减轻其对健康的负面影响。

二、吸烟增加了重症COVID-19的风险

赵千文等荟萃分析了11项总计2002病例的临床研究,结果表明吸烟会增加罹患严重COVID-19的风险($OR=1.98$;$95\%CI$:$1.29\sim3.05$),是不吸烟者的2倍。

Patanavanich等的一项荟萃分析共纳入11 590例COVID-19患者,其中2133例(18.4%)经历了疾病进展,而731例(6.3%)有吸烟史。共有218名有吸烟史的患者(29.8%)经历了疾病进展,相比之下,非吸烟患者仅为17.6%。荟萃分析显示吸烟与COVID-19进展之间存在关联(OR 1.91,95%CI 1.42～2.59,$P=0.001$),从而证实吸烟是导致COVID-19恶化的危险因素,吸烟者的COVID-19严重程度发展的概率是从未吸烟者的1.91倍。该项荟萃分析提到,有学者认为报道的COVID患者吸烟率低于一般人群,以此作为吸烟有保护作用的证据。该项荟萃分析认为这可能与吸烟评估不足从而导致在COVID患者中报道的患病率较低有关。但该项荟萃分析也存在一定局限性,例如①纳入荟萃分析的一些研究对于吸烟的定义不明确,有时包含既往者,有时则不包含;②纳入荟萃分析的一些研究对于一些临床数据未进行多元校正。

Farsalinos的另一项回顾性观察病例系列的荟萃分析发现,住院的COVID-19患者中当前吸烟的发生率出乎意料的低。与非当前吸烟者相比,住院的当前吸烟者发生不良后果的概率更高。因此吸烟不能被视为COVID-19的保护措施。但该项荟萃分析也存在局限性,即未对混杂因素(如合并症情况)进行分析调整。纳入该项荟萃分析的许多研究报道了吸烟史而不是当前吸烟史,其中可能包括

以前的吸烟者,因此高估了住院的COVID-19患者的当前吸烟率。同时由于这些混杂因素存在,导致尼古丁对COVID-19的保护作用可能部分被吸烟相关毒性和吸烟者住院后突然停止尼古丁摄入所掩盖,但这一假设应在使用药物尼古丁产品的实验室研究和临床试验中进行探索。鉴于涉及心血管、呼吸和癌症的发病率和病死率,因此吸烟不能被视为针对COVID-19(或任何其他疾病)的保护措施。因此,仍应鼓励吸烟者戒烟。

三、吸烟增加COVID-19严重程度的病理生理机制

COVID-19是由SARS-CoV-2病毒感染所引起。SARS-CoV-2表面具有高度糖基化的蛋白,其包含两个不同的功能域(S1和S2)。S1结构域包含血管紧张素转化酶2(ACE2)受体结合结构域,并负责第一阶段宿主细胞的进入。S2结构域促进细胞渗透所需的细胞膜和病毒膜之间的融合。S蛋白经过酶修饰,使融合位点暴露于细胞黏附上,这可以通过被称为"弗林蛋白酶"的蛋白质转化酶介导的细胞蛋白酶裂解来实现。弗林蛋白酶在肺中大量表达,SARS-CoV-2病毒也利用该系统转化其表面蛋白。ACE2受体为SARS-CoV-2病毒的S蛋白提供了人类细胞结合位点。最近的研究发现,经修饰的SARS-CoV-2的S蛋白与ACE2有非常高的亲和力,与人体内ACE2结合的可能性比以前的SARS-CoV的S蛋白高10~20倍。这种亲和力的增加使病毒更容易在人与人之间传播,因此,与以前的SARS病毒相比,SARS-CoV-2的估计R0更高。ACE2蛋白在肺泡Ⅱ型上皮细胞表面表达,而且其中调节病毒增生和传播的基因高度表达,在吸烟者(可能包括电子烟烟民)和使用ACE阻断剂的个体(高血压和糖尿病患者)中,ACE2的表达水平很高,从而使他们易患该疾病。病毒附着在细胞表面ACE2上,可保护其免受免疫监视机制的侵害,其在宿主细胞表面留在时间较长,使宿主细胞成为高效的载体,以备将来感染和传播。ACE2的最终吞噬进一步为病毒提供了进入宿主细胞系统的通道,不仅使病毒可以增生,还可以进行突变,影响宿主的免疫系统从而产生逃避机制。

此外,男性中循环的ACE2增多,这为疾病严重程度基于性别的差异提供了证据。ACE2可能在生殖细胞中高表达,即在成年男性和女性中表达更多。ACE2可能与烟碱乙酰胆碱受体(nAChRs)有关,特别是与alpha7nAChR受体有关,进一步支持吸烟(尼古丁)状态可能对COVID-19的病理生理至关重要。ACE2受体(受发育调节)在肺上皮细胞中丰富,特别是肺泡Ⅱ型上皮细胞、杯状细胞、鼻上皮/纤毛和口腔黏膜细胞。吸烟削弱了免疫系统,使其易于进入宿主细胞进行快速增生,继而由宿主体内的"细胞因子风暴"触发的过度炎症反应,最终导致肺组织受损。研究表明,在吸烟者和患有与吸烟相关的疾病如COPD和IPF的患者的小气道上皮中,ACE2表达上调。尽管未经测试,但雾化(尼古丁)可能具有相似的作用,因此使该人群更容易受到该疾病的影响。

Samuel研究发现,慢性阻塞性肺疾病患者和健康肺功能吸烟者的切除肺组织中ACE2表达增强,尽管后者少得多,而健康的非吸烟者却完全不存在。在肺泡Ⅱ型上皮细胞、肺泡巨噬细胞和小气道上皮细胞的顶端,ACE2的表达非常明显。慢性阻塞性肺疾病患者显示出明显更高的ACE2水平,表明慢性阻塞性肺疾病进一步强化了ACE2和潜在的SARS-CoV-2黏附位点,从而也说明吸烟患者更易罹患COVID-19。

中国COVID-19患者中,吸烟的流行率低于预期,这与当时现实的救治情况有很大关系。吸烟增加COVID-19严重程度并与COVID-19进展有关,可能是因为吸烟和电子烟上调气道ACE2受体的表达、增加肺部炎症,使新冠病毒更容易感染气道细胞。

参 考 文 献

[1] Konstantinos Farsalinos, et al. Systematic Review of the Prevalence of Current Smoking Among Hospitalized COVID-19 Patients in China: Could Nicotine Be a Therapeutic Option? Emerg Med, 2020: 1-8.

[2] Statista. Population in China from 2008 to 2018, by gender. https://www.stati sta.com/stati stics/25112 9/popul ation-in-china-by-gende r/. Accessed 9 Apr 2020.

[3] Guan WJ, Liang WH, Zhao Y, et al. Comorbidity and its impact on 1590 patients with Covid-19 in China: a nationwide analysis. Eur Respir J, 2020, 55(5): 2000547.

[4] Zhou F, Yu T, Du R, et al. Clinical course and risk factors for mortality of adult inpatients with COVID-19 in Wuhan, China: a retrospective cohort study. Lancet, 2020, 395(10229): 1054-1062.

[5] Liu W, Tao ZW, Lei W, et al. Analysis of factors associated with disease outcomes in hospitalized patients with 2019 novel coronavirus disease. Chin Med J (Engl), 2020.

[6] Guo T, Fan Y, Chen M, et al. Cardiovascular implications of fatal outcomes of patients with coronavirus disease 2019 (COVID-19). JAMA Cardiol, 2020, 5(7): 811-818.

[7] Nicotine Tob Res, Panagiotis Tsigaris, et al. Smoking Prevalence and COVID-19 in Europe. Nicotime Tob Res, 2020, 22(9): 1646-1649.

[8] Lutchman D. Could the smoking gun in the fight against Covid-19 be the (rh)ACE2? Eur Respir J, 2020, 56(1): 2001560.

[9] Zitek T. The appropriate use of testing for COVID-19. West J Emerg Med, 2020, 21(3): 470-472.

[10] Qianwen Zhao, et al. The impact of COPD and smoking history on the severity of COVID-19: A systemic review and meta-analysis. J Med Virol, 2020.

[11] Roengrudee Patanavanich, et al. Smoking Is Associated With COVID-19 Progression: A Meta-Analysis. Nicotine Tob Res, 2020, 22(9): 1653-1656.

[12] Konstantinos Farsalinos, et al. CurrentSmoking, Former

Smoking, and Adverse Outcome Among Hospitalized COVID-19 Patients: A Systematic Review and Meta-Analysis. Ther Adv Chronic Dis, 2020, 11:2040622320935765.

[13] Li F, Li W, Farzan M, et al. Structure of SARS Coronavirus Spike Receptor-Binding Domain Complexed with Receptor. Science(N. Y.), 2005, 309:1864-1868.

[14] Coutard B, Valle C, de Lamballerie X, et al. The spike glycoprotein of the new coronavirus 2019-nCoV contains a furin-like cleavage site absent in CoV of the same clade. Antivir. Res, 2020, 176:104742.

[15] Follis KE, York J, Nunberg JH. Furin cleavage of the SARS coronavirus spike glycoprotein enhances cell-cell fusion but does not affect virion entry. Virology, 2006, 350:358-369.

[16] National Institutesof Health, U. S.; Department of Healthand Human Services. Novel Coronavirus Structure Reveals Targetsfor Vaccinesand Treatments. 2020. Availableonline: www. nih. gov/news-events/nih-researchmatters/novel-coronavirus-structure-reveals-targets-vaccines-treatments(accessed on 11 March 2020).

[17] Wrapp D, Wang N, Corbett KS, et al. Cryo-EM structure of the 2019-nCoV spike in the prefusion conformation. Science (N. Y.), 2020, 367(6483):1260-1263.

[18] Hamming I, Timens W, Bulthuis ML, et al. Tissue distribution of ACE2 protein, the functional receptor for SARS coronavirus. A first step in understanding SARS pathogenesis. J Pathol, 2004, 203:631-637.

[19] Brake SJ, Barnsley K, Lu W, et al. Smoking upregulates angiotensin-converting Enzyme-2 receptor: a potential adhesion site for novel coronavirus SARS-CoV-2 (Covid-19). J Clin Med, 2020, 9(3):841.

[20] Sama IE, Ravera A, Santema BT, et al. Circulating plasma concentrations of angiotensin-converting enzyme 2 in men and women with heart failure and effects of renin-angiotensin-aldosterone inhibitors. Eur Heart J, 2020, 41:1810-1817.

[21] Xu H, Zhong L, Deng J, et al. High expression of ACE2 receptor of 2019-nCoV on the epithelial cells of oral mucosa. Int J Oral Sci, 2020, 12(1):8.

[22] Ziegler CGK, Allon SJ, Nyquist SK, et al. SARS-CoV-2 Receptor ACE2 Is an Interferon-Stimulated Gene in Human Airway Epithelial Cells and Is Detected in Specific Cell Subsets across Tissues [published online ahead of print, 2020 Apr 27]. Cell. 2020; S0092-8674(20)30500-305006.

[23] Sungnak W, Huang N, Becavin C, et al. SARS-CoV-2 entry factors are highly expressed in nasal epithelial cells together with innate immune genes. Nat Med, 2020, 26(5):681-687.

[24] Yao H, Rahman I. Current concepts on oxidative/carbonyl stress, inflammation and epigenetics in pathogenesis of chronic obstructive pulmonary disease. Toxicol Appl Pharmacol, 2011, 254(2):72-85.

[25] Hwang JH, Lyes M, Sladewski K, et al. Electronic cigarette inhalation alters innate immunity and airway cytokines while increasing the virulence of colonizing bacteria. J Mol Med (Berl), 2016, 94(6):667-679.

[26] Samuel James Brake, et al. Smoking Upregulates Angiotensin-Converting Enzyme-2 Receptor: A Potential Adhesion Site for Novel Coronavirus SARS-CoV-2 (Covid-19). J Clin Med, 2020, 9(3):841.

第二部分

慢性阻塞性肺疾病

1 慢性阻塞性肺疾病年度研究进展（2019—2020）

王凤燕　梁振宇　陈荣昌

慢性阻塞性肺疾病（COPD）发病率高，疾病负担重，严重影响居民特别是老年人的健康和生活质量。其发病机制尚未完全明确，关于疾病亚型、生物标志物、吸入药物选择、急性加重期治疗策略的探讨方兴未艾。2019 年，健康中国行动（2019—2030 年）正式启动，慢性呼吸系统疾病防治行动是十五项重大行动之一，而 COPD 被列为慢呼疾病的代表病种。掌握国内外相关领域的新发现、新观点，对 COPD 防治具有重要意义。

一、发病机制、生物标志物

遗传风险基因位点为疾病发病机制提供了新的见解。国际 COPD 遗传学联盟对英国生物库中的 35 735 名 COPD 患者和 222 076 名对照者进行了全基因组关联研究，确定了 82 个 COPD 基因位点，在 35 个新基因位点中，有 13 个与肺功能相关。利用基因表达和调控数据，该研究确定了 COPD 风险基因位点与肺组织、平滑肌和几种肺细胞的功能富集，还发现有 14 个 COPD 与哮喘或肺纤维化共享的基因位点，不同类别的 COPD 遗传风险基因位点与定量影像学特征和合并症有不同关联。这项研究为 COPD 的遗传易感性和异质性提供了进一步的支持。

2019 年，Cell 介绍了一种新型的病原体——活化中性粒细胞（PMN）衍生的外泌体。这些外泌体具备 α_1-抗胰蛋白酶抗体，并通过整合素 Mac-1 和中性粒细胞弹性蛋白酶（NE）结合并降解细胞外基质（ECM），从而引起 COPD。这种 PMN 衍生的外泌体存在于 COPD 患者的临床标本中，但不存在于健康对照者中，并且能够以 NE 驱动的方式将 COPD 样表型从人转移到小鼠。这些发现揭示了外泌体在 COPD 发病机制中的重要作用。

肺和全身炎症是 COPD 的主要特征。已有多项研究证明了具有生物活性的细胞外基质成分与 COPD 发病机制之间的关系。Wells 等用质谱法测量了 SPIROMICS 队列中受试者的痰和血浆中的细胞外基质乙酰基脯氨酸-甘氨酸脯氨酸（AcPGP），调整已知的危险因素后，发现在 COPD 中，痰液（而非血浆）AcPGP 的浓度与气流受限、小气道疾病、肺气肿的严重程度及随访 1 年时发生严重 AECOPD 的风险有关。这提示 AcPGP 有可能作为 COPD 的生物标志物，也强调了局部炎症在 COPD 发病机制的重要性。

二、评估与分型

COPD 是一种吸烟相关疾病，特征在于气道阻塞和炎症，并且对糖皮质激素的反应不同。IL-17A 参与中性粒细胞炎症和糖皮质激素抵抗，因此在 COPD 分子表型中可能尤其重要。有文献报道，COPD 和吸烟对照组的支气管气道上皮中 IL-17A 反应的基因表达特征与 IL-17 反应的炎症特征相关，包括气道中性粒细胞和巨噬细胞增多；在 SPIROMICS 中，该特征与定量胸部 CT 上气道阻塞增加和功能性小气道疾病相关；在 GLUCOLD 中，无论气道嗜酸性或 Th 2 型炎症反应如何，IL-17 基因表达特征均与对糖皮质激素的反应降低有关。这些数据表明 IL-17 气道上皮反应的基因标志区分了一个生物学上、放射学上和临床上都截然不同的 COPD 亚型，该亚型患者可能受益于个性化治疗。

多项研究已经通过 CT 图像的视觉或定量评估确定 COPD 亚型，但缺乏 CT 影像的视觉和定量相结合的系统评估。COPDGene 研究中，研究者将视觉上定义的肺气肿模式与定量成像特征和肺活量数据相结合，生成了 10 个不重叠的 CT 成像亚型，包括无 CT 影像学异常、肺旁型肺气肿（PSE）、支气管疾病、小气道疾病、轻度肺气肿、上叶为主的小叶中央型肺气肿（CLE）、下叶为主 CLE、弥漫性 CLE、可见无定量肺气肿和定量不可见肺气肿。各组间病死率差异显著（$P<0.01$），在 3 个中度至重度 CLE 组中病死率最高。可见无定量肺气肿和定量不可见肺气肿是轻度 COPD 独有的 2 个亚型，存在进展风险，可能具有不同的潜在机制。与没有 CT 影像学异常的受试者相比，PSE 和（或）中度至重度 CLE 的受试者在 5 年内出现了严重的肺气肿进展（$P<0.01$）。视觉和定量 CT 影像特征的结合反映了异质性 COPD 综合征中不同的潜在病理过程，为 COPD 的重新分类提供了一种有用的方法。

COPD 急性加重（AECOPD）加剧疾病进展、影响患者生存质量，其风险的有效预测与评估一直是临床研究的重点，截至 2019 年文献报道了约 40 多个 AECOPD 预测模型，但大多缺乏有效的外部验证。2020 年 3 月，Lancet Respiratory Medicine 报道了一个汇集 3 项 COPD 试验数据（2380 例）开发的混合效应模型（ACCEPT 模型），来预测 1 年内的急性加重。预测因素包括急性加重史、年龄、性别、体重指数、吸烟状况、家庭氧疗、肺功能、症状负担和目前药物使用情况。ECLIPSE队列被用于外部验证时,≥2次加重的AUC为0.81(95% CI 0.79~0.83),≥1次重度加重的AUC为0.77(95% CI 0.74~0.80)。预测的加重率和观察到的加重率相似(全部加重率为1.31次/年 vs. 1.20次/年;重度加重率为0.25次/年 vs. 0.27次/年)。在有既往加重病史的患者中,风险模型预测重度加重和所有加重同样是准确的。因此,该风险模型有潜力作为COPD个体化治疗和预防急性加重的决策工具。

三、吸入药物的方案选择

ICS/LABA、双支扩与三联疗法的选择仍然是COPD治疗领域的研究热点。

(一)双支扩剂的使用

对于没有使用ICS的COPD低加重风险患者,长效双支扩剂相比单支扩剂在改善症状和预防短期疾病恶化或治疗失败方面的递增效益,此前缺乏前瞻性证据。EMAX试验是一项为期24周的随机双盲对照试验,纳入不用ICS的低加重风险患者,随机分配至乌美溴铵/维兰特罗62.5/25μg 1次/d、乌美溴铵62.5μg 1次/d或沙美特罗50μg 2次/d。在第24周,乌美溴铵/维兰特罗组的谷值FEV_1较基线的改善值大于乌美溴铵组(差值66 ml,95% CI 43~89,$P<0.001$)和沙美特罗组(差值141 ml,95%CI 118~164,$P<0.001$)。相比两种单一疗法,乌美溴铵/维兰特罗在24周内所有时间点均显示出短暂呼吸困难指数(TDI)持续改善,并显著降低首次临床重要恶化的风险。治疗组之间的安全性相似。这些发现表明,早期使用双支气管扩张剂有助于优化不用ICS的低加重风险患者组的治疗。

老年和气道限制较严重的COPD患者,吸入性支气管扩张药的疗效下降,尤其是干粉吸入器。由于合并症和衰弱风险增加、联合用药的可能性及药代动力学或药效学的差异,老年患者对药物安全性的担忧也在增加。一项事后汇总分析对7个≥12周的随机研究进行了调查,发现乌美溴铵/维兰特罗62.5/25μg在不同年龄和气流受限严重程度亚组中,始终显示出相对于噻托溴铵18μg或丙酸氟替卡松/沙美特罗250/50μg更加明显的肺功能改善,同时治疗组之间的安全性相似。这表明乌美溴铵/维兰特罗对老年患者和重度/极重度气道受限的患者均没有疗效下降,可在改善肺功能方面明显获益,且不必增加安全性方面的担忧。

(二)三联疗法与双重疗法

2019年,Chest 一项Meta分析探讨了将LAMA加入ICS/LABA组合的疗效与安全性。该研究纳入了13项随机对照试验,包括15 519例COPD患者。分析发现,相比ICS/LABA,ICS/LABA/LAMA可改善谷值FEV_1(平均差值104.86 ml,95%CI 86.74~122.99;证据等级:高质量),并预防AECOPD($R^2=0.78$,95% CI 0.71~0.85;证据等级:高质量)。在ICS/LABA治疗中添加LAMA不会影响心血管严重不良事件的风险(证据等级:中等质量)。因此,将ICS/LABA升级为三联治疗时,患者可明显临床获益,且不增加心血管严重不良事件的风险。

近年来,已有不少研究评估单剂量水平下吸入糖皮质激素(ICS)、长效毒蕈碱拮抗剂(LAMA)和长效$β_2$受体激动剂(LABA)的三重固定剂量方案对COPD的疗效,但尚缺乏双倍剂量水平的研究。The New England Journal of Medicine 在2020年6月发表的一篇文章中介绍了一项为期52周的3期随机试验,评估了不同ICS剂量水平的两种三联疗法对过去1年有至少1次急性加重史的中度至极重度COPD患者的疗效和安全性。患者随机分配至以下4个组中:两种2次/d的三联疗法(320μg 布地奈德或160μg布地奈德+18μg格隆溴铵+9.6μg福莫特罗)或两种双重疗法(18μg格隆溴铵+9.6μg福莫特罗,320μg布地奈德+9.6μg福莫特罗)。研究结果显示,在320μg布地奈德的三联疗法组、160μg的布地奈德三联疗法组、格隆溴铵-福莫特罗组和布地奈德-福莫特罗组,中度或重度急性加重频率分别是1.08次/年、1.07次/年、1.42次/年、1.24次/年。320μg布地奈德的三联疗法组,其急性加重发生率显著低于格隆溴铵-福莫特罗(降低24%,$R^2=0.76$)或布地奈德-福莫特罗(降低13%,$R^2=0.87$)。同样,采用160μg的布地奈德三联疗法的患者,急性加重发生率显著低于格隆溴铵-福莫特罗(降低25%,$R^2=0.75$)组或布地奈德-福莫特罗(降低14%,$R^2=0.86$)组。各治疗组中不良事件发生率相似。因此,该研究证实,相比两种双重疗法,每日2次的三联疗法可以显著降低中到重度AECOPD频率。

(三)嗜酸性粒细胞与ICS

近年的研究强调了COPD患者基线(EOS)计数与ICS降低急性加重频率之间的关系。IMPACT试验显示,与双重疗法相比,每日1次单吸入三联疗法显著减少了急性加重。2019年 Lancet Respiratory Medicine 报道了IMPACT研究的事后分析,探索血液EOS计数和吸烟状况对ICS治疗反应的影响。该分析通过多种建模方式,发现与不含ICS的双支扩剂组(乌美溴铵-维兰特罗)相比,含ICS方案(糠酸氟替卡松-乌美溴铵-维兰特罗,糠酸氟替卡松-维兰特罗)降低中重度急性加重频率的获益幅度与血液EOS计数成正比。血EOS计数少于90/μl时,三联疗法与双支扩剂之间中重度急性加重率比为0.88(95% CI 0.74~1.04);血EOS计数≥310/μl时,该率比为0.56(95%CI 0.47~0.66);在这2种EOS水平,糠酸氟替卡松-维兰特罗与乌美溴铵-维兰特罗的相应率比分别为1.09(95%CI 0.91~1.29)和0.56(95%CI 0.47~0.66)。不同水平的血EOS,三联疗法与双支扩剂组在FEV_1、TDI和SGRQ总评分等方面的差异类似。吸烟状态改变了EOS计数与疗效(包括中重度急性加重,TDI和FEV_1)之间的关系,在任何EOS水平,既往吸烟者对ICS的治疗反应都比正在吸烟者更敏感。这表明,对于有急性加重病史的COPD患者,血液EOS计数和吸烟状况有潜力在临床实践中优化ICS的使用。

四、急性加重期的药物治疗

全身性糖皮质激素治疗AECOPD有许多不良反应,

迫切需要减少全身性糖皮质激素暴露的策略,并且需要个性化生物标志物指导。2019 年 Lancet Respiratory Medicine 发表了一项多中心随机对照、开放标签的非劣效性试验的结果。该试验中,COPD 患者在入院后 24h 内随机分配至 EOS 引导疗法组或全身性糖皮质激素标准疗法组。所有患者在第 1 天静脉注射 80 mg 甲泼尼龙。EOS 引导组:从第 2 天开始,当血液 EOS 计数≥0.3×10^9/L 时,每天给予泼尼松龙口服片剂 37.5 mg(最多长达 4d)。当 EOS 计数较低时,不给予泼尼松龙。对照组:从第 2 天开始,每天接受 37.5 mg 泼尼松龙片,共 4d。意向治疗分析发现,14d 内存活并出院的天数之间没有组间差异:EOS 引导组平均 8.9d(95%CI 8.3~9.6),而对照组为 9.3d(8.7~9.9)(绝对差 -0.4, 95%CI -1.3~0.5;P = 0.34)。两组间 30d 治疗失败(即因 AECOPD 急诊就诊,入院或需要加强药物治疗)、病死率没有显著差异。EOS 引导组中全身性激素治疗的中位时间较短[2(IQR 1.0~3.0) vs 5(5.0~5.0)d, P <0.001]。该研究提示 EOS 引导疗法在生存和出院天数方面均不逊于标准疗法,并且减少了全身糖皮质激素暴露的持续时间。仍需更大型的研究以确定此策略的全面安全性及其在 AECOPD 管理中的作用。

尽管存在争议,抗生素是仍是目前治疗 AECOPD 的常用手段。如何避免抗生素滥用,也是 COPD 研究领域的难点。在医院研究中,约 80%的 AECOPD 由非感染性因素引起。但在基层医疗,抗生素处方通常仅基于临床特征(痰量增加和脓性增加等),较为主观,不能准确预测哪些患者无须抗生素即可安全治疗。C 反应蛋白(CRP)快速检测可能有助于减少不必要的抗生素使用同时不损害患者安全。一项多中心、开放标签的随机对照试验,将 653 例 AECOPD 患者随机分为 CRP 指导组或常规护理组。与常规治疗组相比,CRP 指导组中 4 周内使用抗生素治疗 AECOPD 患者更少(57.0% vs. 77.4%;调整后 R^2 0.31;95%CI 0.20~0.47),2 周时临床 COPD 问卷(CCQ 评分)的校正平均差异为 -0.19 分(双侧 90%CI, -0.33~-0.05),提示 CRP 指导组健康状况倾向于更好。该研究证实,在初级保健诊所中,CRP 指导抗生素使用可以降低抗生素处方的比例,并且对患者没有额外的损害。

阿奇霉素可预防 AECOPD,但在需要住院治疗的 AECOPD 中的价值仍有待确定。BACE 试验是一项多中心、随机,双盲、安慰剂对照试验,研究了低剂量阿奇霉素对治疗失败率(TF)的影响。吸烟史≥10 包/年,上一年至少 1 次急性加重史的 301 名 AECOPD 住院患者,在入院后 48h 内随机(1:1)接受阿奇霉素或安慰剂。在对全身糖皮质激素和抗生素进行标准化急性治疗的基础上,给予研究药物 500 mg/d,持续 3 d;随后 250 mg/2 d,持续 3 个月;此后随访 6 个月。TF 定义为全身性糖皮质激素和(或)抗生素强化治疗、因呼吸原因加强住院治疗或再次入院,或全因死亡。阿奇霉素组 3 个月内的 TF 率为 49%,安慰剂组为 60%(HR 0.73;95%CI 0.53~1.01;P = 0.0526)。阿奇霉素和安慰剂组的强化治疗率、加强住院治疗率及 3 个月内的病死率分别为 47% vs. 60%(P = 0.027 2)、13% vs. 28%(P = 0.002 4)和 2% vs. 4%(P = 0.507 5)。停药后 6 个月失去临床益处。因此,对于需要住院治疗的传染性 AECOPD,使用阿奇霉素 3 个月可能会在最高风险期间显著降低 TF,而延长治疗似乎对于维持临床获益很有必要。为确定最可能受益的临床亚组,研究者对 BACE 试验进行事后分析,发现在入院时 CRP 高(>50 mg/L, R^2 = 0.18, 95%CI 0.05~0.60, P = 0.005)或血液 EOS 减少(<300cells/μl, R^2 = 0.33, 95%CI 0.17~0.64, P = 0.001)的患者中,阿奇霉素可显著降低 3 个月内再住院率,表明这些生物标志物在指导阿奇霉素治疗中具有潜在作用。

五、其他治疗方式

此前有观察性研究表明,β 受体阻滞剂可以降低中度或重度 COPD 患者急性加重和死亡的风险,但尚未在随机试验中得到证实。BLOCK COPD Trial Group 开展了一项前瞻性随机试验,532 例 40~85 岁的中度气流受限、有较高急性加重风险的 COPD 患者随机接受美托洛尔缓释剂或安慰剂治疗,随访约 1 年,发现到首次急性加重的中位时间没有显著组间差异(202d vs.222d, P = 0.66)。美托洛尔导致住院的急性加重风险更高(HR 1.91,95%CI 1.29~2.83),两组非呼吸性严重不良事件的总发生率相似。因此,或许需要更多的随机试验确定 β 受体阻滞剂对 COPD 患者的总的风险获益比。

高达 40%的 COPD 稳定患者可能患有嗜酸性粒细胞炎症,这与加重风险和糖皮质激素反应性增加有关。减少血液中 EOS 的针对性治疗方法可能会降低 COPD 加重的风险。贝那利珠单抗(benralizumab)是一种 IL-5 受体 α 定向溶细胞单克隆抗体,可通过依赖抗体的细胞毒性作用诱导 EOS 直接、快速和大量消耗。在一项 2 期试验中,发现基线血 EOS≥200/mm^3 的患者,贝那利珠单抗治疗后急性加重率低于安慰剂组,虽然差异不显著。2019 年,The New England Journal of Medicine 报道了两项 3 期临床试验(GALATHEA 和 TERRANOVA)的结果,以评估贝那利珠单抗在预防中重度 COPD 患者的急性加重方面的功效和安全性。接受规范吸入治疗后仍经常发生急性加重的 COPD 患者被纳入研究。患者随机接受贝那利珠单抗(在 GALATHEA 中为 30 mg 或 100 mg;在 TERRANOVA 中为 10 mg、30 mg 或 100 mg)或安慰剂治疗,前 3 剂量每 4 周 1 次,后续治疗每 8 周 1 次,观察基线血 EOS≥220/mm^3 的患者在第 56 周时的年 COPD 加重率比。在 GALATHEA 队列,相比于安慰剂组,30 mg、100mg 贝那利珠单抗组的年化急性加重率比分别为 0.96(P = 0.65)、0.83(P = 0.05);在 TERRANOVA 队列,贝那利珠单抗 10 mg、30 mg 和 100 mg 和安慰剂的年均急性加重率比为 0.85(P = 0.06)、1.04(P = 0.66)和 0.93(P = 0.40),差异均未达到显著水平。这表明,在中度至极重度、有频繁的中重度急性加重史以及血 EOS≥220/mm^3 的 COPD 患者中,贝那利珠单抗治疗不会降低急性加重频率。这与贝那利珠单抗治疗严重 EOS 性哮喘患者的结果相反,提示 EOS 的耗竭可能不会改善大多数伴有 EOS 增多的 COPD

患者的急性加重结果。需要进行进一步的调查,以确定可能受益于抗 IL-5 受体抗体治疗的 COPD 患者亚型。

2019 年以来,关于 COPD 的研究报道较多,涵盖了发病机制、疾病亚型、生物标志物、急性加重预测、吸入药物方案选择和其他治疗方式等。最主要的研究热点仍然是围绕着稳定期药物治疗的选择和相关的因素。几个大型临床研究探索了 β 受体阻滞剂、IL-5 受体抗体等药物在 COPD 治疗领域的的应用。血 EOS、CRP 和吸烟史等对于个体化治疗的指导作用日益凸显。仍需要更多的研究促进 COPD 的分型评估和精准治疗。

参 考 文 献

[1] 健康中国行动推进委员会. 健康中国行动(2019—2030 年). http://www. gov. cn/xinwen/2019-07/15/content_5409694. htm(2019-07-15).

[2] Sakornsakolpat P,Prokopenko D,Lamontagne M,et al. Genetic landscape of chronic obstructive pulmonary disease identifies heterogeneous cell-type and phenotype associations. Nat Genet,2019,51(3):494-505.

[3] Genschmer KR,Russell DW,Lal C,et al. Activated PMN exosomes:pathogenic entities causing matrix destruction and disease in the lung. Cell,2019,176(1-2):113-126.

[4] Wells JM,Xing D,Viera L,et al. The matrikine acetyl-proline-glycine-proline and clinical features of COPD:findings from SPIROMICS. Respir Res,2019,20(1):254.

[5] Christenson SA,van den Berge M,Faiz A,et al. An airway epithelial IL-17A response signature identifies a steroid-unresponsive COPD patient subgroup. J Clin Invest,2019,129(1):169-181.

[6] Park J,Hobbs BD,Crapo JD,et al. Subtyping COPD by using visual and quantitative CT imaging features. Chest,2020,157(1):47-60.

[7] Bellou V,Belbasis L,Konstantinidis AK,et al. Prognostic models for outcome prediction in patients with chronic obstructive pulmonary disease:systematic review and critical appraisal. BMJ,2019,367:l5358.

[8] Adibi A,Sin DD,Safari A,et al. The acute COPD exacerbation prediction tool(ACCEPT):a modelling study. Lancet Respir Med,2020,8(10):1013-1021.

[9] Maltais F,Bjermer L,Kerwin EM,et al. Efficacy of umeclidinium/vilanterol versus umeclidinium and salmeterol monotherapies in symptomatic patients with COPD not receiving inhaled corticosteroids:the EMAX randomised trial. Respir Res,2019,20(1):238.

[10] Ray R,Tombs L,Naya I,et al. Efficacy and safety of the dual bronchodilator combination umeclidinium/vilanterol in COPD by age and airflow limitation severity:a pooled post hoc analysis of seven clinical trials. Pulm Pharmacol Ther,2019,57:101802.

[11] Calzetta L,Cazzola M,Matera MG,et al. Adding a LAMA to ICS/LABA therapy:a Meta-analysis of triple combination therapy in COPD. Chest,2019,155(4):758-770.

[12] Rabe KF,Martinez FJ,Ferguson GT,et al. Triple inhaled therapy at two glucocorticoid doses in moderate-to-very-severe COPD. N Engl J Med,2020,383(1):35-48.

[13] Pascoe S,Barnes N,Brusselle G,et al. Blood eosinophils and treatment response with triple and dual combination therapy in chronic obstructive pulmonary disease:analysis of the IMPACT trial. Lancet Respir Med,2019,7(9):745-756.

[14] Sivapalan P,Lapperre TS,Janner J,et al. Eosinophil-guided corticosteroid therapy in patients admitted to hospital with COPD exacerbation(CORTICO-COP):a multicentre,randomised,controlled,open-label,non-inferiority trial. Lancet Respir Med,2019,7(8):699-709.

[15] Papi A,Bellettato CM,Braccioni F,et al. Infections and airway inflammation in chronic obstructive pulmonary disease severe exacerbations. Am J Respir Crit Care Med,2006,173(10):1114-1121.

[16] Anthonisen NR,Manfreda J,Warren CP,et al. Antibiotic therapy in exacerbations of chronic obstructive pulmonary disease. Ann Intern Med,1987,106(2):196-204.

[17] Miravitlles M,Moragas A,Hernández S,et al. Is it possible to identify exacerbations of mild to moderate COPD that do not require antibiotic treatment? Chest,2013,144(5):1571-1577.

[18] Butler CC,Gillespie D,White P,et al. C-reactive protein testing to guide antibiotic prescribing for COPD exacerbations. N Engl J Med,2019,381(2):111-120.

[19] Vermeersch K,Gabrovska M,Aumann J,et al. Azithromycin during acute chronic obstructive pulmonary disease exacerbations requiring hospitalization(BACE). A multicenter,randomized,double-blind,placebo-controlled trial. Am J Respir Crit Care Med,2019,200(7):857-868.

[20] Vermeersch K,Belmans A,Bogaerts K,et al. Treatment failure and hospital readmissions in severe COPD exacerbations treated with azithromycin versus placebo-a post-hoc analysis of the BACE randomized controlled trial. Respir Res,2019,20(1):237.

[21] Gottlieb SS,McCarter RJ,Vogel RA. Effect of beta-blockade on mortality among high-risk and low-risk patients after myocardial infarction. N Engl J Med,1998,339(8):489-497.

[22] Du Q,Sun Y,Ding N,et al. Beta-blockers reduced the risk of mortality and exacerbation in patients with COPD:a meta-analysis of observational studies. PLoS One,2014,9(11):e113048.

[23] Dransfield MT,Voelker H,Bhatt SP,et al. Metoprolol for the prevention of acute exacerbations of COPD. N Engl J Med,2019,381(24):2304-2314.

[24] Agusti A,Fabbri LM,Singh D,et al. Inhaled corticosteroids in COPD:friend or foe? Eur Respir J,2018,52(6):1801219.

[25] Yun JH,Lamb A,Chase R,et al. Blood eosinophil count thresholds and exacerbations in patients with chronic obstructive pulmonary disease. J Allergy Clin Immunol,2018,141(6):2037-2047.

[26] Pavord I D,Chanez P,Criner GJ,et al. Mepolizumab for eosinophilic chronic obstructive pulmonary disease. N Engl J

Med,2017,377(17):1613-1629.
[27] Brightling CE, Bleecker ER, Panettieri RJ, et al. Benralizumab for chronic obstructive pulmonary disease and sputum eosinophilia: a randomised, double-blind, placebo-controlled, phase 2a study. Lancet Respir Med,2014,2(11):891-901.
[28] Criner GJ, Celli BR, Brightling CE, et al. Benralizumab for the prevention of COPD exacerbations. N Engl J Med,2019, 381(11):1023-1034.

2 从 GOLD2020 更新看慢性阻塞性肺疾病个体化治疗

文富强　申永春

慢性阻塞性肺疾病（简称慢阻肺，COPD）是一种通常是由于暴露于有毒颗粒或气体引起的气道和（或）肺泡异常所导致、以持续呼吸症状和气流受限为主要临床特征、常见的、可以预防和治疗的异质性疾病。慢阻肺发病率、致残率、病死率高，给患者和社会带来较大的经济与社会负担，慢阻肺已成为世界范围内危害公众健康的严重公共卫生问题。王辰院士领衔的大规模人群研究"中国成人肺部健康研究"发现，我国 20 岁以上成人的慢阻肺患病率为 8.6%，40 岁以上则达 13.7%，60 岁以上人群患病率已超过 27%，据此估算我国慢阻肺总患病人数为 9990 万（即约 1 亿人），慢阻肺已构成我国重大疾病负担。来自中国疾控中心的数据显示，慢阻肺位列 2017 年中国人群死亡损失健康生命年的第 4 名，位列 2017 年中国人群死亡原因的第 3 名，病死率高达 68/10 万人，慢阻肺已成为严重危害人民生命安全的疾病。围绕慢阻肺领域内的一系列问题，慢阻肺全球创议（Global Initiative for Chronic Obstructive Lung Disease，GOLD）组织世界范围的慢阻肺领域专家，逐年度更新慢阻肺领域的研究进展，为慢阻肺的诊断、评估、治疗提供一系列指导性文件。2020 年度 GOLD 更新为慢阻肺的治疗提供了更详细的研究证据，指导慢阻肺的治疗更加个体化、精准化，现就 2020 年 GOLD 更新中慢阻肺的个体化治疗进行临床解读。

一、慢阻肺的个体化治疗始于初治阶段

GOLD2020 仍然延续了上一年度的 ABCD 分组方案，根据呼吸困难评分、慢阻肺评估评分（COPD Assessment Test，CAT）、既往的急性家族史/住院史将慢阻肺患者分为 A、B、C、D 共 4 组，并为每一组患者提供了初始治疗推荐方案（图 2-2-1）。根据推荐，根据患者临床特征 D 组患者初始治疗推荐使用长效胆碱能受体拮抗剂（long-acting muscarine anticholinergic，LAMA），对于临床症状明显（如 CAT 评分>20 分），可联用 LAMA+长效 β_2 受体激动剂（long acting beta-agonists，LABA）双支扩剂，对于嗜酸性粒细胞计数超过 300/μl 的 D 组患者，可以考虑 LABA+吸入糖皮质激素（inhaled corticosteroid，ICS）联合使用。GOLD2020 为慢阻肺患者的初始治疗提供了一个初步的建议，避免了慢阻肺患者初始治疗无据可循的境况。需要注意的是，目前没有包括随机对照研究之类的高质量研究证据支持这个初始治疗方案，慢阻肺初始治疗的个体化之路还在探索之中。

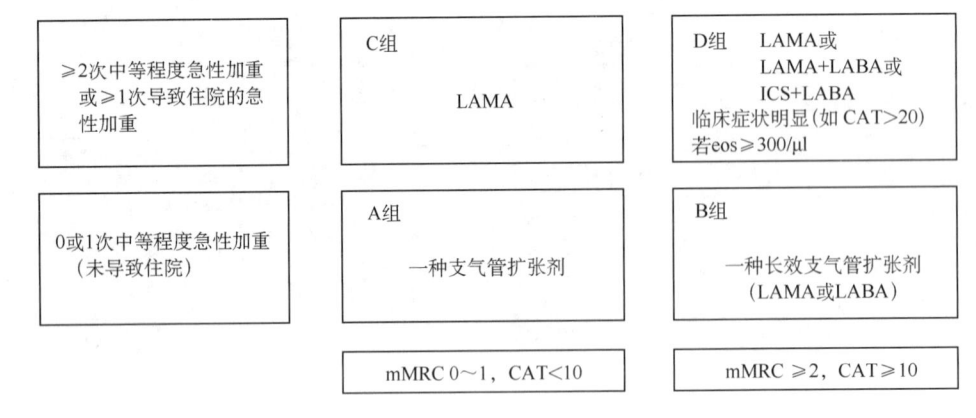

≥2次中等程度急性加重或≥1次导致住院的急性加重	C组 LAMA	D组　LAMA或 LAMA+LABA或 ICS+LABA 临床症状明显（如 CAT>20） 若 eos≥300/μl
0或1次中等程度急性加重（未导致住院）	A组 一种支气管扩张剂	B组 一种长效支气管扩张剂 （LAMA或LABA）
	mMRC 0~1，CAT<10	mMRC ≥2，CAT≥10

图 2-2-1　慢阻肺初始治疗推荐方案

注：CAT. COPD Assessment Test；LABA. Long acting beta-agonists；LAMA. Long-acting muscarine anticholinergic；mMRC. modified British medical research council.

二、慢阻肺治疗的再评估：探索中寻找到治疗慢阻肺的最佳方案

慢阻肺临床表型复杂、患者对不同治疗药物治疗的反应和效果存在较大的差异。如果当前的治疗方案疗效欠佳，慢阻肺的治疗如何调整？GOLD2019尝试对此做了回答：通过评估患者的临床症状与急性加重情况，对治疗方案进行调整。GOLD 2020延续了上一年度的推荐，比如对于初治疗单用LABA或LAMA后呼吸困难缓解不明显的患者，可考虑联合LABA和LAMA双支气管扩张剂治疗；初始治疗选用LABA＋ICS后呼吸困难缓解不明显的患者，可考虑加用LAMA。对于初始治疗后仍有持续的急性加重的患者，GOLD2020也做了相应的治疗调整方案推荐（图2-2-2）。GOLD2020强调慢阻肺治疗全程的反复评估，根据不同的治疗反应调整相应的治疗方案，让个体化治疗的原则贯穿于慢阻肺患者的全程治疗。

1. 若起始治疗合适，则维持原治疗方案
2. 若起始治疗不合适：
  ✓ 针对最主要的症状治疗（呼吸困难或急性加重；若两个症状同时存在，则首先解决急性加重）
  ✓ 根据患者现有治疗将其放入下图中相应位置，并遵循流程图进行下一步治疗
  ✓ 评估治疗反应，调整用药，并回顾疗效
  ✓ 该治疗建议与患者诊断时的ABCD分组无关

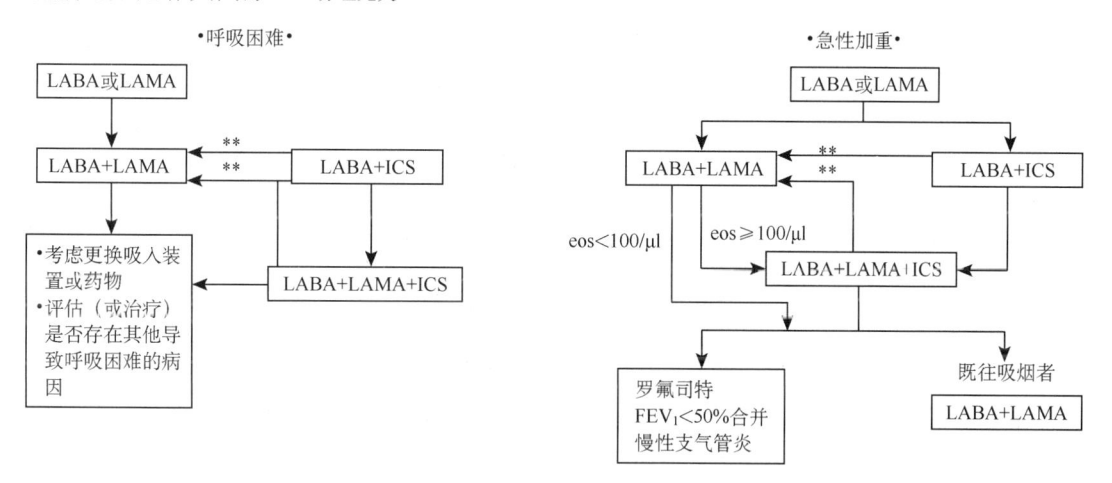

· 呼吸困难 ·

· 急性加重 ·

*如果嗜酸性粒细胞≥300/μl或者嗜碱性粒细胞≥100/μl且≥2次中等程度急性加重/1次住院
**若发生肺炎、无恰当适应证或对ICS治疗无反应，则考虑ICS降级治疗或改用其他治疗

图2-2-2 慢阻肺治疗调整

三、ICS的使用临床精准化

ICS通过发挥其抗感染作用在慢阻肺的治疗中发挥着重要作用，但是ICS的使用如何更加精准，慢阻肺患者可以通过ICS的治疗达到最大的临床获益，之前还没有更好的临床推荐。GOLD2020对此给出了详细的推荐意见：对于有慢阻肺急性加重住院病史、中度慢阻肺急性加重≥2次/年（均在适当的长效支气管扩张剂维持治疗后），外周血嗜酸性粒细胞（eosinophils，EOS）＞300/μl，具有哮喘病史或者合并哮喘的患者，强烈支持在慢阻肺的初始治疗中包含ICS，对于每年1次中度慢阻肺急性加重期的患者、外周血EOS在100～300/μl的患者，可考虑使用ICS，如果患者有反复的肺炎，外周血EOS＜100/μl，存在结核分枝杆菌感染史，则反对使用ICS。既往的研究报道使用ICS可能会增加慢阻肺患者的肺炎发生率，增加结核感染的风险。GOLD2020首次对ICS的使用与否提出了临床推荐，为慢阻肺的个体化治疗提供了进一步的参考建议。鉴于中国慢阻肺患者人群既往多有不规则使用全身糖皮质激素而影响外周血常规结果，临床见到急性加重频繁具有严重气道炎症特征的患者EOS并不高。因此，中国患者可以尝试以100/μl为使用ICS的界值，更精确的中国慢阻肺患者EOS临界值还在探索研究中。

四、EOS在运用ICS治疗慢阻中的标志物作用

近年来的研究关注到EOS计数在慢阻肺治疗中的潜在标志物价值，可用于指导患者是否使用ICS治疗，然而目前关于EOS在慢阻肺中的指导地位仍有争论。GOLD2020就这个问题进行了进一步的总结。一般而言，ICS对于外周血EOS＜100/μl的慢阻肺患者可能效果欠佳，对于外周血EOS＞300/μl的慢阻肺患者可能效果较好，这2个阈值可初步预测患者是否会从ICS的治疗中获得临床获益。同时GOLD2020也指出，将外周血EOS计数用于预测ICS时还需要与患者的临床特征相结合，比如

既往的急性加重病史。其他影响因素比如吸烟、人种、地域等的影响还需要进一步研究。关于 EOS 在慢阻肺急性加重的指导作用，GOLD2020 总结了来自丹麦的一项随机对照研究，该研究发现糖皮质激素治疗外周血 EOS 较低的慢阻肺急性加重患者的临床疗效可能较差，嗜酸性粒细胞指导的治疗有助于减少系统性糖皮质激素使用的持续时间。目前的研究关于外周血 EOS 计数与 ICS 疗效的关系仍存在不同的结果，ICS 用于慢阻肺患者一定要进行个体化评估，进行个体化治疗。

五、C 反应蛋白指导慢阻肺急性加重期的抗生素使用

如何评估与选择抗感染治疗在慢阻肺急性加重中的时间与用量仍然是临床工作的难题，GOLD2020 总结了将 C 反应蛋白(C-reactive protein，CPR)运用于指导慢阻肺急性加重患者抗生素使用的价值。来自英国的一项多中心、随机对照研究评估了采用 CRP 及时检测能否安全减少初级保健机构慢阻肺急性加重患者的抗生素使用，该研究遵循指南建议对患者进行评估指导抗生素使用：对于 CRP 水平＜20 mg/L 者，抗感染治疗无益，不使用；对于 CRP 水平为 20～40 mg/L 者，抗生素治疗可能有益；对于 CRP 水平＞40 mg/L 者，抗生素治疗可能有益。研究发现 CRP 指导组的抗生素使用率显著低于常规治疗组，基于 CRP 的抗感染策略可以减少初级保健机构慢阻肺急性加重患者抗生素的使用。来自荷兰的针对住院慢阻肺急性加重患者的研究表明，根据 CRP 指导可显著降低抗生素的使用率，并且同时对 30d 治疗失败率、至下次急性加重时间、住院天数的影响无差异，在临床实践中将 CRP 作为指导慢阻肺急性加重抗生素治疗的生物标志物可明显降低抗生素使用频率，GOLD2020 中对此进行了总结，对于慢阻肺急性加重期的抗生素使用提出了更加精准的个体化要求。

六、口服类药物的个体化运用

罗氟司特是一种磷酸二酯酶Ⅳ抑制剂，其抗感染机制在慢阻肺的治疗中发挥着潜在的作用。罗氟司特可以降低慢阻肺急性加重风险，给患者带来临床获益。GOLD2020 总结：罗氟司特可能对具有住院史的重度慢阻肺患者带来更大的临床受益，为罗氟司特在慢阻肺的临床个体化治疗带来了进一步的研究证据。大环内酯类抗生素不仅具有抗菌活性，还有免疫调节活性，临床研究已证明阿奇霉素可用于稳定期慢阻肺患者的治疗，降低其急性加重频率。研究发现，阿奇霉素或红霉素一年期的干预可显著降低慢阻肺急性加重高风险的患者急性加重风险，亚组分析显示这种临床获益对于正在吸烟的患者疗效较差。他汀类药物也具有一定的抗感染活性，在慢阻肺的治疗中具有潜在的价值。虽然随机对照研究未能证实辛伐他汀(40 mg/d)干预能给高急性加重风险的慢阻肺患者带来降低急性加重频率方面的获益，但是来自大样本的临床随访研究发现，他汀类药物可能会降低合并心血管疾病的慢阻肺患者的急性加重风险。循证医学的研究证据表明，补充维生素 D 疗效安全，但是只降低了基线 25-羟基维生素 D 水平＜25 nmol/L 这部分慢阻肺患者中/重度慢阻肺急性加重的比例，不能降低基线 25-羟基维生素 D 水平较高的患者中/重度慢阻肺急性加重的比例。GOLD2020 对这些研究进行了总结，口服类药物的临床使用可能存在其优势人群，在特定的慢阻肺患者中可能才发挥作用，这也是慢阻肺治疗的个体化需探索之处。

总体来说，GOLD2020 在延续上一年度的基础上，继续对慢阻肺的诊断、治疗等策略进行了临床更新，将个体化治疗的思维贯穿于慢阻肺治疗的初始阶段、全程再评估再治疗之中，对 ICS 的精准使用、外周血 EOS 在 ICS 疗效预测、慢阻肺急性加重抗生素使用生物标志物、口服类药物的优势人群选择进行了系统总结与推荐。慢阻肺是一种异质性疾病，具有不同的临床特征与表型，不同的表型对临床治疗的反应不尽一致，为慢阻肺的治疗提出了个体化的需求。未来的研究需要进一步探索慢阻肺的个体化临床特征，为药物的精准使用提供更多的研究证据。随着个体化治疗方案越来越多地运用在慢阻肺患者中，将为慢阻肺患者带来最大程度的临床获益。

参 考 文 献

[1] Lareau SC, Fahy B, Meek P, et al. Chronic obstructive pulmonary disease(COPD). Am J Respir Crit Care Med, 2019, 199(1):1-2.

[2] Wang C, Xu J, Yang L, et al. Prevalence and risk factors of chronic obstructive pulmonary disease in China (the China Pulmonary Health [CPH] study): a national cross-sectional study. Lancet, 2018, 391(10131):1706-1717.

[3] Zhou M, Wang H, Zeng X, et al. Mortality, morbidity, and risk factors in China and its provinces, 1990-2017: a systematic analysis for the Global Burden of Disease Study 2017. Lancet, 2019, 394(10204):1145-1158.

[4] Global Strategy for the Diagnosis, Management, and Prevention of Chronic Obstructive Lung Disease: 2020 report. https://goldcopd.org/wp-content/uploads/2019/12/GOLD-2020-FINAL-ver1.2-03Dec19_WMV.pdf.

[5] 陈亚红. 2020 年 GOLD 慢性阻塞性肺疾病诊断、治疗及预防全球策略解读. 中国医学前沿杂志(电子版), 2019, 11(12):32-50.

[6] Yang IA, Clarke MS, Sim EH, et al. Inhaled corticosteroids for stable chronic obstructive pulmonary disease. Cochrane Database Syst Rev, 2012(7):CD002991.

[7] Agusti A, Fabbri LM, Singh D, et al. Inhaled corticosteroids in COPD: friend or foe? Eur Respir J, 2018, 52(6):1801219.

[8] Yang M, Du Y, Chen H, et al. Inhaled corticosteroids and risk

of pneumonia in patients with chronic obstructive pulmonary disease: A meta-analysis of randomized controlled trials. Int Immunopharmacol,2019,77:105950.

[9] Dong YH,Chang CH,Wu FL,et al. Use of inhaled corticosteroids in patients with COPD and the risk of TB and influenza: A systematic review and meta-analysis of randomized controlled trials. Chest,2014,145(6):1286-1297.

[10] Bafadhel M,Peterson S,De Blas MA,et al. Predictors of exacerbation risk and response to budesonide in patients with chronic obstructive pulmonary disease: a post-hoc analysis of three randomised trials. Lancet Respir Med,2018,6(2):117-126.

[11] Sivapalan P,Lapperre TS,Janner J,et al. Eosinophil-guided corticosteroid therapy in patients admitted to hospital with COPD exacerbation (CORTICO-COP): a multicentre, randomised, controlled, open-label, non-inferiority trial. Lancet Respir Med,2019,7(8):699-709.

[12] Butler CC,Gillespie D,White P,et al. C-reactive protein testing to guide antibiotic prescribing for COPD exacerbations. N Engl J Med,2019,381(2):111-120.

[13] Prins HJ,Duijkers R,van der Valk P,et al. CRP-guided antibiotic treatment in acute exacerbations of COPD in hospital admissions. Eur Respir,2019,53(5):1802014.

[14] Rabe KF,Calverley PMA,Martinez FJ,et al. Effect of roflumilast in patients with severe COPD and a history of hospitalisation. Eur Respir J,2017,50(1):1700158.

[15] Albert RK,Connett J,Bailey WC,et al. Azithromycin for prevention of exacerbations of COPD. N Engl J Med,2011,365(8):689-698.

[16] Han MK,Tayob N,Murray S,et al. Predictors of chronic obstructive pulmonary disease exacerbation reduction in response to daily azithromycin therapy. Am J Respir Crit Care Med,2014,189(12):1503-1508.

[17] Criner GJ,Connett JE,Aaron SD,et al. Simvastatin for the prevention of exacerbations in moderate-to-severe COPD. N Engl J Med,2014,370(23):2201-2210.

[18] Ingebrigtsen TS,Marott JL,Nordestgaard BG,et al. Statin use and exacerbations in individuals with chronic obstructive pulmonary disease. Thorax,2015,70(1):33-40.

[19] Jolliffe DA,Greenberg L,Hooper RL,et al. Vitamin D to prevent exacerbations of COPD: systematic review and meta-analysis of individual participant data from randomised controlled trials. Thorax,2019,74(4):337-345.

3 慢性阻塞性肺疾病及其主要合并症的机制关联研究进展

张 静 孙永昌

慢性阻塞性肺疾病(简称慢阻肺,COPD)气流受限进行性发展,与气道和肺对有毒颗粒或气体的慢性炎性反应增强有关,同时也伴随着显著的肺外效应,这些伴随疾病,被称为慢阻肺合并症。研究资料显示,几乎所有患者都至少患有一种合并症,而超过50%的患者患有4种以上合并症。慢阻肺最常见的合并症是心血管疾病(CVD)、代谢综合征(MS)、骨质疏松、骨骼肌功能障碍等。慢阻肺与这些合并症之间存在共同的风险因素,如吸烟、社会经济状况、肺功能低下和职业接触、衰老等。研究表明,慢阻肺与某些合并症之间存在独特的相互作用,而不是简单地合并存在。这些合并症的存在可能影响慢阻肺的结局,导致疾病快速进展,反复出现急性加重,增加病死率,也可能影响慢阻肺治疗过程中的用药决策。因此,慢阻肺及其合并症的关联机制成为近年来关注的热点问题。

一、概述

慢阻肺合并症可以出现于慢阻肺的任何阶段。目前研究发现,合并症与慢阻肺之间相关联的机制主要与全身炎症反应、氧化应激、衰老及吸烟相关。这几方面机制之间也相互影响,相互促进,导致慢阻肺多种合并症的出现。吸烟是慢阻肺最重要的危险因素,当呼吸道黏膜暴露于烟草烟雾或其他有害颗粒后,即引发呼吸道的炎症和氧化应激反应。氧化应激与肺部炎症相互促进,加重组织损伤,放大的炎症反应"溢出",可能是慢阻肺全身炎症的机制之一。吸烟和氧化应激的增加会损害端粒酶的活性,直接导致端粒缩短。端粒缩短导致衰老诱导途径 p21 激活,引起细胞衰老和促炎介质(如 IL-6 和 CXCL8)的释放。当然,不同系统的合并症也存在不同的关联机制。

二、心血管疾病

心血管疾病是慢阻肺患者最常见的致死原因。研究证实,第一秒用力呼气容积(FEV_1)每下降10%,则增加28%的心血管死亡风险和20%非致命心血管事件风险。慢阻肺患者并发心血管疾病的风险明显增加(*OR* 2.46,95% *CI* 2.02～3.0),其中包括缺血性心脏病、心律失常、心力衰竭、肺循环疾病及动脉血管疾病的风险较对照组高2～5倍。而慢阻肺与心血管疾病之间的关联,还可能涉及多种机制参与其中。

(一)全身炎症反应

大量研究发现,除了肺部的炎症,慢阻肺患者还普遍出现循环中炎症标志物的明显升高,如 CRP、IL-6、IL-8、TNF-α、纤维蛋白原、白细胞计数等,提示患者存在全身性的炎症反应,而这种全身性炎症反应,是来自肺部炎症介质的"溢出"还是慢阻肺并发症的一种全身性反应,现在尚未有定论。全身性炎症反应参与慢阻肺的肺外表现,尤其是增加患者的心血管疾病风险。促进动脉粥样硬化的发展是全身性炎症反应增加心血管疾病发生的一个重要途径。动脉粥样硬化的过程启始于炎症所致的血管内皮细胞损伤,活化的 T 淋巴细胞和巨噬细胞刺激细胞因子的释放,诱导内皮细胞黏附分子表达增加,促使循环中白细胞附壁并迁移至血管内膜;炎症环境中单核/巨噬细胞清道夫受体表达增加,增加脂质的摄取,促进泡沫细胞的发育;细胞因子如 IL-1、IL-6、TNF-α 还能促进粥样斑块形成物质的沉积,共同推动动脉粥样硬化的发展。此外,还有研究发现,炎症因子 CRP 可通过对一氧化氮复合酶抑制作用影响血管内皮功能,并抑制纤溶酶原激活物生成,损害内皮细胞的纤溶功能,进一步促进动脉粥样硬化斑块破裂后血栓形成。

(二)氧化应激

氧化应激水平的持续增高被认为是影响慢阻肺患者气道和全身炎症反应持续的主要因素。氧化应激与肺部炎症有相互促进:氧化剂可减弱中性粒细胞的变形能力,通过激活组蛋白乙酰转移酶解开染色质结构,促进多个炎症基因的表达,以及激活核因子-κB 和激活蛋白-1(AP-1)等胞内信号通路调节炎症介质释放,进一步放大炎症反应,而募集、活化的中性粒细胞释放氧自由基(ROS)加重组织损伤。氧化应激的增强除了可直接造成肺损伤或诱导各种细胞反应,还影响细胞外基质和血管的重塑,抗蛋白酶失活、细胞早衰、黏液分泌增加、激素抵抗增强,以及促进血管内皮功能障碍和动脉粥样硬化的发展,导致心肌细胞凋亡及心肌收缩力降低,影响左心室重构。

(三)缺氧

慢阻肺患者均存在不同程度的缺氧,尤其是在重度慢阻肺患者及慢阻肺急性加重期患者更明显。在缺氧条件下,血管内膜巨噬细胞中泡沫细胞的生成增加,同时缺氧诱导转录因子 HIF-1α 过表达,增加巨噬细胞的脂质含量,促进动脉粥样硬化斑块的形成和发展。另外,缺氧还可以增强全身炎症和氧化应激反应,促进凝血激活,上调细胞表面黏附分子,促进血栓形成。

(四) 交感神经过度激活

慢阻肺患者交感神经过度激活,最直接的原因可能源于低氧对外周化学感受器敏感性的影响,以及神经体液机制的激活。交感神经过度兴奋可促进左心室肥厚、动脉硬化、高血压及动脉粥样硬化性疾病的发生。在正常生理条件下,内皮细胞释放的舒张因子和交感神经末梢释放的收缩因子共同作用于血管平滑肌细胞,以维持适当的血管张力。交感神经过度激活破坏该平衡,导致血管内皮功能障碍。不仅如此,交感神经的过度激活还可能会通过升高的儿茶酚胺诱发巨噬细胞进入血管腔,以及增加内皮细胞摄取低密度脂蛋白等,共同促进内皮细胞介导的动脉粥样硬化的发展。此外,交感神经递质的浓度增加,加剧心肌细胞电重构的空间异质性,出现心肌电活动的不稳定;交感神经过度活跃还增强动脉收缩和血小板聚集,心肌细胞缺血影响其电活动,导致心律失常的发生。

(五) 衰老

衰老的标志包括端粒缩短、基因组不稳定、表观遗传改变、蛋白稳态丧失、线粒体功能障碍、营养感应失调和干细胞衰竭。吸烟和氧化应激通过其对DNA的损伤作用,激活mTOR信号转导和端粒缩短而加速衰老的过程。慢阻肺患者的肺内皮细胞和外周血白细胞端粒酶活性降低,端粒缩短,细胞衰老和衰老相关分泌表型(SASP)反应增强,导致衰老加速。在动脉粥样硬化斑块血管内皮细胞和外周血白细胞中也检测到端粒长度的缩短,而内皮细胞增生极低,其根本上来源于造血干细胞(HSC)内端粒的缩短。全身性炎症和氧化应激所致血管内皮细胞受损后,内皮祖细胞即从造血干细胞(HSC)中分化,迁移至血管损伤部位进行修复,故HSC端粒的缩短反映了内皮祖细胞储备的修复能力下降。血管内皮细胞损伤与祖细胞修复能力之间的失衡共同促进了血管内皮细胞功能障碍的发生,导致动脉硬化的进展。因此,细胞的加速老化也参与了慢阻肺患者心血管风险的发生。

三、骨质疏松和骨折

慢阻肺是继发性骨质疏松的首要病因。慢阻肺患者骨质疏松的发生率各项研究不尽一致,为8.7%~69%,平均35.1%。慢阻肺患者骨密度减低、骨小梁疏松、骨皮质宽度减低,均可导致骨脆性增加和骨折的发生。在吸烟者中,肺气肿是骨密度减低的独立预测因素,骨组织连接密度与吸烟(包年数)呈负相关,提示肺气肿与骨质疏松症之间可能存在机制上的关联。

目前研究表明全身炎症反应是慢阻肺合并骨质疏松的重要机制。烟草烟雾导致上皮细胞损伤后,局部炎症反应激活,除了基本的先天免疫过程外,后续的慢性炎症反应还涉及Th1、Th2、Th17系统的激活和肺内干细胞的持续激活。这种局部炎症过程的"溢出"可能是各种系统性炎症变化和并发症(包括骨质疏松症)的始动因素。Evelyn等采用调节性脂质磷酸酶SH2结构域的肌醇5′磷酸酶-1(SHIP-1)缺陷型小鼠建立自发性发展为明显的炎症性肺病的动物模型,其特征类似人类慢阻肺表现,伴有明显的气道和全身炎症、小气道纤维化及肺气肿表现。研究发现SHIP-1$^{-/-}$小鼠除了中性粒细胞、IL-6升高的全身炎症表现外,还出现了骨质减少的合并症。另一组同时敲除粒细胞集落刺激因子(G-CSF)和SHIP-1的小鼠,不但肺内炎症和全身炎症较轻,骨质疏松也明显改善。研究结果一方面说明中性粒细胞在慢阻肺发病机制中的重要作用,另一方面说明慢阻肺炎症与骨质疏松之间确实存在机制上的关联。临床研究也发现,骨密度较低的慢阻肺患者血中CRP和炎性细胞因子(TNF-α、IL-1和IL-6)水平较高。这三种细胞因子在体内外都是破骨细胞诱导分子,一直被认为与骨质疏松的发病机制有关。孙永昌等的研究显示,与骨密度正常患者相比,骨密度较低的COPD患者血清骨质疏松相关蛋白RANK配体水平较高,RANK配体/骨保护素的比例也更高。表达RANKL的中性粒细胞及RANKL阳性CD4T细胞和RANKL-和IL-17双阳性CD4 T细胞在男性慢阻肺患者中增加并且与BMD和肺功能相关。这些结果都提示全身性炎症在COPD相关性骨质疏松症的作用。

免疫机制在骨质疏松发生中的作用是近年来关注的热点。Th17细胞产生的白介素17(IL-17)在慢阻肺的发病机制中发挥重要作用,同时IL-17也是影响破骨细胞的重要细胞因子。孙永昌等观察了长期烟草烟雾(CS)暴露的野生型和IL-17A$^{-/-}$小鼠,与野生型小鼠相比,IL-17A$^{-/-}$小鼠的骨质流失和肺气肿较少;与CS暴露的野生型小鼠相比,CS暴露的IL-17A$^{-/-}$小鼠TRAP+破骨细胞数量减少,RANKL表达降低,血中IL-6和IL-1β等炎症细胞因子减少。表明IL-17A参与了CS引起的骨质丢失和全身炎症反应的发生,可能是慢阻肺与骨质疏松症之间的内在关联机制之一。

长期糖皮质激素(简称激素)治疗是骨质疏松症的常见原因。激素诱导的骨质疏松症(GIO)的发展依赖于每日剂量,曾有研究认为吸入激素(ICS)的使用大大减少了骨折的风险。最近的一项包括16项随机对照试验(RCT)的荟萃分析共纳入17 513名受试者和7项观察性研究与69 000名受试者,研究结果仍表明ICS与骨折风险弱相关(RCT中$OR=1.27$,观察性研究中1.21)。然而,在一项针对251名慢阻肺男性的研究中,ICS被证明可延缓每年骨密度丢失,最有可能的机制是由于减轻炎症反应的发生。因此,ICS的总体作用似乎取决于其局部抗炎作用的益处与其全身作用引起的骨折风险之间的平衡。

维生素D缺乏在慢阻肺患者中非常普遍,晚期慢阻肺患者维生素D水平更低,可能与阳光照射减少、食欲减退和吸烟有关。有推测维生素D的状态可能会影响慢阻肺发展和恶化。对维生素D浓度低于20 ng/ml的慢阻肺患者补充维生素D,发现确实可以使患者获益。维生素D缺乏会导致骨密度下降,骨质疏松的发生。一项纵向研究还发现,在100例稳定期慢阻肺患者中,基线维生素D缺乏会在3年随访期间使骨质疏松症发展的风险增加7.5倍。

四、骨骼肌功能障碍

骨骼肌功能障碍作为慢阻肺的全身效应之一，严重影响慢阻肺患者的生活质量及预后。目前的研究表明，FEV_1与慢阻肺患者运动耐力无显著相关性，20%～40%的慢阻肺患者肺功能没有严重受损，但表现为明显的骨骼肌萎缩或功能障碍导致活动耐力受限。骨骼肌功能障碍的发生是由多因素诱导、多种分子生物学机制参与的复杂过程，如前所述炎症、氧化应激、活动减少均可导致该合并症的发生。各种因素最终导致骨骼肌蛋白降解和合成之间的不平衡，蛋白降解增加大于蛋白合成，致使骨骼肌萎缩。

全身慢性炎症反应可以导致慢阻肺患者骨骼肌功能障碍。研究发现血中升高的炎症因子TNF-α、IL-6、CRP等均与慢阻肺患者肌肉的质量、体积和肌力下降密切相关。TNF-α通过骨骼肌细胞内泛素-蛋白酶体途径激活核转录因子NF-κB增强大鼠骨骼肌蛋白的分解代谢，引起骨骼肌萎缩。在慢阻肺急性发作期间，血清淀粉样蛋白A高度升高，引发Toll样受体2（TLR2）引起的强烈促炎反应，继而导致骨骼肌萎缩。

氧化应激是导致慢阻肺患者骨骼肌功能障碍的重要原因，氧化应激可抑制肌肉收缩力、加速蛋白分解、促进肌肉疲劳及萎缩。线粒体呼吸链是细胞内产生活性氧（ROS）的主要部位，也是活性氧的主要靶点，线粒体DNA对氧化损伤高度敏感，氧化应激很容易损伤线粒体DNA，从而导致线粒体功能受损。慢阻肺患者骨骼肌线粒体功能异常主要表现为氧化功能减低、线粒体活性（mtROS）氧增多和自噬及凋亡增加。研究表明，中重度慢阻肺患者股外侧肌氧化应激产物如超氧化物歧化酶、谷胱甘肽过氧化物酶增高。这些氧化应激产物损伤线粒体DNA导致离子传输链复合物功能失调，进而导致线粒体活性氧增多。mtROS激活转录因子forkhead box O（FOXOs）及NF-κB，通过泛素-26S蛋白酶体蛋白水解增加了肌丝蛋白降解，导致肌肉萎缩。细胞凋亡、细胞自噬等机制造成肌肉细胞的细胞核丢失，导致肌肉萎缩的发生，此后卫星细胞被激活，进行增生、分化并与肌纤维融合，用以补充细胞库。肌肉生长抑制素（MSTN）是肌生成的负调控因子，有研究显示慢阻肺患者肢体肌肉MSTN mRNA表达显著增加，提示肌肉生成受抑制。

研究发现慢阻肺患者长期慢性缺氧可影响全身的骨骼肌功能，促进膈肌疲劳。处于缺氧状态下的动物和人的体重指数、肌肉体积均有所缩小。机体和组织处于慢性缺氧状态可使骨骼肌纤维数量减少，骨骼肌纤维分型也发生改变，Ⅰ型和Ⅱa型肌纤维的构成比明显降低，而Ⅱb型肌纤维的构成比增加，股四头肌横截面积明显减小，从而表现为运动耐力的下降及对骨骼肌疲劳的高度敏感性。缺氧同样能够诱导瘦素的表达，导致食物摄入减少，肌肉消耗增加。

慢阻肺急性加重期常需要全身激素治疗。全身激素可导致肌肉萎缩和肌力下降，称之为激素相关性肌病。激素可影响肌肉功能的机制包括下调胰岛素样生长因子-1（IGF-1）表达，激活泛素蛋白酶体和溶酶体系统，同时上调肌生成抑制蛋白的表达，从而抑制肌肉蛋白合成，促进肌肉蛋白分解。

五、代谢综合征

代谢综合征（MetS）是一组包括过度肥胖，糖、脂代谢异常的复杂疾病，每种代谢因素相互关联，共同促进动脉粥样硬化的发生。根据国际糖尿病联合会的共识，吸烟和慢阻肺都不是MetS的危险因素，反之亦然。但与普通人群相比，慢阻肺患者中MetS的发病率较普通人群高2倍。慢阻肺和MetS并存时，两种疾病的病情均更重，合并症发生的概率均增加。虽然两种疾病之间没有明确的因果关系，但两者之间可能存在以下关联。

全身性炎症被称为MetS和慢阻肺的共同特征。E-CLIPSE研究发现，大多数表现为全身性炎症的患者，血液IL-8和TNF-α升高与吸烟相关，而不与慢阻肺相关。该研究随访期间，炎症组患者全因病死率较对照组增加了6倍。全身性炎症是导致MetS致病的主要因素。患有不同程度MetS的慢阻肺患者中TNF-α、IL-6、IL-8和CRP的水平均升高，TNF-α和IL-6升高可导致胰岛素抵抗。IL-8可通过抑制其受体信号转导直接减弱胰岛素的代谢作用，也可通过募集和激活单核细胞来加剧炎症反应，导致胰岛素抵抗状态恶化。TNF-α和IL-6等促炎因子释放到全身，介导远处的炎性反应，包括激活编码急性期反应物的基因，如纤维蛋白原、CRP和血清淀粉样蛋白A。CRP刺激进一步的细胞因子释放，以及单核细胞和内皮细胞中细胞黏附分子和组织因子的合成，进而可以激活外在凝血级联反应，加重炎症反应。

脂肪组织是炎性介质的重要来源。脂肪组织能够合成和分泌促炎因子、代谢激素、生长因子和血压调节物质。脂肪组织快速的扩张速度往往超过了血管生成的速度，导致深部组织的氧合不足和局部缺氧。脂肪组织缺氧是一种细胞应激形式，可刺激促炎介质IL-6、TNF-α、巨噬细胞迁移抑制因子、VEGF、金属蛋白酶-1的组织抑制剂、瘦素和单核细胞趋化蛋白的产生；同时下调抗炎脂肪因子脂联素的表达，从而加重炎症反应。慢阻肺急性加重期血清瘦素水平升高和瘦素与脂联素的比例增加伴经典促炎标志物如IL-6、TNF的升高，提示脂肪组织可能是肥胖的慢阻肺患者的重要炎症来源。与瘦素相反，脂联素可能是唯一被证实具有抗炎特性的脂肪细胞衍生因子。脂联素降低上皮细胞和单核细胞-巨噬细胞中TNF-α的产生和活性，抑制IL-6的产生，并诱导产生抗炎细胞因子。脂联素促进全身胰岛素敏感性和葡萄糖稳态。脂联素的血管生成作用还有助于改善脂肪组织扩张期间的血管形成，减少由于缺氧引起的局部炎症反应。脂联素还可能作用于内皮细胞以维持血管的稳态，对血管功能障碍有保护作用。瘦素和脂联素受体在人肺组织中均有表达。脂联素与吸烟和糖尿病的发病率呈负相关，这种脂肪组织与肺组织之间的联系提示脂联素是当前慢阻肺与MetS之间联系的最可能的机制。除局部脂肪组织缺氧外，肺功能下降引起的全身性缺氧也被认为是促炎细胞因子表达的重要始动因素。慢性间歇性缺氧会促进脂质失调和胆固醇生物合成,降低胰岛素敏感性。

慢阻肺患者的氧化应激反应会通过激活 NF-κB 介导的信号传导途径导致促炎介质的产生,产生全身性炎症反应。MetS 中氧化应激主要来自特定生化途径的激活(如线粒体中的氧化代谢)、炎症引起的细胞增生、细胞抗氧化机制的耗尽及脂质过氧化。一方面,由于吸烟引起的氧化应激通过胰岛素抵抗而促进糖尿病的发展;另一方面,MetS 的氧化应激通过激活炎症反应而进一步导致肺功能受损。慢性高血糖症可通过过量生成 ROS 触发糖尿病患者血管内皮功能障碍。值得关注的是,高血糖症引起的 ROS 水平升高可导致细胞应激通路(如 MAPK 和 NF-κB 介导的应激通路)激活,从而损害肺功能。在分离的人支气管组织中,高浓度的葡萄糖可通过 Rho 激酶介导的特定细胞途径增强气道平滑肌细胞对收缩剂的反应性。气道高反应性增强是导致慢阻肺患者肺功能加速下降的主要危险因素。此外,高血糖症还会通过在气道分泌物中出现葡萄糖而增加肺部感染的风险。最后,高血糖症引起的氧化应激和炎症反应可能会通过蛋白水解机制的激活而导致肌节损伤,从而使慢阻肺患者的膈肌功能受损。在血糖水平控制不佳的患者中,无论肥胖和年龄如何,其肺功能损害都更为突出。

慢阻肺患者使用激素会影响代谢综合征的发生。首先,激素可通过破坏葡萄糖的摄取和代谢损害胰岛 B 细胞功能。其次,已有研究发现激素在肝、骨骼肌和脂肪组织中发挥抗胰岛素作用:激素可以对抗胰岛素的作用并刺激脂肪组织的分解,引起游离脂肪酸升高,导致外周组织中葡萄糖的吸收受损引起高血糖症;激素的脂解作用还促进体内脂肪向内脏贮库的异常分布,造成中枢/腹部肥胖。最后,激素可能会干扰脂肪组织衍生的细胞因子(例如脂联素、瘦素)的表达和活性,导致胰岛素敏感性减低。除了外源性使用,烟草含有 11β-羟基甾体 2 型脱氢酶抑制剂-甘草酸,它可以抑制皮质醇转化为非活性可的松,从而延长内源性皮质醇的生物利用度及活性。此外,持续性缺氧可能会增加儿茶酚胺的产生,从而通过抑制胰岛素的作用导致高血糖症发生。

参 考 文 献

[1] Negewo NA, Gibson PG, McDonald VM. COPD and its co-morbidities: Impact, measurement and mechanisms. Respirology, 2015, 20(8):1160-1171.

[2] Tsantikos E, Lau M, Castelino CM, et al. Granulocyte-CSF links destructive inflammation and comorbidities in obstructive lung disease. J Clin Invest, 2018, 128(6):2406-2418.

[3] Taivassalo T, Hussain SN. Contribution of the mitochondria to locomotor muscle dysfunction in patients with COPD. Chest, 2016, 149(5):1302-1312.

[4] Inoue D, Watanabe R, Okazaki R. COPD and osteoporosis: links, risks, and treatment challenges. Int J Chron Obstruct Pulmon Dis, 2016, 11:637-648.

[5] Lehouck A, Boonen S, Decramer M, et al. COPD, bone metabolism, and osteoporosis. Chest, 2011, 139(3):648-657.

[6] Barnes PJ. Senescence in COPD and its comorbidities. Annu Rev Physiol, 2017, 79:517-539.

[7] Chan SMH, Selemidis S, Bozinovski S, et al. Pathobiological mechanisms underlying metabolic syndrome(MetS)in chronic obstructive pulmonary disease(COPD): clinical significance and therapeutic strategies. Pharmacol Ther, 2019, 198:160-188.

[8] Xiong J, Tian J, Zhou L, et al. Interleukin-17A deficiency attenuated emphysema and bone loss in mice exposed to cigarette smoke. Int J Chron Obstruct Pulmon Dis, 2020, 15:301-310.

[9] Testelmans D, Crul T, Maes K, et al. Atrophy and hypertrophy signalling in the diaphragm of patients with COPD. Eur Respir J, 2010, 35(3):549-556.

[10] Carter P, Lagan J, Fortune C, et al. Association of cardiovascular disease with respiratory disease. J Am Coll Cardiol, 2019, 73(17):2166-2177.

[11] Kameyama N, Chubachi S, Sasaki M, et al. Predictive and modifying factors of bone mineral density decline in patients with COPD. Respir Med, 2019, 148:13-23.

[12] André S, Conde B, Fragoso E, et al. COPD and cardiovascular disease. Pulmonology, 2019, 25(3):168-176.

[13] Wouters EFM. Obesity and metabolic abnormalities in chronic obstructive pulmonary disease. Ann Am Thorac Soc, 2017, 14(Suppl5):S389-S394.

[14] Graumam RQ, Pinheiro MM, Nery LE, et al. Increased rate of osteoporosis, low lean mass, and fragility fractures in COPD patients: association with disease severity. Osteoporos Int, 2018, 29(6):1457-1468.

[15] Piazzolla G, Castrovilli A, Liotino V, et al. Metabolic syndrome and chronic obstructive pulmonary disease(COPD): The interplay among smoking, insulin resistance and vitamin D. PLoS One, 2017, 12(10):e0186708.

4 肺纤维化合并肺气肿综合征的最新认识

蔡柏蔷

过去一直认为肺气肿(emphysema)和特发性肺纤维化(idiopathic pulmonary fibrosis,IPF)是临床上两类截然不同的疾病,然而近10余年发现部分吸烟者影像学上同时存在上肺野为主的肺气肿和下肺野为主的纤维化表现。2005年《欧洲呼吸杂志》首次报道了61例病例,称为肺纤维化合并肺气肿(combined pulmonary fibrosis and emphysema,CPFE)综合征,并提出CPFE是一种独立疾病。目前认为CPFE包括:吸烟相关肺纤维化合并肺气肿(smoking-associated CPFE)综合征与结缔组织疾病相关肺纤维化合并肺气肿(CTD-associated CPFE,CTD-CPFE)综合征两大类。由于CPFE具有特征性的临床表现、病理生理特点和影像学改变,近年来CPFE越来越受到关注,成为新的临床热点。CPFE的定义和诊断标准需要进一步明确,现在国际上ATS/ERS/JRS正在成立工作组,准备出台CPFE专家共识。近年来国内已有不少关于CPFE的研究,提供了中国人自己的临床资料。

一、肺纤维化合并肺气肿(CPFE)综合征的发病率、病因和发病机制

目前CPFE的发病率不详。在IPF队列研究中,CPFE发生率为8%~50.9%。但是慢性阻塞性肺疾病(慢阻肺)/肺气肿患者、吸烟者或者普通人群中CPFE的发生率仍有待进一步调查。大部分学者认为吸烟是吸烟相关CPFE的主要病因。吸烟分别与慢阻肺/肺气肿和IPF有明确相关性。98%的CPFE患者有吸烟史,提示吸烟在其发病中具有重要作用。其他与CPFE相关因素有:①职业环境因素:肺气肿合并纤维化可见于接触矿物粉尘(如石棉沉着病、硅沉着病)的患者和过敏性肺炎(农民肺)患者,以及轮胎工业的工人。②自身免疫因素:例如,类风湿关节炎、系统性硬化和显微镜下多血管炎,其他疾病包括混合型结缔组织病、干燥综合征和皮肌炎。另外,CPFE患者血浆抗核抗体增高比IPF更常见,部分患者伴有血p-ANCA阳性。③遗传因素。

吸烟相关CPFE的发病机制不明。CPFE与IPF患者的支气管肺泡灌洗液(BALF)细胞分类无显著差异。和单纯肺纤维化患者相比,CPFE患者BALF中CXCL5和白介素(IL)-8/CXCL8显著增高。基质金属蛋白酶、TNF-α、IL-1β及TGF-β等信号途径参与CPFE的发病机制。肺提前衰老和细胞衰老与IPF和慢阻肺/肺气肿的发生有关,可能参与CPFE的发病机制。

二、吸烟相关CPFE

(一)吸烟相关CPFE的临床特点

90%的CPFE患者为男性。发病年龄多在60~70岁。98%的CPFE患者有吸烟史,多为重度吸烟者。主要症状为活动后呼吸困难,伴或不伴咳嗽及咳痰。43%患者有杵状指,87%患者肺部听诊可闻及双下肺爆裂音,CPFE症状体征与IPF类似。

(二)吸烟相关CPFE的影像学特点

高分辨CT(HRCT)对于诊断CPFE是必需的。CPFE的HRCT表现为同时存在上肺肺野为主的肺气肿和下肺肺野为主的纤维化病变。CPFE的肺气肿特点为,41%~97%为小叶中心性肺气肿,54.2%~93%为旁间隔肺气肿,部分有肺大疱。旁间隔肺气肿在CPFE患者中很常见。CPFE的肺间质病变特点为肺外周和下肺肺野为主的网格影,蜂窝肺,牵张性支气管扩张等。约50%的患者HRCT符合典型的IPF,约1/3的患者HRCT提示可能为IPF或纤维化型非特异性间质性肺炎(NSIP),有少部分患者间质病变难以分类。部分患者有磨玻璃影,病理证实为脱屑性间质性肺炎(DIP)。

(三)吸烟相关CPFE肺功能特点

CPFE病理生理特点不同于单纯的慢阻肺/肺气肿或者IPF。CPFE患者肺容积相对正常或轻度异常,仅有20%的患者肺总量(TLC)降低,TLC平均值为64%~98%;无气流受限或者仅有轻度气流受限,仅有约50%的患者$FEV_1/FVC<70\%$,FEV_1/FVC平均值为65%~91%;弥散功能障碍常见而显著,97%~98%的患者一氧化碳弥散量(DLco)降低,DLco平均值为24%~65%。同IPF相比,CPFE患者HRCT纤维化评分更轻,而FVC更高。因此,CPFE的肺功能特点为弥散功能显著下降,与气流受限程度和肺容量不成比例。这是由于肺气肿所致的过度充气与纤维化所致的肺容积下降互相抵消,肺纤维化有助于维持气道开放,同时两者对弥散能力的影响相互叠加所致。值得注意的是,CPFE可以表现为单纯弥散功能障碍,因此单纯弥散功能障碍的鉴别诊断应包括CPFE。

(四)吸烟相关 CPFE 病理表现

CPFE病理研究资料有限。上肺野的病理改变主要为小叶中心型肺气肿。CPFE肺间质病变的病理表现包括寻常型间质性肺炎(UIP)和NSIP、DIP，以及不能分类的间质性肺炎。

(五)吸烟相关 CPFE 的诊断

诊断采用Cottin的诊断标准，主要根据HRCT表现，包括两方面：①肺气肿。定义为边界清楚的低密度影，无壁或者薄壁(<1mm)，或者肺大疱(直径>1cm)，病变以上肺野为主。②肺纤维化。表现为肺外周和下肺野为主的网格影、蜂窝肺，肺组织结构破坏、牵张性支气管扩张；可以有局部、少许磨玻璃影和(或)实变影。尽管多数患者HRCT符合IPF，但是IPF不是诊断CPFE的必要条件。另外，吸烟的IPF患者中肺气肿比较常见，但是目前并没有统一标准定义肺气肿范围多大即可诊断CPFE，有文献认为IPF患者HRCT上肺气肿范围大于5%或10%则诊断CPFE。

(六)吸烟相关 CPFE 的合并症

1. 肺动脉高压 是吸烟相关CPFE的最重要的合并症。和IPF、慢阻肺、肺气肿相比，吸烟相关CPFE的CPFE更容易发生肺动脉高压，且发生率更高、肺动脉高压程度更为严重，并且如果有肺动脉高压的CPFE患者预后更差。47%患者在诊断时即有肺动脉高压，心脏超声测量的肺动脉收缩压为(48±19) mmHg。右心导管测定CPFE患者的平均肺动脉压力为(40±9) mmHg。

2. 肺癌 吸烟相关CPFE综合征患者容易合并肺癌。CPFE合并肺癌风险显著高于单纯肺气肿，但与IPF相似。肺癌患者中CPFE比单纯肺纤维化更常见。CPFE增加癌发病。CPFE患者肺癌发生率为42%，明显高于单纯肺气肿和肺纤维化的肺癌发病率。由于合并肺癌，CPFE病死率显著高于IPF，与肺气肿合并癌相比，CPFE合并癌的生存率更低。CPFE中慢性肺损伤可能影响肺癌的进展，这与吸烟、肺气肿和肺纤维化的三重效应相关。癌基因易感性可能也与CPFE综合征相关。

3. 急性肺损伤 吸烟相关CPFE的CPFE增加外科肺切除术后急性肺损伤的风险。肺叶切除后易发生ARDS。与单纯肺气肿相比，CPFE患者在肺减容手术后，其胸腔引流时间和住院时间延长。CPFE合并肺癌的患者易产生化疗后的肺损伤。19.8%患者在治疗中发展为严重急性肺损伤，其治疗措施包括手术、放疗和化疗。提示CPFE对急性肺损伤的易感性。对于CPFE患者，应在外科手术前或相应治疗前充分评估其急性肺损伤的风险。

(七)吸烟相关 CPFE 的临床上尚未解决的问题

1. 诊断方面存在的问题 现有诊断标准缺少量化指标及明确界限。吸烟相关疾病是一个疾病谱(图2-4-1)，包括位于两端的慢阻肺/肺气肿和IPF/吸烟相关ILD，以及位于中间的CPFE。因为在病理生理特点、治疗和预后的不同，临床上需要识别CPFE患者与以肺纤维化或肺气肿为主的患者。将来诊断标准是否应有量化指标，是否纳入多个临床指标(如男性、吸烟史、肺功能特点及肺动脉高压等)仍有待商榷。符合现有诊断标准的CPFE患者仍存在异质性。临床上观察到吸烟患者，影像学上肺气肿或者纤维化病变可能大致相仿或者轻重有所不同，因此CPFE可能存在不同亚型。

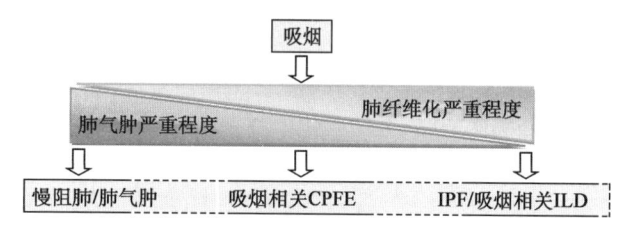

图 2-4-1 吸烟引起的肺疾病谱

注：包括单纯性慢阻肺(COPD)/肺气肿，肺纤维化合并肺气肿(CPFE)，以及特发性肺纤维化(IPF)/吸烟相关肺间质病(ILD)

2. 吸烟与吸烟相关CPFE之间的关系 研究吸烟相关CPFE具有很现实的意义，中国是烟草消费大国，因此可能有不少潜在的吸烟相关CPFE患者尚未被诊断。吸烟相关CPFE临床处理不同于慢阻肺/肺气肿和IPF，CPFE更容易合并肺动脉高压并且预后更差。另外用于评价慢阻肺或者IPF严重程度和疗效的指标(FEV_1、FVC、FEV_1/FVC、TLC等)并不适用于CPFE。因此，在慢阻肺或IPF的临床试验中应排除CPFE患者。临床实践中应该积极识别CPFE患者，如果慢阻肺或IPF患者有显著的呼吸困难、低氧或者弥散功能障碍，与肺功能阻塞程度或肺容积不成比例，或者肺动脉高压显著，应该警惕CPFE。

3. 吸烟相关CPFE的确切发病率 今后临床研究的方向：吸烟人群和普通人群中的吸烟相关CPFE的确切发病率；完善和统一CPFE的定义，将之与肺气肿为主或者纤维化为主的患者更好地区分开来；CPFE不同临床表型及严重程度分级；病因及发病机制；有效的治疗手段及预后判断指标等。

4. 需进一步阐明吸烟相关CPFE与慢阻肺、吸烟相关ILD之间的关系 吸烟相关CPFE影像上表现为上肺为主的肺气肿和下肺为主的纤维化，而肺功能特点为肺容积相对正常而弥散能力显著下降，肺动脉高压发生率显著升高并与预后不良相关，目前缺少有效治疗手段。因此CPFE与慢阻肺或IPF有着显著不同，应该作为一种独立的疾病深入研究。

吸烟相关CPFE的自然病史和预后：CPFE患者的FVC、VC及DLCO每年下降速度比慢阻肺更快。CPFE比肺气肿死亡风险更高，CPFE患者预后比IPF差，CPFE患者5年生存率35%~80%，中位生存期2.1~8.5年。合并肺动脉高压的患者预后更差，1年生存率60%。

三、结缔组织疾病相关肺纤维化合并肺气肿(CTD-associated CPFE, CTD-CPFE)综合征

(一)CTD-CPFE 的发病率

CPFE综合征可发生在任何结缔组织疾病中，与存在的系统性疾病或抗体的类型无明显的关系。CTD相关肺纤维化合并肺气肿综合征的主要基础疾病是类风湿关节

炎和系统性硬化病。临床研究发现：①类风湿关节炎患者如吸烟则易发生肺气肿。②CT发现8.4%的系统性硬化病患者合并肺气肿。③系统性硬化病是肺气肿发生的重要原因。④CPFE可见于多发性肌炎、混合结缔组织病和重迭结缔组织病。表2-4-1显示34例结缔组织病（CTD）患者中相关性CPFE的发生率。

CPFE综合征也可发生在间质性肺炎伴随自身免疫性疾病的患者，即：ILD伴随未分化结缔组织病，或ILD伴随自身免疫特征的疾病，ILD伴随肺部优势结缔组织病等。也可以发生在临床提示结缔组织病，但不能满足任何诊断标准的疾病—间质性肺炎伴自身免疫特征；(interstitial pneumonia with autoimmune features, IPAF)。

CPFE综合征如果发生在系统性血管炎，尤其是显微镜下多血管炎（MPA），患者既往无吸烟史，如果现在诊断为CPFE，应怀疑结缔组织病的可能性。

表2-4-1 34例结缔组织病(CTD)患者中相关性CPFE的发病率

结缔组织病(CTD)	CPFE的发生率
类风湿关节炎	18(53)
系统性硬化病	10(29))
弥漫型	3(9)
局限型	7(20)
混合结缔组织病	2(6)
重叠结缔组织病	2(6)
干燥综合征	1(3)
多发性肌炎	1(3)

典型病例：女性，28岁，患有严重的系统性硬化病，anti-Ul-RNP自身抗体显著升高。曾经有5年吸烟史。胸部CT见图2-4-2。

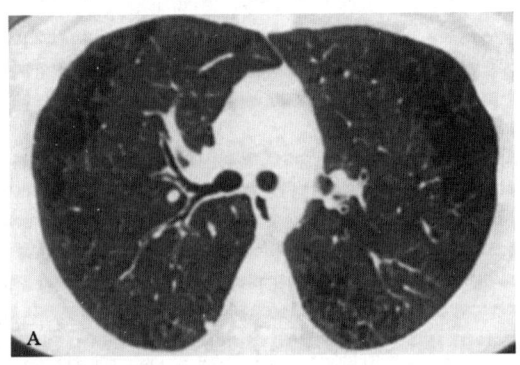

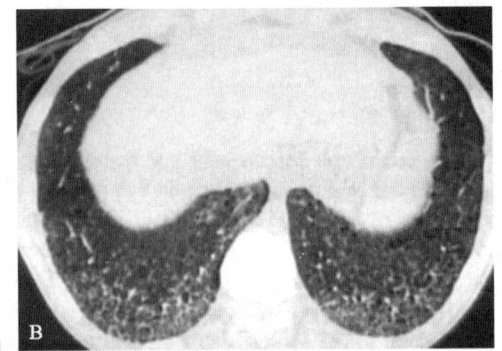

图2-4-2 患者胸部CT
注：A.胸部CT上叶示小叶中心性肺气肿和旁间隔气肿；B.胸部CT肺下带显示非特异性间质肺炎和网状阴影、磨玻璃样改变和牵拉性支气管扩张

（二）CTD相关CPFE与吸烟相关CPFE

CTD相关CPFE患者的年龄显著小于吸烟相关CPFE；CTD相关CPFE患者以女性多见；两类患者的肺容量变化没有差异，但是CTD相关CPFE患者的弥散功能损害比吸烟相关CPFE，相对较轻。

四、CPFE的治疗

吸烟相关CPFE和CTD相关CPFE都缺乏有效治疗手段。吸烟相关CPFE首先应该戒烟。糖皮质激素和免疫抑制剂效果不佳。对于HRCT符合IPF或者终末期肺纤维化的患者，不宜使用免疫抑制治疗。对于某些患者，影像学有磨玻璃改变，有证据提示其他非UIP病理类型，或者合并结缔组织病，可以试用免疫抑制治疗，但是治疗需谨慎并且个体化。支气管扩张药效果不佳，但可以酌情试用。抗纤维化药物吡非尼酮和nintebanib也可试用。低氧和肺动脉高压的患者可以给予氧疗。终末期患者可以考虑肺移植。CPFE合并肺动脉高压不推荐药物治疗。

参 考 文 献

[1] Wong AW, Liang J, Cottin V, et al. Diagnostic features in combined pulmonary fibrosis and emphysema(CPFE): a systematic review. Ann Am Thorac Soc, 2020, 17 (10): 1333-1336.

[2] 彭敏,蔡丰,田欣伦,等.肺纤维化合并肺气肿综合征8例并文献复习.中华结核和呼吸杂志,2010,33(7):515-518.

[3] 马汪伟,李振华,许慧.特发性肺间质纤维化合并肺气肿与未合并肺气肿患者的临床对比研究.中华结核和呼吸杂志,2013,36:173-176.

[4] Ryerson CJ, Hartman T, Elicker BM, et al. Clinical features and outcomes in combined pulmonary fibrosis and emphysema in idiopathic pulmonary fibrosis. Chest, 2013, 144: 234-240.

[5] Champtiaux N, Cottin V, Chassagnon G, et al. Combined pulmonary fibrosis and emphysema in systemic sclerosis: A syndrome associated with heavy morbidity and mortality. Semin Arthritis Rheum, 2019, 49: 98-104.

[6] Jankowich MD, Rounds SI. Combined pulmonary fibrosis and

emphysema syndrome:a review. Chest,2012,141:222-231.
[7] Akagi T,Matsumoto T,Harada T,et al. Coexistent emphysema delays the decrease of vital capacity in idiopathic pulmonary fibrosis. Respir Med,2009,103:1209-1215.
[8] Jankowich MD,Polsky M,Klein M,et al. Heterogeneity in combined pulmonary fibrosis and emphysema. Respiration,2008,75:411-417.
[9] Aduen JF,Zisman DA,Mobin SI,et al. Retrospective study of pulmonary function tests in patients presenting with isolated reduction in single-breath diffusion capacity:implications for the diagnosis of combined obstructive and restrictive lung disease. Mayo Clin Proc,2007,82:48-54.
[10] Cottin V,Nunes H,Brillet PY,et al. Combined pulmonary fibrosis and emphysema:a distinct underrecognised entity. Eur Respir J,2005,26:586-593.
[11] Mejia M,Carrillo G,Rojas-Serrano J,et al. Idiopathic pulmonary fibrosis and emphysema:decreased survival associated with severe pulmonary arterial hypertension. Chest,2009,136:10-15.
[12] Cottin V,Le Pavec J,Prévot G,et al. Pulmonary hypertension in patients with combined pulmonary fibrosis and emphysema syndrome. Eur Respir J,2010,35:105-111.
[13] Jacob J,Bartholmai BJ,Rajagopalan S. et al. Likelihood of pulmonary hypertension in patients with idiopathic pulmonary fibrosis and emphysema. Respirology,2018,23:593-599.
[14] Kwak N,Park CM,Lee J,et al. Lung cancer risk among patients with combined pulmonary fibrosis and emphysema. Respir Med,2014,108(3):524-530.
[15] 彭敏,施举红,蔡柏蔷.肺纤维化合并肺气肿综合征:呼吸内科临床的"新问题".中国实用内科杂志,2014,34(8):744-747.
[16] Cottin V,Nunes H,Mouthon L,et al. Combined pulmonary fibrosis and emphysema syndrome in connective tissue ddisease. Arthritis Rheum,2011,63:295-304.
[17] Cottin V,Cordier JF. The syndrome of combined pulmonary fibrosis and emphysema//Cottin V,Cordier JF,Richeldi L. Orphan lung diseases. London:Springer Press,2015:327-347.

5 慢性阻塞性肺疾病频繁急性加重的对因治疗

赵 立

慢性阻塞性肺疾病（简称慢阻肺），是慢性气道疾病中的一种重要类型。与其他的慢性气道病一样，慢阻肺也具有急性加重的临床特征，称为慢阻肺急性加重。慢阻肺急性加重的定义是呼吸道症状的急性恶化，导致患者需要附加的治疗措施。慢阻肺急性加重的诊断可能是症状驱动，也可以能是事件驱动。需识别的主要症状包括呼吸困难、咳嗽、痰量和痰的性状出现恶化；伴随的医疗事件包括稳定期用药剂量和用药种类增加，乃至需要加用抗菌药物和（或）全身性激素，严重病例可能需要机械通气等辅助治疗。根据慢阻肺急性加重伴随医疗事件的严重程度不同，将慢阻肺急性加重分为轻度、中度和重度。轻度指只需以短效支气管扩张剂附加治疗；中度是指在短效时气管扩张剂的之基础上，还需合并抗菌药物和（或）加用全身激素；重度是指患者需住院治疗或紧急门诊就诊，重度急性加重常伴有呼吸衰竭。每年≥2次中度急性加重或≥1次重度急性加重，被定义为慢阻肺频繁急性加重。慢阻肺频繁急性加重作为慢阻肺的一种独立表型在2010年被首次提出。对这一表型的关注，源于慢阻肺频繁急性加重人群具有显著的生活质量下降、预期生存周期缩短、医疗负担严重等特点。研究表明病毒感染、细菌感染、空气污染、气道嗜酸细胞性炎症等都可成为慢阻肺急性加重的诱因，而这一表型人群与慢阻肺非频繁急性加重表型人群多个蛋白基因表达的不同，应该是其对上述因素易感的内因所在。本文就慢阻肺频繁急性加重不同诱因及其干预措施的疗效加以综述。

一、病毒因素

病毒感染是慢阻肺急性加重最常见的诱因，其中鼻病毒、呼吸道合胞病毒和流感病毒最为重要。注射流感疫苗，可以有效降低慢阻肺患者急性加重的频度和程度，无需住院治疗的比例和急性加重相关的病死率显著下降，因此多个国家慢阻肺诊治指南，流感疫苗都推荐作为预防急性加重的有效措施。遗憾的是，抗流感的有效药物（如奥司他韦）并未在良好设计的减低慢阻肺急性加重频度或程度的临床试验中获得疗效。这可能与以下因素有关：①流感病毒的传播具有明显的季节性，而慢阻肺频繁急性加重并无显著的季节相关，在整个研究项目实施周期中，导致非流感季的急性加重患者无法从抗流感药物中获得疗效。②在病毒感染的早期阶段（急性加重初期）没有入组的受试者，有可能继发/合并细菌感染，这种情况下，抗流感治疗也难以达到理想效果。2019年初，我们启动了国内多中心、随机、双盲、安慰剂对照的临床试验（NCT03851991，ChiCTR1900022146），旨在研究广谱口服抗病毒药物盐酸阿比多尔对于慢阻肺患者急性加重频度和程度的有效性和安全性；该项研究预计2022年会有结果，期待中国民族企业的优秀抗病毒药物，能够为有效阻断慢阻肺患者的频繁加重带来福音。

二、细菌因素

有20%~60%稳定期慢阻肺患者的下呼吸道标本中可以分离出诸如流感嗜血杆菌、肺炎链球菌、肺炎克雷伯杆菌、铜绿假单胞菌等常见呼吸道致病菌。呼吸道细菌负荷的增加，不仅是持续气道炎症导致慢阻肺病情进展的原因，也是长期使用吸入激素易于诱发肺部细菌感染的理论基础。2010年一项有关莫西沙星预防慢阻肺急性加重的随机对照研究表明，连续5 d每日一次口服400 mg莫西沙星，每8周为一个周期，重复6个周期，受试者急性加重比例较安慰剂对照者下降25%。由于长期反复使用莫西沙星可能带来细菌高耐药风险，临床医生还不接受莫西沙星作为预防慢阻肺急性加重的干预措施。另一项为期一年、安慰剂对照、以频繁急性加重患者为研究对象的抗菌药物预防慢阻肺急性加重的研究显示，大环内酯类药物——阿奇霉素250 mg每日一次口服，显著减少患者的急性加重、改善生活质量。该项研究奠定了阿奇霉素长期口服在慢阻肺患者急性加重预防中的地位。随着肺肠轴微生态研究的兴起，有学者发现慢阻肺人群中具有较高比例的幽门螺杆菌感染，这一细菌也构成急性加重的高危因素，阿奇霉素可以显著延长幽门螺杆菌血清型阳性患者下一次急性加重的间隔时间。此外，阿奇霉素还具有调强Th1反应、减低肿瘤坏死因子生成等免疫调节作用。因而多个国家在指南中推荐阿奇霉素长期使用预防慢阻肺急性加重。由于阿奇霉素长期口服可能带来的耳毒性、肝毒性和心脏毒性，在该预防方案选择时应侧重考虑频繁或重度加重的患者，特别是伴有支扩或呼吸道标本分离出铜绿假单胞菌的患者，并注意避免用于伴有肝功损害、QT间期延长、听力下降的患者。在疫苗预防上，13价和23价肺炎疫苗，被推荐用于所有大于65岁的慢阻肺人群。对于伴有严重心肺疾患的小于65岁的慢阻肺人群,肺炎疫苗也可有效减低肺炎和急性加重的发生风险。

三、针对支气管炎型药物

以支气管炎型为主要临床特征的患者,可以从磷酸二酯酶4(PDE4)抑制剂和黏液溶解剂的治疗中获益。一项为期一年、安慰剂对照、多中心、双盲临床试验显示,PDE4抑制剂罗氟司特可以减低17%中至重度急性加重。N-乙酰半胱氨酸兼具黏液溶解和抗氧化作用。钟南山教授团队牵头开展的国内多中心研究显示,与安慰剂比较,长期口服N-乙酰半胱氨酸(600 mg每日2次)可以显著减少慢阻肺患者急性加重。该项研究成果成为慢阻肺诊治重要指南中的推荐依据。

四、吸入药物

吸入药物制剂为稳定慢阻肺患者病情、改善生活质量、降低病死率带来了显著的临床成效。目前国内用于慢阻肺稳定期治疗的吸入制剂主要包括长效抗胆碱能药物(LAMA)、吸入激素(ICS)/长效β_2受体激动剂(LABA)复合制剂、LAMA/LABA复合制剂,以及ICS/LAMA/LABA复合制剂。对于具有嗜酸性粒细胞性气道炎症特质的慢阻肺患者,ICS/LABA具有减低急性加重风险的明显优势。ICS长期使用提高肺炎发生风险,对外周血嗜酸性粒细胞分数低于3%的慢阻肺患者获益/风险比也明显减低。临床试验显示,在ICS+LAMA+LABA稳定6周治疗后撤除ICS的患者人群中,中度或重度急性加重的风险与继续维持三联药物的对照组并无差异,但肺功能下降程度显著高于对照组。有效预防和减缓慢阻肺急性加重的频度和程度是慢阻肺患者管理的重中之重,近年有关慢阻肺的临床试验设计,更侧重于将预防急性加重、延长生存周期作为主要终点事件观察。LAMA/LABA复合制剂的临床试验显示,在以减低急性加重为终点事件的疗效评价中,单一装置的LAMA/LABA复合制剂疗效优于ICS/LABA,大大提升了LAMA/LABA作为慢阻肺稳定期用药的重要地位。两项单一装置的ICS/LAMA/LABA临床试验也都显示了显著优于LAMA/LABA的临床疗效:IMPACT研究(氟替卡松/乌美溴铵/维兰特罗)和ETHOS研究(布地奈德/格隆溴铵/福莫特罗)均较单一装置的LAMA/LABA使用显著降低中度或重度急性加重。同时具有重要临床意义的是,两项研究中ICS都采用较低剂量,从而有可能减低肺炎的发生风险。

五、生物药物的研发

吸烟、生物燃料、空气污染等危险因素暴露是慢阻肺发生发展的共同危险因素,但慢阻肺作为高度异质性疾病,不同表型之间,乃至不同个体之间的发病机制有着显著的差异。众多细胞因子和趋化因子在外界因素刺激和内在信号调控失衡的共同作用下,在慢阻肺急性加重中发挥作用。近年来,包括中国多家医疗机构在内的全球多个研究中心针对多种炎性介质开发的生物或小分子制剂开展临床试验,针对的分子靶点包括IL-1、IL-5、IL-13、IL-17A、TNF、上皮生长因子受体(EGFR)、上皮钠通道等。不同于以往的慢阻肺临床试验,这些研究设计更加聚焦特定的慢阻肺患者人群(亚群),具有鲜明的个体化治疗理念。以IL-5为例,其广泛参与了嗜酸性粒细胞的分化、募集、成熟、活化和脱颗粒,针对IL-5研发的单克隆抗体在减缓慢阻肺病情、预防急性发作中被寄予厚望。2017年抗循环IL-5单克隆抗体药物mepolizumab Ⅲ期临床试验结果发布。Mepolizumab 100mg或300mg每4周1次皮下注射,连续52周并维持三联吸入药物基础治疗,100 mg组、300 mg组和安慰剂组年中度或重度急性加重次数分别为1.19、1.27和1.49;在嗜酸性粒细胞增高的亚组患者,结果更好一些;不过这一试验结果显然低于研究者预期。在以慢阻肺频繁急性加重患者为受试人群、以预防急性加重为主要终点事件的临床试验中,另一抗IL-5受体α单克隆抗体药物benralizumab研究结果失败,在嗜酸性粒细胞增高亚组人群中也失败。慢阻肺在多重因素相互作用下发生和发展,又因众多不同的内在特质(endotype),使疾病趋于不同的表型(包括频繁急性加重表型),各个表型之间又展现出比例不同的重叠和融合,在机体内部则是一张庞大而复杂的细胞—分子网络。单纯针对某种特定的明星分子进行阻断或调强的生物治疗,是否能够为慢阻肺急性加重有效的个体化预防开启里程碑式的篇章,还有待于临床实践的检验。

综上所述,近10年来对于慢阻肺异质性所表现出多种不同表型的认识有了显著进步,频繁急性加重表型作为慢阻肺患者危害最大的一种类型,受到临床研究、基础科研及药物研发的多重关注。这些研究成果为有效减低和预防慢阻肺急性加重带来了显著成效。然而,我们必须充分认识到各表型之间会存在"你中有我,我中有你"的复杂局面。目前定义的"频发急性加重表型"中,即可再分化为嗜酸性粒细胞增多为主、肺气肿为主、支气管炎为主等等不同亚群,因此,对于这一疾病的广泛和深入研究,将有助于实现对于不同个体的有效预防和治疗。

参考文献

[1] Global Strategy for the Diagnosis, Management and Prevention of COPD, Global Initiative for Chronic Obstructive Lung Disease(GOLD)2020. Available from: http://goldcopd.org.

[2] Hurst J R, Vestbo J, Anzueto A, et al. Susceptibility to exacerbation in chronic obstructive pulmonary disease. N Engl J Med, 2010, 363(12):1128-1138.

[3] Kim V, Aaron S D. What is a COPD exacerbation? Current definitions, pitfalls, challenges and opportunities for improve-

ment. Eur Respir J,2018,52(5).

[4] Sun P,Ye R,Wang C,et al. Identification of proteomic signatures associated with COPD frequent exacerbators. Life Sci,2019,230:1-9.

[5] Matsumoto K, Inoue H. Viral infections in asthma and COPD. Respir Investig,2014,52(2):92-100.

[6] Wang H, Anthony D, Selemidis S, et al. Resolving Viral-Induced Secondary Bacterial Infection in COPD:A Concise Review. Front Immunol,2018,9:2345.

[7] Miravitlles M,Anzueto A. Antibiotic prophylaxis in COPD:Why,when,and for whom? Pulm Pharmacol Ther,2015,32:119-123.

[8] Mammen MJ,Sethi S. COPD and the microbiome. Respirology,2016,21(4):590-599.

[9] Sethi S,Jones PW,Theron MS,et al. Pulsed moxifloxacin for the prevention of exacerbations of chronic obstructive pulmonary disease:a randomized controlled trial. Respir Res,2010,11(1):10.

[10] Albert RK, Connett J, Bailey WC, et al. Azithromycin for prevention of exacerbations of COPD. N Engl J Med,2011,365(8):689-698.

[11] Ra SW,Sze MA,Lee E C,et al. Azithromycin and risk of COPD exacerbations in patients with and without Helicobacter pylori. Respir Res,2017,18(1):109.

[12] Baines KJ,Wright TK,Gibson PG,et al. Azithromycin treatment modifies airway and blood gene expression networks in neutrophilic COPD. ERJ Open Res,2018,4(4).

[13] Taylor SP,Sellers E,Taylor BT. Azithromycin for the Prevention of COPD Exacerbations:The Good,Bad,and Ugly. Am J Med,2015,128(12):1362.

[14] Miravitlles M, D′urzo A, Singh D, et al. Pharmacological strategies to reduce exacerbation risk in COPD:a narrative review. Respir Res,2016,17(1):112.

[15] Zheng JP,Wen FQ,Bai CX,et al. Twice daily N-acetylcysteine 600 mg for exacerbations of chronic obstructive pulmonary disease(PANTHEON):a randomised,double-blind placebo-controlled trial. Lancet Respir Med, 2014, 2 (3):187-194.

[16] Magnussen H,Disse B,Rodriguez-Roisin R,et al. Withdrawal of inhaled glucocorticoids and exacerbations of COPD. N Engl J Med,2014,371(14):1285-1294.

[17] Wedzicha JA,Banerji D,Chapman KR,et al. Indacaterol-Glycopyrronium versus Salmeterol-Fluticasone for COPD. N Engl J Med,2016,374(23):2222-2234.

[18] Lipson DA, Barnhart F, Brealey N, et al. Once-Daily Single-Inhaler Triple versus Dual Therapy in Patients with COPD. N Engl J Med,2018,378(18):1671-1680.

[19] Rabe KF, Martinez FJ, Ferguson GT, et al. Triple Inhaled Therapy at Two Glucocorticoid Doses in Moderate-to-Very-Severe COPD. N Engl J Med,2020,383(1):35-48.

[20] Lakshmi SP, Reddy AT, Reddy RC. Emerging pharmaceutical therapies for COPD. Int J Chron Obstruct Pulmon Dis,2017,12:2141-2156.

[21] Yousuf A, Brightling CE. Biologic Drugs: A New Target Therapy in COPD? Copd,2018,15(2):99-107.

[22] Murray LA, Grainge C, Wark PA, et al. Use of biologics totreat acute exacerbations and manage disease in asthma, COPD and IPF. Pharmacol Ther,2017,169:1-12.

[23] Narendra DK, Hanania NA. Targeting IL-5 in COPD. Int J Chron Obstruct Pulmon Dis,2019,14:1045-1051.

[24] Pavord ID,Chanez P,Criner GJ,et al. Mepolizumab for Eosinophilic Chronic Obstructive Pulmonary Disease. N Engl J Med,2017,377(17):1613-1629.

[25] Criner GJ,Celli BR,Brightling CE,et al. Benralizumab for the Prevention of COPD Exacerbations. N Engl J Med,2019,381(11):1023-1034.

6 基于气道炎症的COPD精准化治疗探讨

彭丽萍

慢性阻塞性肺疾病(COPD)是一种常见的、可以预防和治疗的疾病,以持续呼吸症状和气流受限为特征,通常是由于明显暴露于有毒颗粒或气体引起的气道和(或)肺泡异常所导致。目前认为COPD从本质上是气道局部尤其是小气道的慢性炎症。COPD患者的炎症由肺部"溢出"至全身,是COPD全身炎症的可能机制之一。研究表明COPD患者的气道炎症和全身炎症与疾病的进展和病死亡率相关,因此有效控制COPD患者气道局部炎症对于改善COPD患者的预后至关重要。本文结合相关文献,对COPD有关的炎症细胞、亚型和精准化治疗策略进行探讨。

一、与COPD有关的炎症细胞

炎症机制是COPD发生发展过程中最重要的机制,与COPD炎症机制有关的细胞包括中性粒细胞、嗜酸性粒细胞、巨噬细胞和淋巴细胞等,中性粒细胞和嗜酸性粒细胞作为诱导炎症机制的终极细胞,主要通过巨噬细胞和淋巴细胞发挥作用。

(一)中性粒细胞

中性粒细胞是机体固有免疫系统的第一道防线,在吸烟、空气污染物等刺激物的作用下,中性粒细胞活化,迁移至肺部,中性粒细胞在保护宿主的同时,释放多种炎症介质导致组织损伤,中性粒细胞凋亡延迟、气道内过多的中性粒细胞胞外诱捕网(NETs)形成是COPD炎症持续表现的重要原因,中性粒细胞炎症几乎贯穿了COPD发生发展的全过程,活化的中性粒细胞可以释放活性氧代谢产物、细胞因子、脂质介质、抗菌肽等,诱导黏液高分泌、气道重塑和肺气肿形成。杯状细胞化生及黏液过度分泌是COPD患者气道慢性炎症的重要病理改变,而黏蛋白基因表达是控制上皮细胞分化为杯状细胞的主要因素。在体外,中性粒细胞弹性蛋白酶(NE)和活性氧(ROS)可以独立增加上皮细胞黏蛋白mRNA和蛋白的表达,也提示中性粒细胞气道炎症是COPD患者关键的疾病特征。在气道壁内,中性粒细胞气道炎症的确认是难以达到的,不同的研究结果不一,这可能反映了组织中浸润的中性粒细胞寿命较短。有研究对气道平滑肌的分析发现中性粒细胞浸润与空气潴留的CT测量值和气流阻塞的严重程度有关,也提示中性粒细胞在COPD患者气道重塑中的作用,中性粒细胞促进气道重塑的作用可能与NE有关。NE/抗NE失衡是肺气肿发生的主要机制,中性粒细胞是肺部蛋白酶/抗蛋白酶失衡的主要原因。动物模型研究表明,注射纯化NE会产生肺气肿,而内源性NE缺乏可预防暴露于香烟烟雾后的肺气肿。COPD患者尿液和血浆中NE活性产物增加,其肺气肿严重程度与外周血NE水平之间具有相关性,在体外,肺气肿患者的外周血中性粒细胞比对照组的外周血中性粒细胞消化更多的细胞外蛋白。

(二)嗜酸性粒细胞

嗜酸性粒细胞是一种先天的固有免疫细胞,可以合成、储存和分泌多种细胞因子、趋化因子和增长因子,以往认为其主要在变态反应性疾病的宿主免疫防御和寄生虫感染后免疫中发挥作用。越来越多的证据表明,嗜酸性粒细胞在COPD患者的病程中也发挥了重要作用,COPD患者嗜酸性粒细胞炎症的病因尚不清楚,可能是机体固有免疫和适应性免疫结合的结果。由于不同的研究采用了不同的标准,嗜酸性粒细胞为主的COPD患者的患病率目前尚不明确,但在两个COPD队列研究中,嗜酸性粒细胞性COPD患者的患病范围跨度较大,在10%~40%,这除了源于患者群体差异外,还与痰中(>2%或>3%嗜酸性粒细胞)或血液(2%或>250、300、400嗜酸性粒细胞/μl)的阈值设置不同有关。以往的研究认为COPD患者嗜酸性粒细胞浸润的机制似乎与哮喘不同,因为关键的趋化因子IL-4、IL-5和嗜酸性粒细胞趋化因子并没有在COPD患者气道中过度表达。新近研究表明,在嗜酸性粒细胞增多的COPD患者体内存在着T2转录组标签。Th2细胞产生白细胞介素(IL)-4、IL-5和IL-13,其中IL-5是嗜酸性粒细胞生存和成熟的一种专一性细胞因子。嗜酸性粒细胞炎症也可通过激活ILC2细胞而发生,ILC2细胞也是体内IL-5和IL-13来源之一。嗜酸性粒细胞向肺黏膜的募集主要通过由上皮细胞衍生的CCR3趋化因子和其他嗜酸粒细胞趋化剂[如肥大细胞衍生的前列腺素(PG)D2]介导。PGD2通过激活PGD2 2型受体(DP2或CRTH2)来增强T2免疫。还有一种可能的介质是趋化因子IL-8,虽然IL-8通常与中性粒细胞趋化有关,但IL-8同样也展现了对嗜酸性粒细胞的趋化作用,并与慢性支气管炎患者肺泡灌洗液中嗜酸性阳离子蛋白(ECP)水平相关。

(三)巨噬细胞

巨噬细胞是人肺泡灌洗回收的主要炎性细胞,巨噬细胞可以释放各种活性氧、趋化因子、炎性细胞因子、平滑肌收缩剂、基质金属蛋白酶(MMPs)等,这些物质共同作用可以将一系列相似的蛋白质降解为 NE,有助于白细胞向受损组织的迁移和浸润。以往认为,巨噬细胞主要在在肺气肿蛋白持续分解的过程中发挥作用,进一步破坏肺实质,刺激气道内过度分泌黏液。其在肺实质中的密度与肺破坏的严重程度具有明显的相关性。巨噬细胞分泌的 MMP 尤其是 MMP12 是肺气肿的主要原因之一。COPD 患者气道和肺泡巨噬细胞 MMP-12 的表达增加,小鼠中 MMP-12 的缺乏似乎对香烟烟雾引起的肺损伤具有保护作用,使用广谱 MMP 抑制剂可降低暴露于香烟烟雾的豚鼠肺气肿的严重程度。MMP12 除在肺气肿的发生过程中发挥重要作用外,在 COPD 的炎症反应中也具有重要的作用,动物实验证明对于香烟烟雾诱导的小鼠模型中性粒细胞向肺部的浸润也需要 MMP12 的存在,这可能与其释放肿瘤坏死因子 α(TNF-α)及上调血管黏附分子 VCAM-1 有关。巨噬细胞释放的炎症因子在保护机体的同时,也对肺组织造成了损伤,糖皮质激素可以调节炎性因子引起的机体损伤,然而 COPD 患者糖皮质激素对巨噬细胞的调控能力减退。用同等量的糖皮质激素作用于吸烟和 COPD 患者的肺泡巨噬细胞,结果发现 COPD 患者的 IL-8 水平明显增高,IL-8 可进一步促进中性粒细胞趋化、聚集和激活及嗜酸性粒细胞的气道黏膜聚集,导致 COPD 的发生与发展。

(四)淋巴细胞

COPD 患者的肺部存在 CD8$^+$ T 细胞、Th1 和 Th17 CD4$^+$ T 细胞参与的适应性免疫反应。COPD 患者肺气肿肺泡壁中的总 T 细胞增加,但以 CD8$^+$ T 细胞为主,在 COPD 患者的大气道壁、小气道平滑肌和外周气道平滑肌中也有类似的发现。肺 CD8$^+$ T 细胞的数量与气流受限和肺气肿的严重程度有关。CD8$^+$ T 细胞活化后,可以释放穿孔素和颗粒酶等蛋白水解酶,导致结构细胞因凋亡或坏死而死亡。COPD 患者体内 Th1/Th2 比例失衡,以 Th1 细胞占优势,表现为 Th1 型细胞因子数量增多而 Th2 型细胞因子数量减少。Th17 细胞在 COPD 的发病过程中也发挥了重要作用,Th17 细胞的主要效应因子是 IL-17,可以介导中性粒细胞动员的兴奋过程,导致组织炎症反应的发生。COPD 患者 Th17 细胞及其分泌的细胞因子 IL-17A 明显增高,靶向阻断 IL-17A 通路可以减轻 COPD 小鼠的肺组织炎症。Treg 是一类具有免疫抑制作用的 CD4$^+$ T 细胞,可以分泌 IL-10、IL-35、TGF-β 等抗炎因子。COPD 发生过程中 Treg 细胞可以抑制免疫细胞的活性,发挥免疫抑制作用,使 COPD 患者免疫功能受损,导致感染的发生。另外,Treg 细胞分泌的 IL-35 可以抑制效应性 T 细胞的增生分化,是发挥其最大抑制效应的必需因子,也可能参与了 COPD 的发病机制,但具体机制还需进一步研究。B 淋巴细胞作为机体内提呈抗原、介导体液免疫应答的主要细胞也参与了 COPD 的发病过程。研究表明,COPD 患者大气道 B 淋巴细胞明显增多,COPD 患者淋巴滤泡的形成可能是 B 细胞由 CXCL13 依赖性的机制驱动的,应用 CXCL3 抗体可以完全阻止香烟诱导的小鼠淋巴滤泡的形成。

二、与炎症细胞有关的 COPD 亚型

COPD 是一种异质性的疾病,因此有学者提出了 COPD 亚型的概念,根据炎症细胞的类型,COPD 可分为中性粒细胞和嗜酸性粒细胞为主的气道炎症亚型,两者在症状、急性加重、病死率等方面具有明显的差异。

(一)以中性粒细胞为主的炎症亚型

中性粒细胞亚型是 COPD 患者最常见的炎症亚型,气道中性粒细胞的水平与患者的肺功能下降存在明显的相关性,痰中性粒细胞计数的升高与提示吸烟者外周气道功能障碍的 CT 指标相关。增加的中性粒细胞炎症是 COPD 急性加重的特征性表现,然而 COPD 患者存在中性粒细胞功能的受损,在感染的情况下,由于吞噬细胞水平上的宿主-病原体相互作用紊乱,即使中性粒细胞及时招募到肺部,仍无法消除入侵的病原体。即使是明显稳定的 COPD 患者也存在着气道微生物组的高度紊乱,随着疾病严重程度的加重,这些紊乱会表现的更为严重。一部分 COPD 患者还可能存在持续的致病菌如嗜血杆菌属和卡他莫拉菌的定植,导致患者气道炎症加重,频繁地出现急性加重,肺功能进行性下降。有研究发现以中性粒细胞为主的 COPD 患者一旦出现急性加重,通常表现比较严重,合并细菌感染的比例更多,痰量、痰及血清炎性介质水平也明显增高,对标准治疗反应不佳,一部分患者尤其是对于感染了耐药菌的患者需要更长的住院时间和强化药物治疗,定期使用抗生素治疗对其预防可能具有一定的价值。

(二)以嗜酸性粒细胞为主的炎症亚型

嗜酸性粒细胞升高目前被认为是 COPD 加重的潜在危险因素,少部分 COPD 患者可以表现为以嗜酸性粒细胞为主的严重表型,此类患者气道中存在嗜酸性粒细胞的活化和脱颗粒,其发生机制主要与 T2 细胞介导的免疫反应相关。COPD 患者的气道上皮细胞释放上游细胞因子胸腺基质淋巴细胞生成素(TSLP)和 IL-33,这些因子进一步募集分泌 IL-5 的 Th2 细胞和 ILC2 细胞,导致嗜酸性粒细胞炎症,嗜酸性粒细胞在趋化因子 CCL5 的介导下被吸引到肺部,并在 IL-5 和粒细胞-巨噬细胞集落刺激因子(GM-CSF)的作用下在肺部维持浸润状态。有研究发现在部分 COPD 急性加重的患者中,嗜酸性粒细胞数量和细菌感染呈负相关。Ajmal 等对比斯佩伯格大学医院因 COPD 急性加重而入院的所有患者进行单中心回顾性研究,并随访三年,发现嗜酸性粒细胞组 COPD 患者对无创通气的需求更少,住院时间更短,住院病死率、3 年病死率更低。外周血嗜酸性粒细胞是 AECOPD 合并肺炎患者病死率的一种独立的预测因子,有研究发现嗜酸性粒细胞>2% 的 COPD 急性加重患者较<2% 的患者预后更好。

三、基于气道炎症的药物治疗策略

COPD 气道炎症的异质性提示对于不同患者采用精准个体化治疗的必要性,中性粒细胞和嗜酸性细胞作为

COPD气道炎症机制的核心细胞,是目前COPD药物治疗研究的重点和热点。

(一)针对中性粒细胞的治疗

中性粒细胞炎症是COPD的主要炎症途径,针对中性粒细胞的治疗可能是未来COPD治疗的方向,然而迄今为止针对中性粒炎症的治疗研究结果却不尽人意。苦参碱是从苦参中提取的生物碱类化合物,具有抗感染作用,动物实验表明苦参碱可以通过诱导中性粒细胞的凋亡显著降低香烟诱导的小鼠BALF中中性粒细胞和NE的活性,提示其可能在COPD的肺部炎症中具有治疗潜力,但还需进一步进行临床相关研究。Galectin(Gal)-9是一种β-半乳糖苷凝集素蛋白,在猪胰腺弹性蛋白酶(PPE)诱发的肺气肿模型中,Gal-9能抑制PPE诱导的肺气肿病理变化,降低BALF中中性粒细胞数量和MMP-2和MMP-9的水平,在体外也能抑制中性粒细胞的趋化活性,Gal-9缺陷的小鼠肺气肿的严重程度要明显重于野生型小鼠,外源性的Gal-9可能是治疗COPD的潜在药物。IL-8在中性粒细胞所致的炎症中发挥了非常重要的作用,其水平与中性粒细胞的数量相关,同时COPD患者痰液中存在高浓度的TNF-α,可启动NF-κB的转录,随之转向IL-8基因的转录。一项针对COPD的临床试验发现,给予患者IL-8单克隆抗体,患者呼吸困难指数下降,但呼吸状态、肺功能、6min步行距离(6MWT)及对快速缓解药物的需求上没有变化。IL-8的趋化因子受体抗体(抗CXCR2抗体,MK-7123)可以改善患者,特别是目前吸烟患者6个月后的FEV_1,但其可引起剂量依赖性的白细胞绝对值的下降。一项针对抗TNF-α的临床研究发现,对于中重度COPD患者,给予抗TNF-α抗体治疗,尽管患者总体耐受性良好,在研究的主要结果(慢性呼吸系统问卷总分)和次要结果($FEV_1\%$、6WMT、SF-36评分、呼吸困难指数、中重度COPD急性加重次数)上没有改善,但肺炎和恶性肿瘤的发生率明显增加。以IL-17和IL-1为靶点的治疗在COPD的治疗上也无疗效。针对中性粒细胞炎症通路的治疗没有获得满意的临床效果,在某些情况下还可能增加感染的风险。长期应用阿奇霉素可能主要是通过影响气道微生态改善气道炎症,并不具有直接的抗感染作用。

(二)针对嗜酸性粒细胞的治疗

糖皮质激素是目前针对嗜酸粒细胞性COPD比较公认的药物。痰嗜酸性粒细胞计数升高与稳定期COPD患者对激素的治疗反应有关,血嗜酸粒细胞计数可用于预测稳定期和急性加重期COPD患者对激素的反应。大剂量吸入型糖皮质激素可降低嗜酸粒细胞性COPD患者诱导痰嗜酸性粒细胞水平,减少重度急性加重风险。2020年GOLD指南明确推荐嗜酸性粒细胞作为评估吸入糖皮质激素预防COPD急性加重疗效的生物标志物,对于高血嗜酸性粒细胞计数患者(>300个/μl),使用吸入型糖皮质激素疗效显著。糖皮质激素对嗜酸性粒细胞性COPD的益处是否仅限于对嗜酸性粒细胞的作用,还是其他更广泛的抗感染作用尚不确定。T2介导的嗜酸性粒细胞炎症机制也进入了COPD的临床实践,但总体上T2定向的COPD临床试验结果让人失望。贝那利珠单抗是针对IL-5R的单克隆抗体,Brightling等于2010年11月18日至2013年7月13日,在英国、波兰、德国、加拿大、美国、丹麦和西班牙的26个地点进行了一项随机、双盲、安慰剂对照的Ⅱa期研究,发现尽管贝那利珠单抗可以降低血和痰中嗜酸性粒细胞数量、改善患者FEV_1绝对值,但并不能减少中到重度急性加重和患者健康状态。在尚未完全报道的COPD的贝那利珠单抗Ⅲ期试验中,也未观察到可以减少血嗜酸性粒细胞计数增加(≥220个/μl)的患者病情急性加重。抗IL-5R的单克隆抗体美宝利单抗可以降低痰嗜酸性粒细胞计数,但并没有改善肺功能或健康状况及至患者第一次急性加重发生的时间。其他T2定向治疗如GATA 3抑制剂可降低COPD患者痰中嗜酸性粒细胞计数,但与抗IL-5R一样,对临床终点没有影响,抗IL-13、抗IL-4Rα药物在以嗜酸性粒细胞炎症为主的COPD患者是否有益还须进一步研究。

气道炎症是COPD发生与发展的主要机制,糖皮质激素对嗜酸性粒细胞性炎症最有效,然而T2和中性粒细胞靶向的生物制剂治疗在COPD的作用上不尽人意,有必要进行进一步的COPD机制和干预措施的研究。只有不断加深对COPD多元化机制的认识,才能实现COPD的抗感染精准治疗,改善疾病预后。

参 考 文 献

[1] Global Initiative for Chronic Obstructive Lung Disease (GOLD): Global Strategy for the Diagnosis, Management and prevention of Chronic Obstructive Pulmonary Disease. (2020 REPORT).

[2] Celli BR, Locantore N, Yates J, et al. Inflammatory biomarkers improve clinical prediction of mortality in chronic obstructive pulmonary disease. Am J Respir Crit Care Med, 2012, 185(10):1065-1072.

[3] Liu T, Wang FP, Wang G, et al. Role of neutrophil extracellular traps in asthma and chronic obstructive pulmonary disease. Chin Med J, 2017, 130(6):730-736.

[4] Hiemstra PS, van Wetering S, Stolk J. Neutrophil serine proteinases and defensins in chronic obstructive pulmonary disease: effects on pulmonary epithelium. Eur Respir J, 1998, 12:1200-1208.

[5] Dubravec DB, Spriggs DR, Mannick JA, et al. Circulating human peripheral blood granulocytes synthesize and secrete tumor necrosis factor alpha. Proc Natl Acad Sci USA, 1990, 87:6758-6761.

[6] Tetley TD. New perspectives on basic mechanisms in lung disease. 6. Proteinase imbalance: its role in lung disease. Thorax, 1993, 48:560-565.

[7] Rogers DF. Airway goblet cells: responsive and adaptable front-line defenders. Eur Respir J, 1994, 7:1690-1706.

[8] Takeyama K, Dabbagh K, Jeong Shim J, et al. Oxidative stress causes mucin synthesis via transactivation of epidermal

growth factor receptor:role of neutrophils. J Immunol,2000, 164:1546-1552.

[9] Voynow JA, Young LR, Wang Y, et al. Neutrophil elastase increases MUC5AC mRNA and protein expression in respiratory epithelial cells. Am J Physiol,1999,276:835-843.

[10] Fischer B, Voynow J. Neutrophil elastase induces MUC5AC messenger RNA expression by an oxidant-dependent mechanism. Chest,2000,117(50 Suppl1):317-320.

[11] Panzner P, Lafitte JJ, Tsicopoulos A, et al. Marked up-regulation of T lymphocytes and expression of interleukin-9 in bronchial biopsies from patients with chronic bronchitis with obstruction. Chest,2003,124:1909-1915.

[12] O'Shaughnessy TC, Ansari TW, Barnes NC, et al. Inflammation in bronchial biopsies of subjects with chronic bronchitis: inverse relationship of $CD8^+$ T lymphocytes with FEV_1. Am J Respir Crit Care Med,1997,155:852-857.

[13] O'Donnell RA, Richter A, Ward J, et al. Expression of ErbB receptors and mucins in the airways of long term current smokers. Thorax,2004,59:1032-1034.

[14] Snider GL, Lucey EC, Stone PJ. Animal models of emphysema. Am Rev Respir Dis,1986,133:149-169.

[15] Shapiro SD, Goldstein NM, Houghton AM, et al. Neutrophil elastase contributes to cigarette smoke-induced emphysema in mice. Am J Pathol,2003,163:2329-2335.

[16] O'Donnell R, D Breen, S Wilson, et al. Inflammatory cells in the airways in COPD. Thorax,2006,61:448-454.

[17] George L, Brightling CE. Eosinophilic airway inflammation: role in asthma andchronic obstructive pulmonary disease. Ther Adv Chronic Dis,2016,7(1):34-51.

[18] Hardin M, Cho M, McDonald ML, et al. The clinical and genetic features of COPD-asthma overlap syndrome. Eur Respir J,2014,44:341-350.

[19] Singh D, Kolsum U, Brightling CE, et al. Eosinophilic inflammation in COPD:prevalence and clinical characteristics. Eur Respir J,2014,44(6):1697-1700.

[20] Christenson SA, Steiling K, van den Berge M, et al. Asthma-COPD overlap. Clinical relevance of genomic signatures of type 2 inflammation in chronic obstructive pulmonary disease. Am J Respir Crit Care Med,2015,191(7):758-766.

[21] Brightling C, Greening N. Airway inflammation in COPD-progress to precision medicine. Eur Respir J, 2019, 54(2):1900651.

[22] Shapiro SD. The macrophage in chronic obstructive pulmonary disease. Am J Respir Crit Care Med,1999,160:29-32.

[23] Molet SBC, Lena H, Germain N, et al. Increase in macrophage elastase(MMP-12)in lungs from patients with chronic obstructive pulmonary disease. Inflamm Res, 2005, 54:31-36.

[24] Montano M, Beccerril C, Ruiz V, et al. Matrix metalloproteinases activity in COPD associated with wood smoke. Chest,2004,125:466-472.

[25] Selman M, Cisneros-Lira J, Gaxiola M, et al. Matrix metalloproteinases inhibition attenuates tobacco smoke-induced emphysema in guinea pigs. Chest,2003,123:1633-1641.

[26] Churg A, Zay K, Shay S, et al. Acute cigarette smoke-induced connective tissue breakdown requires both neutrophils and macrophage metalloelastase in mice. Am J Respir Cell Mol Biol,2002,27:368-374.

[27] Dhami R, Gilks B, Xie C, et al. Acute cigarette smoke-induced connective tissue breakdown is mediated by neutrophils and prevented by alpha 1-antitrypsin. Am J Respir Cell Mol Biol,2000,22:244-252.

[28] Churg A, Wang RD, Tai H, et al. Macrophage metalloelastase mediates acute cigarette smoke-induced inflammation via tumor necrosis factor-a release. Am J Respir Crit Care Med, 2003,167:1083-1089.

[29] Culpitt SV, Rogers DF, Shah P, et al. Impaired inhibition by dexamethasone of cytokine release by alveolar macrophages frompatients with chronic obstructive pulmonary disease. Am J Respir Crit Care Med,2003,167(1):24-31.

[30] T. Hoshino, S. Kato, N. Oka, et al. Pulmonary inflammation and emphysema:role of the cytokines IL-18 and IL-13. Am J Respir Crit Care Med,2007,176(1):49-62.

[31] Cosio MG, Saetta M, Agusti A. Immunologic aspects of chronic obstructive pulmonary disease. N EnglJ Med, 2009, 360(23):2396-2454.

[32] Rovina N, Koutsoukou A, Kouloris NG. Inflammation and immune response in COPD:where do we stand?. Mediat Inflamm,2013,2013:413735.

[33] Yadava K, Pattaroni C, Sichelstiel AK, et al. Microbiota promotes chronic pulmonary inflammation by enhancing IL-17A and autoantibodies. Am J Respir Crit Care Med, 2016, 193(9):975-987.

[34] Collison LW, Workman CJ, Kuo TF, et al. The inhibitory eytokine IL-35 contributes to regulatory T cell function. Nature,2007,450(7169):566-569.

[35] Belgium KB. Role of CXCL13 in cigarette smoke-induced lymphoid follicle formation and chronic obstructive pulmonary disease. Am J Respir Crit Care Med, 2013, 188 (3):343-355.

[36] O'Donnell RA, Peebles C, Ward JA, et al. Relationship between peripheral airway dysfunction, airway obstruction, and neutrophilic inflammation in COPD. Thorax, 2004, 59:837-842.

[37] Hoenderdos K, Condliffe A. The neutrophil in COPD:too little too late, or too Much too Soon? Am J Respir Cell Mol Biol,2013,48(5):531-539.

[38] Patel IS, Seemungal TA, Wilks M, et al. Relationship between bacterial colonisation and the frequency, character, and severity of COPD exacerbations. Thorax,2002,57:759-764.

[39] Wilkinson TMA, Patel IS, Wilks M, et al. Airway bacterial load and FEV1 decline in patients with chronic obstructive pulmonary disease. Am J Respir Crit Care Med,2003,167:1090-1095.

[40] Hill AT, Campbell EJ, Hill SL, et al. Association between airway bacterial load and markers of airway inflammation in patients with stable chronic bronchitis. Am J Med, 2000, 109:288-295.

[41] Gao P, Zhang J, He X, et al. Sputum inflammatory cell-based classification of patients with acute exacerbation of chronic

obstructive pulmonary disease. PLoS One, 2013, 8 (5):e57678.
[42] Barnes PJ. Inflammatory endotypes in COPD. Allergy,2019, 74(7):1249-1256.
[43] Kolsum, Donaldso, GC, Singh R, et al. Blood and sputum eosinophils in COPD: relationship with bacterial load. Respir Res,2017,18:88.
[44] Jabarkhil A, Moberg M, Janner J, et al. Elevated blood eosinophils in acute COPD exacerbations: better short-and long-term prognosis. Eur Clin Respir J,2020,7:1757274.
[45] Bafadhel M, Greening NJ, Harvey-Dunstan TC, et al. Blood eosinophils and outcomes in severe hospitalized exacerbations of COPD. Chest,2016,150(2):320-328.
[46] Yu X, Seow HJ, Wang H, et al. Matrine reduces cigarette smoke-induced airway neutrophilic inflammation by enhancing neutrophil apoptosis, Clin Sci,2019,133(4):551-564.
[47] Yuko H, Hidenori I, Keisuke K, et al. Protective effect of Galectin-9 in murine model of lung emphysema: involvement of neutrophil migration and MMP-9 production. PLoS One, 2017,12(7):e0180742.
[48] 蔡柏强,李龙芸. 协和呼吸病学. 北京:中国协和医科大学出版社,2010.
[49] Mahler DA, Huang S, Tabrizi M, et al. Efficacy and safety of a monoclonal antibody recognizing interleukin-8 in COPD: a pilot study. Chest,2004,126(3):926-934.
[50] Rennard SI, Dale DC, Donohue JF, et al. CXCR2 antagonist MK-7123. A phase 2 proof-of-concept trial for chronic obstructive pulmonary disease. Am J Respir Critic Care Med, 2015,191(9):1001-1011.
[51] Rennard SI, Fogarty C, Kelsen S, et al. The safety and efficacy of infliximab in moderate to severe chronic obstructive pulmonary disease. Am J Respir Crit Care Med, 2007, 175 (9):926-934.
[52] Siva R, Green RH, Brightling CE, et al. Eosinophilic airway inflammation and exacerbations of COPD, a randomised controlled trial. Eur Respir J,2007,29(5):906-913.
[53] Brightling CE, Bleecker ER, Panettieri RA Jr, et al. Benralizumabfor chronic obstructive pulmonary disease and sputum eosinophilia: a randomised, double-blind, placebo-controlled, phase 2a study. Lancet Respir Med,2014,2(11):891-901.
[54] Greulich T, Hohlfeld JM, Neuser P, et al. A GATA3-specific DNAzyme attenuates sputum eosinophilia in eosinophilic COPD patients: a feasibility randomized clinical trial. Respir Res,2018,19(1):54.

7 经典与旁路炎症通路与COPD

谢俊刚

多种炎症通路在介导慢性阻塞性肺疾病（COPD）患者呼吸道的慢性炎症和结构变化中发挥重要作用。炎症通路激活，导致气道平滑肌收缩和炎症介质释放（如细胞因子、趋化因子、生长因子），以及细胞迁移、激活和增生。此外，COPD患者普遍对糖皮质激素治疗不敏感，这些原因，使人们对作为抗炎疗法的炎症通路抑制剂的开发产生了极大的兴趣。然而，口服后既有效又安全的选择性炎症通路抑制剂研制困难，虽然许多通路与气道疾病的炎症和重构有关，但在这些疾病中很少有药物达到临床研究阶段。本文就COPD常见的炎症通路及近年来研究的旁路做一综述。

一、介绍

慢性阻塞性肺疾病（COPD）是世界范围内发病率和病死率提高的主要原因，引起严重的经济和社会负担，这一负担目前还在不断增加。吸烟是COPD的主要危险因素，此外，暴露于生物燃料、空气污染，个体易感性（基因异常、肺发育异常、衰老）也是发病因素。炎症已被认为是COPD发生和发展中最重要的机制，炎症细胞和介质可通过介导黏液分泌增多、支气管收缩、小气道塌陷和肺泡破坏等过程促进气流阻塞。在COPD中，由于组蛋白去乙酰化酶HDAC2活性的降低，以及AP1、JNK、STAT5、JAK3等促炎因子的增加，使得糖皮质激素（GCs）敏感性下降，因此在糖皮质激素受体（GRs）发挥作用的上游寻找抑制炎症通路的靶点，有望解决糖皮质激素抵抗性的问题。

二、经典炎症通路与COPD

（一）NF-κB通路

核因子-κB（NF-κB）控制许多炎症基因的表达，在COPD的发病机制和严重程度及治疗反应中发挥关键作用。COPD患者痰液、肺组织巨噬细胞和支气管上皮细胞中NF-κB活化增加。NF-κB在调节气道细胞的炎性基因的表达中起着核心作用，包括细胞因子、趋化因子、蛋白酶和凋亡抑制剂，导致炎症反应放大。COPD的炎症主要涉及中性粒细胞、巨噬细胞、气道上皮细胞。气道黏膜下层的中性粒细胞浸润是慢性阻塞性肺病气道炎症的主要原因之一。由中性粒细胞产生的IL-8是一种NF-κB调控基因，中性粒细胞炎症与类固醇抵抗有关。肺泡巨噬细胞在COPD气道炎症中起关键作用。暴露于香烟烟雾（CS）提取物刺激肺泡巨噬细胞多种细胞因子分泌显著增加，这些炎症介质中，许多都是中性粒细胞的趋化剂，增加了它们在肺和气道中的浸润，是COPD发病的关键因素之一。CS引起巨噬细胞内炎症反应放大的分子基础包括氧化应激和随后的NF-κB通路的激活和信号转导。上皮细胞在气道病理中也起着关键作用，是气道与环境的重要界面。上皮细胞通过产生大量由NF-κB调节的免疫/炎症介质协调对各种侵袭性损伤的反应，这些介质大多是趋化剂，它们促进炎症细胞的招募，进而影响上皮功能。气道平滑肌（ASM）细胞是生长因子、细胞因子和其他炎症介质的强大生产者，其在气道阻塞性疾病中也有重要的炎症作用。凝血酶和白介素-1（IL-1）以糖皮质激素（GCs）敏感的方式刺激ASM细胞中的NF-κB活性。在ASM细胞中，NF-κB调节许多在COPD病理中重要的基因，例如TSLP、CD38、VCAM-1、ICAM-1、cyclooxygenase-2、IL-6、IL-8、CXCL10、GM-CSF等。

糖皮质激素可通过抑制NF-κB应答基因的转录发挥抗炎作用。但在COPD中，糖皮质激素敏感性下降，原因之一是糖皮质激素对NF-κB的转录抑制作用减弱，这是组蛋白去乙酰化酶（HDAC）表达和活性降低的结果。由吸烟、严重炎症、细菌定植和（或）病毒感染等损伤引起的氧化应激和硝化应激增加与HDAC异常有关。HDAC缺陷导致组蛋白高乙酰化，染色质结构松弛，从而使原本沉默的炎症基因得以转录。HDAC表达和活性降低的另一个后果是与配体结合的GR乙酰化时间延长，阻止其与细胞核中NF-κB的关联。

针对NF-κB活化或功能的治疗是糖皮质激素抵抗型气道疾病的潜在解决办法，但鉴于NF-κB的广泛表达以及它在细胞生存、凋亡等重要生理过程中有重要作用，抑制NF-κB的活化可能会产生严重的不良反应。

（二）MAPK通路

MAPK是一个高度保守的丝氨酸/苏氨酸蛋白激酶家族，参与信号转导。它可以被有丝分裂原、细胞因子、生长因子和各种压力（渗透压、氧化应激、热休克）等激活，导致不同的细胞反应，如增生、分化、有丝分裂、细胞存活、凋亡和炎症基因表达。MAPK在COPD中被激活，在慢性炎症和皮质类固醇不敏感中发挥重要作用。MAPK参与炎性疾病的主要通路包括ERK、p38 MAPK和JNK。

p38 MAPK是研究最多的通路。P38 MAPK靶向许多蛋白，包括其他激酶、转录因子和细胞骨架蛋白，导致多种炎症作用。p38 MAPK家族由α、β、γ和δ亚基组成。P38 MAPK激活60多个下游靶点，因此可能是抑制作用的关键点。p38α和p38β异构体分布广泛，作用于下游的map活化蛋白激酶2(MAPKAPK2或MK2)，介导生物学作用。p38γ和p38δ亚型的分布较为局限，主要在巨噬细胞，靶向转录因子。磷酸化的p38α在COPD患者肺泡巨噬细胞、上皮细胞、$CD4^+$和$CD8^+$淋巴细胞中表达增加。p38α可以通过稳定细胞因子转录促进炎症，还可通过磷酸化促炎细胞因子和趋化因子基因启动子位点的组蛋白H3，以增加NF-κB与启动子区域的结合，增强NF-κB的促炎作用。p38α还可能在COPD肺中性粒细胞炎症中发挥重要作用，并在糖皮质激素不敏感方面发挥作用。TNF-α和IL-1β通过激活p38α导致糖皮质激素受体(GRα)Ser211位点的磷酸化，防止其转位到细胞核。在COPD患者的PBMC中，使用p38α抑制剂可以逆转对皮质类固醇反应性的降低。选择性p38抑制剂在COPD体外细胞和动物免疫模型中相当有效，一些p38抑制剂已用于临床。为了解决糖皮质激素抵抗性疾病的治疗问题，这些药物已经在一些临床疾病包括COPD进行了试验，但因为它们的不良反应限制了剂量，并且由于代偿信号通路的发展，大多数已经停止开发。

JNK是促炎转录因子激活蛋白-1(AP-1)的重要激酶因子，在COPD中调控许多炎症基因。JNK也可能在气道重塑中发挥作用，JNK的激活参与了皮质类固醇抵抗，原因是AP-1与GRα竞争，且JNK的激活导致GR-α的Ser226磷酸化，从而阻止其核定位。JNK抑制剂可降低皮质类固醇耐药，JNK和IKK-b抑制剂的结合可完全逆转皮质类固醇耐药。JNK活化在COPD中发挥作用。香烟烟雾对气道上皮细胞的细胞毒性可通过JNK的激活介导。

ERK1/2在COPD中也是激活的，研究显示香烟烟雾通过ERK1/2 MAPK信号传导诱导MMP-1产生，在肺气肿形成中起关键作用。

针对这三种通路的抑制剂的抑炎效果明显，但毒性很大，因此临床应用受限。

(三) PI3K通路

根据其结构和脂质底物特异性磷脂酰肌醇3-激酶(PI3Ks)被分为三类(Ⅰ、Ⅱ、Ⅲ类)。研究较多的是Ⅰ类PI3Ks，它是由催化亚基和调节亚基组成的异源二聚体，又分为两类。IA类由催化亚基(p110α/β/δ)和调节亚基(p85α、p55α、p50α、p85β、p55γ)组成，被受体酪氨酸激酶(RTKs)如生长因子、胰岛素激活。IB类由催化亚基(p110γ，主要表达在髓系的中性粒细胞、巨噬细胞、肥大细胞)和调节亚基(p101或p84)组成，被G蛋白偶联受体激活。激活后，Ⅰ类PI3K将PIP2催化为PIP3，作为一种广泛的第二信使，PIP3具有pleckstrin同源结构域的下游信号分子的靶点，如蛋白丝氨酸/苏氨酸激酶(蛋白激酶B/Akt)、磷酸化肌醇依赖性激酶1(PDK1)或蛋白激酶C和MAPK信号通路。这些信号蛋白积极参与调节细胞生长、增生和形状，凋亡(阻止/增强)，细胞运动和细胞激活。

鉴于PI3K信号通路在细胞增生中的关键作用，以往PI3K的研究主要集中在癌症领域，有关PI3K与炎症的研究较少。近年来研究表明，PI3K通路的许多成分在炎症介质的表达和激活、炎症细胞募集、免疫细胞功能、气道重塑和皮质类固醇的不敏感性在慢性炎症呼吸疾病中发挥关键作用。研究显示，PI3K通路还与加速衰老的慢性退行性疾病，以及炎症和免疫疾病的治疗相关。PI3K的激活在COPD中也很重要，p-Akt水平的PI3K总活性在COPD患者外周血和巨噬细胞中显著升高，提示PI3K在COPD发病机制中的潜在作用。越来越多的证据表明，PI3K通过激活炎症、皮质类固醇抵抗和细胞衰老，导致衰老加速，在COPD中发挥关键作用。有研究表明，与肺气肿发病机制有关的MMP9的表达除了受到NF-κB的调控，也受到PI3K信号通路的调控。此外，一些证据表明PI3K在激活巨噬细胞和中性粒细胞中的重要性，它们是COPD炎症的关键因素。

以上效应是通过Ⅰ类PI3Ks介导的，Ⅱ类和Ⅲ类PI3Ks的潜在作用尚不清楚。人们对Ⅰ类PI3K通路抑制剂在治疗COPD中的潜力非常感兴趣。吸入非选择性PI3K催化亚基抑制剂LY294002可抑制致敏小鼠对变应原的过敏性炎症反应，减少嗜酸性粒细胞、Th2细胞因子和气道高反应性。

尽管糖皮质激素在控制轻、中度哮喘方面非常有效，但COPD和严重哮喘患者对皮质类固醇的反应并不好。Ito等报道COPD患者中HDAC2的表达和总HDAC活性的降低，而HDAC2的降低是COPD中皮质类固醇不敏感的原因之一。体外实验也表明，PI3K催化亚基非选择性抑制剂LY294002和Akt抑制剂SH-5恢复了细胞中缺陷的HDAC2表达和活性。茶碱就是通过选择性抑制PI3Kδ活性，恢复HDAC2的活动，从而逆转皮质类固醇耐药。这说明PI3K可以通过降低HDAC活性参与皮质类固醇敏感性，有望作为糖皮质激素抵抗性疾病的替代疗法的重要突破口。

(四) 其他通路

其他经典炎症通路比如Janus激酶(JAK)信号转导和转录激活因子(STAT)途径(JAK-STAT信号通路)也与COPD炎症相关，许多COPD炎症相关的关键细胞因子通过JAK-STAT途径信号产生。因此，作为COPD的潜在治疗手段，JAK-STAT抑制剂的开发也是研究热点之一。目前，所有STAT家族成员在COPD患者组织中的激活情况还不完全清楚。脾酪氨酸激酶(STK)通路可作为NF-κB和PI3K通路的上游参与COPD的炎症过程中。

三、旁路炎症通路与COPD

近年来陆续发现了其他分子可作为经典炎症通路的上下游，调节炎症过程。

(一) NF-κB旁路

核激素受体Nur77活化可通过抑制NF-κB通路抑制炎症，而COPD患者肺组织和气道上皮细胞Nur77表达下调，香烟烟雾可通过下调Nur77加重COPD炎症。FSTL-1(卵泡抑制素-like 1)可通过Nr4a1(一种孤儿核激素受体)负调NF-κB通路，有望减缓肺气肿和炎症进展。过氧化物

酶增生体激活受体 γ(PPARγ)被认为是 COPD 抗炎治疗的潜在靶点,研究显示它可能通过抑制 NF-κB 发挥作用。

此外,有关糖皮质激素抵抗方面的研究显示其他乙酰转移酶和去乙酰酶对 NF-κB 和 IκBα 翻译后的修饰可能参与了 COPD 的 GC 耐药。Sirtuins,即具有组蛋白和非组蛋白去乙酰化酶活性的蛋白,在 COPD 个体的组织和炎症细胞或 CS 暴露的肺泡巨噬细胞中下调。Sirtuin 1 活性降低与吸烟者和 COPD 患者肺泡巨噬细胞中 NF-κB 乙酰化增加和随后的 IL-8 释放有关。Sirtuin 4 也被证明可以保护肺内皮细胞抵抗 CS 体外诱导的细胞因子和细胞黏附分子(CAM)的表达,从而防止 IκBα 的降解,进而抑制 NF-κB 的激活,因此它在 COPD 中的下调也参与了糖皮质激素抵抗。另外,一些糖皮质激素诱导表达的基因也可调节 NF-κB 信号。例如,GCs 可以上调 NF-κB 抑制亚基 IκBα 的表达;糖皮质激素诱导亮氨酸拉链(GILZ)直接通过结合 NF-κB 亚基抑制 NF-κB 信号转导;MKP-1,另一种 GCs 诱导表达的基因,可以抑制气道上皮细胞的 NF-κB 信号,但机制未明。

(二)MAPK 旁路

对 PM2.5 和香烟烟雾在 COPD 的炎症中的作用研究发现,PM2.5 可能通过 Wnt5a-ERK 途径加重香烟烟雾诱导的在 COPD 的炎症。在香烟烟雾诱导的氧化应激下,TGF-β 激活激酶 1 结合蛋白(TAB1)可通过介导人羊膜上皮细胞 p38 MAPK 自磷酸化激活 MAPK 通路,这是一种罕见的激活方式。MAPK(ERK1/2,JNK 和 p38)可能通过抑制 Foxa2 通路介导香烟烟雾诱导的支气管上皮细胞鳞状上皮化生。IL-33 可介导 p38 MAPK 通路的活化。香烟烟雾可以通过 p38 MAPK 活化抑制电压依赖性 K^+ 通道(BK),导致气道黏膜纤毛清除障碍,损害气道防御,加重气道炎症。

(三)PI3K 旁路

目前对于 PI3K 旁路的研究主要集中在催化亚基,抑制剂也多针对催化亚基,而关于调节亚基的功能,以及它们与催化亚基结合的偏好性等机制尚未阐明。有研究显示调节亚基 p85 可能通过影响 Th1 细胞因子向 Th2 细胞因子的转换调节炎症,表明 IA 类 PI3Ks 的调节亚基也可能参与炎症过程,有望作为抗炎治疗的新靶点。由于 PI3K 在正常细胞发育中的关键作用,使用催化亚基抑制剂虽然表现出明显的抑制效果,但导致的不良反应也不容忽视。因此,开发特异性针对其他调节亚基的抑制剂有望降低非选择性抑制剂的毒性,提供新的治疗思路。对 p55γ(IA 类 PI3K 的一种调节亚基,由 *PIK3R3* 基因编码)研究发现,与正常肺功能的人相比,COPD 患者肺组织表达更高水平的 p55γ,在支气管上皮细胞系中敲减 p55γ 的表达,可以减弱香烟烟雾提取物诱导的炎症因子的水平和一些炎症通路的活化,利用 p55γ 的独特 N 端合成重组蛋白对气道上皮细胞进行预处理,也可以抑制香烟烟雾提取物诱导的气道上皮炎症,提示了 p55γ 可能参与香烟烟雾诱导的气道炎症和 COPD 的发生发展,而 p55γ 的 N 端衍生物作为其抑制剂,有望为 COPD 的抗炎治疗提供新靶点。

(四)非编码 RNA

近年来研究发现很多非编码 RNA 参与 COPD 的炎症调节。非编码 RNA 包括 miRNAs、LncRNAs 等。很多 miRNA 通过负调炎症通路组分来调控炎症,例如 microRNA-149-3p 可能通过抑制 TLR4/NF-κB 通路的活化减弱吸烟相关 COPD 的炎症,Let-7 通过靶向 TNF 受体Ⅱ对 CS 诱导的炎症和肺气肿具有保护作用,在 COPD 发病机制中已被证明其重要性。长非编码 RNA(lncRNAs),可能在调节肺对慢性吸入有毒物质的反应和 COPD 的发展方面发挥重要作用。LncRNA 可以作为炎症的诱导剂和抑制剂,参与多种水平的免疫细胞发育和对病原体的应答。

四、结　语

炎症在 COPD 的发病发展中起着核心作用,鉴于 COPD 的糖皮质激素抵抗性,学者们热衷于研究和开发针对炎症通路的特异性抑制剂,许多临床前研究和早期临床试验正在进行中,因此该领域有望取得进展。如何开发出特异性强的抑制剂、开发有效的吸入型炎症通路抑制剂以避免全身暴露,都是需要解决的难题。机体内各种信号通路都不是完全独立的,它们之间有着复杂的联系,经典炎症通路和旁路通过互相影响和协作共同调控炎症过程,因此抑制某个炎症通路可能会导致其他分子通路的反馈性激活,这也是需要关注的难题。此外,还有很多其他分子信号通路可能影响 COPD 的发生发展,这都需要对此进一步研究。

参 考 文 献

[1] Cundall M, et al. Neutrophil-derived matrix metalloproteinase-9 is increased in severe asthma and poorly inhibited by glucocorticoids. J Allergy Clin Immunol, 2003, 112(6):1064-1071.

[2] Yang SR, et al. Cigarette smoke induces proinflammatory cytokine release by activation of NF-kappaB and posttranslational modifications of histone deacetylase in macrophages. Am J Physiol Lung Cell Mol Physiol, 2006, 291(1):46-57.

[3] Lee HC, SF Ziegler. Inducible expression of the proallergic cytokine thymic stromal lymphopoietin in airway epithelial cells is controlled by NFkappaB. Proc Natl Acad Sci U S A, 2007, 104(3):914-919.

[4] Redhu NS, et al. Essential role of NF-κB and AP-1 transcription factors in TNF-α-induced TSLP expression in human airway smooth muscle cells. Am J Physiol Lung Cell Mol Physiol, 2011, 300(3):479-485.

[5] Clarke DL, et al. TNFα and IFNγ synergistically enhance transcriptional activation of CXCL10 in human airway smooth muscle cells via STAT-1, NF-κB, and the transcriptional coactivator CREB-binding protein. J Biol Chem, 2010, 285(38):29101-29110.

[6] Barnes PJ. Corticosteroid resistance in patients with asthma and chronic obstructive pulmonary disease. J Allergy Clin Im-

munol,2013,131(3):636-645.
[7] Ito K,et al. Histone deacetylase 2-mediated deacetylation of the glucocorticoid receptor enables NF-kappaB suppression. J Exp Med,2006,203(1):7-13.
[8] Langereis JD,et al. Abrogation of NF-κB signaling in human neutrophils induces neutrophil survival through sustained p38-MAPK activation. J Leukoc Biol,2010,88(4):655-664.
[9] Chung KF. p38 mitogen-activated protein kinase pathways in asthma and COPD. Chest,2011. 139(6):1470-1479.
[10] Trempolec N, N Dave-Coll AR. Nebreda, SnapShot: p38 MAPK substrates. Cell,2013,152(4):924.
[11] Brook M,et al. Posttranslational regulation of tristetraprolin subcellular localization and protein stability by p38 mitogen-activated protein kinase and extracellular signal-regulated kinase pathways. Mol Cell Biol,2006,26(6):2408-2418.
[12] Dean JL,et al. The involvement of AU-rich element-binding proteins in p38 mitogen-activated protein kinase pathway-mediated mRNA stabilisation. Cell Signal, 2004, 16(10): 1113-1121.
[13] Saccani SS. Pantano, G Natoli. p38-Dependent marking of inflammatory genes for increased NF-kappa B recruitment. Nat Immunol,2002,3(1):69-75.
[14] Szatmáry Z,MJ Garabedian, J Vilcek,et al. Inhibition of glucocorticoid receptor-mediated transcriptional activation by p38 mitogen activated protein (MAP) kinase. J Biol Chem, 2004,279(42):43708-43715.
[15] Khorasani N,et al. Reversal of corticosteroid insensitivity by p38 MAPK inhibition in peripheral blood mononuclear cells from COPD. Int J Chron Obstruct Pulmon Dis,2015,10:283-291.
[16] Charron CE,et al. RV568,a narrow-spectrum kinase inhibitor with p38 MAPK-α and-γ selectivity,suppresses COPD inflammation. Eur Respir J,2017,50(4):1700188.
[17] Eynott PR,et al. Allergen-induced inflammation and airway epithelial and smooth muscle cell proliferation:role of Jun N-terminal kinase. Br J Pharmacol,2003,140(8):1373-1380.
[18] Kobayashi Y,et al. Increased corticosteroid sensitivity by a long acting β2 agonist formoterol via β2 adrenoceptor independent protein phosphatase 2A activation. Pulm Pharmacol Ther,2012,25(3):201-207.
[19] Papi A,et al. Rhinovirus infection causes steroid resistance in airway epithelium through nuclear factor κB and c-Jun N-terminal kinase activation. J Allergy Clin Immunol, 2013, 132 (5):1075-1085.
[20] Lee YC,et al. TRX-ASK1-JNK signaling regulation of cell density-dependent cytotoxicity in cigarette smoke-exposed human bronchial epithelial cells. Am J Physiol Lung Cell Mol Physiol,2008,294(5):921-931.
[21] Mercer BA. JM D'Armiento, Emerging role of MAP kinase pathways as therapeutic targets in COPD. Int J Chron Obstruct Pulmon Dis,2006,1(2):137-150.
[22] Johnson SC,PS Rabinovitch, M. Kaeberlein. mTOR is a key modulator of ageing and age-related disease. Nature, 2013, 493(7432):338-345.
[23] Marwick JA,et al. A role for phosphoinositol 3-kinase delta in the impairment of glucocorticoid responsiveness in patients with chronic obstructive pulmonary disease. J Allergy Clin Immunol,2010,125(5):1146-1153.
[24] Duan W, et al. An anti-inflammatory role for a phosphoinositide 3-kinase inhibitor LY294002 in a mouse asthma model. Int Immunopharmacol,2005,5(3):495-502.
[25] Ito K,et al. Decreased histone deacetylase activity in chronic obstructive pulmonary disease. N Engl J Med, 2005, 352 (19):1967-1976.
[26] Kozikowski AP,et al. Novel PI analogues selectively block activation of the pro-survival serine/threonine kinase Akt. J Am Chem Soc,2003,125(5):1144-1145.
[27] Ito K,et al. A molecular mechanism of action of theophylline:Induction of histone deacetylase activity to decrease inflammatory gene expression. Proc Natl Acad Sci U S A, 2002,99(13):8921-8926.
[28] Schindler C, I. Strehlow, et al. Cytokines and STAT signaling. Adv Pharmacol,2000,47:113-174.
[29] Reddy AT,et al. Cigarette smoke downregulates Nur77 to exacerbate inflammation in chronic obstructive pulmonary disease(COPD). PLoS One,2020,15(2):e0229256.
[30] Henkel M,et al. FSTL-1 Attenuation Causes Spontaneous Smoke-Resistant Pulmonary Emphysema. Am J Respir Crit Care Med,2020,201(8):934-945.
[31] Li Q, et al. Curcumin inhibits cigarette smoke-induced inflammation via modulating the PPARγ-NF-κB signaling pathway. Food Funct,2019,10(12):7983-7994.
[32] Yuan J,et al. Curcumin Attenuates Airway Inflammation and Airway Remolding by Inhibiting NF-κB Signaling and COX-2 in Cigarette Smoke-Induced COPD Mice. Inflammation, 2018,41(5):1804-1814.
[33] Rajendrasozhan S,et al. SIRT1,an antiinflammatory and antiaging protein,is decreased in lungs of patients with chronic obstructive pulmonary disease. Am J Respir Crit Care Med, 2008,177(8):861-870.
[34] Chen Y, et al. SIRT4 inhibits cigarette smoke extracts-induced mononuclear cell adhesion to human pulmonary microvascular endothelial cells via regulating NF-κB activity. Toxicol Lett,2014,226(3):320-327.
[35] Eddleston J,et al. The anti-inflammatory effect of glucocorticoids is mediated by glucocorticoid-induced leucine zipper in epithelial cells. J Allergy Clin Immunol, 2007, 119 (1): 115-122.
[36] Ayroldi E,et al. Modulation of T-cell activation by the glucocorticoid-induced leucine zipper factor via inhibition of nuclear factor kappaB. Blood,2001,98(3):743-753.
[37] King EM,et al. Inhibition of NF-kappaB-dependent transcription by MKP-1: transcriptional repression by glucocorticoids occurring via p38 MAPK. J Biol Chem,2009,284(39):26803-26815.
[38] Wang Z, et al. Fine-particulate matter aggravates cigarette smoke extract-induced airway inflammation via Wnt5a-ERK pathway in COPD. Int J Chron Obstruct Pulmon Dis, 2019, 14:979-994.
[39] Richardson L, et al. Oxidative stress-induced TGF-beta/

TAB1-mediated p38MAPK activation in human amnion epithelial cells. Biol Reprod,2018,99(5):1100-1112.

[40] Du C,et al. MAPK/FoxA2-mediated cigarette smoke-induced squamous metaplasia of bronchial epithelial cells. Int J Chron Obstruct Pulmon Dis,2017,12:3341-3351.

[41] Xie C,et al. Tobacco smoke induced hepatic cancer stem cell-like properties through IL-33/p38 pathway. J Exp Clin Cancer Res,2019,38(1):39.

[42] Sailland J,et al. Role of Smad3 and p38 Signalling in Cigarette Smoke-induced CFTR and BK dysfunction in Primary Human Bronchial Airway Epithelial Cells. Sci Rep,2017,7(1):10506.

[43] Myou S,et al. Blockade of inflammation and airway hyperresponsiveness in immune-sensitized mice by dominant-negative phosphoinositide 3-kinase-TAT. J Exp Med,2003,198(10):1573-1582.

[44] Shen W,et al. Repression of Toll-like receptor-4 by microRNA-149-3p is associated with smoking-related COPD. Int J Chron Obstruct Pulmon Dis,2017,12:705-715.

[45] D'Hulst AI,et al. Role of tumour necrosis factor-alpha receptor p75 in cigarette smoke-induced pulmonary inflammation and emphysema. Eur Respir J,2006,28(1):102-112.

[46] Marchese FP,I Raimondi,M Huarte. The multidimensional mechanisms of long noncoding RNA function. Genome Biol,2017,18(1):206.

8 气道黏液高分泌是慢性阻塞性肺疾病一个新表型吗?

曹 洁

慢性阻塞性肺疾病(COPD)在全球范围内很常见,主要特征为进行性气流受限,主要症状为长期咳嗽、咳痰和呼吸困难。2015年,COPD在世界范围内年龄标化病死率中排名第三,全球约有320万人死于COPD,造成了巨大的社会经济负担。COPD急性加重及多种合并症常常伴随病程始终,严重影响患者的治疗及预后。慢性气道黏液高分泌(CMH)是COPD的主要病理生理特征,临床上表现为慢性咳嗽和排痰。黏液产生增加和纤毛清除功能障碍可能导致呼吸道黏液堆积,从而导致COPD患者形成痰栓,严重痰阻常危及患者生命。COPD被认为是存在共同特征(不完全可逆性气流受限)但具有多种表型的异质性疾病,COPD表型是指具有一种或多种疾病属性,且与临床有意义的结果相关的患者特征(如症状、肺功能、疾病进展或病死率等),用来描述COPD患者之间的差异。气道黏液高分泌是COPD的一个新表型吗?越来越多的证据表明,CMH是COPD患者的重要危险因素,CMH会影响一些重要的结果,如导致气流受限、肺功能下降、呼吸道反复感染、COPD急性加重,住院和病死率增加,以及影响患者整体健康状况。因此关注CMH会加深我们对COPD的认识,有利于COPD的早期发现、早期预防,也有利于COPD患者的个体化治疗。

一、CMH的定义

在COPD患者中,气道上皮黏液腺和杯状细胞分泌黏液过度被描述为"慢性气道黏液高分泌""慢性痰液产生"或"慢性支气管炎(CB)"。黏液清除吸入的微粒和微生物等,也是防止水分流失的屏障,对维持肺部健康起重要作用,黏蛋白(特别是MUC5AC)是其重要成分。含有细菌或炎性细胞碎屑的气道黏液排出时称为"痰",黏液通常可以与痰液互换使用。一些研究定义CMH为慢性排痰或慢性排痰伴咳嗽;也有研究将CMH具体定义为"每天痰液排出量大于30ml,每年至少3个月,持续时间至少1年"。

二、CMH的流行病学

目前关于CMH流行病学的研究较少。对哥本哈根市人群的研究报道表明,CMH在普通人群中患病率约为10.1%,男性为12.5%,女性为8.2%。气道黏液的分泌随着年龄的增长和吸烟量的增加而显著增多。中国一项采用多阶段整群抽样调查的研究发现,30%的COPD受试者曾有慢支炎病史;另一项研究显示接近50%的COPD患者有气道黏液分泌过多。另有研究报道咳嗽咳痰的受试者患COPD的概率是健康人群的近3倍。

三、CMH的机制

正常情况下,分泌至呼吸道的黏液可捕获沉积的物质并通过纤毛运输和咳嗽从肺部清除,起着保护气道和润湿空气的作用,然而黏液分泌过多不能有效清除时会造成各种病理后果。COPD发病过程始终贯穿着CMH现象,其机制较为复杂,涉及多种因素。

(一)表皮生长因子受体(EGFR)

目前针对EGFR信号通路的研究较为广泛,EGFR必须激活才能诱导黏蛋白生成。EGFR与配体(TNF-α和双调蛋白)的结合激活其内在的蛋白激酶,进而诱导下游的磷脂酰肌醇-3-激酶(PI3K)和丝苏氨酸蛋白激酶(AKT)通路,联合IL-13信号途径,增加MUC5AC基因表达和纤毛细胞凋亡,导致COPD患者气道黏液分泌过多、清除困难,从而阻塞气道、限制气流。此外,在炎症介质、细胞因子、细菌产物和病毒等刺激下,可以经由非配体依赖性激活机制使EGFR酪氨酸磷酸化,引起丝裂原活化蛋白激酶(MAPK)级联反应,激活ERK1/2、JNK和P-38,从而激活NF-κB,诱导MUC5ACmRNA的表达。

(二)炎症反应

COPD的炎症反应以中性粒细胞浸润为主。活化的中性粒细胞可分泌多种细胞因子,通过上调EGFR的表达而直接刺激黏蛋白合成。同时,中性粒细胞弹性蛋白酶(NE)可增加MUC5AC的基因表达,还可通过诱导杯状细胞的分化和黏液性质的改变促进CMH。此外,炎症反应会损伤气道上皮细胞,使呼吸道黏膜下腺肥大、杯状细胞增生及纤毛功能障碍,导致黏液堆积、气道感染、气道阻塞和重塑,造成恶性循环,加重COPD。

(三)香烟烟雾暴露

吸烟也是导致COPD患者CMH的重要因素。香烟烟雾中主要含有丙烯醛、乙醛、尼古丁及其代谢产物,其中丙烯醛、乙醛等经上呼吸道吸收而刺激黏液高分泌,而尼古丁可阻碍黏膜水化,导致黏液黏度增加。Innes等研究表明习惯性吸烟者存在大气道杯状细胞肥大和增生,从而导致气道黏蛋白储存量明显高于正常水平。吸烟时大量的活性氧(ROS)和脂多糖(LPS)可促进杯状细胞数量增加,增加黏蛋白及其基因的表达,这种效应依赖于EGFR和氧化应激的参与。

四、CMH 与 COPD 的关系

COPD 被认为是存在共同特征(不完全可逆性气流受限)但具有多种表型的异质性疾病,COPD 的发病机制、临床表现、疾病进展等方面都存在明显差异,影响其治疗及预后。COPD 表型是指一种或多种疾病属性,被定义为与临床有意义的结果相关的患者特征(如症状、肺功能、疾病进展或病死率等),用来描述 COPD 患者之间的差异。1989 年,Snider 最先提出概念化不同的表型,引入 COPD 3 个经典的亚组:慢支炎、肺气肿和哮喘。2012 年,西班牙 COPD 指南根据急性加重频率和主要临床表现对 COPD 进行分型,提出了非急性加重型、哮喘-COPD 重叠综合征、急性加重伴肺气肿表型和急性加重伴慢性支气管炎表型。随着研究深入,COPD 出现了很多新兴表型,如 COPD 合并支气管扩张表型、肺功能快速下降表型、全身炎症表型和全身合并症表型等。COPD 可能存在更多的表型,目前缺乏关于 COPD 表型确切的普遍共识。CMH 会是 COPD 的一个新表型吗?首先必须了解 CMH 与 COPD 的关系。

(一)CMH 与 COPD 患者临床表现的关系

研究发现,在 1025 例有症状的 COPD 患者中,咳嗽最常见(73.6%),其次是咳痰(68.8%)和呼吸困难(61.4%)。伴有 CMH 的 COPD 患者有更多更严重的呼吸系统症状,咳嗽咳痰源于 CMH 和黏膜炎症,当咳嗽咳痰超过 2 年且每年持续 3 个月被定义为"慢性支气管炎"。一项对 COPD 受试者的多因素分析显示,慢支炎与喘息($P=0.002$)和呼吸困难($P=0.003$)等呼吸道症状显著相关。Kim 等发现患有慢支炎的 COPD 受试者症状更明显,例如喘息(86.5% vs 67.6%,$P<0.0001$),鼻塞、鼻漏等上呼吸道症状(69.3% vs 53.4%,$P<0.0001$),继发于咳嗽的夜间觉醒(45.9% vs 19.1%,$P<0.0001$),以及继发于呼吸困难或胸闷的夜间觉醒(39.3% vs 24.4%,$P<0.0001$)。此外,CMH 导致的气道管腔堵塞(如痰栓)与 COPD 患者的肺气肿直接相关。

(二)CMH 与 COPD 患者肺功能的关系

CMH 引起的黏液积聚阻塞会促进支气管感染,从而加剧气道和肺泡损害,并导致气流受限。研究表明患有慢支炎的 COPD 受试者比无慢性支气管炎者的肺功能更差。一项大型队列研究纳入了 972 名 COPD 受试者,包括 220 名慢性咳痰者(其中 172 名符合慢支炎的经典定义)和 752 名无慢性咳痰者,结果发现与无慢性咳痰的 COPD 患者相比,有慢性咳痰的患者基线时的肺功能更差,且在随访期间肺功能下降更严重($P=0.004$)。Vestbo 等研究表明 CMH 与 FEV_1 下降显著相关;并发现校正年龄、身高、体重和吸烟等混杂因素后,与非 CMH 的同性别人群相比,CMH 的男性 FEV_1 每年多下降 22.8 ml,CMH 女性 FEV_1 额外下降为 12.6 ml/年。Sherman 等对 1757 名男性和 2191 名女性随访了 12 年,也证明了 CMH 与 FEV_1 的关系在男性中更为显著。

(三)CMH 与 COPD 患者疾病进展的关系

COPD 加重的特征是黏液分泌过多和急性气道炎症,占 COPD 总负担的最大百分比。研究表明,与无 CMH 的 COPD 患者相比,CMH 患者每年至少出现 2 次急性加重的情况更常见(40% vs 52.6%,$P=0.002$);在该研究的多元回归模型中,CMH 与 COPD 频繁急性加重显著相关($OR:1.54,95\%CI:1.11\sim2.14$)。Kim 发现慢性咳嗽咳痰的 COPD 受试者病情加重及严重加重是无咳嗽咳痰者的 2 倍。一些研究还发现长期咳嗽咳痰与 COPD 病情进展和死亡风险增加有关。COPD 患者存在 CMH 时,死亡风险将增加 3.5 倍。Prescott 等研究发现,CMH 是 COPD 肺部感染死亡的重要预测因子,但不是无肺部感染死亡的预测因素。有研究表明,CMH 的存在增加了所有原因的病死率。此外,患有 CMH 的 COPD 患者的精神状态和生活质量更差。

在一项较大的纵向研究中,虽然慢性排痰的 COPD 患者生活质量较差,但并未发现其呼吸困难更严重,FEV_1 和 COPD 加重次数也没有显著差异。在 COPDGene 研究中($n=1061$),慢性支气管炎与 COPD 病情加重之间有很强的关联,且患有慢性支气管炎的 COPD 患者生活质量更差,但肺功能无差异。在 ECLIPSE 研究中($n=2138$),随访的第一年发现慢性咳嗽与 COPD 加重相关,但未发现慢支炎或慢性痰液生成与 COPD 病情加重的关联。一项多因素分析显示,在 COPD 患者中,呼吸困难严重程度、肺功能和生活质量按以下顺序恶化:无咳嗽咳痰,仅咳痰,仅咳嗽和慢性支气管炎。Mannino 等的研究显示 CMH 与 COPD 死亡风险之间也无统计学意义上的相关性。然而,直接比较 CMH、慢性咳嗽、慢性咳嗽和慢性咳痰伴咳嗽与 COPD 之间关联的研究很少,因此很难比较这些研究报道的结果。

五、COPD 中 CMH 的靶向治疗

鉴于 CMH 对 COPD 重要的临床影响,减少气道黏液堆积对 COPD 患者的治疗很重要。

戒烟可以通过改善黏液纤毛功能、减少杯状细胞增生,从"源头"阻止 CMH。其次,祛痰剂通过阻止黏液的过度分泌和(或)促进黏液溶解清除,不仅缓解 COPD 患者咳嗽、咳痰和呼吸困难等症状,减少气道阻塞,延缓肺功能下降,还可以避免反复感染和急性加重,改善疾病的预后。胸背部拍打、体位排痰可促进痰液引流;吸入疗法可湿润气道、稀释黏液,防止痰栓形成;高频胸壁振荡可增加 COPD 患者的气道黏液清除率,显著改善生活质量。

通过调控黏液细胞分化、黏蛋白基因表达、蛋白加工和胞吐作用,可能直接靶向治疗 CMH。许多研究发现丹参酮ⅡA磺酸钠可能是 COPD 中气道黏液高分泌的新治疗靶点,它可以抑制黏液分泌过多、过度的炎症反应和肺功能下降,明显抑制 COPD 加重的程度。EGFR 抑制剂是典型的靶向治疗药物,通过抑制 EGFR mRNA 的上调来减少黏液合成,同时可防止 IL-13 诱导的杯状细胞增生和中性粒细胞聚集,但在 COPD 的治疗上有大量不良反应。

六、总结与展望

CMH 与 COPD 的关系在各研究中的结果并不一致,存在这些差异的原因还有待确定,可能与目前尚无用于量化 CMH 的标准有关,也与所研究的人群不同等有关。患者对慢性咳嗽咳痰、COPD 加重史、治疗反应等的认知及回忆可能会使研究结果产生偏差。自我评估报告时可能受到多种因素的影响,包括地理区域、文化水平和社会行为等。

CMH 在 COPD 的发生发展中具有重要作用,CMH 会限制气流、降低肺功能,增加 COPD 患者急性加重和预后不良的风险,增加住院率和病死率。鉴于 CMH 与 COPD 疾病进展的密切关系,CMH 可能为 COPD 一种新的表型。

参 考 文 献

[1] Shen Y, Huang S, Kang J, et al. Management of airway mucus hypersecretion in chronic airway inflammatory disease: Chinese expert consensus(English edition). Int J Chron Obstruct Pulmon Dis, 2018, 13:399-407.

[2] GBD 2015 Chronic Respiratory Disease Collaborators. Global, regional, and national deaths, prevalence, disability-adjusted life years, and years lived with disability for chronic obstructive pulmonary disease and asthma, 1990-2015: a systematic analysis for the Global Burden of Disease Study 2015. Lancet Respir Med, 2017, 5(9):691-706.

[3] Vestbo J, Hurd SS, Agusti AG, et al. Global strategy for the diagnosis, management, and prevention of chronic obstructive pulmonary disease: GOLD executive summary. Am J Respir Crit Care Med, 2013, 187(4):347-365.

[4] Jv F, Bf D. Airway mucus function and dysfunction. N Engl J Med, 2010, 363(23):2233-2247.

[5] Kim V, Evans CM, Dickey BF. Dawn of a new era in the diagnosis and treatment of airway mucus dysfunction. Am J Respir Crit Care Med, 2019, 199(2):133-134.

[6] Ramos FL, Krahnke JS, Kim V. Clinical issues of mucus accumulation in COPD. Int J Chron Obstruct Pulmon Dis, 2014, 9:139-150.

[7] Ma J, Rubin BK, Voynow JA. Mucins, mucus, and goblet cells. Chest, 2018, 154(1):169-176.

[8] Voynow JA, Rubin BK. Mucins, mucus, and sputum. Chest, 2009, 135(2):505-512.

[9] Martinez-Rivera C, Crespo A, Pinedo-Sierra C, et al. Mucus hypersecretion in asthma is associated with rhinosinusitis, polyps and exacerbations. Respir Med, 2018, 135:22-28.

[10] de Oca MM, Halbert RJ, Lopez MV, et al. The chronic bronchitis phenotype in subjects with and without COPD: the PLATINO study. Eur Respir J, 2012, 40(1):28-36.

[11] Prescott E, Lange P, Vestbo J. Chronic mucus hypersecretion in COPD and death from pulmonary infection. Eur Respir J, 1995, 8(8):1333-1338.

[12] Lange P, Groth S, Nyboe J, et al. Chronic obstructive lung disease in Copenhagen: cross-sectional epidemiological aspects. J Intern Med, 1989, 226(1):25-32.

[13] Lu M, Yao WZ, Zhong NS, et al. Chronic obstructive pulmonary disease in the absence of chronic bronchitis in China. Respirology, 2010, 15(7):1072-1078.

[14] Miravitlles M, Guerrero T, Mayordomo C, et al. Factors associated with increased risk of exacerbation and hospital admission in a cohort of ambulatory COPD patients: a multiple logistic regression analysis. The EOLO Study Group. Respiration, 2000, 67(5):495-501.

[15] de Marco R, Accordini S, Cerveri I, et al. Incidence of chronic obstructive pulmonary disease in a cohort of young adults according to the presence of chronic cough and phlegm. Am J Respir Crit Care Med, 2007, 175(1):32-39.

[16] Curran DR, Cohn L. Advances in mucous cell metaplasia: a plug for mucus as a therapeutic focus in chronic airway disease. Am J Respir Cell Mol Biol, 2010, 42(3):268-275.

[17] Shim JJ, Dabbagh K, Ueki IF, et al. IL-13 induces mucin production by stimulating epidermal growth factor receptors and by activating neutrophils. Am J Physiol Lung Cell Mol Physiol, 2001, 280(1):L134-L140.

[18] Wang J, Zhu M, Wang L, et al. Amphiregulin potentiates airway inflammation and mucus hypersecretion induced by urban particulate matter via the EGFR-PI3Kalpha-AKT/ERK pathway. Cell Signal, 2019, 53:122-131.

[19] Shin IS, Park JW, Shin NR, et al. Melatonin inhibits MUC5AC production via suppression of MAPK signaling in human airway epithelial cells. J Pineal Res, 2014, 56(4):398-407.

[20] Gray T, Nettesheim P, Loftin C, et al. Interleukin-1beta-induced mucin production in human airway epithelium is mediated by cyclooxygenase-2, prostaglandin E2 receptors, and cyclic AMP-protein kinase A signaling. Mol Pharmacol, 2004, 66(2):337-346.

[21] Mx S, Ja N. Neutrophil elastase induces MUC5AC mucin production in human airway epithelial cells via a cascade involving protein kinase C, reactive oxygen species, and TNF-{alpha}-converting enzyme. J Immunol, 2005, 175(6):4009-4016.

[22] Kirkham S, Sheehan JK, Knight D, et al. Heterogeneity of airways mucus: variations in the amounts and glycoforms of the major oligomeric mucins MUC5AC and MUC5B. Biochem J, 2002, 361(Pt 3):537-546.

[23] Allinson JP, Hardy R, Donaldson GC, et al. The presence of chronic mucus hypersecretion across adult life in relation to chronic obstructive pulmonary disease development. Am J Respir Crit Care Med, 2016, 193(6):662-672.

[24] Gensch E, Gallup M, Sucher A, et al. Tobacco smoke control of mucin production in lung cells requires oxygen radicals AP-1 and JNK. J Biol Chem, 2004, 279(37):39085-39093.

[25] Deshmukh HS, Case LM, Wesselkamper SC, et al. Metalloproteinases mediate mucin 5AC expression by epidermal growth factor receptor activation. Am J Respir Crit Care Med, 2005, 171(4): 305-314.

[26] Rubin BK, Priftis KN, Schmidt HJ, et al. Secretory hyperresponsiveness and pulmonary mucus hypersecretion. Chest, 2014, 146(2): 496-507.

[27] Innes A L, Woodruff PG, Ferrando RE, et al. Epithelial mucin stores are increased in the large airways of smokers with airflow obstruction. Chest, 2006, 130(4): 1102-1108.

[28] Takeyama K, Jung B, Shim JJ, et al. Activation of epidermal growth factor receptors is responsible for mucin synthesis induced by cigarette smoke. Am J Physiol Lung Cell Mol Physiol, 2001, 280(1): L165-L172.

[29] Barnes PJ. Inflammatory endotypes in COPD. Allergy, 2019, 74(7): 1249-1256.

[30] Han MK, Agusti A, Calverley PM, et al. Chronic obstructive pulmonary disease phenotypes: the future of COPD. Am J Respir Crit Care Med, 2010, 182(5): 598-604.

[31] Snider GL. Chronic obstructive pulmonary disease: a definition and implications of structural determinants of airflow obstruction for epidemiology. Am Rev Respir Dis, 1989, 140 (3 Pt 2): S3-S8.

[32] Miravitlles M, Soler-Cataluna JJ, Calle M, et al. Spanish COPD Guidelines(GesEPOC): pharmacological treatment of stable COPD. Spanish Society of Pulmonology and Thoracic Surgery. Arch Bronconeumol, 2012, 48(7): 247-257.

[33] Corlateanu A, Mendez Y, Wang Y, et al. Chronic obstructive pulmonary disease and phenotypes: a state-of-the-art. Pulmonology, 2020, 26(2): 95-100.

[34] Lu M, Wang X, Cai B, et al. Perception of circadian variation of symptoms in Chinese patients with chronic obstructive pulmonary disease. J Thorac Di, 2017, 9(10): 3888-3895.

[35] Kim V, Han MLK, Vance GB, et al. The chronic bronchitic phenotype of COPD: an analysis of the COPDGene study. Chest, 2011, 140(3): 626-633.

[36] Okajima Y, Come CE, Nardelli P, et al. Luminal plugging on chest CT: association with lung function, quality of life, and COPD clinical phenotypes. Chest, 2020, 158(1): 121-130.

[37] Anthonisen NR. The British hypothesis revisited. Eur Respir J, 2004, 23(5): 657-658.

[38] Lahousse L, Seys L, Joos GF, et al. Epidemiology and impact of chronic bronchitis in chronic obstructive pulmonary disease. Eur Respir J, 2017, 50(2): 1602470.

[39] Vestbo J, Prescott E, Lange P. Association of chronic mucus hypersecretion with FEV1 decline and chronic obstructive pulmonary disease morbidity. Copenhagen City Heart Study Group. Am J Respir Crit Care Med, 1996, 153(5): 1530-1535.

[40] Sherman CB, Xu X, Speizer FE, et al. Longitudinal lung function decline in subjects with respiratory symptoms. Am Rev Respir Dis, 1992, 146(4): 855-859.

[41] Ta S, Ja W. COPD exacerbations: defining their cause and prevention. Lancet, 2007, 370(9589): 786-796.

[42] Miravitlles M, Guerrero T, Mayordomo C, et al. Factors associated with increased risk of exacerbation and hospital admission in a cohort of ambulatory COPD patients: a multiple logistic regression analysis. The EOLO Study Group. Respiration, 2000, 67(5): 495-501.

[43] Kim V, Zhao H, Regan E, et al. The St. George's respiratory questionnaire definition of chronic bronchitis may be a better predictor of COPD exacerbations compared with the classic definition. Chest, 2019, 156(4): 685-695.

[44] Pelkonen M, Notkola IL, Nissinen A, et al. Thirty-year cumulative incidence of chronic bronchitis and COPD in relation to 30-year pulmonary function and 40-year mortality: a follow-up in middle-aged rural men. Chest, 2006, 130(4): 1129-1137.

[45] Hogg JC, Chu FS, Tan WC, et al. Survival after lung volume reduction in chronic obstructive pulmonary disease: insights from small airway pathology. Am J Respir Crit Care Med, 2007, 176(5): 454-459.

[46] Lange P, Nyboe J, Appleyard M, et al. Relation of ventilatory impairment and of chronic mucus hypersecretion to mortality from obstructive lung disease and from all causes. Thorax, 1990, 45(8): 579-585.

[47] Meek PM, Petersen H, Washko GR, et al. Chronic bronchitis is associated with worse symptoms and quality of life than chronic airflow obstruction. Chest, 2015, 148(2): 408-416.

[48] Agusti A, Calverley PM, Celli B, et al. Characterisation of COPD heterogeneity in the ECLIPSE cohort. Respir Res, 2010, 11: 122.

[49] Hurst JR, Vestbo J, Anzueto A, et al. Susceptibility to exacerbation in chronic obstructive pulmonary disease. N Engl J Med, 2010, 363(12): 1128-1138.

[50] Koo HK, Park SW, Park JW, et al. Chronic cough as a novel phenotype of chronic obstructive pulmonary disease. Int J Chron Obstruct Pulmon Dis, 2018, 13: 1793-1801.

[51] Mannino DM, Buist AS, Petty TL, et al. Lung function and mortality in the United States: data from the First National Health and Nutrition Examination Survey follow up study. Thorax, 2003(5): 388-393.

[52] Song Y, Wang W, Xie Y, et al. Carbocisteine inhibits the expression of Muc5b in COPD mouse model. Drug Des Devel Ther, 2019, 13: 3259-3268.

[53] Chakravorty I, Chahal K, Austin G. A pilot study of the impact of high-frequency chest wall oscillation in chronic obstructive pulmonary disease patients with mucus hypersecretion. Int J Chron Obstruct Pulmon Dis, 2011, 6: 693-699.

[54] Evans CM, Koo JS. Airway mucus: the good, the bad, the sticky. Pharmacol Ther, 2009, 121(3): 332-348.

[55] Li D, Sun D, Yuan L, et al. Sodium tanshinone IIA sulfonate protects against acute exacerbation of cigarette smoke-induced chronic obstructive pulmonary disease in mice. Int Immunopharmacol, 2020, 81: 106261.

[56] Ha EV, Rogers DF. Novel therapies to inhibit mucus synthesis and secretion in airway hypersecretory diseases. Pharmacology, 2016, 97(1-2): 84-100.

9 嗜酸性粒细胞在慢性阻塞性肺疾病不同时期的意义

陈 燕 崔亚楠

慢性阻塞性肺疾病(以下简称慢阻肺)是一种常见的可以预防和治疗的疾病,以持续的呼吸道症状和气流受限为特征。慢阻肺作为影响人类健康的"四大慢病"之一,其病因和发病机制尚未完全阐明。嗜酸性粒细胞是关键的免疫效应和炎症细胞,在多种疾病中发挥重要作用。近年研究发现部分慢阻肺患者存在气道嗜酸性粒细胞(eosinophil,EOS)炎症,以 EOS 升高为特征的 EOS 型慢阻肺是一种重要的慢阻肺表型。慢性阻塞性肺疾病全球倡议(global initiative for chronic obstructive lung disease,GOLD)2017 首次推荐将血 EOS 作为生物标志物指导稳定期患者治疗。但 EOS 在预测慢阻肺临床特征、治疗反应性及预后等方面的价值仍存在争议。本文将针对 EOS 在慢阻肺炎症中的作用及 EOS 在慢阻肺不同时期的意义介绍相关领域的研究进展,旨在加深对 EOS 指导慢阻肺临床实践的认识。

一、EOS 与慢阻肺气道炎症

(一)气道 EOS 炎症

在慢阻肺中,主要的炎症细胞包括 $CD8^+$ T 细胞、中性粒细胞和巨噬细胞,但一些患者表现为 EOS 参与的炎症反应。已有研究报道,通过支气管镜检、肺泡灌洗液和痰标本检测等手段,发现慢阻肺患者的中央和外周气道中均可存在 EOS 计数增加。Bafadhel 等研究发现,20%~40%的稳定期慢阻肺患者存在气道 EOS 炎症,接近 1/3 的急性加重期慢阻肺患者存在痰 EOS 增高。来源于骨髓造血干细胞的 EOS 成熟后被释放到血液中,在 CCL5 和 CCL11 等趋化因子的作用下,EOS 被招募并迁移至气道中。同时,气道上皮细胞在香烟烟雾、污染物或病原微生物等毒性因子的刺激下释放上游细胞因子 IL-25、IL-33 和 TSLP 等,引起 Th2 辅助细胞和固有淋巴细胞浸润,分泌 IL-5,诱导 EOS 分化、激活和释放。在肺组织中,EOS 衍生的促炎介质,包括多种碱性蛋白、细胞因子和生长因子等,能够促进持续的肺部炎症和组织损伤,导致病情加重。

(二)血 EOS 与气道 EOS

在临床实践中,很少有医疗中心会对慢阻肺患者进行常规的痰 EOS 计数检测。有学者提出在慢阻肺急性加重期,以 2%的外周血 EOS 百分比为阈值预测痰 EOS 增多的敏感度达 90%,特异度为 60%。此外,有研究表明,血 EOS 计数升高的慢阻肺患者的痰液、支气管肺泡灌洗液和肺组织中 EOS 计数明显高于血 EOS 计数低的患者。这提示血 EOS 可能是一个判断气道 EOS 炎症的敏感指标。但是,一项多中心观察性研究报道单独的血 EOS 并不是评估慢阻肺严重程度、急性加重风险或预测痰 EOS 的可靠生物标志物。Turato 等在其纳入不同严重程度慢阻肺患者的前瞻性研究中甚至发现组织 EOS 和血 EOS 之间没有相关性。以上研究结果的差异可能是由于不同研究中心检测气道 EOS 的设备和能力不同,研究纳入的患者严重程度也不相同。我们建议尽可能利用痰 EOS 检测结果进行判定。

(三)血 EOS 升高的阈值

血 EOS 水平可以表示为绝对值计数或白细胞百分比。在 WISDOM 事后分析中,血 EOS≥2%、4%、5%、6%或≥150/μl、300/μl、400/μl 均被用作阈值,研究者发现基线血 EOS≥4% 或 300/μl 预测慢阻肺患者未来急性加重风险的能力最佳。然而,TRISTAN、INSPIRE 和 ISOLDE 的事后分析则认为血 EOS≥2%是一个有效的阈值。最近的一项研究表明,慢阻肺患者的血 EOS 至少为 340/μl 时,其急性加重发生率降低 50%,为 270/μl 时患者有显著的肺功能改善,为 480/μl 时使用吸入性糖皮质激素(inhaled corticosteroids,ICS)可明显提高生活质量。因此,研究终点不同,相应的血 EOS 阈值可能也不相同。尽管 GOLD 2020 推荐在稳定期慢阻肺患者中启动 ICS 治疗时将血 EOS≥300/μl 作为考虑因素,但也强调将此数值视为一个估计值,而非能够预测患者不同治疗获益率的精确阈值。我们认为仅评估单一的阈值在临床实践中是不可行的。

二、EOS 与稳定期慢阻肺

有证据表明 EOS 水平可以预测慢阻肺患者的某些临床特征,并可预测患者对激素治疗的反应性及预后情况,然而 EOS 作为生物标志物的能力仍存在争议,目前研究结果不尽相同,并且多为事后分析和回顾性研究。

(一)临床特征

EOS 计数与患者的临床特征(如症状、呼吸困难评分、肺功能和细菌负荷等)之间可能存在相关性。2014 年,ECLIPSE 队列研究报道持续 EOS≥2%的慢阻肺患者具有以下特征:第 1 秒用力呼气容积(forced expiratory volume in one second,FEV_1)占预计值百分比较高、症状较少、呼吸困难评分较低及 BODE(体重指数、气流阻塞、呼吸困难、运动能力)指数较低。最近 Contoli 等进行的纵向概念验证性研究发现痰 EOS 计数与呼吸困难的严重程度正相关，尤其是在痰 EOS≥2% 的受试者中。这与 SPIROMICS 研究结果一致，该研究指出血 EOS≥200/μl 的患者喘息更重且症状更多。此外，这项大型多中心研究还表明，具有高浓度痰或血 EOS 的慢阻肺患者的 FEV_1 占预计值百分比显著降低。这些研究结果的不同可能归因于纳入患者病情严重程度不同及纳入前治疗方法的差异。

有研究报道 EOS 可能与气道微生物群相关。一项概念验证性前瞻性研究发现，稳定期慢阻肺患者中，仅仅在使用 ICS 治疗的低基线痰或血 EOS 计数(≤2%)的研究对象中观察到气道细菌负荷增加，在高 EOS 水平的患者中并不存在。另外一项为期一年的前瞻性研究报道，稳定期慢阻肺患者若存在 EOS 主导的炎症，则其在急性加重期间感染细菌的风险较低。一项纳入 72 例稳定期慢阻肺患者的横断面研究发现，血 EOS≥2% 与较高的微生物群多样性有关，它们可能抵抗病原菌的存在进而起到保护作用。EOS 与气道微生物群之间可能存在的关系，揭示了慢阻肺发病机制中 EOS 复杂的免疫调控作用。

（二）激素治疗反应性

越来越多的研究报道 EOS 可预测慢阻肺患者对糖皮质激素治疗的反应性。在 TRISTAN 和 INSPIRE 研究的事后分析中，基线高 EOS 水平的慢阻肺患者，是否接受 ICS 治疗在减少急性加重方面存在显著差异，两项研究均发现血 EOS 较高者接受包含 ICS 的治疗方案后未来急性加重率降低。来自三项随机对照试验（randomized controlled trials, RCTs）的事后分析显示，在血 EOS≥100/μl 时，使用 ICS 联合长效 β_2 受体激动剂（long-acting beta2-agonist, LABA）（布地奈德福莫特罗）与单独使用 LABA（福莫特罗）相比，在减少急性加重方面的疗效更为显著。通过分析两项针对中重度慢阻肺患者的大型随机试验中的数据，Pascoe 等发现与单独使用维兰特罗相比，氟替卡松联合维兰特罗可使基线 2%≤血 EOS<4% 的患者的急性加重率降低 24%，而 4%<血 EOS<6% 的患者急性加重率降低了 32%，血 EOS≥6% 的患者降低了 42%。近年，Pascoe 等又对 IMPACT 研究进行了事后分析，IMPACT 研究是一项 3 期、随机、双盲、平行组、52 周的全球性研究，比较每日一次三联疗法，即 ICS 联合 LABA 和长效抗胆碱药（long-acting muscarinic antagonist, LAMA）与双吸入疗法（ICS+LABA 或 LAMA+LABA），该研究招募的患者在过去一年发生了至少一次急性加重。其事后分析共纳入 10 333 例患者，结果发现包含 ICS 的治疗方案在降低急性加重风险方面的获益与血 EOS 成比例增加。此外，在 WISDOM 研究的事后分析中，研究者还发现基线血 EOS>4% 或 300/μl 的患者接受规律三联治疗一段时间后撤除 ICS 会导致其急性加重风险增加。以上研究中的大多数患者都有急性加重的病史。在英国为期 1 年的真实世界队列研究（CPRD）中，Suissa 等也发现使用包含 ICS 方案治疗的血 EOS 升高慢阻肺患者的急性加重风险降低。与上述研究结果不同的是，一项 52 周、随机、双盲、双模拟、非劣效性试验（FLAME）报道，LAMA+LABA 与 LABA+ICS 对急性加重率的影响与基线血 EOS 水平无关。

研究表明 EOS 增高患者的肺功能可能也会从包含 ICS 的治疗方案中获益。Whittaker 等在英国一家大型初级卫生保健机构中招募了 26 675 例慢阻肺患者，平均随访 4.2 年，研究结果发现在 EOS 水平较高的患者中，使用 ICS 可改善 FEV_1（+12 ml/年），而未使用 ICS 则导致 FEV_1 降低（−20.8 ml/年）。IMPACT 的事后分析也显示，血 EOS 水平较高的患者接受包含 ICS 的治疗后肺功能获益更多。然而，在 INSPIRE、TRISTAN 和 SCO30002 研究的事后分析中，以血 EOS 2% 为阈值，研究者并未发现 EOS 与 FEV_1 治疗效果之间具有相关性。Pascoe 等在其二次分析中也报道，与单独使用 LABA 相比，ICS+LABA 治疗后 FEV_1 的改善与血 EOS 无关。

以下几点原因可以在一定程度上解释这些研究结果之间的差异。首先，不同研究选择的治疗方案差异很大。包含 ICS 的治疗可以是单独使用 ICS、三联疗法或 ICS+LABA。不包含 ICS 的治疗可能是 LAMA+LABA、单独的 LAMA、单独的 LABA 或安慰剂。其次，纳入的慢阻肺患者有不同的疾病严重程度和急性加重史。很多事后分析及 RCTs 的研究对象需要有至少一次的急性加重史，但在一些真实世界研究中并无此要求。再次，一些研究纳入了有哮喘病史的慢阻肺患者。实际上，有哮喘病史的患者仍然有可能表现出原发疾病的许多病理生理特征。然后，不同的研究导入期不同。最后，不同的血 EOS 阈值及随访期间 EOS 计数的稳定性对结果均有显著的影响。

（三）临床结局

越来越多的研究显示慢阻肺患者血 EOS 水平与其临床结局之间具有相关性。血 EOS 可能是预测患者未来急性加重风险、病死率和医疗资源利用（health care resource utilization, HCRU）情况的潜在生物标志物。

1. 急性加重风险　Bafadhel 等针对三项 RCTs 中 4528 例慢阻肺患者进行的事后分析显示，血 EOS 水平可作为慢阻肺患者急性加重风险的预测因子。一项大规模、回顾性、观察性队列研究，共纳入 34 268 例有急性加重史的患者，发现与血 EOS<150/μl 的患者相比，血 EOS≥150/μl 者急诊就诊次数增加且未来急性加重风险升高。最近，两项独立的研究分析了中重度慢阻肺患者中血 EOS 与急性加重风险之间的关系。结果显示，在 COPDGene 研究中，血 EOS≥300/μl 的患者急性加重风险增加，这一结论在 ECLIPSE 研究中得到了前瞻性验证。一项回顾性队列研究纳入的患者多数无急性加重史，结果仍显示随访一年期间，血 EOS≥300/μl 的患者急性加重发生率较高，并提出高血 EOS 水平是慢阻肺患者未来急性加重风险的独立危险因素。

与上述结果相反，SPIROMICS 研究并未发现血 EOS 升高和慢阻肺急性加重风险之间的证据。事实上，SPIROMICS 研究招募的患者急性加重发生次数很少，且包括了一些未经肺功能检测证实罹患慢阻肺的吸烟者。此外，分析来自 CHAIN 和 BODE 队列的数据也发现血 EOS≥300/μl 持续至少 2 年并非慢阻肺急性加重的危险因素，但这两个队列中的大多数患者都接受了含有 ICS 的治疗，这可能会影响患者尤其是在EOS增多的患者急性加重的发生率。因此,既往急性加重史和ICS使用情况的不同可能会对研究结果产生一定的影响。

2. 病死率 芬兰的一项非介入性、回顾性研究招募了9042名慢阻肺患者,平均随访时间为3.7～6.5年,结果显示与血EOS＜300/μl的受试者相比,EOS≥300/μl的患者总的及慢阻肺相关的生存率均有所提高。Turato等的研究也显示持续高EOS计数的患者较持续低EOS计数或可变计数的患者具有更好的生存率。CHAIN和BODE队列也报道了高EOS与更好的生存率相关。相反,在一项对一般人群进行的随访超过30年的研究中,Hospers等发现血EOS≥275/μl与全因病死率的增加有关,但在同一人群中,EOS增多与慢阻肺病死率之间的关联仅限于有哮喘病史的患者中。需要包含大样本量的前瞻性研究来进一步评估血EOS作为预测病死率的生物标志物的准确性。

3. HCRU 已有大规模的回顾性研究报道EOS增多与患者的HCRU增加有关。美国的一项横断面研究纳入2832例慢阻肺患者,与EOS＜150/μl的患者相比,EOS≥150/μl的患者每年的全因及慢阻肺相关HCRU更高。EOS增多患者的HCRU较高可能与急性加重风险增加有关。

三、EOS与急性加重期慢阻肺

(一)细菌负荷

EOS水平的高低可能与慢阻肺患者急性加重期细菌负荷有关。Kolsum等研究发现,在急性加重期间,EOS水平与肺炎链球菌、卡他莫拉菌和流感嗜血杆菌的细菌感染率负相关。2019年,Choi等回顾性地分析了韩国住院的急性加重期慢阻肺患者病历资料,共有736次急性加重事件符合纳入标准,将其根据血EOS是否≥2%分为两组,结果发现血EOS＜2%是急性加重事件中细菌感染的潜在指标,EOS可作为急性加重期间抗生素应用的参考因素。EOS在细菌负荷判定中的意义可用其在抗感染固有免疫反应中的一线作用及充当抗原提呈细胞并放大Th1反应等的生物学功能解释。

(二)激素治疗反应性

慢阻肺急性加重期通常需要使用全身性糖皮质激素。已有一些研究对EOS增高的急性加重期患者口服糖皮质激素(oral corticosteroids,OCS)治疗的反应进行分析。在一项前瞻性随机试验中,采用OCS治疗后,存在EOS升高的急性加重患者症状恢复较快且治疗失败(定义为复治、住院或死亡)较少。随后,对三项RCTs的进一步分析发现,与安慰剂相比,急性加重期血EOS≥2%的患者接受泼尼松治疗后,能够显著降低治疗失败率。最近,我们在国内进行了一项针对住院急性加重期慢阻肺患者的观察性研究发现:与无EOS升高者相比,血EOS升高的急性加重期慢阻肺患者接受全身性皮质类固醇治疗后,症状改善率更高,住院时间更短。目前,全身性糖皮质激素在血EOS升高的急性加重期慢阻肺患者中的获益较为明确,提示在住院患者的临床诊治过程中应充分考虑EOS的潜在价值。

(三)临床结局

1. 住院时间及复发情况 MacDonald等对急性加重期住院的慢阻肺患者进行了建模队列和验证队列研究,发现低血EOS患者的平均住院时间较长。在对一家三甲医院住院的急性加重慢阻肺患者进行的前瞻性观察性研究中,使用受试者操作特性曲线计算评估较长住院时间的血EOS阈值。结果显示,入院时血EOS＜144/μl或＜2%与住院时间延长相关。Prins等使用了一项RCT中207例急性加重事件的数据分析血EOS对临床结局的影响,发现急性期患者的血EOS增多与中位住院时间较短有关,但EOS≥2%的患者急性加重复发风险增加。此外,一项纳入479例因慢阻肺急性加重首次入院患者的观察性队列研究也报道,高血EOS与复发风险增加有关。另一项回顾性观察性研究纳入167例急性加重期慢阻肺患者,发现EOS增多与12个月慢阻肺相关再入院风险增加及距首次慢阻肺相关再入院时间缩短有关,这与我们之前针对国内患者进行的研究结果一致。因此,EOS增多患者的短期治疗成功率较高,但这些患者随后可能有更高的复发风险。

2. 病死率 MacDonald等进行的研究同时报道了血EOS与患者病死率之间的关系,研究发现在急性加重期慢阻肺患者中EOS增多与死亡风险较低有关。Li等进行的观察性研究也发现血EOS水平较高的患者死亡风险较低。然而,在国内的一项对890例急性加重期慢阻肺患者进行平均41个月随访的回顾性研究中,血EOS≥300/μl与患者的一年及长期病死率无关。

EOS型慢阻肺是一种重要的慢阻肺表型。虽然不同的研究使用的EOS阈值不同,但具有EOS炎症的慢阻肺患者细菌负荷较低,对皮质类固醇治疗反应较好,尤其是急性加重期患者,更能从全身性激素治疗中获益。此外,对于稳定期患者,EOS升高可能与其病死率降低、急性加重风险及HCRU升高有关,对于急性加重期患者,EOS增多与住院时间缩短有关,但其复发风险升高。EOS在慢阻肺发生发展中发挥复杂的调控作用,其作为生物标志物的应用还需进一步研究。

参考文献

[1] Rutgers SR,Timens W,Kaufmann HF,et al. Comparison of induced sputum with bronchial wash,bronchoalveolar lavage and bronchial biopsies in COPD. Eur Respir J,2000,15(1):109-115.

[2] Bafadhel M,Pavord ID,Russell REK. Eosinophils in COPD: just another biomarker? Lancet Respir Med,2017,5(9):747-759.

[3] Bafadhel M,McKenna S,Terry S,et al. Acute exacerbations of chronic obstructive pulmonary disease:identification of biologic clusters and their biomarkers. Am J Respir Crit Care

Med, 2011, 184(6):662-671.
[4] Yii ACA, Tay TR, Choo XN, et al. Precision medicine in united airways disease: A "treatable traits" approach. Allergy, 2018, 73(10):1964-1978.
[5] Kolsum U, Damera G, Pham TH, et al. Pulmonary inflammation in patients with chronic obstructive pulmonary disease with higher blood eosinophil counts. J Allergy Clin Immunol, 2017, 140(4):1181-1184.
[6] Hastie AT, Martinez FJ, Curtis JL, et al. Association of sputum and blood eosinophil concentrations with clinical measures of COPD severity: an analysis of the SPIROMICS cohort. Lancet Respir Med, 2017, 5(12):956-967.
[7] Turato G, Semenzato U, Bazzan E, et al. Blood Eosinophilia Neither Reflects Tissue Eosinophils nor Worsens Clinical Outcomes in Chronic Obstructive Pulmonary Disease. Am J Respir Crit Care Med, 2018, 197(9):1216-1219.
[8] Watz H, Tetzlaff K, Wouters EF, et al. Blood eosinophil count and exacerbations in severe chronic obstructive pulmonary disease after withdrawal of inhaled corticosteroids: a post-hoc analysis of the WISDOM trial. Lancet Respir Med, 2016, 4(5):390-398.
[9] Barnes NC, Sharma R, Lettis S, et al. Blood eosinophils as a marker of response to inhaled corticosteroids in COPD. Eur Respir J, 2016, 47(5):1374-1382.
[10] Pavord ID, Lettis S, Locantore N, et al. Blood eosinophils and inhaled corticosteroid/long-acting beta-2 agonist efficacy in COPD. Thorax, 2016, 71(2):118-125.
[11] Bafadhel M, Peterson S, De Blas MA, et al. Predictors of exacerbation risk and response to budesonide in patients with chronic obstructive pulmonary disease: a post-hoc analysis of three randomised trials. Lancet Respir Med, 2018, 6(2):117-126.
[12] Singh D, Kolsum U, Brightling CE, et al. Eosinophilic inflammation in COPD: prevalence and clinical characteristics. Eur Respir J, 2014, 44(6):1697-1700.
[13] Contoli M, Baraldo S, Conti V, et al. Airway inflammatory profile is correlated with symptoms in stable COPD: A longitudinal proof-of-concept cohort study. Respirology, 2020, 25(1):80-88.
[14] Contoli M, Pauletti A, Rossi MR, et al. Long-term effects of inhaled corticosteroids on sputum bacterial and viral loads in COPD. Eur Respir J, 2017, 50(4).
[15] Kim VL, Coombs NA, Staples KJ, et al. Impact and associations of eosinophilic inflammation in COPD: analysis of the AERIS cohort. Eur Respir J, 2017, 50(4).
[16] Millares L, Pascual S, Monton C, et al. Relationship between the respiratory microbiome and the severity of airflow limitation, history of exacerbations and circulating eosinophils in COPD patients. BMC Pulm Med, 2019, 19(1):112.
[17] Pascoe S, Locantore N, Dransfield MT, et al. Blood eosinophil counts, exacerbations, and response to the addition of inhaled fluticasone furoate to vilanterol in patients with chronic obstructive pulmonary disease: a secondary analysis of data from two parallel randomised controlled trials. Lancet Respir Med, 2015, 3(6):435-442.

[18] Pascoe S, Barnes N, Brusselle G, et al. Blood eosinophils and treatment response with triple and dual combination therapy in chronic obstructive pulmonary disease: analysis of the IMPACT trial. Lancet Respir Med, 2019, 7(9):745-756.
[19] Suissa S, Dell'Aniello S, Ernst P. Comparative effectiveness of LABA-ICS versus LAMA as initial treatment in COPD targeted by blood eosinophils: a population-based cohort study. Lancet Respir Med, 2018, 6(11):855-862.
[20] Wedzicha JA, Banerji D, Chapman KR, et al. Indacaterol-Glycopyrronium versus Salmeterol-Fluticasone for COPD. N Engl J Med, 2016, 374(23):2222-2234.
[21] Whittaker HR, Mullerova H, Jarvis D, et al. Inhaled corticosteroids, blood eosinophils, and FEV1 decline in patients with COPD in a large UK primary health care setting. Int J Chron Obstruct Pulmon Dis, 2019, 14:1063-1073.
[22] Siddiqui SH, Guasconi A, Vestbo J, et al. Blood Eosinophils: A Biomarker of Response to Extrafine Beclomethasone/Formoterol in Chronic Obstructive Pulmonary Disease. Am J Respir Crit Care Med, 2015, 192(4):523-525.
[23] Mullerova H, Hahn B, Simard EP, et al. Exacerbations and health care resource use among patients with COPD in relation to blood eosinophil counts. Int J Chron Obstruct Pulmon Dis, 2019, 14:683-692.
[24] Yun JH, Lamb A, Chase R, et al. Blood eosinophil count thresholds and exacerbations in patients with chronic obstructive pulmonary disease. J Allergy Clin Immunol, 2018, 141(6):2037-2047.
[25] Zeiger RS, Tran TN, Butler RK, et al. Relationship of Blood Eosinophil Count to Exacerbations in Chronic Obstructive Pulmonary Disease. J Allergy Clin Immunol Pract, 2018, 6(3):944-954.
[26] Casanova C, Celli BR, de-Torres JP, et al. Prevalence of persistent blood eosinophilia: relation to outcomes in patients with COPD. Eur Respir J, 2017, 50(5).
[27] Viinanen A, Lassenius MI, Toppila I, et al. The Burden of Chronic Obstructive Pulmonary Disease(COPD) In Finland: Impact of Disease Severity And Eosinophil Count On Healthcare Resource Utilization. Int J Chron Obstruct Pulmon Dis, 2019, 14:2409-2421.
[28] Hospers JJ, Schouten JP, Weiss ST, et al. Eosinophilia is associated with increased all-cause mortality after a follow-up of 30 years in a general population sample. Epidemiology, 2000, 11(3):261-268.
[29] Ortega H, Llanos JP, Lafeuille MH, et al. Burden of disease associated with a COPD eosinophilic phenotype. Int J Chron Obstruct Pulmon Dis, 2018, 13:2425-2433.
[30] Kolsum U, Donaldson GC, Singh R, et al. Blood and sputum eosinophils in COPD: relationship with bacterial load. Respir Res, 2017, 18(1):88.
[31] Choi J, Oh JY, Lee YS, et al. The association between blood eosinophil percent and bacterial infection in acute exacerbation of chronic obstructive pulmonary disease. Int J Chron Obstruct Pulmon Dis, 2019, 14:953-959.
[32] Bafadhel M, McKenna S, Terry S, et al. Blood eosinophils to direct corticosteroid treatment of exacerbations of chronic ob-

structive pulmonary disease: a randomized placebo-controlled trial. Am J Respir Crit Care Med,2012,186(1):48-55.
[33] Bafadhel M,Davies L,Calverley PM,et al. Blood eosinophil guided prednisolone therapy for exacerbations of COPD: a further analysis. Eur Respir J,2014,44(3):789-791.
[34] Xue J,Cui YN,Chen P,et al. Blood eosinophils: a biomarker of response to glucocorticoids and increased readmissions in severe hospitalized exacerbations of COPD. Zhonghua Jie He He Hu Xi Za Zhi,2019,42(6):426-431.
[35] MacDonald MI,Osadnik CR,Bulfin L,et al. Low and High Blood Eosinophil Counts as Biomarkers in Hospitalized Acute Exacerbations of COPD. Chest,2019,156(1):92-100.
[36] Ko FWS,Chan KP,Ngai J,et al. Blood eosinophil count as a predictor of hospital length of stay in COPD exacerbations. Respirology,2020,25(3):259-266.
[37] Prins HJ,Duijkers R,Lutter R,et al. Blood eosinophilia as a marker of early and late treatment failure in severe acute exacerbations of COPD. Respir Med,2017,131:118-124.
[38] Li Q,Larivee P,Courteau J,et al. Greater eosinophil counts at first COPD hospitalization are associated with more readmissions and fewer deaths. Int J Chron Obstruct Pulmon Dis,2019,14:331-341.
[39] Couillard S,Larivee P,Courteau J,et al. Eosinophils in COPD Exacerbations Are Associated With Increased Readmissions. Chest,2017,151(2):366-373.
[40] Zhang Y,Lin YX. Risk factors analysis for one-year and long-term mortality in patients hospitalized for acute exacerbation of chronic obstructive pulmonary disease. Zhonghua Jie He He Hu Xi Za Zhi,2019,42(12):895-900.

10 靶向诱导粒细胞死亡:慢性气道疾病防治的新靶点?

刘正媛　陈志华

以支气管哮喘(asthma,简称哮喘)和慢性阻塞性肺疾病(chronic obstructive pulmonary disease,简称慢阻肺)为代表的慢性气道疾病是我国最为常见、疾病负担最为严重的慢性疾病种类之一。两项研究显示,截至2015年我国20岁以上成年人哮喘患病人数约4570万,慢阻肺患病人数约9990万。哮喘和慢阻肺已经成为我国严重的经济负担,如何有效推动慢性气道疾病防治工作成为我国亟须解决的公共卫生问题。然而现行的临床治疗方案只能改善哮喘和慢阻肺的症状,很难根治。因此,探索哮喘和慢阻肺的发病机制及开发相关药物具有重要意义。

炎症是机体对病原体入侵的一种保护性反应,也是慢阻肺和哮喘这两种典型的慢性气道炎症性疾病的主要特征,然而过度的炎症反应会导致组织和细胞损伤,引起慢性炎症和组织损伤。粒细胞在哮喘和慢阻肺的气道炎症的发生发展中起着关键作用。粒细胞是在细胞质中具有特殊颗粒的免疫细胞,通常包括中性粒细胞、嗜酸性粒细胞(eosinophil,Eos)和嗜碱性粒细胞。病原体入侵时,中性粒细胞、嗜酸性粒细胞、嗜碱性粒细胞的激活对于清除病原体和促进组织修复维持肺稳态非常重要。在炎症消退期,中性粒细胞和嗜酸性粒细胞通常会经历程序性细胞死亡(凋亡),被巨噬细胞等吞噬细胞吞噬和清除。这一过程的失调被认为是导致慢性炎症性疾病发病和进展的原因。肺组织的粒细胞过度激活或过度募集可导致严重组织损伤,进一步恶化病情。近年来,通过靶向诱导炎症细胞死亡清除炎症细胞是炎症性疾病治疗的重要策略,因此通过靶向诱导粒细胞死亡缓解气道炎症具有非常好的前景。

一、靶向粒细胞死亡作为哮喘治疗靶点

哮喘是一种由多种炎症细胞和细胞组分参与的异质性疾病,由于主导的炎症细胞和细胞组分不同,形成不同的表型和内型。哮喘内型可分为Th2相关性哮喘和非Th2相关性哮喘两大类。粒细胞在哮喘的发展中起着重要作用,不同的粒细胞群似乎与哮喘特定的表型和内型有关。Th2相关性哮喘中,变应性表型的炎症和免疫过程与气道嗜酸性粒细胞密切相关。而在非Th2相关性哮喘中,中性粒细胞是参与发病机制的主要炎症细胞。

Th2相关性哮喘的发病机制主要涉及Th1/Th2细胞免疫失衡,它是一种以嗜酸性粒细胞、肥大细胞、T淋巴细胞、树突状细胞及单核-巨噬细胞等多种炎症细胞及细胞组分共同参与,以气道黏液高分泌、气道高反应性和气道重构为特征的慢性气道炎症性疾病。其中Eos被认为是引起该型哮喘气道炎症最关键的效应细胞之一。研究显示过敏原经树突状细胞等呈递后,可诱导Naïve T细胞分化成为Th2细胞,从而分泌各种Th2型炎症因子如白细胞介素(interleukin,IL)4、IL-5和IL-13等。在骨髓中发育成熟的Eos,可受IL-5的作用迁移入血,进而受到肺内eotaxin的趋化作用入肺。肺内大量募集的Eos可进一步分泌各种炎症因子,从而诱导哮喘慢性气道炎症,气道高反应性和黏液高分泌。在非Th2相关性哮喘中,哮喘患者气道主要以中性粒细胞浸润和募集为主。较多中性粒细胞浸润的患者常产生皮质类固醇药物抵抗,且诱导痰中性粒细胞数量也与重症哮喘发病相关。

靶向诱导Eos凋亡可以缓解哮喘嗜酸性粒细胞性气道炎症,这在哮喘治疗的研究中已受到广泛认可。研究发现在哮喘中,Eos因受粒细胞-巨噬细胞集落刺激因子、IL-5等因子影响,其抗凋亡能力增强、生存周期显著延长,这直接导致在炎症后期Eos消退延迟,活化的Eos在肺部过度募集,释放颗粒蛋白及炎症介质,损伤周围细胞,加重炎症状态并参与炎症维持。因此,Eos的凋亡延迟与哮喘的发生发展及严重程度密切相关,诱导Eos死亡有利于哮喘控制。目前,吸入皮质激素(inhaled corticosteroids,ICS)是控制气道炎症和防止气道损伤/重塑的一线治疗方法,与长效β_2受体激动剂联合使用被认为是治疗哮喘的金标准。研究发现糖皮质激素可通过快速诱导哮喘患者外周血气道组织内Eos凋亡发挥强大的抗炎作用。虽然ICS可以抑制气道炎症,但不能治愈哮喘,并且有部分患者存在激素抵抗,在这部分患者中糖皮质激素诱导Eos凋亡作用比较弱。另外,有部分患者对ICS产生耐药性,他们需要使用更高剂量的糖皮质激素,并且最终需要口服糖皮质激素抑制炎症反应。长期口服糖皮质激素不良反应很多,包括水潴留、脂质和皮质醇代谢功能障碍、白内障、青光眼、骨质疏松症和机会性感染风险增加。值得注意的是,近10%的哮喘患者对糖皮质激素反应不佳或完全没有反应,却约占控制哮喘总医疗费用的50%。

由于长期使用糖皮质激素的不良反应,在相当一部分哮喘患者中存在激素抵抗及以中性粒细胞浸润为主的激素不敏感性哮喘,因此开发新的、有别于激素的靶向诱导粒细胞凋亡、死亡的药物在哮喘防治中具有极大的应用前景,这也成为当前哮喘研究的新热点。凋亡抑制蛋白B淋

巴细胞瘤-2蛋白(B-cell lymphoma-2,Bcl-2)抑制剂就是一种具有较大前景的治疗炎症性疾病的药物。

凋亡抑制蛋白Bcl-2抑制剂可以通过诱导嗜酸性粒细胞和中性粒细胞死亡缓解哮喘气道炎症及气道高反应性。在嗜酸性粒细胞哮喘模型(OVA/Alum)和中性粒细胞哮喘模型(OVA/CFA)中,气道炎症细胞凋亡抑制蛋白Bcl-2出现过表达,这可能是导致在哮喘炎症中炎症细胞凋亡水平下降及存活时间延长的原因。在Bcl-2过表达的哮喘模型小鼠中,中性粒细胞和嗜酸性粒细胞在肺部募集增加、且凋亡水平明显下降进一步验证了这种原因。以上结果提示Bcl-2过表达可能会引起炎症细胞的凋亡及炎症清除过程的阻滞。ABT-199与ABT-737是能够选择性的结合凋亡抑制蛋白Bcl-2家族的小分子抑制剂。利用嗜酸性粒细胞与中性粒细胞型哮喘模型小鼠气道局部给予糖皮质激素地塞米松、ABT-737,发现二者均可以明显增加嗜酸性粒细胞凋亡;但在中性粒细胞型哮喘中糖皮质激素地塞米松则不导致中性粒细胞凋亡增加。地塞米松不能够抑制小鼠的气道高反应,而ABT-737则抑制了乙酰甲胆碱诱导的气道高反应性,逆转哮喘小鼠的气道高反应性。在两种哮喘模型中,新一代的Bcl-2抑制剂ABT-199也得到了与ABT-737一致的结果。为了证明ABT-199及ABT-737对哮喘患者的有效性,进一步在激素治疗无效的重症哮喘患者外周血分离的中性粒细胞中干预ABT-737,同样中性粒细胞凋亡明显增加。此外,将ABT-199制备成纳米颗粒以后,可以在降低最低有效剂量的同时缓解气道炎症。因此,Bcl-2的小分子抑制剂ABT-199及ABT-737是一种具有较好运用价值、极具潜力的哮喘治疗策略。

细胞死亡除了凋亡和坏死两大类以外,Dixon等于2012年还首次提出并命名了一种全新的细胞死亡方式——铁死亡(ferroptosis),这是一种非凋亡性细胞死亡方式,是在小分子物质诱导下发生的氧化性细胞死亡。细胞发生铁死亡时,细胞内谷胱甘肽(glutathione,GSH)耗竭或谷胱甘肽过氧化物酶4(glutathione peroxidase4,GPX4)活性下降,导致脂质过氧化物不能经GPX4催化的谷胱甘肽还原反应代谢,铁依赖的脂质活性氧(reactive oxygen species,ROS)即会在细胞中大量聚集,进而诱导细胞死亡。研究显示哮喘患者气道上皮细胞脂质过氧化与呼出气一氧化氮的含量呈正相关。香烟烟雾、感染等任何可导致GPX4活性下降的因素,均可引起上皮细胞脂质的氧化还原失衡,从而导致气道上皮功能紊乱,加重哮喘气道炎症。因此,哮喘与铁死亡可能存在一定的相关性,通过靶向诱导Eos发生铁死亡,可能是改善哮喘气道炎症的新靶点。

铁死亡诱导剂体内能通过介导Eos铁死亡有效缓解哮喘气道炎症,不管是体外诱导Eos死亡还是体内保护哮喘气道炎症,铁死亡诱导剂与糖皮质激素均显示出良好的协同调控作用。利用哮喘患者及IL-5过表达的NJ.1638小鼠外周血分离纯化Eos体外培养,给予铁死亡诱导剂体外干预,发现铁死亡诱导剂能直接诱导外周血中Eos死亡。另外,铁死亡诱导剂诱导的Eos死亡是由细胞质ROS促发的细胞铁死亡,而不是传统认为的脂质ROS,这可能是一种新的非经典的铁依赖性死亡通路。在卵清清蛋白诱导的哮喘小鼠模型中,体内应用铁死亡诱导剂能通过介导Eos铁死亡有效缓解哮喘气道炎症。

RSL3(ras-selective lethal 3)是一种经典的铁死亡诱导剂,能够直接作用于GPX4,抑制其活性,致细胞抗氧化能力下降,脂质活性氧上升,最终引起铁死亡。铁死亡诱导剂RSL3除了能够诱导Eos死亡,同样能诱导中性粒细胞非经典途径铁死亡,从而对以中性粒细胞浸润为主的哮喘炎症起到很好的保护作用。铁死亡诱导剂RSL3可以在体外诱导哮喘患者外周血中性粒细胞凋亡,这个过程可能与自噬和线粒体ROS水平升高有关。在中性粒细胞为主的OVA/CFA哮喘模型中,腹腔注射给予RSL3明显降低了肺泡灌洗液细胞总数,并降低气道炎症评分。

我们首次在哮喘研究领域引入了铁死亡的概念。我们发现铁死亡诱导剂erastin、RSL3、青蒿琥酯能通过介导Eos铁死亡及RSL3介导中性粒细胞死亡保护哮喘气道炎症,这为哮喘研究提供了一个全新的思路。若铁死亡诱导剂运用成功,不仅能减轻激素不良反应,还能够大大缓解疾病造成的社会经济负担。尽管目前的研究仅表明凋亡抑制蛋白Bcl-2的抑制剂及铁死亡诱导剂可缓解哮喘气道炎症,但是凋亡抑制蛋白Bcl-2的抑制剂及铁死亡诱导剂或许同样可以对其他气道炎症性疾病起到保护作用。

二、靶向粒细胞死亡作为慢性阻塞性肺疾病治疗靶点

中性粒细胞是慢性阻塞性肺疾病发病的主要原因之一,中性粒细胞释放的蛋白酶引起宿主损伤并导致肺气肿,慢阻肺患者气道中性粒细胞的增加与疾病严重程度密切相关。吸烟可引起上皮细胞和巨噬细胞释放粒细胞-巨噬细胞集落刺激因子和粒细胞集落刺激因子,促进粒细胞的产生、释放和存活。中性粒细胞分泌的颗粒蛋白和丝氨酸蛋白酶会加重肺泡破坏、炎症和氧化应激。研究报道,组织蛋白酶G,中性粒细胞弹性蛋白酶和蛋白酶3有助于黏液的高分泌。

中性粒细胞的寿命对中性粒细胞驱动的慢阻肺肺部炎症的强度和持续时间有决定性的影响,因此靶向中性粒细胞死亡同样是非常具有潜力的慢阻肺治疗策略。粒细胞-巨噬细胞集落刺激因子、IL-8和白三烯B4多种促粒细胞因子和炎症介质已被证明在促炎情况下,可以延缓中性粒细胞凋亡,并且这些炎症介质和炎症因子在慢阻肺患者的气道中增加,因此通过恢复中性粒细胞凋亡可能是缓解慢阻肺炎症的潜在靶点。酪氨酸磷酸化抑制剂AG825是一种受体酪氨酸激酶ErbB家族的抑制剂,可以通过减轻粒细胞-巨噬细胞集落刺激因子介导的中性粒细胞抗凋亡效应,促进慢阻肺患者外周血分离的中性粒细胞凋亡。这一点在小鼠中得到了进一步的验证,用脂多糖雾化后,立即腹腔注射给予AG825可以增加中性粒细胞凋亡百分比。苦参碱是苦参的生物活性成分,给吸烟4d的小鼠进行每日苦参碱灌胃,发现苦参碱可以通过促进中性粒细胞凋亡明显降低肺部中性粒细胞活性。虽然慢阻肺主要为中性粒细胞炎症,但在急性加重期间嗜酸性粒细胞炎症增强,

所以通过糖皮质激素诱导嗜酸性粒细胞凋亡可能是控制慢阻肺急性加重的治疗关键。

关于粒细胞的研究可以追溯到18世纪,从那时起,人们就对粒细胞的功能和发展很感兴趣。粒细胞颗粒含量的不同与它们在宿主防御过程中的不同作用密切相关。在宿主防御过程中,粒细胞活化后释放蛋白酶、组胺和抗菌肽,这些物质可以杀死病原体和诱导损伤部位修复。然而,过度的粒细胞募集及激活,以及随之而来的脱颗粒,会导致炎症级联反应的放大和附近组织损伤。因为粒细胞的这些生物学特性及功能,靶向粒细胞是炎症性疾病的有效治疗策略。当过敏原、病原体等物质进入肺时,会被上皮细胞、巨噬细胞识别,从而启动炎症级联反应,招募大量粒细胞到达肺组织,引起组织损伤和呼吸衰竭。因此,开发靶向粒细胞死亡的治疗策略对于缓解气道炎症十分具有潜力。在不同的病理情况下,可能由不同的粒细胞发挥主要致病功能,因此在不同的病理情况下,也需要选择不同的靶向粒细胞死亡的药物。在以后的研究当中,开发能够诱导特定致病表型的粒细胞死亡,而不影响正常宿主防御的粒细胞群可能是一个新的研究方向。

参 考 文 献

[1] Huang K, et al. Prevalence, risk factors, and management of asthma in China: a national cross-sectional study. Lancet, 2019, 394(10196):407-418.

[2] Wang C, et al. Prevalence and risk factors of chronic obstructive pulmonary disease in China(the China Pulmonary Health CPH study): a national cross-sectional study. Lancet 2018, 391(10131):1706-1717.

[3] Yoshikawa T, Naito Y. The role of neutrophils and inflammation in gastric mucosal injury. Free Radical Research, 2000,33(6):785-794.

[4] Barnes PJ. Cellular and molecular mechanisms of asthma and COPD. Clinical Science, 2017, 131(13):1541-1558.

[5] Geering B, et al. Living and dying for inflammation: neutrophils, eosinophils, basophils. Trends in Immunology, 2013, 34(8):398-409.

[6] Haslett C. Granulocyte apoptosis and its role in the resolution and control of lung inflammation. American Journal of Respiratory and Critical Care Medicine, 1999, 160(5):S5-S11.

[7] Aouadi M, et al. Orally delivered siRNA targeting macrophage Map4k4 suppresses systemic inflammation. Nature, 2009, 458(7242).

[8] Wang W, et al. CD8(+)T cells regulate tumour ferroptosis during cancer immunotherapy. Nature, 2019, 569(7755):270-274.

[9] Hallett JM, et al. Novel pharmacological strategies for driving inflammatory cell apoptosis and enhancing the resolution of inflammation. Trends in Pharmacological Sciences, 2008, 29(5):250-257.

[10] Kuruvilla ME, et al. Understanding Asthma Phenotypes, Endotypes, and Mechanisms of Disease. Clinical Reviews in Allergy & Immunology, 2019, 56(2):219-233.

[11] Wenzel SE. Asthma phenotypes: the evolution from clinical to molecular approaches. Nature Medicine, 2012, 18(5): 716-725.

[12] Lambrecht BN, Hammad H. The immunology of asthma. Nature Immunology, 2015, 16(1):45-56.

[13] Fahy JV. Type 2 inflammation in asthma-present in most, absent in many. Nature Reviews Immunology, 2015, 15(1): 57-65.

[14] Denburg JA, Keith PK. Eosinophil Progenitors in Airway Diseases Clinical Implications. Chest, 2008, 134(5): 1037-1043.

[15] Moore WC, et al. Sputum neutrophil counts are associated with more severe asthma phenotypes using cluster analysis. Journal of Allergy and Clinical Immunology, 2014, 133 (6):1557.

[16] Park YM, Bochner BS. Eosinophil Survival and Apoptosis in Health and Disease. Allergy Asthma & Immunology Research, 2010, 2(2):87-101.

[17] Druilhe A, et al. Glucocorticoid-induced apoptosis in human eosinophils: Mechanisms of action. Apoptosis, 2003, 8(5): 481-495.

[18] Fanta CH. DRUG THERAPY Asthma. New England Journal of Medicine, 2009, 360(10):1002-1014.

[19] Barnes PJ. Severe asthma: Advances in current management and future therapy. Journal of Allergy and Clinical Immunology, 2012, 129(1):48-59.

[20] Tian B.-p., et al. Bcl-2 inhibitors reduce steroid-insensitive airway inflammation. Journal of Allergy and Clinical Immunology, 2017, 140(2):418-430.

[21] Tian B.-P., et al. Nanoformulated ABT-199 to effectively target Bcl-2 at mitochondrial membrane alleviates airway inflammation by inducing apoptosis. Biomaterials, 2019, 192: 429-439.

[22] Fuchs Y, Steller H. Live to die another way: modes of programmed cell death and the signals emanating from dying cells. Nature Reviews Molecular Cell Biology, 2015, 16(6): 329-344.

[23] Dixon SJ, et al. Ferroptosis: An Iron-Dependent Form of Nonapoptotic Cell Death. Cell, 2012, 149(5):1060-1072.

[24] Kwon M.-Y., et al. Heme oxygenase-1 accelerates erastin-induced ferroptotic cell death. Oncotarget, 2015, 6(27): 24393-24403.

[25] Daechert J, et al. RSL3 and Erastin differentially regulate redox signaling to promote Smac mimetic-induced cell death. Oncotarget, 2016, 7(39):63779-63792.

[26] Pandey KC, et al. Role of Proteases in Chronic Obstructive Pulmonary Disease. Frontiers in Pharmacology, 2017, 8:512.

[27] Jasper AE, et al. Understanding the role of neutrophils in chronic inflammatory airway disease. F1000Research, 2019,8.

[28] Crisford H, et al. Proteinase 3: a potential target in chronic

obstructive pulmonary disease and other chronic inflammatory diseases. Respiratory Research,2018,19(1):180.

[29] Dey T,et al. Proteases and Their Inhibitors in Chronic Obstructive Pulmonary Disease. Journal of Clinical Medicine, 2018,7(9):244.

[30] Klein JB, et al. Granulocyte-macrophage colony-stimulating factor delays neutrophil constitutive apoptosis through phosphoinositide 3-kinase and extracellular signal-regulated kinase pathways. Journal of Immunology, 2000, 164 (8): 4286-4291.

[31] Petrin D,et al. The anti-apoptotic effect of leukotriene B-4 in neutrophils:A role for phosphatidylinositol 3-kinase, extracellular signal-regulated kinase and Mcl-1. Cellular Signalling,2006,18(4):479-487.

[32] Rahman A, et al. Inhibition of ErbB kinase signalling promotes resolution of neutrophilic inflammation. Elife,2019,8.

[33] Yu X,et al. Matrine reduces cigarette smoke-induced airway neutrophilic inflammation by enhancing neutrophil apoptosis. Clinical Science,2019,133(4):551-564.

[34] Bel EH,ten Brinke. A. New Anti-Eosinophil Drugs for Asthma and COPD Targeting the Trait! Chest, 2017,152(6): 1276-1282.

[35] Kay AB. Paul Ehrlich and the Early History of Granulocytes. Microbiology spectrum,2016,4(4).

11 慢性阻塞性肺疾病合并症与肺康复结局探讨

朱惠莉

慢性阻塞性肺疾病(简称慢阻肺,COPD)是临床常见的呼吸系统疾病之一,患病率高、致残率高、病死率高,是目前全球第三大死亡原因。慢阻肺病程长,老年人患病率高,相关危险因素多,具有合并症的患者比例高。合并症对于慢阻肺的影响明显,而且慢阻肺可加重合并症的严重性,并有相互影响,给患者治疗带来一定困难。

已有证据表明,稳定期慢阻肺患者均可从肺康复中获益,是目前临床推广的重要的非药物治疗手段。肺康复(pulmonary rehabilitation,PR)是一种对慢阻肺确定有效的临床疗法,用于改善患者运动耐力、生活质量,以及与一系列慢性呼吸道疾病相关的肌无力等。肺康复对慢阻肺的有效性临床证据最多。肺康复的方案和有效性与疾病严重程度、合并症、疾病无关的因素(如个人偏好和动机)等有一定关系。某些合并症可以从合适的康复中获益,而有些合并症可能会影响慢阻肺患者肺康复的有效执行和疗效。尽管有大量证据证明康复的益处,但康复治疗的获取和使用仍然非常低。临床上影响开展慢阻肺康复的原因之一是临床医护人员和患者对肺康复的认知度较低,尤其对有一定合并症的患者使用肺康复有效性评估不确定,临床执行有顾虑,导致患者肺康复推广应用存在障碍。

慢阻肺最常见的合并症是冠心病、高血压、骨质疏松、肌萎缩、焦虑和抑郁症等,从当前康复医学的发展来看,这些疾病大多都能从康复治疗中获得改善。Cochrane评价认为,康复的益处超出了运动能力的提高,已证明与健康相关的生活质量的改善、心理疾病的治疗(焦虑和抑郁)和疾病自我管理方面获益。

焦虑和抑郁症是慢阻肺患者非常多见的合并症。有统计,慢阻肺患者发生焦虑为21%~96%,抑郁症发生率为27%~79%。慢阻肺患者合并焦虑或抑郁症状可导致患者急性加重、住院率和病死率增高。研究证实,肺康复是改善慢阻肺稳定期患者焦虑和抑郁症状的有效干预措施。呼吸道康复可能对心血管系统,新陈代谢,肌肉和肺力学产生积极影响。

慢阻肺与合并症的康复管理涉及多个环节。在慢阻肺和其他慢性呼吸道疾病患者中多发合并症很常见,尤其是慢阻肺以老年患者居多,多种合并症共存比例高,其中有些患者会转入康复科进入治疗。虽然没有关于慢阻肺合并症肺康复的正式指南,但美国胸科学会/欧洲呼吸学会(ATS/ERS)关于肺康复的声明建议在肺康复执行前先考虑和评估合并症,并在肺康复期间进行监测和兼顾合并症的康复治疗方案,并确保患者安全。在肺康复的初始治疗前评估非常重。PR患者通常应考虑基线心电图,并建议对COPD患者进行超声心动图检查,其中可有充血性心力衰竭,劳累性头晕,胸痛和(或)呼吸衰竭病史。基于患者以往的症状,在他们的运动训练期间,可以在PR期间新发现一些共病,如心律失常,外周血管疾病,心脏缺血,焦虑,抑郁和认知障碍等。这些疾病应在肺康复的参与者中筛选。通常可以调整运动训练计划以适应一些合并症,如具有显著肺动脉高压的个体可能需要遥测监测,避免可能导致胸内压增加并导致头晕或循环衰竭的活动。

慢阻肺合并症有可能影响患者的运动功能,但也可能参与运动训练并从中获益;患者也可从非体能训练的康复措施中获益。合并症与肺康复之间的关系尚不完全清楚。一项大型回顾性分析发现,多种合并症,如心脏病、代谢疾病等对肺康复后的运动能力和生活质量可能有不利影响。然而,也有不少回顾性和前瞻性研究表明合并症的数量并未明显对肺康复结果产生不利影响。例如,在肺康复患者中,有合并症患者在6MWD、MRC呼吸困难评分和生活质量方面获益;合并肌萎缩和(或)骨质疏松症的患者获益更多;合并心血管疾病的患者,肺康复获益不多。但有临床研究表明,焦虑和抑郁与活动期间呼吸困难的严重程度和肺康复开始前的生活质量差有关,并与肺康复后相对较差的预后相关。因此提倡进行包括心理治疗、体能训练等的综合康复。另外,患者合并症可能影响肺康复的治疗效果部分取决于合并症的特性和疾病严重程度,以及肺康复计划的方案。

由于慢阻肺患者合并症发生率很高,尽管慢阻肺患者某些合并症的存在对肺康复的运动训练带来一些困惑,但从以往的研究与事件中均可见患者可从合理的肺康复治疗中获益,因此合并症的存在不应排除患者参与肺康复治疗。在临床上应建立个体化的肺康复方案,稳定和改善患者肺功能和合并症。目前确认骨骼肌功能障碍。焦虑和抑郁及心血管合并症都可从康复治疗中获益,并最终改善慢阻肺患者的预后。当然有合并症的慢阻肺患者进行肺康复治疗还须制定严格的相关管理流程。

参 考 文 献

[1] Vanfleteren LE, Spruit MA, Groenen M, et al. Clusters of comorbidities based on validated objective measurements and systemic inflammation in patients with chronic obstructive pulmonary disease. Am J Respir Crit Care Med, 2013, 187: 728-735.

[2] Osadnik CR, Singh S. Pulmonary rehabilitation for obstructive lung disease. Respiratory, 24(9): 871-878.

[3] Catherine LG, Norman RM, Anne EH, et al. Practical approach to establishing pulmonary rehabilitation for people with non-COPD diagnoses, 2019, 24(9): 879-888.

[4] Richardson CR, Franklin B, Moy ML, et al. Advances in rehabilitation for chronic diseases: improving health outcomes and function. BMJ, 2019, 365: l2191.

[5] Carla SG, Jacob WW, Rylee MC, et al. Effect of Pulmonary Rehabilitation on Symptoms of Anxiety and Depression in COPD-A Aystematic Review and Meta-Analysis. Chest, 2019, 156(1): 80-91.

[6] Maltais F, Decramer M, Casaburi R. Society statement: update on limb muscle dysfunction in chronic obstructive pulmonary disease. Am J Respir Crit Care Med, 2014, 189: e15-62.

[7] Franssen FME, Rochester CL. Comorbidities in patients with COPD and pulmonary rehabilitation: do they matter? Eur Respir Rev, 2014, 23: 131-141.

[8] Spruit MA, Singh SJ, Garvey C, et al. An official American Thoracic Society/European Respiratory Society statement: key concepts and advances in pulmonary rehabilitation. Am J Respir Crit Care Med, 2013, 188: e13-e64.

[9] Cleutjens FAHM, Spruit MA, Ponds RWHM, et al. The impact of cognitive impairment on efficacy of pulmonary rehabilitation. J Am Med Dir Assoc, 2017, 18: 420-426.

[10] Houben-Wilke S, Spruit MA, Uszko-Lencer NHMK, et al. Echocardiographic abnormalities and their impact on health status in patients with COPD referred for pulmonary rehabilitation. Respirology, 2017, 22: 928-934.

[11] Crisafulli E, Costi S, Luppi F, et al. Role of comorbidities in a cohort of patients with COPD undergoing rehabilitation. Thorax, 2008, 63: 487-492.

[12] Tunsupon P, Lal A, Abo Khamis M, et al. Comorbidities in patients with chronic obstructive pulmonary disease and pulmonary rehabilitation outcomes. J Cardiopulm Rehabil Prev, 2017, 37: 283-289.

[13] Higashimoto Y, Yamagata T, Maeda K, et al. Influence of comorbidities on the efficacy of pulmonary rehabilitation in patients with chronic obstructive pulmonary disease. Geriatr Gerontol Int, 2016, 16: 934-941.

[14] Naz I, Sahin H, Varol Y, et al. The effect of comorbidity severity on pulmonary rehabilitation outcomes in chronic obstructive pulmonary disease patients. Chron Respir Dis, 2018, 16: 1-12.

[15] Hornikx M, Van Remoortel H, Demeyer H, et al. The influence of comorbidities on outcomes of pulmonary rehabilitation programs in patients with COPD: a systematic review. Biomed Res Int, 2013, 2013: 146-148.

[16] von-Leupoldt A, Taube K, Lehmann K, et al. The impact of anxiety and depression on outcomes of pulmonary rehabilitation in patients with COPD. Chest, 2011, 140: 730-736.

[17] Scanlan M, Broderick J. Effect of baseline anxiety and depression symptoms on selected outcomes following pulmonary rehabilitation. J Cardiopulm Rehabil Prev, 2017, 37: 279-282.

12 慢性阻塞性肺疾病合并焦虑抑郁的病因及诊断进展

贺斌峰　王关嵩

慢性阻塞性肺疾病（以下简称慢阻肺）作为慢性病，长期患病会导致患者活动能力及生活质量的下降，也会影响对大脑认识，从而对患者心理产生巨大影响，出现精神异常的状态/障碍，进而影响患者治疗的依从性、病情的进展及预后。焦虑（anxiety）、抑郁（depression）是慢阻肺最常见的精神异常合并症，可单独或混合存在。随着对慢阻肺合并焦虑和（或）抑郁的认识不断加深，人们逐渐了解到慢阻肺合并焦虑和（或）抑郁的发病因素、发病率、临床特征，以及慢阻肺与焦虑、抑郁之间的相互作用。本文就慢阻肺合并焦虑和（或）抑郁的病因、临床特征及诊断等进展进行深入探讨，全面了解慢阻肺合并焦虑和（或）抑郁。

一、慢阻肺合并焦虑和（或）抑郁的临床特征及流行病学

（一）慢阻肺合并焦虑和（或）抑郁的发生率

慢阻肺合并焦虑、抑郁的发生率分别为 8.1%～55%和 8.2%～48.6%，在不同研究报道中有着巨大差异，这可能与流行病学调查人群、患者的疾病状态（稳定期/急性加重期），以及焦虑/抑郁的判断标准有关。中国目前缺乏对慢阻肺患者并发焦虑/抑郁的多中心、大规模的流行病学调查；目前的报道多为区域性流行病学调查结果，慢阻肺并发焦虑/抑郁的发生率也有较大差异。例如：对徐州地区 1100 例 COPD 患者的流行病学调查发现，并发焦虑者占 18.30%，并发抑郁者占 35.70%；上海市某社区 275 例慢阻肺患者中 8.1%并发焦虑，13.4%并发抑郁；对重庆地区 154 例慢阻肺患者的调查发现并发焦虑和（或）抑郁占 26.63%。总体说来，慢阻肺人群并发焦虑/抑郁的发生率明显高于普通人群焦虑/抑郁的发生率（普通人群中抑郁的发生率 2.83%～6.90%；焦虑的发生率 3.60%～7.69%）。

慢阻肺患者亚群分析表明，女性慢阻肺患者并发焦虑和（或）抑郁的发生率高于男性。对 275 例上海某社区慢阻肺患者的调查发现，焦虑、抑郁在女性慢阻肺患者的发生率分别是 12.8%和 15.6%，高于男性慢阻肺患者的 2.2%和 10.5%。Di Marco 的研究表明，女性慢阻肺患者伴有焦虑、抑郁的发生率均高达 38.29%，而男性的仅分别为 25.16%和 12.9%。其他研究也表明，尽管女性慢阻肺的发病率低于男性，但女性慢阻肺患者并发焦虑/抑郁的发生率更高。60～75 岁的慢阻肺患者并发严重抑郁的发生率高于其他年龄段，但并不是传统认为的年龄越大焦虑抑郁的发生率更高。研究表明发现西方和非西方慢阻肺人群并发抑郁/焦虑的比例无明显差异。

（二）慢阻肺合并焦虑和（或）抑郁的临床特征及影响

慢阻肺患者发生焦虑、抑郁可出现一系列的临床症状。抑郁的症状包括是情绪低落沮丧、对外界事物丧失兴趣、疲倦、乏力、明显的睡眠、食欲和体重改变、注意力降低、对未来较为悲观、严重者甚至自杀。焦虑的主要症状包括对事物及未来的焦虑、恐惧、乏力、烦躁不安、易怒、睡眠障碍，注意力和记忆力下降，肌肉紧张等。此外，患者还可能出现胸闷、与病情不符合的呼吸困难、语言急促、过度要求医师给以安慰或保证、警觉性和敏感性增高等。由于焦虑/抑郁所引起呼吸困难、失眠、疼痛、疲倦、乏力等症状疾病特异性不强，常与慢阻肺部分症状重叠，可能导致慢阻肺患者的轻、中度焦虑/抑郁状态被忽视。

焦虑、抑郁对慢阻肺患者和其家庭影响都较大。通过对慢阻肺患者的观察性研究发现，与未并发焦虑（抑郁）的慢阻肺患者相比，并发抑郁（抑郁）的慢阻肺患者的肺功能、活动能力及生活质量明显降低，治疗依从性差，呼吸困难症状更重，进而增加慢阻肺并发焦虑（抑郁）患者的慢阻肺急性发作次数，慢阻肺的急性加重又增加患者的焦虑、抑郁，导致这些患者每次住院天数和每年住院总天数延长，加剧患者及家庭的经济负担，并与患者的预后和病死率相关。

二、慢阻肺合并焦虑和（或）抑郁的病因

持续进展的中重度慢阻肺是发生焦虑、抑郁的最根本原因，其可能通过多种途径诱导患者出现焦虑和（或）抑郁。

（一）吸烟史

长期或大量吸烟是我国慢阻肺患病人群的主要危险因素，并且与焦虑抑郁的发生有着密切的关系。吸烟导致摄取的尼古丁持续激活尼古丁乙酰胆碱受体、直接引起炎症反应或引起大脑及肺组织中生物钟基因表达的改变，并影响皮质醇和 5-羟色胺（5-HT）分泌的节律及水平，从而导致焦虑抑郁的发生；同时，焦虑的人更喜欢吸烟。Agarwal 等发现慢阻肺并发抑郁的患者人均吸烟量为 22.95

包/年,高于慢阻肺未并发抑郁患者的17.66包/年,并且吸烟习惯难戒掉。这样导致吸烟和抑郁形成正反馈环路。临床研究揭示吸烟或既往吸烟的慢阻肺患者更易发生抑郁,并且吸烟或既往吸烟可增加慢阻肺并发焦虑/抑郁患者的死亡风险。此外,由于近年来女性吸烟人数逐年上升,女性慢阻肺患者并发焦虑、抑郁的情况应受到足够重视。

(二)呼吸困难与焦虑、抑郁相互作用

呼吸困难是慢阻肺的常见的症状之一,并随着病情的进展而加重。既往研究表明在慢阻肺患者并发焦虑、抑郁严重程度与呼吸困难程度密切相关。重度的慢阻肺患者发生抑郁症状的风险是正常健康人的2.5倍。在观察性临床研究DEPREPOC(depression in chronic obstructive pulmonary disease)中发现,并发抑郁的慢阻肺患者呼吸困难评分mMRC为2.07,高于未出现抑郁的慢阻肺患者人群(mMRC仅为1.32),慢阻肺并发抑郁的呼吸困难程度明显高于慢阻肺未并发抑郁的患者。另外一项对115例稳定期慢阻肺患者的观察性研究也发现并发抑郁的患者呼吸困难症状较无抑郁的患者更重。慢阻肺患者呼吸困难的严重程度与患者的抑郁程度相关。MRC呼吸困难评分5级的慢阻肺患者其焦虑、抑郁程度明显高于MRC呼吸困难评分1(2)级和3级的患者。此外,呼吸困难更易使女性慢阻肺患者产生焦虑或抑郁情绪。与男性相比,女性慢阻肺患者的评分及焦虑、抑郁发生率明显升高,并发抑郁症状与呼吸困难之间的相关性更强。

(三)全身炎症反应

全身性炎症是慢阻肺的一个重要特征,被称为肺部炎症的"溢出(over-spill)"。既往研究表明炎症细胞因子可导致大脑中小胶质细胞的过度激活,并增加引起神经毒性的活性氧的释放,导致中枢神经系统干细胞功能障碍,损害神经组织的内稳态和修复功能并产生负面情绪。E-CLIPSE队列研究表明,有持续全身炎症反应的慢阻肺患者焦虑评分较无全身炎症反应的患者明显升高。研究表明,TNF-α在慢阻肺进展、急性加重及全身性炎症中的发挥着关键作用,其可溶性受体(soluble tumor necrosis factor receptor-1,sTNFR-1)与慢阻肺患者并发抑郁有密切关系。Lu等的研究表明慢阻肺血清中IL-6和CRP的水平与患者的抑郁程度呈正相关。

(四)认知功能损伤

Pierobon等对慢阻肺患者进行蒙特利尔认知评估(Montreal Cognitive Assessment,MoCA)后发现,9.6%的慢阻肺患者存在不同程度的大脑认识损伤,而慢阻肺患者的大脑认识损伤与抑郁的发生密切相关。大脑认知功能的损害还会大幅度降低患者药物治疗的依从性,导致慢阻肺患者急性加重次数增多,降低生活质量,反过来加重大脑认知功能损伤及焦虑、抑郁。进一步研究表明认知功能损伤的COPD患者脑部海马及白质容量明显减少,进而可能导致抑郁情绪/状态的产生。目前认为慢阻肺患者认知功能的损害可能与吸烟、炎症和慢性低氧有关。长期吸烟除了引起大脑神经的炎症反应外,长期摄入烟碱也导致认知能力的损害。吸烟严重程度与认知功能损伤程度相关,并且开始吸烟年龄越早,损害炎症程度越高。慢性炎症和低氧则是通过改变神经元周围的微环境,诱导神经元及白质损伤,导致大脑认识损伤。

(五)社会经济因素

人的本质是一切社会关系的总和。只有通过参与社会活动和创造社会价值,才能获得个人心理满足。Lustig等在1972年的研究就发现慢阻肺患者发生焦虑与患者社会活动的大幅减少有关。其他研究表明由于慢阻肺进展导致的体力下降明显导致患者社交活动的减少或由于独居得不到家人等较好的照顾,这部分患者的焦虑抑郁发生率和严重程度都较高。反过来,焦虑抑郁进一步损害慢阻肺患者的身体功能,形成恶性循环。此外,经济压力也是导致慢阻肺患者并发焦虑抑郁的重要因素。Kulkarni等研究表明低收入的慢阻肺患者有较高焦虑抑郁的发生率,并且严重程度更高。李建等分析了我国三级慢阻肺患者的经济负担性和经济风险,发现平均每位患者每年的治疗费用在20 107.58元,这对患者及家庭来说都是较重的经济负担。对发达国家的调查同样表明慢阻肺给患者及家庭带来沉重的经济负担。沉重的经济负担可诱使患者发生焦虑、抑郁或加重症状,使慢阻肺患者病情进一步加重,发生急性加重或需入院治疗,加剧患者的经济负担。

三、慢阻肺合并焦虑和(或)抑郁的诊断

(一)慢阻肺合并焦虑抑郁的筛查和诊断

慢阻肺并发焦虑和(或)抑郁中所指的焦虑、抑郁是焦虑抑郁状态和焦虑抑郁障碍等的总称。焦虑抑郁状态指严重程度达中等或以上、超出患者承受或调节能力、对生活和社会功能造成影响、需要医学处理的状况,但严重程度未达到焦虑抑郁障碍的诊断标准。焦虑抑郁障碍是指由精神科或临床心理医生基于精神疾病的诊断和统计手册-Ⅳ(the diagnostic and statistical manual of mental disorders-IV,DSM-IV)标准进行结构化访谈后,符合焦虑抑郁障碍及精神相关疾病诊断标准。

当慢阻肺患者出现失眠、疼痛、疲倦、乏力,以及与病情处境不符的呼吸困难、紧张不安、易怒、心烦、过分担心、坐立不安、语言急促、过度要求医师给以安慰或保证、警觉性和敏感性增高、情绪低落沮丧、对外界事物丧失兴趣、睡眠障碍、注意力和记忆力下降等症状时,可对其进行焦虑抑郁状态的筛查和诊断。焦虑抑郁状态的筛查和诊断可以采用多种量表。抑郁筛查量表包括医院焦虑与抑郁量表(hospital anxiety and depression scale,HADS)、白氏抑郁量表(Beck depression inventory,BDI)、流调中心抑郁量表(centre for epidemiologic studies depression scale,CES-D)、汉密尔顿抑郁量表(Hamilton depression scale,HAMD)、老年抑郁量表(geriatric depression scale,GDS)、患者健康问卷(patient health questionnaire,PHQ)及症状自评量表(symptom checklist-90-revised,SCL-90-R)。焦虑筛查量表包括呼吸系统疾病焦虑量表(anxiety inventory for respiratory disease,AIR)、医院焦虑与抑郁量表(hospital anxiety and depression scale,HADS)、状态特质焦虑量表(state trait anxiety inventory,STAI)、贝克焦虑量表(Beck anxiety inventory,BAI)、汉密尔顿焦虑量表(Hamilton anxiety scale,HAMA)、患者健康问卷(patient health questionnaire,PHQ)。研究表明,上述量表可简便有效地筛查慢阻肺患者是否存在焦虑/抑郁状态,并简单评估焦虑、抑郁严重程度。焦虑/抑郁状态的诊断可由非精神科医师根据患者量表的情况进行诊断。

对于焦虑、抑郁障碍的诊断,中华医学会神经病学分会神经心理学与行为神经病学组的专家共识指出,一般不主张综合医院非精神科医师做出"焦虑/抑郁障碍"的诊断。因此,对于慢阻肺患者焦虑/抑郁障碍的诊断需精神科医师按照其诊断标准进行诊断。

(二)慢阻肺合并焦虑抑郁的筛查和诊断过程中的问题及对策

尽管慢阻肺患者并发焦虑抑郁的比例较高,但在实际临床实践中医师对慢阻肺患者的焦虑、抑郁状态/障碍的筛查和诊断率并不高。这种现状使得此类患者的焦虑抑郁得到进行干预的比例低于33%,可能导致更多慢阻肺并发焦虑抑郁的患者错过最佳的干预时机,降低患者治疗的依从性,加速慢阻肺的病情进展。

慢阻肺合并焦虑抑郁的筛查和诊断过程可能存在以下问题。①医师对慢阻肺并发焦虑抑郁的认识不足,加之焦虑、抑郁所引起呼吸困难、失眠、疼痛、疲倦、乏力等症状疾病特异性不强,常与慢阻肺部分症状重叠,可能导致慢阻肺患者的轻、中度焦虑/抑郁状态可能被忽视而未进行筛查和诊断。②慢阻肺患者对焦虑、抑郁的认识不足。在临床实践中发现,慢阻肺患者对焦虑、抑郁认识模糊或没有正确认识,甚至对关于焦虑、抑郁的问卷调查有抵触情绪。③在慢阻肺患者焦虑、抑郁筛查的过程中,常因医师对调查内容不熟悉、问询话术及问询时机欠妥当导致筛查结果与实际病情有明显的偏差。

对于上述问题,首先,加强医师对慢阻肺并发焦虑抑郁的认识,仔细评估患者的行为并给予进行相关的问卷调查,有效识别慢阻肺患者的焦虑抑郁状态,进而给予有效的干预。其次,在条件允许的情况下最好由受过专业训练的医生来对患者进行问询和量表填写:一方面,尽量排除医师出现诱导性的问询和对结果的干扰;另一方面由于患者自行填写(特别是慢阻肺急性发作时)可能仅仅代表当时一过性的精神状态,不能完全代表者一般情况真实的精神状态。有研究指出HADS作为患者自评估量表,在评估慢阻肺患者是否并发焦虑抑郁时的敏感性和特异性仅为62.1%和62.6%,准确率较低,不适合作为评估慢阻肺患者并发焦虑的标准化诊断工具。最后,加强对慢阻肺患者并发焦虑抑郁的健康宣教工作,让患者能正确认识焦虑、抑郁并参与肺康复训练。

四、结论与展望

焦虑抑郁是慢阻肺的常见合并症,其发生的原因与慢阻肺发生和进展所致的吸烟史、呼吸困难、全身炎症反应、认识损伤及社会经济负担有关。此外,慢阻肺并发焦虑抑郁与患者的生活质量、急性加重次数、住院时间及其病死率的上升有密切相关。在临床实践中医师常常仅关心患者的身体症状,对患者的焦虑抑郁关注不够。因此,迫切需要提高临床医师对慢阻肺合并焦虑和抑郁并发症的认识和诊治能力。建议对慢阻肺患者进行更加详细的焦虑抑郁相关病史记录。在治疗慢阻肺的同时,也要积极关注患者的心理状态及心理疾病对病情的影响。通过对心理状态/疾病的干预,尽可能减轻焦虑抑郁对慢阻肺患者病程的影响,提高患者对慢阻肺治疗的依从性,改善患者的症状和生活质量。

参 考 文 献

[1] Eisner MD, Iribarren C, Blanc PD, et al. Development of disability in chronic obstructive pulmonary disease: beyond lung function. Thorax, 2011, 66(2): 108-114.

[2] Laurin C, Lavoie KL, Bacon SL, et al. Sex differences in the prevalence of psychiatric disorders and psychological distress in patients with COPD. Chest, 2007, 132(1): 148-155.

[3] Xiao T, Qiu H, Chen Y, et al. Prevalence of anxiety and depression symptoms and their associated factors in mild COPD patients from community settings, Shanghai, China: a cross-sectional study. BMC Psychiatry, 2018, 18(1): 89.

[4] Willgoss TG, Yohannes AM. Anxiety disorders in patients with COPD: a systematic review. Respir Care, 2013, 58(5): 858-866.

[5] González-Gutiérrez MV, Guerrero Velázquez J, Morales García C, et al. Predictive model for anxiety and depression in Spanish patients with stable chronic obstructive pulmonary disease. Arch Bronconeumol, 2016, 52(3): 151-157.

[6] Panagioti M, Scott C, Blakemore A, et al. Overview of the prevalence, impact, and management of depression and anxiety in chronic obstructive pulmonary disease. Int J Chron Obstruct Pulmon Dis, 2014, 9: 1289-1306.

[7] Yohannes AM, Baldwin RC, Connolly MJ. Prevalence of subthreshold depression in elderly patients with chronic obstructive pulmonary disease. Int J Geriatr Psychiatry, 2003, 18(5): 412-416.

[8] Yohannes AM, Baldwin RC, Connolly MJ. Depression and anxiety in elderly outpatients with chronic obstructive pulmonary disease: prevalence, and validation of the BASDEC screening questionnaire. Int J Geriatr Psychiatry, 2000, 15(12): 1090-1096.

[9] Lou P, Zhu Y, Chen P, et al. Prevalence and correlations with depression, anxiety, and other features in outpatients with chronic obstructive pulmonary disease in China: a cross-sectional case control study. BMC Pulm Med, 2012, 12: 53.

[10] 陈华萍,尹燕,贺斌峰,等.慢性阻塞性肺疾病合并焦虑抑郁的临床分析.中华肺部疾病杂志(电子版),2019,12(6):677-681.

[11] Halbert RJ, Isonaka S, George D, et al. Interpreting COPD prevalence estimates: what is the true burden of disease? Chest,2003,123(5):1684-1692.

[12] Gabilondo A, Vilagut G, Pinto-Meza A, et al. Comorbidity of major depressive episode and chronic physical conditions in Spain, a country with low prevalence of depression. Gen Hosp Psychiatry,2012,34(5):510-517.

[13] Huang Y, Wang Y, Wang H, et al. Prevalence of mental disorders in China: a cross-sectional epidemiological study. Lancet Psychiatry,2019,6(3):211-224.

[14] Di Marco F, Verga M, Reggente M, et al. Anxiety and depression in COPD patients: The roles of gender and disease severity. Respir Med,2006,100(10):1767-1774.

[15] Ekström MP, Jogréus C, Ström KE. Comorbidity and sex-related differences in mortality in oxygen-dependent chronic obstructive pulmonary disease. PLoS One, 2012, 7(4):e35806.

[16] Agusti A, Calverley PM, Celli B, et al. Characterisation of COPD heterogeneity in the ECLIPSE cohort. Respir Res,2010,11:122.

[17] Naberan K, Azpeitia A, Cantoni J, et al. Impairment of quality of life in women with chronic obstructive pulmonary disease. Respir Med,2012,106(3):367-373.

[18] Al Aqqad S, Tangiisuran B, Hyder Ali IA, et al. Hospitalisation of multiethnic older patients with AECOPD: exploration of the occurrence of anxiety, depression and factors associated with short-term hospital readmission. Clin Respir J,2017,11(6):960-967.

[19] Zhang MW, Ho RC, Cheung MW, et al. Prevalence of depressive symptoms in patients with chronic obstructive pulmonary disease: a systematic review, meta-analysis and meta-regression. Gen Hosp Psychiatry,2011,33(3):217-223.

[20] 中华医学会神经病学分会神经心理学与行为神经病学组.综合医院焦虑、抑郁与躯体化症状诊断治疗的专家共识.中华神经科杂志,2016,49(12):908-917.

[21] Iguchi A, Senjyu H, Hayashi Y, et al. Relationship between depression in patients with COPD and the percent of predicted FEV(1), BODE index, and health-related quality of life. Respir Care,2013,58(2):334-339.

[22] Ivziku D, Clari M, Piredda M, et al. Anxiety, depression and quality of life in chronic obstructive pulmonary disease patients and caregivers: an actor-partner interdependence model analysis. Qual Life Res,2019,28(2):461-472.

[23] Gudmundsson G, Gislason T, Janson C, et al. Depression, anxiety and health status after hospitalisation for COPD: a multicentre study in the Nordic countries. Respir Med,2006,100(1):87-93.

[24] Singh G, Zhang W, Kuo YF, et al. Association of Psychological Disorders With 30-Day Readmission Rates in Patients With COPD. Chest,2016,149(4):905-915.

[25] Iyer AS, Bhatt SP, Garner JJ, et al. Depression is associated with readmission for acute exacerbation of chronic obstructive pulmonary disease. Ann Am Thorac Soc,2016,13(2):197-203.

[26] Long J, Ouyang Y, Duan H, et al. Multiple factor analysis of depression and/or anxiety in patients with acute exacerbation chronic obstructive pulmonary disease. Int J Chron Obstruct Pulmon Dis,2020,15:1449-1464.

[27] Jiang M, Ma JF. Comprehension and recognition of acute exacerbation among chronic obstructive pulmonary disease patients. Zhonghua Liu Xing Bing Xue Za Zhi,2013,34(10):1030-1034.

[28] Pooler A, Beech R. Examining the relationship between anxiety and depression and exacerbations of COPD which result in hospital admission: a systematic review. Int J Chron Obstruct Pulmon Dis,2014,9:315-330.

[29] Dalal AA, Shah M, Lunacsek O, et al. Clinical and economic burden of depression/anxiety in chronic obstructive pulmonary disease patients within a managed care population. COPD,2011,8(4):293-299.

[30] Dahlén I, Janson C. Anxiety and depression are related to the outcome of emergency treatment in patients with obstructive pulmonary disease. Chest,2002,122(5):1633-1637.

[31] Pumar MI, Gray CR, Walsh JR, et al. Anxiety and depression-Important psychological comorbidities of COPD. J Thorac Dis,2014,6(11):1615-1631.

[32] 文富强,陈磊.GOLD 2017更新与中国慢阻肺临床实践.西部医学,2018,30(1):1-2,7.

[33] Brook A, Zhang C. The role of personal attributes in the genesis and progression of lung disease and cigarette smoking. Am J Public Health,2013,103(5):931-937.

[34] Mineur YS, Picciotto MR. Nicotine receptors and depression: revisiting and revising the cholinergic hypothesis. Trends Pharmacol Sci,2010,31(12):580-586.

[35] Sinden NJ, Stockley RA. Systemic inflammation and comorbidity in COPD: a result of 'overspill' of inflammatory mediators from the lungs? Review of the evidence. Thorax,2010,65(10):930-936.

[36] Sundar IK, Yao H, Huang Y, et al. Serotonin and corticosterone rhythms in mice exposed to cigarette smoke and in patients with COPD: implication for COPD-associated neuropathogenesis. PLoS One,2014,9(2):e87999.

[37] Agarwal A, Batra S, Prasad R, et al. A study on the prevalence of depression and the severity of depression in patients of chronic obstructive pulmonary disease in a semi-urban Indian population. Monaldi Arch Chest Dis,2018,88(1):902.

[38] Glassman AH, Helzer JE, Covey LS, et al. Smoking, smoking cessation, and major depression. JAMA,1990,264(12):1546-1549.

[39] Schuler M, Wittmann M, Faller H, et al. The interrelations among aspects of dyspnea and symptoms of depression in COPD patients-a network analysis. J Affect Disord,2018,240:33-40.

[40] Nishimura K, Izumi T, Tsukino M, et al. Dyspnea is a better predictor of 5-year survival than airway obstruction in patients with COPD. Chest,2002,121(5):1434-1440.

[41] Borges-Santos E, Wada JT, da Silva CM, et al. Anxiety and

depression are related to dyspnea and clinical control but not with thoracoabdominal mechanics in patients with COPD. Respir Physiol Neurobiol,2015,210:1-6.

[42] van Manen JG,Bindels PJ,Dekker FW,et al. Risk of depression in patients with chronic obstructive pulmonary disease and its determinants. Thorax,2002,57(5):412-416.

[43] Miravitlles M,Molina J,Quintano JA,et al. Factors associated with depression and severe depression in patients with COPD. Respir Med,2014,108(11):1615-1625.

[44] Martinez RC,Costan GJ,Alcázar NB,et al. Factors associated with depression in COPD:a multicenter study. Lung, 2016,194(3):335-343.

[45] Al-shair K,Dockry R,Mallia-Milanes B,et al. Depression and its relationship with poor exercise capacity,BODE index and muscle wasting in COPD. Respir Med, 2009, 103(10): 1572-1579.

[46] Spruit MA,Pennings HJ,Janssen PP,et al. Extra-pulmonary features in COPD patients entering rehabilitation after stratification for MRC dyspnea grade. Respir Med,2007,101(12): 2454-2463.

[47] Bestall JC,Paul EA,Garrod R,et al. Usefulness of the Medical Research Council(MRC)dyspnoea scale as a measure of disability in patients with chronic obstructive pulmonary disease. Thorax,1999,54(7):581-586.

[48] Tamimi A,Serdarevic D,Hanania NA. The effects of cigarette smoke on airway inflammation in asthma and COPD: therapeutic implications. Respir Med,2012,106(3):319-328.

[49] Reichenberg A,Yirmiya R,Schuld A,et al. Cytokine-associated emotional and cognitive disturbances in humans. Arch Gen Psychiatry,2001,58(5):445-452.

[50] Janssen DJ,Müllerova H,Agusti A,et al. Persistent systemic inflammation and symptoms of depression among patients with COPD in the ECLIPSE cohort. Respir Med, 2014, 108 (11):1647-1654.

[51] Eagan TM,Ueland T,Wagner PD,et al. Systemic inflammatory markers in COPD:results from the Bergen COPD Cohort Study. Eur Respir J,2010,35(3):540-548.

[52] Al-shair K,Kolsum U,Dockry R,et al. Biomarkers of systemic inflammation and depression and fatigue in moderate clinically stable COPD. Respir Res,2011,12:3.

[53] Emoto H,Jacobs G,Chen JF,et al. Intra-right-atrial balloon pumping(IRABP)during a Fontan procedure. ASAIO Trans, 1987,33(3):699-703.

[54] Pierobon A,Sini Bottelli E,Ranzini L,et al. COPD patients' self-reported adherence,psychosocial factors and mild cognitive impairment in pulmonary rehabilitation. Int J Chron Obstruct Pulmon Dis,2017,12:2059-2067.

[55] Vestbo J,Anderson JA,Calverley PM,et al. Adherence to inhaled therapy,mortality and hospital admission in COPD. Thorax,2009,64(11):939-943.

[56] Aras YG,Tunç A,Güngen BD,et al. The effects of depression,anxiety and sleep disturbances on cognitive impairment in patients with chronic obstructive pulmonary disease. Cogn Neurodyn,2017,11(6):565-571.

[57] Shen X,Reus LM,Cox SR,et al. Subcortical volume and white matter integrity abnormalities in major depressive disorder:findings from UK Biobank imaging data. Sci Rep, 2017,7(1):5547.

[58] Kalmijn S,van Boxtel MP,Verschuren MW,et al. Cigarette smoking and alcohol consumption in relation to cognitive performance in middle age. Am J Epidemiol,2002,156(10):936-944.

[59] Razani J,Boone K,Lesser I,et al. Effects of cigarette smoking history on cognitive functioning in healthy older adults. Am J Geriatr Psychiatry,2004,12(4):404-411.

[60] Jacobsen LK,Krystal JH,Mencl WE,et al. Effects of smoking and smoking abstinence on cognition in adolescent tobacco smokers. Biol Psychiatry,2005,57(1):56-66.

[61] Cleutjens F,Spruit MA,Ponds R,et al. Cognitive impairment and clinical characteristics in patients with chronic obstructive pulmonary disease. Chron Respir Dis, 2018, 15 (2): 91-102.

[62] Lustig FM,Haas A,Castillo R. Clinical and rehabilitation regime in patients with chronic obstructive pulmonary diseases. Arch Phys Med Rehabil,1972,53(7):315-322.

[63] Kulkarni RS,Shinde RL. Depression and its associated factors in older Indians:a study based on study of Global Aging and Adult Health(SAGE)-2007. J Aging Health, 2015, 27(4): 622-649.

[64] Maurer J,Rebbapragada V,Borson S,et al. Anxiety and depression in COPD:current understanding,unanswered questions, and research needs. Chest, 2008, 134 (4 Suppl): 43S-56S.

[65] Dueñas-Espín I,Demeyer H,Gimeno-Santos E,et al. Depression symptoms reduce physical activity in COPD patients:a prospective multicenter study. Int J Chron Obstruct Pulmon Dis,2016,11:1287-1295.

[66] 李建,冯月华,崔月颖,等.我国三级医院药物治疗慢阻肺患者的经济负担分析.中国卫生经济,2015,34(9):66-68.

[67] Zhu B,Wang Y,Ming J,et al. Disease burden of COPD in China:a systematic review. Int J Chron Obstruct Pulmon Dis,2018,13:1353-1364.

[68] López-Campos JL, Tan W, Soriano JB. Global burden of COPD. Respirology,2016,21(1):14-23.

[69] Iheanacho I,Zhang S,King D,et al. Economic burden of chronic obstructive pulmonary disease(COPD):a systematic literature review. Int J Chron Obstruct Pulmon Dis, 2020, 15:439-460.

[70] Alwhaibi M,Alhawassi TM. Humanistic and economic burden of depression and anxiety among adults with migraine:A systematic review. Depress Anxiety,2020,37(11):1146-1159.

[71] Vanfleteren L,Spruit MA,Wouters E,et al. Management of chronic obstructive pulmonary disease beyond the lungs. Lancet Respir Med,2016,4(11):911-924.

[72] Schuler M,Strohmayer M,Mühlig S,et al. Assessment of depression before and after inpatient rehabilitation in COPD patients:Psychometric properties of the German version of the Patient Health Questionnaire(PHQ-9/PHQ-2). J Affect Disord,2018,232:268-275.

[73] Yohannes AM, Alexopoulos GS. Depression and anxiety in

patients with COPD. Eur Respir Rev,2014,23(133):345-349.

[74] Nowak C,Sievi NA,Clarenbach CF,et al. Accuracy of the hospital anxiety and depression scale for identifying depression in chronic obstructive pulmonary disease patients. Pulm Med,2014,2014:973858.

13 肺结核与慢性阻塞性肺疾病关系研究进展

李风森

肺结核和慢性阻塞性肺疾病（简称慢阻肺）是呼吸系统常见的两大类疾病，在全球的肺结核和慢阻肺总人数中，中国有占有较大比例，经常可以发现一名患者同时有这两种疾病的患病史。在我国，因肺结核具有传染性，肺结核患者被要求就诊于传染病医院，而综合医院经常收治结核所致的慢阻肺患者，由于不同医院的医师对于二者的关系认知具有局限性，导致结核相关的慢阻肺患者生活质量及治疗效果较差，反复多次住院治疗，为家庭和国家带来了一定的经济负担。

有关肺结核与慢阻肺之间关系及结核相关的慢阻肺的研究报道不断增多。在我国慢阻肺合并肺结核不仅发病率高，而且具有较高的病死率，是公共健康领域面临的严峻挑战。本文评述了近几年国内外关于肺结核与慢阻肺之间关系的研究，希望对这方面研究有越来越多的关注和再认识。

一、肺结核与慢阻肺两者互为因果

最新的流行病学调查结果显示，我国慢阻肺发病率约为 8.6%，40 岁以上群体患病率更是达到 13.7%，我国已有约 1 亿人患有慢阻肺，成为仅次于高血压、糖尿病的中国第三大常见慢性病，每年因慢阻肺死亡的人数达 100 万，占全球该病死亡人数的 1/3。2018 年全球新发结核病患者 1000 万例，其中我国为 80 万例，印度、中国、印度尼西亚分排全球新增结核人数前三位。2019 年 GOLD 报告明确提出，肺结核是慢阻肺的独立危险因素。2014 年，一项对国内 10 个地区的人群调查显示，在中国非吸烟者中（317 000 例）气流阻塞（$FEV_1/FVC<0.7$）的发生率分别为 4%（女性）和 5.1%（男性），既往肺结核在非吸烟者中是气流阻塞发生的独立危险因素。可能由于其自身免疫屏障的受损及使用吸入激素或口服激素等原因，慢阻肺患者也是肺结核的高发人群。慢阻肺是肺结核疾病的高危因素，瑞典的一项队列研究对瑞典的一家医院中 115 867 名 40 岁以上的患者进行观察，最后得出有慢阻肺病史的患者患肺结核的风险程度是无慢阻肺病史的 3 倍。中国台湾省的一项研究显示，应用高剂量 ICS、泼尼松用量≥10 mg/d、既往肺结核病史均为慢阻肺患者发生活动性肺结核的独立危险因素。

二、肺结核与慢阻肺相互影响疾病进程

肺结核和慢阻肺能够相互加速疾病进程，造成较高的致残率和病死率。2017 年国外的一项病例回顾性研究显示，在慢阻肺急性期患者中，既往具有结核病病史的患者外周血白细胞计数、C 反应蛋白、二氧化分压水平均明显高于无结核感染证据者，同时其呼吸功能（FEV_1）下降较快。这一研究更为重要的发现是，尽管两组患者的总体病死率没有统计学意义差异，但既往存在结核病病史的慢阻肺患者表现为更加频繁的住院次数，其慢阻肺的诊断时间平均提前 4 年，死亡时间平均提前 5 年，提示既往结核分枝杆菌感染对慢阻肺的自然病程存在重要影响。2013 年中国台湾省开展了一项关于慢阻肺患者感染肺结核的风险研究，在 23 594 例慢阻肺病例和 47 188 例非慢阻肺对照者中，Cox 回归分析显示慢阻肺是结核病的独立危险因素，危险比为 2.47。感染结核的慢阻肺患者接受了更多的口服糖皮质激素和口服 β 受体激动剂治疗。2010 年来自瑞典的一项大型人群研究，从住院登记中识别出 1987—2003 年在瑞典医院诊断为慢阻肺的患者 115 867 例，进而将其记录与瑞典 1989—2007 年结核病登记库进行连接，通过 Cox 回归将慢阻肺患者与随机选择的对照人群相比，结果发现，慢阻肺患者发生活动性结核病的 HR 增加 3 倍（$95\%CI$ $2.4\sim4.0$），主要是肺结核的风险增加。此外，logistic 回归分析显示，与罹患肺结核的一般人群对照相比，罹患活动性结核病的慢阻肺患者在诊断结核病后的 1 年内，死于各种病因的风险增加 2 倍（$OR=2.2, 95\%CI=1.2\sim4.1$）。对于既往有肺结核病史的慢阻肺患者，使用吸入激素或口服激素能够导致结核菌复燃，因此在 2020 年 GOLD 指南中提出，既往有分枝杆菌病史慢阻肺患者不推荐使用吸入激素。我国目前慢阻肺的患者接近 1 亿，同时也是结核感染人数较多的国家，尚缺乏对二者合并的认识，对既往患肺结核的慢阻肺患者也无大规模的临床观察数据。

三、肺结核与慢阻肺具有共同的危险因素

吸烟、生物燃料污染暴露、社会和经济地位、维生素 D 缺乏、糖尿病病史这些既是慢阻肺的危险因素，也是肺结

核的危险因素，2018年全球新增肺结核的人数前三的国家（印度、中国、印度尼西亚）均为发展中国家，因此在发展中国家，肺结核和慢阻肺的防控显得尤为重要。为避免二者呈相互交错发展，需倡导全民健康，让更多人了解肺结核和慢阻肺之间的关系，这需多部门的参与及配合；同时需要开展多中心的队列研究，观察和总结既往患肺结核的慢阻肺患者的临床特征及非活动性肺结核患者肺功能变化规律，积极预防和干预。

四、结核相关阻塞性肺疾病概念的提出

结核相关阻塞性肺疾病（tuberculosis associated obstructive pulmonary disease，TOPD）是一种以持续的呼吸道症状和气流受限为特点，同时曾感染过肺结核病史的疾病。Allwood等首先在2013年提出了结核相关阻塞性肺疾病的概念，但没有对TOPD进行定义。本文作者认为TOPD仍属于慢阻肺的范畴。肺结核和慢阻肺是两种疾病，TOPD是结核相关的阻塞性肺病，但目前没有界定结核感染的状态和慢阻肺与肺结核（pulmonary tuberculosis，PTB）诊断先后顺序这个两个关键问题。

1. 结核感染的状态　TOPD（tuberculosis associated obstructive pulmonary disease）的英文全称中，"associated"译为"相关"，"相关"一词极为模糊且不准确。TOPD概念本身关注的是患者"气流受限"的状态，而不是"结核杆菌感染"。"associated"一词没有界定结核杆菌的状态是活动期还是非活动期；没有明晰的界定，TOPD可能代表的就是两种疾病，就需要兼顾两种疾病的治疗。本文作者认为TOPD代表慢阻肺合并非活动性肺结核的这类患者，一旦为活动性的肺结核，它应是两种疾病。Allwood关注的也是TOPD气流受限的状态和其疾病发展、转归的特征。

2. 慢阻肺和PTB诊断的先后顺序　慢阻肺患者气道黏膜防御功能状态低下，是肺结核感染的高危人群，若患者有慢阻肺病史，然后感染PTB，进一步加重为TOPD，这一类TOPD患者疾病发生、发展的过程与未有慢阻肺病史的TOPD应有不同。但在临床中我们遇到TOPD时，判定患者是先患慢阻肺，还是先患PTB有一定困难，往往患者患PTB时，未有任何结核中毒症状，完善肺部CT后提示肺部陈旧性病变。患者也可能同时有结核感染病史、环境污染、吸烟等多个因素交织而成，在实际临床研究中这两点对观察TOPD的疾病的发生、发展过程具有一定影响。因此，TOPD更多关注的是非活动性肺结核的慢阻肺患者。在临床中，我们常遇到TOPD患者，对于这类患者的治疗和随访，发现其临床症状及治疗效果与无肺结核病史的慢阻肺患者有所差异，但目前对此类患者的诊治无统一的认识及专家共识方案。

五、既往结核感染造成气流受限的病理机制研究

既往感染肺结核导致气流受限的机制尚不明确，目前有关机制报道为炎症机制、结核杆菌的免疫逃逸及结核感染致肺部结构改变等机制。但支气管扩张、细支气管狭窄、闭塞性支气管炎和肺气肿已经被证实与既往感染肺结核导致气流受限相关。结核病的基本病理变化是炎性渗出、增生和干酪样坏死。其被治愈后，可能会在肺部留下不同的病变表象，如气道狭窄、支气管扩张、肺部空洞和钙化灶等，不同程度上影响到肺功能。肺结核所致慢阻肺是结核杆菌引起的肺实质破坏性改变，导致慢性呼吸道阻塞。有学者通过大量临床研究提出，肺结核所致慢阻肺的特征不是单纯的肺气肿，而是由于小气道周围的纤维化所致，并且弥散能力降低，可能反映了肺血管（小血管）受累。目前关于既往结核感染造成气流受限的过程仅是在根据影像学结果反推得来，缺乏动态演变的病理学依据（图2-13-1）。2019年一篇关于肺结核所致慢阻肺的文章显示：

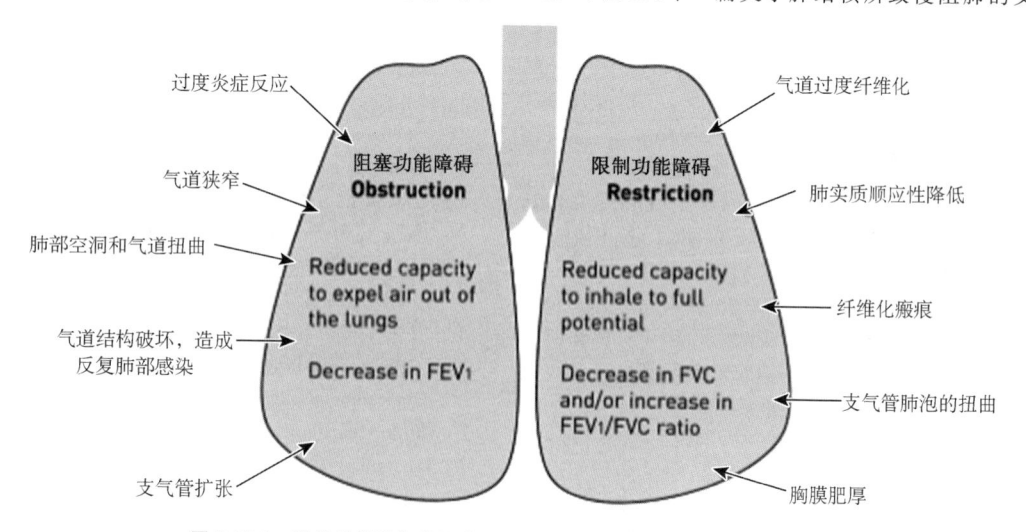

图 2-13-1　肺结核所致气流阻塞和限制性通气障碍的机制和影像学特征

一名年轻患者(既往无吸烟及其他基础病史),使用规范慢阻肺治疗后,症状控制较差,通过经皮肺穿刺获取病理,(吉森)染色结果显示圆形纤维化肉芽肿及扩张,但远端变窄的细支气管及细支气管周围纤维化。与吸烟相关的慢阻肺或支气管扩张的病变不同,这仅是个案,在一定程度上说明了既往单纯肺结核所致气流受限与既往认知病理生理变化有所不同。在临床中遇到的患者往往既有结核感染病史,同时也有吸烟因素及有害气体的暴露因素。既往感染结核与香烟烟雾、生物燃料等致病因素在慢阻肺发病及病情进展中的相互作用与机制有待进行深入研究。

六、肺结核与慢阻肺在临床治疗时的关系

在临床诊治中,肺结核与慢阻肺的关系密切,两者易相互转变,也能合并共存,故需给予足够的重视。有专家提出,慢阻肺患者在应用ICS治疗前,应考虑进行胸部X线片、痰涂片和(或)培养进行结核分枝杆菌检测。本文作者认为,若有条件可将X线胸片调整为肺部CT,这样能更好地观察和对比肺部影像学的变化。结核病患者的抗结核治疗延迟与发生慢阻肺的风险具有"剂量-反应"关系。对于肺部有病变或者病变较明显的患者应进行预防,早期复查肺功能,动态评估患者的病情,及时治疗。肺结核合并慢阻肺的治疗首先需要评估和判定结核感染的状态是活动性还是非活动性,是初治还是复治,是否耐药;然后对慢阻肺的病情评估,关键是吸入激素的使用,若患者症状控制尚可,应尽可能避免使用吸入激素,可以考虑使用单支扩和双支扩。支气管扩张药是否会引起结核杆菌复染目前没有文献报道。若患者症状控制较差,不应顾虑患者有肺结核病史而不使用ICS或全身激素,此时应没有绝对禁忌证;评估患者使用激素所带来风险获益比,若获益大,则使用(尽量使用吸入激素为主)。临床应动态评估病情,避免二者相互交错影响,增加患者家庭及社会的负担。

七、展 望

肺结核与慢阻肺的关系逐渐被重视和再认识,但关于二者的研究多为回顾性的病例研究。研究的国家多为患病人数较少、发病率较低的国家,多为对肺结核与慢阻肺患者临床特征的归纳,缺少大规模的多中心队列研究,对肺结核所致气流受限的机制缺乏深入研究。中国肺结核与慢阻肺的患病率高,同时人口基数大,需从预防、诊断、治疗等多个方面进行研究,如:肺结核所致气流受限的机制,结核感染与香烟烟雾、生物燃料等环境因素在慢阻肺发病及病情进展中的相互作用与机制等,结核相关阻塞性肺病的定义及诊断标准的界定,是否为新的慢阻肺表型或独立的疾病,以及结核所致阻塞性肺疾病的治疗规范等。

参 考 文 献

[1] Wang C, Xu J, Yang L, et al. Prevalence and risk factors of chronic obstructive pulmonary disease in China (the China Pulmonary Health [CPH] study): a national cross-sectional study. Lancet, 2018, 391(10131): 1706-1717.

[2] World Health Organization. Global tuberculosis report 2018. https://www.who.int/tb/publications/global_report/en/. 2019.

[3] Singh D, Agusti A, Anzueto A, et al. Global strategy for the diagnosis, management and prevention of chronic obstructive pulmonary disease: the GOLD Science Committee Report, 2019.

[4] Smith M, Li L, Augustyn M, et al. Prevalence and correlates of airflow obstruction in approximately 317,000 never-smokers in China. Eur Respir J, 2014, 44(1): 66-77.

[5] Inghammar M, Ekbom A, Engstrom G, et al. COPD and the risk of tuberculosis--a population-based cohort study. PLoS One, 2010, 5(4): e10138.

[6] Brassard P, Suissa S, Kezouh A, et al. Inhaled corticosteroids and risk of tuberculosis in patients with respiratory diseases. Am J Respir Crit Care Med, 2011, 183(5): 675-678.

[7] Yakar H I, Gunen H, Pehlivan E, et al. The role of tuberculosis in COPD. Int J Chron Obstruct Pulmon Dis, 2017, 12: 323-329.

[8] Lee CH, Lee MC, Shu CC, et al. Risk factors for pulmonary tuberculosis in patients with chronic obstructive airway disease in Taiwan: a nationwide cohort study. BMC Infect Dis, 2013, 13: 194.

[9] Hung CL, Chien JY, Ou CY. Associated factors for tuberculosis recurrence in Taiwan: a nationwide nested case-control study from 1998 to 2010. PLoS One, 2015, 10(5): e0124822.

[10] Sarkar M, Srinivasa, Madabhavi I, et al. Tuberculosis associated chronic obstructive pulmonary disease. Clin Respir J, 2017, 11(3): 285-295.

[11] Allwood BW, Myer L, Bateman ED. A systematic review of the associationbetween pulmonary tuberculosis and the development of chronic airflow obstruction in adults. Respiration, 2013, 86(1): 76-85.

[12] Kim SJ, Lee J, Park YS, et al. Effect of airflow limitation on acute exacerbations in patients with destroyed lungs by tuberculosis. J Korean Med Sci, 2015, 30(6): 737-742.

[13] Ramandeep S, Mamta S, Garima A, et al. Polyphosphate deficiency in Mycobacterium tuberculosis is associated with enhanced drug susceptibility and impaired growth in guinea pigs. J Bacteriol, 2013, 195(12): 2839-2851.

[14] Jin J, Li S, Yu W, et al. Emphysema and bronchiectasis in COPD patients with previous pulmonary tuberculosis: computed tomography features and clinical implications. Int J Chron Obstruct Pulmon Dis, 2018, 13: 375-384.

[15] Ravimohan S, Kornfeld H, Weissman D, et al. Tuberculosis and lung damage: from epidemiology to pathophysiology. Eur Respir Rev, 2018, 27(147): 170077.

[16] Kim CJ, Yoon HK, Park MJ, et al. Inhaled indacaterol for the treatment of COPD patients with destroyed lung by tuberculosis and moderate-to-severe airflow limitation: results from

the randomized INFINITY study. Int J Chron Obstruct Pulmon Dis,2017,12:1589-1596.
[17] Allwood BW,Rigby J,Griffith-Richards S,et al. Histologically confirmed tuberculosis-associated obstructive pulmonary disease. Int J Tuberc Lung Dis,2019,23(5):552-554.
[18] Shu CC,Wu HD,Yu MC,et al. Use of high-dose inhaled corticosteroids is associated with pulmonary tuberculosis in patients with chronic obstructive pulmonary disease. Medicine (Baltimore),89(1):53-61.
[19] Lee CH,Lee MC,Lin HH,et al. Pulmonary tuberculosis and delay in anti-tuberculous treatment are important risk factors for chronic obstructive pulmonary disease. PLoS One,2012,7(5):e37978.
[20] 孙永昌. 关注肺结核在COPD发生发展中的作用. 国际呼吸杂志,2019(16):1201-1208.

14 慢性阻塞性肺疾病的中枢损害与认知功能障碍最新认识

费广鹤

一、慢性阻塞性肺疾病的中枢损害与认知功能障碍概述

慢性阻塞性肺疾病（chronic obstructive pulmonary disease，COPD，简称慢阻肺）是以气道炎症为核心伴有全身系统性炎症的慢性呼吸系统常见病、多发病。据世界卫生组织统计，目前每年约有300多万人死于慢性阻塞性肺疾病，占全球死亡人数的6%，到2030年COPD将成为全球第三大死亡病因。中国慢阻肺死亡人数约91.1万人，占全世界慢阻肺死亡人数的1/3。最新的调查研究表明，在中国，40岁以上人群中COPD患病率达13.7%，其发病率高、致残率和病死率高，造成了严重的社会危害和经济负担。COPD是以气道慢性炎症为核心，以不可逆性气流受限为特征的慢性呼吸系统疾病，常伴有低氧血症和高碳酸血症。COPD也是一种全身多系统性疾病，COPD患者常有多种合并症，包括心力衰竭、贫血、骨质疏松症和肌肉萎缩等，引起全身的不良效应，这些合并症对患者预后可能会产生重大影响，识别和治疗这些合并症是COPD患者疾病管理中的重要一环，特别值得关注的是COPD引起中枢神经系统明显损害，COPD患者无论是在整体认知功能还是单项认知领域都存在显著的认知功能障碍（CI）。

认知功能障碍在COPD患者中的患病率明显高于正常人，由于研究人群和认知测量工具的差异，各项研究中COPD患者认知功能障碍的发病率差异较大，从12%到88%不等。既往研究报道COPD患者合并轻度至重度的认知功能障碍的平均发病率为32%，而年龄匹配的健康对照组中只有13.3%患有CI。COPD组的平均简易精神状态检查量表（mini-mental state examination，MMSE）评分明显低于对照组，对COPD患者和健康者年龄和性别匹配的个体进行MMSE分析研究表明COPD患者中有44.8%为轻度认知功能障碍（mild cognitive impairment，MCI），6.9%为中度CI，而对照组中分别为33.3%和3.3%。在调整年龄、性别和共病因素后，慢性阻塞性肺疾病患者与非慢性阻塞性肺疾病患者发生痴呆的危险比为1.74。一项大型纵向研究认为COPD重症患者的认知功能随时间推移而恶化，且CI发病率与呼吸系统疾病的严重程度呈正相关。既往研究报道，通过广泛的神经心理学评估认定存在CI的COPD患者有56.7%接受了肺康复疗法，这可能与接受肺康复治疗的患者一般均为COPD中晚期有关。

Meek等研究认为有认知功能障碍的COPD患者更容易出现呼吸困难和疲乏症状。由于认知功能障碍会导致COPD患者吸入装置的不正确使用、医疗过程中的依从性降低，从而增加COPD恶化的风险，并可能导致更差的健康结果。研究表明，神经心理学测试的异常可作为预测COPD人群死亡和致残的指标之一，认知功能障碍严重影响患者的日常生活能力及病死率。认知功能障碍的研究逐渐成为COPD研究的热点领域之一，COPD患者认知能障碍需更加深入的研究。

二、慢性阻塞性肺疾病的认知功能障碍发病模式与评估方式

COPD患者是否存在神经心理功能障碍的特定基本模式，研究结果存在差异，其原因可能是由于研究对象所处的疾病严重程度不同或在不同的研究中使用的神经心理测试量表的组合方式不同等。研究表明，慢性阻塞性肺疾病患者在不同的认知领域表现出相应的损害，主要为执行力、形象记忆力、逻辑推理和抽象推理能力、计划、协调和组织力。因此，慢性阻塞性肺病患者的认知功能损伤的模式是弥漫性的，每个患者表现出不同程度及不同认知领域的认知障碍。这种弥散性损伤类似于年龄增长相关的认知功能减退，而阿尔茨海默病（AD）或其他痴呆症则表现出其他特殊的认知障碍模式，认知功能障碍者往往不伴有注意力、语言等功能的下降，这一点与痴呆患者明显不同，认知功能障碍是正常衰老与轻度AD之间的一种中间过渡状态，因此，相较于AD或者多发梗死性痴呆及健康对照组，COPD患者可能确实存在一个特定的神经心理认知功能障碍模式。

神经心理评估是诊断和研究CI的重要手段，神经心理检查可以实现对COPD患者认知功能的评价，明确认知障碍的特征，对COPD患者进行进一步分类和病因诊断，并监测认知功能的变化。对于认知功能的评估，简易智力状况检查量表（MMSE）简单易行，国内外广泛应用，是痴呆筛查的首选量表，其能全面、准确、迅速地反映受试者智力状态及认知功能缺损程度。然而，Kozora等的研究认为MMSE对于文化背景不同的受试者敏感性差别很大，如文化水平较高者假阴性居多，文化水平较低者假阳性居多，MMSE可能无法发现存在轻微认知功能障碍的COPD患者。蒙特利尔认知量表（Montreal cognitive scale，MoCA

量表)是目前受到关注的新一代临床用来对认知功能异常进行快速筛查的评定工具,它包含了注意与集中、命名、记忆、语言、视空间与执行功能、抽象思维、延迟回忆和定向8个认知领域的11个检查项目,可以较为便捷地判定受试者的认知状态。研究发现,与MMSE相比,MoCA量表可提高认知功能障碍诊断的敏感度,虽然其受教育程度、文化背景的差异、检查的环境及被试者的情绪及精神状态等影响,但对轻度认知功能障碍的筛查更具敏感。其他已证明有效的评估诊断测试方式还包括连线试验(trail making test,TMT)、触摸操作测验(the tactual performance test)、韦氏成人智力量表(the Wechsler adult intelligence scale)、阿尔茨海默病评估量表认知分量表(the Alzheimer's disease assessment scale-cognitive subscale)、画钟试验(CDT)、认知能力筛查量表(CASI)、日常生活能力量表(ADL)和社会活动功能量表(FAQ)等。使用多种诊断测试可以提高对认知缺陷的发现,如Antonellilncalzi等证明,和单独使用任何一种工具相比,MMSE与日常生活能力评估相结合可更准确诊断COPD的认知缺陷。

三、COPD认知障碍的发病机制

脑损伤、吸烟、炎症、低氧血症、动脉粥样硬化、体力活动减少、病情急性加重等都可能是导致慢性阻塞性肺疾病合并认知功能障碍的原因,这归因于中枢神经系统对缺氧和炎症反应最敏感而成为最重要的肺外受累靶器官。结合最新的文献进展及我们前期进行的一系列研究,我们认为慢性缺氧与高碳酸血症、系统性炎症、脑结构损伤及睡眠障碍及精神心理因素等是COPD患者认知障碍发生的本质原因。

(一)慢性缺氧与高碳酸血症

长期慢性缺氧是慢性阻塞性肺疾病重要的病理生理特征,低氧介导的神经损伤是认知受损病理机制的重要一环。关于COPD患者认知功能的早期研究主要集中在低氧血症。大量的研究表明,慢性缺氧和认知能力减退之间有着明确的关联,COPD患者伴低氧血症时,整体认知功能会发生损伤,且主要集中在知觉和运动功能缺陷。Grant等研究发现COPD合并低氧血症患者有认知功能障碍,且低氧血症的程度与认知功能障碍严重程度有关,同时观察到PaO_2与受试者的注意、运动功能和信息处理速度相关。Stuss等研究表明,严重低氧血症的COPD患者在注意、信息处理和记忆任务的得分较轻度低氧血症患者下降。研究发现PaO_2与COPD受试者的MoCA总分呈正相关,同样验证了低氧血症与COPD患者认知功能下降具有相关性(图2-14-1)。接受长期家庭氧疗的COPD患者的认知功能障碍得到部分恢复,未来需要大量的纵向研究来观察低氧及氧疗后脑认知功能改变情况。

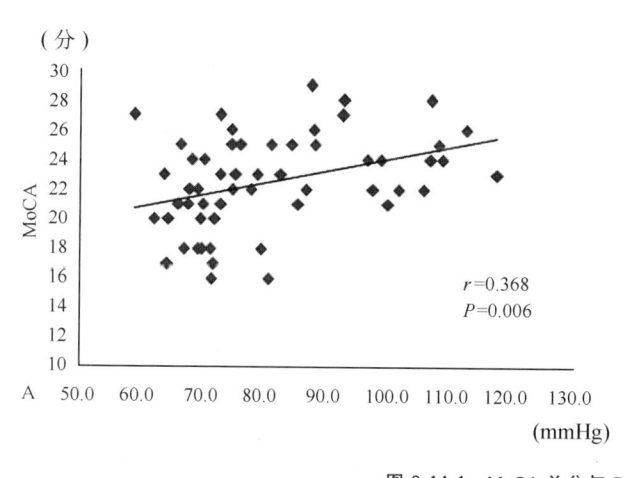

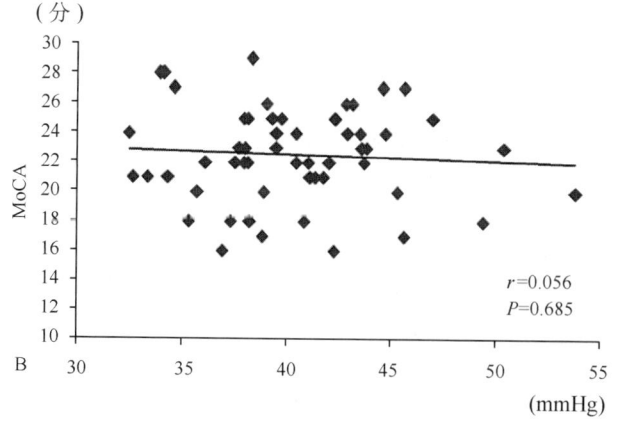

图2-14-1 MoCA总分与PaO_2和$PaCO_2$的相关性分析
注:A. MoCA总分与PaO_2的相关性分析;B. MoCA总分与$PaCO_2$的相关性分析

Heaton等认为缺氧时大脑中氧依赖性酶活性降低,导致神经递质(如乙酰胆碱等)的合成受阻,降低突触间的信息传递,影响神经系统功能,该过程可能是低氧血症损害神经系统功能的病理生理基础。Dodd认为COPD患者由于长期缺氧,机体通过自身调节功能促进红细胞的增生,血液中的红细胞增多将导致血液黏滞度增高,降低血流速度,引起大脑供血不足,同时缺氧时机体内氧自由基增多和一氧化氮(NO)减少,诱导血管内皮细胞损伤,血管收缩,长期作用最终引起动脉硬化及血管狭窄,加重了大脑供血不足,最终影响神经系统结构和功能,并且氧自由基可以直接损伤神经元,促进认知障碍的发生发展。大脑血流灌注不足常见于伴有低氧血症的COPD患者,研究发现该类患者的前额叶灌注显著降低,提示相应脑区的血流量下降,并且预示着额叶调控认知功能的下降。缺氧患者可以发生线粒体循环氧化磷酸化障碍,导致有氧代谢降低,无氧代谢相应增加,产生大量的细胞毒性代谢物,出现脑细胞代谢障碍。缺氧还引起氧自由基产生、神经元损害、炎性反应及神经胶质细胞活化等,改变脑结构和功能。此外,COPD患者低氧血症伴高碳酸血症能够导致脑神经细胞发生变性、坏死及凋亡,而脑神经细胞是认知功能障碍的物质基础。我们首次在非脊椎动物*Lymnaea stagnalis*建立了慢性缺氧动物实验模型,在此模型上分别从分子生物学、细胞学和电生理学及整体动物的水平进行慢性缺氧实验，对慢性缺氧导致认知功能障碍发生机制进行研究，发现慢性缺氧可损害神经元，影响神经突轴和神经生长锥，调控钙及改变钙调蛋白、神经突触蛋白 syntaxin、synaptotagmin、NCS-1 和 SV2，以及与认知功能密切相关的各种蛋白的表达，一定程度上解释了慢性缺氧导致 COPD 患者认知功能减退的机制。

COPD 患者肺实质的破坏及肺血管异常等使肺的气体交换功能降低，逐渐产生低氧血症和高碳酸血症。二氧化碳潴留及血 pH 降低，可以导致颅内血管扩张、血管壁通透性增加，在允许的高碳酸血症情况下，机体通过增加颅脑血流量保证大脑的氧气供应，但是二氧化碳潴留进一步加重将引起颅内压升高及脑水肿，导致脑损伤甚至死亡。同时，高碳酸血症时脑脊液内的氢离子浓度升高，影响颅内神经元的物质代谢，抑制大脑皮质生物活动，并且脑水肿、高碳酸血症、血 pH 降低及缺氧等可增强中枢神经系统内谷氨酸脱羧酶的活性，促进抑制性神经递质的合成，导致患者认知障碍发生。有关高碳酸血症和认知功能之间的相关性研究，结果差异较大。有报道在Ⅱ型呼吸衰竭患者中，$PaCO_2$ 与语言、记忆、复杂注意力和信息处理速度有关，而部分研究结果并未显示出认知功能和高碳酸血症之间的相关性。整体而言，$PaCO_2$ 和认知障碍之间的关系不如 PaO_2 与其之间关系明确。我们的研究结果显示动脉血 $PaCO_2$ 值与 MoCA 总分之间没有相关性（见图 2-14-1），但由于高碳酸血症常存在于危重度患者，危重患者无法配合完成相关检查而导致本次研究中存在高碳酸血症患者数量较少。因此，长期高碳酸血症在 COPD 患者认知功能障碍中扮演的角色需要进一步研究明确。

（二）COPD 认知障碍与系统性炎症反应

有研究发现，即使不伴有低氧血症的 COPD 患者也有明显的认知功能损害，说明慢性缺氧并非认知功能损害的唯一因素。越来越多的证据表明，COPD 作为一种全身性、慢性气道炎性疾病，不仅导致气流阻塞受限，慢性炎症以及肺部受损修复机制的改变还导致气道炎症介质溢出（如细胞因子、IL-6、IL-8、TNF-α）并进入全身血液循环中，引起系统性炎症反应，最终导致 COPD 患者肺外多器官功能受损，如骨骼肌肉萎缩、恶病质、缺血性心脏疾病、心力衰竭、骨质疏松症、正常红细胞性贫血、肺癌、抑郁症、糖尿病等。C 反应蛋白通过直接的神经毒性或致脑动脉粥样硬化作用参与了认知障碍的病理过程，其他炎症介质如 IL-6、IL-1β、TNF-α、$α_1$-抗糜蛋白酶等也与认知受损具有一定的相关性。

重度 COPD 患者及 COPD 急性发作期系统性炎症因子、趋化因子，以及急性时相蛋白，例如 IL-6、IL-8、IL-1β、TNF-α、CRP 等在循环系统中显著增加。此外，吸烟也可以使白细胞升高，导致系统性炎症。若 COPD 患者合并吸烟，其系统性炎症反应将更加严重，长期慢性的系统性炎症可能加重了 COPD 并且最终导致了众多合并症的进一步恶化，尤为重要的是对中枢神经系统的影响。脑部特殊的解剖结构及生理作用使得中枢神经系统对炎症反应十分敏感，其受损后最终导致了认知功能的下降。研究提示 COPD 患者的血凝聚素水平升高与认知功能障碍有关，验证了低水平的全身炎症性反应在 COPD 患者认知功能障碍的病理过程中发挥着重要作用。

（三）COPD 认知障碍与脑结构损伤

认知的基础是大脑皮质的正常功能，任何引起大脑皮质功能和结构异常的因素均可导致认知障碍。有关 COPD 的神经影像学研究也提示，COPD 患者存在脑代谢、结构及功能的改变。Shim 等通过磁共振光谱学检查方法发现 COPD 重症患者的大脑代谢发生显著改变。Ortapamuk 等通过单光子发射计算机断层成像术（single-photon emission computed tomography，SPECT）发现 COPD 组患者的左额上叶、左前额叶、左额中叶、右额上叶、左顶叶区的脑灌注下降显著。Dodd 等通过功能磁共振成像技术发现 COPD 患者存在灰质功能异常和白质微结构受损。Ryu 等研究表明，与对照组相比，重度 COPD 患者显示在灰质和白质中的广泛区域各向异性显著降低（定量衡量大脑组织完整性的指标）和更高的示踪（水跨细胞膜运动的指数）；与正常对照组相比，中度 COPD 患者前额叶的各向异性降低。白质完整性的丧失与 COPD 的严重程度相关，重度 COPD 患者额叶功能显著下降或许可以解释 COPD 患者的病理生理学和心理学变化。

研究表明，在高等哺乳动物及人类中，海马及其相关结构与注意力、记忆力等认知功能密切相关。海马结构影像学能够评价脑部萎缩的程度，海马的结构变化可以作为轻度认知功能障碍的预测指标，海马体积的测定不仅对早期 AD 患者的诊断有重要的意义，还可以作为识别认知功能障碍的一种方法。国内外相关文献报道，轻度认知功能障碍（MCI）及 AD 患者的海马体积较正常人群显著减小，并且与认知功能呈密切相关关系，即患者海马结构萎缩越明显，其认知损害越严重。我们前期研究对 COPD 患者的海马体积进行了划分与分析，应用 MRI 三维重建技术从影像学、形态学上进一步证实 COPD 患者中枢系统的变化，发现轻中度及重度 COPD 患者的左、右侧及双侧整体海马体积均较正常人群均显著减少，萎缩明显，由此表明 COPD 患者发生认知功能障碍与海马受损密切相关（图 2-14-2）。轻中度与重度 COPD 患者的左、右侧及双侧整体海马体积未发现有统计学差异，究其原因，可能是海马对长期慢性缺氧及系统性炎症反应极为敏感，在早期 COPD 患者中即受损发生了萎缩。随着疾病的进展，中枢神经与认知相关的其他结构亦发生了损伤，最终导致了认知水平的进一步降低。

研究表明 COPD 患者的整体脑默认模式网络（default-mode network，DMN）功能调节存在失衡是导致脑认知障碍的神经基础。DMN 在静息状态下激活程度的改变可以作为区分是否认知功能障碍的一个有意义的功能性标志。研究发现，相对于健康受试者，COPD 患者的 DMN 激活是降低的（图 2-14-3），尤其在重度组 COPD 患者，其 DMN 的激活降低更为明显，且 DMN 的激活降低与受试者的 MoCA 总分之间具有相关性，证实了静息态 DMN 脑区激活程度的损害与认知功能障碍有相关性，且 DMN 脑激活区的变化可以作为预测 COPD 患者认知功能损害程度的一个指标。

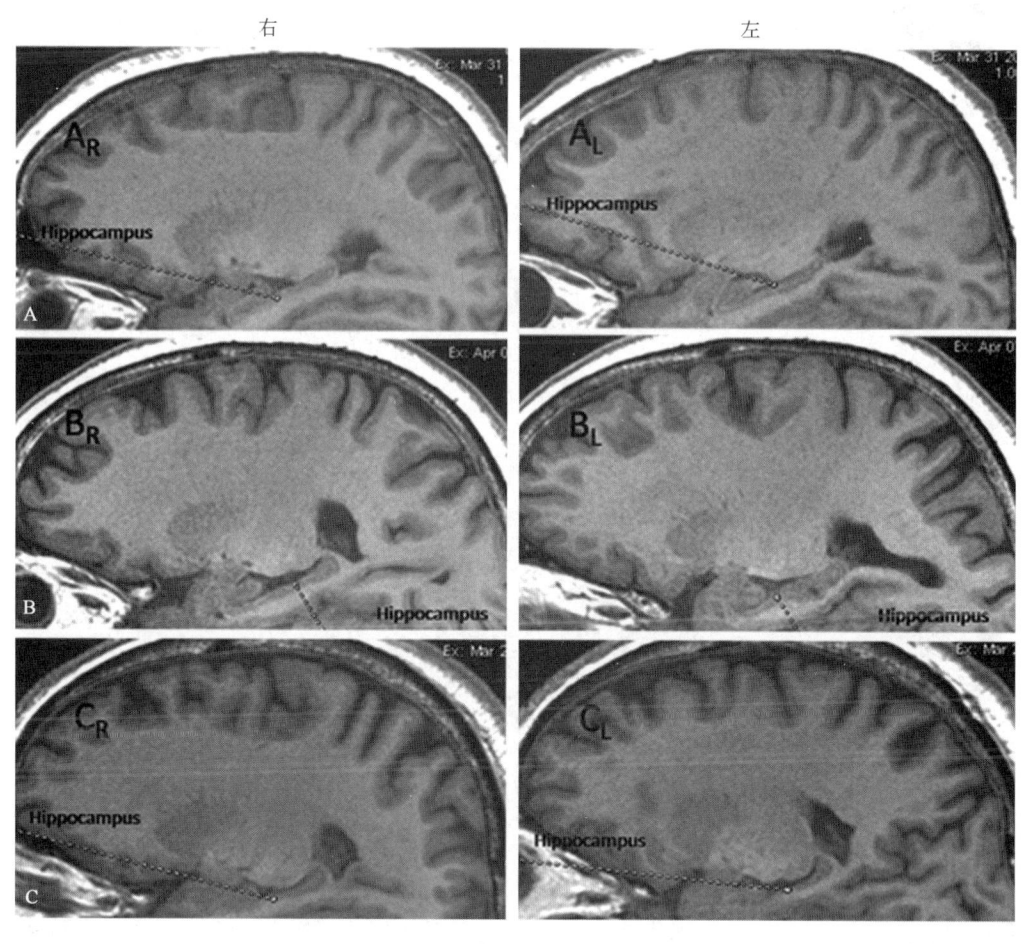

图 2-14-2 COPD 组与对照组 MRI 海马矢状位结构

注：头部磁共振矢状面成像，虚线所示为海马结构。A 组图为正常对照组；B 组图为轻中度 COPD 组；C 组图为重度 COPD 组。可见萎缩的海马

COPD 患者认知功能障碍发生发展的一个重要机制为颅内微小血管病变。研究证实 COPD 是脑出血的一个独立危险因素，该过程与小动脉硬化有关。动脉硬化可使血管顺应性降低，脉压增加，波动的血压降低损害大脑的微小血管，引起脑萎缩和认知障碍，且 COPD 引起的系统性炎症（CRP、IL-6）、氧化应激（基质金属蛋白酶的激活）、生理应激（缺氧、脑感神经系统激活）、蛋白酶/抗蛋白酶失调及加速老化等都可以引起血管病变。因此，COPD 患者导致颅内血管病变在大脑结构损伤及功能障碍中也起到重要作用。

（四）睡眠障碍及精神心理因素

睡眠障碍对 COPD 患者的认知功能也存在影响。研究表明，81.5% 的 COPD 患者存在不同程度的失眠，主要表现为睡眠质量差、睡眠不稳和失眠后反应。夜间频发的咳嗽、咳痰、呼吸困难，同时伴有的睡眠呼吸紊乱，会引起夜间睡眠低氧血症和 CO_2 潴留，影响睡眠质量，从而造成不同程度的认知障碍。另外，我们的研究表明睡眠质量影响 COPD 患者系统性炎症水平，可进一步导致患者认知障碍的发生。

焦虑和抑郁是 COPD 患者的主要合并症，慢阻肺患者中抑郁症状的发生率为 10%～79%，且抑郁症状越严重，MCI 的发生风险越大。在无抑郁症状、轻度抑郁、中重度抑郁患者中，MCI 的发病率分别为 10%、13.3% 和 19.7%。此外，其他不良精神心理因素如焦虑、烦躁、淡漠等均会加速 MCI 向痴呆的转变。

（五）其他

COPD 急性加重、运动、年龄及受教育水平等都与认知障碍发生发展有关。

四、COPD 认知功能障碍的干预措施

目前暂无能显著改善认知功能下降或预防痴呆发生的有效药物，改善认知可以改善患者的临床结果。除针对 COPD 本身的治疗，还应包括氧疗、肺康复治疗、积极治疗和纠正合并症等。非药物干预如科学运动、良好情绪、认知功能训练等是临床上潜在的治疗方法。

（一）氧疗

目前没有研究表明短期的氧疗可以改善 COPD 患者的神经心理状态，长期的氧疗也没有显示出改善认知功能的作用。但是，有纵向研究表明，虽然无法完全阻止认知

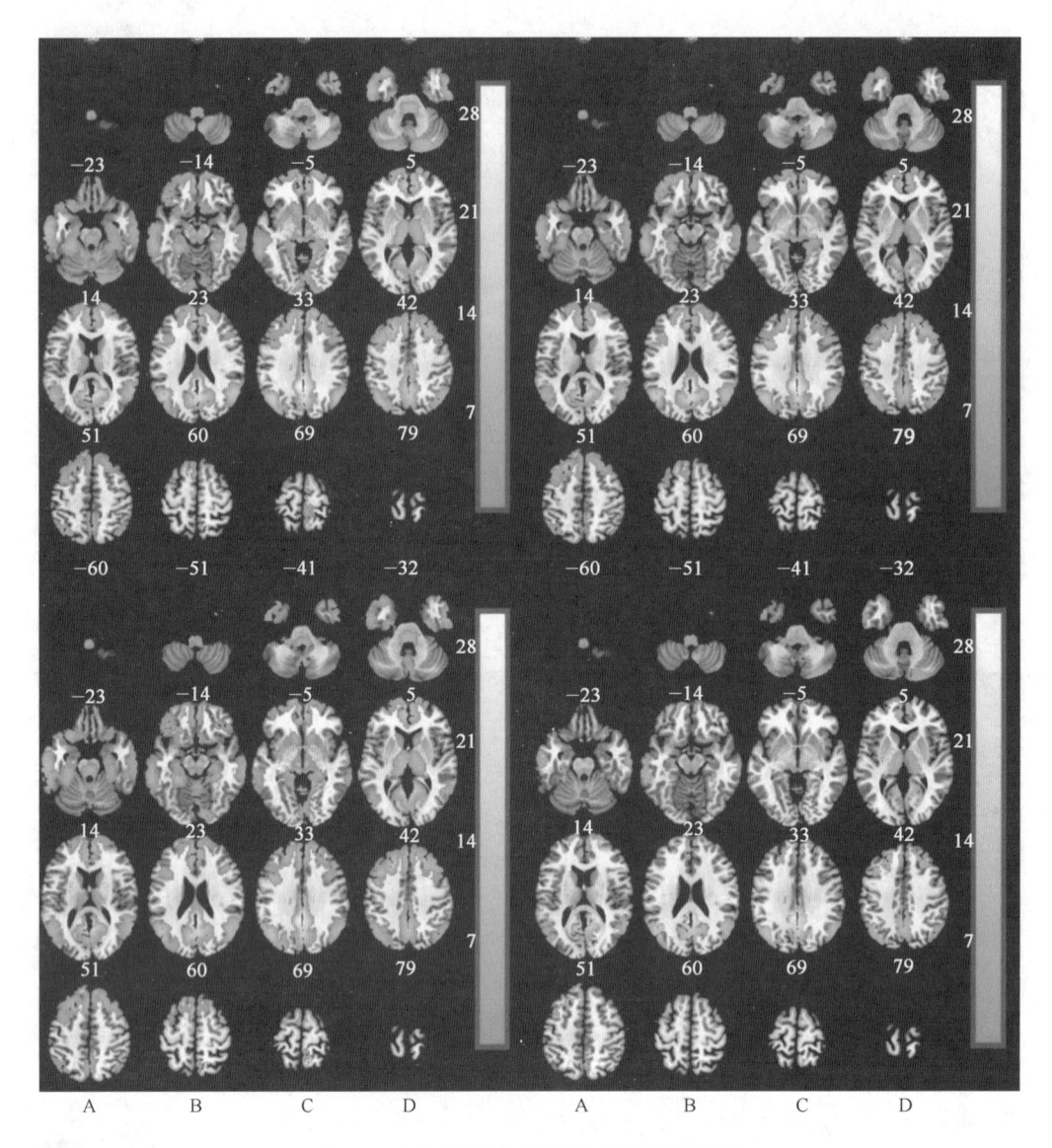

图 2-14-3 四组受试者的脑默认网络的激活脑区

注：四组受试者的静息态功能磁共振的横断面影像，以左后扣带回为种子点，与默认网络中的其他脑区建立功能连接分析，黄色区域为脑激活区域。A 为健康对照组；B 为 COPD 轻度组；C 为 COPD 中度组；D 为 COPD 重度组

功能障碍的发生，但氧疗可能降低发生认知功能障碍的危险性。因此，氧疗对于认知功能的作用尚需要更长期、更大规模及更多人群的研究。

（二）肺康复与运动

一项关于老年人体育活动的临床随机对照试验表明，增加 14% 的有氧运动能够增强老年人的认知能力、运动能力及听觉注意力，同时也能提高语言处理的速度和视觉注意力。但是，目前这一研究结果在 COPD 患者中的研究有限。也有研究表明，进行 3 个月的康复治疗会提高 COPD 患者的语言处理流畅度。由此表明，适当的运动可能会对认知功能产生有益的影响，但是这些益处的长久性还有待进一步研究证实。

（三）认知功能训练

研究表明，在 AD 和血管性痴呆疾病的早期阶段进行认知功能训练，患者的认知功能未表现出改善的迹象。在 COPD 患者中进行认知功能训练也没有显示出认知能力的增强。

（四）合并症的治疗

对糖尿病、高血压、血脂异常、维生素 B_{12} 及叶酸缺乏症等疾病进行干预后，是否影响认知功能还没有确切的结论。此外，合并抑郁症的患者，其认知功能的损伤可能与患者对抗抑郁药物治疗的效果相关。

五、总　结

认知功能障碍是 COPD 患者最常见的合并症之一，与 COPD 患者的预后、致残率和病死率直接相关。认知功能障碍的发展是一个长期的过程，选择在疾病进展后期进行干预,虽然仍可能延缓认知功能衰退的进程,但损害已大多数发展为不可逆的状态,因此,早期干预具有重要意义。在中国,要结合COPD在我国的流行病学特点、病因、发病机制、诊疗方法及合并症的特点及诊治等多方面,对COPD患者合并MCI的早期发现和早干进行深入研究。虽然现代影像医学的快速发展提供了"功能与结构"相结合的模式,降低了该类疾病的发病率,提高了诊断及治疗的准确性,但是针对COPD患者MCI的高危人群,还应进行记忆和智力的测查,以期实现早发现、早治疗。

参 考 文 献

[1] Global Initiative for Chronic Obstructive Lung Disease. Global Strategy for the Diagnosis, Management and Prevention of COPD. 2020. https://goldcopd.org.

[2] Vanfleteren L, LM Fabbri. Self-management interventions in COPD patients with multimorbidity. Eur Respir J, 2019, 54(5):1901850.

[3] Poot B, et al. Cognitive function during exacerbations of chronic obstructive pulmonary disease. Intern Med J, 2019, 49(10):1307-1312.

[4] Dodd JW. Lung disease as a determinant of cognitive decline and dementia. Alzheimers Res Ther, 2015, 7(1):32.

[5] Yohannes AM, et al. Cognitive Impairment in Chronic Obstructive Pulmonary Disease and Chronic Heart Failure: A Systematic Review and Meta-analysis of Observational Studies. J Am Med Dir Assoc, 2017, 18(5):451.e1-451.e11.

[6] Samareh Fekri M, et al. Cognitive Impairment among Patients with Chronic Obstructive Pulmonary Disease Compared to Normal Individuals. Tanaffos, 2017, 16(1):34-39.

[7] Ouellette DR, KL Lavoie. Recognition, diagnosis, and treatment of cognitive and psychiatric disorders in patients with COPD. Int J Chron Obstruct Pulmon Dis, 2017, 12:639-650.

[8] Hung WW, et al. Cognitive decline among patients with chronic obstructive pulmonary disease. Am J Respir Crit Care Med, 2009, 180(2):134-137.

[9] Grant I, et al. Progressive neuropsychologic impairment and hypoxemia. Relationship in chronic obstructive pulmonary disease. Arch Gen Psychiatry, 1987, 44(11):999-1006.

[10] Meek PM, SC Lareau, D. Anderson. Memory for symptoms in COPD patients: how accurate are their reports? Eur Respir J, 2001, 18(3):474-481.

[11] Dodd JW, et al. Cognitive dysfunction in patients hospitalized with acute exacerbation of COPD. Chest, 2013, 144(1):119-127.

[12] Incalzi RA, et al. Construct validity of activities of daily living scale: a clue to distinguish the disabling effects of COPD and congestive heart failure. Chest, 2005, 127(3):830-838.

[13] Antonelli-Incalzi R, et al. Drawing impairment predicts mortality in severe COPD. Chest, 2006, 130(6):1687-1694.

[14] Zhang J, et al. Alteration of spontaneous brain activity in COPD patients. Int J Chron Obstruct Pulmon Dis, 2016, 11:1713-1719.

[15] Schou L, et al. Cognitive dysfunction in patients with chronic obstructive pulmonary disease--a systematic review. Respir Med, 2012, 106(8):1071-1081.

[16] Zhang H, et al. Grey and white matter abnormalities in chronic obstructive pulmonary disease: a case-control study. BMJ Open, 2012, 2(2):e000844.

[17] Andrianopoulos V, et al. Cognitive impairment in COPD: should cognitive evaluation be part of respiratory assessment? Breathe(Sheff), 2017, 13(1):e1-e9.

[18] Kozora E, BJ Make. Cognitive improvement following rehabilitation in patients with COPD. Chest, 2000, 117(5 Suppl 1):249.

[19] Wilke S, et al. One-year change in health status and subsequent outcomes in COPD. Thorax, 2015, 70(5):420-425.

[20] Webb AJ, et al. Validation of the Montreal cognitive assessment versus mini-mental state examination against hypertension and hypertensive arteriopathy after transient ischemic attack or minor stroke. Stroke, 2014, 45(11):3337-3342.

[21] Antonelli-Incalzi R, et al. Screening of cognitive impairment in chronic obstructive pulmonary disease. Dement Geriatr Cogn Disord, 2007, 23(4):264-270.

[22] Dodd JW, SV Getov, PW Jones. Cognitive function in COPD. Eur Respir J, 2010, 35(4):913-922.

[23] Antonelli Incalzi R, et al. Cognitive impairment in chronic obstructive pulmonary disease--a neuropsychological and spect study. J Neurol, 2003, 250(3):325-332.

[24] Kirkil G, et al. The evaluation of cognitive functions with P300 test for chronic obstructive pulmonary disease patients in attack and stable period. Clin Neurol Neurosurg, 2007, 109(7):553-560.

[25] Mikkelsen RL, et al. Anxiety and depression in patients with chronic obstructive pulmonary disease (COPD). A review. Nord J Psychiatry, 2004, 58(1):65-70.

[26] Stuss DT, et al. Chronic obstructive pulmonary disease: effects of hypoxia on neurological and neuropsychological measures. J Clin Exp Neuropsychol, 1997, 19(4):515-524.

[27] Hu X, et al. Alterations of the default mode network and cognitive impairments in patients with chronic obstructive pulmonary disease. Int J Chron Obstruct Pulmon Dis, 2018, 13:519-528.

[28] Heaton RK, et al. Psychologic effects of continuous and nocturnal oxygen therapy in hypoxemic chronic obstructive pulmonary disease. Arch Intern Med, 1983, 143(10):1941-1947.

[29] Incalzi RA, et al. Verbal memory impairment in COPD: its mechanisms and clinical relevance. Chest, 1997, 112(6):1506-1513.

[30] Shim TS, et al. Cerebral metabolic abnormalities in COPD patients detected by localized proton magnetic resonance spectroscopy. Chest, 2001, 120(5):1506-1513.

[31] Ortapamuk H, S. Naldoken. Brain perfusion abnormalities in chronic obstructive pulmonary disease: comparison with cognitive impairment. Ann Nucl Med, 2006, 20(2):99-106.

[32] Dodd JW, et al. Brain structure and function in chronic obstructive pulmonary disease: a multimodal cranial magnetic resonance imaging study. Am J Respir Crit Care Med, 2012, 186(3): 240-245.

[33] Ryu CW, et al. Microstructural change of the brain in chronic obstructive pulmonary disease: a voxel-based investigation by MRI. Copd, 2013, 10(3): 357-366.

[34] Li J, GH Fei. The unique alterations of hippocampus and cognitive impairment in chronic obstructive pulmonary disease. Respir Res, 2013, 14(1): 140.

[35] Yin M, et al. Patterns of brain structural alteration in COPD with different levels of pulmonary function impairment and its association with cognitive deficits. BMC Pulm Med, 2019, 19(1): 203.

[36] Lahousse L, et al. Chronic obstructive pulmonary disease and cerebral microbleeds. The Rotterdam Study. Am J Respir Crit Care Med, 2013, 188(7): 783-788.

[37] Maclay JD, W. MacNee. Cardiovascular disease in COPD: mechanisms. Chest, 2013, 143(3): 798-807.

[38] Barnes DE, et al. Depressive symptoms, vascular disease, and mild cognitive impairment: findings from the Cardiovascular Health Study. Arch Gen Psychiatry, 2006, 63(3): 273-279.

[39] Angevaren M, et al. Physical activity and enhanced fitness to improve cognitive function in older people without known cognitive impairment. Cochrane Database Syst Rev, 2008, (3): Cd005381.

[40] Potter GG, DC Steffens. Contribution of depression to cognitive impairment and dementia in older adults. Neurologist, 2007, 13(3): 105-117.

15 慢性阻塞性肺疾病与肺曲霉菌病疾病管理的挑战和思路转变

马千里

曲霉属真菌是一类环境真菌,其产生的孢子可在空气中弥散,从而被人吸入肺泡。据估测,正常人体每日平均吸入数百个曲霉孢子,但是并不常发生曲霉感染。宿主免疫和基础肺部疾病是决定这种每日常规暴露于曲霉孢子后的结局的关键因素。免疫正常的个体,可以通过咳嗽、气道分泌物、气道纤毛活动、呼吸免疫细胞吞噬等作用清除这些吸入的曲霉孢子。如果人体的免疫异常,例如因为某种原因长期使用大剂量糖皮质激素或免疫抑制剂,或者T细胞功能异常(如获得性免疫缺陷综合征等),或者气道上皮纤毛数量及运动受损、黏膜上皮受损、气道结构性破坏[例如气道内鳞状细胞癌、慢性阻塞性肺疾病(简称慢阻肺)等慢性气道炎症性疾病],曲霉菌可能通过吸入气道或由原有的定植状态转变为侵袭肺组织,造成肺曲霉菌感染。常见肺部致病的曲霉菌主要有烟曲霉、黄曲霉、土曲霉、黑曲霉、构巢曲霉等,其中以烟曲霉感染最为多见,占曲霉感染的80%~90%。曲霉菌甚至可以定植在肺部有结构性改变的宿主体内,是导致气道致敏最常见的类型,这与烟曲霉在自然界中分布最广,生长快速,孢子直径小(2~3μm)有关,临床也常见黄曲霉、烟曲霉、土曲霉等混合感染的情况。

曲霉感染与宿主免疫状态的关系非常密切,其相互作用的结果导致不同的疾病表现类型。其临床特征很大程度上是由呼吸系统结构的完整性和机体固有免疫及在吸入真菌孢子后产生的获得性免疫反应情况所共同决定的。依据患者不同的免疫状态,可分为三大类临床表型:侵袭性肺曲霉病(IPA)、慢性肺曲霉病(CPA)和过敏性支气管肺曲霉病(ABPA)。在明确免疫缺陷(重度免疫抑制),尤其是粒细胞缺乏、HIV感染、实体瘤等患者中,侵袭性肺曲霉菌感染是最常见的类型;在哮喘为代表的免疫亢进的人群中则更多的是引发曲霉致敏性的支气管哮喘发作;更严重的是在哮喘和囊性纤维化患者中导致IgE显著升高的变应性支气管肺曲霉菌病发生;在免疫正常人群,气道黏膜屏障正常的情况,吸入曲霉菌,可能仅仅发现下呼吸道的定植而不致病;在轻度免疫缺陷的非粒细胞缺乏人群,肺曲霉感染表现不典型,更为复杂,往往漏诊、误诊。疾病迁延变化为慢性肺曲霉菌病更为普遍,在有陈旧性结核空洞的患者中表现为单纯曲霉球等多种疾病类型。

慢阻肺是一组以持续性呼吸道症状和气流受限为典型特征的综合征,香烟烟雾、空气污染和生物燃料暴露等是慢阻肺的重要致病因素。其持续存在的气道炎症机制涉及固有免疫与适应性免疫,常以气道内中性粒细胞、巨噬细胞、T淋巴细胞、B淋巴细胞增加伴功能缺陷为特征。一方面,吸入的有害成分激活触发模式识别受体(pattern recognition receptor,PRR),活化各种固有免疫细胞气道内结构细胞,直接或间接的激活炎症相关的损伤相关分子模式(damage associated molecular patterns,DAMP),导致各种细胞因子、趋化因子、生长因子、急性期反应蛋白和抗菌肽的释放,进而引起终末肺组织及呼吸细支气管的结构破坏;另一方面,活化的树突状细胞可诱导适应性免疫应答,包括$CD4^+$ T细胞、$CD8^+$ T细胞和B细胞等的免疫应答,诱发持续性的肺组织慢性炎症,以及免疫失衡。持续的气道炎症、反复的感染导致肺部发生不可逆性的结构改变;气道上皮纤毛数量及功能受损、黏膜屏障破坏、频繁的糖皮质激素和广谱抗生素的使用、气道上皮吞噬细胞功能损害、长期的疾病消耗,导致慢阻肺患者成为非粒缺患者中肺曲霉菌感染位列首位的群体,是慢阻肺漫长的疾病病程管理中容易忽视且必须关注的问题。

一、慢阻肺和并肺曲霉菌感染诊治中的困惑

慢阻肺患者的呼吸道既有明确的结构破坏和以纤毛功能障碍为代表的自洁防护机制缺陷,也具有固有与适应性免疫功能的不同程度损害,同时可能还合并长期糖皮质激素和反复的广谱抗生素治疗,在吸入常规数量曲霉菌孢子时,曲霉与不同状态的慢阻肺宿主之间可以呈现出不同的、比较复杂的关系。①感染类型的复杂:可能为急性侵袭性肺曲霉病、可能为慢性肺曲霉病、也可能表现为定植或致敏。②临床表现的复杂:慢阻肺合并肺曲霉病首先表现出多种交叉重叠难以分辨的临床特征,包括难以与细菌感染导致的AECOPD鉴别的咳嗽、脓痰、呼吸困难等非特异性呼吸道感染表现,难以与结核感染进行鉴别的咯血、发热、消瘦等临床表现。③影像表现的复杂:极不典型的影像学表现也是慢阻肺合并肺曲霉菌病诊断的难点,由于非粒细胞缺乏的轻度免疫受损状态,影像学变化缺乏典型的晕征、实变中心低密度向新月征发展的规律。研究报道提示,气道侵袭性曲霉菌病见于免疫严重抑制或短时间内大量吸入孢子的非粒细胞缺乏患者;气管支气管炎型肺部CT可以无异常,偶见支气管壁增厚伴或不伴阻塞性肺不张;细支气管炎型肺部

CT可见沿支气管播散的小叶中央性的小结节和远端的树芽征；血管侵袭性的肺曲霉菌病影像学表现多样，可有实变、磨玻璃影、空洞、结节影、树芽征、胸腔积液等多种情况。这些不典型的临床和影像学对于痰培养阳性率极低的慢阻肺合并肺曲霉菌感染的诊断造成极大挑战。④确诊技术的缺陷：在现有IPA或CPA的诊断指南中，病理活检依然是金标准，然而在临床病情较重的慢阻肺患者行介入活检的临床实操是很困难的，生物标志物成为最重要的辅助检查手段，包括(1,3)-β-D葡聚糖试验（G试验）、血或肺泡灌洗液（BALF）半乳甘露聚糖抗原试验（GM试验）、曲霉特异性抗体检测等。G试验对曲霉菌特异性低；外周血GM试验特异性高，操作简单快速，但是对于慢阻肺这种非粒细胞缺乏患者敏感性很低。国外指南建议对非粒细胞缺乏患者选择肺泡灌洗液GM试验提高阳性诊断率，但其cut-off折点要高于血清0.5的标准，具体的折点选择目前仍有争议。曲霉特异性抗体IgG对变应性支气管肺曲霉菌病和慢性肺曲霉菌病的诊断敏感性和特异性均在90%，被欧洲指南推荐，但对病程短于10.8d内的IPA的诊断价值有限。这些一系列问题极大地阻碍了慢阻肺合并肺曲霉菌病的早诊断、早治疗；诊断的难以明确，治疗疗程和预后的不确定性对慢阻肺合并曲霉菌病的疾病进展监测的实施也提出了重大挑战。

二、慢阻肺合并肺曲霉菌感染从IPA-CPA的疾病管理

针对慢阻肺合并肺曲霉菌病疾病规律认识的不足，CPA疾病管理的缺乏是我们必须去关注重视的问题。在漫长的疾病诊治过程中，如何早诊断、早治疗、识别停药时机、发现疾病活动在慢阻肺IPA-CPA的疾病管理中需要更多的思考。

(一)识别慢阻肺合并IPA、CPA及重叠综合征高危因素和临床特征

国外报道CPA是慢阻肺合并肺曲霉菌病最常见的类型，但国内研究报道更多的却是慢阻肺合并IPA的情况。国内有学者认为这是由于大家更加关注IPA，本文作者认为还有更多的原因，如：国内数据往往来自于因急性加重住院的患者，其病程时间、临床表现、影像变化更符合IPA的诊断，忽略了既往影像学和病程的追溯，忽视了很多CPA急性加重到IPA、CNPA的情况；当然，由于院外管理缺乏、药物费用昂贵、疗程不足、免疫状态变化等更多方面的原因，IPA迁延到CNPA、CFPA的情况在慢阻肺合并肺曲霉菌病人群中也非常普遍，甚至发生不同类型肺曲霉菌合并存在的重叠综合征，这些情况下由于慢阻肺患者对其咳嗽、咳痰、呼吸困难症状的耐受，及时就医的比例往往较低；各级医疗机构诊治水平、诊疗手段的差异导致无论是慢阻肺合并IPA、CPA、或重叠综合征的情况都被低估，临床报道也很不足。目前，病理活检依然是IPA的诊断金标准，但对于慢阻肺患者并发IPA时很难进行介入有创操作，更多是临床诊断和拟诊。最新2016年IDSA推荐标准中，宿主因素和临床表现非常重要，但其实缺乏特异性；

CPA的诊断标准包括：①慢性肺部或全身症状，包括至少1项如下症状(病程至少3个月)：体重减轻，咳痰或咯血。②影像学发现进展性形成或原有的单一或多个肺部空洞扩大，有空洞壁，可能有胸闷增厚。③血清曲霉菌沉淀素检测阳性，或肺部或胸膜腔样本中分离出曲霉菌属真菌。④炎症综合征生物学指标升高，如C反应蛋白、血浆黏度、红细胞沉降率。⑤排除其他能够引起类似症状的疾病(支气管肺癌、TB和非典型分枝杆菌感染)。⑥无明显的免疫缺陷(HIV感染、白血病和慢性肉芽肿性疾病)。每条标准的表现也常见于肺癌或其他慢性呼吸道感染的患者，如肺结核(TB)或非结核分枝杆菌感染，因此也并不具有特异性。现有观点认为，如果临床慢阻肺合并肺部感染经充分抗生素治疗、糖皮质激素及支气管舒张药这三联AECOPD标准治疗方案无好转的患者，需要考虑肺曲霉菌感染可能，但迄今没有指南或专家共识推荐应用经验性治疗。具体结合到慢阻肺人群，识别高危因素，关注临床表现的差异性变化依然是及时考虑合并曲霉感染可能的首要问题。现有研究发现：除了粒细胞缺乏、血液系统肿瘤、实体器官移植、HIV感染等情况，慢阻肺合并IPA的高危因素主要还包括：口服或静脉使用糖皮质激素、急性加重期入住重症监护室(ICU)及机械通气和广谱抗生素使用、肝硬化失代偿、T淋巴细胞免疫抑制剂治疗、严重流感。慢阻肺合并CPA的高危因素没有入住ICU，但增加了酗酒、大量吸烟、糖尿病、营养不良。我们的研究(尚未发表)进一步发现：近1年≥3次以上AECOPD急性加重使用全身激素(加或不加抗生素治疗病史)、慢性贫血、合并血糖控制不佳的糖尿病史是有别于IPA的高危因素。在临床特征上，慢阻肺患者出现咯血是考虑合并结核或曲霉感染的重要线索；血液的TSPOT检查阴性有利于及时排除结核感染，聚焦曲霉感染可能；既往结核感染陈旧性空洞病灶基础上并发曲霉球是另一重要的CPA诊断线索。CPA的典型表现为无血管侵犯，最多会出现菌丝对空洞壁的中度侵犯(与存在免疫抑制的患者的侵犯形式恰好相反)，转移和慢性型肉芽反应的发生率也低。研究发现：咯血，特别是间断痰血在CPA患者中CNPA这一类型中更为常见；体重减轻、慢性贫血等也较IPA更为明显；而发热、脓痰、发作性喘息在IPA则更为常见。因此，病史、合并症、既往1年急性加重史、用药史、有别于单纯AECOPD的咯血、发热、发作性呼吸困难等临床特征是识别慢阻肺合并IPA、CPA和重叠综合征的重要线索。

(二)关注慢阻肺合并IPA、CPA及重叠综合征病程中肺部影像学的演变

以慢阻肺为代表的非粒细胞缺乏患者的肺曲霉菌病影像学特点最大的特点是：没有特异性。往往观察不到典型的晕轮征到低密度坏死进展到新月征的过程，随真菌负荷以及宿主免疫状态的不同，可以出现实变、树芽征、磨玻璃、结节+晕轮、空洞+絮状物填充、支气管扩张等2种及2种以上混合病灶，但结核、放线菌病和肺癌患者也可出现类似的表现，因此没有特异性。疾病监管过程必须转变思路。慢阻肺合并IPA和CPA的诊疗过程也往往伴随延误、误诊、漏诊过程中影像学的动态变化，具备以下规律和

特征：①关于曲霉菌感染播散的过程：双肺多发结节、空洞、沿支气管播散、支气管壁增厚及局限性扩张、远端黏液栓这些表现是CPA与结核鉴别的难点，但短时间内结核病灶不易改变，而曲霉菌感染容易出现病灶的多种变化，甚至表现为消失或新生病灶游走，且这些特征常为单侧且不对称出现，主要存在于肺部或出现空腔的肺组织。②关于空洞的动态变化：不同于肿瘤的厚壁空洞和单发规律，CPA曲霉感染的空洞多发，也不同于结核空洞周围容易形成卫星灶，曲霉感染的空洞周围多伴有不同程度的实变或磨玻璃影表现，而伴随实变坏死，邻近又形成新的空洞，其内壁不同于结核，往往并不光整，空洞内可见絮状物填充，这个过程可以持续发生在CPA病程的任何阶段；而空洞的新月征表现也是伴随宿主的免疫状态变化病灶周围坏死物重吸收的结果，因此，空洞的动态特点伴随着治疗贯穿疾病监管始终。③关于不同类型的CPA影像表现的差异：CPA是非粒缺慢阻肺患者自身免疫、疾病延误、肺部结构改变程度、基础疾病、激素及抗生素使用多种因素混合、病程迁延导致的最终结果，因此，病程的不同、宿主免疫状态的不同、真菌负荷的不同，不同的类型特征性演变也不同。依据影像学的改变，CPA分为单纯曲霉肿（SA）、亚急性坏死型肺曲霉菌病（CNPA）、慢性空洞型肺曲霉菌病（CCPA）、慢性纤维型肺曲霉菌病（CFPA），CNPA被认为是IPA的亚急性表现，但依然归属CPA范畴。单纯曲霉肿为圆形或类圆形致密阴影，位于肺内空洞或空腔内，上缘与空洞（腔）上壁之间有一半月形空隙，称为空气半月征，空洞内可见有重力的球，仰卧位及俯卧位时可见球在空洞内移动，具备特征性表现，容易识别；CNPA常表现为单侧或双侧边界不清的实变和纤维化，常伴有1个或多个含气空腔或扩张的支气管，免疫状态不同，可以不经过IPA的过程，直接出现，往往是慢阻肺治疗过程中短时间大量激素和广谱抗生素治疗后出现；CCPA影像学与CNPA相似，但发展更为缓慢，可持续数月，即使手术切除后也易出现复发，若不进行治疗，随着时间的推移，这些空洞会逐渐变大、融合，会出现曲霉球，也可能原有的曲菌球消失，若此时仍不治疗曲霉菌病，肺部形成慢性瘢痕和肺纤维化范围扩大，CCPA最终出现纤维化，变为CFPA。④关于曲霉球：50%的曲霉感染病例患者肺部空洞中可出现典型的曲菌球，曲霉球常发生于既往空洞性疾病基础上，其中结核最为多见，陈旧性结核空洞并发曲霉球病程中可以一直保持不变，也可能随免疫抑制的发生导致曲霉菌的播散，导致重叠综合征。⑤关于曲霉感染治疗有效过程中的病灶增大：这在临床中并不罕见，免疫重建炎症综合征是可能的原因，但存在争议，需要在疾病监管过程中通过更多的临床表现、炎症指标、真菌特异性检测指标综合判定治疗的有效性，并坚定维持原方案继续治疗的决心。综上，了解慢阻肺合并IPA、CPA影像学在病程中的演变特点，动态的CT观察能够为我们细化监测病情变化提供更多有用的信息。

（三）监管慢阻肺合并IPA、CPA及重叠综合征病程中生物学标志物变化的重要性

介入活检操作在慢阻肺感染肺曲霉病患者中的难以实施，加上烟曲霉痰标本检出的假阳性（定植）和假阴性（漏检）问题，在慢阻肺合并IPA和CPA的真实临床中我们不得不一边反复痰培养，一边更多地关注其他实验室检测技术提供诊断帮助。目前应用临床的检测技术有半乳甘露聚糖（GM）试验、（1,3）-β-D葡聚糖（G试验）、PCR技术、免疫层析侧流装置（LFD）技术。血G试验无法区分种类，在非粒细胞缺乏患者灵敏性和特异性都很低，受干扰因素也很多，因此，目前对非粒细胞缺乏患者不推荐用于检测；血GM试验在粒细胞缺乏患者的诊断灵敏度和特异性均已得到临床证实，然而，在非粒细胞缺乏患者的诸多研究发现虽然特异性在80%以上，但是灵敏度均不足50%，且波动范围大，容易受到使用过哌拉西林三唑巴坦后的假阳性干扰（这个药物在慢阻肺急性加重期患者中使用频繁），因此，敏感性和特异性更高的BALF的GM试验被推荐为非粒细胞缺乏患者的首选，然而，其结果要求2次以上阳性（在慢阻肺患者，用药前的连续2次纤支镜检查获取标本在临床是很难实现的），且最佳折点依然没有公论；PCR技术是捕获曲霉菌的最灵敏的方式，但受干扰因素较多，受到真菌负荷的影响，血液标本在非粒细胞缺乏患者阳性率依然很低，目前关注最多的依然是BALF中PCR技术，灵敏性比血液最高，尤其是目前采用RT-PCR技术以后，能够更好地区分定植和感染。2016年的一项采用RT PCT法检测BAL液中曲霉菌的研究提示，qPCR的敏感性高达90%，特异性也高于BALF的GM试验，可以高达92.5%。但是目前尚无痰液中qPCR诊断价值的报道，这显然对慢阻肺罹患肺曲霉病的人群具有更重要的价值，有待进一步研究。LFD技术在不同的研究中存在争议，使用的标本也限于血液和BALF，并仅限于定性试验，在疾病监测中受限。不同于IPA，CPA的检测技术中曲霉特异性抗体具有很高的价值，被认为是CPA诊断最有效的方法，只要阳性（与疑似的临床和影像学表现相联系）就足以诊断CPA。虽然这些辅助检测技术用于诊断曲霉菌感染尚存在灵敏性及特异性不足、漏诊误诊、甚至折点不确定的争议，但是，如将这些检测指标应用于慢阻肺合并IPA、CPA及重叠综合征治疗病程中疾病活动度的监测，可能会更有意义。现有研究已经证实在CPA中，曲霉特异性抗体滴度在治疗后较治疗前明显降低，可以反映治疗的疗效。而血清GM检测在识别不同的CPA中也有一定价值，由于CNPA的半侵袭特性，GM检测抗原时可呈阳性，而极少在单纯曲霉肿或CFPA中出现阳性，CNPA患者GM的转阴也提示曲霉侵袭性的减弱或消失。所以，即使折点存在争议，同一患者前后检测指标的比较依然对疾病活动的判断，指导药物治疗的调整具有有益的提示意义。

（四）慢阻肺合并IPA、CPA及重叠综合征病程中治疗策略的更新

具体治疗方式、药物组合、给药途径和疗程的选择与患者的疾病特征密切相关。尽管目前主要依赖于一些队列研究的数据，少量随机对照研究的数据及部分病例报告的数据，而且这些研究多数还未区分CPA的各种临床亚型，造成证据相对欠缺，但根据患者临床表型、是否适合手术、高危因素的识别与控制等，仍然可以指引临床决策的过程。

1. 是否使用糖皮质激素　慢阻肺患者在稳定期使用吸入型糖皮质激素或者在慢阻肺急性加重期联合或单独使用全身糖皮质激素治疗非常常见，然而无论是吸入型糖皮质激素还是全身糖皮质激素均是 CPA 的主要危险因素，且显著增加疾病进展或播散的风险。在没有充分、有效的抗真菌治疗基础上，盲目采用糖皮质激素治疗会加速 CPA 的进展，因此只有在充分使用抗真菌药物的情况下，才可谨慎使用泼尼松龙 5～30 mg/d 或等效其他糖皮质激素的治疗，以进行症状控制。

2. 抗真菌治疗　目前认为口服三唑类抗真菌药对于进行性和(或)有症状的 CPA 提供治疗获益，且是 CCCP 的标准治疗方案。口服伊曲康唑可用于预防或治疗危及生命的咯血。口服伏立康唑对 CCPA 也是有效的，且耐受性良好，亦可被用于伊曲康唑治疗失败或不耐受后的替代治疗。一项回顾性队列研究则支持口服泊沙康唑，这是一种潜在的替代治疗方案。长期口服伊曲康唑可延缓患者发展为 CFPA，并延缓呼吸困难症状的进展。对长期呼吸困难的患者产生有益的影响。

对于 SAIA 的治疗更多可以参照 IPA 的治疗思路，在一些队列研究中长期口服伏立康唑能够取得获益，且在一项前瞻性多中心研究中，初步证实伏立康唑在 SAIA 患者中的疗效显著高于 CCPA 患者。

静脉给药治疗更多用于暴发进展的患者或是口服治疗失败的患者。此外，一些研究也证实，通过早期静脉给药控制感染，续贯口服维持治疗也是可选的治疗策略之一。两性霉素 B 和棘白菌素类抗真菌药是三唑类药物的可靠替代药物。在一个小样本双盲研究中，短期治疗 CPA（2～4 周），米卡芬净相对于伏立康唑安全性更好。CPA 患者接受两性霉素 B 脂质体静脉给药 17d 的研究发现 32% 患者出现肾衰竭，因此，两性霉素 B 静脉给药治疗 CPA 的风险过大，获益有限。

治疗周期的确定与患者个体的治疗应答和疾病临床表型密切相关。对于 CCPA，抗真菌治疗的应答缓慢，但大多数有反应的患者在 6 个月内展示出治疗应答，因此初始治疗建议持续 4～6 个月口服三唑类药物，如果在此期间病情恶化，应被视为治疗失败，应该采用替代方案。在 4～6 个月的初始治疗期中，如果治疗应答不理想，可以延长到 9 个月。对于所有治疗反应良好的患者，为了取得远期获益，尤其为避免或延缓进展到 CFPA 及咯血，建议长期维持治疗，因此这个治疗期事实上是不确定的。终止治疗以后的复发较为常见，需要警惕并适当监测。

综上所述，肺曲霉菌感染是慢阻肺患者漫长的疾病病程中需要被特别关注的感染类型，由于诊断困难，其发病率一直被低估，直接影响到慢阻肺患者出现更多更重的临床症状、更为迅速恶化的肺功能损害、甚至长期用药的调整(包括吸入激素、全身激素、抗生素治疗、预防性抗生素使用)。不同于粒细胞缺乏患者，又有别于免疫正常人群，高危因素的识别、不同类型肺曲霉菌病不同的临床表现和影像学演变、检测技术手段的局限性都给临床实操提出了挑战。由于免疫状态的变化和慢阻肺本病药物治疗的影响，我们必须转变思路，加强疾病的全程监管，寻找识别慢阻肺合并不同类型肺曲霉菌的不同高危因素，认识不同疾病阶段的临床表现差异，动态比较影像学变化规律，灵活应用现有争议的检测技术辅助评价疾病活动状态，正确选择不同疾病类型、严重程度肺曲霉菌病的药物及给药方式，进一步开展更多的临床研究为临床实践提供更多的证据，指导这一特殊群体肺曲霉感染的全程诊疗监管。

参 考 文 献

[1] HospenthalDR, K. J. Kwon-Chung, and J. E. Bennett, Concentrations of airborne Aspergillus compared to the incidence of invasive aspergillosis: lack of correlation. Med Mycol, 1998, 36(3): 165-168.

[2] Dagenais TR and NP Keller, Pathogenesis of Aspergillus fumigatus in Invasive Aspergillosis. Clin Microbiol Rev, 2009, 22(3): 447-465.

[3] Patterson TF, et al. Practice Guidelines for the Diagnosis and Management of Aspergillosis: 2016 Update by the Infectious Diseases Society of America. Clin Infect Dis, 2016, 63(4): e1-e60.

[4] Baddley JW. Clinical risk factors for invasive aspergillosis. Med Mycol, 2011, 49 Suppl 1: S7-S12.

[5] Saraceno JL, et al. Chronic necrotizing pulmonary aspergillosis: approach to management. Chest, 1997, 112(2): 541-548.

[6] Lowes D, et al. Predictors of mortality in chronic pulmonary aspergillosis. Eur Respir J, 2017, 49(2).

[7] Kosmidis C, DW Denning. The clinical spectrum of pulmonary aspergillosis. Thorax, 2015, 70(3): 270-277.

[8] From the Global Strategy for the Diagnosis, Management and Prevention of COPD, Global Initiative for Chronic Obstructive Lung Disease (GOLD). 2020; Available from: http://www.goldcopd.org/.

[9] Balloy V, et al. Differences in patterns of infection and inflammation for corticosteroid treatment and chemotherapy in experimental invasive pulmonary aspergillosis. Infect Immun, 2005, 73(1): 494-503.

[10] Ullmann AJ, et al. Diagnosis and management of Aspergillus diseases: executive summary of the 2017 ESCMID-ECMM-ERS guideline. Clin Microbiol Infect, 2018, 24 Suppl 1: e1-e38.

[11] Denning DW, et al. Chronic pulmonary aspergillosis: rationale and clinical guidelines for diagnosis and management. Eur Respir J, 2016, 47(1): 45-68.

[12] Jenks JD, H. J. F. Salzer, and M. Hoenigl, Improving the rates of Aspergillus detection: an update on current diagnostic strategies. Expert Rev Anti Infect Ther, 2019, 17(1): 39-50.

[13] Guo Y, et al. Evaluation of Aspergillus IgG, IgM antibody for diagnosing in chronic pulmonary aspergillosis. Medicine, 2019, 98(16): e15021.

[14] Yoshimura K, et al. Utility of serum Aspergillus-galactomannan antigen to evaluate the risk of severe acute exacerbation

in chronic obstructive pulmonary disease. PLoS One, 2018, 13(6):e0198479.
[15] Yao Y, et al. Evaluation of a quantitative serum Aspergillus fumigatus-specific IgM assay for diagnosis of chronic pulmonary aspergillosis. The Clinical Respiratory Journal, 2018, 12(11):2566-2572.
[16] Bhimji A, et al. Aspergillus galactomannan detection in exhaled breath condensate compared to bronchoalveolar lavage fluid for the diagnosis of invasive aspergillosis in immunocompromised patients. Clin Microbiol Infect, 2018, 24(6):640-645.
[17] Lahmer T, et al. Comparison of 1,3-beta-d-glucan with galactomannan in serum and bronchoalveolar fluid for the detection of Aspergillus species in immunosuppressed mechanical ventilated critically ill patients. J Crit Care, 2016, 36:259-264.
[18] Dandachi D, et al. Invasive pulmonary aspergillosis in patients with solid tumours: risk factors and predictors of clinical outcomes. Ann Med, 2018, 50(8):713-720.
[19] Guinea J, et al. Pulmonary aspergillosis in patients with chronic obstructive pulmonary disease: incidence, risk factors, and outcome. Clin Microbiol Infect, 2010, 16(7):870-877.
[20] Garnacho-Montero J, et al. Isolation of Aspergillus spp. from the respiratory tract in critically ill patients: risk factors, clinical presentation and outcome. Crit Care, 2005, 9(3):191-199.
[21] Poh TY, et al. Evaluation of Droplet Digital Polymerase Chain Reaction (ddPCR) for the Absolute Quantification of Aspergillus species in the Human Airway. Int J Mol Sci, 2020, 21(9).
[22] 王琴, 等. PCR检测痰曲霉菌在慢性阻塞性肺疾病合并侵袭性肺曲霉菌病中的诊断价值. 中国临床医学. 2019, 26(2):238-241.
[23] Aquino VR, et al. The Performance of Real-Time PCR, Galactomannan, and Fungal Culture in the Diagnosis of Invasive Aspergillosis in Ventilated Patients with Chronic Obstructive Pulmonary Disease(COPD). Mycopathologia, 2012, 174(2):163-169.
[24] Heldt S, et al. Diagnosis of invasive aspergillosis in hematological malignancy patients: Performance of cytokines, Asp LFD, and Aspergillus PCR in same day blood and bronchoalveolar lavage samples. J Infect, 2018, 77(3):235-241.
[25] Prattes J, et al. Novel tests for diagnosis of invasive aspergillosis in patients with underlying respiratory diseases. Am J Respir Crit Care Med, 2014. 190(8):922-929.
[26] Buchheidt D, et al. Biomarker-based diagnostic work-up of invasive pulmonary aspergillosis in immunocompromised paediatric patients--is Aspergillus PCR appropriate? Mycoses, 2016, 59(2):67-74.
[27] Barberan J, FJ Candel, A. Arribi. How should we approach Aspergillus in lung secretions of patients with COPD? Rev Esp Quimioter, 2016, 29(4):175-182.
[28] Zhang S, et al. Quantitative Real-Time PCR and Platelia Galactomannan Assay for the Diagnosis of Invasive Pulmonary Aspergillosis: Bronchoalveolar Lavage Fluid Performs Better Than Serum in Non-neutropaenic Patients. Mycopathologia, 2016, 181(9-10):625-629.
[29] Rafferty P, et al. What happens to patients with pulmonary aspergilloma? Analysis of 23 cases. Thorax, 1983, 38(8):579-583.
[30] Hafeez I, et al. Non-tuberculous mycobacterial lung infection complicated by chronic necrotising pulmonary aspergillosis. Thorax, 2000, 55(8):717-719.
[31] Agarwal R, et al. Itraconazole in chronic cavitary pulmonary aspergillosis: a randomised controlled trial and systematic review of literature. Mycoses, 2013. 56(5):559-570.
[32] Dupont B, Itraconazole therapy in aspergillosis: study in 49 patients. J Am Acad Dermatol, 1990, 23(3 Pt 2):607-614.
[33] Jain LR, DW Denning. The efficacy and tolerability of voriconazole in the treatment of chronic cavitary pulmonary aspergillosis. J Infect, 2006, 52(5):133-137.
[34] Felton, TW, et al. Efficacy and safety of posaconazole for chronic pulmonary aspergillosis. Clin Infect Dis, 2010, 51(12):1383-1391.
[35] Denning DW, et al. Chronic cavitary and fibrosing pulmonary and pleural aspergillosis: case series, proposed nomenclature change, and review. Clin Infect Dis, 2003, 37 Suppl 3:265-280.
[36] Cadranel J, et al. Voriconazole for chronic pulmonary aspergillosis: a prospective multicenter trial. Eur J Clin Microbiol Infect Dis, 2012, 31(11):3231-3239.
[37] Sambatakou H, et al. Voriconazole treatment for subacute invasive and chronic pulmonary aspergillosis. Am J Med, 2006, 119(6):527 e17-e24.
[38] Kohno S, et al. Intravenous micafungin versus voriconazole for chronic pulmonary aspergillosis: a multicenter trial in Japan. J Infect, 2010, 61(5):410-418.
[39] Newton PJ, et al. Impact of liposomal amphotericin B therapy on chronic pulmonary aspergillosis. J Infect, 2016, 73(5):485-495.

16 免疫治疗在慢性阻塞性肺疾病合并肺癌治疗中的进展

周 敏

近年来,免疫治疗在非小细胞肺癌的一线及二线治疗领域取得了突破性的进展,甚至正在逐渐成为包括小细胞肺癌、间皮瘤等其他肺部恶性肿瘤的治疗新选择。同时,50%以上的肺癌患者同时合并存在慢性阻塞性肺疾病(chronic obstructive pulmonary disease,COPD)等慢性肺部疾病,这一群体早期确诊难度较大,因肺功能受损对手术耐受程度低,对放、化疗等传统治疗手段效果欠佳,且更易并发感染、急性肺损伤等相关合并症。然而,近期临床研究显示,合并 COPD 的肺癌患者接受免疫治疗效果显著,是此类患者抗肿瘤治疗的有效策略之一。本文主要从免疫治疗在 COPD 合并肺癌治疗中的进展、优势及不良反应相关处理与预防等角度进行分析和探讨。

一、免疫检查点抑制剂治疗肺癌的作用机制

肿瘤的免疫治疗旨在激活人体免疫系统,依靠自身免疫功能杀灭癌细胞和肿瘤组织,近年来这种治疗方式在肺癌领域已广泛应用,并成效显著。免疫治疗有多种分类方法,各类之间又有交叉:根据对机体免疫功能的影响,可分为免疫增强疗法和免疫抑制疗法;根据治疗的特异性,可分为特异性免疫治疗和非特异性免疫治疗;根据免疫制剂的作用特点,可分为主动免疫治疗和被动免疫治疗。

免疫检查点抑制剂(immune checkpoint inhibitor,ICIs)是阻断免疫细胞上免疫检查点的一类单抗类药物,而免疫检查点抑制剂疗法(checkpoint inhibitor therapy,CIT)是针对免疫检查点的免疫调节器,当免疫系统受到刺激时,可降低免疫系统对免疫刺激的反应,阻止肿瘤逃逸的发生。其中,程序性死亡受体 1(programmed death 1,PD-1)通路抑制剂是目前肺癌治疗常用的一种免疫疗法。

PD-1 受体是一种在 T 细胞与初级 B 细胞表面表达,并在细胞分化与凋亡过程中发挥作用的受体。PD-L1、PD-L2 是它的 2 个配体,前者可广泛表达于活化 T 细胞、B 细胞与巨噬细胞,参与免疫负向调控;后者可能具有维持正常组织免疫稳态的潜在作用。正常情况下,当机体受到外来抗原或病原体侵犯时,抗原提呈细胞(antigen-presenting cells,APC)可捕获抗原并对其进一步加工为可识别的抗原表位,与主要组织相容性复合体(major histocompatibility complex,MHC)结合并呈现于细胞外侧,供 T 细胞识别。同时,表达于 T 细胞表面的 CD28 受体与 APC 上的 B7.1(CD80)或 B7.2(CD86)结合,产生协同刺激信号,对 T 细胞进行正向调控,促使其活化为效应 T 细胞,启动免疫应答。当机体遭受持续抗原刺激时,为避免过度应答造成的组织损伤,活化 T 细胞表面可持续表达 PD-1,与 APC 细胞表面的 PD-L1 结合,导致 T 细胞增生抑制甚至凋亡,以及 IL-2、IFN-γ 和 IL-10 的产生,对机体免疫应答起负性调节作用。

PD-1/PD-L1 通路可在两种不同水平下调抗肿瘤免疫应答。一方面,PD-L1 表达可阻断淋巴结中 T 细胞的启动与活化,通过正常免疫环境中的负向调控,削弱机体免疫能力;另一方面,肿瘤微环境可诱导肿瘤细胞表面的 PD-L1 表达,通过与 CD8$^+$ T 细胞表面的 PD-1 受体结合,抑制 T 细胞的活化,诱导抗肿瘤 T 细胞凋亡,通过对 T 细胞的负向调控辅助肿瘤细胞实现免疫逃逸。在这种情况下,PD-1/PD-L1 通路抑制剂,即 PD-1 或 PD-L1 抗体,可通过直接选择性作用于相应靶点,阻断二者结合,阻断负向调控信号,增强 T 细胞的免疫应答;另外,由于 PD-1/PD-L1 通路受到抑制,CD28 与 B7.1 结合的共刺激作用相对强化,可进一步增强淋巴结中 T 细胞启动和活化,从而对抗肿瘤进展。两种免疫抑制剂作用靶点效果相似,其中抗 PD-1 抑制剂由于同时阻断了 PD-1 与 PD-L2 的交互作用,可能存在增加自身免疫反应的潜在风险,具体差异仍待进一步研究。

目前肺癌常见的 PD-1/PD-L1 通路抑制剂包括以 PD-1 为靶点的纳武单抗(nivolumab)和帕博利珠单抗(pembrolizumab),以及以 PD-L1 为靶点的阿特珠单抗(atezolizumab)、度伐利尤单抗(durvalumab)等。此外,以细胞毒 T 淋巴细胞相关抗原 4(cytotoxic T lymphocyte-associated antigen-4,CTLA-4)为靶点的免疫治疗如易普利姆玛(ipilimumab)已被临床应用于肺癌患者治疗。

二、免疫治疗在 COPD 合并肺癌疗效中的影响因素

慢性阻塞性肺疾病和肺癌均为全球性高发病率、高病死率疾病,严重增加社会经济负担。既往研究表明,40%~70%的肺癌患者合并 COPD,尤其是非小细胞肺癌患者。烟雾暴露、遗传易感性和慢性炎症等是二者发病的共同易感因素。针对慢性肺部疾病与肺癌发病关系的多篇 Meta 分析研究提示,COPD 可能是肺癌发病的危险因

素之一。异常炎症免疫反应在两种疾病的发生、发展中均有作用,在免疫应答过程中逐渐产生有利于血管生成和免疫抑制的肿瘤微环境(tumor microenvironment,TME),最终使肿瘤细胞发生免疫逃逸,导致肿瘤形成;此外,COPD与肺癌发病存在共同的基因异常有关,如p53、MMP-1、CYP1A1等。

非小细胞肺癌(non-small cell lung cancer,NSCLC)合并COPD患者具有特殊的临床特点,除患病率较高外,该人群具有复杂的免疫微环境,慢性炎症反应与肿瘤免疫混杂。既往认为COPD合并NSCLC是接受传统治疗预后较差的危险因素之一,因此,这类患者是免疫治疗的潜在获益人群。对一组NSCLC患者接受PD-1/PD-L1免疫抑制剂后的治疗效果的临床研究回顾显示:合并COPD组患者有更多OS及PFS获益。另一项针对东亚人群NSCLC合并COPD的研究结果也表明合并COPD组患者接受帕博利珠单抗单药治疗后OS及PFS较单纯NSCLC组显著延长,进一步证实了免疫治疗的作用。多项研究表明,免疫治疗为合并COPD的肺癌患者带来更多治疗选择,而影响治疗效果的相关因素及COPD和肺癌的共同免疫机制成为目前的重点研究方向。

(一)吸烟对免疫治疗疗效的影响

肺癌合并COPD患者的吸烟状态与疾病发生及预后均密切相关。

从免疫环境角度,长期吸烟会对机体T细胞水平产生显著影响。既往临床血清学分析及动物模型结果均显示,吸烟会促进$CD4^+$ T细胞向Th17的分化过程,Th17表达水平与吸烟指数呈正相关,戒烟后其水平可逐渐下降,而Th17分化过程与COPD并无显著关联。这一结果提示吸烟状态可通过改变T细胞水平对机体产生影响,成为COPD患者罹患肺癌后治疗及预后的独立危险因素之一。

吸烟对COPD合并肺癌肿瘤突变负荷(tumor mutation burden,TMB)存在影响。尽管免疫组化技术可以检测肿瘤细胞PD-L1的表达水平,作为生物标志物之一来预测免疫治疗的反应,但多种因素如肿瘤组织的异质性、抗体种类、染色方法等均可能影响结果判定。作为一个新的潜在生物标志物,TMB指的是肿瘤细胞基因组中所评估基因编码区发生体细胞突变的总数,TMB越高,免疫治疗疗效愈佳。研究发现,非小细胞肺癌患者中有吸烟史者TMB较非吸烟患者明显升高,说明烟草暴露可导致高负荷肿瘤基因突变。

在PD-L1高表达患者中,吸烟状态与肿瘤预后存在相关性。研究纳入了283名接受免疫抑制剂治疗且PD-L1高表达(TPS≥50%)的NSCLC患者,通过对重度吸烟者(>10包/年)与其余患者的对比研究发现,在PD-L1表达状态基线均衡的情况下,重度吸烟组患者的TMB水平更高,其接受免疫治疗后的缓解持续时间(duration of overall response,DoR)也相对更长。其他研究也表明有吸烟史的患者接受免疫治疗往往疗效更佳,这一关联或许与长期烟草暴露下突变负荷的升高相关。此外,Checkmate003研究分析了89例吸烟史及肿瘤组织学资料完整的患者,评估应用纳武单抗治疗后,患者吸烟史与肿瘤客观缓解率(ob-jective response rate,ORR)之间的相关性,结果显示有长期吸烟史者ORR更高,>5包/年组的ORR率明显高于≤5包/年组,且PFS显著延长(2.2个月 vs. 1.7个月)。对于接受免疫治疗的肿瘤患者而言,烟草暴露程度是重要的影响因素之一,具体相关机制尚待研究。

吸烟状态对免疫治疗疗效存在影响。有吸烟相关慢性肺部疾病史的患者,无论PD-L1表达水平如何,都呈现出更高的肿瘤突变负荷,是PD-1/PD-L1免疫抑制剂治疗的靶向人群。既往临床研究也证实了这一免疫治疗的效果,有长期吸烟史者治疗后ORR、PFS及DoR都有更长的趋势,疗效更佳。

(二)COPD免疫微环境对免疫治疗疗效的影响

近年来,关于COPD和NSCLC潜在免疫微环境的研究取得了新的成果。以往认为这些疾病仅由固有免疫及相关炎症因子蛋白所驱动,随着相关研究进展,获得性免疫在其中的作用得到重视。研究表明,对于小气道狭窄或合并肺气肿的COPD患者而言,$CD4^+$ T细胞及Th1极化程度明显升高,同时其体内可产生IFN-γ的$CD8^+$ T细胞水平显著增加,对细胞毒性T细胞介导的细胞免疫存在促进作用,同时AECOPD可上调溶酶体相关膜蛋白1(CD107a)水平,是目前公认的细胞毒性T细胞脱颗粒的标志。此外,COPD等慢性肺部疾病可对肺癌患者体内的巨噬细胞水平产生影响。在肿瘤微环境中,巨噬细胞可极化为1型(M1)与2型(M2)两种亚型,通过调节细胞黏附、凋亡和衰老等功能在肿瘤发生中发挥相关作用,M1巨噬细胞主要出现于肿瘤发生的初始过程中,而肿瘤组织中的巨噬细胞主要为M2型。研究发现,COPD合并肺癌患者的M1/M2水平高于单纯肺癌组,这可能与肿瘤患者预后存在相关性,需要进一步研究证实。COPD免疫环境对PD-1/PD-L1通路也有一定影响。研究显示,COPD患者体内的$CD8^+$ T细胞表达PD-1受体的水平高于普通对照人群,而对于由流感病毒感染引发的AECOPD患者,其PD-1水平可进一步升高。

COPD患者体内免疫微环境的改变,同时也作用于免疫治疗的效果。COPD严重程度与T细胞表达水平相关,$CD8^+$ T细胞的升高可增强NSCLC对PD-1抑制剂治疗的敏感性,而Th1细胞的进一步极化会加强NSCLC对免疫治疗的反应,通过分泌IFN-γ介导巨噬细胞的激活,并通过产生IL-2介导$CD8^+$ T细胞增生,介导B细胞向免疫球蛋白分化,从而增强机体对肿瘤细胞的清除作用。

三、免疫治疗在COPD合并肺癌的不良反应及处理

与传统化疗相比,免疫治疗是一种相对更加高效且低毒性的治疗选择,但也会导致一系列不良反应。免疫相关不良反应(irAEs)可见于全身各个组织和器官,根据临床出现频率,irAEs主要分为常见毒性和罕见毒性。常见毒性包括皮肤、胃肠、内分泌、呼吸和肌肉骨骼等器官;罕见毒性包括心血管、血液、肾、神经和眼。不同免疫抑制剂治疗的不良反应亦存在一定差异,如阻断PD-1通路的不良

反应多为器官特异性自身免疫性疾病,而阻断 CTLA-4 的不良反应通常为多系统多器官自身免疫性疾病。此外,既往关于应用于 NSCLC 患者抗 PD-1 与抗 CTLQ-4 联合免疫治疗的研究显示,相对于单药免疫治疗,联合治疗发生 3 级以上 irAEs 的风险明显升高,因此在免疫治疗的选择上,应充分平衡其有效性与毒性,谨慎制订方案。

大多数 irAEs 具有可逆性,但也存在某些 irAEs 易累及多脏器,甚至威胁生命。PD-1/PD-L1 通路免疫抑制剂治疗临床常见的不良反应主要包括疲劳、皮疹、肝毒性、内分泌紊乱、腹泻或结肠炎等,少数患者可出现肺炎、急性肾功能不全、心肌炎、三系下降等毒性症状。NCCN 指南根据毒性程度可将 irAEs 分为 1 级至 5 级,根据等级情况决定处理方案。

免疫检查点抑制剂相关性肺炎(checkpoint inhibitor-related pneumonitis,CIP)是最常见的严重致死性 irAE,占 ICIs 相关死亡原因的 35%,具体发生机制目前尚不明确。根据一项回顾性临床研究分析,不同肺癌类型发生 CIP 的可能性存在差异,相对腺癌而言,鳞癌及其他类型肺癌发生 CIP 的风险更高。另外,有 Meta 分析显示,接受 PD-L1 抑制剂的患者,其严重 CIP 发生率低于 PD-1 治疗(1.3% vs. 3.6%,$P=0.001$)。目前暂不清楚不同的 PD-1 配体在肺炎中的作用,一种假说认为 PD-L1 抑制剂不影响 PD-1 与 PD-L2 的相互作用,可介导免疫耐受。一小鼠模型试验也佐证了这一假说:抑制 PD-1 受体可能会改变 PD-L2 与其他结合配体间相互作用的平衡,增加 PD-L2 与排斥性引导分子 b 结合的可能性,从而导致 CIP 发生。尽管有研究认为,腺癌患者或使用抗 PD-L1 治疗发生 CIP 的风险较低,但这些结论缺乏充分的循证依据。

在接受免疫治疗的肺癌患者中,吸烟和罹患 COPD 可增加发生免疫相关肺炎的风险。尽管免疫相关性肺炎发生率不高,第 5 级肺炎发生率仅为 0.1%,但因其严重性与致死性,临床应重点关注患者是否存在相关危险因素,并对高危人群加强随访。目前针对发生免疫相关性肺炎的危险因素已开展相关研究,KEYNOTE-001 研究对比了使用帕博利珠单抗治疗的肺癌人群,发现曾有胸部放疗史的患者较无胸部放疗史者更易出现治疗相关肺损伤(13% vs. 1%),其他潜在的危险因素包括基础肺部疾病、肺部感染、吸烟等。

除关注危险因素外,免疫治疗安全性管理需要明确并遵守常规处理流程及原则,在临床过程中应做好预防、评估、检测、治疗和监测五大支柱。IrAEs 的早期预防至关重要,对于临床工作者而言,应充分知悉免疫不良反应毒性谱,早期识别免疫相关危险因素并告知患者,治疗期间规范随访评估;一旦发生免疫不良反应,则应及时处理、密切监测,根据情况及时停止免疫治疗,预防其进一步发展成为严重的不良反应。

呼吸科在 irAE 管理中,尤其是免疫治疗过程中出现免疫相关性肺炎时存在优势:①早期发现,对相关呼吸道症状如咳嗽、呼吸困难、胸痛等敏感,能及时发现患者异常。②早期诊断,擅长肺部影像学解读,需要时可及时采取支气管镜等介入手段完善检查。③明确诊断,呼吸科对于肺部感染、间质性肺炎等拥有更丰富的诊治经验,能及时明确鉴别是否为 CIP。④及时处理,呼吸与危重症学科对于重症患者的治疗及激素使用经验丰富,临床判断更为准确及时。

四、小 结

免疫治疗对于合并 COPD 的肺癌患者而言无疑是新的机遇,但治疗道路仍存在诸多挑战。给药时机、是否联合用药、特异性预测标志物及性价比等问题也待进一步探索。未来需结合 COPD 合并肺癌人群的特点,验证这一群体作为免疫治疗优势人群的可行性,同时在发病机制、生物标志物探索及临床治疗策略等领域开展深层次研究。

参 考 文 献

[1] Pardoll DM. The blockade of immune checkpoints in cancer immunotherapy. Nat Rev Cancer,2012,12(4):252-264.

[2] Chen DS,Irving BA,Hodi FS. Molecular pathways:next-generation immunotherapy—inhibiting programmed death-ligand 1 and programmed death-1. Clin Cancer Res,2012,18(24):6580-6587.

[3] O'Donnell JS,Smyth MJ,Teng MWL. PD1 functions by inhibiting CD28-mediated co-stimulation. Clin Transl Immunol,2017,6(5):e138.

[4] Merelli B,Massi D,Cattaneo L,et al. Targeting the PD1/PD-L1 axis in melanoma:biological rationale,clinical challenges and opportunities. Crit Rev Oncol Hematol,2014,89(1):140-165.

[5] Rozali EN,Hato SV,Robinson BW,et al. Programmed death ligand 2 in cancer-induced immune suppression. Clin Dev Immunol,2012,2012:656340.

[6] Proto C,Ferrara R,Signorelli D,et al. Choosing wisely first line immunotherapy in non-small cell lung cancer(NSCLC):what to add and what to leave out. Cancer Treat Rev,2019,75:39-51.

[7] Calles A,Aguado G,Sandoval C,et al. The role of immunotherapy in small cell lung cancer. Clin Transl Oncol,2019,21(8):961-976.

[8] Young RP,Hopkins RJ,Christmas T,et al. COPD prevalence is increased in lung cancer,independent of age,sex and smoking history. Eur Respir J,2009,34(2):380-386.

[9] Brenner DR,McLaughlin JR,Hung RJ. Previous lung diseases and lung cancer risk:a systematic review and meta-analysis. PLoS One,2011,6(3):e17479.

[10] Wang H,Yang L,Zou L,et al. Association between chronic obstructive pulmonary disease and lung cancer:a case-control study in Southern Chinese and a meta-analysis. PLoS One,

2012,7(9):e46144.
[11] Adcock IM, Caramori G, Barnes PJ. Chronic obstructive pulmonary disease and lung cancer: new molecular insights. Respiration, 2011, 81(4): 265-284.
[12] Houghton AM. Mechanistic links between COPD and lung cancer. Nat Rev Cancer, 2013, 13(4): 233-245.
[13] Mark NM, Kargl J, Busch SE, et al. Chronic obstructive pulmonary disease alters immune cell composition and immune checkpoint inhibitor efficacy in non-small cell lung cancer. Am J Respir Crit Care Med, 2018, 197(3): 325-336.
[14] Shin SH, Park HY, Im Y, et al. Improved treatment outcome of pembrolizumab in patients with nonsmall cell lung cancer and chronic obstructive pulmonary disease. Int J Cancer, 2019, 145(9): 2433-2439.
[15] Gibbons DL, Byers LA, Kurie JM. Smoking, p53 mutation, and lung cancer. Mol Cancer Res, 2014, 12(1): 3-13.
[16] Justin F, et al. Response and durability of checkpoint blockade in never-or light-smokers with NSCLC and high PD-L1 expression, 2018.
[17] Reck M, Rodriguez-Abreu D, Robinson AG, et al. Pembrolizumab versus chemotherapy for PD-L1-positive non-small-cell lung cancer. N Engl J Med, 2016, 375(19): 1823-1833.
[18] Freeman CM, Han MK, Martinez FJ, et al. Cytotoxic potential of lung CD8(+)T cells increases with chronic obstructive pulmonary disease severity and with in vitro stimulation by IL-18 or IL-15. J Immunol, 2010, 184: 6504-6513.
[19] Hogg JC, Chu F, Utokaparch S, et al. The nature of small-airway obstruction in chronic obstructive pulmonary disease. N Engl J Med, 2004, 350: 2645-2653.
[20] Grumelli S, Corry DB, Song LZ, et al. An immune basis for lung parenchymal destruction in chronic obstructive pulmonary disease and emphysema. PLoS Med, 2004, 1: e8.
[21] Mateu-Jimenez M, Curull V, Pijuan L, et al. Systemic and tumor Th1 and Th2 inflammatory profile and macrophages in lung cancer: influence of underlying chronic respiratory disease. J Thorac Oncol, 2017, 12(2): 235-248.
[22] McKendry RT, Spalluto CM, Burke H, et al. Dysregulation of antiviral function of CD8(+)T cells in the chronic obstructive pulmonary disease lung. Role of the PD-1-PD-L1 axis. Am J Respir Crit Care Med, 2016, 193(6): 642-651.
[23] Hellmann MD, Rizvi NA, Goldman JW, et al. Nivolumab plus ipilimumab as first-line treatment for advanced nonsmall-cell lung cancer (CheckMate 012): results of an open-label, phase 1, multicohort study. Lancet Oncol, 2017, 18: 31-41.
[24] NCCN Guidelines Version 1. 2018. Management of Immunotherapy-Related Toxicities (Immune Checkpoint Inhibitor-Related Toxicities).
[25] Wang DY, Salem JE, Cohen JV, et al. Fatal toxic effects associated with immune checkpoint inhibitors: A systematic review and meta-analysis. JAMA Oncol, 2018, 4(12): 1721-1728.
[26] Suresh K, Voong KR, Shankar B, et al. Pneumonitis in non-small cell lung cancer patients receiving immune checkpoint immunotherapy: incidence and risk factors. J Thorac Oncol, 2018, 13(12): 1930-1939.
[27] Khunger M, Rakshit S, Pasupuleti V, et al. Incidence of pneumonitis with use of programmed death 1 and programmed death-ligand 1 inhibitors in non-small cell lung cancer: a systematic review and Meta-analysis of trials. Chest, 2017, 152(2): 271-281.
[28] Xiao Y, Yu S, Zhu B, et al. RGMb is a novel binding partner for PD-L2 and its engagement with PD-L2 promotes respiratory tolerance. J Exp Med, 2014, 211: 943-959.
[29] Shaverdian N, Lisberg AE, Bornazyan K, et al. Previous radiotherapy and the clinical activity and toxicity of pembrolizumab in the treatment of non-small-cell lung cancer: a secondary analysis of the KEYNOTE-001 phase 1 trial. Lancet Oncol, 2017, 18(7): 895-903.
[30] Remon J, Mezquita L, Corral J, et al. Immune-related adverse events with immune checkpoint inhibitors in thoracic malignancies: focusing on non-small cell lung cancer patients. J Thorac Dis, 2018, 10(Suppl 13): S1516-S1533.

17 低风险慢性阻塞性肺疾病的早期干预

赵丽敏　唐学义

慢性阻塞性肺疾病（简称慢阻肺）是一种以持续气流受限和慢性呼吸系统症状为特征的慢性呼吸道疾病，具有高发病率、高致残率和高病死率等特点。全球疾病负担显示，2016年中国死于慢阻肺的患者达87万之多，占中国总死亡人数的9%，成为中国部分地区的第三大死亡原因，这也使慢阻肺成为中国的重大疾病负担之一。2018年《柳叶刀》报道了中国40岁以上人群中慢阻肺患病率为13.7%，60岁以上超过27%，远高于2007年的8.2%。随着吸烟人数的增多及人口老龄化的加剧，慢阻肺发病率可能再创新高，因此，明确慢阻肺的诊断标准并给予及时有效的治疗措施至关重要。目前我们对慢阻肺，尤其是对早期低风险无症状慢阻肺的认识、诊断和治疗仍存在很大不足。2011年版的慢阻肺全球策略对慢阻肺的综合评估，将FEV_1%占预计值的百分比（FEV_1%pred）的50%作为高风险和低风险的界值，并以前一年住院次数≥1次作为急性加重高、低风险的分层标准，即上一年急性加重≥1次或FEV_1%pred<50%的患者急性加重的风险增加。处于早期慢阻肺的人群FEV_1%pred≥50%，一般处于低风险状态。中国关于早期慢阻肺的研究多取GOLD Ⅰ~Ⅱ级慢阻肺患者，GOLD Ⅰ~Ⅱ级慢阻肺肺功能损害较轻，一般为低风险慢阻肺。低风险慢阻肺病情一般较为稳定，病程较短，多为早期慢阻肺，因此早期慢阻肺与低风险慢阻肺很大程度上是相互重叠的。人群流行病学研究发现，在中国，70%的GOLD Ⅰ~Ⅱ级慢阻肺患者无明显的活动受限或者呼吸困难、慢性咳嗽咳痰等症状，由于缺乏临床症状，加之患者一般为中老年患者，病情容易被误认为是机体衰老、吸烟所致，导致低就诊率、低诊断率。早期慢阻肺占比较大，症状少，漏诊率高，同时肺功能下降比中晚期慢阻肺更为迅猛，一旦发展至出现呼吸困难症状，患者大都被确诊为慢阻肺中晚期，此时大部分患者的肺功能严重受损，降低了30%~50%，甚至更多。一旦发展为重度功能障碍，病情往往不可逆转，气流受限严重影响患者的活动耐量和生活质量，预后不佳。由于慢阻肺早期肺功能下降速度较快，因此需要早期干预，减缓肺功能的下降。越早干预慢阻肺的疾病进展，肺功能可恢复的程度越大；慢阻肺越早干预，获益越大。研究表明，肺功能正常的吸烟者与GOLD Ⅰ级慢阻肺患者的异常气道结构及支气管内光学相干断层扫描（EB-OCT）结果相似，表明早期慢阻肺可能仅显示气道结构异常，而无临床症状，甚至肺功能也正常。因此，钟南山院士推荐，对长期暴露在危险因素的人群，即使无症状，也应及早筛查，尽早干预，以有效防止低风险慢阻肺急性加重，延缓病情发展，甚至逆转肺部结构和功能的病理改变。

慢阻肺的早防早治关键在于早期诊断。2020年GOLD指南建议凡有呼吸困难、慢性咳嗽、咳痰症状和（或）有慢阻肺危险因素接触史者，均应该考虑慢阻肺的诊断，肺功能检查是确诊慢阻肺的必备条件。吸入支气管扩张剂后FEV_1/FVC<70%可确诊存在气流受限。研究表明，FEV_1下降速率可以作为COPD高危人群患病率的一个可靠指标。另外，肺功能受损程度与慢阻肺严重程度呈正相关，肺功能分级在慢阻肺急性加重、病死率等远期风险评估中具有重要地位。作为人口大国，基层医疗机构仍然是中国慢阻肺初筛的重要基地，但基层医院对肺功能尚未普查、基层医生对慢阻肺诊断标准认识不足、健康宣教不到位等导致基层医疗机构对早期慢阻肺的漏诊率较高，因此建立基层慢阻肺防控体系是慢阻肺早筛早诊的关键。这需要对基层医生进行规范化配训，培养其对慢阻肺的全面认识，大力推广肺功能检查规范化建设。另外，积极开展对慢阻肺患者的筛查：对出现慢性呼吸道症状的患者进行详细问诊，肺功能检查仍然是诊断慢阻肺的金标准，必要时给予肺功能等相关检查；对于长期吸烟、生活在工业区的高危因素暴露者给予肺功能检查；结合病史，可疑慢阻肺患者填写慢性阻塞性肺疾病筛查问卷，这对缺乏肺功能仪的基层医院有很大帮助；近期流行病学调查显示，40~50岁的慢阻肺人群中女性患者占比较大，40岁以上女性患病率高达7.5%，女性气道更为敏感，室内被动吸烟及生物燃料的使用是女性罹患慢阻肺的重要危险因素，因此要重视女性慢阻肺的早期诊断。随着烟民年轻化态势，慢阻肺发病年龄正在逐步提前，我国20岁以上慢阻肺发病率高达8.6%。来自上海的一项研究表明，FEV_1/FVC<70%或FEV_1/FVC%pred<80%作为年轻人群阻塞性通气功能障碍和慢阻肺的诊断标准，漏诊率较高，而FEV_1/FVC%pred<95%可考虑作为年轻人早期通气功能障碍和慢阻肺的诊断标准，可有效预防慢阻肺在年轻人群中诊断的不足，在早期慢阻肺的年轻患者中值得推广。刘亚男等发现，当呼气峰流速（PEF）占预计值的百分比PEF%pred=95%时，PEF对GOLD Ⅰ级、症状轻、慢阻肺综合评估A级的早期低风险慢阻肺筛查灵敏性较低；当PEF%pred=80%时，峰流速筛查对早期慢阻肺的敏感性大幅度提高；PEF仪相对便宜，操作方便，又能反映气道通

畅性,因此是早期慢阻肺筛查的良好方法。

慢阻肺最主要的危险因素是吸烟,吸烟损害气道黏膜纤毛系统,激发气道炎症反应,严重损害了肺组织的结构和功能。范木英等的研究表明,吸烟量大、烟龄长的慢阻肺患者的大小气道功能都会受到不同程度的影响,且吸烟更加明显地降低了反映小气道指标的 MEF 和反映气道阻塞的 $FEV_1\%/Vcmax$,表明吸烟对慢阻肺小气道功能的影响更大。研究表明,戒烟是轻度慢阻肺患者的重要治疗选择,尤其是在联合支气管扩张药治疗时效果更佳。戒烟组慢阻肺患者的各项肺功能参数显著增高,戒烟 3 个月后的患者,FEV_1 较未戒烟组升高超过 200 ml,同时 FEF 25%~75%和慢阻肺评估测试评分等均有显著改善,表明戒烟在功能改变和症状缓解方面有很大益处。有研究表明肺功能正常的重度吸烟者存在气道壁增厚和肺气肿等气道重塑现象,这类患者慢阻肺早期大多表现为小气道功能受损,随着病程进展,弥散功能障碍逐渐加重,3 年后患慢阻肺的风险为 22%。对于未确诊的慢阻肺患者,其急性加重和罹患肺炎的风险都明显增加,2018 年 GOLD 指南指出,慢阻肺急性加重住院的患者 5 年内病死率高达 50%,因此临床医师需要对慢阻肺给予足够的重视,尽早进行干预,而戒烟正是慢阻肺早期干预最有效和最具有成本效益的治疗措施。研究表明,轻度慢阻肺患者戒烟后获得的 FEV_1 改善程度较重度慢阻肺患者更明显,戒烟 3 个月后的早期慢阻肺患者较继续吸烟者 FEV_1 增加 230 ml,占预计值的百分比由基线水平的 75%增至 95%,其他肺功能指标(如 FVC,FEF 25%~75%,呼出气 CO 等指标)也显著提升,同时 CAT 评分也明显改善;而那些减少吸烟量但并未完全戒烟者,其肺功能改善情况不如完全戒烟者好;戒烟 5 年后还能进一步改善肺功能;提示早发现、早戒烟对早期低风险慢阻肺患者的预后至关重要。因此要重视健康教育以加强民众对慢阻肺的认识,促使其积极配合治疗,建立基于社区的综合干预策略。对于戒烟困难的患者,药物治疗和尼古丁替代疗法可以提高患者成功戒烟的概率。大气污染、粉尘、有毒有害物质的接触、生物燃料、下呼吸道感染等也是慢阻肺的危险因素,减少危险因素暴露史,积极接种疫苗防治呼吸道疾病也是预防慢阻肺的重要举措。

支气管扩张药是慢阻肺治疗的核心药物,但是药物治疗在早期慢阻肺的治疗中存在一定的争议。有学者提出,并非所有的轻度慢阻肺均能发展为重度慢阻肺,药物治疗并不能有效改善肺功能下降,现有的证据并不足以推荐无症状患者使用长效支气管扩张药。近年来很多临床研究结果支持使用长效支气管扩张药干预早期阶段慢阻肺。UPLIFT 研究结果表明,长效 M_3 受体拮抗剂(LAMA)噻托溴铵可以减缓 GOLD2 级慢阻肺患者 FEV_1 下降速率,提高波谷值和健康相关生活质量评分(HRQoL),延缓圣乔治呼吸调查问卷(SGRQ)总分下降速度,减少急性发作频率,改善 SGRQ 评分,与未接受治疗的慢阻肺患者相比,噻托溴铵明显延缓了疾病的进展。2017 年,钟南山等在《新英格兰医学杂志》上发表的一篇关于噻托溴铵干预早期慢阻肺的文章指出,治疗 2 年后,噻托溴铵显著改善了轻中度慢阻肺的 FEV_1,降低了肺功能的年下降速率,显著改善了患者的生活质量;在预防急性加重方面,噻托溴铵组第一次出现急性加重的时间长于安慰剂组;与安慰剂组相比,噻托溴铵组降低了急性加重的发作频率及患者的住院风险;两组的不良事件发生率基本相似。这篇文章强调了噻托溴铵对早期慢阻肺的临床疗效和安全性问题,提示尽早对慢阻肺进行药物干预也许能逆转慢阻肺气流受限引起的临床症状。研究表明,茚达特罗能明显改善 FEV_1,早期低风险慢阻肺患者虽然无明显的呼吸困难症状,但是可能已经出现轻微的肺功能异常,如果得不到及时治疗,肺功能继续下降就可能出现呼吸困难症状,此时大部分患者的肺功能可能已经低至 30%~50%,甚至更低。茚达特罗可以通过提升早期慢阻肺的 FEV_1,延缓肺功能下降速率,有效抑制慢阻肺的进展。也有学者认为 LABA/LAMAL 联用是治疗早期低风险慢阻肺最适合的疗法。LABA/LAMA 联合治疗明显改善了慢阻肺患者的肺功能、症状负担和生活质量等,可有效降低 GOLD Ⅱ 级慢阻肺加重的风险。既往研究表明,早期使用双支气管扩张药对肺功能的疗效优于单用 LAMA 噻托溴铵,LABA/LAMA 联合应用于早期慢阻肺有症状的患者,能更大程度上提升 FEV_1 和 SGRQ 评分,显著降低短期恶化风险。LABA/ICS 固定剂量组合应用于早期慢阻肺明显降低轻中度慢阻肺患者 FEV_1 年下降速率,这一益处不仅仅归功于 LABA,TORCH 的数据也提示我们应该适度权衡激素对慢阻肺的潜在益处和不良反应。早期慢阻肺肺功能下降速度较晚期重度慢阻肺下降速度更快,早期干预可有效阻断早期慢阻肺向晚期慢阻肺的进展,减少不必要的医疗花费,有效减轻社会负担。

虽然早期低风险慢阻肺病情稳定,但其治疗不仅仅局限于药物治疗,还应积极开展肺康复锻炼。慢阻肺肺康复是一种比较全面的多学科康复措施,首先要对患者的运动负荷量做一个综合的评估,然后再通过肢体运动训练、呼吸生理治疗、营养支持等多项锻炼手段,增强呼吸机、膈肌的肌力,缓解呼吸困难、气促等症状,有效改善患者活动耐力和生活质量。肺康复过程中,一定要注意补充足够的营养,增强患者免疫力,改善慢阻肺患者营养不良的状态,提升患者活动能力和生活质量;同时症状的改善也会减轻患者的心理压力,提高患者参加体育锻炼的兴趣,进而改善睡眠,从身体和心理两方面促进了患者病情的恢复。慢阻肺作为不可逆性呼吸系统疾病,肺康复对肺功能严重受损的重度慢阻肺患者的效果有限,肺康复应用于早期慢阻肺患者,甚至是肺功能正常的慢阻肺患者,疗效更显著,能有效延缓肺功能下降速率,减轻症状,改善活动耐力,延缓病情进展,并明显减少慢阻肺急性加重的风险,这正是慢阻肺治疗的主要方向。鉴于吸烟、血脂异常、合并焦虑抑郁状态等在轻中度慢阻肺患者中比较多见,因此,健康教育、社会心理支持等肺康复项目也占有重要地位。

2020 年 GOLD 指南指出,慢阻肺患者老年人居多,大多数患者都存在重大的共患慢性疾病,如心血管疾病、肺动脉高压、癌症、骨骼肌功能障碍等,这些共患疾病极大程度上影响了患者的气道阻塞程度,增加了慢阻肺的致残率和病死率。最新研究表明，慢阻肺患者的症状可能与增加的肺动脉压力及伴随的心血管疾病相关，呼吸系统疾病和心血管系统疾病均是导致FEV_1下降的危险因素，因此临床应该重视对早期慢阻肺患者合并的调查。

虽然早期慢阻肺临床症状轻，甚至没有症状，但同样需要长期规范化管理。在规范化管理过程中，应该重视患者的依从性。临床调查显示，接近50%的慢阻肺患者在症状缓解后自行停药，因此，早期慢阻肺患者也需定时随访，定期进行肺功能检查以评估肺功能变化情况，对戒烟不成功等依从性较差的患者进行健康宣教，或者督促其通过药物治疗等方法戒烟，积极配合治疗，尽早防止肺功能继续下降。

慢阻肺在全球具有发病率高、致残率高、病死率高等特点，其治疗花费较高，成为全球的重大疾病负担之一。

中国是一个发展中国家，人口基数大，慢阻肺患者占比较大，死亡人数占全球慢阻肺死亡人数的30%，可见中国慢阻肺防控形式严峻。慢阻肺是一种可防、可治的疾病，疾病的严重程度与患者年龄、病程长短等密切相关。一旦错过早期诊断，病程拖延越久，肺功能也越差，疾病也就越严重，因此，对无症状患者及高危人群进行慢阻肺筛查是非常重要的一项任务。对早期慢阻肺的治疗目标应该转为早期诊断、早期干预，如果能早期诊断可以阻断疾病向重度慢阻肺发展甚至逆转病情。早期慢阻肺的早期诊断需要基层医院逐步普及肺功能检查，不断提高临床医师对早期慢阻肺指南的认识。治疗方面，做好健康教育，脱离危险因素，辅以药物治疗和非药物治疗，增强患者依从性。目前，早期慢阻肺的定义及分型等仍未形成一致意见，早期低风险慢阻肺的早期诊断和早期干预也需要继续研究。

参 考 文 献

[1] 姚婉贞,路明.慢性阻塞性肺疾病病情严重程度评估系统在中国应用的专家共识.中华结核和呼吸杂志,2013,36(6):476-478.

[2] 郑劲平.肺功能检查临床意义和诊断思路.中国实用内科杂志,2012,32(08):569-574.

[3] Ding M, Chen Y, Guan WJ, et al. Measuring airway remodeling in patients with different COPD staging using endobronchial optical coherence tomography. Chest, 2016, 150: 1281-1290.

[4] 刘海波,商田歌,林颖,等.FEV1下降速率与COPD高危人群患病率的相关性及其危险因素.中国医药科学,2016,6(14):147-150.

[5] 竺文静.第一秒率<LLN评价不同阻塞性通气障碍诊断方法.上海:复旦大学出版社,2010.

[6] 刘亚男,许文兵,孟淑珍,等.探究峰流速仪呼气峰流速检测对慢性阻塞性肺疾病的筛查效力.中国呼吸与危重监护杂志,2015,14(03):250-254.

[7] 范木英,黄金梅,业秀林.吸烟与肺部疾病患者的肺功能参数状况的分析.昆明医科大学学报,2020,41(6):77-79.

[8] Aldo P, Marco S, Giovanna C, et al. Short-term benefit of smoking cessation along with glycopirronium on lung function and respiratory symptoms in mild COPD patients: a retrospective study. J Breath Res, 2018, 12: 046007.

[9] 赵海金,赵文驱,彭显如.重视慢性阻塞性肺疾病的早期诊断和早期干预.实用医学杂志,2018,34(21):3493-3495.

[10] Troosters T, Celli B, Lystig T, et al. Tiotropium as a first maintenance drug in COPD: secondary analysis of the UPLIFT trial. Eur Respir J, 2010, 36: 65-73.

[11] Zhou YM, Zhong NS, Li XC, et al. Tiotropium in early-stage chronic obstructive pulmonary disease. N Engl J Med, 2017, 377: 923-935.

[12] Patel HJ. An update on pharmacologic management of chronic obstructive pulmonary disease. Curr Opin Pulm Med, 2016, 22: 119-124.

[13] Ritwick A, Shahram M, Uma A, et al. Update on management of stable chronic obstructive pulmonary disease. J Thorac Dis, 2019, 11: S1800-S1809.

[14] Reza MYM, Dave S, Antonio A, et al. Assessing short-term deterioration in maintenance-naïve patients with COPD receiving umeclidinium/vilanterol and tiotropium: a pooled analysis of three randomized trials. Adv Ther, 2017, 33: 2188-2199.

[15] 李怀东,李报春.慢性阻塞性肺病早期干预研究现状.中国医药导刊,2019,21(12):727-730.

[16] 沈露,王红卫.肺康复训练联合健康教育在稳定期COPD患者中的应用效果观察.当代护士(下旬刊),2019,26(10):47-49.

[17] 胡进锋.肺康复治疗在慢性阻塞性肺疾病稳定期患者中的应用分析.中国医药指南,2019,17(23):110-111.

[18] 史丽秋.肺康复治疗对慢阻肺稳定期患者肺功能及生活质量影响研究进展.国际感染病学(电子版),2020,9(2):252-253.

[19] 杜飞,张李,陈代刚,等.不同程度的慢性阻塞性肺疾病患者合并心血管疾病及其危险因素的比较.中国呼吸与危重监护杂志,2017,16(4):311-313.

[20] Onur Y, Sule TG, Ufuk E, et al. The evaluation of cardiac functions according to chronic obstructive pulmonary disease groups. Aging Male, 2020, 23: 106-111.

18 慢性阻塞性肺疾病表观遗传研究进展

王舟 陈平

慢性阻塞性肺疾病（COPD）是世界上最常见的慢性呼吸道疾病，目前尚无有效的治疗策略。目前其发病机制主要包括：弹性蛋白酶-抗弹性蛋白酶假说、慢性炎症、氧化剂-抗氧化剂平衡和细胞凋亡。近年来表观遗传学发展迅猛，它是研究在不直接改变 DNA 序列情况下的基因表达变化。在肺部疾病包括 COPD 的发病机制中已经确定了许多表观遗传过程，其中 DNA 甲基化、组蛋白修饰和非编码 RNA（ncRNA）是研究最多的表观遗传机制。

一、DNA 甲基化和 COPD

DNA 甲基化是染色质修饰的最典型类型。在哺乳类动物中，DNA 甲基化涉及甲基从 S-腺苷甲硫氨酸到 CG 二核苷酸中胞嘧啶残基的 59 个位点的共价转移。哺乳类动物的 DNA 甲基化机制与 DNA 甲基转移酶（DNMT）和甲基结合蛋白（MBP）密切相关。现已明确基因启动子中 CpG 岛的超甲基化通常会导致基因沉默，而低甲基化则会导致主动转录。

根据呼吸领域的最新研究，DNA 甲基化改变与吸烟关系密切。Joehanes 等对来自 16 个队列近 16 000 名参与者血液来源的 DNA 样本进行了全基因组荟萃分析，发现与吸烟有关的 DNA 甲基化位点涉及超过 7000 个基因（约占人类基因的 1/3），大多数 DNA 甲基化位点在戒烟 5 年期之内恢复到从未吸烟者的水平；然而，有一些 DNA 甲基化位点的变化能持续长达 30 年。体内、外试验均表明，增加 ROS 负荷能通过上调细胞内的 DNMT1 表达导致基因出现高甲基化改变，而在抗氧化干预后 DNMT1 表达及基因甲基化水平均回落，提示吸烟可能通过引氧化应激上调 DNMT1 的表达，进而引起基因甲基化。

在 COPD 患者的肺泡巨噬细胞和上皮细胞中，发现了促炎基因启动子的 DNA 甲基化，使促炎因子 NF-κB 表达增加。特定细胞中与炎症相关的基因（如 TLR2、RUNX3、JAK3 和 KRT1 等）高甲基化，可调节炎症因子（如 TNF-α、IL-1β、IL-6 和 IL-10 等）的表达。以上研究均表明 DNA 甲基化可能在肺部炎症中起作用。除了炎症外，DNA 甲基化还参与了 COPD 的细胞凋亡。我们既往通过吸烟小鼠模型研究发现，吸烟可以引起小鼠肺组织细胞凋亡，而给予去甲基化处理的吸烟小鼠，其细胞凋亡率则显著下降，提示吸烟可能通过诱导基因高甲基化引起肺组织细胞凋亡。同时我们研究证实香烟烟雾提取物（CSE）可诱导 COX Ⅱ 异常甲基化，与人脐静脉内皮细胞（HUVEC）凋亡相关。除 COX Ⅱ 外，COPD 患者线粒体转录因子 A（mtTFA）启动子区域 CpG 岛甲基化状态也发生改变，mtTFA 通过结合线粒体 DNA（mtDNA）的重链启动子 1（HSP1）和轻链启动子（LSP）的上游来调节 mtDNA 的复制和起始翻译，这一改变与 COPD 的内皮细胞凋亡相关，脱甲基处理则可以逆转这些变化。Song 等发现 COPD 患者 FoxA2 和 SP-DEF 的启动子均低甲基化，而 FoxA2 和 SPDEF 对黏液产生和杯状细胞分化至关重要，这提示 DNA 甲基化可能与 COPD 杯状细胞化生及过多的黏液分泌相关。综上，DNA 甲基化在 COPD 的发病机制中似乎是必不可少的。

二、组蛋白修饰和 COPD

（一）组蛋白乙酰化/脱乙酰化

组蛋白是染色质的重要蛋白质成分。组蛋白尾巴中赖氨酸残基的 ε-氨基可经历可逆的乙酰化和脱乙酰化，在调节炎症基因表达中起重要作用。组蛋白的乙酰化作用激活了炎症基因，而组蛋白的脱乙酰化作用则抑制了炎症基因。调节组蛋白乙酰化/去乙酰化平衡的酶包括组蛋白乙酰转移酶（HATs）和组蛋白去乙酰化酶（HDACs）。现已鉴定出多种 HAT，其中 CBP/p300 的研究最为广泛。CBP/p300 增加组蛋白（H3/H4）和 NF-κB 的乙酰化水平，与香烟烟雾介导的促炎细胞因子释放有关，这导致了 COPD 中持续的炎症反应。HDAC 通过逆转核心组蛋白的过度乙酰化，在抑制基因表达中起关键作用。据报道，慢性氧化应激（如在 COPD 患者的肺部观察到的）与 HDAC2 活性和表达降低有关。抑制 HDAC 可以通过增加组蛋白乙酰化状态来促进 NF-κB 的核保留，从而增加促炎基因的转录。COPD 患者肺泡巨噬细胞中 HDAC2 的敲除不仅影响炎症反应，而且影响皮质类固醇反应性，导致皮质类固醇耐药性发生。Ito 等报道，HDAC2 的过表达可以使糖皮质激素不敏感的 COPD 肺泡巨噬细胞恢复对糖皮质激素的敏感性。现已发现在 COPD 和其他对内固醇反应较差的疾病中 HDAC2 表达降低。COPD 的皮质类固醇耐药性应该是可逆的，相关研究对 COPD 新疗法开发具有重要意义。

（二）组蛋白甲基化

组蛋白甲基化最早是在 40 多年的基因表达控制中发现的。组蛋白甲基化修饰通常发生在组蛋白的赖氨酸和精氨酸残基上。组蛋白 H3 的第 4、36、9、27 和 79 位及 H4 的第 20 位赖氨酸，H3 的第 2、17、26 位及 H4 的第 3 位精氨酸都是甲基化的常见位点。分别由组蛋白赖氨酸甲基转移酶(HKMT)和组蛋白精氨酸甲基转移酶(HRMT)介导。吸烟相关的赖氨酸甲基转移酶中 EZH2 及精氨酸甲基转移酶 PRMT 家族研究较为广泛。PRMT 可以特异地甲基化精氨酸残基，以产生蛋白质结合的单甲基-精氨酸(MMA)、对称的二甲基精氨酸(SDMA)或不对称的二甲基精氨酸(ADMA)。由于 COPD 与吸烟密切相关，因此有研究调查了吸烟与 ADMA 水平之间的关系。与不吸烟者相比，吸烟者的 ADMA 水平较高，尽管结果存在争议，但吸烟者 ADMA 水平的改变可能与 PRMT 活动失调有关。研究表明，COPD 肺组织标本中 PRMT4、5、6、9 和 10 的 mRNA 表达水平被上调。Kohse 等发现 PRMT2、4 和 6 可能在 Th17 细胞分化中起调节作用，因此可能与 COPD 中发生的炎症过程有关。Yildirim 等证实，慢性缺氧小鼠的肺中 PRMT2 mRNA 和蛋白水平上调。同样，PRMTs 响应人类内皮细胞的氧化应激而被上调，这在 COPD 的发病机制中起着关键作用。我们既往研究发现 CSE 可以诱导细胞凋亡，并且证实这与 CSE 引起的细胞精氨酸甲基转移酶 PRMT6 表达下降相关；过表达 PRMT6 可以显著逆转 CSE 引起的细胞凋亡，而阻断 PRMT6 后细胞凋亡则显著增加。目前关于 COPD 中组蛋白甲基化的数据有限，因此需要进一步的体外和体内研究来阐明其潜在机制。

（三）组蛋白磷酸化

组蛋白磷酸化在有丝分裂，细胞死亡，DNA 修复、复制和重组中起直接作用。组蛋白在丝氨酸，苏氨酸和酪氨酸上的磷酸化作用主要但非唯一地发生在 N 端组蛋白尾巴上。H3 磷酸化由核糖体 S6 激酶(RSK)-2，有丝分裂原，应激激活激酶(MSK)1 和 MAPK 介导，诱导早期基因表达。已经证明了 H3S10 磷酸化在 NF-κB 调控基因的激活中的作用。Sundar 等证明 MSK1 是一种重要的下游激酶，参与香烟烟雾诱导的 H3 磷酸乙酰化和 NF-κB 活化，进而调控 COPD 的炎症反应。肺泡巨噬细胞通过释放细胞因子、趋化因子、活性氧(ROS)和弹性蛋白酶在 COPD 的发生发展中起关键作用。有研究表明，吸烟者 COPD 肺泡巨噬细胞中 MAPKs p38 亚基的磷酸化形式增加，这可能与吸烟引起的氧化应激增强有关。因此，香烟烟雾可通过上调激酶诱导的组蛋白磷酸化水平诱导炎性基因表达。这些激酶可能是控制香烟烟雾介导的 COPD 慢性炎症反应的潜在靶标。

（四）组蛋白泛素化

组蛋白泛素化探索已经有 30 多年的历史，但对它功能的理解仍然不如其他组蛋白修饰深入。泛素是在所有真核生物中高度保守的 76 个氨基酸的调节蛋白。许多细胞过程(蛋白降解、细胞周期控制、应激反应、DNA 修复、免疫反应、信号转导、转录调节、胞吞作用和囊泡运输)受靶蛋白的泛素化翻译后修饰的控制。泛素-蛋白酶体系统(UPS)是一个组织良好的破坏机器，多种成分相互配合，以确保及时有效地对目标底物进行蛋白水解。泛素化组蛋白的主要形式是单泛素化的 H2A(H2Aub)和 H2B (H2Bub)，其中单分子的泛素被添加到高度保守的赖氨酸残基上。据报道，组蛋白泛素化或去泛素化的畸变导致多种人类疾病，包括癌症。UPS 参与许多生物过程，例如氧化应激、炎症和细胞凋亡。在 COPD 中，UPS 对收缩蛋白降解起着至关重要的作用，并且该系统参与重要的细胞过程，例如对低氧的反应。轻度至中度 COPD 患者中，促炎性细胞因子的局部表达增加 UPS 触发的隔膜中肌球蛋白的丢失。CSE 暴露可通过 UPS 诱导 Akt 蛋白降解，密切影响细胞的存活和增生。CSE 暴露还可以显著诱导小鼠肺中上皮细胞和巨噬细胞 HDAC2 的泛素化，导致 HDAC2 丰度降低，这与 COPD 患者的类固醇耐药性有关。所有这些研究表明，UPS 的异常激活在 COPD 的发病机制中起着重要的作用。

三、非编码 RNA 和 COPD

仅约 2% 的哺乳类动物转录本被翻译成功能蛋白，其余的转录本被定义为非编码 RNA(ncRNA)，并在基因调控中起关键作用。具有表观遗传功能的调控型 ncRNA 包括小干扰 siRNA(18～30 nt)，piwiRNA(24～30 nt)和 miRNA(20～24 nt)，其中，以 miRNA 的研究最为深入。

MiRNA 调节许多细胞过程，可能在肺癌、肺纤维化、哮喘和 COPD 等肺部疾病的发病机制中起作用。很多研究报道了吸烟对 miRNA 丰度的下调，miRNA 表达的下调可能与 Dicer 磺酰化后 Dicer 活性降低有关，烟龄较常的个体中丰度降低更为明显，这表明 miRNA 下调的数量与吸烟史之间存在相关性。与非吸烟 COPD 患者相比，吸烟 COPD 患者痰中 let-7c 和 miR-126a 的表达降低。CSE 下调了许多参与 NF-κB 途径激活的 miRNA，例如 miR-30、miR-146、miR-132 和 miR-155。COPD 成纤维细胞中较低的 miR-146a 表达导致环氧合酶-2mRNA(miR-146a 的靶标)的降解降低和半衰期延长，最终导致环氧合酶 2 的过表达和前列腺素 E_2 产量的增加。在 COPD 患者肺部和香烟烟雾暴露的小鼠中 miR-101 的表达升高，miR-101 的表达升高与 COPD 中 CFTR 的表达降低有关，这可能导致黏液积聚和慢性炎症。在 COPD 患者中，miR-424-5p 的表达可通过调节聚合酶Ⅰ预起始复合物的形成来抑制 rRNA 的合成，从而抑制蛋白质的合成，导致肌肉量下降。

miRNA 不仅在特定的细胞内起作用，而且通过细胞外囊泡(EVs)可在细胞间主动转运。EVs 除了具有细胞稳态和细胞间通讯功能外，还可能参与表观遗传调控。暴露在香烟烟雾中可以诱导支气管上皮细胞 EVs 的分泌，这些 EVs 富含 miR-210，后者可以抑制自噬，促进成肌纤维细胞分化，在 COPD 中引起病理性气道重塑。Serban 等发现 CSE 暴露后，内皮细胞 EVs 的货物发生改变，其中富含 let-7d、miR-191、miR-126 和 miR-125a，这些 miRNA 传递至肺部巨噬细胞后会影响其对凋亡细胞的清除能力。Ismail 等的一项研发现活化的肺泡巨噬细胞 EVs 能够将 miR-223 转移到各种靶细胞，并提出巨噬细胞产生的 EVs miRNA 可诱导单核巨噬细胞分化，同时激活骨髓中的造血细胞产生且释放更多的微泡，导致局部及全身的炎症反应放大，形成瀑布样效应。这些靶向作用在 COPD 内皮损伤和炎症机制中占据重要位置。

多种潜在因素会影响表观遗传调节的水平。DNA 甲基化改变、组蛋白修饰及 ncRNA 可影响多种分子和细胞过程,如炎症介质的基因表达、DNA 复制、重组、修复、细胞凋亡、衰老、自噬等。表观遗传调节在慢性阻塞性肺疾病中的作用逐步得到认识,并且越来越多的证据证明表观遗传变化可能是吸烟引起的遗传效应的一部分。有关表观遗传学的知识帮助我们更好地理解 COPD 的分子基础,可能为 COPD 早期诊断提供一些新思路,加快 COPD 新疗法的开发。

参 考 文 献

[1] Bayarsaihan D. Epigenetic mechanisms in inflammation. J Dent Res,2011,90(1):9-17.

[2] Joehanes R, Just AC, Marioni RE, et al. Epigenetic signatures of cigarette smoking. Circ Cardiovasc Genet, 2016, 9: 436-447.

[3] Liu F, Killian J, Yang M, et al. Epigenomic alterations and gene expression profiles in respiratory epithelia exposed to cigarette smoke condensate. Oncogene, 2010, 29 (25): 3650-3664.

[4] Siedlinski M, Klanderman B, Sandhaus RA, et al. Association of cigarette smoking and CRP levels with DNA methylation in α-1 antitrypsin deficiency. Epigenetics, 2012, 7 (7): 720-728.

[5] Fabre C, Grosjean J, Tailler M, et al. A novel effect of dna methyltransferase and histone deacetylase inhibitors:nfkb inhibition in malignant myeloblasts. Cell Cycle, 2008, 7 (14): 2139-2145.

[6] Zhang H, Chen P, Zeng H, et al. Protective effect of demethylation treatment on cigarette smoke extract-induced mouse emphysema model. Pharmacol Sci,2013,123(2):159-166.

[7] Zeng H, Shi Z, Kong X, et al. Involvement of b-cell cll/lymphoma 2 promoter methylation in cigarette smoke extract-induced emphysema. Exper Biol Med,2016,241(8):808-816.

[8] Peng H, Yang M, Chen ZY, et al. Expression and methylation of mitochondrial transcription factor A in chronic obstructive pulmonary disease patients with lung cancer. PLoS One, 2013,8:e82739.

[9] Song J, Heijink I, Kistemaker L, et al. Aberrant DNA methylation and expression of SPDEF and FOXA2 in airway epithelium of patients with COPD. Clin Epigenetics,2017,9(1): 42.

[10] Park KS, Korfhagen TR, Bruno MD, et al. SPDEF regulates goblet cell hyperplasia in the airway epithelium. J Clin Invest,2007,117(4):978-988.

[11] Tang X, Liu XJ, Tian C, et al. Foxa2 regulates leukotrienes to inhibit Th2-mediated pulmonary inflammation. Am J Respir Cell Mol Biol,2013,49(6):960-970.

[12] Barnes PJ. Targeting the epigenome in the treatment of asthma and chronic obstructive pulmonary disease. Proc Am Thorac Soc,2009,6:693-696.

[13] Wang YL, Faiola F, Martinze E. Purification of multi-protein histone acetyltransferase complexes. Methods Mol Biol, 2012,809:427-443.

[14] Bedford DC, Brindle PK. Is histone acetylation the most important physiological function for CBP and p300? Aging(Albany NY),2012,4:247-255.

[15] Clarke D, Sutcliffe A, Deacon K, et al. PKCbetaII augments NF-kappaB-dependent transcription at the CCL11 promoter via p300/CBP-associated factor recruitment and histone H4 acetylation. J Immounl,2008,181:3503-3514.

[16] Meja KK, Rajendrasozhan S, Adenuga D, et al. Curcumin restores corticosteroid function in monocytes exposed to oxidants by maintaining HDAC2. Am J Respir Cell Mol Biol, 2008,39:312-323.

[17] Rahman I, Marwick J, Kirkham P. Redox modulation of chromatin remodeling:impact on histone acetylation and deacetylation, NF-kappaB and pro-inflammatory gene expression. Biochem Pharmacol,2004,68:1255-1267.

[18] Adcock IM, Tsaprouni L, Bhavsar P, et al. Epigenetic regulation of airway inflammation. Curr Opin Immunol,2007,19: 694-700.

[19] Ito K, Yamamura S, Essilfie-Quare S, et al. Histone deacetylase 2mediated deacetylation of the glucocorticoid receptorenables NF-kappaB suppression. J Exp Med,2006,203:7-13.

[20] Sakao S, Tatsumi K. The importance of epigenetics in the development of chronic obstructive pulmonary disease. Respirology,2011,16(7):1056-1063.

[21] Zakrzewicz D, Eickelberg O. Fromarginine methylation to ADMA: a novel mechanism with therapeutic potential in chronic lung diseases. BMC Pulm Med,2009,9:5.

[22] Onat A, Hergenc G, Can G, et al. Serum asymmetric dimethylarginine levels among Turks: association with metabolic syndromein women and tendency to decrease in smokers. Turk Kardiyol Dern Ars,2008,36:7-13.

[23] Yildirim AQ, Konigshoff M, Wang Q, et al. Expressionprofiling of protein arginine methyl-transferase(Prmt)isoforms in chronic obstructive pulmonary disease(COPD). Am J Respir Crit Care Med,2010,181:A4954.

[24] Kohse K, Wang Q, StiitzkeS, et al. Proteinarginine methyl-trans-ferases(prmt)are involved in Th17 cell differentiation. Am J Respir Crit Care Med,2011,183:A4399.

[25] Yildirim AO, Bulau P, Zakrzewicz D, et al. Increased protein arginine methylation in chronic hypoxia: role of protein arginine methyl-transferases. Am J Respir Cell Mol Biol,2006, 35:436-443.

[26] Boger RH, Sydow K, Borlak J, et al. LDL cholesterol upregulates synthesis of asymmetrical di-methylarginine in human endothelial cells: involvement of Sadenosylmethionine-dependent methyltransferases. Circ Res,2000,87:99-105.

[27] Kang N, Chen P, Chen Y, et al. PRMT6 mediates CSE induced inflammation and apoptosis. Int Immunopharmacol, 2015,24(1):95-101.

[28] Oki M, Aihara H, Ito T. Role of histone phospho-rylation in chromatin dynamics and its implications in diseases. Subcell Biochem, 2007, 41:319-336.

[29] Sugiyama K, Sugiura K, Hara T, et al. Aurora-B associated protein phosphatases as negative regulators of kinase activation. Oncogene, 2002, 21:3103-3111.

[30] Kuzarides T. Chromatin modifications and their function. Cell, 2007, 128:693-705.

[31] Sundar IK, Chung S, Hang JW, et al. Mitogen-and stress-activatedkinase 1(MSK1) regulates cigarette smoke-induced histone modifications on NF-κB-dependent genes. PLoS One, 2012, 7:e31378.

[32] Renda T, Baraldo S, Pelaia G, et al. Increased activation of p38 MAPK in COPD. Eur Respir J, 2008, 31:62-69.

[33] Rahman I. Oxidative stress in pathogenesis of chronic obstructive pulmonary disease: cellular and molecular mechanisms. Cell Biochem Bio-phy, 2005, 43:167-188.

[34] Ottenheijm CA, Heunks LM, Li YP, et al. Activation of the ubiquitin-proteasome pathway in the diaphragm in chronic obstructive pulmonary disease. Am J Respir Crit Care Med, 2006, 174:997-1002.

[35] Kim SY, Lee JH, Huh JW, et al. Cigarette smoke induces Akt protein degradation by the ubiquitin-proteasome system. J Biol Chem, 2011, 286:31932-31943.

[36] Adenuga D, Yao H, March TH, et al. Histone deacetylase 2 is phosphorylated, ubiquitinated, and degraded by cigarette smoke. Am J Respir Cell Mol Biol, 2009, 40:464.

[37] Gross TJ, Powers LS, Boudreau RL, et al. A microRNA processing defect in smokers' macrophages is linked to SUMOylation of the endonuclease DICER. J Biol Chem, 2014, 289:12823-12834.

[38] Van Pottelberge GR, Mestdagh P, Bracke KR, et al. MicroRNA expression in induced sputum of smokers and patients with chronic obstructive pulmonary disease. Am J Respir Crit Care Med, 2011, 183:898-906.

[39] Sato T, Liu X, Nelson A, et al. Reduced miR-146a increases prostaglandin E2 in chronic obstructive pulmonary disease fibroblasts. Am J Respir Crit Care Med, 2010, 182:1020-1029.

[40] Humbert M, Busse W, Hanania NA, et al. Omalizumab in asthma: an update on recent developments. J Allergy Clin Immunol Pract, 2014, 2:525-536.

[41] Connolly M, Paul R, Farre-Garros R, et al. miR-424-5p reduces ribosomal RNA and protein synthesis in muscle wasting. J Cachexia Sarcopenia Muscle, 2018, 9(2):400-416.

[42] Kadota T, Fujita Y, Yoshioka Y, et al. Extracellular vesicles in chronic obstructive pulmonary disease. Int JMol Sci, 2016, 17:1801.

[43] Serban KA, Rezania S, Petrusca DN. Structural and functional characterization of endothelial microparticles released by cigarette smoke. Sci Rep, 2016, 6:31596.

[44] Sundar IK, Li D, Rahman I. Small RNA-sequence analysis of plasma-derived extracellular vesicle miRNAs in smokers and patients with chronic obstructive pulmonary disease as circulating biomarkers. J Extracell Vesicles, 2019, 8(1):1684816.

19 肌肉评估在慢性阻塞性肺疾病治疗中的重要性

李雯 邹义敏

中国慢性阻塞性肺疾病(简称慢阻肺)流行病学研究显示,中国40岁以上人群患病率高达13.7%,患者人数约1亿。随着吸烟人群增加和人口老龄化进一步加剧,慢阻肺患病率在未来30年中将持续升高,慢阻肺防治形势非常严峻。慢阻肺以持续气流受限为特征,最常见的呼吸系统症状包括呼吸困难、咳嗽和(或)咳痰,此外,慢阻肺本身也可以有明显的肺外(全身)效应,包括体重下降、营养不良、骨骼肌功能障碍等。虽然骨骼肌功能障碍可能会同时影响呼吸肌群和四肢肌肉,但后者受到的影响通常更严重。有研究显示股四头肌功能障碍对慢阻肺患者的生存率和病死率有显著负面影响。

一、骨骼肌结构和功能

(一)骨骼肌结构

骨骼肌由肌肉纤维束组成,每根肌纤维由数千根肌原纤维组成,并含有数十亿根肌丝。肌丝组合在一起形成肌节,肌节是骨骼肌的基本收缩单位。最丰富的两种肌丝成分是肌动蛋白和肌球蛋白。各种刺激,如运动训练、衰老及各种神经肌肉病变,都会导致肌细胞的结构成分和功能发生显著变化。成人肢体肌肉纤维常分为3种纤维类型:Ⅰ型(慢、氧化、抗疲劳)、ⅡA型(快速、氧化、中间代谢特性)和ⅡX型(最快、糖酵解、疲劳)。一般来说,肌肉质量取决于蛋白质合成与降解之间的平衡,这两个过程对营养状况、激素平衡、体力活动/运动、损害或疾病等因素都很敏感。

(二)骨骼肌生理功能

肌肉最主要的生理功能特性是力量和耐力。从力学的角度来看,骨骼肌的主要功能是将化学能转化为机械能,以产生力量和耐力,保持姿势,进行运动。肌肉激活的生理学兴奋-收缩耦合是力产生所需的两个过程的协调;神经刺激传递到三联体,然后从肌质网池释放钙,肌动蛋白和肌球蛋白相互作用形成交叉桥。只要肌动蛋白上的活性部位暴露,就可以使肌球蛋白分子的头部与肌动蛋白结合,最终结果是肌动蛋白和肌球蛋白丝的滑动和力的产生。收缩速度与肌质网发育程度相关,而疲劳耐受性和氧化能力与线粒体含量相关。

(三)线粒体功能

线粒体通过氧化磷酸化在ATP产生中起着重要作用,所有的肌肉活动都需要消耗能量,人体运动过程中,为骨骼肌提供能量的系统包括3个:①ATP-CP供能系统,由ATP和CP(磷酸肌酸)以水解分子内高能磷酸键的方式供能。②糖酵解供能系统,由糖原或葡萄糖无氧分解生成乳酸,并合成ATP供能。③有氧供能系统,由糖类、脂肪及蛋白质等能源物质在氧气充足的情况下,通过有氧分解合成ATP供能。需要注意的是,这些代谢途径的利用并不是一种"全有或无"的现象。在一次运动中,根据运动强度的不同,在不同的时间点可以激活不同通路。

二、慢阻肺骨骼肌功能障碍流行病学

慢阻肺患者常见的肺外效应是骨骼肌功能障碍,呼吸肌群和四肢肌肉通常会受到影响,慢阻肺呼吸肌肉功能障碍的发生率在大型队列研究中没有完全阐明。一项前瞻性研究采用超声波测量技术评估慢阻肺急性加重期膈肌功能障碍的患病率,结果显示在接受无创正压通气治疗的慢阻肺急性加重住院患者中,近1/4的患者出现严重膈肌功能障碍。此外,与年龄匹配的健康对照组相比,重度慢阻肺患者膈肌功能下降20%~30%。在肢体肌肉功能方面,欧洲一项研究显示,英国和荷兰的慢阻肺患者中有32%和33%出现股四头肌无力。在GOLD 1级、GOLD 2级或呼吸困难评分为1分、2分的患者中,有较大比例的股四头肌肌无力发生(分别为28%和26%);在GOLD 4级患者中该值上升到38%,而在MRC评分为4或5的患者中上升到43%。对45岁以上的慢阻肺患者,采用数字手持式测量仪评估股四头肌肌肉强度进行横断面研究,结果显示92%的慢阻肺患者有股四头肌肌无力发生;即使在慢阻肺早期且年龄较轻的患者中,股四头肌无力的比例也很高。这些结果表明,慢阻肺中肌无力的发生可能比气急症状出现的时间还要早。

采用大腿中部横截面积和股四头肌肌力进行评估,显示出肌肉质量下降和下肢肌肉功能障碍强烈影响运动能力和生活质量,增加医疗费用,并预测慢阻肺患者的生存率和病死率。

三、慢阻肺骨骼肌功能障碍临床特点

(一)呼吸肌肉功能障碍

慢阻肺患者膈肌障碍导致跨膈压下降,这在很大程度上是由于肺过度充气所致,因为膈肌肌肉处于拉伸状态机械上的劣势。经过校正肺容积,实际上慢阻肺膈肌的收缩强度相比健康对照组并没有降低,甚至在某些情况下是增强的,维持该肌肉的力量可能是由于持续的非自主运动继而增加了呼吸功。研究发现,膈肌中Ⅰ型肌纤维的比例增加了20%~50%,而ⅡX型纤维减少,从而重塑成抗疲劳表型来适应膈肌运动。其他辅助呼吸肌的情况似乎也以相同的方式适应呼吸功的增加,在重症患者的胸骨旁肋间肌中也可见到肌纤维类型从Ⅱ型到Ⅰ型的转变,抗疲劳慢纤维比例明显增多;相对于股四头肌,保存了胸大肌和背阔肌的力量,而且腹肌力量也得以保留,这可能是由于慢阻肺中呼气肌肉的额外活动所致。

慢阻肺患者呼吸肌肉尽管经历了积极的重塑适应使其更耐疲劳,但这些肌肉的最大吸气压、最大呼气压及耐力仍逐渐降低。呼吸肌肉功能障碍对患者造成通气功能受限,可加重慢阻肺患者潜在呼吸衰竭,尤其是在疾病晚期。此外,呼吸肌肉需克服由慢阻肺急性加重期增加的通气需求所产生的吸气负荷,进一步损害患者的呼吸肌功能。

(二)肢体肌肉功能障碍

慢阻肺患者的肢体肌肉功能障碍表现为肌无力和耐力下降,大部分数据来自于股四头肌的研究。慢阻肺患者的股四头肌力量平均每年下降4.3%,而在健康老龄化人群中每年1%~2%,下降速度明显加快。轻度至中度慢阻肺患者中有20%的患者出现肌肉无力,相比之下,超过50%的预期患有下肢肌无力的重度慢阻肺患者却并未表现出股四头肌强度降低。这些数据表明,在慢阻肺患者中可能存在与肌无力有关的特殊表型。部分研究显示采用大腿肌肉横截面积量化股四头肌强度,慢阻肺患者与健康对照者之间无显著差异,推测减小的股四头肌力量可能主要来自损失的肌肉质量;然而,在一些患者中肌力损失与肌肉质量下降并不成比例。肌无力在肌群之间分布并不均匀,尽管上肢肌肉也出现肌无力,但肌力保留的程度明显好于下肢肌肉;与上肢近端肌肉相比,上肢远端肌肉的力量得到了更好的保留。

在耐力方面,慢阻肺患者股四头肌耐力下降的幅度(32%~77%)变化很大,在低氧血症的情况下,耐力会更严重地降低。慢阻肺患者在正常行走时表现出腓肠肌和胫骨前肌更容易疲劳;6 min步行距离测试显示锻炼能力明显下降。与健康对照组相比,慢阻肺患者的肢体肌肉耐力降低,即使是轻中度气流阻塞患者,也与肺功能或体力活动参数无关;然而,上肢肌肉的耐力得到了较好的保留,这表明慢阻肺患者的肢体肌肉异常似乎是异质的,并且可能与肌肉群的活动有关。

总之,在慢阻肺中,呼吸肌的变化与股四头肌形成鲜明对比,膈肌重塑为抗疲劳的轮廓,Ⅰ型纤维相对增加,最终增加氧化能力;股四头肌的特点是质量减轻,抗疲劳的Ⅰ型纤维和氧化能力降低,从而削弱强度和耐力。这些支持肌肉失用是导致慢阻肺肢体和呼吸肌群差异适应的主要病因。尽管肌耐力的评估可能更为敏感,有助于设计针对慢阻肺患者的干预措施,但目前在临床中的应用却较有限,可能是由于缺乏标准化的方案或参考值。肌力并不是评估肌肉功能最敏感的指标,但它在临床应用中的有效性被证明是可行的,这有助于临床医生更容易地诊断慢阻肺患者的骨骼肌功能障碍。

四、病因及生物学机制

(一)病因

许多因素已被证明参与了慢阻肺呼吸和肢体肌肉功能障碍的发生,包括烟草烟雾、缺氧、高碳酸血症和酸中毒、代谢改变、营养不良、遗传、全身性炎症、衰老、合并症、伴随治疗、急性加重和缺乏运动等。

(二)生物学机制

1. 内在机制　主要包括①泛素-蛋白酶和溶酶体-自噬途径:通过以上两个分子途径,分解代谢活化导致蛋白质净损失增加,最终导致蛋白质降解加速,这是肌肉萎缩的标志。②合成代谢抑制:包括两个主要的信号传导途径控制骨骼肌生长:胰岛素样生长因子途径和肌肉生长抑制素途径,调节肌成纤维细胞增生。③氧化应激与线粒体功能障碍:不平衡的氧化应激可能会改变肌肉蛋白的完整性,从而增强其降解。受损的线粒体功能障碍导致能量失衡,引起肌肉萎缩和肌肉无力。

2. 外在机制　主要包括①胸壁结构重塑:慢阻肺患者通气功能障碍明显,主要是由胸壁几何形状的改变引起的。过度充气所致膈肌拉长,导致通气工作效率降低。②乳酸过度产生,运动耐力下降:由于外周肌肉纤维转变,在急性运动过程中慢阻肺患者会产生更多的乳酸和二氧化碳,这需要增加呼吸代偿做功,并可能耗尽呼吸生理储备,导致运动耐力进一步下降。

五、慢阻肺骨骼肌功能障碍评估手段

(一)肌肉质量评估

1. 直接测量　肌肉活检是评估肢体肌肉形态和生化特性的最有价值的工具,但是该技术是侵入性的,具有潜在的合并症,包括不适和轻微瘢痕、出血等。

2. 间接测量　间接测量包括:①生物电阻抗法(BIA):该技术基于非脂肪组织的电导率高于脂肪原理,测量是非侵入性的,价格便宜,只需几分钟,并且不需要主动协作,该技术测量准确性已通过使用氘稀释空间法进行了验证。②双能X线吸收法(DEXA):尽管比BIA更昂贵,但DEXA被认为是一种准确,安全且无创的方法。③影像技术:计算机断层摄影、磁共振成像、超声检查已经用于评估慢阻肺患者股四头肌肌肉质量,用这些技术测量的局部肌肉量与慢阻肺患者肌肉力量和病死率等有关。

(二)力量评估

1. 呼吸肌肉力量测试　非侵入性测量技术有肺量计(最大吸气压和最大呼气压)和最大鼻吸气压。侵入性测试技术有食管电极测压法。此外,已开发出膈神经电磁波刺激测量膈肌功能的方法。

2. 肢体肌肉测试　常用的方法有肌电图、握力计、股四头肌的最大等距收缩法。其中肌电图不需要患者主动配合，握力计测试用于上肢肌力评估，简单、可靠有效。股四头肌最大主动收缩力测量用于评估下肢肌力非常有用，但需要患者主动配合，已有参考值可用。

（三）耐力评估

由于没有标准化和参考值，肌肉耐力测试一般不用于慢阻肺评估。静态耐力测试方法有电磁刺激法、以10%的股四头肌的最大等距收缩法测试耐力时间，而动态耐力测试方法有6 min步行距离测试。

六、慢阻肺肌肉功能障碍与预后

慢阻肺肌肉功能障碍除了影响患者日常活动能力之外，更与患者预后较差有关。

肢体肌肉功能障碍并非慢阻肺终末期现象，而是在慢阻肺早期患者中即有发生，与健康受试者相比，GOLD 1级患者日常体育活动水平明显下降，而并不完全与肺功能下降水平相关联。采用BIA法测量慢阻肺患者非脂肌肉质量，发现原始BIA变量是慢阻肺患者2年病死率的强有力的独立预测因子。大腿中部肌肉横截面积减少和股四头肌强度降低可较好地预测病死率。同样，6 min步行距离测试表现不佳和握力测试结构也可以预测病死率；肺康复治疗恢复肌肉力量可改善患者症状、运动能力、生活质量。慢阻肺患者呼吸肌无力表现为最大吸气压和跨膈压下降，呼吸肌肉功能障碍造成通气限制，加重慢性呼吸衰竭，也是导致急性加重再入院的一个重要因素。吸气肌训练可改善患者吸气肌力量和耐力，减少呼吸困难症状，但并不能提高6 min步行距离。

七、展　望

骨骼肌功能障碍是慢阻肺相关的合并症，与较差的预后有关，包括较高的住院率、较差的生活质量和较低的生存率，目前不适合使用任何单一手段来测量和监测骨骼肌功能。由于骨骼肌功能障碍的临床和预后价值，骨骼肌功能评估应成为慢阻肺患者常规评估的一部分。为了实现这一目标，需要标准化的临床可行性测量方案，这也有助于为患者制定个体化康复训练方案或评估各种干预措施的疗效。慢阻肺患者肌肉功能障碍应被视为慢阻肺的系统性反应，需要针对运动耐受能力和营养状况尽早发现肌肉功能障碍，采取整体干预方法预防疾病进展并改善预后。

参 考 文 献

[1] Wang C, Xu J, Yang L, et al. Prevalence and risk factors of chronic obstructive pulmonary disease in China (the China Pulmonary Health [CPH] study): a national cross-sectional study. Lancet, 2018, 391:1706-1717.

[2] Jaitovich A, Barreiro E. Skeletal Muscle Dysfunction in Chronic Obstructive Pulmonary Disease. What We Know and Can Do for Our Patients. Am J Respir Crit Care Med, 2018, 198:175-186.

[3] Swallow EB, Reyes D, Hopkinson NS, et al. Quadriceps strength predicts mortality in patients with moderate to severe chronic obstructive pulmonary disease. Thorax, 2007, 62:115-120.

[4] Greising SM, Gransee HM, Mantilla CB, et al. Systems biology of skeletal muscle: fiber type as an organizing principle. Wiley Interdiscip Rev Syst Biol Med, 2012, 4:457-473.

[5] Frontera WR, Ochala J. Skeletal muscle: a brief review of structure and function. Calcif Tissue Int, 2015, 96:183-195.

[6] Rebbeck RT, Karunasekara Y, Board PG, et al. Skeletal muscle excitation-contraction coupling: who are the dancing partners? Int J Biochem Cell Biol, 2014, 48:28-38.

[7] Antenora F, Fantini R, Iattoni A, et al. Prevalence and outcomes of diaphragmatic dysfunction assessed by ultrasound technology during acute exacerbation of COPD: A pilot study. Respirology, 2017, 22:338-344.

[8] Barreiro E, Gea J. Respiratory and Limb Muscle Dysfunction in COPD. COPD, 2015, 12:413-426.

[9] Seymour JM, Spruit MA, Hopkinson NS, et al. The prevalence of quadriceps weakness in COPD and the relationship with disease severity. Eur Respir J, 2010, 36:81-88.

[10] Kharbanda S, Ramakrishna A, Krishnan S. Prevalence of quadriceps muscle weakness in patients with COPD and its association with disease severity. Int J Chron Obstruct Pulmon Dis, 2015, 10:1727-1735.

[11] Puente-Maestu L, Stringer WW. Hyperinflation and its management in COPD. Int J Chron Obstruct Pulmon Dis, 2006, 1:381-400.

[12] Levine S, Kaiser L, Leferovich J, Tikunov B. Cellular adaptations in the diaphragm in chronic obstructive pulmonary disease. N Engl J Med, 1997, 337:1799-1806.

[13] Levine S, Nguyen T, Friscia M, et al. Parasternal intercostal muscle remodeling in severe chronic obstructive pulmonary disease. J Appl Physiol (1985), 2006, 101:1297-302.

[14] Donaldson AV, Maddocks M, Martolini D, Polkey MI, Man WD. Muscle function in COPD: a complex interplay. Int J Chron Obstruct Pulmon Dis, 2012, 7:523-535.

[15] Hopkinson NS, Tennant RC, Dayer MJ, et al. A prospective study of decline in fat free mass and skeletal muscle strength in chronic obstructive pulmonary disease. Respir Res, 2007, 8:25.

[16] Maltais F, Decramer M, Casaburi R, et al. An official American Thoracic Society/European Respiratory Society statement: update on limb muscle dysfunction in chronic obstructive pulmonary disease. Am J Respir Crit Care Med, 2014, 189:15-62.

[17] Koechlin C, Maltais F, Saey D, et al. Hypoxaemia enhances peripheral muscle oxidative stress in chronic obstructive pul-

monary disease. Thorax,2005,60:834-841.

[18] Gagnon P,Maltais F,Bouyer L,et al. Distal leg muscle function in patients with COPD. COPD,2013,10:235-242.

[19] Beaumont M,Losq A,Peran L,et al. Comparison of 3-minute Step Test(3MStepT)and 6-minute Walk Test(6MWT)in Patients with COPD. COPD,2019,16:266-271.

[20] Marklund S,Bui KL,Nyberg A. Measuring and monitoring skeletal muscle function in COPD:current perspectives. Int J Chron Obstruct Pulmon Dis,2019,14:1825-1838.

[21] Barreiro E,Gea J. Molecular and biological pathways of skeletal muscle dysfunction in chronic obstructive pulmonary disease. Chron Respir Dis,2016,13:297-311.

[22] Elliott B,Renshaw D,Getting S,Mackenzie R. The central role of myostatin in skeletal muscle and whole body homeostasis. Acta Physiol(Oxf),2012,205:324-340.

[23] Abrigo J,Elorza AA,Riedel CA,et al. Role of Oxidative Stress as Key Regulator of Muscle Wasting during Cachexia. Oxid Med Cell Longev,2018,2018:2063179.

[24] Saey D,Michaud A,Couillard A,et al. Contractile fatigue, muscle morphometry,and blood lactate in chronic obstructive pulmonary disease. Am J Respir Crit Care Med,2005,171: 1109-1115.

[25] Hayot M,Michaud A,Koechlin C,et al. Skeletal muscle microbiopsy:a validation study of a minimally invasive technique. Eur Respir J,2005,25:431-440.

[26] Rutten EP,Spruit MA,Wouters EF. Critical view on diagnosing muscle wasting by single-frequency bio-electrical impedance in COPD. Respir Med,2010,104:91-98.

[27] Barreiro E,Bustamante V,Cejudo P,et al. Guidelines for the evaluation and treatment of muscle dysfunction in patients with chronic obstructive pulmonary disease. Arch Bronconeumol,2015,51:384-395.

[28] Shrikrishna D,Patel M,Tanner RJ,et al. Quadriceps wasting and physical inactivity in patients with COPD. Eur Respir J, 2012,40:1115-1122.

[29] de Blasio F,Scalfi L,Di Gregorio A,et al. Raw Bioelectrical Impedance Analysis Variables Are Independent Predictors of Early All-Cause Mortality in Patients With COPD. Chest, 2019,155:1148-1157.

[30] Beaumont M,Mialon P,Le Ber C,et al. Effects of inspiratory muscle training on dyspnoea in severe COPD patients during pulmonary rehabilitation: controlled randomised trial. Eur Respir J,2018,51(1):1701107.

[31] O'Donnell DE,Elbehairy AF,Berton DC,Domnik NJ,Neder JA. Advances in the Evaluation of Respiratory Pathophysiology during Exercise in Chronic Lung Diseases. Front Physiol, 2017,8:82.

[32] Charususin N,Gosselink R,Decramer M,et al. Randomised controlled trial of adjunctive inspiratory muscle training for patients with COPD. Thorax,2018,73:942-950.

[33] Langer D,Ciavaglia C,Faisal A,et al. Inspiratory muscle training reduces diaphragm activation and dyspnea during exercise in COPD. J Appl Physiol(1985),2018,125:381-392.

[34] Zeng Y,Jiang F,Chen Y,et al. Exercise assessments and trainings of pulmonary rehabilitation in COPD: a literature review. Int J Chron Obstruct Pulmon Dis, 2018, 13: 2013-2023.

20 从队列研究认识慢性阻塞性肺疾病诊断标准的争议

刘耘充　陈亚红

1998年慢性阻塞性肺疾病(简称慢阻肺)全球倡议(global initiative for chronic obstructive lung disease, GOLD)启动,其目标是根据已发表的最佳研究结果制定慢阻肺的管理推荐。2001年第1版GOLD倡议发布至今已有20年,回顾GOLD20年的变迁,伴随慢阻肺研究的深入,围绕着慢阻肺的评估和个体化治疗定期进行更新。目前慢阻肺的诊断要满足①存在呼吸困难、慢性咳嗽或咳痰,有复发性下呼吸道感染史和(或)有接触该疾病危险因素史。②存在持续气流受限,即吸入支气管扩张药后$FEV_1/FVC<0.7$。但是,随着慢阻肺人群队列研究结果发布,对目前慢阻肺的诊断标准提出了新的挑战。

一、大型队列研究发现的问题

Genetic epidemiology of COPD(COPD gene)研究由美国国立心、肺、血液研究所(NHLBI)资助,2008年在美国21家临床中心正式开展,该研究共募集受试者12 000例,包括不同肺功能分级(Ⅰ～Ⅳ)的慢阻肺患者6000例、吸烟但肺功能正常的对照者4500名,以及不吸烟且肺功能正常的对照者1500例。受试者年龄45～80岁,非西班牙裔白种人占2/3,非洲裔美国人占1/3。该研究在对受试者进行详细问卷调查、6 min步行测试、肺量计检测的基础上进行全基因关联(GWA)及吸气、呼气相胸部CT影像学检查。2012年,NHLBI再次资助COPD gene研究,继续开展随访追踪。该项目的主要研究目的是识别慢阻肺发生、发展的易感基因及关键因子,并通过整合临床、遗传学、CT影像学数据等创建慢阻肺新的分类体系。基于该研究的一项结果发现,临床上有明显呼吸系统症状的现症吸烟者和戒烟者肺功能检查可能正常,但胸部CT却显示存在一定程度的气道壁增厚、肺气肿及气体陷闭,这一比例在FEV_1/FVC正常的吸烟者中达到了42.3%。受试者FEV_1也出现轻度下降,但尚未达到慢阻肺的肺功能诊断标准。

SPIROMICS研究是在美国6个临床中心开展的一项纵向队列研究。该研究入组受试者3200名,年龄为40～80岁,其中77%为白种人,19%为非洲裔美国人,3%亚洲人。分别纳入严重慢阻肺(600例)、轻/中度慢阻肺(1500例)、吸烟(>20包/年)无气流阻塞(900例),以及非吸烟(<1包/年)无气流阻塞者(200例),基线信息包括肺量计数据、6 min步行距离、吸气呼气相胸部CT及一些标准问卷,生物样本的收集包括血清、血浆、DNA、尿样及诱导痰,随访3年,并记录受试者在随访期间的急性加重、住院及死亡信息。2016年,基于该研究的"吸烟肺功能正常人群症状的临床意义"一文发表于《新英格兰医学杂志》,文章表明临床上有明显呼吸系统症状的现症吸烟者和戒烟者肺功能检查可能正常,但存在急性加重、活动受限、高分辨率CT下气道增厚,以及FEV_1、FVC轻度降低等现象,在目前没有任何循证医学证据支持的情况下,这部分患者已在长期使用一些治疗呼吸道疾病的药物。

以上两项大型队列研究提示,现症吸烟者存在与慢阻肺相似的临床症状或影像学表现,但其肺功能不存在持续气流受限,对这类人群目前没有推荐的药物干预治疗方案,药物干预能否获益尚不可知,但确实会增加个人与国家的医疗支出;若不对其进行干预管理,这类人群的FEV_1逐年下降,最终会进展为慢阻肺。目前没有太多关于这类人群的队列研究,原因之一在于这类人群的诊断定位不明确,研究设计难以被批准。

一项丹麦人群队列研究纳入108 246名年龄为20～100岁的受试者,慢性呼吸系统症状包括呼吸困难、慢性黏液分泌过多、喘息和咳嗽,评估肺量计正常伴慢性呼吸系统症状因气道疾病加重和肺炎而住院的风险及呼吸系统疾病相关死亡风险和全因死亡风险。2003—2018年随访,有52 999人肺量计正常但无慢性呼吸系统症状,30 890人肺量计正常同时伴有慢性呼吸系统症状。随访期间,1037例因呼吸系统疾病加重住院,5743例因肺炎住院,8750例死亡,其中463例死于呼吸系统疾病。与肺量计正常无慢性呼吸系统症状者相比,肺量计正常有慢性呼吸系统症状增加了呼吸系统疾病住院率(校正风险比:1.62,95%CI:1.20～2.18)、肺炎住院率(校正风险比:1.26,95%CI:1.17～1.37)、呼吸道死亡率(校正风险比:1.59,95%CI:1.2～2.06)和全因死亡率(校正风险比:1.19,95%CI:1.13～1.25)。

一项对2个北美前瞻性随访队列[肺健康研究队列(lung health study,LHS),5861例,随访5年;加拿大阻塞性肺疾病研究队列(Canadiancohort of obstructive lung disease,CanCOLD),1561例,随访4年]的研究观察到慢阻肺诊断存在不稳定性(包括2种情况:患者初始诊断为慢阻肺,随访肺功能正常,然后又出现肺功能下降;或患者初始正常,随访肺功能下降达到慢阻肺诊断标准,然后肺功能又正常)和逆转性(患者初始诊断为慢阻肺,随访结束后恢复正常)。该研究发现,轻-中度慢阻肺患者经常会出现诊断波动,LHS 研究约占 19.5%,CanCOLD 研究占 6.4%。部分慢阻肺发生逆转,LHS 占 12.6%,CanCOLD 占 27.2%。可见慢阻肺的诊断不能仅依赖一次肺功能检查,而需要动态随访。GOLD 倡议组也发现诊断中存在的"漏洞",因此 GOLD 2018 指出,评估是否存在气流受限时,单次使用支气管扩张药后 FEV_1/FVC 为 0.6~0.8 时,应在另一场所重复肺功能检查以确诊。在某些情况下,间隔一段时间后,由于个体差异,FEV_1/FVC 可能会发生改变。若初始使用支气管扩张剂后,$FEV_1/FVC<0.6$,则不太可能升至 0.7 以上。

FEV_1/FVC 的比值会随着年龄的增加而自然下降,正常人在 50 余岁时此比值在 0.7 附近,如以固定的比值作为单一确诊慢阻肺的标准,在年龄小于 50 岁的人群中存在漏诊可能,在大于 50 岁的人群中则存在过诊的可能。有学者建议以各年龄的正常值下限(LLN)作为气流受限的标准来诊断慢阻肺,但临床应用上会稍烦琐,不是最好的选择。NHLBI 整合了来自 4 项基于美国人群的队列研究(社区动脉粥样硬化风险研究,心血管健康研究,健康、衰老和体质研究,动脉粥样硬化多种族研究),比较了基线 FEV_1/FVC<固定阈值范围(0.75~0.65)或<LLN 对于慢阻肺相关事件的识别。研究从 1987—2000 年纳入 45~102 岁共 24 207 例受试者,平均随访 15 年。超过 340 757 人/年随访中,3925 例受试者发生慢阻肺相关事件(每 1000 人/年发病密度为 11.5),其中包括 3563 例慢阻肺相关住院和 447 例慢阻肺相关死亡。与其他固定阈值和 LLN 相比,$FEV_1/FVC<0.70$ 识别慢阻肺相关住院和死亡事件差异均无统计学意义,甚至更加准确,这一研究结果在识别有慢阻肺风险的个体方面又支持了以固定比值作为气流受限的标准。

目前慢阻肺诊断标准的争议在于是否应该将慢阻肺的诊断前移,在受试者未达到慢阻肺的持续气流受限之前确定慢阻肺高危人群,进行干预。

二、诊断的更新实为大势所趋

早在 GOLD 2001 中,便出现了 GOLD 0 期的概念,是指患者肺功能无气流受限,但有慢性咳嗽、咳痰症状,旨在预测这些患者未来很可能会发展为慢阻肺。然而,由于缺少足够的证据显示 GOLD 0 期患者极有可能发展为慢阻肺,于是 2007 年 GOLD 取消了这一分期概念。但近年来大规模的队列研究发现肺通气功能正常者也可存在反复的急性加重,肺部结构性改变及肺功能其他指标异常。部分学者提出 GOLD 0 级应该再回到慢阻肺分级中;但有反对者指出,从肺功能轨迹来看,即使 40 岁前 FEV_1 低于 80%预计值的个体,仅有 1/4 在 22 年后发展为慢阻肺。相比 GOLD 0 概念而言,吸烟仍是慢阻肺的主要危险因素,GOLD 0 患者并不稳定,多达 40%的人 5 年后症状消失,对发展为慢阻肺的预测价值有限;慢性咳嗽、咳痰是许多慢性呼吸系统疾病的共同或前驱症状,将有慢性咳嗽、咳痰症状而无气流受限的群体作为 GOLD 0 期,容易局限人们的思维,可能延误其他呼吸疾病的诊断。在原有 GOLD 0 期定义的基础上进一步丰富内容,可能更具有价值。

COPD gene 2019 研究中建议重新定义慢阻肺的诊断,通过使用危险因素(吸烟)、症状、CT 和肺功能这 4 个疾病特征,按参与者满足特征的数量不同分成 8 类,分别对应无慢阻肺(noCOPD)、疑诊慢阻肺(possible COPD)、拟诊慢阻肺(probable COPD)、确诊慢阻肺(definite COPD)四种诊断。在参与研究的 8784 名受试者中,以目前慢阻肺诊断标准可诊断 46%的慢阻肺患者,而以此研究推荐的诊断标准可诊断出 82%的疑诊、拟诊和确诊慢阻肺患者。建议中摆脱了以单一的气流受限为诊断标准,有助于对受试者进行个性化、精准化治疗,尤其适合无法配合肺功能检查的患者,是慢阻肺早期干预的重大进程,但这种观点能否被学界广泛纳仍有待进一步讨论。

与上述 GOLD 0 期、疑诊及拟诊慢阻肺的概念类似,作为慢阻肺自然病程的起始阶段,"早期慢阻肺"的概念近年来越来越被提及。不同于轻度慢阻肺,早期慢阻肺是指慢阻肺自然病程的初期,即疾病发生之前或尚未产生全部临床影响的时期,是一个时间概念,而非程度概念。研究发现,早期慢阻肺在出现明显症状和肺功能下降前,已存在小气道的严重破坏,导致气道狭窄和增厚。因此,早期识别和诊断对于慢阻肺患者的全病程管理具有重要意义。但由于慢阻肺临床表现的异质性,早期慢阻肺的诊断也存在争议。目前国际对于早期慢阻肺的诊断主要依据 Martinez 等提出的早期慢阻肺可操作性定义:在吸烟史超过 10 包/年、年龄小于 50 岁的人群中,具有至少一项以下标准:①早期气流受限(支气管扩张剂后第 1 秒用力呼气容积/用力肺活量(FEV_1/FVC)小于正常值下限)。②CT 异常(肉眼可见的轻度或中度肺气肿、空气滞留或支气管增厚)。③FEV_1 快速下降(>60ml/年),排除其他已知的慢性肺病,包括间质性肺病等,但不包括哮喘。我国郑劲平教授提出的早期慢阻肺定义则认为症状、肺功能及影像学特征任意符合一条即可诊断:①$FEV_1/FVC<0.7$。②有持续呼吸症状。③胸部 CT 或胸部 X 线片显示肺大疱或肺过度充气。早期慢阻肺对于慢阻肺自然病程的管理和干预存在重要作用,慢阻肺的诊断中若涉及早期的概念,则可更加有效地规范慢阻肺的预防和管理,提高患者生活质量。

三、小 结

尽管学者们对慢阻肺的诊断定义存在争论,但最终目的都是更好地对患者进行分层、个体化管理。慢阻肺疾病本身也具有不同临床表型,不应以单独的检验手段对其进行框定。对于还不能被确诊为慢阻肺的患者,临床医生需要早期关注,密切随访并及时给予干预。同时,可以通过扩大适应证用药等临床试验,对早期疾病机制、药物疗效等进行更深入的研究,以提供循证医学证据,支持慢阻肺诊断标准的更新和完善。

参 考 文 献

[1] 陈亚红. 2020年GOLD慢性阻塞性肺疾病诊断、治疗及预防全球策略解读. 中国医学前沿杂志(电子版),2019,11(12):32-50.

[2] Keener A. Redefining the diagnostic criteria for COPD. Nature,2020,581(7807):S4-S6.

[3] 黄克武,王辰. 慢性阻塞性肺疾病队列研究的概况与思考. 中华结核和呼吸杂志,2016,39(11):910-912.

[4] Regan EA, Lynch DA, Curran-Everett D, et al. Clinical and radiologic disease in smokers with normal spirometry. JAMA Intern Med,2015,175(9):1539-1549.

[5] Woodruff PG, Barr RG, Bleecker E, et al. Clinical significance of symptoms in smokers with preserved pulmonary function. N Engl J Med,2016,374(19):1811-1821.

[6] Çolak Y, Nordestgaard BG, Vestbo J, et al. Prognostic significance of chronic respiratory symptoms in individuals with normal spirometry. Eur Respir J,2019,54(3).

[7] Aaron SD, Tan WC, Bourbeau J, et al. Diagnostic instability and reversals of chronic obstructive pulmonary disease diagnosis in individuals with mild to moderate airflow obstruction. Am J Respir Crit Care Med,2017,196(3):306-314.

[8] 陈亚红. 2018年GOLD慢性阻塞性肺疾病诊断、治疗及预防全球策略解读. 中国医学前沿杂志(电子版),2017,9(12):15-22.

[9] Rennard SI, Drummond MB. Early chronic obstructive pulmonary disease: definition, assessment, and prevention. The Lancet,2015,385(9979):1778-1788.

[10] Jian W, Gao Y, Hao C, et al. Reference values for spirometry in Chinese aged 4-80 years. J Thorac Dis,2017,9(11):4538-4549.

[11] Bhatt SP, Balte PP, Schwartz JE, et al. Discriminative accuracy of FEV1:FVC thresholds for COPD-related hospitalization and mortality. JAMA,2019,321(24):2438-2447.

[12] Lange P, Celli B, Agusti A, et al. Lung function trajectories leading to chronic obstructive pulmonary disease. N Engl J Med,2015,373(2):111-122.

[13] Vestbo J, Lange P. Can GOLD Stage 0 provide information of prognostic value in chronic obstructive pulmonary disease?. Am J Respir Crit Care Med,2002,166(3):329-332.

[14] Lowe KE, Regan EA, Anzueto A, et al. COPDGene® 2019: Redefining the diagnosis of chronic obstructive pulmonary disease. Chron Obstr Pulm Dis,2019,6(5):384-399.

[15] Agusti A, Celli B. Natural history of COPD: gaps and opportunities. ERJ Open Res,2017,3(4).

[16] Martinez FJ, Han MK, Allinson JP, et al. At the Root: Defining and halting progression of early chronic obstructive pulmonary disease. Am J Respir Crit Care Med,2018,197(12):1540-1551.

[17] Zheng J. Early diagnosis and treatment of chronic obstructive pulmonary disease(in Chinese). Chin J Gener Pract,2018,17(7):504-507.

21 HFNC 及 NPPV 在慢性阻塞性肺疾病急性加重期治疗中的地位与选择

李亚清

慢性阻塞性肺疾病急性加重(acute exacerbation of chronic obstructive pulmonary disease,AECOPD)是慢性阻塞性肺疾病(简称慢阻肺)病程中的重要事件,其特征是呼吸困难、咳嗽、咳痰等呼吸道症状急性恶化,需要增加额外的治疗。慢阻肺急性加重导致患者肺功能恶化、生活质量下降、病情急剧进展及死亡风险显著增加。无创正压通气(non-invasive positive pressure ventilation,NPPV)是目前慢阻肺急性加重合并Ⅱ型呼吸衰竭患者首选的呼吸支持方式,可改善患者呼吸性酸中毒,降低 $PaCO_2$、呼吸频率、呼吸困难程度,缩短住院时间,降低气管插管率和病死率等,同时也能避免气道损伤、减低呼吸机相关性肺炎的发生及镇静剂的使用等。尽管如此,部分患者由于幽闭恐惧、焦虑不安、皮肤破损或皮疹、排痰障碍、口鼻咽干燥、眼睛刺激、胃胀气等因素仍拒绝或不能耐受 NPPV,其失败率达 16%～20%。经鼻高流量湿化氧疗(high-flow nasal cannula oxygen therapy,HFNC)是指一种通过高流量鼻塞持续为患者提供可以调控并相对恒定吸氧浓度(21%～100%)、温度(31～37℃)和湿度的高流量(8～80 L/min)吸入气体的治疗方式。该治疗设备主要包括空氧混合装置、湿化治疗仪、高流量鼻塞及连接呼吸管路。因此,与传统氧疗相比,HFNC 供氧浓度更精确,加温湿化效果更好。2000 年 HFNC 开始应用于临床,2014 年进入中国内地,至今短短 6 年时间,HFNC 已得到快速普及推广。目前 HFNC 临床应用的适应证和禁忌证尚无统一的标准。已有临床研究证明了 HFNC 在轻中度单纯低氧性呼吸衰竭(Ⅰ型呼吸衰竭)的治疗价值,其对轻中度Ⅰ型呼吸衰竭患者具有明确的治疗效果。但 HFNC 在慢阻肺急性加重治疗中的作用需要进一步研究,因此,临床上如何把握 HFNC 的适应证和禁忌证需要认真考虑。

一、慢阻肺急性加重期病理生理改变

慢阻肺的基本肺功能改变包括气流受限、肺容积最大和换气功能减退等,小气道结构病变及周围弹性纤维组织破坏,产生气体陷闭。慢阻肺急性加重期由于气道分泌物潴留、气道阻力增加,肺弹性回缩力下降、呼吸期气道陷闭,形成动态肺过度充气,导致内源性呼气末气道正压(iPEEP)升高。

二、HFNC 治疗慢阻肺急性加重的生理学机制

(一)呼气末正压(positive end expiratory pressure,PEEP)效应

HFNC 通过输送高流速气体的方式维持一定水平的 PEEP,从而对抗慢阻肺急性加重患者由于 DPH 肺泡内产生的 iPEEP,使吸气阻力明显下降,有效地减低呼吸做功,缓解呼吸疲劳,降低氧耗量。Corley 等研究发现心脏术后患者使用 HFNC 组平均口咽部的压力为 4.4 cmH_2O,HFNC 通过高流量产生的 PEEP 作用促进肺复张。HFNC 流速每增加 10 L/min,患者咽腔 PEEP 就增加 0.5～1 cmH_2O。流速增加到 60 L/min 时,闭口的女性受试者咽腔 PEEP 可达到 8.7 cmH_2O 左右,男性为 5.4 cmH_2O,张口呼吸情况下女性为 3.1 cmH_2O,男性为 2.6 cmH_2O 左右。因此,HFNC 的 PEEP 效应与流量、是否闭口相关。

(二)生理无效腔冲刷效应,促进二氧化碳(CO_2)排出

HFNC 通过为患者提供恒定的、可调节的高流速空氧混合气体,冲刷慢阻肺急性加重患者呼气末残留在鼻腔、口腔及咽部的气体,减少生理性无效腔。Moller 等采用红外二氧化碳吸收光谱放射性氚 γ 相机成像技术证实了 HFNC 对于 CO_2 清除,并且随着流量的增加,CO_2 清除率增加。

(三)降低患者上气道阻力和呼吸功

HFNC 全过程高流量恒温恒湿,提供满足患者吸气需求流速的高流量氧气。患者在吸气时不需要用力吸气及对吸入气体进行加温加湿。因此,HFNC 不仅可以降低吸气阻力,同时为患者提供精确稳定的吸氧浓度,有利于改善慢阻肺急性加重患者氧合,使患者呼吸更舒适,避免患者对吸入气体进行温化湿化所需的代谢消耗,从而降低患者呼吸功。

(四)维持黏液纤毛清除系统功能

HFNC 精确的恒温和恒湿的高流量氧疗,可降低干冷气体对上下呼吸道黏液纤毛系统功能和黏膜的影响,有助于慢阻肺急性加重患者稀释痰液和排痰,修复和维持其呼吸道上皮细胞和纤毛的结构和功能,不仅提高了其舒适度,同时降低了患者下呼吸道感染的发生概率。

三、HFNC 和 NPPV 的异同点

HFNC 和 NPPV 都是电动涡轮机驱动形成高速气流，通过电磁阀实现流量控制、气流加温加湿，并维持一定水平的 PEEP，实现气道开放，减少无效腔，改善通气。HFNC 和 NPPV 的不同点如表 2-21-1。

表 2-21-1 HFNC 和 NPPV 的不同点对比

项目	HFNC	NPPV
连接方式	主要通过鼻塞进行氧疗	口鼻面罩、鼻罩、全脸罩
压力支持	高流量,不稳定的气道正压,辅助通气效果有限	通气模式及参数多且稳定,如 BiPAP、PCV 等
漏气	允许较低漏量,漏气较多会影响治疗效果	允许一定量漏气,漏气多会严重影响人机同步
人机配合	基本不需要人机配合及吸呼切换	同步性、协同性要求高,尤其重症患者对呼吸机的要求高,呼吸之间人机同步直接决定治疗成败
舒适度	舒适感较好	舒适感较差,有幽闭感
气道保护	有利于患者咳痰和气道保护	重症患者要注意气道保护和湿化问题
治疗目标	恒温、恒湿、恒流、恒氧	主要关注于改善患者通气与换气功能,解决低氧和高碳酸血症,缓解呼吸肌疲劳
适应患者	主要适用于轻中度Ⅰ型呼吸衰竭患者,对Ⅱ型呼吸衰竭患者应用需把握适应证	Ⅰ型和Ⅱ型急慢性呼吸衰竭患者

注：HFNC：经鼻高流量湿化氧疗；NPPV：无创正压通气；BiPAP：双水平正压通气；PCV：压力控制通气

四、HFNC 在慢阻肺急性加重期治疗中临床研究进展

（一）HFNC 治疗慢阻肺急性加重的时机选择

目前 HFNC 治疗慢阻肺合并Ⅱ型呼吸衰竭缺乏大样本、多中心随机研究。对于意识清楚的急性低氧血症合并高碳酸血症患者，可在密切监测下使用 HFNC，若患者病情加重，建议立即更换 NPPV 或气管插管。Yuste 等针对 HFNC 治疗急性Ⅱ型呼吸衰竭患者的有效性、安全性进行研究，其招募 95 名患者，根据病情分为中度呼吸衰竭 75 例及重度呼吸衰竭 20 例。重度呼吸衰竭患者需满足 MOD>2,pH<7.25 的条件，可直接给予有创机械通气治疗；中度呼吸衰竭患者应满足 pH 7.25~7.35、SpO₂ 88%~92%，其中 35 例给予 HFNC 治疗，40 例给予 NPPV 治疗。35 例 HFNC 治疗患者中有 5 例被排除，30 例进入临床研究，其中 26 例 HFNC 治疗成功，患者 pH 从 7.28±0.02 改善为 7.37±0.01,4 例患者治疗无效，其中 1 例调整为 NPPV 治疗,3 例接受气管插管有创机械通气治疗。因此，作为 NPPV 及有创机械通气的替代方案，HFNC 治疗中度急性Ⅱ型呼吸衰竭是安全、有效的，且与 NPPV（气管插管率 18%~28%；住院病死率 10%~13%）相比，其气管插管率（10%）及住院病死率（6.6%）更低。HFNC 为慢阻肺患者在普通氧疗与 NPPV 治疗之间提供了更多的选择。HFNC 治疗慢阻肺急性加重的时机选择非常重要。对于 pH>7.35、PCO₂>45 mmHg 的慢阻肺急性加重患者可以常规给予 HFNC 治疗。对于轻中度呼吸性酸中毒（7.25<pH<7.35）和存在显著呼吸困难（辅助呼吸肌参与、呼吸频率>25 次/min）慢阻肺急性加重患者，可以在密切观察下给予 HFNC 治疗，如患者临床表现无明显改善或病情加重需及时调整为 NPPV 或有创机械通气治疗。对于慢阻肺急性加重合并严重高碳酸性呼吸衰竭（pH<7.25）患者可直接有创机械通气治疗，应避免使用 HFNC 延误治疗时机。

（二）HFNC 治疗慢阻肺急性加重的临床证据

Pilcher 等将 24 例慢阻肺急性加重患者随机分为 HFNC 及普通鼻导管氧疗两组。HFNC 组给予 35 L/min HFNC 氧疗，两组 SpO₂ 维持在 94% 左右，两组均治疗 30 min 后测经皮 CO₂ 分压等，结果表明 HFNC 组经皮 PCO₂ 较普通鼻导管吸氧组显著下降，两组 SpO₂ 无显著性统计学差异。Lee 等对比研究 HFNC 和 NPPV 在 88 例慢阻肺急性加重合并中度Ⅱ型呼吸衰竭患者中的治疗作用，其研究发现：HFNC 和 NPPV 治疗 24h 后，两组患者在 pH、PaO₂、PaCO₂ 等方面均无显著性差异，且 HFNC 和 NPPV 两组患者在 30d 病死率和气管插管率方面无显著性统计学差异。Plotnikow 等报道了一位慢阻肺急性加重合并Ⅱ型呼吸衰竭患者由于面部畸形使用 NPPV 治疗失败，改为流量 50 L/min HFNC 治疗后，患者高碳酸血症及呼吸性酸中毒均得到改善。Bräunlich 等运用 HFNC 治疗 38 例慢阻肺急性加重合并Ⅱ型呼吸衰竭、且不耐受 NPPV 治疗的患者。治疗期间吸气流量为 (25.8±8.2) L/min，治疗时间为 (195±23) min；治疗后 PaCO₂ 水平从 (67.6±12.9) mmHg 降至 (58.5±9.7) mmHg，pH 水平从 7.339±0.041 升至 7.392±0.048。其结果表明 HFNC 对轻到中度慢阻肺急性加重合并Ⅱ型呼吸衰竭患者具有一定的积极治疗作用。在序贯撤机方面，Fernandez 等研究发现：与普通吸氧相比，HFNC 应用于慢阻肺急性加重患者序贯撤机明显降低膈肌电活动和呼吸功耗，更有利于慢阻肺患者康复，显著降低了再次气管插管

风险。Thille 等研究表明：与 NPPV 序贯治疗组相比，不合并高碳酸血症的慢阻肺急性加重患者在应用 HFNC 序贯撤机再插管风险上的差异无统计学意义，但对于高碳酸血症患者，HFNC 治疗再次气管插管风险增加。

五、HFNC 治疗慢阻肺急性加重的注意事项

对于慢阻肺急性加重患者，HFNC 流量初始设置可为 20～30 L/min，根据其耐受性和依从性调节。如果患者二氧化碳潴留明显，流量可设置在 45～55 L/min 甚至更高，达到患者能耐受的最大流量；FiO_2 设置的目标是使 SpO_2 维持在 88%～92%，结合血气分析动态调整；温度设置范围 31～37℃，依据患者舒适性和耐受度，以及痰液黏稠度适当调节。当原发病控制后逐渐降低 HFNC 参数，如果达到吸气流量 < 20 L/min、FiO_2 < 30% 时可考虑撤离 HFNC。制订合理的气道管理方案：HFNC 上机前应和患者充分交流，患者应尽量闭口呼吸，半卧位或头高位（> 20°）。在 HFNC 治疗过程中应重视温湿化、痰液引流、胸部物理治疗和雾化吸入等方法的联合应用。避免湿化过度或湿化不足而发生痰堵窒息，按需吸痰。鼻塞位置高度应高于机器和管路水平，及时发现并处理管路积水现象，警惕误入气道引起呛咳和误吸。HFNC 相关院感预防控制：HFNC 附件一人一用。HFNC 装置使用前后需终末消毒。HFNC 鼻导管、湿化罐及管路为一次性物品，按医疗垃圾丢弃。HFNC 的空气过滤纸片应定期更换，建议 3 个月或 1000 h 更换 1 次。

六、小 结

对慢阻肺合并轻中度急性低氧性呼吸衰竭患者，HFNC 可作为普通氧疗或 NPPV 的替代治疗方案，其耐受性好。HFNC 能改善慢阻肺患者肺通气、改善高碳酸血症。对于慢阻肺急性加重合并轻中度呼吸性酸中毒（pH：7.25～7.35）者，HFNC 临床疗效不劣于 NPPV。目前仍需要大样本、多中心、随机研究以阐明 HFNC 与普通氧疗、NPPV 在慢阻肺合并急性低氧性或高碳酸血症呼吸衰竭治疗中的疗效。

参 考 文 献

[1] Global strategy for the diagnosis, management and prevention of chronic obstructive pulmonary disease 2020 report. https://goldcopd.org/gold-reports/.

[2] Suissa S, Dell'Aniello S, Ernst P. Long-term natural history of chronic obstructive pulmonary disease: severe exacerbations and mortality. Thorax, 2012, 67: 957-963.

[3] de Miguel-Diez J, Jiménez-García R, Hernández-Barrera V, et al. Trends in the use and outcomes of mechanical ventilation among patients hospitalized with acute exacerbations of COPD in Spain, 2001 to 2015. J Clin Med, 2019, 8(10): 1621.

[4] Wedzicha JAEC-C, Miravitlles M, Hurst JR, et al. Management of COPD exacerbations: a European Respiratory Society/American Thoracic Society guideline. Eur Respir J, 2017, 49: 1600791.

[5] Crisafulli E, Barbeta E, Ielpo A, et al. Management of severe acute exacerbations of COPD: an updated narrative review. Multidiscip Respir Med, 2018, 13: 36.

[6] Keenan SP, Sinuff T, Burns KE, et al. Clinical practice guidelines for the use of noninvasive positive-pressure ventilation and noninvasive continuous positive airway pressure in the acute care setting. CMAJ, 2011, 183(3): 195-214.

[7] Shah NM, D'Cruz RF, Murphy PB. Update: non-invasive ventilation in chronic obstructive pulmonary disease. J Thorac Dis, 2018, 10(Suppl 1): S71-S79.

[8] 中华医学会呼吸病学分会呼吸危重症医学学组. 成人经鼻高流量湿化氧疗临床规范应用专家共识. 中华结核和呼吸杂志, 2019, 42(2): 83-91.

[9] Frat JP, Thille AW, Mercat A, et al. High-flow oxygen through nasal cannula in acute hypoxemic respiratory failure. N Engl J Med, 2015, 372: 2185-2196.

[10] Ischaki E, Pantazopoulos I, Zakynthinos S. Nasal high flow therapy: a novel treatment rather than a more expensive oxygen device. Eur Respir Rev, 2017, 26(145): 170028.

[11] Spoletini G, Alotaibi M, Blasi F, et al. Heated humidified high-flow nasal oxygen in adults: mechanisms of action and clinical implications. Chest, 2015, 148: 253-261.

[12] Corley A, Caruana LR, Barnett AG, et al. Oxygen delivery through high-flow nasal cannulae increase end-expiratory lung volume and reduce respiratory rate in post-cardiac surgical patients. Br J Anaesth, 2011, 107: 998-1004.

[13] Moller W, Celik G, Feng S, et al. Nasal high flow clears anatomical dead space in upper airway models. J Appl Physiol (1985), 2015, 118: 1525-1523.

[14] Yuste ME, Moreno O, Narbona S, et al. Efficacy and safety of high-flow nasal cannula oxygen therapy in moderate acute hypercapnic respiratory failure. Rev Bras Ter Intensiva, 2019, 31(2): 156-163.

[15] Pilcher J, Eastlake L, Richards M, et al. Physiological effects of titrated oxygen via nasal high-flow cannulae in COPD exacerbations: a randomized controlled cross-over trial. Respirology, 2017, 22: 1149-1155.

[16] Lee MK, Choi J, Park B, et al. High flow nasal cannulae oxygen therapy in acute-moderate hypercapnic respiratory failure. Clin Respir J, 2018, 12: 2046-2056.

[17] Plotnikow G, Thille AW, Vasquez D, et al. High-flow nasal cannula oxygen for reverting severe acute exacerbation of chronic obstructive pulmonary disease: A case report. Med Intensiva, 2017, 41(9): 571-572.

[18] Bräunlich J, Wirtz H. Nasal high-flow in acute hypercapnic exacerbation of COPD. Int J Chron Obstruct Pulmon Dis, 2018, 30(13): 3895-3897.

[19] Fernandez R, Subira C, Frutos-Vivar F, et al. High-flow nasal

cannula to prevent postextubation respiratory failure in high-risk non-hypercapnic patients: a randomized multicenter trial. Ann Intensive Care, 2017, 7:47.

[20] Thille AW, Muller G, Gacouin A, et al. Effect of postextubation high-flow nasal oxygen with noninvasive ventilation vs high-flow nasal oxygen alone on reintubation among patients at highrisk of extubation failure: a randomized clinical trial. JAMA, 2019, 322(15):1465-1475.

第三部分

支气管哮喘

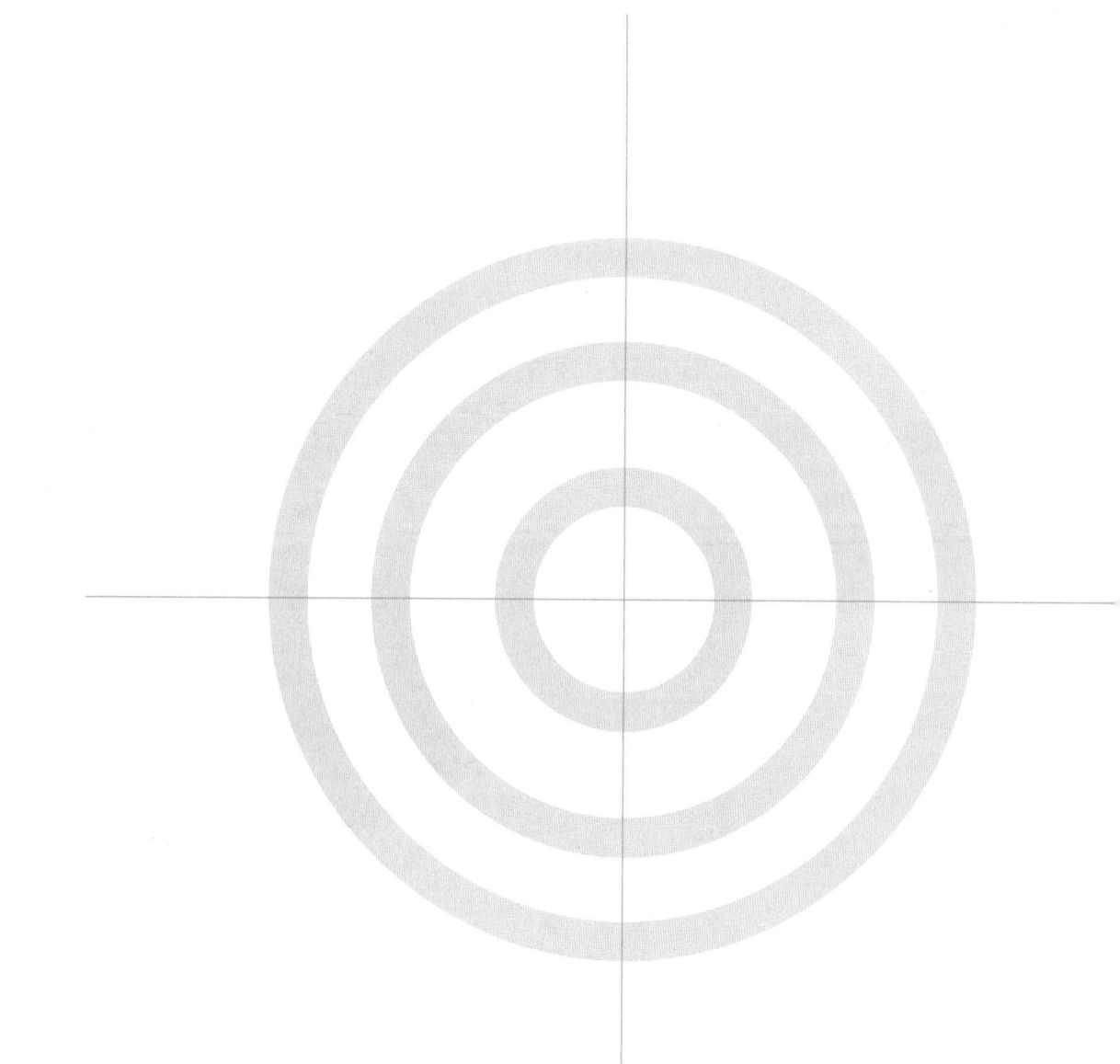

1 《成人和青少年咳嗽型哮喘和嗜酸性粒细胞性支气管炎(NAEB)》——ACCP指南解读

詹 晨　陈玥晗　许婷婷　蒋紫玉　詹文志　赖克方

美国胸科医师协会(ACCP)颁布的咳嗽指南是目前最具有权威、普及度最广的指南。其内容十分丰富,不仅从整体上阐述了咳嗽的诊断和治疗方法,还对不同病因的咳嗽设立了独立的章节进行阐述,包括咳嗽型哮喘、嗜酸粒细胞性支气管炎、胃食管反流性咳嗽、难治性慢性咳嗽等。同时指南持续更新,从2006年起至今已经先后颁布70余篇。指南采用循证医学法产生循证建议,并进行分级。咳嗽型哮喘和嗜酸性粒细胞性支气管炎(NAEB)是成人及青少年慢性咳嗽的常见病因,2006年版ACCP已经对两种病因进行了阐述。随着相关研究的开展,为对咳嗽型哮喘和NAEB的诊断治疗意见修订提供了参考。本篇主要解读2019年版ACCP《成人和青少年咳嗽型哮喘和嗜酸粒性支气管炎(NAEB)》指南提出的热点问题。

一、定 义

哮喘是由多种细胞及细胞组分参与的气道慢性炎症性疾病,临床表现为反复发作的咳嗽、胸闷、气急或喘息等症状,同时伴有可变的气流受限和气道高反应性。咳嗽伴随喘息、呼吸困难、胸闷等症状,但是咳嗽也可以作为哮喘的唯一症状(咳嗽变异性哮喘,CVA)或主要症状。

Gibson在1989年报道了7例慢性咳嗽患者,诱导痰嗜酸性粒细胞增生、对糖皮质激素治疗反应良好,但肺通气功能正常、无气道高反应性,因无法诊断为哮喘,被称之为非哮喘性嗜酸粒细胞性支气管炎(NAEB)。

二、流行病学与发病机制

哮喘被认为是慢性咳嗽的主要病因之一,多项研究显示24%~32%的非吸烟慢性咳嗽患者的咳嗽与哮喘相关。鉴于大多数慢咳流行病学调查研究中未应用诱导痰细胞学检查,无法明确NAEB的诊断,因此NAEB的人群患病率尚不明确。在呼吸专科门诊的慢性咳嗽患者中,NAEB的患病率为10%~30%。

哮喘和NAEB的病因尚未清楚,基因与环境的相互作用起重要作用,可能与吸入性变应原或职业性环境暴露有关。两种疾病的病理生理学改变相似,包括相似的诱导痰、肺泡灌洗液及气道黏膜嗜酸性性细胞炎症程度和一定的气道基底膜增厚。然而肥大细胞在两者气道平滑肌束中的浸润程度不同,哮喘患者气道平滑肌束中肥大细胞浸润程度较NAEB更重,这可能部分解释了为何虽然两者存在相似的气道嗜酸性粒细胞性气道炎症,但NAEB无气道高反应性和可变性气流受限。

关于哮喘和NAEB的自然病程尚缺乏全面的研究。对143例EB患者进行长达10年的临床观察,发现高达60%的患者曾出现复发,有的患者甚至出现多次复发。过敏性鼻炎和持续性气道嗜酸性粒细胞炎症是复发的高危因素。5.7% NAEB患者发展为轻度哮喘,但这一比例与普通人群的哮喘患病率基本接近。所有随访患者没有出现明显的进行性或不可逆的肺功能下降,FEV_1长期保持稳定,但小气道功能有所下降,提示NAEB可能是一种独立性的呼吸道疾病。成年及青少年群体的CVA患者中17%~31%的患者会发展为典型哮喘,但目前针对CVA预后的研究样本量较小,后续仍需要大样本研究以探究CVA的预后。

三、制订方法

2006版ACCP咳嗽指南推荐抗炎治疗作为两种疾病的主要治疗方法。该指南推荐对于疑似NAEB或激素治疗咳嗽无改善的哮喘患者,应进行无创性气道炎症检查,但是该推荐证据等级较低。此次更新的ACCP指南旨在评价无创性气道炎症检查,包括外周血细胞计数、诱导痰细胞学分类和呼出一氧化氮(FeNO)在评估咳嗽型哮喘及NAEB方面的作用。此次更新的ACCP指南继续沿用循证医学法,遵循PICOS原则提出临床问题,经过文献检索、质量评估,最终针对"咳嗽型哮喘患者的气道炎症的无创性评估方法""咳嗽型哮喘的最佳治疗手段""嗜酸性粒细胞性支气管炎的最佳治疗手段"三个临床问题分别筛选出3篇、53篇、6篇研究并进行系统评价。证据参考GRADE方法分为"A高,B中,C低或极低"3个质量等级。推荐意见综合考虑患者获益与风险分为"1-强推荐"和"2-弱推荐"2个级别。对于证据质量极低或者缺乏证据支持的问题可参考专家组共识,但是其并不归为推荐意见。

四、主要推荐意见与解析

(一)无创性气道炎症检查在评估咳嗽型哮喘中的作用

在成人及青少年哮喘相关慢性咳嗽患者中进行无创性气道炎症检查,存在气道嗜酸性粒细胞性炎症的哮喘相关慢性咳嗽患者对糖皮质激素可能具有更好的治疗反应(Grade 2B)。

既往研究已证实无创性气道炎症检查在哮喘尤其是重症哮喘中的作用,其可以预测哮喘患者对糖皮质激素治疗的反应性,证据评级为中等。但是关于无创性气道炎症检查在咳嗽型哮喘的研究报道较少。本次系统评价最终仅纳入3项研究,偏倚风险小,但纳入研究样本量小,提示这一临床问题仍缺乏高质量的证据。现有结果提示无创性气道炎症检查有助于预测咳嗽患者对糖皮质激素治疗的反应性。诱导痰高嗜酸性粒细胞水平、高嗜酸性粒细胞阳离子蛋白浓度、高FeNO值均提示咳嗽型哮喘患者对吸入型糖皮质激素(ICS)的治疗反应性更好。而无创性气道炎症检查结果对孟鲁司特、扎鲁司特等药物的疗效无明显预测作用。虽然国内外哮喘指南将无创性气道炎症检查纳入诊疗规范中,但是受限于技术、成本等因素,无创性气道炎症检查,尤其是诱导痰细胞学检查,仍未被广泛应用。另外,在典型哮喘人群中建立的评估气道炎症无创性检查的临界值能否适用到咳嗽型哮喘人群仍值得探讨。不同于之前版本指南中所推荐的"对吸入性激素治疗效果不佳的患者需进一步进行气道炎症检查",本次ACCP指南推荐"在成人及青少年哮喘相关慢性咳嗽患者中进行无创性气道炎症检查,存在气道嗜酸性粒细胞性炎症的哮喘相关慢性咳嗽患者对糖皮质激素可能具有更好的治疗反应(Grade 2B)"。进一步突出了无创气道炎症检测的地位。

(二)咳嗽型哮喘的最佳治疗方案

推荐在成人及青少年咳嗽型哮喘患者中,如果以咳嗽作为唯一症状,建议使用ICS作为一线治疗。若CVA对ICS治疗反应不佳或哮喘患者经过ICS治疗后胸闷、喘息症状缓解但是咳嗽仍在持续,重新评估并排除了慢性咳嗽的其他病因后,推荐升级ICS剂量,或联合白三烯受体拮抗剂治疗,或联合β受体激动剂(Grade 1B)。

旧版ACCP咳嗽型哮喘指南指出若咳嗽症状经过糖皮质激素治疗明显改善,则可明确咳嗽型哮喘诊断。新版ACCP指南在旧版基础上纳入了更多的研究,然而纳入研究存在较高的偏倚风险,样本量中等(共53篇)。现有结果显示ICS及白三烯受体拮抗剂能够降低哮喘患者治疗前后的咳嗽评分或咳嗽次数,且各项研究结果具有一致性。另有2项研究观察到哮喘患者使用吸入性β受体激动剂获益。既往有研究报道茶碱类药物、肥大细胞稳定剂亦可不同程度改善咳嗽症状,但为很多年前的研究,证据评级低。而对于抗组胺类药物是否能改善哮喘患者咳嗽症状,研究结果则不一致。在一项对哮喘患者的单中心小样本研究中,相较于安慰剂组,使用美泊利单抗并不能有效降低VAS评分,然而本研究未说明纳入的哮喘患者本身是否有慢性咳嗽。对于生物制剂在咳嗽型哮喘的疗效仍需要更多研究。对比之前指南推荐的ICS+支气管扩张剂治疗咳嗽型哮喘,本次ACCP指南推荐在成人及青少年咳嗽型哮喘患者中,如果以咳嗽作为唯一症状,建议使用ICS作为一线治疗。若CVA对ICS治疗反应不佳或者哮喘患者经过ICS治疗后胸闷、喘息症状缓解但是咳嗽仍在持续,推荐升级ICS剂量,同时重新评估并排除了慢性咳嗽的其他病因后,可联合白三烯拮抗剂治疗,或联合β受体激动剂治疗(Grade 1B)。因此,新版指南没有强调ICS与β受体激动剂的联合治疗。

(三)NAEB咳嗽的最佳治疗方案

在成人及青少年NAEB患者中使用ICS作为首选治疗(Grade 2B)。

在成人及青少年NAEB患者中,若患者对ICS治疗反应不佳,在经重新评估并排除了慢性咳嗽的其他病因后,建议升级ICS剂量,或联合白三烯受体拮抗剂治疗。

目前关于NAEB治疗的研究较少,本次系统评价共纳入6篇研究,纳入研究存在较高的偏倚风险,样本量偏小。现有研究结果显示ICS及白三烯受体拮抗剂可显著改善NAEB患者咳嗽症状。一项研究显示抗组胺药物对于NAEB患者咳嗽有一定改善。目前未有对于NAEB的生物免疫治疗的研究报道。本次指南推荐在成人及青少年NAEB患者中使用ICS作为首选治疗(Grade 2B),若治疗反应不佳,建议在升级ICS剂量,经重新评估并排除了慢性咳嗽的其他病因后可联合白三烯拮抗剂治疗。新版指南肯定了白三烯受体拮抗剂对NAEB的治疗作用(Grade 2C)。

五、与中国指南、ERS咳嗽指南的异同

《中国慢性咳嗽诊治指南(2015版)》及《ERS成人和儿童慢性咳嗽诊治指南(2019版)》针对ACCP提出的3点临床问题也进行了部分阐述。中国咳嗽指南和ERS咳嗽指南均肯定了无创性气道炎症检查在评估咳嗽型哮喘中的作用,认为所有的慢性咳嗽患者需要评估是否存在嗜酸性粒细胞性炎症,诱导痰嗜酸性粒细胞是反映慢性咳嗽患者是否存在嗜酸性粒细胞性炎症最精准的指标并且能够指导治疗。同时,ERS咳嗽指南也指出FeNO、外周血嗜酸性粒细胞计数能够作为在无法开展诱导痰检查时评估气道嗜酸性粒细胞性炎症的替代检查,但是关于FeNO、外周血嗜酸性粒细胞计数能否预测慢性咳嗽患者对激素或白三烯受体拮抗剂的反应性,目前缺乏高质量的证据,需要开展更多的RCT研究,另外FeNO在慢性咳嗽患者的界值也需要建立。关于咳嗽型哮喘、NAEB的最佳治疗方案,中国咳嗽指南与ACCP咳嗽指南建议基本相符,其中中国指南建议咳嗽型哮喘患者使用ICS和支气管扩张剂联用(1B),除了白三烯受体拮抗剂,短期口服糖皮质激素(10~20 mg/d,3~5 d)也可用于对ICS治疗不敏感的咳嗽型哮喘患者(2C)。ICS仍然作为NAEB的一线用药。ERS咳嗽指南依据治疗特征的相似性将NAEB与咳嗽变异性哮喘、典型哮喘统一归为咳嗽型哮喘,指出单用ICS或ICS联

合支气管扩张药在治疗咳嗽型哮喘的疗效需要进一步评估。建议对成人慢性咳嗽尤其是咳嗽型哮喘患者进行短疗程(2～4周)抗白三烯治疗(推荐,低质量)。由于ERS指南建议主要针对所有慢性咳嗽患者,因此没有专门针对NAEB、咳嗽型哮喘的治疗推荐意见。

六、结 语

在过去的10年间,关于哮喘尤其是重症哮喘治疗的国际指南在循证医学上有很大的更新。无创性气道炎症检查,尤其是呼出气一氧化氮(FeNO)和诱导痰细胞学检查在各项更新指南中被推荐应用于哮喘的辅助诊断,但更多是为了确定炎症表型,以便精准治疗。相较于典型哮喘研究中有大量高质量研究支持嗜酸性气道炎症指标对哮喘的诊断及治疗有着极好的指导作用,目前对于无创性气道炎症检查在咳嗽型哮喘和NAEB中的诊断及治疗的指导地位仍缺少高质量研究支持。虽然近年已逐渐将咳嗽症状纳入了哮喘研究中,但咳嗽始终作为与其他呼吸道症状如呼吸困难、喘息、气促的伴随症状而提及,且在哮喘控制问卷和哮喘控制评分中并无单独针对咳嗽的评估条目。目前仍缺乏针对咳嗽型哮喘人群的高质量研究以及将咳嗽特异性检查作为观察指标的临床干预性研究。

本次ACCP指南更新了无创性气道炎症检查手段在咳嗽型哮喘和NAEB的评估作用及对咳嗽型哮喘和NAEB的治疗建议。但值得注意的是,目前缺乏高质量的研究,现有的建议更多是参考了对典型哮喘管理的证据,本次推荐建议的证据等级偏低。因此,希望针对国内外同行积极开展高质量的多中心咳嗽型哮喘、NAEB相关的气道炎症与治疗研究,为咳嗽指南的更新提供更多高质量的循证依据。

附:《成人和青少年咳嗽型哮喘和嗜酸性粒细胞性支气管炎(NAEB)》—ACCP指南撰写专家: Andreanne Côté, Richard J Russell, Louis-Philippe Boulet, Peter G Gibson, Kefang Lai, Richard S. Irwin, Christopher E. Brightling, on behalf of the CHEST Expert Cough Panel。

参 考 文 献

[1] Gibson PG, et al. Chronic cough: eosinophilic bronchitis without asthma. Lancet, 1989. 1(8651):1346-1348.

[2] Brightling CE, et al. Eosinophilic bronchitis is an important cause of chronic cough. Am J Respir Crit Care Med, 1999. 160(2):406-410.

[3] Carney IK, et al. A systematic evaluation of mechanisms in chronic cough. Am J Respir Crit Care Med, 1997, 156(1): 211-216.

[4] Ayik SO, et al. Eosinophilic bronchitis as a cause of chronic cough. Respir Med, 2003, 97(6): 695-701.

[5] Irwin RS, FJ Curley, CL French. Chronic cough. The spectrum and frequency of causes, key components of the diagnostic evaluation, and outcome of specific therapy. Am Rev Respir Dis, 1990. 141(3): 640-647.

[6] McGarvey LP, et al. Evaluation and outcome of patients with chronic non-productive cough using a comprehensive diagnostic protocol. Thorax, 1998, 53(9): 738-743.

[7] Lai K, et al. A prospective, multicenter survey on causes of chronic cough in China. Chest, 2013, 143(3): 613-620.

[8] Lemiere C, A. Efthimiadis, FE Hargreave. Occupational eosinophilic bronchitis without asthma: an unknown occupational airway disease. J Allergy Clin Immunol, 1997, 100(6 Pt 1): 852-853.

[9] Brightling CE, et al. Comparison of airway immunopathology of eosinophilic bronchitis and asthma. Thorax, 2003, 58(6): 528-532.

[10] Gibson PG, et al. Chronic cough resembles asthma with IL-5 and granulocyte-macrophage colony-stimulating factor gene expression in bronchoalveolar cells. J Allergy Clin Immunol, 1998, 101(3): 320-326.

[11] Brightling CE, et al. Mast-cell infiltration of airway smooth muscle in asthma. N Engl J Med, 2002, 346(22): 1699-1705.

[12] Siddiqui S, et al. Airway hyperresponsiveness is dissociated from airway wall structural remodeling. J Allergy Clin Immunol, 2008, 122(2): 335-341.

[13] Lai K, et al. Will nonasthmatic eosinophilic bronchitis develop into chronic airway obstruction?: a prospective, observational study. Chest, 2015, 148(4): 887-894.

[14] Matsumoto H, et al. Prognosis of cough variant asthma: a retrospective analysis. J Asthma, 2006, 43(2): 131-135.

[15] Fujimura M, et al. Predictors for typical asthma onset from cough variant asthma. J Asthma, 2005, 42(2): 107-111.

[16] Lewis SZ, et al. Methodologies for the development of CHEST guidelines and expert panel reports. Chest, 2014, 146(1): 182-192.

[17] Lewis SZ, et al. Methodologies for the development of the management of cough: CHEST guideline and expert panel report. Chest, 2014, 146(5): 1395-1402.

[18] Takemura M, et al. Clinical, physiological and anti-inflammatory effect of montelukast in patients with cough variant asthma. Respiration, 2012, 83(4): 308-315.

[19] Tamaoki J, et al. Comparable effect of a leukotriene receptor antagonist and long-acting beta (2)-adrenergic agonist in cough variant asthma. Allergy Asthma Proc, 2010, 31(5): 78-84.

[20] Chaudhuri R, et al. Effect of inhaled corticosteroids on symptom severity and sputum mediator levels in chronic persistent cough. J Allergy Clin Immunol, 2004, 113(6): 1063-1070.

[21] Boyd G, S. Abdallah, R. Clark. Twice or four times daily beclomethasone dipropionate in mild stable asthma? Clin Allergy, 1985, 15(4): 383-389.

[22] Fyans PG, PC Chatterjee, SS Chatterjee. A trial comparing nedocromil sodium (Tilade) and placebo in the management of bronchial asthma. Clin Allergy, 1986, 16(6): 505-511.

[23] Boe J, O. Thulesius. Treatment of steroid-dependent asthma with beclomethaxone dipropionate administered by aerosol. Curr Ther Res Clin Exp, 1975, 17(5): 460-466.

[24] Clancy L, S. Keogan. Treatment of nocturnal asthma with nedocromil sodium. Thorax, 1994, 49(12): 1225-1227.

[25] Rafferty P, et al. Terfenadine, a potent histamine H1-receptor antagonist in the treatment of grass pollen sensitive asthma. Br J Clin Pharmacol, 1990, 30(2): 229-235.

[26] Kubavat AH, et al. A randomized, comparative, multicentric clinical trial to assess the efficacy and safety of zileuton extended-release tablets with montelukast sodium tablets in patients suffering from chronic persistent asthma. Am J Ther, 2013, 20(2): 154-162.

[27] Murali PM, et al. Plant-based formulation for bronchial asthma: a controlled clinical trial to compare its efficacy with oral salbutamol and theophylline. Respiration, 2006, 73(4): 457-463.

[28] Bergmann KC, CP Bauer, A. Overlack. A placebo-controlled, blind comparison of nedocromil sodium and beclomethasone dipropionate in bronchial asthma. Curr Med Res Opin, 1989, 11(8): 533-542.

[29] Lal S, et al. Nedocromil sodium: a new drug for the management of bronchial asthma. Thorax, 1984, 39(11): 809-812.

[30] Bone MF, et al. Nedocromil sodium in adults with asthma dependent on inhaled corticosteroids: a double blind, placebo controlled study. Thorax, 1989, 44(8): 654-659.

[31] Blumenthal MN, et al. A multicenter evaluation of the clinical benefits of cromolyn sodium aerosol by metered-dose inhaler in the treatment of asthma. J Allergy Clin Immunol, 1988, 81(4): 681-687.

[32] Foresi A, MC Morelli, E. Catena. Low-dose budesonide with the addition of an increased dose during exacerbations is effective in long-term asthma control. On behalf of the Italian Study Group. Chest, 2000, 117(2): 440-446.

[33] Mullarkey MF, JK Lammert, BA Blumenstein. Long-term methotrexate treatment in corticosteroid-dependent asthma. Ann Intern Med, 1990, 112(8): 577-581.

[34] Irwin RS, et al. Interpretation of positive results of a methacholine inhalation challenge and 1 week of inhaled bronchodilator use in diagnosing and treating cough-variant asthma. Arch Intern Med, 1997, 157(17): 1981-1987.

[35] Mann JS, et al. Inhaled lodoxamide tromethamine in the treatment of perennial asthma: a double-blind placebo-controlled study. J Allergy Clin Immunol, 1985, 76(1): 83-90.

[36] Dorow P, W Schiess. The influence of ketotifen and aminophylline on the central and peripheral airways. Arzneimittelforschung, 1983, 33(2): 265-268.

[37] Malo JL, et al. Influence of inhaled steroids on recovery from occupational asthma after cessation of exposure: an 18-month double-blind crossover study. Am J Respir Crit Care Med, 1996, 153(3): 953-960.

[38] Moeller M, S. Grimmbacher, and U. Munzel. Improvement of asthma therapy by a novel formoterol multidose dry powder inhaler. Arzneimittelforschung, 2008, 58(4): 168-173.

[39] van As A, et al. A group comparative study of the safety and efficacy of nedocromil sodium (Tilade) in reversible airways disease: a preliminary report. Eur J Respir Dis Suppl, 1986, 147: 143-148.

[40] Malo JL, et al. Four-times-a-day dosing frequency is better than a twice-a-day regimen in subjects requiring a high-dose inhaled steroid, budesonide, to control moderate to severe asthma. Am Rev Respir Dis, 1989, 140(3): 624-628.

[41] Abidi A, et al. Evaluation of Efficacy of Curcumin as an Add-on therapy in Patients of Bronchial Asthma. J Clin Diagn Res, 2014, 8(8): 19-24.

[42] Aaronson DW. Evaluation of cetirizine in patients with allergic rhinitis and perennial asthma. Ann Allergy Asthma Immunol, 1996, 76(5): 440-446.

[43] Bao W, et al. Efficacy of procaterol combined with inhaled budesonide for treatment of cough-variant asthma. Respirology, 2013, 18 Suppl 3: 53-61.

[44] Etter RL, RH Jackson, WJ Raymer. Effects of theophylline-alcohol with potassium iodide in asthmatic patients. Ann Allergy, 1969, 27(2): 70-78.

[45] Callaghan B, NC Teo, L. Clancy. Effects of the addition of nedocromil sodium to maintenance bronchodilator therapy in the management of chronic asthma. Chest, 1992, 101(3): 787-792.

[46] Tagaya E, et al. Effects of regular treatment with combination of salmeterol/fluticasone propionate and salmeterol alone in cough variant asthma. J Asthma, 2015, 52(5): 512-518.

[47] Di Franco A, et al. Effects of inhaled corticosteroids on cough threshold in patients with bronchial asthma. Pulm Pharmacol Ther, 2001, 14(1): 35-40.

[48] Fyans PG, PC Chatterjee, SS Chatterjee. Effects of adding nedocromil sodium (Tilade) to the routine therapy of patients with bronchial asthma. Clin Exp Allergy, 1989, 19(5): 521-528.

[49] Bianco S, et al. Effectiveness of nedocromil sodium versus placebo as additions to routine asthma maintenance therapy: a multicentre, double-blind, group comparative trial. Respiration, 1989, 56(3-4): 204-211.

[50] Spector SL, RA Tan. Effectiveness of montelukast in the treatment of cough variant asthma. Ann Allergy Asthma Immunol, 2004, 93(3): 232-236.

[51] Yokoyama A, et al. Effect of pranlukast, a leukotriene receptor antagonist, in patients with severe asthma refractory to corticosteroids. J Asthma, 1998, 35(1): 57-62.

[52] Tukiainen P, A. Lahdensuo. Effect of inhaled budesonide on severe steroid-dependent asthma. Eur J Respir Dis, 1987, 70(4): 239-244.

[53] Pavord I, et al. Effect of 443c81, an inhaled mu-opioid receptor agonist in asthma. Clin Exp Allergy, 1994, 24(2): 144-148.

[54] Fink JN, et al. A double-blind study of the efficacy of nedocromil sodium in the management of asthma in patients using high doses of bronchodilators. J Allergy Clin Immunol, 1994, 94(3 Pt 1): 473-481.

[55] A double-blind multicenter group comparative study of the

efficacy and safety of nedocromil sodium in the management of asthma. North American Tilade Study Group. Chest,1990,97(6):1299-1306.

[56] Fairfax AJ, M Allbeson. A double-blind group comparative trial of nedocromil sodium and placebo in the management of bronchial asthma. J Int Med Res,1988,16(3):216-224.

[57] Monie RD,et al. A double-blind clinical trial of ketotifen and disodium cromoglycate in bronchial asthma. Br J Dis Chest,1982,76(4):383-389.

[58] Petty TL,et al. Cromolyn sodium is effective in adult chronic asthmatics. Am Rev Respir Dis,1989,139(3):694-701.

[59] Fairfax AJ,et al. Controlled-release theophylline in the treatment of nocturnal asthma. J Int Med Res,1990,18(4):273-281.

[60] Hedman J,et al. Controlled trial of methotrexate in patients with severe chronic asthma. Eur J Clin Pharmacol,1996,49(5):347-349.

[61] Tukiainen H,et al. Comparison of twice-daily and four-times daily administration of beclomethasone dipropionate in patients with severe chronic bronchial asthma. Eur J Clin Pharmacol,1986,30(3):319-322.

[62] Wells A,et al. Comparison of nedocromil sodium at two dosage frequencies with placebo in the management of chronic asthma. Respir Med,1992,86(4):311-316.

[63] Wolstenholme RJ,SP Shettar. Comparison of a combination of fenoterol with ipratropium bromide(Duovent)and salbutamol in young adults with nocturnal asthma. Respiration,1989,55(3):152-157.

[64] Schwartz HJ,et al. A comparative study of the clinical efficacy of nedocromil sodium and placebo. How does cromolyn sodium compare as an active control treatment? Chest,1996,109(4):945-952.

[65] Nierop G,et al. Auranofin in the treatment of steroid dependent asthma: a double blind study. Thorax,1992,47(5):349-354.

[66] Wasserman SI,et al. Asthma symptoms and airway hyperresponsiveness are lower during treatment with nedocromil sodium than during treatment with regular inhaled albuterol. J Allergy Clin Immunol,1995,95(2):541-547.

[67] Kita T,et al. Antitussive effects of the leukotriene receptor antagonist montelukast in patients with cough variant asthma and atopic cough. Allergol Int,2010,59(2):185-192.

[68] Dicpinigaitis PV, JB Dobkin, J Reichel. Antitussive effect of the leukotriene receptor antagonist zafirlukast in subjects with cough-variant asthma. J Asthma,2002,39(4):291-297.

[69] Rebuck AS,et al. A 3-month evaluation of the efficacy of nedocromil sodium in asthma: a randomized, double-blind, placebo-controlled trial of nedocromil sodium conducted by a Canadian multicenter study group. J Allergy Clin Immunol,1990,85(3):612-617.

[70] Connolly KC,et al. Challenging Current Asthma Treatment Guidelines,2000,7(4):225.

[71] Nishimura K,et al. Additive effect of oxitropium bromide in combination with inhaled corticosteroids in the treatment of elderly patients with chronic asthma. Allergology International,1999,48(1):85-88.

[72] Morice A, M. Taylor. A randomised trial of the initiation of asthma treatment,1999,7(1):9.

[73] Cai C,et al. Add-on montelukast vs double-dose budesonide in nonasthmatic eosinophilic bronchitis: a pilot study. Respir Med,2012,106(10):1369-1375.

[74] Brightling CE,et al. Airway inflammation, airway responsiveness and cough before and after inhaled budesonide in patients with eosinophilic bronchitis. Eur Respir J,2000,15(4):682-686.

[75] Shioya T,et al. Antitussive effects of the H1-receptor antagonist epinastine in patients with atopic cough (eosinophilic bronchitis). Arzneimittelforschung,2004,54(4):207-212.

[76] Gibson PG,et al. Chronic cough with eosinophilic bronchitis: examination for variable airflow obstruction and response to corticosteroid. Clin Exp Allergy,1995,25(2):127-132.

[77] Bao W,et al. Efficacy of add-on montelukast in nonasthmatic eosinophilic bronchitis: the additive effect on airway inflammation, cough and life quality. Chin Med J(Engl),2015,128(1):39-45.

[78] National Institute for Health and Care Excellence (NICE). Asthma: diagnosis, monitoring and chronic asthma management. 2017. https://www.nice.org.uk/guidance/ng80/resources/asthmadiagnosismonitoring-and-chronic-asthma-management-pdf-1837687975621(accessed 22nd June 2019).

[79] 赖克方.咳嗽的诊断与治疗指南(2015)中华结核和呼吸杂志,2016,39(05):323-354.

[80] AHM,et al. ERS guidelines on the diagnosis and treatment of chronic cough in adults and children,2020,55(1).

2 重度激素抵抗型哮喘新型治疗方法探索及机制

褚淑媛 莫碧文

一、前 言

难治性哮喘是指尽管采用了大剂量吸入性糖皮质激素治疗或其他控制剂治疗仍无法控制的哮喘,或需要这些治疗以保持疾病控制良好的哮喘。重度哮喘是难治性哮喘的一个亚类,指的是虽然在过去一年内采用大剂量吸入性糖皮质激素联合长效 β_2 受体激动剂(long-acting β_2-agonist,LABA)、白三烯调节剂(leukotriene modifier)或茶碱,或至少之前 6 个月内采用全身性糖皮质激素治疗,仍然无法控制的哮喘;或者需要这些治疗以保持疾病良好控制的哮喘。虽然重度哮喘患者仅占成人哮喘患者中的 3%~10%,但却占哮喘相关医疗支出的 60%,并且平均每例重度哮喘患者的医疗支出比 2 型糖尿病、卒中或慢性阻塞性肺疾病更高。由此可见,重度激素抵抗型哮喘的控制目前仍然是临床的难点,该疾病给患者和社会均带来极大的疾病负担,也是值得重点关注的卫生问题。

重度激素抵抗型哮喘的发病机制比普通哮喘更为复杂,除了与气道持续的 Th2 免疫炎症有关外,还与多种机制有关,包括激素受体 α(glucocorticoid receptor α,GRα)的表达和活性发生缺陷,气道重塑,气道中性粒细胞炎症、Th2-Th17 混合性免疫炎症等。目前对于重度激素抵抗型哮喘的治疗在临床上也有诸多尝试,例如在临床上尝试采用多学科评估和治疗的方法进行干预,对于改善患者的生活质量、缓解焦虑有疗效,但仍未从根本上解决治疗的难点。此外,目前也有已上市或准备上市的多种靶向细胞因子的单克隆抗体药物,例如抗 IL-5 单克隆抗体(美泊利单抗、瑞利珠单抗、benralizumab 单抗)、抗 IL-13 单克隆抗体(金珠单抗、tralokinumab 单抗),以及抗 IL-4 受体 α 亚基单克隆抗体(dupilumab)等。但这些药物在临床上的疗效仍有待长期和进一步的观察,并且此类药物主要针对 Th2 相关炎症,对于机制更为复杂的重度难治性哮喘而言,仍需进一步探索和研发新的治疗方法。

随着对重度难治性哮喘发病机制在细胞、蛋白、基因等多层面的不断探究和分子生物学技术的不断进步,某些新型的治疗方法成为探索的方向,未来有可能突破重度难治性哮喘治疗难点。本文主要从干细胞治疗、针对表观遗传靶点的治疗以及 siRNA 技术相关的治疗三个方面进行介绍。

二、干细胞治疗

干细胞是未充分分化,并具有再生成各种组织器官的潜力的一类细胞。在哺乳类动物体内的干细胞主要是胚胎干细胞和成体干细胞。干细胞可以从血液、骨髓和脂肪组织中分离获得,主要包括内皮祖细胞和间充质干细胞(mesenchymal stem cells,MSCs)。近年来,干细胞逐渐成为多种疾病治疗的新希望,干细胞治疗也成为重度难治性哮喘研究的新热点。

目前对哮喘治疗的研究,主要集中在 MSCs 细胞。MSCs 细胞属于基质细胞,目前该细胞主要包括以下几种类型,即表达 $CD105^+$/$CD90^+$/$CD73^+$、$CD34^-$/$CD45^-$/$CD11b^-$、$CD14^-$/$CD19^-$ 或 $CD79a^-$/$HLA-DR1^-$ 的细胞,这些细胞具有体外分化为骨、软骨和脂肪组织等多种组织的能力。在哮喘小鼠模型中,从尾静脉注入人 MSCs 细胞后,哮喘小鼠的气道高反应性、气道炎症、气道重塑都得到缓解,气道灌洗液(bronchoalveolar lavage fluid,BALF)中的 IL-4、IL-5、IL-13 等 Th2 炎症因子水平均降低,并且血中嗜酸性粒细胞的数量减少,血清 IgE、IgG、IgG1 和 IgG2a 的水平都降低。

近年来,研究者对 MSCs 细胞治疗哮喘的机制也做了多方面的探索。通过体内实验发现,MSCs 细胞对哮喘的保护作用与多方面机制有关,包括 MSCs 细胞参与减少细胞外基质的沉积,改变透明质酸的合成,减少胶原沉积,减少气道黏液分泌,减少肺部炎症细胞的浸润,改变 T 细胞向 Th2 和 Th1 极化的方向,减少气道 IL-5、IL-13、IL-17 的表达,Th2 和 Th17 细胞减少,调节性 T 细胞(regulatory T cells,Tregs)增多等。值得关注的是,哮喘患者牙囊间充质干细胞可以抑制过敏原诱导的 Th2 细胞极化,有利于 Th1 反应,并减弱抗原提呈细胞共刺激的活性。

对 MSCs 细胞与 Treg 细胞相关炎症的研究发现 MSCs 细胞诱导的 Treg 增加与血红素加氧酶-1(heme oxygenase-1,HO-1)有关。HO-1 是细胞内限速酶,其过表达会刺激 Treg 细胞的增生,若抑制 HO-1 表达则可减少 Treg 细胞的数量。但在消解 Treg 细胞后,MSCs 细胞的作用被阻断。尽管 MSCs 对 Treg 细胞的作用有限,但仍然明显减轻了哮喘模型的病理改变。MSCs 细胞还可以诱导半成熟的树突状细胞(dendritic cell,DC)通过 Notch 信号促进 Treg 细胞的增生。除此之外,MSCs 细胞对 DC 也有影响。MSCs细胞可以通过增加IL-1受体拮抗剂的水平，抑制尘螨诱导哮喘小鼠的气道上皮细胞活化；并且，IL-1受体拮抗剂水平的增高会损害IL-1α的自分泌环，降低下游HMGB1和IL-25等细胞因子的表达，从而抑制DC的募集、抗原提呈功能和细胞的成熟。

目前的研究均表明MSCs细胞在哮喘治疗方面的获益，以及其临床应用的潜力。但是目前的研究局限于动物实验阶段，未来需要更多的临床研究验证。除了研究较多的MSCs细胞，其他类型的干细胞，例如内皮祖细胞、脐带血干细胞和诱导多能干细胞等，在哮喘治疗中的作用尚有待探索。此外，干细胞在预防哮喘急性发作方面的作用也需要更多的研究来证实。

三、针对表观遗传靶点的治疗

尽管哮喘与遗传关系密切，但是近年来全基因组分析研究发现，基因突变只能有限地解释哮喘的发病机制。遗传学不能解释的因素，主要与环境和发育有关。多年来对哮喘的研究发现，哮喘发病与环境因素和生活方式密切相关，甚至生命早期的环境暴露也与哮喘发病的风险密切相关。因此，目前研究逐渐聚焦在了遗传与环境的交互作用方面，其中表观遗传修饰是重要的研究突破口。表观遗传机制是指在基因的DNA不发生改变的情况下，基因的功能发生了可以遗传的改变，并最终导致表型的改变。表观遗传机制主要包括DNA CpG甲基化、组蛋白修饰、非编码RNA、染色质重塑和核小体定位等。围绕哮喘的研究主要涉及在DNA CpG甲基化和组蛋白修饰。

（一）DNA甲基化

在表观遗传修饰中，由于DNA甲基化与基因表达存在着密切的功能关系，并且DNA甲基化是较为稳定的表观遗传标记，定量检测甲基化的方法便于操作，并且技术也越来越成熟，因此，对哮喘的大量表观遗传学研究都集中在DNA甲基化上，因此获得的表观遗传靶点也较多。目前大部分研究关注寻找哮喘的表观遗传成分，寻找哮喘患者的DNA甲基化特征。Stefanowicz等在哮喘儿童的气道上皮细胞中，发现了8个DNA甲基化差异化表达的位点，分别位于8个基因上，这些基因的功能涉及细胞的分裂、分化、增生以及细胞黏附功能；其中STAT5A-E42-F和CRIP1-P874-R位点的DNA甲基化程度比过敏儿童更高，并且与过敏儿童相比，健康儿童STAT5A基因表达明显降低，而CRIP1基因的表达增强。另一项儿童哮喘的研究发现，与健康对照组相比，在患有持续性特应性哮喘的儿童中发现了81个差异化的DNA甲基化区域；其中包括IL-13、RUNX3和TIGIT等免疫相关基因在哮喘中发生低甲基化，并且有11个差异甲基化区域与较高的血清IgE浓度相关，16个区域与FEV_1预测值百分比相关。以上研究结果提示这些DNA甲基化位点作为治疗靶点的可能性。

虽然哮喘患者的DNA甲基化改变与临床表型之间具有显著的临床相关性，但是仍然难以确定这些甲基化改变是哮喘相关改变的原因还是结果，动物实验可以提供更直接的证据。在屋尘螨致敏的哮喘小鼠肺组织中，全局甲基化和羟甲基化都增加，提示在哮喘中，外来抗原的刺激可以改变DNA甲基化。另一方面，在卵清蛋白（ovalbumi, OVA）致敏的哮喘小鼠中，DNMT1胞嘧啶残基启动子区域调控的位点发生甲基化改变，同时发现肺组织、气管和肺泡灌洗液细胞中的DNMT1的表达都较正常小鼠降低。DNMT1是一种甲基转移酶，在Th1和Th2细胞的发育、分化和调节中，发挥重要的维持甲基化的作用。另一个DNMT家族成员DNMT3A可以限制OVA致敏小鼠的Th2细胞表达IL-13，并减轻气道过敏性炎症反应。可见甲基转移酶可能是治疗哮喘的重要的表观遗传学靶点。Wu等利用DNA甲基转移酶抑制剂5-氮胞苷（5-azacytidine, Aza）干预OVA致敏的哮喘小鼠后，小鼠的气道高反应性、肺泡灌洗液的嗜酸性粒细胞数量、循环中的OVA特异性IgG1和IgE、Th2细胞因子的水平，都随着Aza剂量的增加而明显降低；同时，Treg细胞明显增多。因此，DNMT家族成员的甲基化改变可能与重度激素抵抗型哮喘的T细胞混合炎症有关，未来可从T细胞混合炎症的角度着手，对治疗重度激素抵抗型哮喘进行探索。

（二）组蛋白乙酰化与去乙酰化

组蛋白乙酰化有助于DNA与组蛋白的解离，使核小体的结构松弛，有助于转录因子与DNA结合，激活基因转录。组蛋白乙酰转移酶（histone acetyltransferases, HAT）催化组蛋白乙酰化，而组蛋白去乙酰化酶（histone deacetylase, HDAC）则发挥相反的作用。在对哮喘患者的研究中发现哮喘的炎症反应与外周血单核细胞、肺泡巨噬细胞中，HDAC活性降低、HAT活性增强有关，其中HDAC活性降低与重度激素抵抗型哮喘密切相关；利用人气道上皮细胞系研究证实，糖皮质激素和茶碱可以通过调节HAT和HDAC活性，进而下调哮喘的炎症反应。进一步的研究发现，HDAC-2对糖皮质激素发挥活性有重要作用，并且在激素抵抗的哮喘中发现HDAC-2活性降低；甲基黄嘌呤茶碱和多酚姜黄素可以恢复HDAC的活性，从而恢复糖皮质激素的作用，但是其机制目前尚不清楚。

气道平滑肌细胞增生与气道重塑密切相关，参与重度激素抵抗型哮喘的发病。气道平滑肌的表观遗传修饰，尤其是组蛋白乙酰化修饰，在驱动哮喘气道重塑中发挥重要作用。在对哮喘患者气道平滑肌细胞的研究中发现，CXCL8基因组蛋白H3乙酰化增强，尤其是H3K18，HAT p300的结合力增强；并且乙酰化读取蛋白Brd3和Brd4与CXCL8启动子结合，可以促进气道平滑肌细胞分泌CXCL8，Brd抑制剂则抑制该效应。因此，Brd抑制剂可能是重度激素抵抗型哮喘治疗的新方法。对哮喘患者气道平滑肌细胞的体外研究进一步发现，H3K9me可以降低Sp1和RNA转移酶Ⅱ与VEGF启动子的结合，从而使VEGF过度分泌，参与哮喘气道重塑。

在针对HDAC为治疗靶点的探索中，Banerjee等尝试用HDAC的1类和2类抑制剂曲古他汀A（trichostatin A, TSA）来治疗烟曲菌抗原致敏的哮喘小鼠。该研究发现，TAS可以降低哮喘小鼠的气道高反应性，减少气道平

滑肌细胞 Ca^{2+} 动员,减少肺组织的收缩性;但并未明显改变气道的 IL-4 水平和嗜酸性粒细胞数。由此可见,HDAC 抑制剂主要对非 Th2 相关哮喘有作用。

尽管目前动物实验发现靶向抑制 HDAC 可能对激素抵抗型哮喘有作用,但在哮喘中,HDAC 活性降低可以增强促炎因子基因的表达,因此 HDAC 抑制剂能否减轻肺部的慢性炎症,目前尚不清楚。此外,目前也缺乏对 HAT 抑制剂在重度激素抵抗型哮喘中的研究,未来需要在动物实验和临床研究中进行探索。

四、siRNA 技术相关的治疗

RNA 干扰(RNA interference,RNAi)是指当细胞中导入与内源性 mRNA 编码区同源的双链 RNA 时,使该 mRNA 发生降解,阻碍基因的转录或翻译,从而导致基因表达沉默,抑制基因的表达。由于 RNAi 技术在剔除或关闭特定基因表达方面具有高度特异性,因此 RNAi 技术在通过基因沉默治疗多种慢性炎症性疾病方面受到关注。目前研究中应用较多的是小干扰 RNA 技术(small-interfering RNAs,siRNA)。RNAi 通过引入合成双链 RNA(double-stranded RNA,dsRNA),dsRNA 进入细胞,宿主细胞对 dsRNA 产生反应,RNaseIII 核酶家族的 Dicer 与 dsRNA 结合,并将 dsRNA 剪切成长度为 21~23 bp 及 3'端突出的 siRNA,siRNA 在细胞内 RNA 解旋酶的作用下解链成正义链和反义链,其中反义 siRNA 与内切酶、外切酶、解螺旋酶等结合形成 RNA 诱导的沉默复合体(RNA-induced silencing complex,RISC)。RISC 被激活后,激活型 RISC 受已成单链的 siRNA 引导(guide strand),序列特异性地结合在标靶 mRNA 上并切断标靶 mRNA,引发靶 mRNA 的特异性分解。由于 RNAi 在基因沉默方面具有高效性和高度特异性,是一种具有潜力的新型治疗方法。

在哮喘等呼吸疾病的治疗方面,由于可以通过鼻腔、气管和肺内途径使 siRNA 进入体内,因此基于 siRNA 的治疗方法越来越受到关注。siRNA 主要针对哮喘相关发病机制中的重要因子。随着近年来对哮喘相关基因易感性和变态反应相关病理生理学关键分子的深入认识,研究者发现了多种与 Th2 细胞分化和变应性炎症等与哮喘发病机制相关的 RNAi 靶点,涉及细胞表面受体(包括 G 蛋白偶联受体、细胞因子和趋化因子受体)、黏附分子、离子通道、细胞因子、去化因子、生长因子、信号转导受体、以及非受体蛋白激酶或转录因子。例如,Khaitov 等用呼吸道合胞病毒(respiratory syncytial virus,RSV)诱导 OVA 致敏的哮喘小鼠急性发作,然后利用 siRNA 同时靶向阻断 IL-4 和 RSV。在 siRNA 成功阻断肺部的 IL-4 和 RSV 后,小鼠气道高反应性降低,气道炎症减轻,肺泡灌洗液中的

嗜酸性粒细胞数量减少,但是会上调肺部 IFN-γ 的水平。该研究表明在动物模型中,利用 siRNA 靶向阻断疾病相关因子来治疗哮喘是可行的。由于哮喘的临床表现与 T 细胞亚型密切相关,因此利用 siRNA 靶向抑制控制 T 细胞分化的关键因子值得关注。

在哮喘相关的因子中,细胞因子信号转导抑制物(suppressors of cytokine signaling,SOCS)家族的 SOCS1 和 SOCS3,在 T 细胞分化成 Th1,Th2,Th17 和 Treg 细胞亚型的过程中,发挥重要的调节作用。Zafra 等利用 SOCS3-siRNA 鼻腔给药治疗 OVA 致敏的哮喘小鼠,发现 SOCS3 经 siRNA 阻断后,哮喘小鼠的气道高反应性降低,气道灌洗液中的嗜酸性粒细胞数减少,气道的黏液分泌和肺部胶原沉积均减少,气道重塑也减轻。该研究还进一步发现,此 SOCS3-siRNA 的治疗效应与下调 JAK/STAT 和 RhoA/Rho-kinase 信号通路有关。

以上研究是利用 siRNA 靶向 Th2 细胞的相关因子来进行干预,多年来已建立了多种 siRNA 靶向转运进入特点类型的细胞的系统,包括 T 细胞、巨噬细胞、树突状细胞等。但是有效地转染 T 细胞仍然是技术上的难点,尤其是针对特异性的 T 细胞亚型。Keil 等发明了一种新技术直接对活化的 Th2 细胞进行干预:利用转铁蛋白-聚乙烯亚胺(transferrin-polyethyleneimine,PEI)与 siRNA 结合,用 siRNA 干扰 Th2 细胞转录因子 GATA3,实现了对 Th2 细胞的抑制,突破 siRNA 转染特异性 T 细胞亚型的难点,并改善了内源性逃逸和基因沉默效应。该研究对于利用 siRNA 技术治疗哮喘具有方法学上的突破意义,使利用 siRNA 直接靶向 T 细胞亚型治疗哮喘的治疗方法成为可能,通过直接抑制目标细胞,治疗效果将比单纯抑制细胞因子更明显。

目前利用 siRNA 技术治疗哮喘的探索仅限于动物实验,并且主要聚焦于 T 细胞等免疫细胞。在对气道上皮细胞、气道平滑肌细胞等气道结构型细胞的干预和治疗方面,仍有待未来的探索。此外,临床方面的研究要注意伦理问题和治疗的安全性问题。

五、总结及展望

目前针对重度激素抵抗型哮喘的新型治疗方法,主要聚焦于辅助性 T 细胞和调节性 T 细胞相关的慢性炎症机制及气道重塑方面,而对于激素抵抗方面的研究仍然较少,未来可在此方面进行更多的探索。随着对重度激素抵抗型哮喘疾病机制的认识不断加深,以及生物医学技术的发展,不同于传统治疗方案的新型治疗方法逐步出现,并具备在未来进行临床应用的可能性。但是,距离真正实现临床应用,为患者解除痛苦,仍然任重道远,还需要研究者们不懈的探索和努力。

参 考 文 献

[1] Hekking PP, Wener RR, Amelink M, et al. The prevalence of severe refractory asthma. J Allergy Clin Immunol, 2015, 135(4): 896-902.

[2] Chung KF, Wenzel SE, Brozek JL, et al. International ERS/ATS guidelines on definition, evaluation and treatment of severe asthma. Eur Respir J, 2014, 43(2): 343-373.

[3] Sadatsafavi M, Lynd L, Marra C, et al. Direct health care costs associated with asthma in British Columbia. Can Respir J, 2010, 17: 74-80.

[4] O'Neill S, Sweeney J, Patterson CC, et al. The cost of treating severe refractory asthma in the UK: an economic analysis from the British Thoracic Society Difficult Asthma Registry. Thorax, 2015, 70: 376-378.

[5] Wadhwa R, Dua K, Adcock IM, et al. Cellular mechanisms underlying steroid-resistant asthma. Eur Respir Rev, 2019, 28(153): 190096.

[6] Saglani S, Lui S, Ullmann N, et al. IL-33 promotes airway remodeling in pediatric patients with severe steroid-resistant asthma. J Allergy Clin Immunol, 2013, 132(3): 676-685. e13.

[7] Israel E, Reddel HK. Severe anddifficult-to-treat asthma in adults. N Engl J Med, 2017, 377(10): 965-976.

[8] Gibeon D, Heaney LG, Brightling CE, et al. Dedicatedsevere asthma services improve health-care use and quality of life. Chest, 2015, 148: 870-876.

[9] van der Meer AN, Pasma H, Kempenaar-Okkema W, et al. A 1-day visit in a severe asthma centre: effect on asthma control, quality of life and healthcare use. Eur Respir J, 2016, 48: 726-733.

[10] Kajstura J, Rota M, Hall SR, et al. Evidence for human lung stem cells [retracted in: N Engl J Med, 2018, 379(19): 1870]. N Engl J Med, 2011, 364(19): 1795-1806.

[11] Huertas A, Palange P. Circulating endothelial progenitor cells and chronic pulmonary diseases. Eur Respir J, 2011, 37(2): 426-431.

[12] Rankin S. Mesenchymal stem cells. Thorax, 2012, 67(6): 565-566.

[13] Trounson A, Thakar RG, Lomax G, et al. Clinical trials for stem cell therapies. BMC Med, 2011, 9: 52.

[14] Dominici M, Le Blanc K, Mueller I, et al. Minimal criteria for defining multipotent mesenchymal stromal cells. The International Society for Cellular Therapy position statement. Cytotherap, 2006, 8(4): 315-317.

[15] Sun YQ, Deng MX, He J, et al. Human pluripotent stem cell-derived mesenchymal stem cells prevent allergic airway inflammation in mice. Stem Cells, 2012, 30(12): 2692-2699.

[16] Wang CY, Chiou GY, Chien Y, et al. Induced pluripotent stem cells without c-Myc reduce airway responsiveness and allergic reaction in sensitized mice. Transplantation, 2013, 96(11): 958-965.

[17] Firinci F, Karaman M, Baran Y, et al. Mesenchymal stem cells ameliorate the histopathological changes in a murine model of chronic asthma. Int Immunopharmacol, 2011, 11(8): 1120-1126.

[18] Kavanagh H, Mahon BP. Allogeneic mesenchymal stem cells prevent allergic airway inflammation by inducing murine regulatory T cells. Allergy, 2011, 66(4): 523-531.

[19] Ge X, Bai C, Yang J, et al. Effect of mesenchymal stem cells on inhibiting airway remodelingand airway inflammation in chronic asthma. J Cell Biochem, 2013, 114(7): 1595-1605.

[20] Goodwin M, Sueblinvong V, Eisenhauer P, et al. Bone marrow-derived mesenchymal stromal cells inhibit Th2-mediated allergic airways inflammation in mice. Stem Cells, 2011, 29(7): 1137-1148.

[21] Bonfield TL, Koloze M, Lennon DP, et al. Human mesenchymal stem cells suppress chronic airway inflammation in the murine ovalbumin asthma model. Am J Physiol Lung Cell Mol Physiol, 2010, 299(6): L760-L770.

[22] Goldstein BD, Lauer ME, Caplan AI, et al. Chronic asthma and Mesenchymal stem cells: Hyaluronan and airway remodeling. J Inflamm(Lond), 2017, 14: 18.

[23] Park HK, Cho KS, Park HY, et al. Adipose-derived stromal cells inhibit allergic airway inflammation in mice. Stem Cells Dev, 2010, 19(11): 1811-1818.

[24] Lathrop MJ, Brooks EM, Bonenfant NR, et al. Mesenchymal stromal cells mediate Aspergillus hyphal extract-induced allergic airway inflammation by inhibition of the Th17 signaling pathway. Stem Cells Transl Med, 2014, 3(2): 194-205.

[25] Li Y, Li H, Cao Y, et al. Placenta-derived mesenchymal stem cells improve airway hyperresponsiveness and inflammation in asthmatic rats by modulating the Th17/Treg balance. Mol Med Rep, 2017, 16(6): 8137-8145.

[26] Genç D, Zibandeh N, Nain E, et al. Dental follicle mesenchymal stem cells down-regulate Th2-mediated immune response in asthmatic patients mononuclear cells. Clin Exp Allergy, 2018, 48(6): 663-678.

[27] Li JG, Zhuan-sun YX, Wen B, et al. Human mesenchymal stem cells elevate CD4+CD25+CD127low/-regulatory T cells of asthmatic patients via heme oxygenase-1. Iran J Allergy Asthma Immunol, 2013, 12(3): 228-235.

[28] Kavanagh H, Mahon BP. Allogeneic mesenchymal stem cells prevent allergic airway inflammation by inducing murine regulatory T cells. Allergy, 2011, 66(4): 523-531.

[29] Cahill EF, Tobin LM, Carty F, et al. Jagged-1 is required for the expansion of CD4+ CD25+ FoxP3+ regulatory T cells and tolerogenic dendritic cells by murine mesenchymal stromal cells. Stem Cell Res Ther, 2015, 6(1): 19.

[30] Duong KM, Arikkatt J, Ullah MA, et al. Immunomodulation of airway epithelium cell activation by mesenchymal stromal cells ameliorates house dust mite-induced airway inflammation in mice. Am J Respir Cell Mol Biol, 2015, 53(5): 615-624.

[31] Manolio TA, Collins FS, Cox NJ, et al. Finding the missing heritability of complex diseases. Nature, 2009, 461(7265): 747-753.

[32] Martinez FD, Vercelli D. Asthma. Lancet, 2013, 382(9901): 1360-1372.

[33] von Mutius E, Vercelli D. Farm living: effects on childhood asthma andallergy. Nat Rev Immunol, 2010, 10(12): 861-868.

[34] Ober C, Vercelli D. Gene-environment interactions in human disease: nuisance or opportunity? Trends Genet, 2011, 27(3):107-115.

[35] Jaenisch R, Bird A. Epigenetic regulation of gene expression: how the genome integrates intrinsic and environmental signals. Nat Genet, 2003, 33 Suppl:245-254.

[36] Jirtle RL, Skinner MK. Environmental epigenomics and disease susceptibility. Nat Rev Genet, 2007, 8(4):253-262.

[37] Reddington JP, Pennings S, Meehan RR. Non-canonical functions of the DNA methylome in gene regulation. Biochem J, 2013, 451(1):13-23.

[38] Stefanowicz D, Hackett TL, Garmaroudi FS, et al. DNA methylation profiles of airway epithelial cells and PBMCs from healthy, atopic and asthmatic children. PLoS One, 2012, 7(9):e44213.

[39] Yang IV, Pedersen BS, Liu A, et al. DNA methylation and childhood asthma in the inner city. J Allergy Clin Immunol, 2015, 136(1):69-80.

[40] Cheng RY, Shang Y, Limjunyawong N, et al. Alterations of the lung methylome in allergic airway hyper-responsiveness. Environ Mol Mutagen, 2014, 55(3):244-255.

[41] Shang Y, Das S, Rabold R, et al. Epigenetic alterations by DNA methylation in house dust mite-induced airway hyper-responsiveness. Am J Respir Cell Mol Biol, 2013, 49(2):279-287.

[42] Verma M, Chattopadhyay BD, Paul BN. Epigenetic regulation of DNMT1 gene in mouse model of asthma disease. Mol Biol Rep, 2013, 40(3):2357-2368.

[43] Yu Q, Zhou B, Zhang Y, et al. DNA methyltransferase 3a limits the expression of interleukin-13 in T helper 2 cells and allergic airway inflammation. Proc Natl Acad Sci U S A, 2012, 109(2):541-546.

[44] Wu CJ, Yang CY, Chen YH, et al. The DNA methylation inhibitor 5-azacytidine increases regulatory T cells and alleviates airway inflammation in ovalbumin-sensitizedmice. Int Arch Allergy Immunol, 2013, 160(4):356-364.

[45] Hew M, Bhavsar P, Torrego A, et al. Relative corticosteroid insensitivity of peripheral blood mononuclear cells in severe asthma. Am J Respir Crit Care Med, 2006, 174(2):134-141.

[46] Ito K, Lim S, Caramori G, et al. A molecular mechanism of action of theophylline: Induction of histone deacetylase activity to decrease inflammatory gene expression. Proc Natl Acad Sci U S A, 2002, 99(13):8921-8926.

[47] Cosío BG, Mann B, Ito K, et al. Histone acetylaseand deacetylase activity in alveolar macrophages and blood mononocytes in asthma. Am J Respir Crit Care Med, 2004, 170(2):141-147.

[48] Marwick JA, Ito K, Adcock IM, Kirkham PA. Oxidative stress and steroid resistance in asthma and COPD: pharmacological manipulation of HDAC-2 as a therapeutic strategy. Expert OpinTher Targets, 2007, 11(6):745-755.

[49] Kaczmarek KA, Clifford RL, Knox AJ. Epigeneticchanges in airway smooth muscle as a driver of airway inflammation and remodeling in asthma. Chest, 2019, 155(4):816-824.

[50] Clifford RL, Patel JK, John AE, et al. CXCL8 histone H3 acetylation is dysfunctional in airway smooth muscle in asthma: regulation by BET. Am J Physiol Lung Cell Mol Physiol, 2015, 308(9):L962-L972.

[51] Clifford RL, John AE, Brightling CE, et al. Abnormal histone methylation is responsible for increased vascular endothelial growth factor 165a secretion from airway smooth muscle cells in asthma. J Immunol, 2012, 189(2):819-831.

[52] Banerjee A, Trivedi CM, Damera G, et al. Trichostatin A abrogatesairway constriction, but not inflammation, in murine and human asthma models. Am J Respir Cell Mol Biol, 2012, 46(2):132-138.

[53] Fire A, Xu S, Montgomery MK, et al. Potent and specific genetic interference by double-stranded RNA in Caenorhabditis elegans. Nature, 1998, 391(6669):806-811.

[54] Bagasra O, Prilliman KR. RNA interference: the molecular immune system. J Mol Hist, 2004, 35(6):545-553.

[55] Ali HM, Urbinati G, Raouane M, Massaad-Massade L. Significance and applications of nanoparticles in siRNA delivery for cancer therapy. Expert Rev Clin Pharmacol, 2012, 5(4):403-412.

[56] Rana TM. Illuminating the silence: understanding the structure and function of small RNAs. Nat Rev Mol Cell Biol, 2007, 8(1):23-36.

[57] Fuchs U, Damm-Welk C, Borkhardt A. Silencing of disease-related genes by small interfering RNAs. Curr Mol Med, 2004, 4(5):507-517.

[58] Denli AM, Hannon GJ. RNAi: an ever-growing puzzle. Trends Biochem Sci, 2003, 28(4):196-201.

[59] Dykxhoorn DM, Novina CD, Sharp PA. Killing the messenger: short RNAs that silence gene expression. Nat Rev Mol Cell Biol, 2003, 4(6):457-467.

[60] Kupferschmidt K. A lethal dose of RNA. Science, 2013, 341(6147):732-733.

[61] Bumcrot D, Manoharan M, Koteliansky V, et al. RNAi therapeutics: a potential new class of pharmaceutical drugs. Nat Chem Biol, 2006, 2(12):711-719.

[62] Fujita Y, Takeshita F, Kuwano K, et al. RNAi therapeutic platforms for lung diseases. Pharmaceuticals(Basel), 2013, 6(2):223-250.

[63] Ball HA, Sandrasagra A, Tang L, et al. Clinical potential of respirable antisense oligonucleotides (RASONs) in asthma. Am J Pharmacogenomics, 2003, 3(2):97-106.

[64] Popescu FD. Pharmacological modulation of gene expression in asthma(review inJapanese and English). Inter Rev Asthma (Japan), 2005, 7:74-90.

[65] Popescu FD. Antisense- and RNA interference-based therapeutic strategies in allergy. J Cell Mol Med, 2005, 9(4):840-853.

[66] Khaitov MR, Shilovskiy IP, Nikonova AA, et al. Small interfering RNAs targeted to interleukin-4 and respiratory syncy-

tial virus reduce airway inflammation in a mouse model of virus-induced asthma exacerbation. Hum Gene Ther,2014,25(7):642-650.

[67] Yoshimura A,Suzuki M,Sakaguchi R,et al. SOCS,inflammation,and autoimmunity. Front Immunol,2012,3:20.

[68] Zafra MP,Mazzeo C,Gámez C,et al. Gene silencing of SOCS3 by siRNA intranasal delivery inhibits asthma phenotype in mice PLoS One,2014,9(3):e91996.

[69] Xie Y,Merkel OM. Pulmonarydelivery of siRNA via polymeric vectors as therapies of asthma. Arch Pharm(Weinheim),2015,348(10):681-688.

[70] Keil TWM,Baldassi D,Merkel OM. T-cell targeted pulmonary siRNA delivery for the treatment of asthma. Wiley Interdiscip Rev Nanomed Nanobiotechnol,2020.

3 EGPA 的肺部表现带来的临床挑战

张清玲

嗜酸性肉芽肿性多血管炎（eosinophilic granulomatosis with polyangiitis,EGPA）是一种可累及全身多个脏器并伴有高嗜酸性粒细胞（eosinophil,Eos）血症和肉芽肿性炎症的自身免疫性疾病,主要表现为外周血及组织中嗜酸粒细胞增多及中小血管的坏死性肉芽肿性,属于抗中性粒细胞胞质抗体（anti-neutrophil cytoplasmic antibodies,ANCA）相关性系统血管炎。EGPA 发病年龄在 30~40 岁,无明显性别差异。目前,国外报道 EGPA 总患病率为 10.7~13.0 例/百万人,每年的新发病率为 0.5~6.8 例/百万人,而在哮喘患者的人群中,EGPA 每年的新发病率是 34.6~64.4 例/百万人,超出总人群中 EGPA 发病率。

EGPA 可累及全身多个脏器,包括鼻窦、肺、心脏、胃肠道、肾、皮肤、眼睛、神经系统等,其中大部分患者首发症状为喘息、咳嗽、胸闷等哮喘样症状。EGPA 主要临床表现可以概括为与呼吸道过敏性疾病密切相关的综合征,其典型的三联征为:①呼吸道过敏,表现为过敏性鼻炎、鼻息肉和哮喘等;②外周血 Eos 增多,常大于 10%;③组织 Eos 浸润,最常见为肺组织 Eos 浸润,其次为胃肠道。EGPA 全身症状主要表现为全身不适、发热、乏力、食欲缺乏、体重减轻等,可持续数月至数年不等,无特异性。与其他血管炎不同,EGPA 最早且最易累及呼吸道和肺,绝大多数首发表现为喘息样发作和鼻-鼻窦炎症状,因此首诊于呼吸内科,常被误诊为难治性哮喘。随着病情进展,全身多系统均可受累并造成不可逆的器官损害。大部分 EGPA 患者在出现多器官损害后才得以确诊,给治疗带来困难,并影响预后。

一、EGPA 肺部受累的临床及影像特征

肺是 EGPA 最常累及的器官。多数 EGPA 患者肺部病变按前驱期-嗜酸性粒细胞浸润期-血管炎期的顺序发展,部分阶段重叠。不同阶段的病理表现有其相应的临床及影像特征。前驱期嗜酸性粒细胞在支气管管壁及小叶间隔浸润,形成支气管炎和小叶间隔增厚。症状表现为支气管哮喘,影像学上以小叶中心性结节、树枝发芽征、支气管管壁增厚及管腔扩张等细支气管炎表现多见,也可出现以小叶间隔增厚为突出改变的间质网格影,提示嗜酸性粒细胞、中性粒细胞在前驱期分别向小叶中心及小叶周边趋化。嗜酸性粒细胞浸润期支气管管壁和小叶间隔的浸润更加突出,同时出现嗜酸性粒细胞肺炎,影像学上多表现为游走性片状影、磨玻璃样浸润影、实变影。一旦进入血管炎期,往往是致命的,病理表现为坏死性肉芽肿累及中小动脉、静脉和毛细血管,临床上多表现为发热、胸痛、咯血,影像学表现为多发外周实变,伴或不伴有空洞。

胸部 HRCT 可清晰显示 EGPA 的肺内外病变,EGPA 胸部影像表现多种多样,归纳如下:①肺内病变:双肺磨玻璃密度影,最常见,占 40%~400%,双侧多发、边界不清,可散在分布;肺实变影,占 32%~75%,多呈双侧多灶性、非节段性、游走性,常位于肺外周或散在分布;肺结节影,占 23.5%~88.9%,多见于 p-ANCA 阳性的 EGPA 患者,结节大小不等,形态可规则或不规则,分布无明显特征,小叶中心结节多见,大结节影相对少见;小叶间隔增厚,占 22.2%~66.6%,多累及肺外周;支气管壁增厚,占 35.3%~77.8%,多见于严重哮喘的患者,可伴管腔扩张,病变程度与患者哮喘病程长短有关,哮喘病程长者,支气管病变较重,但有研究者认为,支气管壁增厚对 EGPA 的诊断作用不大。②肺外病变:纵隔或肺门淋巴结肿大,占 0.7%~50%;单侧或双侧胸腔积液,占 11.8%~57.1%;心影增大、心包增厚、心包积液等旧例。此外,肺气腔或气道受累程度的不同,影像表现也会有所差别。EGPA 累及肺气腔时,CT 主要表现为肺实变、肺磨玻璃密度影、结节等,累及气道时可见支气管壁增厚、支气管扩张、小叶中心结节、树芽征、马赛克征等征象。

二、EGPA 肺部受累的诊断及鉴别诊断

EGPA 的诊断标准目前比较普遍认可的仍是 1990 年美国风湿病协会制定的 CSS/EGPA 分类标准:即至少符合以下标准中的 4 条:①哮喘样症状（或喘息发作）;②外周血嗜酸性粒细胞≥10%（或绝对值≥$1.5×10^9$/L）;③单发或多发性神经病变;④胸部影像学表现为非固定性肺浸润;⑤鼻窦病变;⑥活检提示血管外嗜酸性粒细胞浸润。此诊断标准的敏感性与特异性分别为 85% 和 99.7%。病理是 EGPA 诊断"金标准",且能够与其他肺部浸润的嗜酸性粒细胞增多性疾病相鉴别。

EGPA 的病理诊断①典型表现:嗜酸性肺炎,坏死血管炎和肉芽肿性炎症;②高度提示性表现:嗜酸性肺炎和坏死性血管炎;③提示性表现:嗜酸性粒细胞性肺炎与实质坏死;④常见但非诊断性表现:嗜酸性肺炎。与其他器

官一样,典型的发现包括嗜酸性粒细胞组织浸润、坏死性血管炎和血管外肉芽肿。值得注意的是肺受累的EGPA,经纤维支气管镜肺活检(TBLB)病理发现典型坏死性肉芽肿性病变的阳性率不高,电视胸腔镜手术(VATS)肺活检的临床价值要大于TBLB,但由于是有创性检查,需要十分慎重。

EGPA肺部组织学改变需与其他嗜酸性粒细胞浸润或嗜酸性粒细胞与肉芽肿性炎症疾病相鉴别。

(一)喘息样发作疾病

1. 支气管哮喘　EGPA可以先有支气管哮喘的病史。两者鉴别的要点为:哮喘极少出现累及其他器官的表现,外周血Eos比例一般为轻度增高或正常,弥散功能多正常,无游走性肺部炎性浸润等胸部X线表现,ANCA阴性,活检多以支气管黏膜膜及黏膜下Eos浸润为主,偶可见肺组织少量Eos浸润,无血管Eos浸润特征的表现。

2. ABPA　参照变应性支气管曲霉病诊治专家共识(2017年)进行鉴别诊断。鉴别要点:ABPA不累及肺外器官(不包括上呼吸道),胸部CT常见中心性支气管扩张,烟曲霉特异性IgE水平增高,或烟曲霉皮试速发反应阳性,血清烟曲霉抗原沉淀抗体阳性等特点可以与EGPA相鉴别。

(二)Eos增多相关性疾病

Eos升高患者要和Eos增多相关性疾病进行鉴别诊断,鉴别诊断包括遗传性(家族性)高嗜酸粒细胞增多症、继发性(反应性)高嗜酸粒细胞增多症、原发性(克隆性)高嗜酸粒细胞增多症和意义未定(特发性)高嗜酸粒细胞增多症等,建议参照嗜酸粒细胞增多症诊断与治疗中国专家共识(2017年版)相应诊断标准进行鉴别诊断。

(三)其他ANCA相关性血管炎及其他血管炎

1. GPA　既往称为韦格纳肉芽肿(Wegener's granulomatosis,WG),是一种坏死性肉芽肿性血管炎,病变累及全身小动脉、静脉及毛细血管,上下呼吸道及肾最常受累。该病无喘息样症状,外周血Eos增高不明显,主要是c-ANCA和(或)抗PR3-ANCA阳性,胸片特征表现包括结节、空洞,多形、多变,活检组织表现为少量Eos。

2. MPA　主要累及小血管的系统性坏死性血管炎,可侵犯肾、皮肤和肺等脏器的小动脉、微动脉、毛细血管和小静脉。常表现为坏死性肾小球肾炎和肺毛细血管炎。无明显喘息症状,外周血Eos无明显增高,p-ANCA和(或)抗MPO-ANCA阳性,且阳性率较EGPA高。活检组织无Eos浸润和肉芽肿病变。

3. 结节性多动脉炎　是一种累及中、小动脉的坏死性血管炎,多以皮疹和周围神经系统损害为主,几乎不累及肺部,无哮喘的典型临床表现。肾受累以肾动脉受损为主,肾小球几乎不受累,因此临床无肾小球肾炎的表现。外周血Eos比例增高不明显,ANCA阴性,病理活检以非肉芽肿性血管炎表现为主。

4. 其他　感染是最重要的,尤其是球虫病,会引起类似的肺部浸润改变,通过特殊染色寻找病原体可鉴别,并且通常是孤立的结节性病变,尽管血管炎症可能存在,坏死性血管炎不会发生。此外,蠕虫在坏死区的血管腔内应该很容易看到;椎间盘结节常类似坏死性肉芽肿,周围可见明显的嗜酸性粒细胞浸润,但通常为孤立性结节,且不会发生坏死性血管炎。

三、EGPA肺部受累的治疗及预后

正确评估临床预后对于确定最合适的治疗策略至关重要。目前评估标准主要参考法国血管炎研究组织(French Vasculitis Study Group,FVSG)基于1996年5因子评分(five-factor score,FFS),在2011年修改后,提出的5因子评分评价体系:①胃肠道受累;②心脏受累;③肾功能不全(血肌酐>150 μmol/L);④年龄>65岁;⑤缺乏耳鼻喉受累证据。每1项计1分,总分5分。分数越高,预后越差。不存在影响预后的因素时,5年生存率为88%,存在1项影响预后因素时,5年生存率为74%,≥2项时,5年生存率为54%。糖皮质激素是EGPA治疗基础,FFS=0分时,可用糖皮质激素治疗,93%患者可获得缓解,35%患者复发;FFS≥1分,需糖皮质激素联合免疫抑制剂治疗,时间不少于18个月。

EGPA患者的预后与最初治疗的方案相关。制定治疗方案前要先进行FFS评分以评估是否存在预后不良因素。FFS评分=0的EGPA患者可使用糖皮质激素治疗来症状控制,FFS评分≥1的患者建议糖皮质激素和免疫抑制剂联合治疗。总体治疗方案分为诱导缓解和维持治疗2个阶段。缓解的定义为临床表现[除外哮喘和(或)耳鼻喉表现]消失。诱导缓解治疗方案主要包括糖皮质激素和(或)免疫抑制剂(如环磷酰胺),诱导缓解治疗的疗程目前尚无定论;病情达到缓解后,维持治疗推荐使用硫唑嘌呤或甲氨蝶呤,维持治疗疗程尚无定论,2015年EULAR推荐治疗时间为疾病达到缓解后至少24个月。

(一)糖皮质激素治疗

糖皮质激素是EGPA的基础治疗药物。有危及生命的脏器受累患者建议采用甲泼尼龙冲击治疗(500~1000 mg,静脉注射,连续3d)。对有严重器官受累表现的患者,建议糖皮质激素的剂量为1 mg/(kg·d)泼尼松或等效剂量的其他糖皮质激素。对于无危及生命及无严重器官受累表现的EGPA患者可考虑单用糖皮质激素治疗。诱导治疗阶段建议糖皮质激素如泼尼松的起始剂量1 mg/(kg·d),4~6周后逐渐减量[理想状态3个月后减至0.3 mg/(kg·d),6个月后减至0.15 mg/(kg·d)]至最小有效剂量,若有可能,直至停用。

(二)糖皮质激素联合免疫抑制剂治疗

对危及生命和(或)FFS≥1(或)有严重器官受累的患者(如严重心脏、胃肠道、中枢神经系统、严重外周神经病变、严重眼部病变、肺泡出血和(或)肾小球肾炎等)应采用糖皮质激素联合免疫抑制剂如环磷酰胺(cyclophosphamide,CTX)进行诱导缓解治疗。需要注意的是,严重肺泡出血、眼病变、暴发性的多发性单神经炎等可危及生命和(或)导致严重功能障碍,因此尽管这些表现没有被列入FFS,但仍建议联合免疫抑制剂如CTX治疗。CTX连续口服[2mg/(kg·d)]或静脉冲击治疗可能同样有效。静脉冲击的建议疗法为前3次每2周给药一次，每次15 mg/kg或0.6g/m²，最大剂量每次1.2g；以后每3周冲击一次，每次15 mg/kg或0.7g/m²，共3～6次。使用时要注意根据肾功能调节CTX剂量及其不良反应，如对卵巢功能的抑制、粒细胞减少等。

在诱导缓解治疗后建议给予维持治疗（推荐使用硫唑嘌呤或甲氨蝶呤）以避免复发及减少糖皮质激素的用量。硫唑嘌呤的建议剂量为每日2mg/kg，甲氨蝶呤剂量建议为每周10～20mg并每周10～30mg补充叶酸。维持治疗的疗程尚无定论，根据2015年EULAR推荐至少24个月。

对于无危及生命和（或）严重器官受累表现者可单用糖皮质激素治疗若患者不能在3～4个月将激素减量至<7.5mg/d可考虑添加免疫抑制剂；对于疾病复发的EGPA患者也要考虑添加免疫抑制剂。

（三）靶向治疗药物

1. 利妥昔单抗（rituximab） 抗CD-20嵌合单克隆抗体rituximab被认为是诱导ANCA相关性血管炎缓解的一线治疗选择，尤其是对GPA和MPA患者。Rituximab也对ANCA相关性血管炎的维持治疗有效。利妥昔单抗对EGPA有一定疗效，并导致泼尼松用量减少，但哮喘和耳鼻咽喉炎复发率较高。

2. 奥马珠单抗（omalizumab） 抗人源化IgE单克隆抗体omalizumab已在美国被批准用于治疗中度至重度持续性过敏性哮喘，它可能通过与嗜酸性粒细胞膜上的IgE受体直接相互作用诱导细胞凋亡减少嗜酸性粒细胞数量。由于EGPA也存在高嗜酸性粒细胞血症和高水平IgE，Omalizumab已被研究作为这种类型的ANCA相关性血管炎的靶向治疗。

3. 美泊利单抗（mepolizumab） Mepolizumab是人源化单克隆抗体IgG1-k类型，它能阻止IL-5与IL-5受体（IL-5R）的α链相互作用。它首次是用于治疗伴有嗜酸性粒细胞增多的哮喘患者，并取得了良好的效果。Mepolizumab治疗EGPA的初步研究发现，其可以减少糖皮质激素用量，减少嗜酸性粒细胞数，并且还可以缓解症状。

4. 贝那利珠单抗（benralizumab） 贝那利单抗是一种完全人源化的无糖基化抗IL-5受体抗体，与人IL-5Rα链结合，阻断其活化和信号转导。此外，磺酰化增强了抗体依赖性细胞介导的细胞毒性（ADCC）功能，增加了贝那利珠单抗减少与炎症反应有关的循环嗜酸性粒细胞（以及定居在不同组织中的嗜酸性粒细胞）数量的能力。与其他抗IL-5单抗相比，苯那利单抗具有不同的作用机制，它能够通过增强ADCC减少嗜酸性粒细胞的数量，这决定了其在EGPA治疗方面具有潜在优势。目前正在进行nct0300436的临床试验，探讨贝那利珠单抗治疗嗜酸性粒细胞性巨球增多症伴多发性脉管炎的疗效和安全性。

（四）其他及吸入药物治疗

EGPA具有和支气管哮喘相似的呼吸道临床表现和病理生理学特点，需要同时给予局部治疗。通常按照重症哮喘的治疗方案（GINA4-5级的治疗）；推荐使用高剂量吸入糖皮质激素和支气管舒张剂（β₂受体激动剂）的复方制剂，如布地奈德/福莫特罗、倍氯米松/福莫特罗、氟替卡松/沙美特罗等，大部分患者需要维持吸入治疗。对于有呼吸道哮喘表现的患者还可以考虑联合白三烯受体拮抗剂（如孟鲁司特钠等）、茶碱缓释制剂、抗胆碱能药物（如噻托溴铵等）治疗，有助于缓解喘息症状及改善肺通气功能。有报道白三烯受体拮抗剂的使用与EGPA发病相关，但研究缺乏严谨的设计，暂不作为限制EGPA患者使用白三烯受体拮抗剂的理论依据。

（五）免疫球蛋白、血浆置换及其他

根据EULAR/EDTA关于ANCA相关性血管炎治疗的建议，血浆置换适用于危及生命的患者，例如继发于急进型肾小球肾炎（证据水平1B）或严重肺泡弥漫性出血的肾衰竭（水平证据3C）患者。Danieli等研究了在18例EGPA患者中静脉注射免疫球蛋白（IVIG）和血浆置换的有效性，每月2g/kg的IVIG加血浆置换6个月，然后每隔1个月进行一次IVIG超过3个月，1年后患者队列的总体诱导缓解率达50%。鼓励患者接种灭活疫苗和抗流行性感冒、肺炎球菌疫苗；服用免疫抑制剂和（或）≥20 mg/d泼尼松的患者禁忌接种活疫苗。有周围神经受累或运动功能障碍的患者应常规接受物理治疗。

综上所述，肺是EGPA最常受累的脏器之一，病变特征与血管炎的不同阶段密切相关，是呼吸科医师面临的重要挑战。呼吸科医师需掌握EGPA肺部受累临床表现、各阶段影像学特征及病理特征，以早发现、早干预，提高疾病的治疗效果。

参 考 文 献

[1] Ormerod AS, Cook MC. Epidemiology of primary systemic vasculitis in the Australian Capital Territory and south-eastern New South Wales. Intern Med J, 2008, 38(11): 816-823.

[2] Comarmond C, Pagnoux C, Khellaf M, et al. Eosinophilic granulomatosis with polyangiitis (Churg-Strauss): clinical characteristics and long-term followup of the 383 patients enrolled in the French Vasculitis Study Group cohort. Arthritis Rheum, 2013, 65(1): 270-281.

[3] Mahr A, Guillevin L, Poissonnet M, et al. Prevalences of polyarteritis nodosa, microscopic polyangiitis, Wegener's granulomatosis, and Churg-Strauss syndrome in a French urban multiethnic population in 2000: a capture-recapture estimate. Arthritis Rheum, 2004, 51(1): 92-99.

[4] Berti A, Dejaco C. Update on the epidemiology, risk factors, and outcomes of systemic vasculitides. Best Pract Res Clin Rheumatol, 2018, 32(2): 271-294.

[5] Cottin V, Khouatra C, Dubost R, et al. Persistent airflow obstruction in asthma of patients with Churg-Strauss syndrome and long-term follow-up. Allergy, 2009, 64(4): 589-595.

[6] Kim YK, Lee KS, Chung MP, et al. Pulmonary involvement in Churg-Strauss syndrome: an analysis of CT, clinical, and pathologic findings. Eur Radiol, 2007, 17(12): 3157-3165.

[7] Silva CI, Muller NL, Fujimoto K, et al. Churg-Strauss syndrome: high resolution CT and pathologic findings. J Thorac Imaging, 2005, 20(2): 74-80.

[8] Feng RE, Xu WB, Shi JH, et al. Pathological and high resolution CT findings in Churg-Strauss syndrome. Chin Med Sci J, 2011, 26(1): 1-8.

[9] Szczeklik W, Sokolowska B, Mastalerz L, et al. Pulmonary findings in Churg-Strauss syndrome in chest X-rays and high resolution computed tomography at the time of initial diagnosis. Clin Rheumatol, 2010, 29(10): 1127-1134.

[10] Castaner E, Alguersuari A, Gallardo X, et al. When to suspect pulmonary vasculitis: radiologic and clinical clues. Radiographics, 2010, 30(1): 33-53.

[11] Groh M, Pagnoux C, Baldini C, et al. Eosinophilic granulomatosis with polyangiitis (Churg-Strauss) (EGPA) Consensus Task Force recommendations for evaluation and management. Eur J Intern Med, 2015, 26(7): 545-553.

[12] Cottin V. Eosinophilic lung diseases. Clin Chest Med, 2016, 37(3): 535-556.

[13] Tazelaar HD, Linz LJ, Colby TV, et al. Acute eosinophilic pneumonia: histopathologic findings in nine patients. Am J Respir Crit Care Med, 1997, 155(1): 296-302.

[14] Curtis C, Ogbogu P. Hypereosinophilic syndrome. Clin Rev Allergy Immunol, 2016, 50(2): 240-251.

[15] Ueki S, Hebisawa A, Kitani M, et al. Allergic bronchopulmonary aspergillosis-A luminal hypereosinophilic disease with extracellular trap cell death. Front Immunol, 2018, 9: 2346.

[16] Almouhawis HA, Leao JC, Fedele S, et al. Wegener's granulomatosis: a review of clinical features and an update in diagnosis and treatment. J Oral Pathol Med, 2013, 42(7): 507-516.

[17] Quan MV, Frankel SK, Maleki-Fischbach M, et al. A rare case report of polyangiitis overlap syndrome: granulomatosis with polyangiitis and eosinophilic granulomatosis with polyangiitis. BMC Pulm Med, 2018, 18(1): 181.

[18] Sobonya RE, Yanes J, Klotz SA. Cavitary pulmonary coccidioidomycosis: pathologic and clinical correlates of disease. Hum Pathol, 2014, 45(1): 153-159.

[19] Katzenstein AA, Askin FB. Surgical pathology of non-neoplastic lung disease. Major Probl Pathol, 1982, 13: 1-430.

[20] Pagnoux C, Guilpain P, Guillevin L. Churg-Strauss syndrome. Curr Opin Rheumatol, 2007, 19(1): 25-32.

[21] Groh M, Pagnoux C, Baldini C, et al. Eosinophilic granulomatosis with polyangiitis (Churg-Strauss) (EGPA) Consensus Task Force recommendations for evaluation and management. Eur J Intern Med, 2015, 26(7): 545-553.

[22] Cartin-Ceba R, Keogh KA, Specks U, et al. Rituximab for the treatment of Churg-Strauss syndrome with renal involvement. Nephrol Dial Transplant, 2011, 26(9): 2865-2871.

[23] Wechsler ME, Akuthota P, Jayne D, et al. Mepolizumab or placebo for eosinophilic granulomatosis with polyangiitis. N Engl J Med, 2017, 376(20): 1921-1932.

[24] Jones RB, Ferraro AJ, Chaudhry AN, et al. A multicenter survey of rituximab therapy for refractory antineutrophil cytoplasmic antibody-associated vasculitis. Arthritis Rheum, 2009, 60(7): 2156-2168.

[25] Bagnasco D, Ferrando M, Varricchi G, et al. Anti-interleukin 5(IL-5) and IL-5Ra biological drugs: efficacy, safety, and future perspectives in severe eosinophilic asthma. Front Med (Lausanne), 2017, 4: 135.

[26] Menzella F, Biava M, Bagnasco D, et al. Efficacy and steroid-sparing effect of benralizumab: has it an advantage over its competitors?. Drugs Context, 2019, 8: 212580.

[27] Coppola A, Flores KR, De Filippis F. Rapid onset of effect of benralizumab on respiratory symptoms in a patient with eosinophilic granulomatosis with polyangiitis. Respir Med Case Rep, 2020, 30: 101050.

[28] Wechsler ME, Finn D, Gunawardena D, et al. Churg-Strauss syndrome in patients receiving montelukast as treatment for asthma. Chest, 2000, 117(3): 708-713.

[29] Donohue JF. Montelukast and Churg-Strauss syndrome. Chest, 2001, 119(2): 668.

[30] Yates M, Watts R, Bajema I, et al. Validation of the EULAR/ERA-EDTA recommendations for the management of ANCA-associated vasculitis by disease content experts. RMD Open, 2017, 3(1): e449.

[31] Danieli MG, Cappelli M, Malcangi G, et al. Long term effectiveness of intravenous immunoglobulin in Churg-Strauss syndrome. Ann Rheum Dis, 2004, 63(12): 1649-1654.

4 ABPA 激素、抗真菌、靶向药物之争

黄丹辉 蔡绍曦

变应性支气管肺曲霉病(allergic bronchopulmonary aspergillosis, ABPA)是烟曲霉致敏引起的一种变应性肺部疾病,表现为慢性哮喘和反复出现的肺部阴影,可伴有支气管扩张。该病相对少见,临床上常被误诊为支气管哮喘(以下简称哮喘)、支气管扩张等。少见情况下,其他真菌也可引起与 ABPA 相似的表现,统称变应性支气管肺真菌病(allergic bronchopulmonary mycosis, ABPM)。ABPA 的治疗目标包括控制症状,预防急性加重,防止或减轻肺功能受损。虽然 Hinson 等早在 1952 年就初步描述了 ABPA,但目前仍缺少统一的 ABPA 治疗标准。迄今为止,临床专家开展了一系列研究探讨采用不同方案治疗不同时期 ABPA 患者的获益情况。总体来说,糖皮质激素(以下简称激素)是治疗 ABPA 的基础药物;抗真菌药物通常与激素联合使用治疗活动期或激素依赖期 ABPA,或单独应用在缓解期 ABPA;而 IgE 单抗,抗 IL-5 单抗可能对于激素依赖及反复复发 ABPA 患者具有一定疗效。现将激素、抗真菌药物及靶向药物治疗 ABPA 的相关研究进展进行总结,以梳理目前关于 ABPA 治疗已经明确的和存在争议的地方。

一、ABPA 的发病机制

目前认为 ABPA 发生是由于遗传易感的哮喘或囊性纤维化个体产生了高频率或强度的曲霉特异性 $CD4^+$ Th2 细胞反应。ABPA 发病始于易感个体吸入曲霉菌孢子。直径 3～5μm 的曲霉菌孢子被吸入进支气管深部,在此生长为菌丝。烟曲霉可以产生多种蛋白,包括过氧化氢酶、磷脂酶、蛋白酶、溶血素等多种物质,多种曲霉蛋白可以破坏上皮完整性并引起单核炎性反应。上皮细胞炎性因子释放所引起的炎性反应同样可以导致上皮完整性遭到破坏。支气管上皮的受损可以导致机体对一种以上曲霉蛋白产生以曲霉特异性 $CD4^+$ Th2 为主的过敏反应,主要分为 IgE 介导的 I 型变态反应或 IgG 介导的 III 型变态反应。IL-4 可能在这一过程中发挥了重要作用。有研究者在哮喘合并 ABPA 患者中发现特异性增生的 T 细胞群表型为 Th2 细胞($IL-4^+$, $IFN-\gamma^-$)或 Th0 细胞($IL-4^+$, $IFN-\gamma^+$)。T 细胞产生的 IL-4 与 B 细胞表面的 IL-4 受体结合,导致 IgE 抗体同种型转换及 B 细胞增生。此外 IL-4 还可增强气道嗜酸粒细胞炎性反应及抗原暴露引起的气道高反应性相关。激活的免疫反应、真菌的水解酶一方面引起哮喘症状,另一方面加重气道损伤,导致支气管壁增厚、组织重构,支气管扩张乃至支气管纤维化。

二、激素

(一) 口服激素

口服激素是 ABPA 的基础治疗,不仅抑制过度免疫反应,同时可减轻曲霉引起的炎症损伤。早期应用口服激素治疗,可防止或减轻支气管扩张及肺纤维化造成的慢性肺损伤。绝大多数 ABPA 患者对口服激素治疗反应良好,短时间内症状缓解、肺部阴影吸收。目前临床上对口服激素治疗 ABPA 的初始方案存在争议。临床实践中有 3 种常用的泼尼松起始治疗方案。方案 1:0.5 mg/kg,口服,1～2 周,之后隔日服用该剂量泼尼松 6～8 周,之后每 2 周减量 5～10 mg,疗程持续 3～5 个月。方案 2:0.75 mg/kg,6 周,之后 0.5 mg/kg,6 周,之后每 2 周减量 5 mg,疗程持续 8～10 个月。方案 3:0.5 mg/kg,每日 1 次,2 周;继以 0.25 mg/kg,每日 1 次,4～6 周,之后每 2 周减量 5 mg,疗程持续 4 个月。近期的一项研究比较了方案 1 和方案 2 治疗 ABPA 患者的获益及不良反应情况。该研究共纳入了 92 位 ABPA 患者,结果显示两组患者在治疗结束 1 年后出现急性加重的次数以及治疗结束 2 年后进展为激素依赖性 ABPA 的比例相似;两组肺功能改善情况及距离治疗结束到发生第 1 次急性加重的时间也相似。不良反应方面,方案 2 不良反应发生率显著高于另一组患者。因此方案 1 适用于治疗大多数新发 ABPA 患者。然而该研究发现在方案 1 组,13% 的患者在治疗 6 周后没有获得早期应答。基于此,该研究作者提倡在治疗 ABPA 患者的过程中要定期监测疗效,及时发现无应答者并调整激素剂量。此外,未来临床研究需要进一步探究对于方案 1 无应答的 ABPA 患者的临床特征。该研究团队在后续的 2 项研究中采用方案 3 治疗活动期 ABPA 患者,2 项研究的结果显示方案 3 可以使 100% 的患者获得早期应答,且不良反应发生率较低。中国 ABPA 专家共识也推荐采用方案 3 对 ABPA 患者进行初始治疗。然而这 2 项研究的主要目的是比较激素与单用抗真菌药物治疗活动期 ABPA 的疗效差异,并没有直接对比方案 1 及方案 2 疗效及不良反应发生率。因此,目前关于方案 1 及方案 2 的选择仍存在争议。此外,除了上述 3 种常用方案,是否还存在更优的治疗方案,未来也需要进一步探索。

(二)吸入激素(inhaled corticosteroids, ICS)

ICS可以有效沉积在肺支气管树。与口服激素相比,其不良反应更少,因此临床专家推论ICS可以作为口服激素的替代治疗方案。然而早期的一项纳入了32个ABPA患者的研究显示每日吸入400μg二丙酸倍氯米松并没能显著改善ABPA患者的肺功能及症状。之后也有一些小样本病例研究及病例报道尝试探讨ICS在ABPA的作用。然而这些研究的样本量不足,患者使用ICS剂量不一致,大部分患者同时联合使用了口服激素,因此难以准确评价ICS的作用。近期的一项研究纳入了21位ABPA血清型(ABPA-S)患者,患者接受高剂量福莫特罗/布地奈德(24/1600 mg/d)治疗,在6个月的随访时间里,患者哮喘症状均未达到完全控制,并且患者6个月血清IgE水平较基线值增加了99%。因此单独使用ICS可能无法有效控制ABPA患者的症状、急性加重风险及改善肺功能。中国ABPA专家共识认为当全身激素减量至≤10mg/d(泼尼松当量)的患者,联合ICS可能有助于哮喘症状的控制,同时减少全身激素用量。对于已经经过口服激素后停用,长期病情缓解的ABPA-S患者,使用ICS可以有效延缓其进展为支气管扩张型ABPA(ABPA-B)。

(三)激素冲击治疗

少量研究显示采用激素冲击疗法也可有效治疗ABPA患者。早期的一项病例研究纳入了4位口服激素抵抗或不良反应严重的儿童ABPA患者,结果显示激素冲击疗法可以有效治疗ABPA。后续的一项病例研究显示对于口服激素[0.5mg/(kg·d)]无应答的急性期ABPA患者,激素冲击治疗可以有效缓解ABPA患者症状。这些研究提示激素冲击疗法可用于治疗口服激素依赖性或口服激素抵抗的ABPA患者。其作用机制主要在于长期使用口服激素治疗会导致激素受体下调,进而导致激素抵抗;而激素冲击疗法主要通过非基因效应发挥作用。考虑到长期服用口服激素对儿童生长发育的影响,激素冲击疗法更适用于儿童ABPA患者。目前关于激素冲击疗法均为系列病例报道或者小样本研究,也缺乏关于激素冲击治疗远期疗效的评价,因此关于激素冲击疗法的作用还有待进一步证实。此外,对于激素抵抗或激素依赖性ABPA患者,临床上还可选择联合抗真菌药物或使用靶向药物如奥马珠单抗,未来也需要进一步比较不同方案的优劣。

三、抗真菌药物

抗真菌药物可能通过减少真菌定植、减轻炎症反应而发挥作用。早在1967年就有临床医生采用吸入性制霉菌素有效治疗ABPA患者的病例报道。此后有文献报道利用酮康唑治疗ABPA疗效不佳,并且有较高的不良反应发生率。目前三唑类抗真菌药物因其较低的不良反应发生率及治疗ABPA的有效性而被广泛应用在临床实践中。

(一)伊曲康唑

伊曲康唑是最常用的治疗ABPA的抗真菌药物。目前有许多小样本的研究探讨伊曲康唑治疗ABPA患者的作用,但仅有2项研究为随机对照前瞻性研究。其中一项纳入了55个激素依赖ABPA患者的随机对照研究显示给予ABPA患者16周伊曲康唑(400 mg/d)治疗后,患者有临床缓解的可能性显著增加。临床缓解包括口服激素用量至少减少50%,血清IgE浓度至少下降25%,以及下述情况之一:运动耐量或肺功能检查显示至少改善25%,或肺部浸润影部分或完全消失。基于这项研究,中国ABPA专家共识提倡将伊曲康唑用于激素依赖、激素治疗后复发患者。另一项随机对照研究纳入了29位缓解期ABPA患者,其中15位患者接受了16周伊曲康唑(400 mg/d)治疗,结果显示伊曲康唑可以显著减少ABPA复发活动次数,降低痰液嗜酸性粒细胞、血清IgE及血清抗曲霉IgG抗体水平。对于缓解期患者何时需启用抗真菌治疗、哪些缓解期ABPA患者可能从抗真菌治疗获益仍需进一步探索。此外,这2项研究均未对接受伊曲康唑治疗的ABPA患者进行超过1年的随访,因此关于伊曲康唑治疗激素依赖性ABPA或缓解期ABPA的长期疗效还有待进一步证实。

关于抗真菌药物在治疗新发活动期ABPA的地位还有待进一步探索。近期发表的1项随机对照前瞻研究纳入了131例急性ABPA伴哮喘患者,旨在比较单用伊曲康唑(200 mg,2次/天)及泼尼松龙(按照方案3开始给药)治疗新发活动期ABPA疗效差异。结果显示两组在1年和2年时发作次数、治疗结束后首次发作的时间、6周及3个月血清总IgE下降百分比以及6周后肺功能改善情况均无差异。然而泼尼松组在治疗6周时的临床缓解率更高(100% vs 88%)。临床缓解指临床症状改善,影像学提示病灶部分或完全消失,IgE较基线值下降25%。不良反应方面,泼尼松组的不良反应发生率显著高于伊曲康唑组。基于以上结果,研究者认为对于存在激素治疗禁忌的ABPA活动期患者,伊曲康唑是良好的替代药物。然而该研究存在一些缺陷:例如研究为非盲研究,在治疗第6周有8例伊曲康唑治疗无效者更换为泼尼松龙治疗,以及两组2年时均有约25%的失访率。因此关于单用抗真菌药物治疗ABPA急性期的疗效还有待进一步验证。此外,为了减少长期激素治疗的剂量及疗程并改善ABPA患者的长期预后,在临床实践中常采用激素联合抗真菌药物治疗急性期ABPA的患者,然而该治疗方案尚缺乏循证医学证据。目前正在进行的一项临床研究(clinicaltrials.gov: NCT02440009)旨在比较联合用药与单用激素治疗活动期ABPA患者的疗效及不良反应差异。

中国ABPA专家共识推荐成人的伊曲康唑治疗剂量为200 mg,2次/天,疗程为4~6月。然而关于伊曲康唑治疗ABPA的治疗剂量多沿用侵袭性肺曲霉菌病的推荐剂量,缺乏循证医学证据。也有文献报道采用低剂量伊曲康唑(200 mg/d)也可有效治疗ABPA。考虑到抗真菌药物费用及治疗长疗程问题,低剂量方案优势显而易见,但其临床疗效仍需进一步明确。

(二)新三唑类药物

相比于伊曲康唑,伏立康唑及泊沙康唑在治疗ABPA也具有一定疗效。目前只有少量研究探索伏立康唑及泊沙康唑治疗ABPA的疗效。其中的一项研究回顾性分析了20个曾接受伊曲康唑治疗但因疗效欠佳或不良反应而停药的ABPA患者，结果显示伏立康唑(300~600 mg/d)或泊沙康唑(800 mg/d)治疗后，70%~75%患者在3个月及6个月的时间获得临床缓解(包括激素减量，症状控制，血清IgE下降)。但因样本量较少，这项研究无法明确新三唑类药物治疗ABPA的长期疗效。与伊曲康唑相比，伏立康唑及泊沙康唑具有明显的优势，如胃肠道耐受性和生物利用度均较高，但仍不清楚在ABPA的治疗中，伏立康唑及泊沙康唑是否优于伊曲康唑，未来需要前瞻性随机对照研究比较伊曲康唑与新三唑类药物之间的疗效及不良反应差异。

四、靶向治疗

ABPA是一种严重的炎症性肺病，其病因包括真菌孢子刺激呼吸道上皮细胞引发强烈的Th2型炎症，因此针对Th2型细胞因子IgE和IL-5的靶向治疗可能对ABPA有效。

(一) 抗IgE

奥马珠单抗(omalizumab)是一种针对IgE的人源化单克隆抗体，全球哮喘防治倡议推荐奥马珠单抗用于4级治疗无法控制的中至重度过敏性哮喘，可降低哮喘急性加重的频率、减少糖皮质激素的使用。ABPA患者的血清总IgE水平显著升高，因此，奥马珠单抗对ABPA患者可能有一定疗效。一篇对30篇已发表文献中的102例奥马珠单抗治疗ABPA患者的系统评价表明，奥马珠单抗对于ABPA患者具有良好的安全性，可降低FeNO、急性加重率、激素用量及血清IgE，并能显著改善症状，但对肺功能无明显改善作用。另一篇对于14例ABPA合并囊性纤维化患者临床研究的系统评价则表明，奥马珠单抗治疗ABPA合并囊性纤维化的有效性和安全性缺乏证据，有必要进行抗IgE治疗的大型前瞻性随机对照研究。在用药剂量方面，相较于哮喘患者，ABPA患者血清总IgE水平较高，按照标准计算的剂量要求给药可能达不到疗效，既往报道中ABPA患者使用奥马珠单抗的剂量从225mg到750mg不等，给药频率从每周一次到每月一次不等，而最常用的给药方法为375mg皮下注射，每两周一次，疗程从3个月到60个月不等，平均疗程为13.4个月，疗程长短取决于药物疗效。因此奥马珠单抗作为靶向抗IgE的生物制剂，对于ABPA患者可能是一种安全而有效的治疗选择，但用药剂量、给药频率及疗程长短目前仍无统一标准，未来仍需要进行大规模临床试验以进一步明确。

(二) 抗IL-5

美泊利单抗(mepolizumab)是抗IL-5的人源化单克隆抗体，可有效减少过敏性哮喘患者外周血嗜酸性粒细胞，降低急性加重率，减少口服激素使用，改善肺功能和生活质量。一例病例报告报道了一名58岁女性ABPA患者，在接受激素、抗真菌、奥马珠单抗治疗后症状均无改善，但在治疗方案中加用美泊利单抗，一次100 mg，4周1次，治疗3个月后成功撤除口服激素、活动耐量明显提高、外周血嗜酸性粒细胞计数显著降低。一项对20例ABPA患者的前瞻性研究表明应用美泊利单抗可显著减少口服糖皮质激素的使用、急性加重率、血嗜酸性粒细胞计数，并显著改善患者生活质量和FEV_1，但FeNO无明显变化。同奥马珠单抗一致，目前针对美泊利单抗治疗ABPA的数据尚不全面，仍有必要进行更大规模的随机试验探究疗效及其安全性。

五、小结及展望

当前中国哮喘患病率呈明显上升趋势，但临床控制率不容乐观，重症哮喘仍属常见。ABPA是重症哮喘的重要原因。由于ABPA发病率相对较低，目前关于ABPA的临床研究相对较少，治疗缺乏规范可循。口服激素是ABPA患者的一线治疗方案；然而关于口服激素治疗活动期ABPA的初始剂量、缓解期维持方案及疗程仍缺乏统一规范。抗真菌药物是重要的辅助药物，其可有效治疗激素依赖期ABPA患者；也可减轻缓解期ABPA患者气道炎症水平，减少急性加重次数；然而关于抗真菌药物治疗的初始剂量、疗程及长期疗效仍有待进一步探讨。此外，目前迫切需要了解抗真菌药物联合口服激素治疗新发活动期ABPA患者的疗效。奥马珠单抗、美泊利珠单抗治疗激素依赖期ABPA患者可以实现临床缓解，但文献多为个例报道及小样本研究，其疗效也有待深入研究。

参 考 文 献

[1] Agarwal R. Allergic bronchopulmonary aspergillosis. Chest, 2009,135(3):805-826.

[2] Hinson KF, Moon AJ, Plummer NS. Broncho-pulmonary aspergillosis: a review and a report of eight new cases. Thorax, 1952,7(4):317-333.

[3] 张鼎,胡建,廖纪萍,等. 变应性支气管肺曲霉菌病的免疫机制与诊治. 中华临床免疫和变态反应杂志,2015(2):142-147.

[4] Hogan C, Denning DW. Allergic bronchopulmonary aspergillosis and related allergic syndromes. Semin Respir Crit Care Med,2011,32(6):682-692.

[5] Agarwal R, Aggarwal AN, Dhooria S, et al. A randomised trial of glucocorticoids in acute-stage allergic bronchopulmonary aspergillosis complicating asthma. Eur Respir J,2016,47(2):490-498.

[6] Agarwal R, Dhooria S, Sehgal IS, et al. A randomised trial of voriconazole and prednisolone monotherapy in acute-stage allergic bronchopulmonary aspergillosis complicating asthma. Eur Respir J,2018,52(3).

[7] Agarwal R, Dhooria S, Singh SI, et al. A randomized trial of itraconazole vs prednisolone in acute-stage allergic bronchopulmonary aspergillosis complicating asthma. Chest,2018,153(3):656-664.

[8] 中华医学会呼吸病学分会哮喘学组. 变应性支气管肺曲霉病诊治专家共识. 中华医学杂志,2017,97(34):2650-2656.

[9] Report to the Research Committee of the British Thoracic Association. Inhaled beclomethasone dipropionate in allergic bronchopulmonary aspergillosis. Br J Dis Chest,1979,73(4): 349-356.

[10] Heinig JH,Weeke ER,Groth S,et al. High-dose local steroid treatment in bronchopulmonary aspergillosis. A pilot study. Allergy,1988,43(1):24-31.

[11] Imbeault B,Cormier Y. Usefulness of inhaled high-dose corticosteroids in allergic bronchopulmonary aspergillosis. Chest,1993,103(5):1614-1617.

[12] Seaton A,Seaton RA,Wightman AJ. Management of allergic bronchopulmonary aspergillosis without maintenance oral corticosteroids: a fifteen-year follow-up. QJM,1994,87(9): 529-537.

[13] Agarwal R,Khan A,Aggarwal AN,et al. Role of inhaled corticosteroids in the management of serological allergicbronchopulmonary aspergillosis (ABPA). Intern Med, 2011, 50 (8):855-860.

[14] Thomson JM,Wesley A,Byrnes CA,et al. Pulse intravenous methylprednisolone for resistant allergic bronchopulmonary aspergillosis in cystic fibrosis. Pediatr Pulmonol, 2006, 41 (2):164-170.

[15] Singh SI, Agarwal R. Pulse methylprednisolone in allergic bronchopulmonary aspergillosis exacerbations. Eur Respir Rev,2014,23(131):149-152.

[16] Karst H,Berger S,Turiault M,et al. Mineralocorticoid receptors are indispensable for nongenomic modulation of hippocampal glutamate transmission by corticosterone. Proc Natl Acad Sci U S A,2005,102(52):19204-19207.

[17] Stark JE. Allergic pulmonary aspergillosis successfully treated with inhalations of nystatin. Report of a case. Dis Chest, 1967,51(1):96-99.

[18] Shale DJ,Faux JA,Lane DJ. Trial of ketoconazole in non-invasive pulmonary aspergillosis. Thorax,1987,42(1):26-31.

[19] Fournier EC. Trial of ketoconazole in allergic bronchopulmonary aspergillosis. Thorax,1987,42(10):831.

[20] Wark PA, Gibson PG, Wilson AJ. Azoles for allergic bronchopulmonary aspergillosis associated with asthma. Cochrane Database Syst Rev,2004(3):D1108.

[21] Stevens DA,Schwartz HJ,Lee JY,et al. A randomized trial of itraconazole in allergic bronchopulmonary aspergillosis. N Engl J Med,2000,342(11):756-762.

[22] Wark PA, Hensley MJ, Saltos N, et al. Anti-inflammatory effect of itraconazole in stable allergic bronchopulmonary aspergillosis: a randomized controlled trial. J Allergy Clin Immunol,2003,111(5):952-957.

[23] Germaud P,Tuchais E. Allergic bronchopulmonary aspergillosis treated with itraconazole. Chest,1995,107(3):883.

[24] Salez F,Brichet A,Desurmont S,et al. Effects of itraconazole therapy in allergic bronchopulmonaryaspergillosis. Chest, 1999,116(6):1665-1668.

[25] Skov M,Hoiby N,Koch C. Itraconazole treatment of allergic bronchopulmonary aspergillosis in patients with cystic fibrosis. Allergy,2002,57(8):723-728.

[26] Glackin L,Leen G,Elnazir B,et al. Voriconazole in the treatment of allergic bronchopulmonary aspergillosis in cystic fibrosis. Ir Med J,2009,102(1):29.

[27] Chishimba L, Niven RM, Cooley J, et al. Voriconazole and posaconazole improve asthma severity in allergic bronchopulmonary aspergillosis and severe asthma with fungal sensitization. J Asthma,2012,49(4):423-433.

[28] Agarwal R,Sehgal IS,Dhooria S,et al. Developments in the diagnosis and treatment of allergic bronchopulmonary aspergillosis. Expert Rev Respir Med,2016,10(12):1317-1334.

[29] Li JX,Fan LC,Li MH,et al. Beneficial effects of Omalizumab therapy in allergic bronchopulmonary aspergillosis: A synthesis review of published literature. Respir Med, 2017, 122: 33-42.

[30] Jat KR,Walia DK,Khairwa A. Anti-IgE therapy for allergic bronchopulmonary aspergillosis in people with cystic fibrosis. Cochrane Database Syst Rev,2018,3:D10288.

[31] Altman MC,Lenington J,Bronson S,et al. Combination omalizumab and mepolizumab therapy for refractory allergic bronchopulmonary aspergillosis. J Allergy Clin Immunol Pract,2017,5(4):1137-1139.

[32] Schleich F,Vaia ES,Pilette C,et al. Mepolizumab for allergic bronchopulmonary aspergillosis:Report of 20 cases from the Belgian Severe Asthma Registry and review of the literature. J Allergy Clin Immunol Pract,2020.

5 非 Th2 相关性支气管哮喘的研究进展

于化鹏 陈丽嫦

自从嗜酸性粒细胞被发现以来，气道嗜酸性粒细胞炎症一直是哮喘的一个关键特征。过去的30年，随着分子生物学和成像技术的发展，确立了在哮喘中嗜酸性粒细胞的作用和辅助性T淋巴细胞（T helper，Th）的功能。目前普遍认为哮喘是一种Th2免疫性疾病。然而许多重症哮喘并非以嗜酸性粒细胞和Th2型细胞因子为特征，而是低Th2型细胞因子或无Th2细胞因子。Wenzel等研究表明，哮喘病理学可能表现为嗜酸性粒细胞型气道炎症，也可能表现出中性粒细胞型气道炎症或混合细胞型气道炎症。TENOR、SARP及BSAR等重症哮喘相关研究表明，随着时间的推移，一些嗜酸性粒细胞表型的哮喘患者可转换为非嗜酸性粒细胞或混合性粒细胞表型。

糖皮质激素联合支气管扩张剂可延长重症哮喘急性发作的时间间隔，减少急性发作的次数，是重症哮喘治疗的基础。然而非Th2相关性哮喘患者对糖皮质激素不敏感，且不适合使用如抗总免疫球蛋白E（immunoglobulin E，IgE）或抗白细胞介素（interleukin，IL）-5等靶向治疗。因此，探索非Th2相关性哮喘的发病机制，寻找合适的生物标志物和有效的治疗方案具有重要的现实意义。本文综述了非Th2相关性支气管哮喘的定义、机制，总结了迄今用于非Th2相关性哮喘的治疗方法。

一、Th2和非Th2相关性哮喘的定义

哮喘是一种异质性疾病，Th2相关性哮喘与Th2型细胞因子如IL-4、IL-5和IL-13等表达增加有关。这一类型主要是基于嗜酸性粒细胞气道炎症的存在，其通常根据痰或血嗜酸性粒细胞的数量来确定，但目前尚无公认的用于诊断Th2相关性哮喘的嗜酸性粒细胞界值，大部分研究将痰液中嗜酸性粒细胞比例≥3%作为界定嗜酸性粒细胞型哮喘的标准。非Th2相关性哮喘占哮喘的一大部分，其主要包括中性粒细胞型哮喘、混合细胞型哮喘及寡细胞型哮喘等，然而目前人们对这一类型及其分子机制都知之甚少。在大多数情况下，非Th2相关性哮喘的定义是Th2炎症标志物的缺失，主要以气道内嗜中性粒细胞或少量粒细胞浸润为特征。目前对于定义中性粒细胞型哮喘表型所需痰中性粒细胞的百分比并没有统一的规定，文献中使用的切点值范围在40%~76%。值得注意的是，这一指标不包括细胞总数升高。中性粒细胞升高伴总细胞计数很高通常表示气道感染。

二、非Th2相关性哮喘的临床特征

非Th2相关性哮喘具有迟发性、对糖皮质激素不敏感等特征。研究表明，随着年龄的增长，痰液中中性粒细胞数量增加。对于非嗜酸性粒细胞表型的肥胖哮喘患者，其特征主要是中年女性、迟发性哮喘及哮喘症状反复发作。这些哮喘患者控制不佳，且病情加重的风险较高。非Th2相关性哮喘的另一个特征是对糖皮质激素不敏感。研究表明，中性粒细胞气道炎症与吸烟、空气污染及病毒/细菌感染等相关。气道微生物群中的莫拉氏菌，链球菌和嗜血杆菌与哮喘患者痰液中中性粒细胞增多及IL-8浓度升高有关。此外，剧烈运动和寒冷是中性粒细胞型哮喘的诱因。

三、非Th2相关性哮喘的生物标志物

非Th2相关性哮喘在哮喘中，尤其是重症哮喘中并不罕见。比利时的一项重症哮喘研究表明：嗜酸性粒细胞型哮喘（痰液中嗜酸性粒细胞≥3%）是主要表型，约为55%，中性粒细胞型哮喘（痰液中中性粒细胞≥76%）和寡细胞型哮喘（痰液中嗜酸性粒细胞<3%且中性粒细胞<76%）分别占22%和17%。

除痰细胞计数外，目前尚无其他特异性生物标志物可用于鉴别Th2和非Th2相关性哮喘。一些非Th2相关性哮喘的气道和血液生物标志物正处于研究阶段。IL-8激活中性粒细胞，促使其脱颗粒，产生超氧阴离子，引起呼吸暴发。Gibson等研究发现，非嗜酸性粒细胞哮喘患者痰液中的IL-8的水平更高，且其与痰中性粒细胞计数相关。IL-8以及其他中性粒细胞趋化剂，如趋化因子配体1（chemokine ligand 1，CXCL1）和趋化因子配体5（chemokine ligand 5，CXCL5），通过与趋化因子受体1（chemokine receptor 1，CXCR1）和趋化因子受体2（chemokine receptor 2，CXCR2）相互作用以调节它们的趋化活性。这两种受体在中性粒细胞哮喘患者痰液中的表达均显著增加。髓过氧化物酶（myeloperoxidase，MPO）和中性粒细胞弹性蛋白酶（neutrophil elastase，NE）是哮喘中性粒细胞活化的另外两个重要的生物标志物。研究表明，在中性粒细胞相关的重症哮喘中，痰液中MPO和NE的水平升高。肿瘤坏死

因子α(tumor necrosis factor-α,TNF-α)是一种促炎细胞因子，其与重症难治性哮喘及非Th2相关性哮喘均相关。然而，TNF-α抑制剂在重症持续性哮喘患者的临床研究中并未达到预期的治疗效果。IL-17是导致非Th2型气道炎症的Th17通路的生物标志物，其与IL-8在中性粒细胞哮喘中均升高。

在临床诊治过程中并不是依靠上述非Th2相关的生物标志物对非Th2相关性哮喘进行识别，而是通过Th2相关的生物标志物进行排除。呼出气一氧化氮、血嗜酸性粒细胞、总IgE和血清骨骼肌肌球蛋白是良好的Th2相关性哮喘的生物标志物。在Busse等最近的一项研究中，用于定义高Th2气道炎症的生物标志物及其临界点为：IgE≥100 IU/ml、嗜酸性粒细胞≥300/ml、呼出气一氧化氮≥30 ppb，其中符合两个或两个以上的生物标志物升高为Th2相关性哮喘，否则为非Th2相关性哮喘。这种分类方法简单易行，可以在临床实践中使用。

四、Th2/非Th2相关性哮喘气道炎症的机制

根据哮喘免疫病理学可将其分为嗜酸性粒细胞型哮喘(过敏性和非过敏性)、非嗜酸性粒细胞型哮喘(中性粒细胞型哮喘和寡细胞型哮喘)和混合粒细胞型哮喘。Th2相关性哮喘(嗜酸性粒细胞型哮喘)可以是过敏性的，也可以是非过敏性的。在过敏性哮喘患者中，树突状细胞识别过敏性抗原决定簇，呈递抗原并诱导T细胞分化为Th2细胞，Th2细胞释放IL-4和IL-13等Th2细胞因子，导致B细胞生成IgE增加。此外，Th2细胞释放的IL-5促进嗜酸性粒细胞的募集和增生。在非过敏性哮喘患者中，环境污染物、细菌/病毒感染使得支气管上皮产生胸腺基质淋巴生成素(thymic stromallymphopoietin,TSLP)、IL-25和IL-33，促使2型先天淋巴细胞(innate lymphoid cell 2,ILC2)产生效应细胞因子IL-5、IL-13和IL-9。两种途径最终都导致嗜酸性气道炎症及气道重塑。一些迟发、重症非Th2相关性哮喘是嗜中性粒细胞型的，而不是嗜酸性粒细胞型的。目前对于非Th2相关性哮喘的具体机制尚不清楚。气道平滑肌异常、IL-8和(或)IL-17介导的炎症过程被认为是可能的机制。此外，非Th2相关性哮喘可能与有害刺激物有关，如职业暴露、吸烟和细菌/病毒感染。以中性粒细胞气道炎症为主的重症哮喘患者表现出混合的Th1和Th17炎症特征。活化的Th17细胞和3型先天淋巴样细胞(innate lymphoid cell 3,ILC3)释放IL-17和IL-22，刺激支气管上皮细胞合成和释放促中性粒细胞趋化因子，例如IL-8和CXCL1。Gibson等报道了IL-8在非Th2相关性哮喘通路中的作用。该研究小组还发现，在中性粒细胞哮喘患者中，IL-8受体(包括IL-8RA和IL-8RB)增加。动物实验研究表明，IL-8通过NF-κB途径导致糖皮质激素耐受性中性粒细胞气道炎症的发生。此外，支气管上皮受损也可能与中性粒细胞炎症的建立直接相关。中性粒细胞释放的炎性介质造成气道损伤、气道高反应性和气道重塑。

五、非Th2相关性哮喘的管理

目前尚缺乏有效的药物治疗非Th2相关性哮喘。戒烟和避免接触环境/职业污染物可改善哮喘患者的病情，是一项重要但常常被忽视的低成本干预措施。吸烟不仅加重哮喘的症状，使得哮喘难以控制，而且还与难治性哮喘有关。此外，戒烟3个月可改善哮喘症状，降低哮喘患者气道高反应性。另一方面，臭氧和氮氧化物等污染物可诱导气道高反应性和中性粒细胞气道炎症，引起气道损伤和气道重塑。

尽管目前尚无治疗非Th2相关性哮喘的有效药物，然而一些新的药物正处于研发或临床试验阶段，如CXCR2拮抗剂、5-脂氧合酶激活蛋白(5-lipoxygenase activating protein,FLAP)抑制剂、前列腺素E3/E4和多种蛋白激酶抑制剂。研究表明，CXCR2拮抗剂可能在治疗非Th2相关性哮喘方面具有良好的效果。然而关于阻断Th17和Th1介导的气道炎症相关药物的临床研究，如抗IL-17和抗TNF-α药物并未取得令人满意的结果，甚至增加了患者严重感染和恶性肿瘤的风险。Brusselle等的研究表明，使用阿奇霉素显著降低非Th2相关性哮喘患者的病情恶化率。此外，在难治性哮喘患者的治疗中添加噻托溴铵可改善患者气道阻塞，降低恶化率。支气管热成形术是一项高安全性的显著减少气道平滑肌的支气管镜下治疗技术，其可改善哮喘的临床控制，减少急性加重次数。非Th2相关性哮喘治疗方法的选择应考虑每个患者的特性，如气道炎症的类型(中性粒细胞性、少粒细胞性)及对糖皮质激素的敏感程度等。

六、小 结

尽管对于嗜酸性粒细胞驱动的Th2相关性哮喘的机制研究比较深入，但目前对于非Th2相关性哮喘的了解仍然不足。IL-8和IL-17似乎在非Th2相关性哮喘的发病中具有一定的作用，但目前尚无有力的研究证据证明它们可以作为治疗非Th2相关性哮喘的靶点，因此当前的治疗方法仍然是非特异性的。由于目前对关于非Th2相关性哮喘的研究仍不充分，许多问题并未达成共识，因此今后需进一步深入研究非Th2相关性哮喘的发病机制，进而寻找合适的生物标志物和有效的治疗方案，以提高哮喘疗效、减少急性发作及降低病死率。

参 考 文 献

[1] Wenzel SE, Schwartz LB, Langmack EL, et al. Evidence that severe asthma can be divided pathologically into two inflammatory subtypes with distinct physiologic and clinical characteristics. Am J Respir Crit Care Med, 1999, 160 (3):

1001-1008.

[2] The ENFUMOSA cross-sectional European multicentre study of the clinical phenotype of chronic severe asthma. European Network for Understanding Mechanisms of Severe Asthma. Eur Respir J,2003,22(3):470-477.

[3] Jarjour NN,Erzurum SC,Bleecker ER,et al. Severe asthma: lessons learned from the National Heart,Lung,and Blood Institute Severe Asthma Research Program. Am J Respir Crit Care Med,2012,185(4):356-362.

[4] Schleich F,Brusselle G,Louis R,et al. Heterogeneity of phenotypes in severe asthmatics. The Belgian Severe Asthma Registry(BSAR). Respir Med,2014,108(12):1723-1732.

[5] Selroos O. A smarter way to manage asthma with a combination of a long-acting beta(2)-agonist and inhaled corticosteroid. Ther Clin Risk Manag,2007,3(2):349-359.

[6] Tan R,Liew MF,Lim HF,et al. Promises and challenges of biologics for severe asthma. Biochem Pharmacol, 2020:114012.

[7] Schleich F,Brusselle G,Louis R,et al. Heterogeneity of phenotypes in severe asthmatics. The Belgian Severe Asthma Registry(BSAR). Respir Med,2014,108(12):1723-1732.

[8] Katz LE,Gleich GJ,Hartley BF,et al. Blood eosinophil count is a useful biomarker to identify patients with severe eosinophilic asthma. Ann Am Thorac Soc,2014,11(4):531-536.

[9] Ortega HG,Yancey SW,Mayer B,et al. Severe eosinophilic asthma treated with mepolizumab stratified by baseline eosinophil thresholds:a secondary analysis of the DREAM and MENSA studies. Lancet Respir Med,2016,4(7):549-556.

[10] Simpson JL,Scott R,Boyle MJ,et al. Inflammatory subtypes in asthma:assessment and identification using induced sputum. Respirology,2006,11(1):54-61.

[11] Green RH,Brightling CE,Woltmann G,et al. Analysis of induced sputum in adults with asthma:identification of subgroup with isolated sputum neutrophilia and poor response to inhaled corticosteroids. Thorax,2002,57(10):875-879.

[12] Moore WC,Hastie AT,Li X,et al. Sputum neutrophil counts are associated with more severe asthma phenotypes using cluster analysis. J Allergy Clin Immunol,2014,133(6):1557-1563.

[13] Thomas RA,Green RH,Brightling CE,et al. The influence of age on induced sputum differential cell counts in normal subjects. Chest,2004,126(6):1811-1814.

[14] Ducharme ME,Prince P,Hassan N,et al. Expiratory flows and airway inflammation in elderly asthmatic patients. Respir Med,2011,105(9):1284-1289.

[15] Telenga ED,Tideman SW,Kerstjens HA,et al. Obesity in asthma:more neutrophilic inflammation as a possible explanation for a reduced treatment response. Allergy, 2012, 67 (8):1060-1068.

[16] McGrath KW,Icitovic N,Boushey HA,et al. A large subgroup of mild-to-moderate asthma is persistently noneosinophilic. Am J Respir Crit Care Med,2012,185(6):612-619.

[17] Berry M,Morgan A,Shaw DE,et al. Pathological features and inhaled corticosteroid response of eosinophilic and non-eosinophilic asthma. Thorax,2007,62(12):1043-1049.

[18] Chalmers GW,MacLeod KJ,Thomson L,et al. Smoking and airway inflammation in patients with mild asthma. Chest, 2001,120(6):1917-1922.

[19] McCreanor J,Cullinan P,Nieuwenhuijsen MJ,et al. Respiratory effects of exposure to diesel traffic in persons with asthma. N Engl J Med,2007,357(23):2348-2358.

[20] Nightingale JA,Rogers DF,Barnes PJ. Effect of inhaled ozone on exhaled nitric oxide,pulmonary function,and induced sputum in normal and asthmatic subjects. Thorax,1999,54 (12):1061-1069.

[21] Guarnieri M,Balmes JR. Outdoor air pollution and asthma. Lancet,2014,383(9928):1581-1592.

[22] Green BJ, Wiriyachaiporn S, Grainge C, et al. Potentially pathogenic airway bacteria and neutrophilic inflammation in treatment resistant severe asthma. PLoS One, 2014, 9 (6):e100645.

[23] Seys SF,Daenen M,Dilissen E,et al. Effects of high altitude and cold air exposure on airway inflammation in patients with asthma. Thorax,2013,68(10):906-913.

[24] Sue-Chu M. Winter sports athletes:long-term effects of cold air exposure. Br J Sports Med,2012,46(6):397-401.

[25] Schleich F,Demarche S,Louis R. Biomarkers in the Management of Difficult Asthma. Curr Top Med Chem, 2016, 16 (14):1561-1573.

[26] Sadik CD, Kim ND, Luster AD. Neutrophils cascading their way to inflammation. Trends Immunol, 2011, 32 (10): 452-460.

[27] Baines KJ,Simpson JL,Wood LG,et al. Sputum gene expression signature of 6 biomarkers discriminates asthma inflammatory phenotypes. J Allergy Clin Immunol,2014,133(4): 997-1007.

[28] Sanchez-Ovando S, Baines KJ, Barker D, et al. Six gene and TH2 signature expression in endobronchial biopsies of participants with asthma. Immun Inflamm Dis,2020,8(1):40-49.

[29] Wright TK,Gibson PG,Simpson JL,et al. Neutrophil extracellular traps are associated with inflammation in chronic airway disease. Respirology,2016,21(3):467-475.

[30] Jatakanon A, Uasuf C, Maziak W, et al. Neutrophilic inflammation in severe persistent asthma. Am J Respir Crit Care Med,1999,160(5 Pt 1):1532-1539.

[31] Vroman H,Bergen IM,van Hulst J,et al. TNF-alpha-induced protein 3 levels in lung dendritic cells instruct TH2 or TH17 cell differentiation in eosinophilic or neutrophilic asthma. J Allergy Clin Immunol,2018,141(5):1620-1633.

[32] Meteran H, Meteran H, Porsbjerg C, et al. Novel monoclonal treatments in severe asthma. J Asthma, 2017, 54 (10): 991-1011.

[33] Kivihall A,Aab A,Soja J,et al. Reduced expression of miR-146a in human bronchial epithelial cells alters neutrophil migration. Clin Transl Allergy,2019,9:62.

[34] Gao W,Han GJ,Zhu YJ,et al. Clinical characteristics and biomarkers analysis of asthma inflammatory phenotypes. Biomark Med,2020,14(3):211-222.

[35] Parulekar A D,Diamant Z,Hanania N A. Role of T2 inflammation biomarkers in severe asthma. Curr Opin Pulm Med,

2016,22(1):59-68.
[36] Busse WW, Holgate ST, Wenzel SW, et al. Biomarker profiles in asthma with high vs low airway reversibility and poor disease control. Chest,2015,148(6):1489-1496.
[37] Simpson JL, Guest M, Boggess MM, et al. Occupational exposures, smoking and airway inflammation in refractory asthma. BMC Pulm Med,2014,14:207.
[38] Gibson PG, Simpson JL, Saltos N. Heterogeneity of airway inflammation in persistent asthma: evidence of neutrophilic inflammation and increased sputum interleukin-8. Chest, 2001,119(5):1329-1336.
[39] Wood LG, Baines KJ, Fu J, et al. The neutrophilic inflammatory phenotype is associated with systemic inflammation in asthma. Chest,2012,142(1):86-93.
[40] Liu R, Bai J, Xu G, et al. Multi-allergen challenge stimulates steriod-resistant airway inflammation via NF-kappaB-mediated IL-8 expression. Inflammation,2013,36(4):845-854.
[41] Kiljander T, Poussa T, Helin T, et al. Symptom control among asthmatics with a clinically significant smoking history: a cross-sectional study in Finland. BMC Pulm Med,2020, 20(1):88.
[42] Shimoda T, Obase Y, Kishikawa R, et al. Influence of cigarette smoking on airway inflammation and inhaled corticosteroid treatment in patients with asthma. Allergy Asthma Proc,2016,37(4):50-58.
[43] Westergaard CG, Porsbjerg C, Backer V. The effect of smoking cessation on airway inflammation in young asthma patients. Clin Exp Allergy,2014,44(3):353-361.
[44] Nishimura KK, Galanter JM, Roth LA, et al. Early-life air pollution and asthma risk in minority children. The GALA II and SAGE II studies. Am J Respir Crit Care Med,2013,188 (3):309-318.
[45] Nair P, Gaga M, Zervas E, et al. Safety and efficacy of a CX-CR2 antagonist in patients with severe asthma and sputum neutrophils: a randomized, placebo-controlled clinical trial. Clin Exp Allergy,2012,42(7):1097-1103.
[46] Chaudhuri R, Norris V, Kelly K, et al. Effects of a FLAP inhibitor, GSK2190915, in asthmatics with high sputum neutrophils. Pulm Pharmacol Ther,2014,27(1):62-69.
[47] Thomson NC. Novel approaches to the management of noneosinophilic asthma. Ther Adv Respir Dis, 2016, 10 (3): 211-234.
[48] Busse WW, Holgate S, Kerwin E, et al. Randomized, double-blind, placebo-controlled study of brodalumab, a human anti-IL-17 receptor monoclonal antibody, in moderate to severe asthma. Am J Respir Crit Care Med, 2013, 188 (11): 1294-1302.
[49] Brusselle GG, Vanderstichele C, Jordens P, et al. Azithromycin for prevention of exacerbations in severe asthma (AZ-ISAST): a multicentre randomised double-blind placebo-controlled trial. Thorax,2013,68(4):322-329.
[50] Gibson PG, Yang IA, Upham JW, et al. Effect of azithromycin on asthma exacerbations and quality of life in adults with persistent uncontrolled asthma (AMAZES): a randomised, double-blind, placebo-controlled trial. Lancet, 2017, 390 (10095):659-668.
[51] Kerstjens HA, Engel M, Dahl R, et al. Tiotropium in asthma poorly controlled with standard combination therapy. N Engl J Med,2012,367(13):1198-1207.
[52] Madsen H, Henriksen DP, Backer V, et al. Efficacy of bronchial thermoplasty in patients with severe asthma. J Asthma, 2019:1-7.
[53] Wechsler ME, Laviolette M, Rubin AS, et al. Bronchial thermoplasty: Long-term safety and effectiveness in patients with severe persistent asthma. J Allergy Clin Immunol, 2013, 132 (6):1295-1302.

6 酷似哮喘的 VCD 研究进展

郑青松　戴　威　戴元荣

声带功能障碍(vocal cord dysfunction,VCD),又称声带矛盾运动(paradoxical vocal fold movement disorder,PVFM)或诱导性喉梗阻(inducible laryngeal obstruction,ILO),是一种由吸气时声带矛盾性内收运动导致气道阻塞而出现相应症状的综合征。发作时主要表现为喘息、呼吸困难、喉头或胸部紧迫感等。与哮喘的症状极为相似,因此极易误诊为哮喘,从而误诊误治,导致严重后果。因此,正确认识、诊断 VCD,无论是对患者,还是对临床医师来说都很有必要。

一、病因及其机制

VCD 的确切发病机制目前仍未十分清楚,但是许多学者认为它是一种多种病因因素引起的疾病,目前研究多倾向于强调易感因素而不是具体机制,如精神心理因素、药物因素、胃食管反流、运动及咽喉部的高反应性等,最近 Bardin 等认为在易感个体中,如焦虑、呼吸功能障碍等因素可激活喉反射,此反射又可因胃食管反流、慢性鼻炎、精神因素或运动因素等增强,而使 VCD 进展,如果不治疗,会加重患者的焦虑、呼吸失调,进而形成恶性循环。

根据病因及高危因素,将 VCD 分为以下 4 个亚型。

(一)精神因素型 VCD

Christopher 等认为 VCD 是一种精神心理因素导致的疾患,患者对心理治疗能产生显著的反应。既往研究提示此类 VCD 患者具有突发性。

(二)刺激物诱发型 VCD

根据刺激物来源不同,又可分为内源性刺激物型 VCD 和外源性刺激物型 VCD。前者诱发因素如胃食管反流、鼻炎等。Woolnough 等研究的 77 例 VCD 患者中,被诊断胃食管反流的占 83.9%($n=62$),经过 8 周的抑酸治疗,仅 24.2% 的患者症状稍有改善,提示其与 VCD 关系复杂,反流仅是 VCD 形成的部分原因。后者诱发因素还包括香烟烟雾、化学制剂、香水产品和空气污染物等外源性刺激物。此类患者通常有明显的触发因素,在职业环境中接触后 24h 内出现症状,当暴露到同样的刺激物时症状可复发。

(三)运动诱导型 VCD

又称运动性喉梗阻(exercise-induced laryngeal obstruction,EILO),常见于年轻的运动员和军人,他们可能有相似的性格特征,如特强的竞争力或过于追求完美。Rundell 推测运动诱导型 VCD 患者的发作与该类患者处于高度精神紧张的竞技状态有关,具体机制还需进一步研究探讨。

(四)自发型 VCD(spontaneous VCD)

是一类原因未明的 VCD。

二、临床表现

主要是由上呼吸道阻塞所引起的症状。Morris 和 Christopher 总结了 1020 例 VCD 患者,发现临床表现主要以呼吸困难(73%)为主,其次为喘息(36%)、喘鸣(28%)和咳嗽(25%)。患者也可感颈部疼痛、声音嘶哑、喉和胸部发紧、有时吞咽困难症状。喘鸣可与气促并存、也可单独存在。有时仅表现为慢性咳嗽。VCD 症状常因睡眠而缓解,但少数患者可因夜间发作而惊醒。无发作时无阳性体征。发作时于吸气期或呼气期出现喘鸣或喘息,声门产生的高调喘息音在全肺均可闻及而以喉部和大气道附近最响。有时最响部位不在喉部和大气道附近,喘息也不具有高调的特点,这时极似哮喘。

另外,VCD 患者常常伴有精神症状,如焦虑、抑郁、失眠等。

三、辅助检查

诊断 VCD 的金标准是喉镜检查,可直观观察声带运动情况。其他检查还有肺功能检查、支气管激发试验、血气分析、胸部 X 线片、喉部高分辨率 CT 等。

(一)喉镜

发作时喉镜示声带矛盾性运动是诊断 VCD 的金标准,表现为吸气时因声带内收而使声门前 2/3 闭合,声门后部呈钻石状裂隙(图 3-6-1)。

但无此征象不能排除 VCD 的诊断。有时可以观察到吸气期和呼气期两期声门均内收,即双相 VCD,运动期间连续喉镜检查(continuous laryngoscopy with exercise,CLE)可以提高诊断敏感性,需提前安装好喉镜,然后让患者在自行车或跑步机上锻炼直至出现典型症状,通常是 8~12min,届时可看到声带矛盾性运动。喉镜结合闪频观测仪(闪频喉镜)不仅能观察声带运动,还可评价声带振动,在无症状时可观察到黏膜波动减弱、声带振幅降低等微细的改变,这提示 VCD 可能是在不稳定持续状态下由诱发因素刺激产生的急性发作。喉镜检查时最好能录像,可让患者观察其声带的异常运动,有利于宣教。同时为更

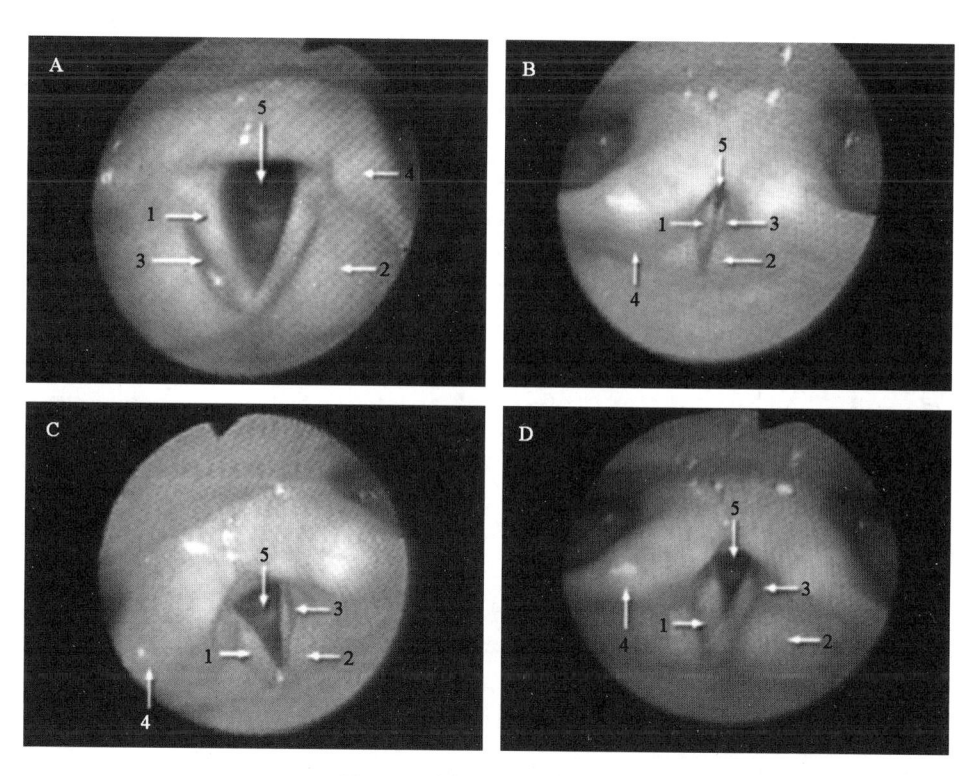

图 3-6-1 喉镜示声带矛盾性运动

真实地观察到声门异常活动,喉镜检查时应避免使用镇静药和麻醉剂。用于治疗哮喘的异丙托溴铵因能抑制迷走神经而干扰声带活动,故也应避免使用。

(二)肺功能检查

肺功能检查可评估上呼吸道的通气状况。患者无症状时肺功能检查通常正常。患者发作时表现为可变的胸腔外气道阻塞,吸气相流速-量环变得扁平(图 3-6-2)。

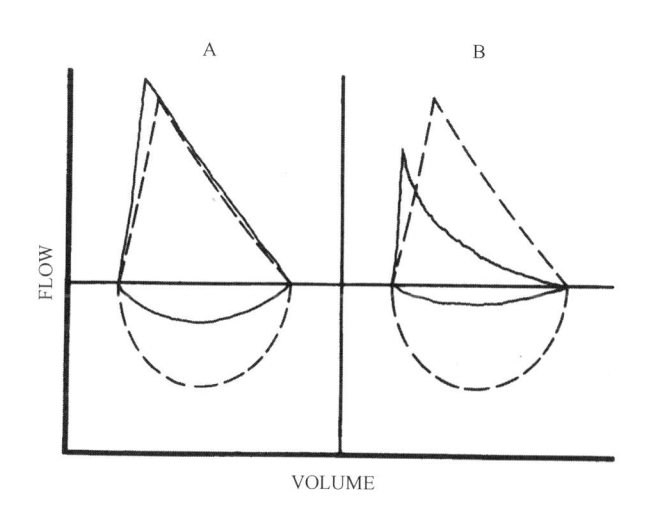

图 3-6-2 肺功能检查可评估上呼吸道的通气状况

如果伴有呼气期声门关闭(即双相 VCD)或同时伴有哮喘则可见流速-量环下降支凹向横轴。流速-容量曲线是 VCD 的主要检查之一,即使在无症状时仍有 23% 异常。VCD 单独存在时 FEV_1、FVC、FEV_1/FVC、PEF 正常,合并哮喘时则下降。正常情况下,50% 肺活量位时呼气流量与吸气流量之比(FEF50/FIF50)≤1,VCD 发作时由于吸气相声带反常内收,使声门变小,FEF50/FIF50≥1。

(三)激发试验

对于喉镜或肺功能检查未见异常的患者,可借助激发试验(如高渗盐水、组胺、乙酰甲胆碱、运动等)提高诊断阳性率。然而,当疑似 VCD 的患者激发试验阳性时,应谨慎,因为本身吸气量的减少有可能导致 FEV_1 和用力肺活量的平行下降,若怀疑有 VCD,在激发试验中 FEV_1 从基线下降到 20% 以下,如果患者的临床条件允许,应在使用支气管扩张药之前进行吸气和呼气流量-容积曲线检查。同时,哮喘的激发试验也可呈阳性。故两者间的鉴别也极为重要。Schulze 等以气雾化的乙酰胆碱作为激发剂,由低剂量开始依次激发并在每次激发后 2 min 做肺功能检查,研究发现 VCD 患者在低剂量的乙酰胆碱激发下 FEV_1 即可显著下降(图 3-6-3)。

非 VCD 患者 FEV_1 则随着乙酰胆碱的剂量逐渐升高而逐渐下降(图 3-6-4)。

值得注意的是,虽然二者的阳性表现皆是 FEV_1 的下降,但其发生机制则不一样:哮喘患者激发试验阳性的发生机制是刺激物致使下呼吸道痉挛;VCD 患者则可能为刺激物直接作用于声带引起声带痉挛,具体机制还有待进一步的探讨,但这也许将成为鉴别 VCD 和哮喘的另一方法。

(四)其他检查

血气分析:尽管有上气道阻塞的表现,但 PaO_2、SaO_2、$P_{(A-a)}O_2$ 均正常,虽然也有报道存在高碳酸血症或低碳酸血症,但大多数患者 $PaCO_2$ 正常。

X 线检查:与哮喘不同,X 线检查往往提示肺部无通气过度。

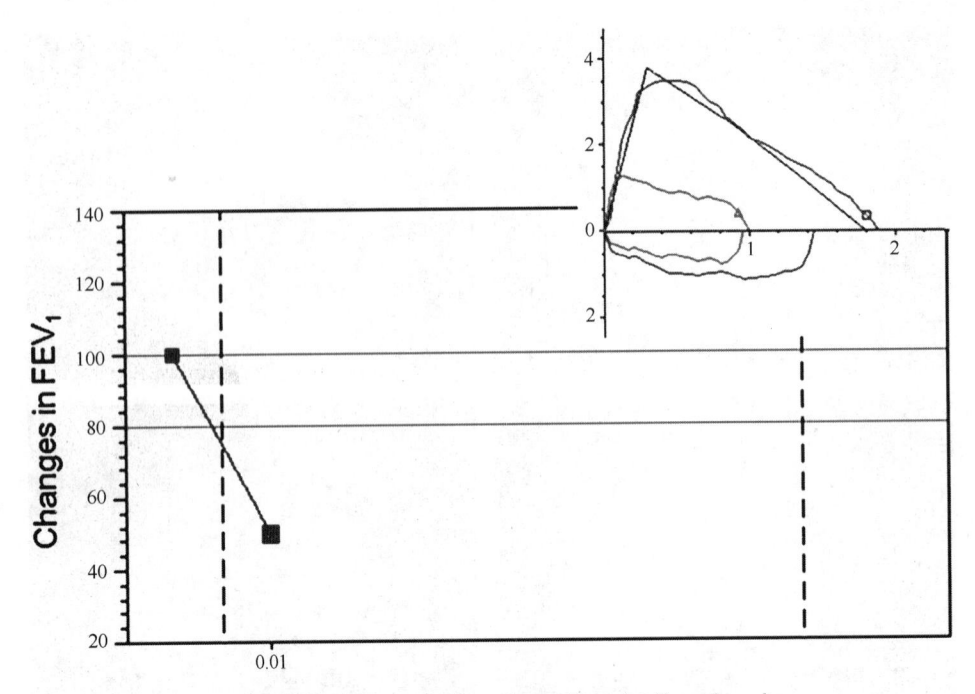

图 3-6-3　VCD 患者在低剂量的乙酰胆碱激发下 FEV₁

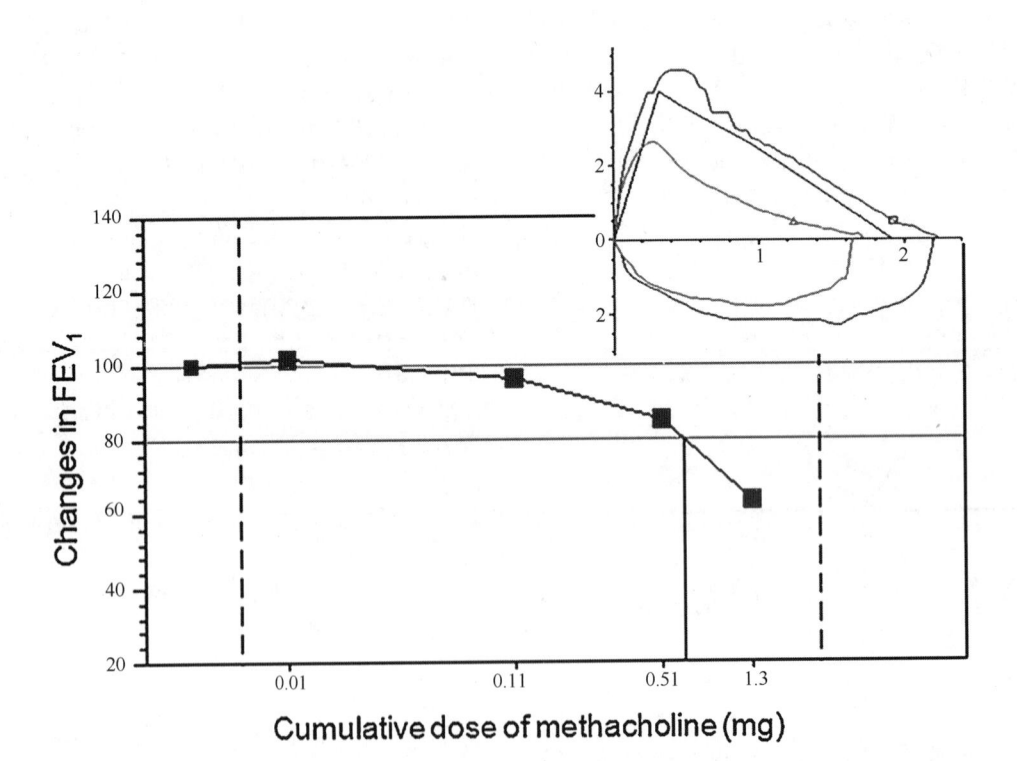

图 3-6-4　非 VCD 患者 FEV₁ 随着乙酰胆碱剂量变化情况

现有学者在做小样本研究使用高分辨率螺旋CT进行检查声带的内收,有望成为新的非侵入性诊断方法。近期有学者使用喉部动态 CT 诊断伴有哮喘急性发作期的 VCD 患者,提示此无创性检测可成为一种有效的协助诊断方法。Bardin 等也验证 46 例患者其喉部动态 CT 与喉镜检查结果具有一致性。

有研究团队使用了一些调查问卷,如匹兹堡声带功能障碍指数问卷,但其准确性还有待进一步评估。

四、诊断标准

1. 喘息、呼吸困难等临床症状。
2. 喉镜下可见声带矛盾性内收。
3. 肺功能检查流速容量异常(大多数见于吸气相)。

其中临床症状和喉镜检查是诊断 VCD 的必需条件。

五、鉴别诊断

所有能引起气道阻塞症状的疾病均需鉴别,首先需除外上气道器质性病变,如喉头水肿和肿瘤、声门下狭窄、双侧喉返神经麻痹、重症肌无力等。譬如,声门下狭窄通常表现为上气道阻塞的逐渐恶化,这类患者可能报告有近期插管史。双侧喉返神经麻痹的患者通常不会有明显的喉咙紧绷感,更常见于手术合并症、神经系统性疾病或风湿免疫性疾病等。肺功能检查有利于鉴别诊断,若吸气和呼气流速容量环持续变平,提示有固定的上气道阻塞,VCD 患者吸气流速容量环提示胸腔外气道阻塞且具有可变性,气道阻力正常,结合全面细致的咽喉部和神经系统检查有助于与无此类疾病的鉴别诊断。

(一)与慢性咳嗽的关系

Perkner 等报道 44 例 VCD 患者中 95% 具有咳嗽症状,Morrison 等则通过"喉易激综合征"的概念把慢性咳嗽和 VCD 联系起来,他们认为脑干中枢神经网络受到持续的刺激,使控制喉部的脑干处于持续的过度兴奋状态,出现咽喉部的高反应性,最后导致喉部肌肉痉挛或声带矛盾运动。慢性咳嗽和 VCD 患者均普遍存在类似的声带发声异常,Vertigan 等发现超过 1/3 的慢性咳嗽和 VCD 患者存在中到重度的发声紧张,声音粗糙和附加呼吸音。通过声门电图检测发现,相对于健康对照组,慢性咳嗽及 VCD 患者发声时间更短,和谐音/噪音比下降,发声范围更小,声带振动时关闭过程更短。

(二)与哮喘的关系

VCD 发作时主要表现为喘息、呼吸困难、喉头或胸部紧迫感等,与哮喘极为相似,极易误诊为哮喘,Maturo 研究显示,44%VCD 的患儿被误诊为哮喘。最近的一项系统分析回顾了 1637 例哮喘患者,成年哮喘患者中合并 VCD 的患病率为 25%(95%CI:15%~37%);同时,VCD 本身可使哮喘加重,Bardin 曾报道 46 例难治性哮喘患者中 50% 伴有 VCD。VCD 与哮喘鉴别诊断时需注意:①既往史:哮喘患者常有家族史,而 VCD 缺少,两者发作皆与情绪压力、运动和外部或内在刺激物有关。②临床表现:哮喘患者常有胸部紧迫感,常夜间或凌晨发作至夜间憋醒、咳痰等,而 VCD 患者常感喉部紧迫感。③哮鸣音:哮喘患者哮鸣音往往来自于小气道,以呼气相较为明显;VCD 患者则是由于胸腔外大气道的阻塞或痉挛,听诊为喉源性喘息或喘鸣。④肺功能流速容量曲线:哮喘患者的流速容量环常表现为呼气相的内凹;VCD 患者则常常表现为吸气相曲线的扁平。但非典型的 VCD 患者喉镜下可观察到呼气相的声带内收,从而导致肺功能流速容积曲线在呼气相的内凹,此时究竟是双相 VCD 还是哮喘合并 VCD 难以鉴别。对此,本研究团队曾发表文章建议:对怀疑为哮喘的患者,若使用哮喘常规药物治疗后疗效不明显,应及时行喉镜检查以排除 VCD 可能;而对诊断哮喘明确的患者,出现突发的哮喘发作并且使用哮喘药物疗效不如之前明显的,需考虑合并 VCD 可能。有少数哮喘合并 VCD 的患者,VCD 的急性发作恰恰是由于吸入哮喘治疗药物诱发的,如果没有认识到这种情况,进而加大或更换哮喘治疗药物,会导致患者预后不良,并造成医疗资源浪费。

六、治 疗

(一)急性发作期

急性发作时可喷入利多卡因来缓解患者声带的反常运动,针对有症状的 VCD 患者,吸入氦氧混合气可以减少急诊就诊次数,发挥类似于 β 受体激动剂对哮喘的缓解作用。通过鼻导管或面罩吸入氦氧混合气(70:30 或 80:20)能有效解除发作,因为氦气在空气中比氮密度低,氦氧混合气通过狭窄的声门时较少产生湍流,所以能减轻呼吸困难,有时吸氧也能缓解症状。异丙托溴铵为常用于哮喘治疗的抗胆碱能类药物,该类药物通过阻断支气管上的 M 受体,降低迷走神经张力而舒张支气管,有报道认为称异丙托溴铵可提高支气管激发试验阳性 VCD 患者的 FEV_1 及改善呼吸道症状。也有报道称无创正压通气可成功解决声带运动异常。

(二)行为干预治疗

行为干预治疗一直被认为是治疗 VCD 的主要方法。而语言病理学疗法(speech pathology treatment,SPT)是行为干预的重要组成部分。Vertigan 等研究提示言语病理治疗有效率可达 88%,该疗法的核心是教会患者如何控制喉部并且保持呼吸过程中气道足够通畅,包括劝导患者减少一些坏习惯例如咳嗽和清嗓,尽量放松以减少肌肉紧张等。Vertigan 团队近期的研究把语言病理学疗法提炼为以下四个方面:①教育;②止咳策略;③减少喉部刺激;④心理辅导。

(三)药物疗法

阿米替林为临床常用的三环类抗抑郁药,常用于焦虑或抑郁症患者。而 90%VCD 患者伴有焦虑、抑郁、失眠等精神症状,Varney 等发现低剂量阿米替林(10~20mg 睡前服用)能有效控制 VCD 的发作,他们观察了 62 例 VCD 患者,发现 90% 的患者可用低剂量阿米替林控制症状,且大多数患者在 1 周内即可起效,若联合心理治疗和行为治疗则疗效更为显著。同时 Vertigan 的一项前瞻性随机对照研究显示语言病理学疗法联合普瑞巴林比单纯 SPT 更有疗效。

(四)肉毒杆菌毒素治疗

Baxter 研究了 24 例伴有异常声带运动的顽固性哮喘患者,评估其单侧声带注射肉毒杆菌毒素前后的反应,发现患者哮喘控制测试评分(ACT)提高,喉部 CT 扫描气道大小也有所改善,表明局部注射肉毒杆菌毒素可能是治疗伴有异常声带运动的顽固性哮喘的有效方法,但具体仍待研究证实。

(五)个体化管理

VCD 患者需长期管理。针对 VCD 的分型采取相对应的治疗能更好地提高治疗的有效率。精神因素型 VCD 患者以行为干预治疗为主,辅以一定的精神类药物;刺激物诱导型患者可采取回避刺激物的方法来减少发作的次数,如胃食管反流物刺激型的患者给予质子泵抑制剂,对于合并哮喘的 VCD 患者因吸入抗哮喘药物诱发 VCD 急性发作的,则可以考虑减少剂量或是改变给药途径,有研究称在运动前吸入抗胆碱能药物(如异丙托溴铵)能预防运动诱发型 VCD 患者的发作。

VCD 是一种较为常见但易被临床医师忽视的的疾病,近年来随着研究的深入,逐渐认识到 VCD 是一个多因素疾病,体征和症状复杂,诊断和治疗较为困难,需要多学科合作,方可取得满意疗效。

参 考 文 献

[1] Bardin PG, Low K, Ruane L, et al. Controversies and conundrums in vocal cord dysfunction, 2017, 5(7):546-548.

[2] Christopher KL, Wood RP, Eckert RC, et al. Vocal-cord dysfunction presenting as asthma, 1983, 308(26):1566-1570.

[3] Mobeireek A, Alhamad A, Alsubaei A, et al. Psychogenic vocal cord dysfunction simulating bronchial asthma. 1995, 8(11):1978-1981.

[4] Niggemann BJPA, Immunology. Functional symptoms confused with allergic disorders in children and adolescents, 2002, 13(5):312-318.

[5] Niggemann BJPA, Immunology. How to diagnose psychogenic and functional breathing disorders in children and adolescents, 2010, 21(6):895-899.

[6] Woolnough K, Blakey JD, Pargeter N, et al. Acid suppression does not reduce symptoms from vocal cord dysfunction, where gastro-laryngeal reflux is a known trigger, 2013, 18(3):553-554.

[7] Newman KB, Mason UG, Schmaling KBJAJoR, et al. Clinical features of vocal cord dysfunction, 1995, 152(4):1382-1386.

[8] Petrov AAJI, America ACoN. Vocal Cord Dysfunction: The Spectrum Across the Ages, 2019, 39(4):547-560.

[9] Fan E, Olin JT. Exercise-induced Laryngeal Obstruction. Am J Respir Crit Care Med, 2019, 199(12):23-24.

[10] Rundell KW, Spiering BA. Inspiratory stridor in elite athletes. Chest, 2003, 123(2):468-474.

[11] Morris MJ, Christopher KLJC. Diagnostic Criteria for the Classification of Vocal Cord Dysfunction, 2010, 138(5):1213-1223.

[12] Olin JT, Clary MS, Fan EM, et al. Continuous laryngoscopy quantitates laryngeal behaviour in exercise and recovery, 2016, 48(4):1192-1200.

[13] Bahrainwala AH, Simon MR. Wheezing and vocal cord dysfunction mimicking asthma. Curr Opin Pulm Med, 2001, 7(1):8-13.

[14] Schulze J, Weber S, Rosewich M, et al. Vocal cord dysfunction in adolescents. Pediatr Pulmonol, 2012, 47(6):612-619.

[15] Daley CP, Ruane L, Leong P, et al. Vocal Cord Dysfunction in Patients Hospitalized with Symptoms of Acute Asthma Exacerbation. 2019, 200(6):782-785.

[16] Low K, Lau KK, Holmes P, et al. Abnormal vocal cord function in difficult-to-treat asthma, 2011, 184(1):50-56.

[17] Traister RS, Fajt ML, Landsittel D, et al. A Novel Scoring System to Distinguish Vocal Cord Dysfunction From Asthma, 2014, 2(1):65-69.

[18] Perkner JJ, Fennelly KP, Balkissoon R, et al. Irritant-associated vocal cord dysfunction. J Occup Environ Med, 1998, 40(2):136-143.

[19] Morrison M, Rammage L, Emami AJ. The irritable larynx syndrome. J Voice, 1999, 13(3):447-455.

[20] Vertigan AE, Theodoros DG, Winkworth AL, et al. Perceptual voice characteristics in chronic cough and paradoxical vocal fold movement. Folia Phoniatr Logop, 2007, 59(5):256-267.

[21] Vertigan AE, Theodoros DG, Winkworth AL, et al. Acoustic and electroglottographic voice characteristics in chronic cough and paradoxical vocal fold movement. Folia Phoniatr Logop, 2008, 60(4):210-216.

[22] 黎志雄. 声带功能障碍研究进展. 国际呼吸杂志, 2014.

[23] Maturo S, Hill C, Bunting G, et al. Pediatric Paradoxical Vocal-Fold Motion: Presentation and Natural History, 2011, 128(6).

[24] Tay TR, Hew MJA. Comorbid "treatable traits" in difficult asthma: Current evidence and clinical evaluation, 2018, 73(7):1369-1382.

[25] Mcdonald VM, Hiles SA, Godbout K, et al. Treatable traits can be identified in a severe asthma registry and predict future exacerbations, 2019, 24(1):37-47.

[26] Lee J, Tay TR, Paddle P, et al. Diagnosis of concomitant inducible laryngeal obstruction and asthma, 2018, 48(12):1622-1630.

[27] Benninger C, Parsons JP, Mastronarde JG. Vocal cord dysfunction and asthma. Curr Opin Pulm Med, 2011, 17(1):45-49.

[28] Reisner C, Borish L. Heliox therapy for acute vocal cord dysfunction. Chest, 1995, 108(5):1477.

[29] Weir M. Vocal cord dysfunction mimics asthma and may respond to heliox. Clin Pediatr(Phila), 2002, 41(1):37 41.

[30] Goldman J, Muers M. Vocal cord dysfunction and wheezing. Thorax, 1991, 46(6):401-404.

[31] Doshi DR, Weinberger MJ, AoAA, Immunology. Long-term outcome of vocal cord dysfunction, 2006, 96(6):794-799.

[32] Denipah N, Dominguez CM, Kraai EP, et al. Acute Management of Paradoxical Vocal Fold Motion(Vocal Cord Dysfunction), 2017, 69(1):18-23.

[33] Vertigan AE, Theodoros D, Gibson PG, et al. Efficacy of speech pathology management for chronic cough: a randomised placebo controlled trial of treatment efficacy, 2006, 61(12):1065-1069.

[34] Vertigan AE, Haines J, Slovarp LJTJoA, et al. An Update on Speech Pathology Management of Chronic Refractory Cough, 2019, 7(6):1756-1761.

[35] Varney V, Parnell H, Evans J, et al. The successful treatment of vocal cord dysfunction with low-dose amitriptyline-including literature review. J Asthma Allergy, 2009, 2:105-110.

[36] Vertigan AE, Kapela SL, Ryan NM, et al. Pregabalin and Speech Pathology Combination Therapy for Refractory Chronic Cough: A Randomized Controlled Trial. Chest, 2016, 149(3):639-648.

[37] Baxter M, Uddin AKMN, Raghav S, et al. Abnormal vocal cord movement treated with botulinum toxin in patients with asthma resistant to optimised management, 2014, 19(4):531-537.

[38] Hull JHJR. Multidisciplinary team working for vocal cord dysfunction: Now it's GO time, 2019, 24(8):714-715.

[39] Baxter M, Ruane L, Phyland D, et al. Multidisciplinary team clinic for vocal cord dysfunction directs therapy and significantly reduces healthcare utilization, 2019, 24(8):758-764.

7 趋化因子与哮喘

张 超 杜旭菲 邵喆婳 张 岩 应颂敏 沈华浩

趋化因子是一类由细胞分泌的小细胞因子或信号蛋白，因具有定向的细胞趋化作用而得名。支气管哮喘（哮喘）是一种过敏原引起的由嗜酸性粒细胞、肥大细胞、T淋巴细胞等多种细胞和细胞组分参与的气道慢性炎症性疾病。目前已经有大量研究表明趋化因子及其受体在哮喘的发病过程中发挥着极其重要的作用，本团队也做了大量的工作来补充和完善趋化因子对哮喘气道炎症的调控作用，阐明哮喘气道炎症发生发展的分子机制，从而为哮喘的临床治疗提供新的靶点。

一、趋化因子及受体与哮喘

(一) 趋化因子的功能

趋化因子的基本功能是定向趋化表达有相应趋化因子受体的细胞。至今已发现 40 多种人的趋化因子，属细胞因子中的最大家族。根据靠近分子氨基端（N端）的前两个C之间是否插入其他氨基酸，可将趋化因子分为 4 个亚类：CXC 类（插入 1 个氨基酸残基）、CC 类（不插入其他氨基酸残基）、C 类（N端仅 1 个 C）和 CX3C 类（插入 3 个其他氨基酸）。趋化因子受体是在白细胞表面发现的含有 7 个跨膜结构域的 G 蛋白偶联受体，目前已经鉴定出的趋化因子受体约有 19 种，根据它们结合的趋化因子的类型被分为四个家族：与 CXC 趋化因子结合的 CXCR，与 CC 趋化因子结合的 CCR，唯一与 CX3C 趋化因子（CX3CL1）结合的 CX3CR1，与两个 C 类趋化因子（XCL1 和 XCL2）结合的 XCR1。趋化因子与其受体的相互作用，控制着各种免疫细胞在循环系统和组织器官间的定向迁移，对清除病原体、促进创伤愈合、消灭异常增生细胞及维持组织细胞平衡起到关键作用。此外，有研究表明趋化因子还具有控制和调节 DCs 的迁移及成熟过程、参与 T、B 淋巴细胞活化及 T 细胞定向分化、抑制和清除病原体，以及调节器官及细胞发育、血管生成等功能。

(二) 趋化因子与哮喘

哮喘是一个典型的 Th2 型免疫反应介导的气道炎症性疾病，其中嗜酸性粒细胞是哮喘的主要炎症效应细胞。哮喘的主要病理改变是大量的嗜酸性粒细胞在骨髓分化并向肺部趋化，而后嗜酸性粒细胞在肺局部活化并释放大量炎症因子进而导致气道局部的炎症浸润。研究发现，趋化因子 CCL11、CCL24 和 CCL27 即 eotaxin 可通过与其受体 CCR3 结合定向诱导嗜酸性粒细胞和 Th2 细胞迁移入肺从而介导哮喘炎症的发生发展；趋化因子 CCL17 和 CCL22 则可通过与其受体 CCR4 结合促进 Th2 型免疫反应的发生。

除了定向趋化嗜酸性粒细胞和 Th2 细胞和促进 Th2 型免疫反应外，趋化因子是否还能够通过其他途径介导哮喘的发生目前尚不清楚。

二、CCL6-CCR1 轴调控哮喘气道炎症

(一) 嗜酸性粒细胞分泌 CCL6 调控哮喘

本研究团队发现哮喘小鼠骨髓干/祖细胞数目增多，但造血重建能力下降，其中干/祖细胞数目的增多主要表现为各阶段的 HSC 及粒-单核系的祖细胞 GMP 的增多，而造血重建能力的下降则表现为体外克隆形成能力的下降。哮喘小鼠的外周血、脾及骨髓中均有较高水平的嗜酸性粒细胞，那么 HSC 的数目增加和造血重建功能的降低是否与高水平的嗜酸性粒细胞有关呢？于是我们在研究中引入了 Cd3-IL5 Transgenic 的小鼠，因为 IL5 是嗜酸性粒细胞分化的重要细胞因子，所以 IL5 过表达会导致该小鼠体内存在大量成熟的嗜酸性粒细胞，经检测我们发现：该小鼠成年后骨髓中嗜酸性粒细胞比例超过 80%。进一步分析发现：其骨髓 HSC 的数目和功能都呈现出显著的耗竭，表现为 HSC 数目和体内外造血重建功能的显著下降。将其与 Eos 缺失的小鼠进行杂交，产生的子代小鼠虽然体内有高水平 IL5，但仍缺乏嗜酸性粒细胞，该品系小鼠骨髓 HSC 的数目和功能耗竭的表型可被明显的挽救，提示导致 HSC 功能耗竭的主要原因是嗜酸性粒细胞，而非 IL-5。

为了探究其中的分子机制，我们对各品系小鼠的骨髓上清进行了蛋白组学分析，发现在 IL5 过表达小鼠骨髓上清中存在大量的 CCL6，我们也通过一系列的体内、外试验证实了 CCL6 是来源于高水平的嗜酸性粒细胞，而且利用 CCL6 的中和抗体和 CCR1 的抑制剂 BX471 特异性的阻断 CCL6 都可以缓解嗜酸性粒细胞对 HSC 功能的损伤。到此我们建立了如下模型来解释哮喘气道炎症的发生发展：嗜酸性粒细胞分泌的 CCL6 作用于骨髓 HSC，使其活化、增生，并在 IL5 的作用下定向分化成嗜酸性粒细胞，然后在趋化因子 eotaxin 的作用下被募积到肺局部发挥炎症效应，不断的正反馈调控最终导致哮喘病理反应（图 3-7-1）。该研究证明了嗜酸性粒细胞分泌的 CCL6 能够调控哮喘炎症，为气道炎症及 HSC 稳态的研究领域带来了新的概念，提供了新的思路。

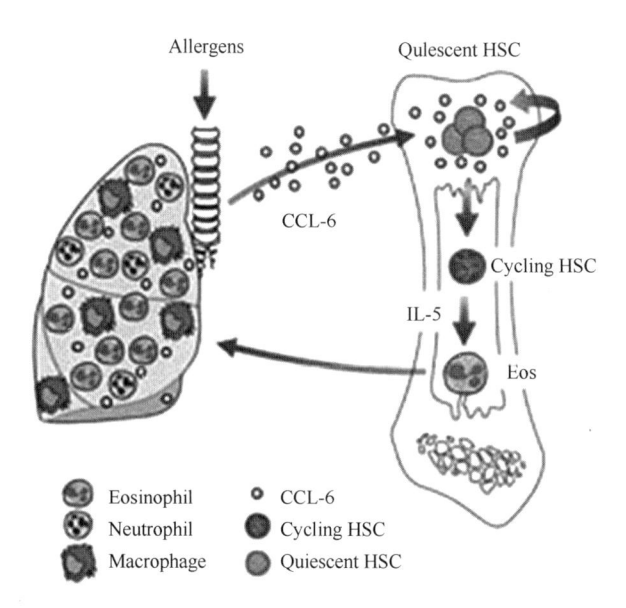

图 3-7-1 嗜酸性细胞及其分泌的 CCL6 在哮喘气道炎症过程中对干细胞的调控作用

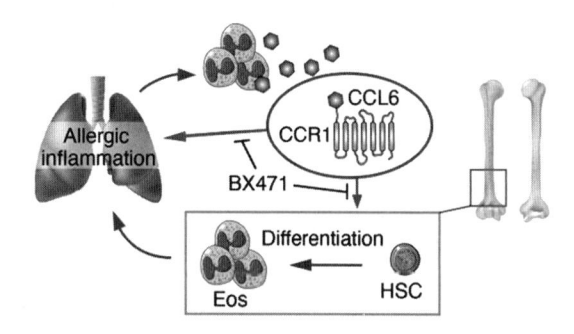

图 3-7-2 CCL6-CCR1 轴通过嗜酸性粒细胞的分化调控哮喘气道炎症

润情况,提示 CCL6-CCR1 轴可以调控嗜酸性粒细胞分化和哮喘气道炎症(图 3-7-2)。

通过以上研究,我们发现了嗜酸性粒细胞分泌的趋化因子 CCL6 及其受体在哮喘发病过程中发挥着极其重要的作用,对趋化因子介导哮喘的分子机制研究进行了有效补充,对哮喘的发病过程有了更进一步的认识。

三、趋化因子受体结构导向药理

既然趋化因子及受体在哮喘发病过程中发挥着如此重要的作用,那么是否可以靶向趋化因子及其受体来治疗哮喘呢?我们团队研究表明:用 CCR3 单克隆抗体阻断 CCR3 可以显著缓解哮喘小鼠的嗜酸性粒细胞炎症及黏液高分泌,从而达到治疗哮喘炎症的目的。2009 年 Allergy 的研究也表明:CCR3 单克隆抗体可以抑制哮喘小鼠中嗜酸性粒细胞的迁移。而 2017 年的一项研究表明:利用 CCR4 拮抗剂阻断 CCR4 可以有效缓解哮喘小鼠的肺部炎症和气道高反应性进而治疗哮喘。基于 CCR3 和 CCR4 在哮喘发病过程中的作用,很多靶向 CCR3 和 CCR4 的药物已经被应用于哮喘的临床研究,但是最终都未能进入到Ⅲ期临床试验阶段,其主要原因在于目前用于临床试验的药物对趋化因子受体的抑制效果不佳,且由于特异性差会造成难以避免的不良反应。

如果能够以趋化因子及其受体的结构为导向来筛选有效且特异性好的药物,是否有助于靶向趋化因子及受体的临床研究呢?

我们的研究已经证实 CCL6-CCR1 轴在哮喘发病过程中发挥着至关重要的作用,成功解析出 CCL6 受体的结构可以为靶向性药物筛选提供依据。我们建立了大量纯化趋化因子的实验体系,包括构建不同形式的截短体,以及添加不同的蛋白纯化标签,成功纯化出趋化因子 CCL6 及其受体的复合物,并利用冷冻电镜技术对其结构进行解析,这也是第一个被解析的趋化因子受体的激活态结构(图 3-7-3)。我们还根据其结构筛选出了受体与配体结合口袋的一些关键位点,进行了针对性的功能实验,为特异性药物的设计提供了依据。

(二)CCL6 对哮喘病理的调控机制

为了进一步明确 CCL6 与嗜酸性粒细胞的关系及其在哮喘发病过程中的具体作用机制,我们进行了更加深入的研究。我们首先检测了哮喘患者外周血白细胞中小鼠 CCL6 同源物 CCL23 和 CCL15 的 mRNA 表达水平及血浆中 CCL23 蛋白水平,发现相较健康对照均有明显升高,且血浆中 CCL23 的蛋白水平和外周血嗜酸性粒细胞数目呈正相关。我们也通过免疫荧光嗜酸性粒细胞特异性颗粒蛋白 EPX 和 CCL23,CCL15 的共染证明了 CCL23 和 CCL15 主要由外周血的嗜酸性粒细胞产生。在哮喘小鼠中我们也得到了同样的结果,哮喘小鼠的血清、肺泡灌洗液、肺组织中的 CCL6 的蛋白水平相较对照小鼠都有明显升高,且嗜酸性粒细胞是 CCL6 的主要分泌来源。

在此基础上我们构建了 CCL6 全身敲除的小鼠,发现敲除 CCL6 对哮喘气道炎症有明显的保护作用,肺泡灌洗液中炎症细胞尤其是嗜酸性粒细胞的浸润,炎症因子的表达和黏液高分泌都在 CCL6 敲除之后得到了显著缓解。同时我们分析了外周血和骨髓中的成熟嗜酸性粒细胞,以及骨髓中的造血干细胞、嗜酸性粒细胞祖细胞等,发现敲除 CCL6 后骨髓造血干细胞的增生、及其向嗜酸性粒细胞的分化均受到明显的抑制,这正是哮喘气道炎症被保护的原因。

CCL6 究竟是通过何种方式参与哮喘病理过程呢?我们利用体外功能实验证实了 CCL6 的受体是 CCR1,而 CCR1 是一种 7 次跨膜的 G 蛋白偶联受体,主要表达在免疫系统中,可以通过招募下游 G 蛋白参与细胞内多种信号通路调控。利用 BX471 特异性的阻断 CCR1 可以抑制骨髓中嗜酸性粒细胞的定向分化过程,同时能够有效缓解 OVA 诱导的哮喘气道炎症,降低肺局部嗜酸性粒细胞的浸

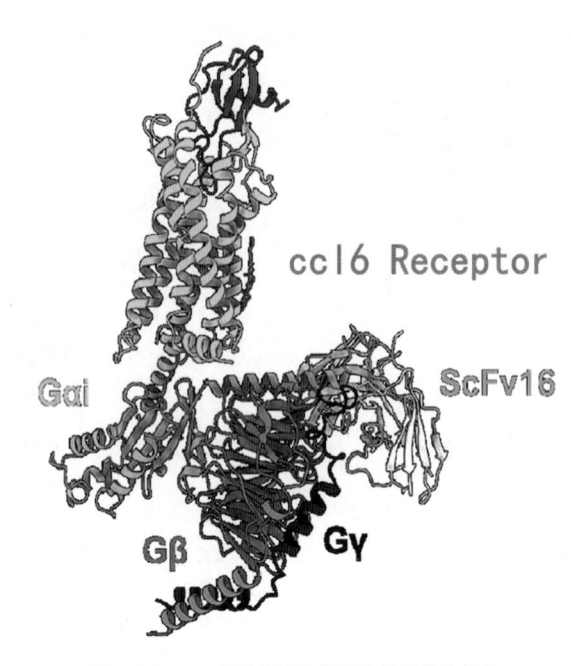

图 3-7-3　CCL6 及其受体复合物的激活态结构

四、总结与展望

我们团队以趋化因子和哮喘为出发点,原创性地研究了 CCL6 及其特异性受体 CCR1 在哮喘病理过程中的调控作用,并首次成功解析了 CCL6 及其受体激活态的结构,为结构导向特异性药物筛选提供了依据。我们期待更多更新的研究成果,更多更有效的生物学靶向药物,给哮喘患者带来更大的帮助。

参 考 文 献

[1] Lazennec G, Richmond A. Chemokines and chemokine receptors: new insights into cancer-related inflammation. Trends Mol Med, 2010, 16(3): 133-144.

[2] Griffith JW, Sokol CL, Luster AD. Chemokines and chemokine receptors: positioning cells for host defense and immunity. Annu Rev Immunol, 2014, 32: 659-702.

[3] Lambrecht BN, Hammad H. The immunology of asthma. Nat Immunol, 2015, 16(1): 45-56.

[4] Zhang C, Yi W, Li F, et al. Eosinophil-derived CCL-6 impairs hematopoietic stem cell homeostasis. Cell Res, 2018, 28(3): 323-335.

[5] Shen HH, Xu F, Zhang GS, et al. CCR3 monoclonal antibody inhibits airway eosinophilic inflammation and mucus overproduction in a mouse model of asthma. Acta Pharmacol Sin, 2006, 27(12): 1594-1599.

[6] Ben S, Li X, Xu F, et al. Treatment with anti-CC chemokine receptor 3 monoclonal antibody or dexamethasone inhibits the migration and differentiation of bone marrow CD34 progenitor cells in an allergic mouse model, Allergy, 2008, 63 (9): 1164-1176.

[7] Zhang Y, Wu Y, Qi H, et al. A new antagonist for CCR4 attenuates allergic lung inflammation in a mouse model of asthma. Sci Rep, 2017, 7(1): 15038.

[8] Pease JE, Horuk R. Recent progress in the development of antagonists to the chemokine receptors CCR3 and CCR4. Expert Opin Drug Discov, 2014, 9(5): 467-483.

8 上皮因子与过敏性哮喘

汤葳

支气管哮喘表型和内型研究是哮喘个体化治疗的基础。2019年开始，GINA指南把重症哮喘的治疗作为单独的章节进行阐述，其中针对这些重症哮喘的内型是区分不同重症哮喘的基础。根据发病机制哮喘分为T2型和非T2型，上皮细胞源性细胞因子胸腺基质淋巴生成素（TSLP）、IL-33和IL-25为典型的T2型免疫的重要调控因子，是过敏性哮喘的重要发生发展促进因子。

上皮细胞衍生的细胞因子（简称上皮因子）通常被认为是屏障上皮应对外界刺激所释放的"警报素"，这些上皮因子警示免疫系统外界的损伤，并参与组织损伤后的调节修复。对于这些细胞因子作用的理解最初主要集中在2型炎症的早期，但近年来的研究发现，这三种细胞因子为固有免疫和适应性免疫细胞群提供了重要的组织特异性信号。例如，出生时IL-33在肺部的释放有助于建立肺免疫环境，可能通过在围生期肺中建立免疫环境而影响哮喘的易感性，从而影响哮喘的风险和发展；TSLP可直接作用于DCs（树突状细胞），促进Th2细胞的发育；IL-25和IL-4也可以直接促进Th2细胞的分化。TSLP、IL-33和IL-25作用于多种天然免疫细胞，在诱导和激活ILC2s（Ⅱ型先天淋巴细胞）中尤为重要；在哮喘的神经源性炎症中，TSLP和IL-33可作用于感觉神经元，刺激瘙痒反应。

上皮因子通过与分布在先天免疫细胞、获得性免疫细胞、结构细胞表面特异性受体结合活化这些细胞，参与哮喘气道的慢性、急性炎症和重塑过程。部分这些细胞也能正反馈，刺激上皮细胞产生更多的上述上皮因子，加剧哮喘气道炎症。在最常见的嗜酸性粒细胞性哮喘的发生发展中，无论是过敏性的还是非过敏性的嗜酸粒细胞性哮喘（即可能以Ⅱ型先天淋巴细胞活化为起始）都有上皮因子作为始动因素的参与。在获得性免疫细胞中，IL-33、IL-25和TSLP均可作用于树突状细胞、嗜酸性粒细胞、嗜碱性粒细胞、Th0细胞、Th2细胞、Th9细胞和NK细胞，促进这些细胞在过敏性炎症中分泌更多的趋化因子和细胞因子，加剧过敏性炎症的反应。总体上，TSLP、IL-33和IL-25可通过记忆性Th2细胞亚群促进适应性2型反应，这些亚群具有TSLP、IL-33和IL-25高受体表达的特征。在过敏性哮喘患者的气道抗原激发研究中发现，吸入过敏原后气道上皮和黏膜下这三种上皮因子的表达均增加。现对这三种上皮因子与过敏性哮喘的关系分述如下。

一、白细胞介素-33

（一）概述

白细胞介素（interleukin, IL）-33是IL-1家族的核细胞因子，组成性表达于上皮屏障组织和淋巴器官，是参与2型免疫和过敏性气道疾病的关键细胞因子。IL-33在肺上皮细胞中大量表达，在黏膜器官的先天性和适应性免疫反应中发挥着重要作用。在先天免疫中，IL-33与ILC2s的相互作用为快速免疫反应和组织稳态提供了一个重要的轴心。在适应性免疫中，IL-33与树突状细胞、Th2细胞、滤泡T细胞和调节性T细胞相互作用，影响慢性气道炎症和组织重塑的发展。IL-33在黏膜免疫反应中的作用机制为：当暴露于过敏原、微生物或环境压力时，上皮细胞会释放IL-33，IL-33激活固有免疫细胞，包括ILC2s、嗜碱性粒细胞、嗜酸性粒细胞和肥大细胞，从而驱动2型炎症。同时，IL-33还激活DCs和$CD4^+$ T细胞，促进Th2、Tfh和Treg细胞增生和分化以及B细胞产生抗体。

（二）IL-33的结构及其细胞外释放机制

人类IL-33蛋白由两个进化保守结构域（核结构域和细胞因子结构域）组成，两者由高度分化的中心结构域分开，包含染色质结合基序和炎性蛋白酶及凋亡蛋白酶的裂解位点。IL-33的释放存在特殊的机制：当上皮损伤和应激时，细胞质膜和核膜失去完整性，白细胞介素-33在坏死过程中被被动释放。当细胞凋亡时，IL-33保留在细胞内，并被凋亡蛋白酶如caspase 3和caspase 7灭活。当暴露于抗原或受外界环境因素刺激时，全长的IL-33会在组织损伤和细胞凋亡（或细胞应激）时在胞外释放，招募并活化上述先天性和获得性免疫细胞，启动气道过敏性炎症反应。炎症反应产生的蛋白酶又可以反向作用于全长的IL-33，降解其中心结构域，释放IL-1样细胞因子域，使其失活。由于IL-33始终处于一个自动调节的稳态，所以以抗体阻断IL-33可导致稳态失衡从而诱发其他疾病，而阻断ST2又可能导致游离ST2被阻断，从而影响其他细胞的功能。这也是目前在开发IL-33靶向治疗中的难点。

（三）IL-33与过敏性哮喘

Gasiunene等2019年的研究观察了IL-33与哮喘表型之间的关系。研究纳入了哮喘患者（$n=115$）和健康受试者（$n=85$），将哮喘患者按表型分为过敏性/非过敏性、嗜酸性/非嗜酸性、肥胖/非肥胖、使用/未使用ICS、严重程度（根据GINA分为轻、中、重度），用ELISA法测定血清中IL-33的浓度。结果显示,在血清 IL-33 水平上,过敏性哮喘患者高于非过敏性哮喘患者和正常对照,嗜酸性粒细胞性哮喘患者高于非嗜酸性粒细胞性哮喘患者,未用 ICS 的哮喘人群高于已经使用了 ICS 的患者;在肥胖与否和严重程度方面结果没有统计学差异。在人群年龄方面,一篇 2019 年发表的临床研究发现非老年性哮喘患者的血清 IL-33 水平低于老年性哮喘患者。

哮喘急性加重的相关研究发现,在急性加重期,患者上呼吸道(鼻咽拭子采样后测定)的 IL-33 水平与上呼吸道 IL-5 和 IL-13 水平相关(R 分别 $= 0.84$ 和 0.76, P 皆 < 0.01),也和下呼吸道(通过诱导痰样本测定)的 IL-13 水平相关($R = 0.49$, $P = 0.03$),都较非急性加重显著增高。mRNA 表达也有同样的相关性。下呼吸道 IL-13 水平与下呼吸道 IL-33 水平也呈正相关($R = 0.84$, $P < 0.01$),IL-13、IL-33 水平与 FeNO 呈正相关,IL-5 水平与嗜酸性粒细胞呈正相关。而且,这种 IL-33 和 T2 型细胞因子之间的相关性即使在急性加重 4 周后仍然存在。另一篇研究证明了支气管纤毛细胞是 IL-33 在病毒驱动下的哮喘恶化过程中一个主要的局部来源。病毒感染时,IL-33 通过抑制固有免疫反应和获得性免疫反应削弱了抗病毒能力,是导致病情恶化的必要因素。通过尘螨致敏小鼠模型发现,IL-33 减弱了哮喘小鼠上皮细胞和树突状细胞产生可以抗病毒的 IFN-β 的水平,也降低了树突状细胞产生 Th1 型抗感染免疫的活性,但对 Th2 型免疫反应没有影响,故导致气道高反应性和过敏性气道炎症的长时间存在,从而促进病毒诱发过敏性哮喘炎症的发生发展。

二、白细胞介素-25

(一)概述

IL-25 是一种多源化的上皮因子。它可以由多种细胞产生,包括结构细胞——上皮细胞、内皮细胞;先天免疫细胞——如嗜酸性粒细胞、嗜碱性粒细胞、肥大细胞和巨噬细胞;获得性免疫细胞——Th2 细胞,是典型的 T2 炎症因子。它的受体也分布在以上这些细胞上,此外还包括一些近年来发现或证实的细胞亚类,如 Th9 细胞,先天淋巴细胞 Ⅱ 型,Ⅱ 型髓样细胞。另外,NKT 细胞、树突状细胞、成纤维细胞上也发现其受体的存在。这些细胞和 IL-25 之间形成互动,导致过敏性炎症和组织过度修复,从而促进 Th2 型气道炎症和气道重构,促进了哮喘的发生发展。

(二)IL-25 与过敏性哮喘

Beale 等研究发现,哮喘恶化时鼻病毒诱导的 IL-25 促进 Th2 型炎症和过敏性肺部炎症的发生。RV(鼻病毒)感染后,健康个体和哮喘患者的鼻黏液中 IL-25 蛋白表达均显著增加,在哮喘患者中,IL-25 表达水平增加更高。研究证实,IL-25 及其受体的两个部分——IL-17RA 和高亲和力受体 IL-17RB 在过敏性哮喘患者嗜酸性粒细胞中较过敏性非哮喘患者和正常无过敏人群的表达增高,抗原激发试验可导致哮喘患者嗜酸性粒细胞表面的 IL-25 受体在抗原刺激 7h 和 24h 后动态增高。研究表明在嗜碱性粒细胞和树突状细胞中也存在同样的情况,而且,随着抗原激发的过程,过敏性哮喘患者的血浆 IL-25 水平也呈动态的增高。我们近期的研究还发现,对尘螨过敏的过敏性鼻炎合并过敏性哮喘患者进行尘螨特异性免疫治疗,血浆 IL-25 水平在治疗后第 12 个月较治疗基线显著下降,同时伴随着尘螨特异性 IgG4 水平(即特异性免疫治疗阻断抗体)的明显增高。

IL-25 作为 T2 炎症的成员之一,也可以作为一种哮喘内型进行患者临床特征的探索。研究发现,哮喘患者支气管黏膜的上皮因子转录水平 IL-25 显著高于对照组,黏膜下 IL-25 阳性的细胞数目在哮喘患者显著增多,支气管刷检标本中 IL-25 特异性高亲和力受体 IL-17RB 的转录本水平也在哮喘患者中较对照组显著增高,两者具有相关性。以支气管黏膜 IL-25 表达中位水平进行划分,将哮喘患者分为 IL-25 高表达内型组和 IL-25 低表达内型组。分析的结果显示,相较于低表达内型,高 IL-25 表达内型组的诱导痰、支气管内膜上皮中嗜酸性粒细胞的比例更高、基底膜增厚更为明显、皮肤点刺试验阳性的过敏原种类更多,血清 IgE 水平和外周血嗜酸性粒细胞计数也更高。但也看到了 IL-25 高表达内型的优点,即患者对吸入激素的治疗敏感性更好:高 IL-25 内型组治疗 4 周后 FEV$_1$ 和气道高反应性(PD20 水平)的改善值较低内型组显著增高,且疗效持续至第 8 周,提示 IL-25 高表达内型是一种更为良性的哮喘内型。

三、胸腺淋巴细胞生成素(TSLP)

(一)概述

TSLP(胸腺淋巴细胞生成素)是一种多效性细胞因子,最初被认为是淋巴细胞生长因子。它是一种上游细胞因子,通过与由 TSLPR 和 IL-7 受体(IL-7R)组成的高亲和力异构体受体复合物结合而发挥其生物学活性。TSLP 主要由活化的肺和肠上皮细胞、角化细胞和成纤维细胞表达。然而,树突状细胞(DCs)、肥大细胞和其他免疫细胞也可能产生 TSLP。

(二)TSLP 在过敏性哮喘中的作用机制

在肺内,不同表型/内型哮喘的发病机制涉及广泛的刺激,如过敏原、细胞因子、呼吸道病毒、细菌和真菌产物、机械应激和香烟烟雾提取物等,这些刺激都可诱导肺上皮细胞释放 TSLP。释放的 TSLP 与效应细胞表面的 TSLP 高亲和力受体 TSLPR 结合,同时与其受体的另一部分 IL-7Rα 形成异二聚体,启动效应细胞的活化。TSLP 的效应细胞和后续的效应反应包括:肥大细胞活化后释放细胞因子和趋化因子;树突状细胞和 ILC2 细胞活化后促进 Th2 型炎症反应的极化;嗜酸性粒细胞和嗜碱性粒细胞活化后促进细胞活化脱颗粒。不同的细胞信号传导途径有所不同,TSLP/TSLPR/IL-7Rα 形成三聚体后,激活 JAK1 和 JAK2 激酶,通过 MAPKS 途径促进嗜酸性粒细胞的趋化和存活;通过 NF-κB 的活化促进树突状细胞的 Th2 细胞极化;通过 STAT 5 和 STAT 3 的磷酸化途径导致细胞增生、抗凋亡和迁移功能。

(三)TSLP 抗体的临床应用研究

上皮因子抗体研究最为成熟的是抗 TSLP 抗体。加拿大 McMaster 哮喘研究中心的 TSLP 抗体临床研究数据显示:治疗前,过敏性哮喘患者在特异性过敏激发后均产生典型的气道速发相和迟发项反应(即吸入过敏原后 7h

和24h内的双向FEV_1的降低),抗TSLP抗体治疗后的第1和第2个月,再次进行过敏原激发后治疗组的FEV_1降低明显减弱,与对照组有显著统计学差异;同时还伴随着外周血嗜酸性粒细胞计数、诱导痰嗜酸性粒细胞计数和FENO的减少。目前,全球有5种抗TSLP抗体进入临床研究阶段,绝大多数都是重组的IgG1单克隆抗体,其中美国FDA已经批准Amgen公司的tezepelumab已经进入Ⅲ期临床研究,属于IgG2γ单克隆抗体。

四、展 望

上皮因子表型的治疗方面目前还处于起步阶段。很多针对T2类型的抗体理论上可以通过负反馈的机制改善上皮因子的过度表达,奥马珠单抗的研究证实了这一点:来自气道上皮因子高表达的患者奥马珠单抗治疗的有效性比低表达患者更好。气道上皮既是哮喘炎症的受累靶点,也是哮喘启动和发生发展的重要源头。上皮因子是各类亚型哮喘的重要始动和促进因子,尤其是过敏性哮喘。上皮因子与过敏性哮喘之间的相关靶细胞(先天免疫细胞和获得性免疫细胞)之间都存在密切的作用,从不同的机制(抗原依赖性和非抗原依赖性)促进过敏性哮喘的发病。分析上皮因子的内型有利于对今后的个体化治疗。目前针对上皮因子内型哮喘的研究主要集中在动物、细胞体外研究和体内前研究阶段,对于不同上皮因子内型在不同哮喘表型中的分布尚不清楚。针对上皮因子的靶向治疗研究也正在不断深入。

参 考 文 献

[1] Global Initiative for Asthma. Global Strategy for Asthma Management and Prevention,2019. Available from:www. ginasthma. org.

[2] Muraro A,Lemanske RF,Jr. Hellings PW,et al. Precision medicine in patients with allergic diseases:Airway diseases and atopic dermatitis-PRACTALL document of the European Academy of Allergy and Clinical Immunology and the American Academy of Allergy,Asthma & Immunology. J Allergy Clin Immunol,2016,137(5):1347-1358.

[3] Roan F,Obata-Ninomiya K,Ziegler SF. Epithelial cell-derived cytokines:more than just signaling the alarm. J Clin Invest,2019,129(4):1441-1451.

[4] Wang W,Li Y,Lv Z,et al. Bronchial Allergen Challenge of Patients with Atopic Asthma Triggers an Alarmin(IL-33,TSLP,and IL-25)Response in the Airways Epithelium and Submucosa. J Immunol,2018,201(8):2221-2231.

[5] Cayrol C,Girard JP. IL-33:an alarmin cytokine with crucial roles in innate immunity,inflammation and allergy. Curr Opin Immunol,2014,31:31-37.

[6] Kamijo S,Takeda H,Tokura T,et al. IL-33-Mediated Innate Response and Adaptive Immune Cells Contribute to Maximum Responses of Protease Allergen-Induced Allergic Airway Inflammation. Journal of Immunology,2013,190(9):4489-4499.

[7] Drake LY,Kita H. IL-33:biological properties,functions,and roles in airway disease. Immunol Rev,2017,278(1):173-184.

[8] Gasiuniene E,Janulaityte I,Zemeckiene Z,et al. Elevated levels of interleukin-33 are associated with allergic and eosinophilic asthma. Scand J Immunol,2019,89(5):e12724.

[9] Ulambayar B,Lee SH,Yang EM,et al. Association Between Epithelial Cytokines and Clinical Phenotypes of Elderly Asthma. Allergy Asthma Immunol Res,2019,11(1):79-89.

[10] Poulsen NN,Bjerregaard A,Khoo SK,et al. Airway Interleukin-33 and type 2 cytokines in adult patients with acute asthma. Respir Med,2018,140:50-56.

[11] Ravanetti L,Dijkhuis A,Dekker T,et al. IL-33 drives influenza-induced asthma exacerbations by halting innate and adaptive antiviral immunity. J Allergy Clin Immunol,2019,143(4):1355-1370 e16.

[12] Yao X,Sun Y,Wang W,et al. Interleukin(IL)-25:Pleiotropic roles in asthma. Respirology,2016,21(4):638-647.

[13] Beale J,Jayaraman A,Jackson DJ,et al. Rhinovirus-induced IL-25 in asthma exacerbation drives type 2 immunity and allergic pulmonary inflammation. Sci Transl Med,2014,6(256):256ra134.

[14] Tang W,Smith SG,Beaudin S,et al. IL-25 and IL-25 receptor expression on eosinophils from subjects with allergic asthma. Int Arch Allergy Immunol,2014,163(1):5-10.

[15] Tang W,Smith SG,Salter B,et al. Allergen-Induced Increases in Interleukin-25 and Interleukin-25 Receptor Expression in Mature Eosinophils from Atopic Asthmatics. Int Arch Allergy Immunol,2016,170(4):234-242.

[16] Salter BM,Oliveria JP,Nusca G,et al. IL-25 and IL-33 induce Type 2 inflammation in basophils from subjects with allergic asthma. Respir Res,2016,17:5.

[17] Tworek D,Smith SG,Salter BM,et al. IL-25 Receptor Expression on Airway Dendritic Cells after Allergen Challenge in Subjects with Asthma. Am J Respir Crit Care Med,2016,193(9):957-964.

[18] Cheng D,Xue Z,Yi L,et al. Epithelial interleukin-25 is a key mediator in Th2-high,corticosteroid-responsive asthma. Am J Respir Crit Care Med,2014,190(6):639-648.

[19] Varricchi G,Pecoraro A,Marone G,et al. Thymic Stromal Lymphopoietin Isoforms,Inflammatory Disorders,and Cancer. Front Immunol,2018,9:1595.

[20] Marone G,Spadaro G,Braile M,et al. Tezepelumab:a novel biological therapy for the treatment of severe uncontrolled asthma. Expert Opin Investig Drugs,2019,28(11):931-940.

[21] Matera MG,Rogliani P,Calzetta L,et al. TSLP Inhibitors for Asthma:Current Status and Future Prospects. Drugs,2020,80(5):449-458.

[22] Gauvreau GM,O'Byrne PM,Boulet LP,et al. Effects of an anti-TSLP antibody on allergen-induced asthmatic responses. N Engl J Med,2014,370(22):2102-2110.

[23] Sy CB,Siracusa MC. The Therapeutic Potential of Targeting Cytokine Alarmins to Treat Allergic Airway Inflammation. Front Physiol,2016,7:214.

9 哮喘气道重塑的免疫标志物和个体化治疗前景

张锦涛 董亮

作为支气管哮喘的主要特征之一,气道重塑一方面在哮喘的病程进展中具有重要作用,另一方面却在当今的治疗与临床分型中占很低的比重。按照现今的哮喘阶梯化诊疗标准,目前对患者临床病情水平的干预多基于其炎症治疗反应。然而,尽管加强了抗炎治疗,许多哮喘患者尤其是重度哮喘患者的病情仍得不到良好控制。作为不可逆性气道损伤的主要表现形式,气道重塑一定程度上决定着哮喘的病情严重程度。尤其对于重症哮喘患者,气道重塑可能严重影响其治疗和预后。早期发现并有效干预气道重塑可以显著降低急性哮喘发作和严重损伤的比例。近年来,随着各种辅助技术的发展,气道重塑的研究有所深入。针对哮喘表型的生物制剂逐渐增多,气道重塑对哮喘治疗的影响逐渐凸显。在个体化治疗的时代,通过寻找可靠的气道重塑生物标志物帮助区分哮喘表型并进一步结合不同表型对患者进行精准治疗,成为哮喘治疗的发展方向之一。本文综述了目前哮喘气道重塑的研究现状,进一步为哮喘的分类和治疗提供了基础。文中还讨论了一些有潜力的气道重塑生物标志物及它们在个体化治疗中应用的可能。我们认为未来在气道重塑方面,不断完善的机制和随之出现的生物标志物能更好地帮助哮喘患者实现个体化治疗。

一、哮喘气道重塑的研究现状

(一)哮喘气道重塑研究的意义

自气道重塑在哮喘中被首次提出已经过了近百年的时间,大量针对气道重塑的研究已经完成或正在进行。基于人类受试者的多项哮喘研究逐渐深入,为之后的扩展及临床应用打下了良好的基础。目前研究认为,虽然气道炎症和重塑之间有不少重叠与联系,但两者仍属于两种不同的系统,有各自的一套病理发生机制并随疾病发展相互影响。而对炎症和气道重塑的合并研究,能够进一步理解哮喘完整的病理生理机制。除与炎症反应机制相互影响外,哮喘气道重塑也与气道高反应性息息相关。气道高反应性的发展和持续一定程度上依赖于气道重塑事件,包括胶原沉积、气道平滑肌质量和收缩能力的增加等。

气道重塑在气道结构的改变中起着关键作用,并可能逐渐导致固定性的气道阻塞,其也被认为是许多严重哮喘患者的重要特征之一。对于哮喘患者来说,固定性的气流受限可能不是一个提示治疗的指征,但为了防止过度治疗,这类特征必须被正确对待。对于公共医疗支出而言,重症哮喘虽然只占哮喘人群的一小部分但却承担了大部分的医疗花销和社会负担,而气道重塑是重症哮喘患者的突出表现。对于儿童哮喘患者来说,多项出生队列研究表明气道结构改变可以出现在儿童患者早期并与永久性肺功能损伤平行,同时研究认为网状基底膜是未来哮喘发展预测因素,而与气道平滑肌厚度或嗜酸性炎症无关。总体来说,目前哮喘患者的气道重塑一个亟待解决的问题。

(二)哮喘气道重塑研究的进展

与许多现存的有效的疾病管理方法相同,要想成功地管理哮喘也取决于对其基本生物学过程及在疾病背景下的功能障碍的理解。虽然气道重塑对人类造成了许多不良后果包括导致肺功能下降和持续进行性气流受限等,但不可否认,尤其对哮喘患者来说,气道重塑确实带来了一些益处包括抑制气道收缩和抵消过度狭窄。到目前为止,我们仍不清楚哮喘气道重塑的完整机制。如何有效预防病理性气道重塑,使其顺利回归到合理修复的轨道,是当前和研究的主要问题。

气道重塑的复杂性体现在多个方面,其涉及不同的组织结构和细胞类型并且与各种机体生物学进程的相互关联。众多未探明的病理生理机制及临床应用方面的困难使气道重塑进展缓慢。过去的几十年,哮喘患者的气道生态特征得到了进一步的阐释,哮喘的不同致病机制和细胞相互作用被广泛地研究(如自噬和衰老)。随着基础研究的不断深入,哮喘气道重塑机制的整体框架不断完善。流行病学研究表明,遗传和环境因素都能降低肺功能,增加气道重塑的可能性。在哮喘相关基因领域,与气道重塑相关的遗传学研究很少。虽然100多个基因已经被证明与哮喘有关,但只有少数基因与哮喘的肺功能下降有关,与气道重塑相关的则更少。

动物模型研究是疾病发病机制研究过程中必不可少的关键环节之一。作为目前最常用的动物模型,小鼠模型在哮喘研究中得到了广泛的应用,但其同时也有许多局限性。首先,小鼠不能自发产生哮喘,人工诱导只能产生某些特定类型的哮喘;其次,小鼠在气道结构和大小与人类有显著差异。这些都影响哮喘,尤其是气道重塑的研究。近年来动物学家越来越关注马哮喘模型。马可以自发产生哮喘,与小鼠相比,其较大的呼吸系统也便于观察和研究气道重塑。有时在马模型中甚至可以分离出炎症和气道重塑,使其成为研究非嗜酸性粒细胞哮喘的合适动物模型。到目前为止，哮喘气道重塑仍存在很多困惑，需要更多深入的纵向或横向研究。

在各种检测手段中，活检通常被认为是评估哮喘患者气道重塑程度最关键的方法。此外，影像学检查，特别是CT检查，也被认为有助于评价哮喘患者的气道重塑，但它们都受到实用性和伦理性的限制。由于技术水平有限，目前对的研究和测量主要集中在大、中气道，但气道重塑也涉及到细支气管和小支气管，甚至它们因为与大气道结构不同发挥不同的作用，但这方面研究还比较困难。另外，现在对哮喘多集中于横断面研究，而气道重塑的突出特征是一个长期演化的纵向过程，这也给气道重塑研究增加了障碍。过去，由于涉及多个细胞及细胞因子在不同时期复杂的连锁反应和多种检测技术的局限性，气道重塑一直难以很好阐释；现在，优化的辅助检验技术，包括成像技术和测量指标的进展，为更深入研究气道重塑提供了可能。

气道重塑不仅是对气道"量"的变化，更是对其"质"的变化，即使目前在多种技术的加持下，我们对气道重塑的测量仍处于粗测阶段。随着新方法的引入和技术的进步，这方面研究将会不断深入。

二、哮喘气道重塑生物标志物

（一）哮喘气道重塑生物标志物的研究意义

近年来，生物标志物在糖尿病、癌症等多种疾病的治疗和控制中受到越来越多的关注。目前已知哮喘相关的生物标志物可以通过多种方式获得，包括尿液、血液、支气管肺泡灌洗液、诱导痰、呼出气体凝集物和支气管活检等。对于损伤最小性和可重复性而言，血液和呼出气体凝集物可能显示出比其他更多的优势。在哮喘，特别是重症哮喘中，许多可能的生物标志物已经或正在研究。目前生物标志物的重叠表明，可能不只需要一个而是一组生物标志物来准确地区分哮喘的内型，从而在哮喘特别是在重症哮喘中的控制和治疗中发挥积极作用。目前临床上在哮喘治疗中广泛应用的炎症相关生物标志物包括血嗜酸性粒细胞、痰嗜酸性粒细胞和中性粒细胞、血清总IgE和呼出气一氧化氮（FeNO）等。

缺乏有效的能用于临床应用的气道重塑生物标志物成为阻碍其研究的一个主要问题，目前大多数哮喘生物标志物的重点在疾病的炎症反应方面。与此同时，已有的研究指出哮喘患者病情程度与气道炎症不完全平行，可能与气道重塑有关。对于低T2型哮喘，先前的研究表明这类哮喘患者通常缺乏环境过敏史，对糖皮质激素的治疗反应较差。由于缺乏有效的生物标志物，临床上通常多使用排除法来诊断这类哮喘。在这种情况下，反映气道重塑的生物标志物可能有助于识别这种疾病。

（二）对哮喘气道重塑相关生物标志物的探索

研究表明，许多蛋白和细胞因子都与哮喘气道重塑有关，但它们所证明的重塑功能都不可避免地与炎症相互重叠。此外由于诸多限制，在基于人类样本的研究中，气道重塑的水平主要反映在对治疗的反应上，如肺功能的改善、FEV_1的提高等。一些学者认为成像技术可作为气道重塑的标志物，包括定量CT和超极化气体磁共振成像技术。研究人员甚至可以利用影像学方法对哮喘患者进行分类，为进一步的治疗提供指导，但由于影像学仅仅局限于粗略生化结构的观察和计算，无法准确区分气道层次，另外，它们在哮喘中的应用也受到实用性和经济性的限制。

到目前为止，支气管镜活检仍是医生检测和分析患者气道重塑水平的一种最直观的测量方法。基于支气管肺泡灌洗和支气管内膜活检的多项研究提出了大量可行的生物标志物。然而，大多数分子需要从气道活检或者肺泡灌洗液中收集，具有损伤性和劳动密集性，从而限制了它们的临床应用。与其他生物标志物不同，三种分子具有很大的潜力，即Galectin-3、YKL40和VitD。活检证实，它们在血液中的含量可以一定程度上揭示气道结构的变化，提示它们可能被实际用于支持哮喘气道重塑的诊断与程度分型。

Galectin-3（Gal-3）可以在血液中释放并测量，是不同器官纤维化形成的共有因子。因此，Gal-3被认为是一种生物标志物，与包括心力衰竭等在内的多种疾病有关。动物实验研究证实，Gal-3可通过分泌多种细胞因子和募集炎性细胞促进气道重塑。通过支气管镜活检分析8例严重哮喘患者的气道平滑肌厚度，嗜酸性粒细胞和中性粒细胞浸润及蛋白质组学特征后，研究人员认为Gal-3作为生物标志物可以有效地反映哮喘患者支气管平滑肌，嗜酸性炎症和肌肉蛋白成分的减少；研究同时排除了骨膜素作为气道重塑的预测性生物标志物的可能性。然而，由于样本量小，其结果有很多局限性，需要更多实验进一步证明。除了哮喘气道重塑，血清中Gal-3的水平还与炎症反应及其他纤维化过程有关，从而限制了它的实际应用。

作为哺乳类动物几丁质酶样蛋白家族的一员，YKL-40是一种炎性糖蛋白，其确切功能尚不完全清楚。目前认为它可以参与炎症、损伤和组织重塑等多种病理生理过程。先前的研究证实，编码YKL-40蛋白的基因 *CHI3L1* 与哮喘气道重塑有关。Bara等对40例哮喘患者的气道活检标本进行了相关研究，报道了YKL-40与气道重塑之间的密切关系。实验结果表明，YKL-40可以通过PAR-2信号通路促进支气管平滑肌细胞的增生和迁移。此外，其在上皮中的表达与哮喘患者气道平滑肌的质量呈正相关。Konradsen等比较了难治性哮喘儿童患者和健康儿童中血清YKL-40的水平，发现难治性哮喘患儿的血清YKL-40水平较高且与气道厚度、哮喘控制水平关系密切。Chupp等通过生化和免疫组织化学分析，认为血清YKL-40水平与气道上皮下基膜厚度有关。与Galectin-3类似，YKL-40的表达也会在其他纤维化疾病中增高，如特发性肺纤维化患者的血液及肺组织中。

过去的几年，维生素D引起了科学界的极大关注。包括支气管哮喘在内的多种气道疾病均被认为与维生素D缺乏有关。回顾性研究表明，一些试验支持维生素D补充剂在降低儿童哮喘严重程度方面发挥积极作用。猜测维生素D可能通过多种免疫途径改善哮喘气道炎症和重塑，包括通过检查点激酶1抑制气道平滑肌细胞的生长等。

研究表明，治疗抵抗的严重哮喘儿童，其维生素 D 的主要循环形式血清 25(OH)D₃ 水平低于轻中度哮喘儿童。在随后的研究中，研究人员收集气道活检证实，患者血清中 25(OH)D₃ 水平的降低与气道平滑肌质量增加、肺功能下降和哮喘控制有关。而且，25(OH)D₃ 水平与气道重塑的其他参数(包括气道炎症)无关。尽管有不少优势，维生素 D 作为生物标志物同样具有一些不足之处。先前的研究报道血清 25(OH)D₃ 水平可能受性别、年龄、季节及慢性疾病的影响。

由于多种限制因素的存在，目前对哮喘气道重塑生物标志物的研究大多局限于较小的样本。而且，对于气道重塑这一呼吸道结构的改变，从痰样本中选择合适的生物标志物可能比于从血液样本中选择更为理想，但相关研究较少。

三、哮喘治疗和气道重塑

尽管哮喘的表型和内型越来越受到重视，但抗感染治疗仍然是哮喘治疗的支柱，目前哮喘治疗方法与内型或表型之间的关联仍较少。在临床实践中，哮喘的抗感染治疗已不断地完善和标准化，而气道重塑目前受药理和生物治疗影响较小。

糖皮质激素作为目前哮喘治疗的主要药物，对炎症有明显的改善作用，但其改善或逆转气道重塑的作用仍有待进一步探讨。有研究认为，糖皮质激素可部分改善哮喘患者的肺功能，降低气道厚度，但也有研究认为糖皮质激素对气道重塑没有任何作用或只有轻微影响，这可能与研究对象、激素剂量等差异有关。一些研究却表明吸入糖皮质激素可能对气道上皮细胞产生有害影响，包括诱导凋亡和破坏上皮细胞迁移，从而抑制其对哮喘的治疗作用。

大量关于单克隆抗体的临床试验表明，多种 IL-5 单克隆抗体，包括美泊利单抗和瑞利珠单抗，可以改善哮喘气道重塑，包括减少网状基底膜蛋白的表达，从而部分抑制气道重塑。然而，对于长期哮喘伴持续气道阻塞的患者，目前的生物制剂效果有限。虽然大规模的临床试验表明，新的抗 IL-4/IL-13 单克隆抗体如 Dupilumab 和 tralokinumab 可以有效地减少哮喘的发生，改善 FEV₁，但它们对气道重塑的确切影响仍需要进一步的研究。

支气管热成形术，为哮喘患者气道重塑治疗带来了新的希望。作为一种新兴的非药物干预手段，支气管热成形术可以通过应用热作用于气道，并主要通过减少过多的气道平滑肌改善患者的症状和生活质量，在临床实践中取得了很好的效果。已有研究证实支气管热成形术对气道上皮、黏液腺和杯状细胞肥大或增生无明显影响。但一些研究指出，单纯气道平滑肌的减少不足以解释其临床结果，气道平滑肌质量的减少不能完全归因于直接的快递加热反应。对于这项新技术，仍需进一步完善其作用机制，降低不良反应的发生率，改善患者预后。

在哮喘气道重塑治疗中，部分非常用药物可能有更广泛的应用前景。加洛帕米作为一种钙离子受体拮抗剂，在体外实验中被证明能够抑制气道平滑肌细胞增生。研究人员进行了为期 12 个月的双盲临床对照试验证明，加洛帕米能在不影响炎症的情况下降低重症哮喘患者气道平滑肌厚度，减少哮喘的急性发作，为气道重塑的治疗提供了可能。Kunzmann 等报道组胺可诱导肺成纤维细胞中结缔组织生长因子(CTGF)的表达，促进慢性气道重塑的发生。另一项研究也证实抗组胺药对哮喘有明显的缓解作用，并能改善肺功能，这在一定程度上为抗组胺药在哮喘中的应用提供了理论依据。作为白三烯受体拮抗剂，孟鲁司特也被发现具有抑制轻度哮喘患者气道成纤维细胞的功能，可能作为改善气道重塑和减轻气道炎症的有效药物。已有证据表明，作用于 PGD2 受体 2(DP2) 的前列腺素 D2(PGD2) 在哮喘气道嗜酸性粒细胞浸润中起重要作用，可能是哮喘治疗中一个有潜力的靶点。一项随机对照试验表明，作为 DP2 拮抗剂，fevipiprant 可以减少哮喘患者气道平滑肌质量。同时研究还证实，在气道平滑肌细胞培养模型中使用 DP2 特异性拮抗剂，气道平滑肌迁移受到明显抑制。然而根据药物公司的最新报道，fevipiprant 因在三期临床试验中未能有效改善肺功能而宣告失败。

四、气道重塑个性化治疗的可能性

多年来，对哮喘的治疗主要是基于"一刀切"的治疗原则，部分患者尤其是一些重症患者的病情未能得到有效控制。在个体化治疗时代，根据哮喘的不同表型制订治疗策略，可以最大限度地控制病情；而进一步了解气道重塑的程度和分类，也有助于哮喘的防治。经过数十年的研究，目前对哮喘气道重塑的认识取得了显著进展，但离实际应用仍存在一定差距。个体化治疗不仅只考虑疾病及其病理生理机制，而将患者视为一个整体，在实施治疗的过程中将多种因素考虑在内，包括患者的心理、经济等方面。然而，作为个体化治疗实施的基础也是第一步，气道重塑的机制仍尚未阐明。我们对气道重塑机制的认识仍处于起步阶段，还需要进一步的阐释与发展。

不同的患者有着独特的重塑类型，这在一定程度上使他们对药物的反应不同，他们的表型应该被明确并精确分类，以便进行适宜的个体化治疗。找到一个或者几个可靠的特征或生物标志物，以准确地区分患者的表型，是个体化治疗实际应用的基础。最近研究人员提出了一种新的哮喘分类方法：他们在拓扑数据分析的基础上融入了气道重塑的特点进行多维数据分析，成功将哮喘患者分为 4 种病理类型，丰富和完善了哮喘各表型的内容。目前，在缺乏有效的气道重塑生物标志物的情况下，通过这种特别的方法对哮喘的表型进行完整的分类，为下一步针对不同病理表型的治疗提供了可能。在临床治疗上，长期以来使用奥马利珠单抗，其次是美伯利珠单抗及陆续产生的其他单克隆抗体。从只有一种单克隆抗体可用到拥有一组具有多种不同靶点和功能的生物制剂，就要求我们从中做出正确的临床选择，这进一步强调了寻找有效的标志物合理、准确进行哮喘分型的重要性，以期对患者更个性化的精准治疗。

五、结 语

迄今为止,有关气道重塑的研究仍存在许多问题。在支气管哮喘中,理想的气道重塑相关生物标志物仍然没有定论。随着越来越多的生物制剂的出现,与寻找更多新而可靠的生物标志物相比,进一步探索气道重塑的完整机制仍然是首先需要解决的问题。相信在病理生理机制逐步改善的过程中,合适的气道重塑标志物将会被发现。在控制哮喘的过程中,必须通过基于生物标志物或其他方法进行精确分类,只有在这个基础上,为不同表型的患者选择个性化的干预措施进行治疗,最终达到理想的状态。

参 考 文 献

[1] Bullone M, Lavoie JP. The equine asthma model of airway remodeling: from a veterinary to a human perspective. Cell Tissue Res, 2020, 380(2): 223-236.

[2] Boulet LP. Airway remodeling in asthma: update on mechanisms and therapeutic approaches. CurrOpinPulm Med, 2018, 24(1): 56-62.

[3] Uwaezuoke SN, Ayuk AC, Eze JN. Severe bronchial asthma in children: a review of novel biomarkers used as predictors of the disease. J Asthma Allergy, 2018, 11: 11-18.

[4] Pavord ID, Beasley R, Agusti A, et al. After asthma: redefining airways diseases. Lancet, 2018, 391(10118): 350-400.

[5] O'Neill S, Sweeney J, Patterson CC, et al. The cost of treating severe refractory asthma in the UK: an economic analysis from the British Thoracic Society Difficult Asthma Registry. Thorax, 2015, 70(4): 376-378.

[6] Jarjour NN, Erzurum SC, Bleecker ER, et al. Severe asthma: lessons learned from the National Heart, Lung, and Blood Institute Severe Asthma Research Program. Am J Respir Crit Care Med, 2012, 185(4): 356-362.

[7] Saglani S, Bush A. Onset of Structural Airway Changes in Preschool Wheezers. A Window and Target for Secondary Asthma Prevention? Am J Respir Crit Care Med, 2015, 192(2): 121-122.

[8] Yadav SK, Shah SD, Penn RB. Give Me a Fork: Can Autophagy Research Solve the Riddle of Airway Remodeling in Asthma? Am J Respir Cell Mol Biol, 2019, 60(5): 494-496.

[9] Durrani SR, Viswanathan RK, Busse WW. What effect does asthma treatment have on airway remodeling? Current perspectives. J Allergy Clin Immunol, 2011, 128(3): 439-448.

[10] Prakash YS, Halayko AJ, Gosens R, et al. An Official American Thoracic Society Research Statement: Current Challenges Facing Research and Therapeutic Advances in Airway Remodeling. Am J Respir Crit Care Med, 2017, 195(2): e4-e19.

[11] Vieira Braga FA, Kar G, Berg M, et al. A cellular census of human lungs identifies novel cell states in health and in asthma. Nat Med, 2019, 25(7): 1153-1163.

[12] Broide DH. Immunologic and inflammatory mechanisms that drive asthma progression to remodeling. J Allergy Clin Immunol, 2008, 121(3): 560-570.

[13] Hur GY, Broide DH. Genes and Pathways Regulating Decline in Lung Function and Airway Remodeling in Asthma. Allergy Asthma Immunol Res, 2019, 11(5): 604-621.

[14] Kianmeher M, Ghorani V, Boskabady MH. Animal Model of Asthma, Various Methods and Measured Parameters: A Methodological Review. Iran J Allergy Asthma Immunol, 2016, 15(6): 445-465.

[15] Shin YS, Takeda K, Gelfand EW. Understanding asthma using animal models. Allergy Asthma Immunol Res, 2009, 1(1): 10-18.

[16] Przybyszowski M, Paciorek K, Zastrzezynska W, et al. Influence of omalizumab therapy on airway remodeling assessed with high-resolution computed tomography (HRCT) in severe allergic asthma patients. Adv Respir Med, 2018.

[17] Kotaru C, Schoonover KJ, Trudeau JB, et al. Regional fibroblast heterogeneity in the lung, implications for remodeling. Am J Respir Crit Care Med, 2006, 173(11): 1208-1215.

[18] Witt CA, Sheshadri A, Carlstrom L, et al. Longitudinal changes in airway remodeling and air trapping in severe asthma. AcadRadiol, 2014, 21(8): 986-993.

[19] Vijverberg SJ, Hilvering B, Raaijmakers JA, et al. Clinical utility of asthma biomarkers: from bench to bedside. Biologics, 2013, 7: 199-210.

[20] Wadsworth S, Sin D, Dorscheid D. Clinical update on the use of biomarkers of airway inflammation in the management of asthma. J Asthma Allergy, 2011, 4: 77-86.

[21] Perry R, Braileanu G, Palmer T, et al. The Economic Burden of Pediatric Asthma in the United States: Literature Review of Current Evidence. Pharmacoeconomics, 2019, 37(2): 155-167.

[22] Stokes JR, Casale TB. Characterization of asthma endotypes: implications for therapy. Ann Allergy Asthma Immunol, 2016, 117(2): 121-125.

[23] Aubier M, Thabut G, Hamidi F, et al. Airway smooth muscle enlargement is associated with protease-activated receptor 2/ligand overexpression in patients with difficult-to-control severe asthma. J Allergy Clin Immunol, 2016, 138(3): 729-739.

[24] Hirota N, Martin JG. Mechanisms of airway remodeling. Chest, 2013, 144(3): 1026-1032.

[25] de Boer RA, Voors AA, Muntendam P, et al. Galectin-3: a novel mediator of heart failure development and progression. Eur J Heart Fail, 2009, 11(9): 811-817.

[26] Ge XN, Bahaie NS, Kang BN, et al. Allergen-induced airway remodeling is impaired in galectin-3-deficient mice. J Immunol, 2010, 185(2): 1205-1214.

[27] Mauri P, Riccio AM, Rossi R, et al. Proteomics of bronchial biopsies: galectin-3 as a predictive biomarker of airway remodelling modulation in omalizumab-treated severe asthma

[28] Riccio AM, Mauri P, De Ferrari L, et al. Galectin-3: an early predictive biomarker of modulation of airway remodeling in patients with severe asthma treated with omalizumab for 36 months. Clin Transl Allergy, 2017, 7:6.

[29] Lee CG, Da Silva CA, Dela Cruz CS, et al. Role of chitin and chitinase/chitinase-like proteins in inflammation, tissue remodeling, and injury. Annu Rev Physiol, 2011, 73:479-501.

[30] Gomez JL, Crisafi GM, Holm CT, et al. Genetic variation in chitinase 3-like 1 (CHI3L1) contributes to asthma severity and airway expression of YKL-40. J Allergy Clin Immunol, 2015, 136(1):51-58 e10.

[31] Bara I, Ozier A, Girodet PO, et al. Role of YKL-40 in bronchial smooth muscle remodeling in asthma. Am J Respir Crit Care Med, 2012, 185(7):715-722.

[32] Konradsen JR, James A, Nordlund B, et al. The chitinase-like protein YKL-40: a possible biomarker of inflammation and airway remodeling in severe pediatric asthma. J Allergy Clin Immunol, 2013, 132(2):328-335 e5.

[33] Chupp GL, Lee CG, Jarjour N, et al. A chitinase-like protein in the lung and circulation of patients with severe asthma. N Engl J Med, 2007, 357(20):2016-2027.

[34] Jiao J, Castro M. Vitamin D and asthma: current perspectives. CurrOpin Allergy Clin Immunol, 2015, 15(4):375-382.

[35] Damera G, Fogle HW, Lim P, et al. Vitamin D inhibits growth of human airway smooth muscle cells through growth factor-induced phosphorylation of retinoblastoma protein and checkpoint kinase 1. Br J Pharmacol, 2009, 158(6):1429-1441.

[36] Gupta A, Sjoukes A, Richards D, et al. Relationship between serum vitamin D, disease severity, and airway remodeling in children with asthma. Am J Respir Crit Care Med, 2011, 184(12):1342-1349.

[37] Das G, Taylor PN, Javaid H, et al. Seasonal Variation of Vitamin D and Serum Thyrotropin Levels and Its Relationship in a Euthyroid Caucasian Population. EndocrPract, 2018, 24(1):53-59.

[38] Niimi A, Matsumoto H, Amitani R, et al. Effect of short-term treatment with inhaled corticosteroid on airway wall thickening in asthma. Am J Med, 2004, 116(11):725-731.

[39] Boulet LP, Turcotte H, Laviolette M, et al. Airway hyperresponsiveness, inflammation, and subepithelial collagen deposition in recently diagnosed versus long-standing mild asthma. Influence of inhaled corticosteroids. Am J Respir Crit Care Med, 2000, 162(4 Pt 1):1308-1313.

[40] Chakir J, Shannon J, Molet S, et al. Airway remodeling-associated mediators in moderate to severe asthma: effect of steroids on TGF-beta, IL-11, IL-17, and type I and type III collagen expression. J Allergy Clin Immunol, 2003, 111(6):1293-1298.

[41] Royce SG, Li X, Tortorella S, et al. Mechanistic insights into the contribution of epithelial damage to airway remodeling. Novel therapeutic targets for asthma. Am J Respir Cell Mol Biol, 2014, 50(1):180-192.

[42] Jiang D, Wang Z, Shen C, et al. Small airway dysfunction may be an indicator of early asthma: findings from high-resolution CT. Ann Allergy Asthma Immunol, 2019, 122(5):498-501.

[43] Hoshino M, Ohtawa J. Effects of adding omalizumab, an anti-immunoglobulin E antibody, on airway wall thickening in asthma. Respiration, 2012, 83(6):520-528.

[44] Brightling CE, Chanez P, Leigh R, et al. Efficacy and safety of tralokinumab in patients with severe uncontrolled asthma: a randomised, double-blind, placebo-controlled, phase 2b trial. Lancet Respir Med, 2015, 3(9):692-701.

[45] Hanania NA, Noonan M, Corren J, et al. Lebrikizumab in moderate-to-severe asthma: pooled data from two randomised placebo-controlled studies. Thorax, 2015, 70(8):748-756.

[46] Castro M, Rubin AS, Laviolette M, et al. Effectiveness and safety of bronchial thermoplasty in the treatment of severe asthma: a multicenter, randomized, double-blind, sham-controlled clinical trial. Am J Respir Crit Care Med, 2010, 181(2):116-124.

[47] Pretolani M, Bergqvist A, Thabut G, et al. Effectiveness of bronchial thermoplasty in patients with severe refractory asthma: Clinical and histopathologic correlations. J Allergy Clin Immunol, 2017, 139(4):1176-1185.

[48] Chernyavsky IL, Russell RJ, Saunders RM, et al. In vitro, in silico and in vivo study challenges the impact of bronchial thermoplasty on acute airway smooth muscle mass loss. Eur Respir J, 2018, 51(5).

[49] Girodet PO, Dournes G, Thumerel M, et al. Calcium channel blocker reduces airway remodeling in severe asthma. A proof-of-concept study. Am J Respir Crit Care Med, 2015, 191(8):876-888.

[50] Trian T, Benard G, Begueret H, et al. Bronchial smooth muscle remodeling involves calcium-dependent enhanced mitochondrial biogenesis in asthma. J Exp Med, 2007, 204(13):3173-3181.

[51] Kunzmann S, Schmidt-Weber C, Zingg JM, et al. Connective tissue growth factor expression is regulated by histamine in lung fibroblasts: potential role of histamine in airway remodeling. J Allergy Clin Immunol, 2007, 119(6):1398-1407.

[52] Simons FE. Advances in H1-antihistamines. N Engl J Med, 2004, 351(21):2203-2217.

[53] Kelly MM, Chakir J, Vethanayagam D, et al. Montelukast treatment attenuates the increase in myofibroblasts following low-dose allergen challenge. Chest, 2006, 130(3):741-753.

[54] Gonem S, Berair R, Singapuri A, et al. Fevipiprant, a prostaglandin D2 receptor 2 antagonist, in patients with persistent eosinophilic asthma: a single-centre, randomised, double-blind, parallel-group, placebo-controlled trial. Lancet Respir Med, 2016, 4(9):699-707.

[55] Saunders R, Kaul H, Berair R, et al. DP2 antagonism reduces airway smooth muscle mass in asthma by decreasing eosinophilia and myofibroblast recruitment. Sci Transl Med, 2019, 11(479).

[56] Canonica GW, Ferrando M, Baiardini I, et al. Asthma: personalized and precision medicine. CurrOpin Allergy Clin Immunol, 2018, 18(1):51-58.

[57] Siddiqui S, Shikotra A, Richardson M, et al. Airway patholog-

ical heterogeneity in asthma: Visualization of disease microclusters using topological data analysis. J Allergy Clin Immunol,2018,142(5):1457-1468.

[58] Brasier AR, Zhou J. Validation of the epigenetic reader bromodomain-containing protein 4(BRD4) as a therapeutic target for treatment of airway remodeling. Drug Discov Today, 2020,25(1):126-132.

10 《支气管哮喘防治指南(2020年更新版)》解读

周 新 张 旻

《支气管哮喘防治指南(2020年更新版)》是在我国既往哮喘防治指南基础上,结合近年来国内外循证医学研究结果,由我国哮喘学组数十位专家集体讨论和重新修订的。本指南旨在为提高我国医务人员对哮喘规范化诊治的认识和水平提供指导性文件。

《支气管哮喘防治指南(2020年更新版)》有十一个部分:哮喘的定义;哮喘的流行病学;诊断;哮喘的评估;哮喘的鉴别诊断;哮喘慢性持续期的治疗;哮喘急性发作期的治疗;重度哮喘;特殊类型哮喘及哮喘的某些特殊问题;哮喘的管理、教育和预防;结束语。

本文主要介绍《支气管哮喘防治指南(2020年更新版)》与2016年版比较有哪些更新的内容,并做一解读。

一、关于我国成人哮喘的流行病学

(一)哮喘的患病率

近年来国内外流行病学调查资料均表明哮喘的患病率在逐年上升。由于流行病学调查采用的抽样方法以及对哮喘的定义差异,不同调查得出的结果差异较大。2010—2011年在我国8个省市进行的"全国支气管哮喘患病情况及相关危险因素流行病学调查(China Asthma and Risk factors Epidemiologic investigation study,CARE研究)",采用多级随机整群抽样入户问卷调查,共调查了164 215名14岁以上人群,结果显示,我国14岁以上人群医生诊断的哮喘患病率为1.24%。

2012—2015年,在中国10个省市进行的"中国肺健康研究(China Pulmonary Health study,CPH研究)",采用多阶段分层抽样方法,在160个城乡调查点,采用曾被GBD等研究用于大型流行病学调查时欧洲社区呼吸健康调查的哮喘问卷。哮喘诊断的定义是:受调查者自我报告曾被医生诊断为哮喘,或过去一年曾有过喘息症状。该研究共纳入57 779名20岁以上受调查者,其中50 991名完成了哮喘调查问卷,并有吸入支气管舒张剂后质控合格的肺功能检测结果,该调查显示我国20岁及以上人群的哮喘患病率为4.2%。按照2015年的全国人口普查数据推算,我国20岁以上人群应该有4570万哮喘患者。

以上二项流行病学调查结果反映了相同时期我国哮喘的患病率,但是差异较大,希望今后能有更大样本量的哮喘流行病学调查数据。

(二)我国哮喘的控制现状

经过多年推广哮喘的规范化治疗,我国哮喘的控制现状有了明显的进步,但仍不够理想。2017年我国30个省市城区门诊支气管哮喘患者控制水平的调查,共纳入3875例患者,根据GINA定义的哮喘控制水平分级,结果显示我国城区哮喘总体控制率为28.5%,其中参与2008年哮喘控制调查的10个城市在本次调查中哮喘的控制率为39.2%,与2008年比较,有较大程度的提高。

二、关于哮喘的分期

2006年版哮喘防治指南根据临床表现哮喘可分为急性发作期、慢性持续期和临床缓解期。在GINA文件中没有临床缓解期,也没有临床控制期的定义。但是GINA文件根据患者过去4周的症状、用药情况、肺功能检查结果等复合指标将患者分为完全控制、部分控制和未控制,并提出治疗目标要达到哮喘控制。因此,《支气管哮喘防治指南(2020年更新版)》将临床缓解期改为临床控制期,临床控制期是指患者无喘息、气促、胸闷、咳嗽等症状4周以上,1年内无哮喘急性发作,肺功能正常。

三、关于哮喘的评估方法

与2006年版哮喘防治指南比较,《支气管哮喘防治指南(2020年更新版)》在本部分中增加了以下检测项目。

(一)血清总IgE和过敏原特异性IgE

有很多因素会影响血清总IgE水平,可以使血清总IgE水平增高,如其他过敏性疾病,寄生虫、真菌、病毒感染,肿瘤和免疫性疾病等。血清总IgE没有正常值,其水平增高缺乏特异性,需要结合临床判断,但可以作为使用抗IgE单克隆抗体治疗选择剂量的依据。过敏原特异性IgE增高是诊断过敏性哮喘的重要依据之一,其水平高低可以反映哮喘患者过敏状态的严重程度。

(二)过敏原检测

有体内皮肤过敏原点刺试验及体外特异性IgE检测,通过检测明确患者的过敏因素,宣教患者尽量避免接触过敏原,以及用于指导过敏原特异性免疫疗法。

四、哮喘的鉴别诊断

这部分内容是《支气管哮喘防治指南(2020年更新版)》新增加的内容。支气管哮喘应注意与左心功能不全、慢性阻塞性肺疾病、上气道阻塞性病变等常见疾病相鉴别,此外还应与嗜酸性粒细胞肉芽肿性多血管炎、变应性支气管肺曲霉病等疾病相鉴别,以上这些疾病在临床上都可以表现有哮喘样症状。

五、药　物

治疗哮喘的药物可以分为控制药物和缓解药物,以及重度哮喘的附加治疗药物。在控制药物中《支气管哮喘防治指南(2020年更新版)》增加了甲磺司特。甲磺司特是一种选择性Th2细胞因子抑制剂,可抑制IL-4、IL-5的产生和IgE的合成,减少嗜酸粒细胞浸润,减轻气道高反应性。该药为口服制剂,安全性好,适用于过敏性哮喘患者的治疗。

近年来发展了几种吸入性糖皮质激素的新药物和新制剂,本文介绍临床上常用的ICS每日低、中、高剂量(表3-10-1)。

对于成人哮喘患者的初始治疗,应根据患者具体情况选择合适的治疗级别,本文参照2019年GINA文件将初始哮喘治疗的推荐方案做了更新(表3-10-2)。

表 3-10-1　临床上常用的ICS每日低、中、高剂量

成人和青少年(12岁及以上)			
药　物	每日剂量(μg)		
	低剂量	中剂量	高剂量
二丙酸倍氯米松(pMDI,标准颗粒,HFA)	200~500	>500~1000	>1000
二丙酸倍氯米松(pMDI,超细颗粒,HFA)	100~200	>200~400	>400
布地奈德(DPI)	200~400	>400~800	>800
环索奈德(pMDI,超细颗粒,HFA)	80~160	>160~320	>320
丙酸氟替卡松(DPI)	100~250	>250~500	>500
丙酸氟替卡松(pMDI,标准颗粒,HFA)	100~250	>250~500	>500
糠酸莫米松(DPI)		200	400
糠酸莫米松(pMDI,标准颗粒,HFA)		200~400	>400
糠酸氟替卡松(DPI)		100	200

注:DPI. 干粉吸入剂;HFA. 氢氟烷烃抛射剂

表 3-10-2　初始哮喘治疗-成人和青少年的推荐选择

存在症状	首选初始治疗
所有患者	不推荐仅用SABA治疗(而无ICS)
哮喘症状不频繁,如,少于每月2次	1. 按需低剂量ICS+福莫特罗(证据B) 2. 其他选择包括使用SABA时同时使用ICS,联合使用或单独的吸入器(证据B)
每月2次或2次以上哮喘症状或需要缓解药物。	1. 低剂量ICS,且按需使用SABA(证据A),或按需低剂量ICS+福莫特罗(证据A) 2. 其他选择包括LTRA(疗效低于ICS,证据A) 3. 使用SABA同时使用ICS,用联合或单独的吸入器(证据B)。如果缓解药物使用的是SABA,需评估患者使用控制药物的依从性
大多数日子有哮喘症状;或每周1次或1次以上因哮喘觉醒,尤其是存在任何危险因素时	1. 低剂量ICS+LABA作为维持治疗,ICS+福莫特罗 2. 按需使用SABA为缓解治疗(证据A),同时联合ICS 3. 中剂量ICS及按需SABA(证据A)
初始哮喘表现伴严重未控制的哮喘,或伴急性发作	1. 短期口服糖皮质激素及开始规律使用控制药物治疗 2. 采用高剂量ICS(证据A)或中剂量ICS+LABA(证据D)
在开始初始控制药物治疗之前 　若可能,记录哮喘诊断证据 　记录患者症状控制水平和风险因素,包括肺功能 　考虑影响治疗方案选择的因素 　确保患者正确使用吸入器 　计划随访预约 在开始初始控制药物治疗之后 　在2~3个月后或更早,评估患者治疗反应 　维持良好控制达3个月以上,可考虑降级治疗	

关于哮喘的长期(阶梯式)治疗方案也按照2019年GINA文件做了更新(表3-10-3)。与2016年哮喘指南治疗方案表相比,表3-10-3主要更新是治疗方案中按需使用SABA时即需要联合低剂量ICS,推荐使用按需ICS-福莫特罗。此外在第5级治疗方案中增加了或加抗IL-5、或加抗IL-5R、或加抗IL-4R单克隆抗体的治疗药物。

表3-10-3 哮喘患者长期(阶梯式)治疗方案

	1级	2级	3级	4级	5级
推荐选择控制药物	按需 ICS-福莫特罗	低剂量 ICS 或按需 ICS+福莫特罗	低剂量 ICS+LABA 或低剂量 ICS+福莫特罗维持缓解治疗	中剂量 ICS+LABA	高剂量 ICS+LABA 加其他治疗,如加 LAMA,或加茶碱或加低剂量口服激素(注意不良反应)
其他选择控制药物	按需使用 SABA 时即联合低剂量 ICS	白三烯受体拮抗剂(LTRA)低剂量茶碱	中剂量 ICS 或低剂量 ICS 加 LTRA 或加茶碱	高剂量 ICS 加 LAMA 或加 LTRA 或加茶碱	参考临床表型加抗 IgE 单克隆抗体,或加抗 IL-5、或加抗 IL-5R、或加抗 IL-4R 单克隆抗体
首选缓解药物	按需使用低剂量 ICS+福莫特罗处方维持和缓解治疗的患者按需使用低剂量 ICS+福莫特罗				
其他可选缓解药物	按需使用 SABA				

六、关于重度哮喘

以往定义为重症、重度哮喘不统一,《支气管哮喘防治指南(2020年更新版)》统一称为重度哮喘,区别于哮喘发作病情为重症。在重度哮喘中增加了临床类型:早发过敏性哮喘;晚发持续嗜酸性粒细胞性哮喘;频繁急性发作性哮喘;持续气流受限性哮喘;肥胖相关性哮喘。区分哮喘的临床表型有助于对患者进行更有针对性的治疗。

在药物治疗中除了生物靶向药物抗IgE单克隆抗体以外,《支气管哮喘防治指南(2020年更新版)》还介绍了抗IL-5单克隆抗体、抗IL-5受体(IL-5R)的单克隆抗体和抗IL-4R单克隆抗体,这些靶向治疗药物已经在国外临床应用,也写入到2019年GINA文件中,作为重度哮喘患者的推荐治疗药物。

美国胸科学会和欧洲呼吸学会2019年颁布了新的难治性哮喘诊治指南,在第5级的成人哮喘患者,经规范治疗后哮喘症状仍然不能控制,有条件的推荐大环内脂类药物治疗,如口服阿奇霉素250～500 mg/d,每周3次,治疗26～48周,可以减少哮喘急性发作。《支气管哮喘防治指南(2020年更新版)》对此也作了介绍,大环内脂类药物主要适应于中性细胞为主的重度哮喘治疗,但长期使用大环内脂类药物可以有腹泻、QT间期延长、听力减退等不良反应,在临床治疗哮喘时需要谨慎使用。

七、特殊类型哮喘及哮喘的某些特殊问题

关于咳嗽变异性哮喘(cough variant asthma,CVA),支气管激发试验阳性是诊断CVA最重要的条件,《支气管哮喘防治指南(2020年更新版)》在本内容中增加了临床上要注意支气管激发试验假阳性和假阴性,需结合治疗反应,抗哮喘治疗有效才能确诊CVA。

关于哮喘合并慢性阻塞性肺疾病,我国2016年版哮喘指南介绍了哮喘-慢性阻塞性肺疾病重叠综合征(asthma-COPD overlap syndrome,ACOS)的概念。2019年GINA文件认为ACO并不是一种病名,是对临床上同时具有哮喘和慢阻肺特征的一种描述性用语,其包含了哮喘和慢性阻塞性肺疾病不同的临床表型,ACO的患病率在15%～20%。《支气管哮喘防治指南(2020年更新版)》特别强调ACO不是一种疾病,而是哮喘和慢性阻塞性肺疾病两种不同的疾病。ACO的治疗推荐联合应用ICS-LABA-LAMA。同时,ACO治疗应包括戒烟、肺康复、疫苗接种和合并症的治疗。

《支气管哮喘防治指南(2020年更新版)》的修订得到了中华医学会呼吸病学分会哮喘学组全体成员以及中国医师协会呼吸病学分会哮喘与变态反应工作委员会部分成员的大力支持,各位专家为新指南的修订提出了许多很好的建议。本指南得到了我国著名呼吸病学专家陈荣昌教授、瞿介明教授、殷凯生教授、陈萍教授的审阅和修改,他们提出了很好的修改意见。本指南通信作者之一钟南山院士亲自参加了二次哮喘指南修订会讨论,并且对稿件作了几次认真地审阅,提出了宝贵的修订意见。大家一致认为本指南的更新基于国内外最新研究证据并结合中国的国情,在编写过程中专家们深感中国的哮喘防治事业还有诸多问题亟待解决,最大的问题在于我们缺乏足够的循证医学证据。将来中国哮喘防治指南更新应建立在更加广泛、深入的研究基础上,积累更多的中国哮喘防治的经验,更好地指导我国哮喘的防治工作。

参 考 文 献

[1] 中华医学会呼吸病学分会哮喘学组.支气管哮喘防治指南(2016年版).中华结核和呼吸杂志,2016,39(9):675-697.

[2] Lin J, Wang W, Chen P, et al. Prevalence and risk factors of asthma in mainland China: The CARE study. Respir Med, 2018,137:48-54.

[3] Huang K, Yang T, Xu J, et al. Prevalence, risk factors, and management of asthma in China: a national cross-sectional study. Lancet, 2019, 394(10196):407-418.

[4] 林江涛,王文巧,周新,等.我国30个省市城区门诊支气管哮喘患者控制水平的调查结果.中华结核和呼吸杂志,2017,40(7):494-498.

[5] Global Initiative for Asthma. Global Strategy for Asthma Management and Prevention: update 2019. Http://www.ginaasthma.org/.

[6] 中华医学会呼吸病学分会哮喘学组.中国哮喘联盟.重症哮喘诊断与处理中国专家共识.中华结核与呼吸杂志,2017,40(11):813-829.

[7] Diagnosis and Management of Difficult-to-Treat and Severe Asthma in adolescent and adult patients. https//ginasthma org.

[8] Holguin F, Cardet JC, Chung KF, et al. Magagement of severe asthma: a European Respiratory Society/American Thoracic Society guideline. Eur Respir J, 2020, 55(1):1900588.

11 哮喘合并胃食管反流性疾病的诊疗

云春梅

哮喘(asthma)是以接触或未接触过敏原后气道高反应性为特征的呼吸道慢性炎症性疾病,影响全球1%～18%的人口,临床表现为可逆性气流受限、间断发作性喘息、气短、胸闷和(或)咳嗽;运动、过敏原或刺激物暴露、气温变化或呼吸道病毒感染等均会诱发哮喘发作。哮喘临床症状个体差异显著,患者可能在几周甚至是几个月间均无症状,但在接触过敏原或暴露有害刺激情况下即可出现症状,严重时甚至可危及生命。1892年Osler首次发现胃膨大与哮喘之间存在相关性,近20年越来越多的临床医师也意识到胃食管反流病(gastroesophageal reflux disease,GERD)是多种呼吸道疾病如慢性支气管炎、吸入性肺炎、支气管扩张、间质性肺疾病发病病因,其中很大一部分研究揭示了GERD与哮喘发病的相关性。

一、流行病学特征

随着近年相关流行病学调查发现,作为临床常见疾病,哮喘和GERD在临床上可以并行发生,与普通人群相比,GERD在哮喘人群中发病率更高。因为胃食管反流评估方式不同,各研究结果差别较大,但初步估算哮喘并发GERD的患病率在34%～89%。2019年Yoshihiro Kanemitsu等发表的一项关于慢性咳嗽病因分析研究显示咳嗽变异性哮喘(cough variant asthma CVA)是GERD最常见的合并症,在慢性咳嗽中CVA合并GERD发病率为68.1%,CVA合并GERD并同时合并其他疾病为6.7%。2009年林江涛发表的一篇研究对2005年10月—2009年2月就诊中日友好医院的慢性咳嗽患者病因进行统计分析发现CVA合并GERD占慢性咳嗽两种病因以上疾病中的48%,提示GERD与CVA关系密切,考虑GERD是CVA发病重要危险因素。

Field等使用详细问卷的方式调查了门诊的109例哮喘患者和两个对照组(68例拜访家庭医生的患者和67例患有其他医学疾病的患者)中的GERD症状的发生率,其中77%哮喘患者有胃灼热症状,55%自述存在反流,24%患者有吞咽困难,上述症状比例均高于两个对照组。在调查前一周41%的哮喘患者曾出现过与反流相关的呼吸道症状,28%出现反流症状的哮喘患者使用了吸入药物控制哮喘症状,37%的哮喘患者至少需要一种抗反流药物(通常是抗酸药或奥美拉唑),是两个对照组的5倍。另一个值得注意的是无症状GERD也常发生在哮喘患者中,Irwin等研究结果提示在24%难治性哮喘患者合并有无症状GERD。同时,哮喘患者伴发很高的食管功能障碍。Kjelle等发现在97例哮喘持续患者中,有38%伴有食管运动障碍,27%患者食管下括约肌(lower esophageal sphincter, LES)压力减低。Sontag等通过内镜检查和食管活检发现在186例成年男性哮喘持续发作患者中有79例(43%)患有食管炎或Barrett's食管炎,且82%哮喘患者存在酸反流异常。与正常对照组相比,哮喘患者LES压力显著降低,反流发作频率更高,食管酸暴露时间也更长。

二、哮喘合并GERD的发病机制

目前学者认为哮喘与GERD的病理生理学改变可相互影响其发病率。一方面,哮喘患者增加的胸腹腔压力梯度会增加胃食管反流的可能性,另一方面,GERD患者的胃酸气道微吸入会增强患者迷走神经调节功能、诱发支气管高反应性进而引起气道狭窄出现喘息、胸闷、咳嗽等症状。食管和支气管胚胎期同源,因此胃酸可通过刺激酸性感受器引起食管和气道迷走神经反射。Wright等对136人进行食管酸注入试验(Bernstein test)测试酸注入前后患者气流和动脉血氧饱和度,发现136人酸食管注入后气流和动脉血氧饱和度均显著降低,使用阿托品进行预处理后这一现象消失。这一试验证明了酸可以通过食管气管迷走神经调节诱发气道反应。Mansfield和Stein对正常对照组,哮喘和GERD及合并发生的四组患者进行Bernstein test双盲对照研究,结果显示Bernstein test阳性的哮喘患者气道阻力比基线增加10%,与此同时哮喘合并GERD患者总呼吸阻力增加更为显著,高达72%。Schan等研究了酸微吸入对哮喘的影响,即对上述研究中同样分组的四类人群进行酸清除后发现哮喘合并GERD呼气峰流速(peak expiratory flow PEF)进一步下降,其他三组均有改善。可见尽管清除了食管胃酸,但因合并GERD哮喘患者的气道酸微吸入与肺功能恶化有关。

哮喘患者因胸闷、喘息、咳嗽等症状会增加胸腹腔压力梯度,增加的压力会传递到食管下括约肌(lower esophageal sphincter LES),同时增加膈肌与食管连接处压力损坏LES功能,进而使酸反流更易发生。其次,影响气管、食管另一重要因素就是哮喘患者β_2受体激动剂的使用,β_2受体激动剂主要因其可松弛支气管平滑肌而应用于哮喘的诊治中,但β_2受体激动剂对LES的作用机制目前还不清楚。有研究显示β₂受体激动剂可降低LES紧张度,吸入性沙丁胺醇治疗哮喘以剂量依赖方式降低LES基础张力和收缩幅度,增加了患者食管酸化程度,食管酸化促进支气管收缩,支气管收缩通过增加胸腹腔压力形成恶性循环。

另外,GERD与无症状BHR(bronchial hyper-responsiveness)之间关系进一步证明哮喘与GERD之间的联系。Bagnato等发现36%的无呼吸道症状的GERD患者存在BHR,提示GERD与无症状BHR升高有关。Lapa等的研究也发表了类似结果,50%成年人GERD发现有BHR,而对照组仅为27%。一项对2600多人进行的横断面研究表明GERD哮喘患者夜间症状明显增加。

三、哮喘合并GERD的诊断

国际指南提出对哮喘患者快速诊断GERD有利于哮喘的控制,对改善患者生活质量和肺功能至关重要。从胃肠病学角度检测方法有三种:①经验性质子泵抑制剂试验(proton pump-inhibitors PPIs);②24h胃食管pH监测;③胃肠内镜检查。对于临床推断可能患有GERD的患者予以PPIs治疗可以作为验证诊断,即PPIs测试。但PPIs准确性与目前GERD客观检查的符合性还不清楚。24h食管pH监测是GERD目前诊断的"金标准",这是一种通过电极测量患者食管上下两端酸暴露情况与呼吸道症状之间关系的检测方法,对于典型和非典型GERD检出有很大的帮助,对于难治性GERD抑酸水平的评估很有作用。最后胃肠镜可用于鉴别糜烂性食管炎,并可对严重程度进行分级。

咽喉检查也可提供相关症状的诊断信息,且可以提供是否有复发的信息。GERD常见喉镜下症状有红斑,后连合肥大,肉芽肿,声带功能障碍,假性沟,水肿,鼻咽部红斑黏膜和舌扁桃体红色黏膜。其次,支气管肺泡灌洗(bronchoalveolar lavage BAL)可以通过将支气管镜插入支气管树中直接抽吸取证,即可从肺泡灌洗液中回收到从胃肠道产生的胃蛋白酶和胆汁酸等物质进行诊断,近期有研究报道100%哮喘患者BAL中发现胃蛋白酶。但在BAL中检测胃蛋白酶不一定是异常发现,也可能是由于上食管括约肌张力下降患者在睡眠期间吸入鼻咽的分泌物。呼出气冷凝物(exhaled breath condensate EBC)是通过使用收集设备对呼吸水蒸气进行冷却(通常在4℃或零以下的温度下),相关研究报道在咳嗽的患者中EBC中发现了胃蛋白酶,在哮喘急性发作的患者其EBCPH值显著降低。

四、哮喘合并GERD的治疗

吸入性激素(inhaled corticosteroids ICS)和β₂受体激动剂是哮喘治疗的基础,β₂受体激动剂对GERD的影响前面已有介绍。ICS对GERD的影响主要是考虑沉积于咽部的ICS通过吞咽动作被胃肠道吸收和肝首过清除效应,目前还没有关于吞咽的ICS对GERD的发生和进展影响的相关研究发表。研究显示,口服激素治疗重症哮喘对合并的GERD有潜在影响,Strickland等研究显示健康人群予以20 mg/d泼尼松龙口服会引起胃酸分泌影响GERD的发生。Lazenby等对口服激素治疗的中度持续性哮喘患者食管pH监测发现其食管下端酸接触时间增加。上述研究结果可见激素对哮喘合并的GERD影响有待进一步研究。

国际指南指出对于有症状的GERD哮喘患者需要PPIs治疗,虽然对哮喘预后无明显作用,但对患者PEF有一定改善。难治性哮喘有反流症状的患者需进行PPIs治疗,Yii等对177例难治性哮喘患者进行临床评估发现GERD是其急性加重的重要风险。在临床上有部分GERD患者表现为哮喘相关症状,因此国际指南就难治性哮喘患者有反流表现者需极积诊治,使其潜在风险降到最低。关于GERD的治疗有药物治疗、体位改变物理疗法、外科手术治疗和外科手术联合药物治疗。

目前相关GERD药物治疗的研究主要涉及抑酸剂、H₂受体拮抗剂和胃肠动力药(西咪替丁、雷尼替丁)。研究结果显示,抑酸剂和体位改变可以改善临床症状但对肺功能无改善,西沙必利对GERD诱发的儿童哮喘有效。而质子泵抑制剂可有效改善哮喘患者症状及肺功能。Meier等对15例合并有GERD哮喘患者进行双盲,安慰剂对照的交叉研究,每天使用两次奥美拉唑20 mg,治疗6周只有4名哮喘患者(27%)第一秒用力肺活量(forced expiratory volume in 1 minute, FEV₁)或PEF改善大于20%。且症状无改善的患者往往合并有更为严重食管炎,24h酸暴露时间是改善者的2～5倍。这一研究也提示常量奥美拉唑可能在治疗该类疾病时抑酸不足,也可能是部分相关研究抑酸制剂对哮喘患者肺功能改善的原因。Teichtahl等报道了一项安慰剂对照交叉试验,该试验对20名夜间哮喘患者进行了试验,每天使用40 mg的奥美拉唑治疗4周,结果表明PEF有轻度改善,但该研究治疗期太短。另一项抑酸研究对30例哮喘和GERD患者进行了前瞻性/前测后评估,采用3个月的酸抑制疗法(每天20～60 mg奥美拉唑)滴定,连续24h通过pH测试控制酸反流,结果显示73%GERD哮喘患者PEF增加20%和(或)喘息症状减少20%。与基线相比酸抑制治疗1个月后,哮喘症状减轻了30%;在2个月时减少了43%;到3个月时,哮喘症状减少了57%。通过24h测试pH的结果提示经常出现反流或食管近端反流过多的患者更可能长期抑酸治疗中获益。Levin等在一项双盲,随机,安慰剂对照的交叉试验中研究了9名哮喘患者经过4周的导入期后,为患者开具每日20 mg的奥美拉唑或安慰剂的处方共8周,然后进行替代治疗。结果显示与安慰剂组比较,接受奥美拉唑治疗的患者早上PEF率增高37.8%,晚上PEF增高31.2%(分别为P 0.025和0.060),且生活质量问卷、症状评分、运动耐力和情绪等均有改善。

相关研究回顾了抗反流手术后GERD哮喘患者预后的研究,抗反流手术涉及的术式有尼森胃底折叠术、贝尔西胃底折叠术和Toupet修复术。虽然大多数研究存在设计缺陷,如缺乏对照组、术前和术后气流障碍相关数据、哮喘严重程度的记录不全,尽管存在这些缺陷,但结合10个研究结果共有318例哮喘和GERD患者,其中253例(80%)哮喘得到改善,GERD组中许多以前使用类固醇的患者手术后超过50%患者"治愈"了哮喘。其中几项研究确定了抗反流手术是良好预后的预测因子。

手术联合药物治疗GERD哮喘的研究共有两项,药物为胃肠动力药。Larrain等随机对照研究发现,与安慰剂组比较手术组(Hill修复)和西咪替丁(300 mg每天4次)的平均症状评分显著改善,药物使用减少。6个月后,随机分为手术组的26例患者中有80%改善了哮喘,西咪替丁组的27例患者中有80%改善了哮喘,而安慰剂组的28例患者中仅有33%改善了哮喘。外科手术患者11名其中8名,西咪替丁患者13名中2名可以停止类固醇激素治疗,而安慰剂组14名患者仍需继续激素治疗。5年后只有外科组患者保持无症状状态,安慰剂和西咪替丁组临床特征恢复到患者治疗前基线状态。另外一项研究是Sontag等将雷尼替丁(150mg,3次/天)与尼森胃底折叠术和药物治疗进行了比较。在5年的随访中,通过症状、肺功能检查和用药需求对患者进行评估,手术组中将近75%的患者治愈或喘息症状得到改善,而雷尼替丁组为10%,对照组5%。

临床上,GERD合并哮喘患病率较高,且有多种病理生理学机制参与。因许多研究存在设计缺陷,哮喘合并GERD治疗的相关研究目前仍有较大争议,但在设计较为合理且研究周期较长的研究中可以看到进行积极的抗反流疗法可改善患者临床症状、肺功能。在总结前期研究经验的基础上,相信有更多可靠的研究数据会为哮喘合并GERD寻找到更加合理的诊治手段。

参 考 文 献

[1] Solidoro P, Patrucco F, Fagoonee S, et al. Asthma and gastroesophageal reflux disease a multidisciplinary point of view. Minerva Medica, 2017, 108(4):350-356.

[2] Global Initiative for Asthma. Global Strategy for asthma management and pPrevention, 2016.

[3] Osler WB. The principles of internal medicine. New York: Appleton, 1892.

[4] Locke GR, Talley NJ, Fett SC, et al. Prevalence and clinical spectrum of gastroesophageal reflux: a population study in Olmsted County, Minnesota. Gastroenterology, 1997, 112:1448-1456.

[5] McFadden ER Jr, Gilbert IA. Asthma. N Engl J Med, 1992, 327:1928-1937.

[6] Harding SM, Richter JE. The role of gastroesophageal reflux in chronic cough and asthma. Chest, 1997, 111:1389-11402.

[7] Kanemitsu Y, Kurokawa R, Takeda N, et al. Clinical impact of gastroesophageal reflux disease in patients with subacute/chronic cough. Allergol Inter, 2019, 68:478-485.

[8] 刘国梁,林江涛. 不明原因慢性咳嗽的病因构成和临床特征分析. 中华结核和呼吸杂志, 2009, 6(32):422-425.

[9] Field SK, Underwood M, Brant R, et al. Prevalence of gastroesophageal reflux symptoms in asthma. Chest, 1996, 109:316-322.

[10] Irwin RS, Curley FJ, French CL. Difficult-to-control asthma: contributing factors and outcome of a systematic management protocol. Chest, 1993, 103:1662-1669.

[11] Kjellen G, Brundin A, Tibbling L, et al. Oesophageal function in asthmatics. Eur J Respir Dis, 1981, 62:87-94.

[12] Sontag SJ, Schnell TG, Miller TQ, et al. Prevalence of oesophagitis in asthmatics. Gut, 1992, 33:872-876.

[13] Sontag SJ, O'Connell S, Khandelwal S, et al. Most asthmatics have gastroesophageal reflux with or without bronchodilator therapy. Gastroenterology, 1990, 99:613-620.

[14] Cazzola M, Calzetta L, Bettoncelli G, et al. asthma and comorbid medical illness. Eur Respir J, 2011, 38:42-49.

[15] Harding SM, Richter Je. The role of gastroesophageal reflux in chronic cough and asthma. Chest, 1997, 111:1389-1402.

[16] Schan CA, Harding SM, Haile JM, et al. Gastroesophageal reflux-induced bronchoconstriction: an intraesophageal acid infusion study using state-of-the-art technology. Chest, 1994, 106:731-737.

[17] Wright RA, Miller SA, Corsello BF. Acid-induced esophagobronchial cardiac reflexes in humans. Gastroenterology, 1990, 99:71-73.

[18] Mansfield LE, Stein MR. Gastroesophageal reflux and asthma: a possible reflex mechanism. Ann Allergy, 1978, 41:224-226.

[19] Zerbib F, Guisset O, Lamouliatte H, et al. Effects of bronchial obstruction on lower esophageal sphincter motility and gastroesophageal reflux in patients with asthma. Am J Respir Crit Care Med, 2002, 166:1206-1211.

[20] Moote DW, Lloyd DA, McCourtie DR, et al. Increase in gastroesophageal reflux during methacho-line-induced bronchospasm. J Allergy Clin immunol, 1986, 78:619-623.

[21] DiMarino AJ Jr, Cohen S. Effect of an oral β_2-adrenergic agonist on lower esophageal sphincter pressure in normal and in patients with achalasia. diagnosis Sci, 1982, 27:1063-1066.

[22] Bagnato GF, Gulli S, Giacobbe O, De, et al. Bronchial hyperresponsiveness in subjects with gastroesophageal reflux. Respiration, 2000, 67:507-509.

[23] LapaMS, Fisse R Jr. Bronchialhyper reactivity in patients with gastroesophageal reflux disease. J Bras Pneumol 2005, 31:286-291.

[24] Gislason T, Janson C, Vermeire P, et al. respiratory symptoms and nocturnal gastroesophageal reflux: a population-based study of young adults in three european countries. Chest, 2002, 121:158-163.

[25] Pellicano R, Astegiano M, Rizzetto M. The epidemiology of gastro-oesophageal reflux disease. A brief review. Minerva Gastroenterol Dietol, 2003, 49:231-234.

[26] Allaix Me, Piatti MG. current status of diagnosis and treatment of Gerd in the United States. Minerva Gastroenterol Dietol, 2013, 59:41-48.

[27] Timms C, Yates dH, Thomas PS. Diagnosing GERD in respiratory medicine. Front Pharmacol, 2011, 22:40.

[28] Reder NP, Davis CS, Kovacs EJ, et al. The diagnostic value of

gastroesophageal reflux disease(GERD) symptoms and detection of pepsin and bile acids in bron-choalveolar lavage fluid and exhaled breath condensate for identifying lung transplantation patients with Gerd-induced aspiration. Surg Endosc, 2014,28:1794-1800.

[29] Timms C, Thomas PS, Yates DH. Detection of gastro-oesophageal reflux disease (GORD) in patients with obstructive lung disease using exhaled breath profling. J Breath Res, 2012,6:016003.

[30] Strugala V, Dettmar PW, Morice AH. Detection of pepsin in sputum and exhaled breath condensate: could it be a useful marker for reflux-related respiratory disease? Gastroenterology,2009,136(5 Suppl. 1):A-287.

[31] Brunetti L, Tesse R, Francavilla R, et al. The pH of exhaled breath condensate (EBC): a non-invasive tool for evaluation of asthma in childhood. J Allergy Clin Immunol, 2004, 113:S266.

[32] Dahl R. Systemic side effects of inhaled corticosteroids in patients with asthma. respiratory Medicine, 2006, 100: 1307-1317.

[33] Ducharme FM, Ni Chroinin M, Greenstone I, et al. Addition of long-acting beta2-agonists to inhaled corticosteroids versus same dose inhaled corticosteroids for chronic asthma in adults and children. Cochrane Database Syst Rev,2010:CD005535.

[34] Strickland RG, Fisher JM, Taylor KB. Effect of prednisolone on gastric function and structure in man. Gastroenterology, 1969,56:675-686.

[35] Lazenby JP, Guzzo Mr, Harding SM, et al. Oral corticosteroids increase esophageal acid contact times in patients with stable asthma. Chest,2002,121:625-634.

[36] Yii AC, Tan JH, Lapperre TS, et al. Long-term future risk of severe exacerbations: distinct 5-years trajectories of problematic asthma. Allergy,2017,72(9):1398-1405.

[37] Kjellen G, Tibbling L, Wranne B. Effect of conservative treatment of oesophageal dysfunction on bronchial dysfunction on bronchial asthma. Eur J Respir Dis,1981,62:190-197.

[38] Meier JH, McNally PR, Punja M, et al. Does omeprazole (Prilosec) improve respiratory function in asthmatics with gastroesophageal reflux? A double-blind, placebo-controlled crossover study. Dig Dis Sci,1994,39:2127-2133.

[39] Teichtahl H, Kronbert IJ, Yeomans ND, et al. Adult asthma and gastroesophageal reflux: the effects of omeprazole therapy on asthma. Aust N Z J Med,1996,26:671-676.

[40] Levin TR, Sperling RM, McQuaid KR. Omeprazole improves peak expiratory flow rate and quality of life in asthmatics with gastroesophageal reflux. Am J Gastroenterol,1998,93: 1060-1063.

[41] Urschel HC, Paulson DL. Gastroesophageal reflux and hiatal hernia: complications and therapy. J Thoracic Cardiovasc Surg,1967,53:21-32.

[42] Kennedy JH. A silent gastroesophageal reflux. Dis Chest, 1962,42:42-45.

[43] Overholt RH, Ashraf MM. Esophageal reflux as a trigger in asthma. N Y State J Med,1966,66:3030-3032.

[44] Lomasney TL. Hiatus hernia and the respiratory tract. Ann Thorac Surg,1977,24:448.

[45] Sontag S, O'Connell SO, Greenlee H, et al. Is gastroesophageal reflux a factor in some asthmatics? Am J Gastroenterol,1987,82:119-126.

[46] Tardif C, Nouvet TG, Denis P, et al. Surgical treatment of gastroesophageal reflux in 10 patients with severe asthma. Respiration,1989,56:110-115.

[47] Perrin-Fayolle M, Gormand F, Braillon G, et al. Long-term results of surgical treatment for gastroesophageal reflux in asthmatic patients. Chest,1989,96:40-45.

[48] DeMeester TR, Bonavina L, Iascone C, et al. Chronic respiratory symptoms and occult gastroesophageal reflux: a prospective clinical study and results of surgical therapy. Ann Surg, 1990,211:337-345.

[49] Johnson WE, Hagan JA, De Meester TR, et al. Outcome of respiratory symptoms after anti-reflux surgery on patients with gastroesophageal reflux disease. Arch Surg, 1996, 131: 489-492.

[50] Wetscher GJ, Glaser K, Hinder RA, et al. Respiratory symptoms in patients with gastroesophageal reflux disease following medical therapy and anti-reflux surgery. Am J Surg, 1997,174:639-643.

[51] Larrain A, Carrasco E, Galleguillos F, et al. Medical and surgical treatment of nonallergic asthma associated with gastroesophageal reflux. Chest,1991,9:1330-1335.

第四部分

呼吸系统感染

1 糖尿病合并肺炎诊治路径中国专家共识

中华医学会呼吸病学分会感染学组

糖尿病是一组由多种原因所致的、以高血糖为特征的慢性代谢性疾病,我国流行病学研究结果显示多达1.139亿中国成年人患有糖尿病,4.934亿人处于糖尿病前期;美国研究结果显示,糖尿病患者的医疗支出是非糖尿病的2.3倍,其中50%的费用用于控制糖尿病并发症。糖尿病患者因宿主免疫受损易合并各种感染,而肺炎是糖尿病人群最常见的感染性并发症之一。在糖尿病患者中因肺炎导致住院者占26%,在糖尿病晚期直接死亡原因中肺炎占8%。我国糖尿病合并肺炎高发、机会性感染病原体致病增多,但检出率低、重症肺炎多见且病死率高,造成严重的医疗和经济负担。因此亟须多学科专家共同探讨、制定规范的诊治路径,以降低患病率、提高诊断率和改善预后。结合国内外文献和我国临床实践,中华医学会呼吸病学分会感染学组特邀内分泌、微生物、感染及临床药学等领域的专家共同撰写了本共识,以供临床医生参考。

一、糖尿病合并肺炎的病原谱

糖尿病合并社区获得性肺炎(community-acquired pneumonia,CAP)的常见病原体包括肺炎链球菌、肺炎支原体、流感嗜血杆菌、肺炎克雷伯杆菌和金黄色葡萄球菌,流感病毒和腺病毒也是糖尿病合并CAP易感的病原体。此外,糖尿病患者合并特殊病原体感染如结核分枝杆菌、军团菌、奴卡菌、放线菌、曲霉、毛霉的概率也显著升高。

糖尿病合并医院获得性肺炎(hospital-acquired pneumonia,HAP)的常见病原体为铜绿假单胞菌和鲍曼不动杆菌,碳青霉烯耐药肺炎克雷伯杆菌(carbapenem-resistant *Klebsiella pneumoniae*,CRKP)和耐甲氧西林金黄色葡萄球菌(methicillin-resistant *Staphylococcus aureus*,MRSA)感染也很常见。

二、糖尿病易感肺炎的机制及高危因素

(一)糖尿病易感肺炎的机制

高糖微环境可使宿主肺泡巨噬细胞(alveolar macrophage,AM)表面伪足减少,膜表面受体及黏附分子表达异常,使AM对病原微生物识别及黏附能力降低,胞内溶菌酶合成减少致杀菌能力下降;另外,AM产生的促炎因子减少且抑炎因子增加,抗原呈递作用下降,最终导致肺局部防御功能缺陷。同时,糖尿病晚期糖基化终末产物(advanced glycation end products,AGESs)显著增加,AGEs导致胶原蛋白降解减少,在肺泡外聚集,从而引起患者肺顺应性降低;AGEs与特异性的AGEs受体结合导致各种炎性因子(如白细胞介素-1和肿瘤坏死因子-α等)的分泌和释放增加,引起血管内皮损伤,从而导致肺血管通透性增加,肺结构和功能的改变使肺通气及弥散功能均受影响,导致病原微生物在肺内易于聚集。此外,糖尿病患者呼吸道黏液纤毛清除功能减弱,自主神经病变可导致副交感神经调节支气管活动能力降低,并引起支气管痉挛,使呼吸道分泌物潴留和病原微生物在局部寄殖。且糖尿病患者因胃动力不足、胃食管反流等误吸风险也增加。

(二)糖尿病罹患肺炎的易感因素

高血糖是引起糖尿病患者发生肺炎的重要因素,长期血糖控制不佳及糖尿病病程≥10年的患者发生肺炎风险明显增加,男性较女性更易出现肺炎;入院后血清白蛋白≤40 g/L增加糖尿病患者HAP发生的风险。此外,糖尿病患者合并神经系统疾病导致反复误吸及合并其他疾病(如慢性呼吸系统疾病、慢性肾功能不全、营养不良、充血性心力衰竭等)都可以增加肺炎风险,医疗干预措施如肾脏透析增加感染MRSA肺炎的风险。

(三)糖尿病合并肺炎的预后相关因素

在合并2型糖尿病的肺炎住院患者中入院血糖过高或过低都会增加肺炎病死率,糖尿病合并CAP的患者入院血糖间隙(即感染后血糖较平均血糖升高的幅度)与不良预后呈明显相关;入院时高糖化血红蛋白(hemoglobin A_{1C},HbA_{1C})水平(>8%)与肺炎严重性相关,预示着高病死率。高龄(≥65岁)是糖尿病合并肺炎患者死亡的独立危险因素,65岁以上糖尿病患者年龄每增加1岁肺炎的死亡风险增加16%,在医院获得性MRSA肺炎患者中年龄每增长10岁死亡风险增加1.4倍;CURB-65评分≥3分是糖尿病合并金黄色葡萄球菌肺炎死亡的独立预测因素;糖尿病合并肺炎克雷伯杆菌肺炎患者死亡的独立预测因素包括男性、白蛋白<35 g/L、合并血流感染及有创机械通气。

三、糖尿病合并肺炎的诊断路径

糖尿病患者出现肺部阴影,伴或不伴有发热或呼吸道症状时,建议按以下思路诊断指导治疗(图4-1-1):

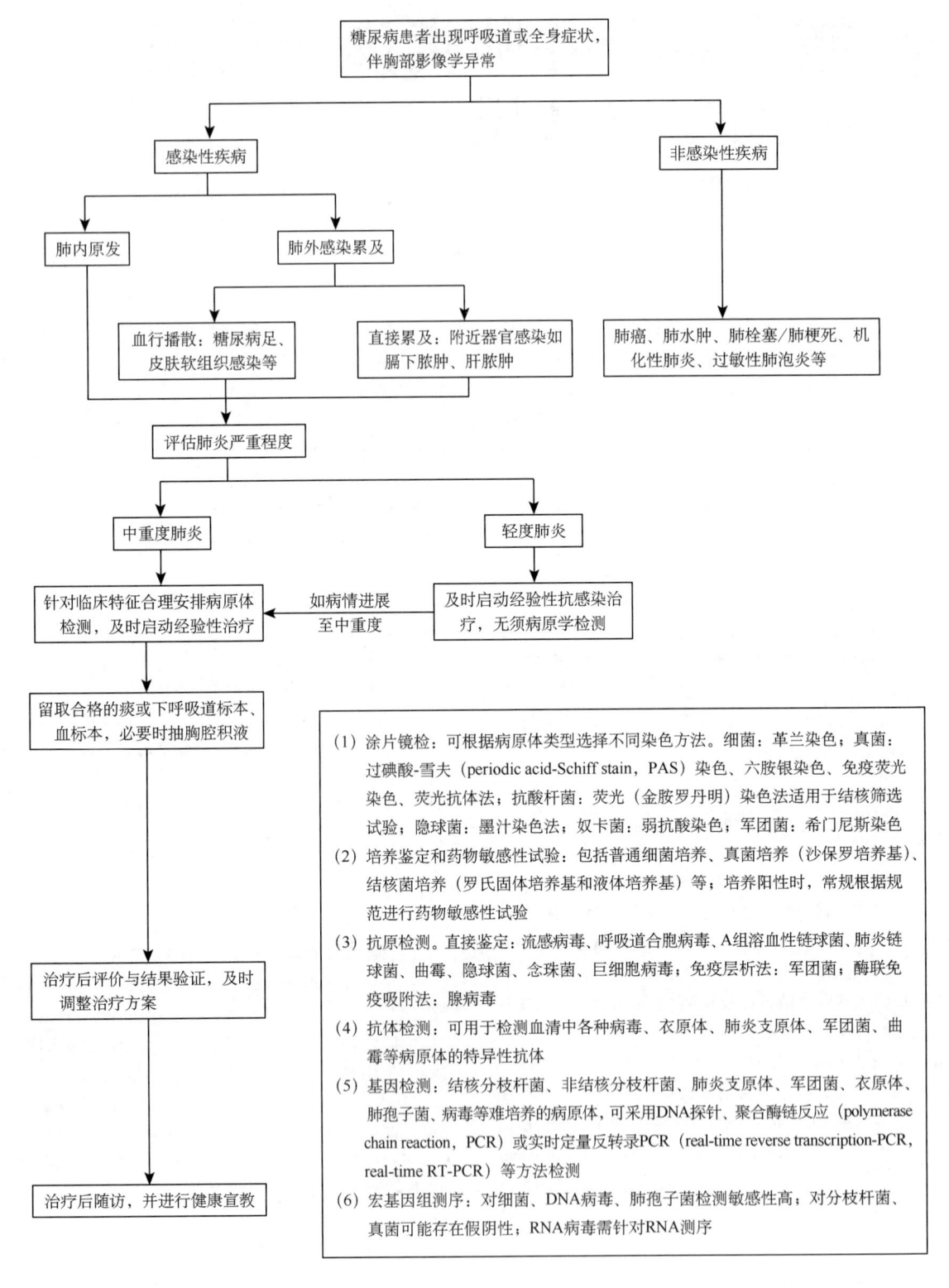

```
                  ┌─────────────────────────────────┐
                  │糖尿病患者出现呼吸道或全身症状,      │
                  │伴胸部影像学异常                   │
                  └──────────────┬──────────────────┘
                    ┌────────────┴────────────┐
              ┌─────┴─────┐             ┌─────┴─────┐
              │ 感染性疾病 │             │非感染性疾病│
              └─────┬─────┘             └─────┬─────┘
           ┌───────┴────────┐                 │
      ┌────┴────┐    ┌──────┴──────┐          │
      │肺内原发 │    │肺外感染累及 │          │
      └────┬────┘    └──────┬──────┘          │
           │         ┌──────┴───────┐          │
           │   ┌─────┴─────┐  ┌─────┴─────┐   ┌─┴─────────────┐
           │   │血行播散:糖 │  │直接累及:附│   │肺癌、肺水肿、肺│
           │   │尿病足、皮肤│  │近器官感染如│   │栓塞/肺梗死、机 │
           │   │软组织感染等│  │膈下脓肿、肝│   │化性肺炎、过敏性│
           │   │           │  │脓肿       │   │肺泡炎等       │
           │   └─────┬─────┘  └─────┬─────┘   └───────────────┘
           └─────────┴──────────────┘
                     │
              ┌──────┴──────┐
              │评估肺炎严重度│
              └──────┬──────┘
              ┌─────┴──────┐
         ┌────┴────┐   ┌───┴────┐
         │中重度肺炎│   │轻度肺炎│
         └────┬────┘   └───┬────┘
```

(1) 涂片镜检:可根据病原体类型选择不同染色方法。细菌:革兰染色;真菌:过碘酸-雪夫(periodic acid-Schiff stain, PAS)染色、六胺银染色、免疫荧光染色、荧光抗体法;抗酸杆菌:荧光(金胺罗丹明)染色法适用于结核筛选试验,隐球菌:墨汁染色法;奴卡菌:弱抗酸染色;军团菌:希门尼斯染色

(2) 培养鉴定和药物敏感性试验:包括普通细菌培养、真菌培养(沙保罗培养基)、结核菌培养(罗氏固体培养基和液体培养基)等;培养阳性时,常规根据规范进行药物敏感性试验

(3) 抗原检测。直接鉴定:流感病毒、呼吸道合胞病毒、A组溶血性链球菌、肺炎链球菌、曲霉、隐球菌、念珠菌、巨细胞病毒;免疫层析法:军团菌;酶联免疫吸附法:腺病毒

(4) 抗体检测:可用于检测血清中各种病毒、衣原体、肺炎支原体、军团菌、曲霉等病原体的特异性抗体

(5) 基因检测:结核分枝杆菌、非结核分枝杆菌、肺炎支原体、军团菌、衣原体、肺孢子菌、病毒等难培养的病原体,可采用DNA探针、聚合酶链反应(polymerase chain reaction, PCR)或实时定量反转录PCR(real-time reverse transcription-PCR, real-time RT-PCR)等方法检测

(6) 宏基因组测序:对细菌、DNA病毒、肺孢子菌检测敏感性高;对分枝杆菌、真菌可能存在假阴性;RNA病毒需针对RNA测序

图 4-1-1 糖尿病合并肺炎的诊断路径

(一)鉴别是感染性疾病还是非感染性疾病

首先需详细询问病史、进行体格检查。感染性疾病的临床特征包括发热、咳嗽伴有脓痰,可有肺实变体征或闻及湿啰音等。实验室检查可有血白细胞升高或降低、中性粒细胞核左移、降钙素原或C反应蛋白升高等。影像学表现为片状影、斑片状影、实变影或结节影伴有空洞或晕征,可伴有胸腔积液;如病毒性感染可表现为间质性渗出。病原学检查有助于鉴别。需注意的是,感染性疾病与非感染性疾病可以合并存在。

(二）鉴别是肺内原发感染，或是肺外感染累及肺

糖尿病患者除易并发肺部感染之外，其他多部位感染也较常见，如糖尿病足、皮肤软组织感染、肝脏及尿道感染等，这些感染均可通过血行播散到肺，或腹腔脏器感染直接累及肺。肺部感染性疾病亦有可能发生播散累及肺外其他脏器。鉴别感染来源的要点是进行详细的病史询问和体格检查，根据症状和阳性体征选择相应的检查。如浅表器官超声鉴别皮肤软组织感染，腹腔脏器超声或CT鉴别深部脏器感染如肝脓肿等，胸腔超声评估是否合并脓胸等，如出现肺外感染需进行积极对症处理，如肝脓肿需要穿刺引流等。

（三）评估病原体类型

肺炎最常见的胸部影像学表现为实质性渗出病变，伴或不伴有胸腔积液。虽然根据影像学表现难以确定是哪种病原体感染，但可以给予临床重要的提示。病毒性肺炎通常表现为磨玻璃样阴影，而腺病毒肺炎可表现为实变影；大片肺实变伴叶间裂下坠、蜂窝状脓肿提示肺炎克雷伯杆菌肺炎可能；肺叶浸润、液气囊腔，早期出现空洞、脓胸，需警惕金黄色葡萄球菌肺炎。糖尿病除了常见病原体感染外，合并机会性感染病原体的概率增加。肺部真菌病以曲霉最常见，多表现为以胸膜为基底的楔形影、结节或团块影，内有空洞，如有"反晕征"需考虑肺毛霉病的可能。糖尿病患者易并发肺结核，其影像学改变可不同于典型肺结核表现，临床抗感染效果欠佳时应进一步完善相关检查以明确病因。

轻症肺炎患者建议尽早经验性抗感染治疗，无须行病原学检测，中重度肺炎患者需根据临床特征选择病原学检测方法，同时行经验性治疗。48～72 h后对初始抗感染治疗反应及病原学检查结果进行评估。当病情无改善、病原学检查阳性时，应仔细评估阳性结果的临床意义、是否合并发症及其他部位感染，必要时调整抗菌药物治疗方案；病情无改善且病原学检查阴性时，需要进一步完善病原学检查及排查非感染性疾病。

四、评估糖尿病合并肺炎的严重程度

糖尿病合并CAP严重程度评估可以采用CRB-65、CURB-65或肺炎严重指数（pneumonia severity index，PSI）评估体系，CURB-65对评估糖尿病合并肺炎严重程度不够全面和特异。糖尿病合并肺炎的严重程度评估可参考我国CAP诊疗指南关于重症肺炎的诊断标准。

在PSI评分系统中，血糖＞14 mmol/L者评分增加10分，合并充血性心力衰竭和脑血管疾病者评分各增加10分，合并血尿素氮＞11mmol/L者评分增加20分。因此当糖尿病患者血糖控制不佳、合并心脑血管疾病和肾功能异常时，PSI评分往往较高，提示发生重症肺炎的风险增加。

HAP常用的病情严重度评分系统有序贯器官衰竭评分（sequential organ failure assessment，SOFA）、急性生理与慢性健康评分（acute physiology and chronic health evaluation，APACHE-Ⅱ）、IBMP-10等。对于非重症监护室（intensive care unite，ICU）患者，快速SOFA评分（quick SOFA，qSOFA）预测住院病死率的效能优于SOFA。

五、糖尿病合并肺炎的治疗路径

（一）糖尿病合并肺炎的经验治疗

1. 糖尿病合并肺炎初始经验性治疗抗感染药物选择的原则：①首先确定患者发病的场所是社区还是院内，然后根据临床及影像学特征推测最有可能的病原体，并根据患者病情严重度及耐药风险进行分层治疗；覆盖常见病原体兼顾患者基础疾病、器官功能状态、药物的药动学/药效学（pharmacokinetics/pharmacodynamics，PK/PD）特性、药物过敏史等选择恰当的抗感染药物和给药方案。②我国不同地区病原流行病学分布和抗感染药物耐药率差异明显，所以治疗推荐仅仅是原则性的。经验性治疗应根据本地区及本医院的病原体分布及耐药特点选择抗感染药物。③选择抗感染药物时还要注意患者糖尿病相关的脏器损害程度，如糖尿病肾病；要注意抗菌药物在肺组织局部的浓度和抗菌活性；注意是否可能与降糖药物产生相互作用，从而导致血药浓度降低或血糖代谢异常等。④如果初始治疗失败或病情反复，需要特别关注糖尿病患者是否伴有肺外感染病灶，如皮肤软组织感染（包括糖尿病足）、肺外脓肿（如肝脓肿）或伴发血流感染形成迁徙性病灶；此外还需要关注机会性病原体感染风险增加（如分枝杆菌、军团菌、曲霉、毛霉及肺孢子菌等）。⑤如经验性选用喹诺酮类药物，需要警惕其可能带来的肺结核诊断的延误及血糖异常波动等问题。

2. 糖尿病合并CAP初始经验性治疗抗感染药物的选择（图4-1-2）

3. 糖尿病合并HAP/呼吸机相关性肺炎（ventilator-associated pneumonia，VAP）初始经验性治疗抗感染药物的选择（图4-1-3）　糖尿病合并HAP/VAP的初始经验性治疗应根据患者病情严重度及耐药危险因素等参数进行分层治疗，糖尿病住院患者尤其要关注长期卧床引起的压疮等皮肤软组织葡萄球菌感染继发血流感染导致全身感染播散，此外由于各种医疗措施导致皮肤黏膜屏障破坏（如气管插管、留置胃管或深静脉导管等）引起肺炎克雷伯杆菌、念珠菌等内源性感染风险增加，肾脏透析增加MRSA感染风险。

（二）目标性抗感染治疗的药物选择及疗程

糖尿病患者对机会性病原体感染及耐药菌感染的风险均增高且常存在多种病原体混合感染，因此在解读基于核酸的分子生物学方法等敏感度较高的检测结果时，需谨慎鉴别区分感染与定植或污染；糖尿病患者目标性抗感染疗程一般为7 d以上，对于初始抗感染治疗无效、病情危重、泛耐药（extensively drug-resistant，XDR）或全耐药（pandrug-resistant，PDR）菌感染、肺脓肿、脓胸或坏死性肺炎者，应酌情延长疗程；金黄色葡萄球菌、铜绿假单胞菌、克雷伯菌属或厌氧菌等容易导致肺组织坏死，抗感染疗程可延长至14～21 d，但可以考虑静脉抗感染药物序贯为同类的口服药物。

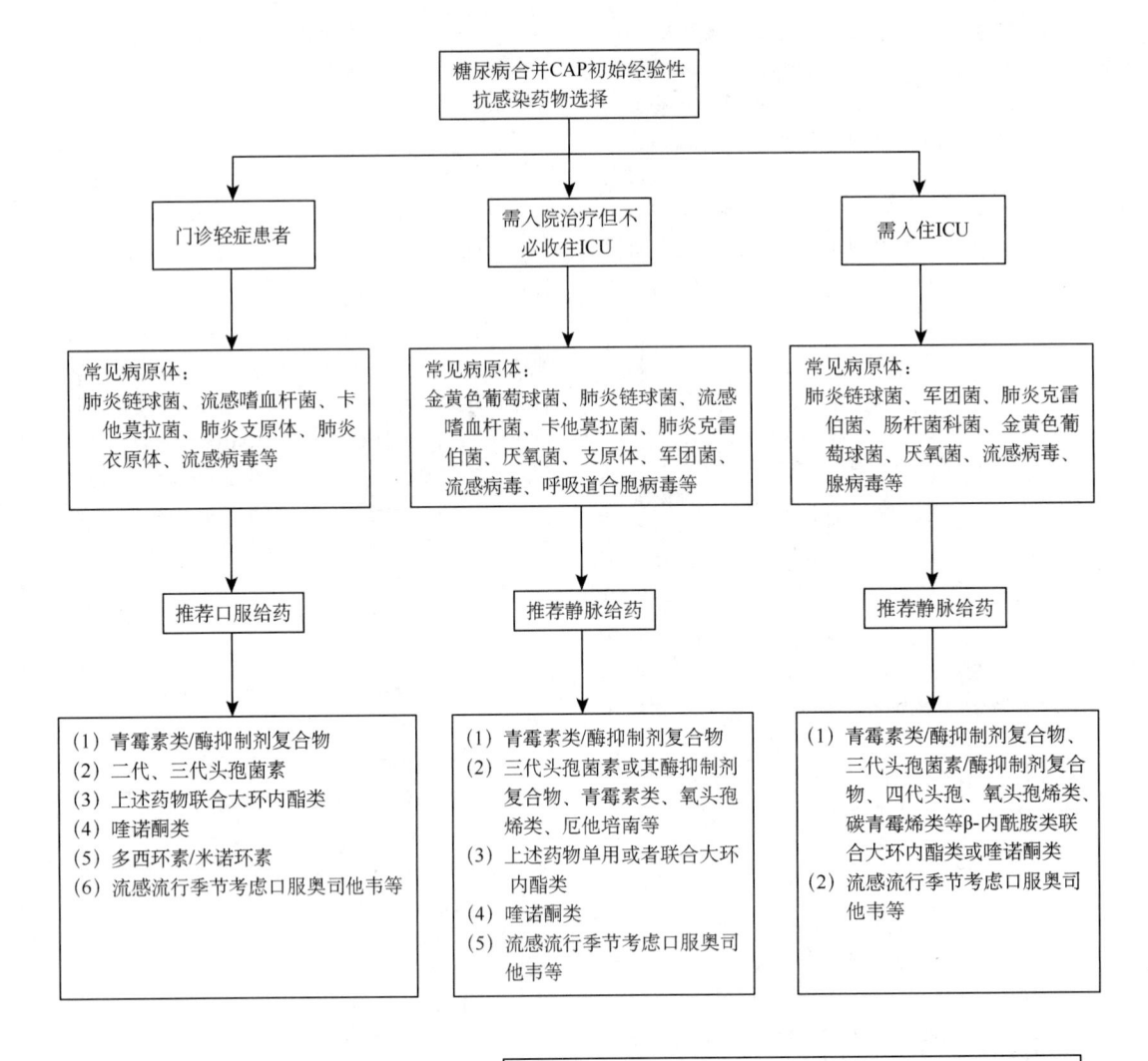

```
                    糖尿病合并CAP初始经验性
                      抗感染药物选择
         ┌──────────────────┼──────────────────┐
    门诊轻症患者        需入院治疗但不          需入住ICU
                       必收住ICU
         │                   │                   │
   常见病原体:          常见病原体:           常见病原体:
   肺炎链球菌、流感嗜血杆菌、卡   金黄色葡萄球菌、肺炎链球菌、流感   肺炎链球菌、军团菌、肺炎克雷
   他莫拉菌、肺炎支原体、肺炎   嗜血杆菌、卡他莫拉菌、肺炎克雷   伯菌、肠杆菌科菌、金黄色葡
   衣原体、流感病毒等         伯菌、厌氧菌、支原体、军团菌、   萄球菌、厌氧菌、流感病毒、
                           流感病毒、呼吸道合胞病毒等    腺病毒等
         │                   │                   │
     推荐口服给药          推荐静脉给药          推荐静脉给药
         │                   │                   │
  (1) 青霉素类/酶抑制剂复合物  (1) 青霉素类/酶抑制剂复合物   (1) 青霉素类/酶抑制剂复合物、
  (2) 二代、三代头孢菌素     (2) 三代头孢菌素或其酶抑制剂       三代头孢菌素/酶抑制剂复合
  (3) 上述药物联合大环内酯类     复合物、青霉素类、氧头孢       物、四代头孢、氧头孢烯类、
  (4) 喹诺酮类               烯类、厄他培南等               碳青霉烯类等β-内酰胺类联
  (5) 多西环素/米诺环素     (3) 上述药物单用或者联合大环       合大环内酯类或喹诺酮类
  (6) 流感流行季节考虑口服奥司他韦等   内酯类                (2) 流感流行季节考虑口服奥司
                        (4) 喹诺酮类                   他韦等
                        (5) 流感流行季节考虑口服奥司
                            他韦等
```

注意:糖尿病患者发生重症流感后继发肺炎链球菌、金黄色葡萄球菌、流感嗜血杆菌、曲霉感染风险增加,需关注混合感染问题;糖尿病患者要考虑产肠杆菌科细菌感染可能,评估产ESBL肠杆菌科细菌感染的风险;有吸入性肺炎风险者需进一步关注吸入风险因素及厌氧菌的药物覆盖

图 4-1-2　糖尿病合并社区获得性肺炎(CAP)初始经验性抗感染药物选择

(三)糖尿病合并肺炎的血糖管理原则

糖尿病合并肺炎患者住院期间的血糖管理尤为重要。中国住院患者血糖管理专家共识建议,住院期间血糖水平持续且明显高于 7.8 mmol/L 则考虑高血糖状态,提示患者有可能需要接受或调整降糖治疗。

1. 糖尿病合并肺炎住院患者的入院评估:患者入院时均应详细询问既往糖尿病病史及降糖药物使用情况;既往有低血糖事件者,评估发生低血糖的风险程度;评估肺炎的病情,包含年龄、预期生存期、是否存在多器官功能不全、精神或智力障碍、心脑血管疾病既往史和(或)风险程度、是否需要重症监护、营养状态及进食情况等。同时需完善全天血糖水平监测,掌握血糖波动情况,必要时检测 HbA_{1c} 水平以明确患者住院前 3 个月是否已经存在血糖控制不佳的情况。

2. 糖尿病合并肺炎患者的个体化血糖管理目标见表 4-1-1。

3. 糖尿病合并肺炎患者血糖管理的主要措施:对于大多数糖尿病合并肺炎患者,胰岛素是控制血糖的首选治疗;需进行重症监护的患者推荐采用持续静脉小剂量胰岛素输注,监护期间可根据血糖波动情况随时调整胰岛素剂量;病情稳定拟改用胰岛素皮下注射时,需在停止静脉输注胰岛素前 1~2 h 开始接受皮下胰岛素注射,同时,每日皮下注射胰岛素的总剂量可以在原每日静脉注射胰岛素的总剂量基础上减少 20%~40%。

不需要进行重症监护的患者推荐皮下注射胰岛素治疗,无法正常进食、需肠内或肠外营养的患者,根据不同营养摄入情况制定血糖管理方案(表 4-1-2)。

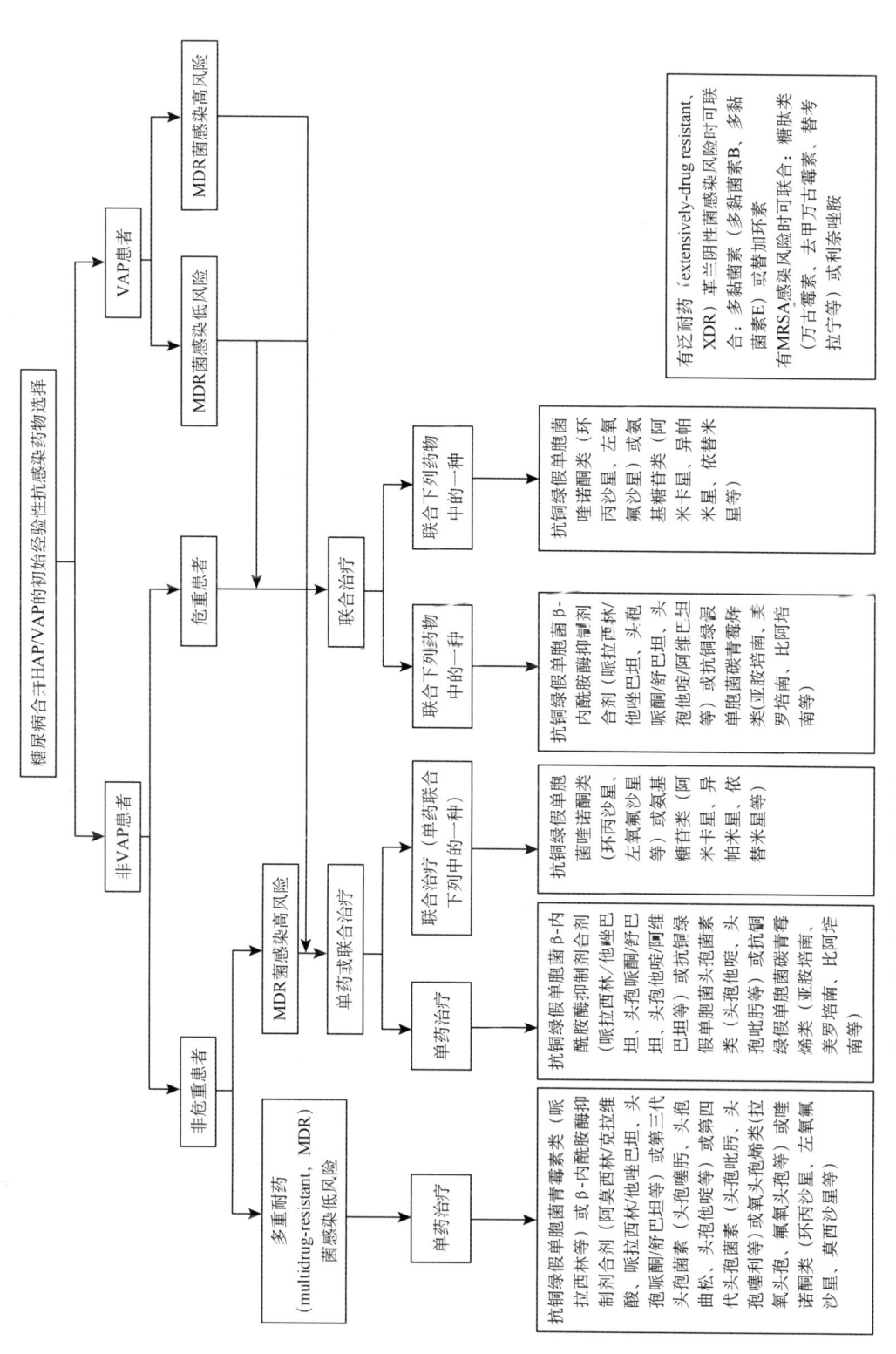

图4-1-3 糖尿病合并医院获得性肺炎（HAP）/呼吸机相关性肺炎（VAP）的初始经验性抗感染药物选择

表 4-1-1 糖尿病合并肺炎患者设定个体化的血糖管理目标

人群	空腹或餐前血糖（mmol/L）	餐后 2h 或随机血糖（mmol/L）
年龄较轻；低血糖发生风险较低	4.4~6.1	6.1~7.8
合并心脑血管疾病，心脑血管疾病高风险，治疗方案中包含糖皮质激素	6.1~7.8	7.8~10.0
高龄、低血糖发生风险较高且无法耐受低血糖，存在多器官功能不全，预期生存期低于5年，需重症监护	7.8~10.0	7.8~13.9

表 4-1-2 不需要进行重症监护的患者血糖管理方案

人群	血糖管理方案
持续肠内营养患者	每日 1~2 次基础胰岛素联合每 4h 给予短效或速效胰岛素皮下注射
分次肠内营养患者	基础胰岛素治疗，同时在每次进行肠内营养时给予短效或速效胰岛素皮下注射
肠外营养患者	全肠外静脉营养液中添加短效或速效胰岛素，同时每 4h 给予短效或速效胰岛素皮下注射
正常进食或营养摄入充足的患者	基础联合餐时胰岛素治疗方案，必要时临时补充短效或速效胰岛素；有条件的也可考虑皮下胰岛素泵治疗
需要糖皮质激素治疗的重症肺炎患者	中效或长效胰岛素控制血糖，并根据血糖监测结果及时调整胰岛素的剂量与使用方法

如糖尿病合并肺炎患者入院前接受口服降糖药物，入院后一般情况良好，血糖较平稳，进食规律，且没有使用口服降糖药物的禁忌证可以考虑继续应用其入院前已经使用的降糖方案，注意密切监测血糖并及时调整方案。建议所有糖尿病合并肺炎患者接受密切随访，出院 1 个月内接受内分泌专科评估，进行适当的降糖方案调整并制订长期随访方案。

（四）抗感染药物与糖尿病治疗药物相互作用

1. 降糖药物与抗菌药物相互作用 由于糖尿病患者平时常规使用降糖药物，有些降糖药物与抗菌药物存在相互作用，从而对患者的血糖造成影响，在抗感染治疗中需要引起注意。①二甲双胍：二甲双胍在体内无须肝脏 CYP450 酶代谢，直接以原型经肾脏排泄，目前尚无与抗菌药物合用出现相互作用的报道。②α-糖苷酶抑制剂：伏格列波糖在胃肠道内几乎不吸收入血，主要以原型经肠道排泄，无药物相互作用的报道。阿卡波糖原型药物在肠道内极少被吸收，口服生物利用度为 1%~2%，其在肠道内的代谢产物 35% 吸收入血，但血药浓度不受抗菌药物影响。③磺脲类：磺脲类药物在体内主要经 CYP2C9 代谢，合并使用 CYP2C9 抑制剂氟康唑、伏立康唑、咪康唑、环丙沙星和氯霉素可能减慢其代谢，增加低血糖风险，合用时需加强血糖监测；中成药消渴丸中含有格列本脲，合并以上抗菌药时应注意。克拉霉素抑制 P-糖蛋白（P-glycoprotein，P-gp）而提高格列本脲的药时曲线下面积（area under the curve，AUC），两药合用可使格列本脲的血药峰浓度升高 1.25 倍，AUC 增加 1.35 倍，临床使用时应加强血糖监测。④格列奈类：瑞格列奈经 CYP2C8 和 CYP3A4 代谢，那格列奈主要经 CYP2C9 和 CYP3A4 代谢，米格列奈直接经 II 相代谢酶 UGT 代谢，极少量经 CYP2C9 代谢。瑞格列奈与 CYP3A4/5 强抑制剂（如酮康唑、伊曲康唑、克拉霉素等）合用时可能导致血药浓度升高，增加低血糖风险。⑤二肽基肽酶 IV（dipeptidyl peptidase-4，DPP-4）抑制剂：沙格列汀主要通过 CYP3A4/5 代谢，与 CYP3A4/5 强抑制剂（如酮康唑、伊曲康唑、克拉霉素等）合用时，能显著升高沙格列汀的血浆药物浓度，合用时沙格列汀的日剂量不超过 2.5mg。西格列汀少量经 CYP3A4 和 CYP2C8 代谢，有临床意义的相互作用比较少。阿格列汀、利格列汀和维格列汀在人体内基本不经 CYP450 酶代谢，不存在药物代谢酶相关的相互作用。⑥噻唑烷二酮类：罗格列酮、吡格列酮主要经 CYP2C8 代谢，与抗菌药物合用相互作用少见。⑦钠-葡萄糖共转运蛋白 2（sodium-glucose cotransporter 2，SGLT-2）抑制剂：达格列净主要经 UGT1A9 代谢为无活性的达格列净 3-O-葡糖苷酸，仅有极少量经 CYP450 酶代谢。恩格列净在体内经 UGT2B7、UGT1A3、UGT1A8、UGT1A9 代谢为无活性的葡糖苷酸，不抑制、诱导 CYP450 酶，不抑制 UGT1A1，药物相互作用少见。卡格列净仅有 7% 经 CYP3A4 代谢，不诱导、抑制 CYP450 酶。

2. 氟喹诺酮类抗菌药物对血糖的影响 多种抗菌药物均可导致血糖紊乱，如氟喹诺酮类和大环内酯类等。其中氟喹诺酮类药物与血糖异常升高或降低有关。其引起血糖紊乱的机制尚不明确，可能通过副交感神经使胰岛细胞中的三磷酸腺苷敏感的钾离子通道受阻，导致胰岛素分泌紊乱而出现胰岛素异常的升高和降低等有关。使用加替沙星、左氧氟沙星、环丙沙星和阿奇霉素的患者低血糖的每千例发生率分别为 0.35、0.19、0.10 和 0.07，而高血糖的每千例发生率分别为 0.45、0.18、0.12 和 0.10。在糖尿病患者中，加替沙星、左氧氟沙星和环丙沙星较之阿奇霉素引起低血糖的相对危险度（odds ratio，OR）依次为 4.3、2.1 和 1.1，引起高血糖的 OR 依次为 4.5、1.8 和 1.0。加替沙星和左氧氟沙星引起严重血糖异常风险显著高于阿奇霉素，而环丙沙星和阿奇霉素相比，差异不大。

氟喹诺酮类药物引起的血糖异常与年龄呈正相关，60 岁以上糖尿病患者发生血糖异常的概率较高，可能与老年人生理功能减退，致垂体前叶、肾上腺皮质功能下降，当发生血糖异常时正常反调节功能减低，不能及时分泌调节血糖的激素有关,治疗过程中要严密监测血糖,最大限度地降低可能出现血糖异常的风险,确保用药安全。

六、糖尿病合并肺炎的预防

预防感染、减少感染相关的并发症,对降低糖尿病相关病死率有重要意义。

(一)疫苗接种

美国糖尿病协会推荐,糖尿病患者须接种肺炎链球菌多糖疫苗。65岁以上的患者如果既往曾经接种过疫苗,接种时间超过5年者则需再接种一次。2～64岁糖尿病患者应接受23价肺炎链球菌多糖疫苗(23-valent pneumococcal polysaccharide vaccine,PPSV23);年龄≥65岁时,无论接种史如何都需要重新接种PPSV23疫苗。流感疫苗接种可显著降低流感流行期糖尿病人群的发病率、住院率和病死率,建议糖尿病患者每年都要接种流感疫苗。

(二)葡萄球菌去定植

保持皮肤清洁,加强口腔卫生,增加自身抵抗力可预防感染的发生。对入住ICU的重症患者研究结果显示:入ICU时及24 h内采集鼻和咽拭子进行MRSA主动筛查,对MRSA阳性患者进行鼻部莫匹罗星软膏涂抹,一日3次,持续5 d,可去定植,从而有效防控MRSA肺炎的发生。对皮肤软组织损伤携带或可能感染MRSA的患者进行治疗或清除细菌时,如果是莫匹罗星敏感的MRSA,推荐在全身应用敏感抗菌药物的前提下,局部使用莫匹罗星。

参与撰写的专家组成员(按姓氏汉语拼音排序):包志瑶(上海交通大学医学院附属瑞金医院呼吸与危重症医学科);毕宇芳(上海交通大学医学院附属瑞金医院内分泌科);陈愉(中国医科大学附属盛京医院呼吸与危重症医学科);程齐俭(上海交通大学医学院附属瑞金医院北院呼吸与危重症医学科);范红(四川大学华西医院呼吸与危重症医学科);方洁(上海交通大学医学院附属瑞金医院药剂科);韩立中(上海交通大学医学院附属瑞金医院临床微生物科);李玉苹(温州医科大学附属第一医院呼吸与危重症医学科);乔洁(上海交通大学医学院附属第九人民医院内分泌科);苏欣(东部战区总医院呼吸与危重症医学科);夏雨(北京大学人民医院药剂科);叶枫(广州医科大学附属第一医院广州呼吸健康研究院呼吸与危重症医学科/呼吸疾病国家重点实验室/国家呼吸系统疾病临床医学中心);张静(复旦大学附属中山医院呼吸与危重症医学科);周华(浙江大学医学院附属第一医院呼吸与危重症医学科)

总执笔:周敏(上海交通大学医学院附属瑞金医院呼吸与危重症医学科)

指导专家组成员(按姓氏拼音排序):

呼吸专业:曹彬(中日友好医院呼吸中心/呼吸与危重症医学科);贺蓓(北京大学第三医院呼吸与危重症医学科);黄怡(海军军医大学第一附属医院呼吸与危重症医学科);瞿介明(上海交通大学医学院附属瑞金医院呼吸与危重症医学科);施毅(东部战区总医院呼吸与危重症医学科);张湘燕(贵州省人民医院呼吸与危重症医学科)

内分泌专业:宁光(上海交通大学医学院附属瑞金医院内分泌科);王卫庆(上海交通大学医学院附属瑞金医院内分泌科)

微生物专业:倪语星(上海交通大学医学院附属瑞金医院临床微生物科)

参 考 文 献

[1] Xu Y,Wang L,He J,et al. Prevalence and control of diabetes in Chinese adults. JAMA,2013,310(9):948-959.

[2] American Diabetes Association. Economic Costs of Diabetes in the U. S. in 2017. Diabetes Care,2018,41(5):917-928.

[3] Korbel L,Spencer JD. Diabetes mellitus and infection:an evaluation of hospital utilization and management costs in the United States. J Diabetes Complications,2015,29(2):192-195.

[4] Fisher-Hoch SP,Mathews CE,McCormick JB. Obesity,diabetes and pneumonia:the menacing interface of non-communicable and infectious diseases. Trop Med Int Health,2013,18(12):1510-1519.

[5] Koskela HO,Salonen PH,Romppanen J,et al. Long-term mortality after community-acquired pneumonia--impacts of diabetes and newly discovered hyperglycaemia:a prospective,observational cohort study. BMJ Open,2014,4(8):e005715.

[6] 赵航,赵洪文.糖尿病患者合并社区获得性肺炎的临床特点及预后分析.国际呼吸杂志,2017,37(13):1013-1017.

[7] 王艳红,岳宗相,刘致勤,等.2型糖尿病合并感染患者感染相关因素及病原菌分析.糖尿病新世界,2017,20(19):1-3.

[8] Liu B,Yi H,Fang J,et al. Antimicrobial resistance and risk factors for mortality of pneumonia caused by Klebsiella pneumoniae among diabetics:a retrospective study conducted in Shanghai,China. Infect Drug Resist,2019,12:1089-1098.

[9] Zhang QR,Chen H,Liu B,et al. Methicillin-resistant Staphylococcus aureus pneumonia in diabetics:a single-center,retrospective analysis. Chin Med J(Engl),2019,132(12):1429-1434.

[10] Nakayama M,Sugiyama Y,Yamasawa H,et al. Effect of hochuekkito on alveolar macrophage inflammatory responses in hyperglycemic mice. Inflammation,2012,35(4):1294-1301.

[11] Sunahara KK,Martins JO. Alveolar macrophages in diabetes:friends or foes?. J Leukoc Biol,2012,91(6):871-876.

[12] Frydrych LM,Fattahi F,He K,et al. Diabetes and Sepsis:Risk,Recurrence,and Ruination. Front Endocrinol(Lausanne),2017,8:271.

[13] Kornum JB,Thomsen RW,Riis A,et al. Diabetes,glycemic control,and risk of hospitalization with pneumonia:a population-based case-control study. Diabetes Care,2008,31(8):1541-1545.

[14] Jimenez-Trujillo I,Jimenez-Garcia R,de Miguel-Diez J,et al.

[14] Incidence, characteristic and outcomes of ventilator-associated pneumonia among type 2 diabetes patients: An observational population-based study in Spain. Eur J Intern Med, 2017, 40: 72-78.

[15] Muller LM, Gorter KJ, Hak E, et al. Increased risk of common infections in patients with type 1 and type 2 diabetes mellitus. Clin Infect Dis, 2005, 41(3): 281-288.

[16] Lopez-de-Andres A, de Miguel-Diez J, Jimenez-Trujillo I, et al. Hospitalisation with community-acquired pneumonia among patients with type 2 diabetes: an observational population-based study in Spain from 2004 to 2013. BMJ Open, 2017, 7(1): e013097.

[17] Di Yacovo S, Garcia-Vidal C, Viasus D, et al. Clinical features, etiology, and outcomes of community-acquired pneumonia in patients with diabetes mellitus. Medicine (Baltimore), 2013, 92(1): 42-50.

[18] Liu J. Impact of diabetes mellitus on pneumonia mortality in a senior population: results from the NHANES III follow-up study. J Geriatr Cardiol, 2013, 10(3): 267-271.

[19] Equils O, da Costa C, Wible M, et al. The effect of diabetes mellitus on outcomes of patients with nosocomial pneumonia caused by methicillin-resistant Staphylococcus aureus: data from a prospective double-blind clinical trial comparing treatment with linezolid versus vancomycin. BMC Infect Dis, 2016, 16: 476.

[20] Chiang CY, Lee JJ, Chien ST, et al. Glycemic control and radiographic manifestations of tuberculosis in diabetic patients. PLoS One, 2014, 9(4): e93397.

[21] Huang LK, Wang HH, Lai YC, et al. The impact of glycemic status on radiological manifestations of pulmonary tuberculosis in diabetic patients. PLoS One, 2017, 12(6): e0179750.

[22] 中华医学会呼吸病学分会. 中国成人社区获得性肺炎诊断和治疗指南(2016年版). 中华结核和呼吸杂志, 2016, 39(4): 253-279.

[23] 中华医学会呼吸病学分会感染学组. 中国成人医院获得性肺炎与呼吸机相关性肺炎诊断和治疗指南(2018年版). 中华结核和呼吸杂志, 2018, 41(4): 255-280.

[24] 中国医师协会内分泌代谢科医师分会, 中国住院患者血糖管理专家组. 中国住院患者血糖管理专家共识. 中华内分泌代谢杂志, 2017, 33(1): 1-10.

[25] American Diabetes Association. 15. Diabetes Care in the Hospital: Standards of Medical Care in Diabetes-2019. Diabetes Care, 2019, 42(Suppl 1): S173-S181.

[26] Balfour JA, McTavish D. Acarbose. An update of its pharmacology and therapeutic use in diabetes mellitus. Drugs, 1993, 46(6): 1025-1054.

[27] Ahr HJ, Boberg M, Krause HP, et al. Pharmacokinetics of acarbose. Part I: Absorption, concentration in plasma, metabolism and excretion after single administration of [14C] acarbose to rats, dogs and man. Arzneimittelforschung, 1989, 39(10): 1254-1260.

[28] 中国老年医学研究会内分泌代谢分会, 中国毒理学会临床毒理专业委员会. 老年人多重用药安全管理专家共识. 中国药物警戒, 2018, 15(10): 627-640.

[29] Chou H-W, Wang J-L, Chang C-H, et al. Risk of severe dysglycemia among diabetic patients receiving levofloxacin, ciprofloxacin, or moxifloxacin in Taiwan. Clinical infectious diseases: an official publication of the Infectious Diseases Society of America, 2013, 57(7): 971-980.

[30] El Ghandour S, Azar ST. Dysglycemia associated with quinolones. Primary Care Diabetes, 2015, 9(3): 168-171.

[31] Aspinall SL, Good CB, Jiang R, et al. Severe dysglycemia with the fluoroquinolones: a class effect?. Clin Infect Dis, 2009, 49(3): 402-408.

[32] 赵陶丽, 胡燕琴, 崔向丽. 氟喹诺酮类药物引起血糖异常71例文献分析. 中国医院用药评价与分析, 2010, 10(9): 839-841.

[33] American Diabetes Association. 4. Comprehensive Medical Evaluation and Assessment of Comorbidities: Standards of Medical Care in Diabetes-2019. Diabetes Care, 2019, 42(Suppl 1): S34-S45.

[34] Goeijenbier M, van Sloten TT, Slobbe L, et al. Benefits of flu vaccination for persons with diabetes mellitus: A review. Vaccine, 2017, 35(38): 5095-5101.

[35] Dadashi M, Nasiri MJ, Fallah F, et al. Methicillin-resistant Staphylococcus aureus (MRSA) in Iran: A systematic review and meta-analysis. J Glob Antimicrob Resist, 2018, 12: 96-103.

[36] Parente DM, Cunha CB, Mylonakis E, et al. The Clinical Utility of Methicillin-Resistant Staphylococcus aureus (MRSA) Nasal Screening to Rule Out MRSA Pneumonia: A Diagnostic Meta-analysis With Antimicrobial Stewardship Implications. Clin Infect Dis, 2018, 67(1): 1-7.

2 新型冠状病毒肺炎特异性免疫治疗的现状与展望

何玉坤 马昕茜 高占成

一、前言

2019年12月31日，中国武汉市卫健委报告湖北省武汉市出现了的一组不明原因肺炎病例，后确认病原体为一种新型冠状病毒，并将其命名为SARS-CoV-2。2020年1月30日，世界卫生组织（WHO）宣布该疫情构成国际关注的突发公共卫生事件。2020年3月11日，世界卫生组织正式宣布全球大流行。截至2020年7月10日，全球已有1200余万确诊病例，超过55万死亡病例。

冠状病毒（coronavirus, CoV）分为四个属，包括α、β、γ、δ。α和β属冠状病毒能够感染哺乳动物，而γ和δ属冠状病毒则倾向于感染鸟类。此前，已有6种冠状病毒被鉴定为人类易感病毒，其中α冠状病毒属的HCoV-229E和HCoV-NL63，以及致病性低的β冠状病毒属HCoV-HKU1和HCoV-OC43，分别引起类似普通感冒的轻微呼吸道症状。而另两种已知的β属冠状病毒，即SARS-CoV和MERS-CoV会导致严重和潜在致命的呼吸道感染。本次疫情中的SARS-CoV-2为β属冠状病毒。全基因组序列比对和系统发育研究表明，SARS-CoV和MERS-CoV属于同一分支，与SARS-CoV-2属姊妹分支；并提示蝙蝠可能作为SARS-CoV-2的天然宿主，经中间宿主穿山甲最终传播至人类。但这仅仅是科学家的推测或假说，彼此之间基因的同源性差异不容忽视，因为人类与黑猩猩之间基因相似度接近99%，人类拥有语言功能的FOX2基因相关蛋白与黑猩猩之间的差异仅仅2个氨基酸。因此，SARS-CoV2究竟源于何方"神圣"？仍有待科学家们寻找更多的线索和证据。

我国临床资料显示，COVID-19住院患者最常见的临床症状为发热（88.7%），其次是咳嗽（67.8%），恶心或呕吐占5%，腹泻患者占3.8%，部分患者伴有头晕。欧美患者相当比例患者显示嗅觉和味觉缺失。约48%的患者有基础疾病，最常见的是心血管疾病和糖尿病。儿童和青少年病例临床表现较轻，但极少数重症儿童病例可发生类川崎病样的多系统炎症综合征（Kawasaki-like multisystem inflammatory sondrome），最常见的实验室检查异常为C反应蛋白升高（68.6%），淋巴细胞计数下降（57.4%）和乳酸脱氢酶升高（51.6%）。总体病死率为3.6%。中国疾控中心一项针对72 314例SARS-CoV-2感染病例的回顾性分析表明，5%新冠患者进展为危重病例，以呼吸衰竭、感染性休克和（或）多器官功能障碍或衰竭为特征。急性呼吸窘迫综合征（acute respiratory distress syndrome, ARDS）是COVID-19危重病例的标志性特征之一，可导致器官衰竭，直接危及生命。

当前COVID-19患者基数庞大，确诊病例数不断攀升，临床医生需要掌握有效干预SARS-CoV-2感染的准确证据。目前，COVID-19患者标准治疗方案主要为一般抗病毒治疗及支持治疗（包括呼吸支持、循环支持等）。危重COVID-19患者的处理与大多数引起呼吸衰竭的病毒性肺炎处理类似。对任何有紧急症状及无紧急症状但血氧饱和度<90%的患者，均应立即给予补充氧气治疗；密切监测患者的临床恶化迹象，如进行性呼吸衰竭和休克，并立即采取支持性护理干预措施；对于呼吸情况进行性恶化、影像学进展迅速、机体炎性反应过度激活状态的患者可考虑短期应用糖皮质激素；对脏器功能受损患者应进行相应的脏器支持治疗。WHO暂行指南推荐对符合条件的ARDS患者行体外膜肺氧合（ECMO）治疗，但该治疗目前仍面临着许多技术挑战和限制。

目前的治疗策略远远不能满足COVID-19患者的需要，全球众多团队纷纷开展研究，探索COVID-19的潜在治疗药物。WHO于2020年3月开展国际COVID-19临床试验，以进一步评估伦地西韦、羟氯喹/氯喹和洛比那韦-利托那韦加联合/不联合干扰素β1的疗效。中期试验结果表明，与标准治疗相比，使用羟氯喹和洛匹那韦/利托那韦没有或几乎没有降低COVID-19住院患者的死亡率。针对住院患者使用羟氯喹和洛匹那韦/利托那的治疗实验于7月4日停止。部分研究将已经被批准用于其他疾病的药物应用于COVID-19患者，但尚无临床试验数据表明这些药物单独使用或联合使用对COVID-19治疗有明确疗效。

结合以往SARS和MERS的治疗经验，COVID-19的潜在治疗方法与靶点众多，包括RAS系统抑制剂、抗疟药、抗生素和抗寄生虫药、抗病毒药物、干扰素、恢复期血浆疗法、类固醇激素、单克隆抗体、天然产品和膳食补充剂、中药治疗、干细胞疗法和疫苗等。特异性免疫治疗作为其中的重要分支，有很大研究价值。目前已有众多针对SASV-CoV和MERS-CoV等病毒的特异性免疫治疗研究，主要集中在疫苗、单克隆抗体级恢复期血浆等方面。此外，先前抗击埃博拉、流感、SARS和MERS等病毒感染的研究显示，血浆置换有可能降低病毒载量和疾病死亡率。本文将着重探讨新冠肺炎免疫治疗的相关机制与研究现状。

二、免疫机制

(一) 病毒侵入

冠状病毒为有包膜的单股正链 RNA 病毒，其大小约为 30kb。SARS-CoV-2 有 4 种主要的结构蛋白，即刺突蛋白(spike,S)、包膜蛋白(envelope,E)、核衣壳蛋白(nucleocapsid,N)和膜蛋白(membrane,M)。其中 S 蛋白是 I 类病毒融合蛋白，需要蛋白酶裂解才能激活其融合潜能。其为病毒最大的结构蛋白，包含病毒的主要抗原决定簇，能够刺激机体产生中和抗体和介导免疫反应，决定病毒的多样性和宿主趋向性。S 蛋白包括 2 个功能亚单位，S1 包含受体结合域(RBD)，负责受体识别和结合。S2 亚单位则具有膜融合机制，负责病毒和细胞膜的融合，包括一个内在的膜融合肽(fusion peptide,FP)，2 个 7 肽重复序列(heptad repeat,HR)，1 个跨膜邻近区(juxamembrane domain,JMD)和 1 个跨膜结构域(transmembrane domain,TMD)。现有研究显示，血管紧张素转换酶 2(angiotensin converting enzyme,ACE2)为 S 蛋白的功能性受体，其他受体尚不清楚。SARS-CoV-2 感染宿主细胞的过程包括 5 个阶段，即附着、渗透、生物合成、成熟与释放。首先，SARS-CoV-2 的 S 蛋白结合宿主细胞表面的 ACE2 受体，随后由蛋白酶(包括 TMPRSS2、furin 蛋白酶和组织蛋白酶 L 等)水解激活。紧接着病毒通过内吞作用或膜融合(渗透)进入宿主细胞，并借助宿主细胞内转录翻译系统进行再合成组装，最终释放合成病毒，开始下一个感染周期。

(二) 宿主免疫反应与细胞因子风暴

随着病毒不断进行上述过程，感染由局部进一步播散，可扩散入血，导致继发性病毒血症，随后广泛攻击表达 ACE2 的靶器官，如胃肠道、肝脏、肾脏等。病毒侵入细胞进行复制增殖，不仅会直接损伤感染细胞，还会激活先天性和适应性免疫反应。气道先天性免疫的 3 个主要成分为上皮细胞、肺泡巨噬细胞和树突状细胞(dendritic cells,DCs)，在获得性免疫中，T 细胞经抗原呈递启动，$CD4^+$ T 细胞可激活 B 细胞促进病毒特异性抗体的产生，而 $CD8^+$ T 细胞可杀伤病毒感染细胞。现有研究认为，疾病晚期机体的众多损伤不仅来源于病毒直接侵入，更来源于免疫介导损伤。

COVID-19 重症和危重患者的显著特征为炎症进行性增加和异常高凝状态。炎症进行性增加可能导致机体免疫失衡，此时免疫系统过度激活，可能诱发由众多细胞因子驱动的"细胞因子风暴 cytokine release syndrome,CRS)"。CRS 在重症患者中表现为血浆促炎细胞因子浓度升高，包括白细胞介素 6(interleukin 6,IL-6)、白细胞介素 10(interleukin 6,IL-10)、粒细胞集落刺激因子(Granulocyte colony stimulating factor,G-CSF)、单核细胞趋化蛋白 1(Monocyte chemoattractant protein,MCP1)、巨噬细胞炎性蛋白 1α(Macrophage inflammatory protein 1α,MIP-1α)和肿瘤坏死因子 α(tumor necrosis factor α,TNF-α)。高水平的促炎细胞因子可使肺组织出现中性粒细胞和巨噬细胞大量浸润，引发弥漫性肺泡损伤，可能导致急性呼吸窘迫综合征，肺纤维化和肺容量降低。CRS 还可能引起休克，心脏、肝脏和肾脏的组织损伤，甚至多器官功能衰竭。免疫系统过度激活可能会引起免疫细胞的耗竭，削弱机体应对感染的能力。淋巴细胞减少是重症 COVID-19 患者的常见特征，表现为 $CD4^+$ T 细胞、$CD8^+$ T 细胞、B 细胞和自然杀伤细胞(NK)细胞数量急剧减少，伴有单核细胞、嗜酸性粒细胞和嗜碱性粒细胞比例降低。此外 COVID-19 患者中还存在细胞毒性淋巴细胞(包括 NK 细胞和 $CD8^+$ T 细胞)耗竭标记物(如 NKG2A)上调。COVID-19 患者凝血功能紊乱可能与多种因素有关，其中重症和危重 COVID-19 患者的持续炎症状态是凝血级联的重要触发因素。内皮功能包括促进血管舒张、纤溶和抗聚集。由于内皮细胞在血栓性调节中起着重要作用，在严重疾病中出现的高凝状态可能表明内皮损伤严重。内皮细胞也表达 ACE2，内皮损伤导致微血管通透性增加，可以促进病毒侵袭。

(三) 免疫治疗机制

免疫功能紊乱的患者往往预后更差，如何平衡生理性免疫反应与病理性 CRS 是治疗过程中亟待解决的问题。由于没有经证实的抗病毒药物，早期干预主要集中在阻止或减缓疾病进展，一旦患者病情恶化，综合性治疗是唯一的选择。针对新冠的潜在免疫治疗措施包括恢复期血浆疗法、大剂量静脉注射免疫球蛋白、多克隆或单克隆抗体，以及抗 IL-6R 抗体(tocilizumab 等)和其他免疫调节剂等。

以患者康复期血浆为例，其中不仅含有中和抗体(neutralizing antibodies,NAbs)，还有其他蛋白质如抗炎细胞因子、凝血因子、天然抗体、防御素、戊聚糖。其可能作用机制包括：直接中和病毒、控制过度活跃的免疫系统(如细胞因子风暴、Th1/Th17 比值、补体激活)和高凝状态的免疫调节。NAbs 与病毒结合为主要作用机制，可直接中和病毒传染性。针对 SARS-CoV 的研究发现，NAbs 通过结合于 S 蛋白，限制其结合域与宿主受体的相互作用，阻止病毒侵入细胞。血浆中除 NAbs 外，还有其他保护性抗体，包括免疫球蛋白 G(immunoglobulin G,IgG)和免疫球蛋白 M(immunoglobulin M,IgM)。而其他抗体介导的途径如补体激活、抗体依赖性细胞毒性和(或)吞噬作用也可能促进恢复期血浆的治疗效果。恢复期血浆还可以发挥免疫调节作用，改善严重的免疫反应，使机体能够控制由几种传染源或败血症引起的过度炎症级联反应。

其他治疗方法如单克隆抗体及免疫球蛋白，获取及加工过程较为复杂，研发及生产有一定难度，但治疗更有针对性，其含有的抗体效价更高，疗效更确切，相比恢复期血浆更具有可控性和安全性。已有研究发现，IL-6 是参与 CRS 的主要细胞因子之一，通过阻断 IL-6 有望减轻过度免疫反应。Tocilizumab 是一种人源化抗 IL-6 受体的单克隆抗体，可能对细胞因子升高的新冠肺炎患者有一定获益。

三、免疫治疗研究及临床应用现状

综上所述，COVID-19 自暴发起，在全球范围内迅速蔓延，传播率高，死亡率高。其症状范围从轻度、自限性呼吸道疾病到严重的进行性肺炎、多器官衰竭,甚至死亡,且目前尚无特效治疗方法。免疫治疗可分为两大类,即主动免疫治疗和被动免疫治疗。对于传染病而言,主动免疫治疗的代表为疫苗,而被动免疫治疗包括恢复期全血、恢复期血浆、静脉注射或肌内注射用混合人免疫球蛋白、高滴度人免疫球蛋白和多克隆或单克隆抗体。受限于研发时间和成本,目前首选的治疗方法是恢复期血浆。

(一)恢复期血浆

恢复期血浆自20世纪初即开始应用于临床,1918年流感、2003年SARS和2009年H1N1流感期间的相关研究,均显示应用恢复期血浆治疗后死亡率有所降低。尽管已有很长的历史,但其确切临床疗效尚未得到有力的研究证实,结论也很薄弱。可能由于恢复期血浆多在大流行暴发期间的危急情况下使用,没有进行严格的临床试验。

恢复期血浆治疗,即被动多克隆抗体(Ab)给药以提供及时免疫,已被用于提高病毒病因学严重急性呼吸综合征患者。目前已有多篇关于SARS-CoV和MERS的恢复期血浆使用的研究,包括综述、观察性研究(回顾性、前瞻性或病例系列)和系统性文献综述等。SARS-CoV-2和SARS-CoV都是高致病性的嗜肺冠状病毒(SARS-CoVs),并且它们都通过与ACE2受体结合进入细胞。研究表明,在SARS患者中,恢复期血浆表现出针对病毒S蛋白的中和抗体反应。这种抗体阻断了SARS-CoVs与ACE2的作用,其至在感染24个月后也可以检测到。2015年进行的一项对恢复期血浆和免疫球蛋白治疗严重急性呼吸道病毒感染进行的系统回顾和探索性事后荟萃分析报告,综合了32项关于SARS和严重流感的研究,这些研究涉及了699名接受治疗的患者和568名未经治疗的"对照组",研究显示,接受治疗后死亡率在统计学上显著降低(75%)。进一步探索性荟萃分析显示,与安慰剂或不接受治疗相比,治疗后的总死亡率也有所降低。另一项研究报道,重症SARS患者接受血清抗体滴度>1:640的恢复期血浆治疗后,成功存活。总结已有研究,发现恢复期血浆疗效因病原体和治疗方案不同而存在差异(如给药时间和剂量等)。

由于COVID-19病例和疾病相关死亡人数正以惊人的速度增长,COVID-19患者使用恢复期血浆疗法是否有效是目前迫切需要解决的问题。现有临床研究发现,COVID-19患者接受恢复期血浆治疗可能获益。在症状出现后不久(14d内)给予恢复期血浆,可能效果最好,保护可持续数周至数月,有效的恢复期血浆应含有高滴度的特异性抗体,这些抗体可与SARS-CoV-2结合,中和病毒颗粒,阻断其感染细胞的路径,并激活有效的免疫效应机制。但如果采集尚未完全康复患者血浆给予治疗,则可能会因其血浆中仍留滞相当水平的炎症因子,导致受试者出现一过性发热,甚或过敏反应。

中国现已有多个使用恢复期血浆治疗COVID-19病例的研究,一些重症患者应用后表现出氧合改善,炎症减轻和病毒载量降低。武汉的一项研究显示,6位实验室确诊COVID-19患者接受恢复期血浆后,有两位患者的抗SARS-CoV-2抗体滴度立即增加,部分患者影像学病灶有所改善,强调了这是一种有效并且特异的治疗方法。但该研究中恢复期血浆治疗的时间在发病4周后,混杂因素较多。另一项研究报道了4名危重型SARS-CoV-2患者的病程,对他们给予了支持治疗和恢复期血浆治疗,并进行了病毒载量或抗体IgM和IgG检测。结果显示,输注恢复期血浆后出现SARS-CoV-2病毒载量显著下降,两例患者在输注后约14d产生抗SARS-CoV-2的IgG抗体。与非严重疾病患者相比,危重病患者可能会出现更高的抗体反应,这种反应可以持续更长的时间。另一项同样针对危重症患者采用恢复期血浆治疗的研究中,在输注血浆后,5例患者中有4例在3d内体温恢复正常,SOFA评分下降,PAO_2/FiO_2在12d内升高。输血后12d内,病毒载量也下降并呈阴性,输血后SARS-CoV-2特异性中和抗体滴度增加。4例患者在12d内ARDS得到缓解,3例在治疗2周内停止机械通气。

这些研究的结果均表明,恢复期血浆可能是SARS-CoV-2感染危重患者的一种潜在治疗方法。然而,这些研究中的抗体水平还可能与其他治疗方法相关,如抗病毒药物、类固醇,支持性护理及患者的免疫反应,其对生存率的相对贡献尚不能确定。因此需在精心设计的临床试验中研究SARS-CoV-2感染患者输注恢复期血浆的确切安全性和有效性。由Li等在JAMA报道的针对危重症COVID-19患者恢复期血浆治疗的第一个随机临床试验表明,在所有随机患者中,接受恢复期血浆输注疗法和标准治疗的患者临床好转时间与仅接受标准治疗的患者之间没有显著差异。从随机分组到出院的28d的临床改善或死亡率也没有显著差异。但是与24 h、48 h和72 h鼻咽拭子的病毒阴性率有较高的相关性,表明恢复期血浆治疗与COVID-19患者的抗病毒活性相关。但是这项研究被提前终止,因此解释的结果有限。

恢复期血浆应用的不良反应多与输血相关不良反应有关。研究显示,在这些受试者中,输注恢复期血浆无严重不良反应。但部分患者存在由血浆输注引起输血相关急性肺损伤(TRALI)的风险。此外,一些病毒性疾病,如登革热病毒和非典型肺炎,可能因存在某些非中和抗体,导致抗体依赖增强现象,反而增强致病性。然而,一系列关于SARS和MERS的数据表明,恢复期血浆有较好的安全性。恢复期血浆在针对245名COVID-19患者的应用研究,安全性也较高。日后研究中,输血相关的不良反应仍不容忽视。

因此,恢复期血浆有可能在评估现有药物和开发新的特异性疫苗和治疗方法的同时,提供一个立即有希望的治疗选择。确定捐赠者标准以选择合格捐赠者、调整血液处理设施和检测能力、开发血清学分析进行筛选,以及确定恢复期血浆的给药方案是应对当前的大流行时最重要的。此外,恢复期血浆还可用于病毒性呼吸道疾病预防。可将恢复期血浆汇集并分离出高免疫性IgG,这已经成功地用于治疗严重的甲型H1N1流感感染。

(二)单克隆抗体疗法

单克隆抗体是被动免疫治疗对抗病毒感染的主要生物治疗方法。单克隆抗体的应用克服了血清疗法和静脉注射免疫球蛋白制剂在特异性、纯度、血源性病原体污染风险和安全性等方面的不足。它能为特定疾病提供高效和高度特异性的治疗干预。近年来已开发了多种针对病毒的单克隆抗体,有些已投入临床应用。

关于COVID-19的单克隆抗体研究尚处在初期,如寻找有效的单克隆中和抗体。目前应用于临床的单克隆抗体药物为Tocilizumab,即IL-6受体单克隆抗体。由于IL-6是参与COVID-19诱导的细胞因子风暴的最重要细胞因子之一,靶向IL-6受体的单克隆抗体Tocilizumab成为最近出现细胞因子风暴风险的COVID-19患者的替代疗法。但是目前关于TCZ对COVID-19患者的炎症活动影响的临床数据比较有限。在意大利的一项将TCZ用于治疗伴有炎性综合征和急性呼吸衰竭的重症COVID-19患者的单中心研究中,发现该治疗与3/4以上患者的临床改善相关。在临床状况改善的患者中CRP、铁蛋白和纤维蛋白原的血清水平下降至正常范围,淋巴细胞计数增加,IL-6血清水平升高,与类风湿关节炎和Castleman病患者TCZ给药后报道的相似。D-二聚体水平仍然很高,这表明TCZ仅能部分作用于炎症级联反应,但是对下调凝血的作用可能很小或没有影响。对于重症COVID-19患者而言,及时诊断高炎症状态及其治疗方法对于中断级联反应导致的不可逆转的肺损伤及死亡可能至关重要。在这些情况下,如果其他治疗失败或无法使用,则可将Tocilizumab视为抢救治疗。

四、展　望

新冠病毒传染性强,病死率高,危害大,但尚无有效治疗措施,且疫苗研发及投入使用周期较长,面临众多困难。此外,患者感染SARS-CoV-2后,抗体产生时间较长,导致病程较长,给COVID-19疫情的控制造成了很大的困难。而当下被动免疫治疗(如恢复期血浆)有较好的应用前景,其获取及处理相对容易,可为患者早期预防及危重症患者的治疗提供一定辅助,但具体疗效及相关的不良反应尚未明确,快速的供给程序也尚未建立,其他治疗方式如单克隆抗体、高效价的免疫球蛋白的具体疗效仍需要进一步探索和研究,因此免疫治疗研究任重道远。

参 考 文 献

[1] Li H, Liu Z, Ge J. Scientific research progress of COVID-19/SARS-CoV-2 in the first five months. J Cell Mol Med, 2020, 24:6558-6570.

[2] WHO. WHO Timeline-COVID-19. https://wwwwhoint/news-room/detail/27-04-2020-who-timeline---covid-19 2020.

[3] Guo YR, Cao QD, Hong ZS, et al. The origin, transmission and clinical therapies on coronavirus disease 2019(COVID-19) outbreak-an update on the status. Mil Med Res, 2020, 7:11.

[4] Dong R, Pei S, Yin C, He RL, Yau SS. Analysis of the Hosts and Transmission Paths of SARS-CoV-2 in the COVID-19 Outbreak. Genes(Basel), 2020, 11.

[5] King MC, Wilson AC. Evolution at two levels in humans and chimpanzees. Science, 1975, 188:107-116.

[6] Guan WJ, Ni ZY, Hu Y, et al. Clinical Characteristics of Coronavirus Disease 2019 in China. N Engl J Med, 2020, 382:1708-1720.

[7] Tong JY, Wong A, Zhu D, Fastenberg JH, Tham T. The Prevalence of Olfactory and Gustatory Dysfunction in COVID-19 Patients: A Systematic Review and Meta-analysis. Otolaryngol Head Neck Surg, 2020, 163:3-11.

[8] Zhou F, Yu T, Du R, et al. Clinical course and risk factors for mortality of adult inpatients with COVID-19 in Wuhan, China: a retrospective cohort study. The Lancet, 2020, 395:1054-1062.

[9] Verdoni L, Mazza A, Gervasoni A, et al. An outbreak of severe Kawasaki-like disease at the Italian epicentre of the SARS-CoV-2 epidemic: an observational cohort study. The Lancet, 2020, 395:1771-1778.

[10] Fu L, Wang B, Yuan T, et al. Clinical characteristics of coronavirus disease 2019(COVID-19) in China: A systematic review and meta-analysis. Journal of Infection, 2020, 80:656-665.

[11] Zunyou Wu JM. Characteristics of and Important Lessons From the Coronavirus Disease 2019(COVID-19) Outbreak in China Summary of a Report of 72 314 Cases From the Chinese Center for Disease Control and Prevention. 2020.

[12] Geier MR, Geier DA. Respiratory conditions in coronavirus disease 2019(COVID-19): Important considerations regarding novel treatment strategies to reduce mortality. Medical Hypotheses, 2020, 140:109760.

[13] Zhang B, Liu S, Tan T, et al. Treatment With Convalescent Plasma for Critically Ill Patients With Severe Acute Respiratory Syndrome Coronavirus 2 Infection. Chest, 2020.

[14] WHO. Clinical management of COVID-19. 2020.

[15] 国家卫生健康委办公厅. 新型冠状病毒肺炎诊疗方案_试行第7版. 2020.

[16] Archived: WHO Timeline-COVID-19. 2019, 2020. at https://www.who.int/news-room/detail/27-04-2020-who-timeline-covid-19.

[17] "Solidarity" clinical trial for COVID-19 treatments. 2020. at https://www.who.int/emergencies/diseases/novel-coronavirus-2019/global-research-on-novel-coronavirus-2019-ncov/solidarity-clinical-trial-for-covid-19-treatments.

[18] Pooladanda V, Thatikonda S, Godugu C. The current understanding and potential therapeutic options to combat COVID-19. Life Sci, 2020, 254:117765.

[19] Triggle CR, Bansal D, Farag E, Ding H, Sultan AA. COVID-19: Learning from Lessons To Guide Treatment and Prevention Interventions. mSphere, 2020, 5(3):e00317-20.

[20] Ou X, Zheng W, Shan Y, et al. Identification of the Fusion Peptide-Containing Region in Betacoronavirus Spike Glycoproteins. Journal of Virology, 2016, 90:5586.

[21] Hoffmann M, Kleine-Weber H, Schroeder S, et al. SARS-

CoV-2 Cell Entry Depends on ACE2 and TMPRSS2 and Is Blocked by a Clinically Proven Protease Inhibitor. Cell,2020, 181:271-280.

[22] Yoshikawa T,Hill T,Li K,Peters CJ,Tseng C-TK. Severe acute respiratory syndrome (SARS) coronavirus-induced lung epithelial cytokines exacerbate SARS pathogenesis by modulating intrinsic functions of monocyte-derived macrophages and dendritic cells. Journal of virology,2009,83:3039-3048.

[23] Cao W,Li T. COVID-19: towards understanding of pathogenesis. Cell Research,2020,30:367-369.

[24] Ye Q,Wang B,Mao J. The pathogenesis and treatment of the 'Cytokine Storm' in COVID-19. J Infect,2020,80(6):607-613.

[25] Qin C,Zhou L,Hu Z,et al. Dysregulation of immune response in patients with COVID-19 in Wuhan,China. Clin Infect Dis,2020,71(15):762-768.

[26] Zhou Y,Fu B,Zheng X,et al. Pathogenic T-cells and inflammatory monocytes incite inflammatory storms in severe COVID-19 patients. National Science Review,2020,7:998-1002.

[27] Huang C,Wang Y,Li X,et al. Clinical features of patients infected with 2019 novel coronavirus in Wuhan,China. Lancet,2020,395(10223):497-506.

[28] Guan W-j,Ni Z-y,Hu Y,et al. Clinical Characteristics of Coronavirus Disease 2019 in China. New England Journal of Medicine,2020,382:1708-1720.

[29] Zheng M,Gao Y,Wang G,et al. Functional exhaustion of antiviral lymphocytes in COVID-19 patients. Cellular & Molecular Immunology,2020,17:533-535.

[30] Marano G,Vaglio S,Pupella S,et al. Convalescent plasma: new evidence for an old therapeutic tool? Blood Transfus,2016,14:152-157.

[31] Benjamin RJ,McLaughlin LS. Plasma components: properties,differences,and uses. Transfusion,2012,52:9S-19S.

[32] Rajendran KA-O,Krishnasamy N,Rangarajan J,et al. Convalescent plasma transfusion for the treatment of COVID-19: Systematic review. J Med Virol,2020,92(9):1475-1483.

[33] Du L,He Y,Zhou Y,et al. The spike protein of SARS-CoV-a target for vaccine and therapeutic development. Nat Rev Microbiol,2009,7(3):226-236.

[34] Garraud O,Heshmati F,Pozzetto B,et al. Plasma therapy against infectious pathogens,as of yesterday,today and tomorrow. Transfus Clin Biol,2016,23(1):39-44.

[35] Wang C,Li W,Drabek D,et al. A human monoclonal antibody blocking SARS-CoV-2 infection. Nature Communications,2020,11:2251.

[36] Chen X,Zhao B,Qu Y,et al. Detectable Serum Severe Acute Respiratory Syndrome Coronavirus 2 Viral Load (RNAemia) Is Closely Correlated With Drastically Elevated Interleukin 6 Level in Critically Ill Patients With Coronavirus Disease 2019. Clinical Infectious Diseases,2020.

[37] Wang D,Hu B,Hu C,et al. Clinical Characteristics of 138 Hospitalized Patients With 2019 Novel Coronavirus-Infected Pneumonia in Wuhan,China. JAMA,2020.

[38] Wu Z,McGoogan JM. Characteristics of and Important Lessons From the Coronavirus Disease 2019 (COVID-19) Outbreak in China: Summary of a Report of 72314 Cases From the Chinese Center for Disease Control and Prevention. JAMA 2020.

[39] Luke TC,Kilbane EM,Jackson JL,Hoffman SL. Meta-analysis: convalescent blood products for Spanish influenza pneumonia: a future H5N1 treatment? Ann Intern Med,2006,145:599-609.

[40] Cheng Y,Wong R,Soo YO,et al. Use of convalescent plasma therapy in SARS patients in Hong Kong. Eur J Clin Microbiol Infect Dis,2005,24:44-46.

[41] Hung IF,To KK,Lee CK,et al. Convalescent plasma treatment reduced mortality in patients with severe pandemic influenza A(H1N1)2009 virus infection. Clin Infect Dis,2011,52:447-456.

[42] Mair-Jenkins J,Saavedra-Campos M,Baillie JK,et al. The effectiveness of convalescent plasma and hyperimmune immunoglobulin for the treatment of severe acute respiratory infections of viral etiology: a systematic review and exploratory meta-analysis. J Infect Dis,2015,211:80-90.

[43] Shen C,Wang Z,Zhao F,et al. Treatment of 5 Critically Ill Patients With COVID-19 With Convalescent Plasma. JAMA,2020.

[44] Kuo-Ming,Yeh T-SC,Siu LK,et al. Experience of using convalescent plasma for severe acute respiratory syndrome among healthcare workers in a Taiwan hospital. J Antimicrob Chemother,2015,56:919-922.

[45] Walls AC,Park YJ,Tortorici MA,et al. Structure,Function,and Antigenicity of the SARS-CoV-2 Spike Glycoprotein. Cell,2020,181:281-292.

[46] K D. The feasibility of convalescent plasma therapy in severe COVID-19 patients: a pilot study. https://doiorg/101101/202003 1620036145 2020.

[47] Chen L XJ,Bao L,Shi Y. Convalescent plasma as a potential therapy for COVID-19. Lancet Infect Dis,2020.

[48] Cunningham AC,Goh HP,Koh D. Treatment of COVID-19: old tricks for new challenges. Crit Care 2020,24:91.

[49] China puts 245 COVID-19 patients on convalescent plasma therapy. News releaseXinhua 2020; Available at: http://www.xinhuanet.com/english/2020-02/28/c_138828177.htm.

[50] Ye M,Fu D,Ren Y,et al. Treatment with convalescent plasma for COVID-19 patients in Wuhan,China. J Med Virol,2020.

[51] Chen J,Zhu H,Horby PW,et al. Specificity,kinetics and longevity of antibody responses to avian influenza A(H7N9) virus infection in humans. J Infect,2020,80:310-319.

[52] Li L,Zhang W,Hu Y,et al. Effect of Convalescent Plasma Therapy on Time to Clinical Improvement in Patients With Severe and Life-threatening COVID-19: A Randomized Clinical Trial. JAMA,2020.

[53] Afessa B,Gajic O,Keegan MT. Severity of illness and organ failure assessment in adult intensive care units. Crit Care Clin,2007,23:639-658.

[54] Casadevall A,Pirofski LA. The convalescent sera option for containing COVID-19. J Clin Invest,2020,130(4):1545-1548.

[55] Hung IFN, To KKW, Lee CK, et al. Hyperimmune IV immunoglobulin treatment: a multicenter double-blind randomized controlled trial for patients with severe 2009 influenza A (H1N1) infection. Chest, 2013, 144: 464-473.

[56] Kaur S, Bansal Y, Kumar R, Bansal G. A panoramic review of IL-6: Structure, pathophysiological roles and inhibitors. Bioorg Med Chem, 2020, 28: 115327.

[57] Toniati P, Piva S, Cattalini M, et al. Tocilizumab for the treatment of severe COVID-19 pneumonia with hyperinflammatory syndrome and acute respiratory failure: A single center study of 100 patients in Brescia, Italy. Autoimmun Rev, 2020, 19: 102568.

[58] Nishimoto N, Terao K, Mima T, Nakahara H, Takagi N, Kakehi T. Mechanisms and pathologic significances in increase in serum interleukin-6 (IL-6) and soluble IL-6 receptor after administration of an anti-IL-6 receptor antibody, tocilizumab, in patients with rheumatoid arthritis and Castleman disease. Blood, 2008, 112: 3959-3964.

3 新型冠状病毒肺炎继发感染的诊断与治疗

施 毅

随着我国抗击新型冠状病毒肺炎(以下简称"新冠肺炎")的决定性胜利,全国人民正在逐渐恢复正常的日常生活,但全球的抗疫斗争并没有结束。所以,总结经验,做好准备,是我们的当务之急。国家卫健委颁布的《新型冠状病毒肺炎诊疗方案》多达7版,说明了对这个疾病的认识还相距甚远。本文对新型冠状病毒肺炎继发细菌性感染的诊治做一初步的讨论,以期为临床提供一定的参考。

一、国家卫健委《新型冠状病毒肺炎诊疗方案》有关抗菌药物合理应用的推荐

国家卫健委在新冠肺炎战役的关键时刻,近2个月内连续修订了第7版《新型冠状病毒肺炎诊疗方案》(以下简称"方案"),既反映了对此种新型疾病的认识尚远远不够,还需要积累更多临床经验,也反映了诊断和治疗手段的长足进步,需要不断更新。

所有的诊疗方案从开始就不断强调原则性的规定,且一直没有大的变化,即"避免盲目或不恰当使用抗菌药物,尤其是联合使用广谱抗菌药物"。在第3、4版"方案"中,曾经加上:加强细菌学监测,有继发细菌感染证据时及时应用抗菌药物。随后删除,并未做抗菌药物使用的详细介绍,推测其目的就是不希望医生把抗菌药物的使用作为新冠肺炎的主要治疗手段,淡化其地位,突出大原则,从而避免盲目使用,特别是不恰当联合使用广谱抗菌药物。

卫健委针对重型危重型患者的诊疗方案中,涉及抗菌药物治疗时略微详细一些:如果无明确细菌感染证据,不建议常规使用抗菌药物。需要注意的是,重型患者往往病程已经超过5~7d,多存在细胞免疫抑制的表现,特别是入住ICU需要有创机械通气的患者,需要注意继发细菌或真菌感染。若条件许可,应积极行呼吸道病原体监测,进行针对性的抗感染治疗。如90d内有抗菌药物应用史、住院时间超过72h,或既往存在结构性肺病,抗菌药物选择应考虑覆盖耐药菌。重症方案强调了重型和危重型患者继发细菌或真菌感染的概率增加,在留取标本行病原学检测后,应积极进行抗感染治疗,并尽量做到针对性治疗,同时给出了覆盖耐药菌的条件。同样对抗感染治疗提倡持谨慎的态度,但明确指出了应该应用的指征。

二、新型冠状病毒肺炎诊疗中抗细菌治疗的现状与问题

国家卫健委有关新冠肺炎的各版诊疗方案中,一直强调"避免盲目或不恰当使用抗菌药物,尤其是联合使用广谱抗菌药物"。病毒感染不需要应用抗菌药物,所以在新冠肺炎早期没有细菌感染征象的情况下不推荐使用抗菌药物,这个定义是有前提的,这也是大多数解读方案或指南的时候经常会有的一些不全面的理解。

我们对新型冠状病毒肺炎诊治的认识,在初始阶段多是参考以往的经验,例如SARS、MERS、禽流感、新型甲型H1N1流感等,这些既往资料可以给我们一定的临床经验,更多的是需要我们深入的思考和灵活的运用。随着临床诊治新冠肺炎经验的积累,开始有文献报道病例诊治经验总结,但总体来说涉及继发感染后抗细菌或真菌治疗的数据很有限,相信以后从大样本的回顾分析里可以了解到更多,如常见哪些细菌感染,具体用了哪些抗菌药物,各自所占的比例,治疗效果等情况,但目前我们还只能从一些已经发表的小样本的病例总结里窥见一些实际情况。目前的临床现状是,有的医生不能准确把握应用抗菌药物的时机和正确地选择合适的抗菌药物和疗程;而更多的是在病毒感染的早期没有评估细菌感染的指征就开始经验性使用抗菌药物,以及一开始就用到顶级的抗菌药物,如见到的最为常见的方案组合是美罗培南+利奈唑胺,同时覆盖耐药的阴性菌和阳性菌。因此,合理应用抗菌药物在新冠肺炎的诊治中仍然是需要探讨的一个问题。

新型冠状病毒感染的病情分为轻型、普通型、重型和危重型病例。结合文献报道及临床实际情况,重型及危重型病例的患者继发感染的概率高,使用抗菌药物的概率会很大。钟南山院士在回答记者问的时候提到:新冠肺炎有个突出的特点:小气道里面有非常多的黏液,阻碍了气道的通畅,气道的不通畅容易导致继发感染;感染又加重了病情,引发脓毒症、全身多脏器功能衰竭。武汉的医生在临床中也发现(武汉同济医学院与金银潭医院团队)疫情早期危重患者的病死率超过了60%,这部分患者有14%继发了院内细菌或真菌感染,需要抗感染药物治疗。武汉收治新冠肺炎的定点医院金银潭医院99例患者报道里,所有患者均进行了9种呼吸道病原体的检测及甲型和乙型

流感病毒核酸检测,同时行细菌和真菌培养。其中71%采用了抗细菌治疗,15%采用了抗真菌治疗。在继发细菌感染时,使用的抗菌药物包括头孢菌素、喹诺酮类、碳青霉烯类、替加环素、利奈唑胺,以及抗真菌药物。武汉中南医院138例患者中,重症患者占比26.1%,所有患者均接受了抗菌药物治疗,使用的抗感染药物主要有莫西沙星、头孢曲松、阿奇霉素。还有一些特殊人群,例如武汉大学中南医院团队报道的9例感染新冠肺炎的孕妇,所有患者也都接受了经验性抗菌药物治疗,估计是考虑到孕妇出现继发感染可能更大,一旦发生继发感染死亡风险更高的原因。而武汉大学人民医院、武汉大学健康学院分析了9例新冠病毒感染的1岁以下住院婴儿都没有使用抗感染药物,因为患儿皆为轻症。

我们总结了江苏省COVID-19患者继发感染的情况,病原诊断为继发细菌感染的发生率是7.7%(45/583),临床诊断为继发细菌感染的发生率是25.0%(146/583)。细菌病原学结果阳性率最高的是肺炎支原体(24例,4.1%),基于病原体培养结果显示较常见的病原体为肺炎克雷伯菌和鲍曼不动杆菌。继发细菌感染加重了COVID-19疾病的严重程度,病情越重抗菌药物,使用疗程越长。COVID-19患者抗菌药物使用率为60.4%(352/583),应用最多的抗菌药物为莫西沙星(297/352,84.38%)。抗菌药物联合治疗(两种及两种以上)的比例为37.2%(131/352)。可以看出,继发细菌感染临床诊断的发生率仅为25.0%,但抗菌药物的使用率却为60.4%,明显高于诊断率,说明临床实践中确实存在抗菌药物不合理使用的状况。

因此,在新冠肺炎的诊治中,是否合并存在或继发细菌及真菌感染,需要结合患者的病情严重程度、当地呼吸道感染的流行病学和耐药情况,进行合并或继发细菌感染的风险评估,在积极留临床标本的同时,根据感染相关的指征,正确的选择抗菌药物进行经验治疗,再根据病原学检查结果和初始治疗反应调整抗感染治疗方案。

三、正确判定新冠肺炎是否合并细菌感染,以及可能的病原菌

冬季是呼吸道感染性疾病的高发季节,即使没有新型冠状病毒肺炎,还会有其他的常见呼吸道感染性肺炎,如细菌性肺炎、支原体肺炎、衣原体肺炎,以及常见病毒性肺炎。文献报道,我国免疫功能正常成人社区获得性肺炎(CAP)患者检测到病毒的比例为15%~34.9%,常见病毒有流感病毒、副流感病毒、鼻病毒、腺病毒、人偏肺病毒及呼吸道合胞病毒等。因此,不能有这样的概念,现患的肺炎就是新型冠状病毒肺炎,就像2003年初期许多人认为只要得肺炎就是SARS(非典)肺炎一样。这就需要尽量做好肺炎的鉴别诊断,特别是在当前疫情严重的情况下。

中华医学会呼吸病学分会制定的《中国成人社区获得性肺炎诊断和治疗指南(2016年版)》在论及CAP诊断时明确告知,当患者符合CAP的诊断标准后,必须除外肺结核、肺部肿瘤、非感染性肺间质性疾病、肺水肿、肺不张、肺栓塞、肺嗜酸性粒细胞浸润症及肺血管炎等后,才可建立临床诊断。而引起CAP最常见的病原学是肺炎支原体和肺炎链球菌,其他常见病原体包括流感嗜血杆菌、肺炎衣原体、肺炎克雷伯菌、金黄色葡萄球菌,少见铜绿假单胞菌和鲍曼不动杆菌。当然,也包括常见呼吸道病毒在内。

新冠病毒肺炎与流感病毒肺炎非常相似。重症流感的并发症中最常见的是肺炎,包括细菌感染和真菌感染,也是导致重症流感患者死亡的重要原因之一。继发感染者分离出的病原体以肺炎链球菌最为多见,其他常见的有流感嗜血杆菌、化脓性链球菌、金黄色葡萄球菌等,但不同地区存在差异。也有报道以金黄色葡萄球菌为主,或是鲍曼不动杆菌、粪肠球菌,而肺炎链球菌比率极低。近年来,重症流感后继发真菌感染也越来越多见,主要是继发曲霉感染,发病率在15%~20%。近日《柳叶刀》报道,武汉99例患者采集痰标本,分离培养到细菌(鲍曼不动杆菌)和真菌(白念珠菌),但这与通常认为的肺部病毒感染后合并的细菌常见病原菌不一样。当然,在武汉疫情这么紧张的情况下,大家更注重救治患者,加上传染病的疫情使平时开展的病原学实验室检查都不做了,所以难以拿到充分的依据。因此,目前的数据非常有限,需要收集更多的循证医学证据。武汉协和医院张劲农教授也认为,此次新冠肺炎和流感肺炎有非常惊人的相似之处,继发性感染病原菌还是以金黄色葡萄球菌或肺炎链球菌等革兰阳性菌为主。使用有创呼吸机的患者更容易出现继发感染,甚至出现耐药菌感染。当然,大家都在摸着石头过河,如患者确认合并感染的比例、病原学的分布状况、实际运用抗菌药物的类型等,我们都还不清楚,相信今后的总结文献一定会让我们有更多的了解。

四、病毒性肺炎之后应该正确地进行肺部感染的病原学检测

新型冠状病毒肺炎实际上就是一种特殊类型的CAP。CAP常见病原体包括细菌、病毒、非典型病原体及真菌等。那么CAP患者何时和应该采集哪些标本进行哪些实验室检查?《中国成人社区获得性肺炎诊断和治疗指南(2016年版)》有非常明确的定义,通常情况下,门诊患者不需要进行病原学检查,但特殊情况下和住院患者,应该进行相关的实验室检查,包括痰等呼吸道标本、血液、胸腔积液病原体培养,血清特异性抗体检测,军团菌或肺炎链球菌尿抗原监测,核酸检测,真菌抗原检测,结核菌相关检查等。表4-3-1给出了具体的建议。需要进行呼吸道病毒筛查有5种情况:群聚性发病、初始经验性治疗无效、重症CAP、双肺多叶病灶和免疫缺陷的患者。

表 4-3-1 CAP 特定临床情况下建议进行的病原学检查

临床情况	痰涂片及培养	血培养	胸腔积液培养	支原体/衣原体/军团菌筛查	呼吸道病毒筛查	LP1尿抗原	SP尿抗原	真菌抗原	结核筛查
群聚性发病				√	√	√			
初始经验性治疗无效	√	√		√	√	√	√		
重症CAP	√	√		√	√	√	√		
特殊影像学表现									
坏死性肺炎或合并空洞	√	√						√	√
合并胸腔积液	√	√	√	√					√
双肺多叶病灶	√	√		√	√	√			
基础疾病									
合并慢性阻塞性肺疾病	√								
合并结构性肺病	√								√
免疫缺陷	√	√		√	√	√	√	√	
发病前2周内外出游旅行史					√				

LP1. 嗜肺军团菌1型；SP. 肺炎链球菌

目前大家都将关注点放在了新冠病毒感染上，觉得只要不是新冠肺炎就好了，其他的就不重要，放松了对新冠病毒感染相关的鉴别诊断，从而忽略了对其他病原菌的实验室检查。其实这个季节还有很多的呼吸道感染性疾病同时存在。武汉金银潭医院报道的99例患者均进行9种呼吸道病原体的检测，以及甲型和乙型流感病毒核酸检测，同时行细菌和真菌培养，做得非常好，应该大力推荐。但湖北地区短时间大量涌现的新冠肺炎患者导致各个不同等级医院间因条件的限制而开展的实验室检查有所不同，确诊的患者送检情况也不尽一样。因此，病原学检查送检的覆盖率、检测率、检测条件、检测类型都是影响实验室检查结果的因素。

前面已经提及了CAP应该做哪些病原学检查，那么当临床高度怀疑病毒性肺炎时，可以考虑进行哪些相关的病毒学检测呢？《中国成人社区获得性肺炎诊断和治疗指南（2016年版）》推荐的病毒学检测方法共有4种（表4-3-2），包括病毒分离培养、血清特异性抗体检测、病毒抗原检测和核酸检测，在甲流的诊断中实际临床应用的主要是病毒抗原检测（如胶体金法的抗原筛查检测）和病毒核酸检测。

表 4-3-2 病毒学检测方法及其诊断意义

检测方法	采用标本	诊断意义	说明
核酸检测	口咽拭子、鼻咽拭子、鼻咽吸引物、气管吸引物、痰等呼吸道标本	1. 可作为病原学确定诊断的检测结果：①口咽/鼻咽拭子、合格下呼吸道标本或肺组织标本中流感病毒、副流感病毒1-4型、呼吸道合胞病毒、腺病毒、冠状病毒、人偏肺病毒等核酸检测阳性；②急性期和恢复期双份血清流感病毒、呼吸道合胞病毒等呼吸道病毒特异性IgG抗体滴度有4倍或4倍以上变化；③口咽/鼻咽拭子或合格下呼吸道标本中流感病毒快速抗原检测阳性（DFA法或胶体金法），并有相关流行病学史支持；④口咽/鼻咽拭子或合格下呼吸道标本中副流感病毒1-4型、呼吸道合胞病毒、腺病毒、人偏肺病毒的快速抗原检测阳性（DFA法）；⑤合格下呼吸道标本中分离到流感病毒、呼吸道合胞病毒等呼吸道病毒 2. 对病原学诊断具有重要参考意义的检测结果：血清流感病毒、呼吸道合胞病毒等呼吸道病毒特异性IgM阳性	1. 病毒分离培养是确诊呼吸道病毒感染的金标准，对新发或突发呼吸道传染病病原的发现和确诊具有重要意义，但需时较长，实验添加要求高，不是临床检测的常规项目 2. Real-time PCR/rRT-PCR（real-time reverse transcriptase PCR）的敏感性和特异性较高，是流感病毒、禽流感病毒等呼吸道病毒感染快速诊断的首选方法 3. 合格下呼吸道标本的病毒抗原检测可作为早期快速诊断的初筛方法，敏感度低于核酸检测方法，对其结果的解释应结合患者的流行病史和临床症状综合考虑，必要时使用核酸检测或病毒分离培养进一步确认 4. 血清特异性病毒抗体检测是回顾性诊断的主要手段
病毒抗原检（DFA、胶体金法）			
血清特异性抗体检测（IFA、ELISA、CF、血凝抑制试验）	急性期及恢复期双份血清		
病毒分离培养	口咽拭子、鼻咽拭子、鼻咽吸引物、气管吸引物、痰等呼吸道标本		

此次新型冠状病毒感染的实验室检测主要推荐特异的病毒核酸检测(PCR或核酸测序),是确诊病例的实验室诊断标准。标本从早期的呼吸道标本,扩展为呼吸道(鼻咽拭子、痰、下呼吸道分泌物)、血液、粪便等标本,阳性指的是标本中可检测出新型冠状病毒核酸。患者确诊的依据就是在疑似病例的基础上,具备以下病原学证据之一者:①实时荧光RT-PCR检测新型冠状病毒核酸阳性。②病毒基因测序,与已知的新型冠状病毒高度同源。③新型冠状病毒血清特异性IgM和IgG抗体阳性。提示新的确诊手段正在不断地应用于临床,将进一步推动诊断率的提高。

深圳市第三人民医院的临床研究证实,新冠病毒核酸检测的阳性率按标本取材的最佳顺序是肺泡灌洗液>痰液>鼻咽拭子>咽拭子。因此,对于轻中症患者来说,应尽量采用痰标本,其次是鼻拭子、咽拭子,而对于重症行气管插管机械通气的患者来说最好取BALF标本。由于80%左右的患者是轻型或普通型患者,只能采集鼻咽拭子,如果方法不正确,就会明显影响检测结果。其他影响核酸检测结果的因素包括标本的保存(应该用病毒专用保存液)、运输(应该4℃以下冷藏)、待检时间(冠状病毒属于RNA病毒,极易降解)、样本的病毒灭活、检测试剂盒的品质(是否为国家批准的产品)、检测实验室条件(2P标准)和检测人员技术(专门培训)等,都可以导致假阳性,特别是假阴性,这也是前段时间核酸检测不及时、阳性率不高、假阴性却太高,以至于要求改进的呼声最高的问题。随着国家批准的合格试剂不断面市,检测点的不断增多,情况已经大为改观。希望新的快速检测方法如抗体检测,抗原检测等尽早进入临床,使诊断手段更为丰富便捷,检测结果更为可靠可信。

关于核酸检测,除了实时荧光RT-PCR之外,另外一个好方法是宏基因二代测序(mNGS),可以弥补RT-PCR的不足,发现病毒可能的变异,确认是否存在混合感染,及时发现继发感染,应该引起大家的关注,不要遗忘了。mNGS唯一的缺点是费用较高,检测时间稍长。今后改善核酸检测的应对策略与发展方向为:①正确地采集、保存和运送标本。②及时检测。③检测结果不一致者,增加检测次数或采用mNGS确认。④采用合格的检测试剂盒,规范检测程序。⑤结合临床实际(临床表现,常规实验室检查,影像学改变等)正确的解读检测结果。

五、新冠肺炎继发感染抗菌药物的优化选择、应用及恰当的管理

在肺炎治疗中使用的抗感染治疗药物并非固定不变的,即并无标准方案。在第7版卫健委《新型冠状病毒肺炎诊疗方案》里明确规定,避免盲目或不恰当使用抗菌药物,尤其是联合使用广谱抗菌药物。但给药的原则,缺乏合理应用抗菌药物的具体指导。WHO疑似新型冠状病毒(2019-nCoV)感染引起的严重急性呼吸道感染(SARI)临床处置指南推荐:应基于临床诊断(社区获得性肺炎、医院获得性肺炎)进行评估,如果病情较轻,根据当地细菌流行病学状况、耐药情况和药物供应情况经验性选择适宜的抗菌药物;如果病情较重,则建议"广覆盖",即应用广谱抗菌药物,再根据病原学检测结果,降阶梯或调整治疗方案。

既往在SARS、MERS等病毒性感染时抗菌药物的应用目的主要有2个:①用于对疑似患者的试验性治疗,以帮助鉴别诊断。②用于治疗和控制继发细菌、真菌感染。未使用糖皮质激素治疗且无合并细菌感染证据的轻症患者,原则上不需要使用抗菌药物。对于重症患者特别是大剂量激素冲击治疗后合并感染的可能性大,可适当应用预防性抗菌药物。总体来说,个体之间合并细菌性感染的概率和时机差异较大,而本次新冠肺炎患者合并细菌感染的比例相对较低。因此,大家的共识是,在病毒感染的早期没有细菌感染的指征时不推荐应用抗菌药物。只有在出现细菌性感染征象的轻中症患者,或重型患者(往往病程已经超过5~7d,多存在细胞免疫抑制的表现,特别是入住ICU需要有创机械通气的患者),需要注意继发细菌或真菌感染。若条件许可,应积极进行临床微生物监测。每天留取患者痰液和尿液进行培养,高热患者及时行血培养。所有留置血管导管的疑似脓毒症患者,均应同时送检外周静脉血培养和导管血培养。所有疑似脓毒症患者可考虑采集外周血进行病原学分子诊断检查,包括实时荧光RT-PCR和mGNS,进行针对性的抗感染治疗。CRP水平升高对诊断细菌和真菌感染引起的脓毒症缺乏特异性,但PCT水平升高对诊断脓毒症/脓毒性休克具有提示意义。若发生脓毒症,则应尽快给予经验性抗感染治疗。重症患者在经验性选择治疗药物时要评估患者感染可能的病原学及其耐药性,以及患者的既往用药史、器官功能状态等来选择适宜的抗菌药物。如90d内有抗菌药物应用史、住院时间超过72h,或既往存在结构性肺病,抗菌药物选择应考虑覆盖耐药菌。

对于脓毒性休克患者可联合使用经验性抗菌药物,覆盖最为常见的肠杆菌科细菌、葡萄球菌和肠球菌感染。住院后发生感染者可选用β-内酰胺酶抑制剂复合物。若治疗效果不佳,或患者为重症感染性休克,则可换用碳青霉烯类药物治疗。如考虑合并肠球菌和葡萄球菌感染,可加用糖肽类药物(万古霉素)进行经验性治疗;血液感染可选用达托霉素;以肺部感染为主,则可选用利奈唑胺。应高度重视危重症患者的导管相关感染,治疗应经验性覆盖甲氧西林耐药的葡萄球菌,可选用糖肽类药物(万古霉素)进行经验性治疗。念珠菌感染在危重症患者中也较为常见,必要时应经验性覆盖抗念珠菌治疗,可加用棘白菌素类药物。随着重症患者住院时间延长,耐药菌感染也会逐渐增加,此时须根据药敏感试验结果调整抗菌药物的使用。

是否增加抗真菌治疗,要视病情需要而定。可以参照流感病毒感染,近年来的研究显示,在流感后期(大概1周以后),有相当一部分患者(15%~20%)继发真菌感染,以曲霉感染为主。新型冠状病毒感染以后也会遇到类似情况,尤其是重症患者。如果重症患者后期继发细菌感染,抗细菌治疗效果不好,且存在真菌感染迹象(如影像学改

变,G试验,GM试验)时,可以经验性覆盖真菌感染(应该覆盖曲霉),但不建议一开始即"广覆盖"真菌。

因此,新型冠状病毒感染后的经验性抗感染治疗,应建立在临床充分评估病情的基础上进行,再根据实验室检测的证据和理性地分析,严格管控和合理应用抗菌药物,在保证充分治疗的同时避免过度治疗,以拯救患者的生命。

参 考 文 献

[1] Chen N, et al. Epidemiological and clinical characteristics of 99 cases of 2019 novel coronavirus pneumonia in Wuhan, China: a descriptive study. Lancet, 2020 Feb 15;395(10223):507-513.

[2] Wang D, et al. Clinical Characteristics of 138 Hospitalized Patients With 2019 Novel Coronavirus-Infected Pneumonia in Wuhan, China. JAMA. 2020,323(11):1061-1069.

[3] Guan W, et al. Clinical characteristics of 2019 novel coronavirus infection in China. MedRxiv. 2020.

[4] 张彦平,等. 新型冠状病毒肺炎流行病学特征分析. 中国流行病学杂志,2020,41(2):145-151.

[5] Wei M, et al. Novel Coronavirus Infection in Hospitalized Infants Under 1 Year of Age in China. JAMA. 2020.

[6] Chen H, et al. Clinical characteristics and intrauterine vertical transmission potential of COVID-19 infection in nine pregnant women: a retrospective review of medical records. The Lancet,2020.

[7] Holshue ML, et al. First Case of 2019 Novel Coronavirus in the United States. N Engl J Med,2020.

[8] Xu Z, et al. Pathological findings of COVID-19 associated with acute respiratory distress syndrome. Lancet Respir Med,2020,S2213-2600.

[9] Guan WJ, et al. Clinical Characteristics of Coronavirus Disease 2019 in China. N Engl J Med,2020.

[10] 张文宏,等. 上海市2019冠状病毒病综合救治专家共识.

[11] 中华医学会呼吸病学分会. 中国成人社区获得性肺炎诊断和治疗指南(2016年版). 中华结核和呼吸杂志,2016,39(4):1-27.

4 当前支原体肺炎诊治中面临的困难和挑战

佘丹阳

肺炎支原体是社区获得性肺炎(community-acquired pneumonia,CAP)最常见的病原体。一项全球性的 CAP 病原学调查结果显示,CAP 中支原体肺炎占 12%,在所有非典型病原体 CAP 中所占的比例超过了 50%。与大多数国外地区相比,我国肺炎支原体肺炎的发病率更高。在迄今为止我国仅有的两项全国性成人 CAP 调查中,支原体肺炎的比例分别达到了 20.7% 和 38.9%,肺炎支原体的感染率已经超过了肺炎链球菌,成为 CAP 最常见的致病原。典型的支原体肺炎表现为发热、干咳、外周血白细胞总数和中性粒细胞比例正常、肺内单发或多发斑片影、大环内酯抗生素治疗有效,既往临床识别和治疗并不困难。但是,近年来,延误诊断或初始治疗失败的支原体肺炎病例日益多见,严重者甚至导致呼吸衰竭、危及生命。

1. 当前支原体肺炎的诊治中主要面临以下四个方面的困难

(1) 影像表现复杂多样。基于普通 X 线胸片的早期研究结果通常将支原体肺炎描述为以多发斑片渗出影为主要影像表现的支气管肺炎或小叶性肺炎,但是,通过病理组织学研究和高分辨 CT 检查发现,支原体肺炎的影像表现其实相当复杂,包括由于支气管周围、血管周围单核细胞浸润导致支气管血管束增厚、小气道细胞性支气管炎伴管腔内渗出物或肉芽组织填充导致的小叶中心性结节(伴或不伴树芽征)、肺泡腔内渗出物和中性粒细胞聚集导致的磨玻璃样斑片影和实变。在这些影像表现中,支气管血管束增厚、小叶中心性结节(伴或不伴树芽征)和磨玻璃密度渗出影等征象由于更具特征性而更受重视,但发生率并不低的实变却往往容易被忽略。有研究显示,61% 的支原体肺炎中存在实变,这一比例在统计学上并不低于肺炎链球菌肺炎,在进展期支原体肺炎中,特征性的支气管管壁增厚、小叶中心性结节等表现并不常见,实变尤其是叶段实变往往是支原体肺炎进展期(重症)的重要影像表现。日本的一项回顾性研究的结果显示,在 52 例暴发性支原体肺炎中,20 例(38.5%)患者有叶段实变表现,其中 13 例(25%)以叶段实变为唯一影像学表现。在韩国最近的一项研究中,5~18 岁的青少年支原体肺炎患者中叶段实变的发生率高达 44%(89/200)。但是,在实际工作中,相当数量的临床医师常常倾向于把叶段实变作为鉴别细菌性肺炎与包括支原体肺炎在内的所谓"非典型肺炎"的重要影像学依据,从而导致此类以叶段实变为主要影像表现的支原体肺炎延误诊断。

(2) 缺乏早期快速诊断技术。目前国内绝大多数医院主要依靠血清特异性抗体检测来诊断支原体肺炎,其弊端是显而易见的,因为只有急性期和恢复期双份血清抗体滴度 4 倍或 4 倍以上变化才有确诊价值,而肺炎支原体感染后出现较早的特异性 IgM 抗体也往往在感染后的 7~10d 才转为阳性,特异性 IgG 抗体阳性的时间则更晚。有学者曾经用 RT-PCR 的检测结果对国际上普遍使用的 12 种商用肺炎支原体 IgM 试剂盒进行了评价,结果发现,在发病后 6d 内,多数肺炎支原体 IgM 试剂盒的阳性率均不到 10%,阳性率最高者也不到 30%,所以,国内的绝大多数医院实际上都不能够实现支原体肺炎的早期确诊。对于临床和影像表现比较经典的病例尚可依据经验早期识别,而对临床和影像表现不典型的病例或者混合感染的病例则很容易出现诊断延误。

(3) 肺炎支原体与其他致病原的混合感染比较普遍。在社区获得性肺炎中,混合感染的比例占 10%~20%,住院患者中混合感染的比例比门诊患者高,重症肺炎中混合感染的比例比轻中症患者高。根据我国成人社区获得性肺炎的流调结果,肺炎支原体与其他致病原的混合感染是社区获得性肺炎中最为常见的混合感染类型。韩国最近的一项研究显示,在流感相关肺炎接受肺炎支原体感染检测的患者中,肺炎支原体的阳性率达到了 16.8%。当肺炎支原体与细菌等其他致病原混合感染时,支原体肺炎的临床特征和影像特征常被掩盖,很容易导致对致病原预判的不全面和初始经验性治疗的失败。

(4) 大环内酯抗生素耐药情况严重。大环内酯抗生素曾经是治疗支原体肺炎的首选药物。但是,自 2001 年日本首先从儿童患者的下呼吸道标本中分离到大环内酯耐药肺炎支原体菌株以来,全球范围内肺炎支原体对大环内酯抗生素的耐药率一直呈逐渐上升的趋势,根据最近的调查结果,北美地区已经超过了 10%,欧洲各国之间差别较大,意大利、英国已经达到了 20% 左右,东亚地区是全球肺炎支原体大环内酯抗生素耐药情况最为严重的地区,其中,日本和中国肺炎支原体对大环内酯抗生素的耐药率均已达到了 90% 左右,而且我国肺炎支原体对大环内酯抗生素的耐药水平普遍为高水平耐药。就经验性治疗而言,如果不了解我国肺炎支原体的这种耐药特点,一旦大环内酯类抗生素初始治疗失败就轻易排除支原体肺炎的诊断,很可能导致诊断和有效治疗的进一步延误。就目标性治疗而言,大环内酯类抗生素治疗失败不仅会导致支原体肺炎的退热时间和抗感染疗程的延长,少数患者也会因为得不到及时有效的治疗而进展为重症肺炎,甚至危及生命。

2. 临床医师应对措施　在实际的临床工作中,上述4个方面的问题常交织在一起,干扰临床医生的判断,不仅影响社区获得性肺炎治疗前的病原学分析和初始治疗方案的选择,增加初始治疗失败的风险,在初始抗感染治疗失败时,还会给分析治疗失败的原因和调整抗感染治疗方案增加难度。对此,临床医生应有充分认识。①要重视支原体肺炎影像表现的复杂性,避免简单地以是否存在叶段实变来鉴别支原体肺炎和细菌性肺炎,要警惕大叶性实变可能是支原体肺炎病情进展的征象。②要正确应用和解读肺炎支原体相关病原学检测的结果,在病程早期不要仅仅根据血清学检测结果阴性就排除支原体肺炎,对于怀疑暴发性支原体肺炎的重症患者应及早进行核酸检测。③要重视社区获得性肺炎中的混合感染问题,警惕细菌感染掩盖肺炎支原体感染的可能,对于抗细菌治疗后一般情况改善或部分改善但退热缓慢的患者,应及时进行肺炎支原体感染相关的病原学检查;在社区获得性肺炎的治疗中,选择初始治疗方案和进行疗效评估时应充分考虑大环内酯类抗生素耐药的影响,大多数情况下,大环内酯类药初治失败并不能排除支原体肺炎。对于大环内酯类药初治失败的支原体肺炎,可用于替换的抗菌药物包括呼吸喹诺酮类药物、四环素类药物(包括替加环素)。与大环内酯类抗生素严峻的耐药形势相比,呼吸喹诺酮类药物和四环素类抗生素对肺炎支原体仍然保持了很好的体外抗菌活性。迄今为止,在国内外现有的研究中尚未发现对这两类抗菌药物耐药的肺炎支原体菌株。对于成人支原体肺炎患者而言,大环内酯类抗生素初治失败者原则上宜及早换用四环素类药物或呼吸喹诺酮类药物;对于儿童或青少年肺炎支原体肺炎患者,8岁以上患者可以优先考虑换用四环素类药物,8岁以下目前国内尚无说明书批准、安全有效的抗菌药物可以替换大环内酯类抗生素,所以应在审慎评估病情进展的风险和药物不良反应的风险后决定是继续大环内酯类抗生素治疗,还是换用其他药物。

参 考 文 献

[1] Waites KB, Xiao L, Liu Y, et al. Mycoplasma pneumoniae from the Respiratory Tract and Beyond. Clin Microbiol Rev, 2017,30(3):747-809.

[2] Sharma L, Losier A, Tolbert T, et al. Atypical Pneumonia: Updates on Legionella, Chlamydophila, and Mycoplasma Pneumonia. Clin Chest Med,2017,38(1):45-58.

[3] Arnold FW, Summersgill JT, LaJoie AS, et al. A worldwide perspective of atypical pathogens in community-acquired pneumonia. Am J Respir Crit Care Med, 2007; 175: 1086-1093.

[4] 刘又宁,赵铁梅,陈民钧,等. 中国城市成人社区获得性肺炎665例病原学多中心调查. 中华结核和呼吸杂志,2006,29(1):3-9.

[5] Tao LL, Hu BJ, He LX, et al. Etiology and antimicrobial resistance of community-acquired pneumonia in adult patients in China. Chin Med J(Engl),2012,125(17):2967-2972.

[6] Miyashita N, Sugiu T, Kawai Y, et al. Radiographic features of Mycoplasma pneumoniae pneumonia: differential diagnosis and performance timing. BMC Med Imaging,2009,9:7.

[7] Izumikawa K, Izumikawa K, Takazono T, et al. Clinical features, risk factors and treatment of fulminant Mycoplasma pneumoniae pneumonia: a review of the Japanese literature. J Infect Chemother,2014,20(3):181-185.

[8] Kim JH, Kwon JH, Lee JY, et al. Clinical features of Mycoplasma pneumoniae coinfection and need for its testing in influenza pneumonia patients. J Thorac Dis, 2018, 10(11): 6118-6127.

[9] Kishaba T. Community-Acquired Pneumonia Caused by Mycoplasma pneumoniae: How Physical and Radiological Examination Contribute to Successful Diagnosis. Front Med (Lausanne),2016,3:28.

[10] Tanaka H. Correlation between Radiological and Pathological Findings in Patients with Mycoplasma pneumoniae Pneumonia. Front Microbiol,2016,7:695.

[11] Cho YJ, Han MS, Kim WS, et al. Correlation between chest radiographic findings and clinical features in hospitalized children with Mycoplasma pneumoniae pneumonia. PLoS One, 2019,14(8):e0219463.

[12] Evaluation of 12 commercial tests and the complement fixation test for Mycoplasma pneumoniae-specific immunoglobulin G(IgG) and IgM antibodies, with PCR used as the "gold standard". J Clin Microbiol,2005,43(5):2277-2285.

[13] Cao B, Qu JX, Yin YD, et al. Overview of antimicrobial options for Mycoplasma pneumoniae pneumonia: focus on macrolide resistance. Clin Respir J,2017,11(4):419-429.

5 支气管镜技术在肺部感染的应用进展

姜淑娟

近年来,随着造血干细胞移植(HSCT)、实体器官移植的广泛开展、高强度免疫抑制剂和大剂量化疗药物的应用及各种导管的体内介入与留置等,肺部感染如侵袭性真菌感染、难治性细菌感染、病毒感染及结核感染等的发病率逐年上升。传统的痰镜检及培养已不能满足临床精准诊治的要求。

支气管镜技术是呼吸专业的看家本领,但是在肺部感染领域尚有较大进步空间,其优势在于可直视下发现气道内病变并进行活检或刷检、吸引病变部位气道内炎性分泌物或保护毛刷、支气管肺灌洗检查等。支气管镜在肺部感染中的应用不仅限于诊断,在与非感染性疾病的鉴别诊断及感染的治疗方面也发挥着不可替代的作用。

一、支气管镜在肺部感染中的诊断价值

传统的病原微生物检测方法主要包括形态学检测、培养分离、生化检测、免疫学和核酸检测。这些方法收到诸多内在和外在因素的影响,导致其阳性率较低。宏基因组新一代测序技术(mNGS)直接对临床样本中的核酸进行高通量测序,然后与数据库进行比对分析,根据比对到的序列信息来判断样本包含的病原微生物种类(包括病毒、细菌、真菌、寄生虫),且无须特异性扩增。

宏基因组学(metagenomics)最早是在 1998 年由 Handelsman 等提出的。临床也称之为二代测序、宏基因组测序、高通量测序。其主要优势:没有偏移性、广覆盖,高效率。主要用于临床的标本病原学检测,定植还是感染,预测耐药等几个方面。

规范留取标本主要是痰液和肺泡灌洗液(BALF)的留取。BALF 的留取可参考《肺部感染性疾病支气管肺泡灌洗病原体检测中国专家共识(2017 年版)》。其中有几点注意事项:①充分麻醉,适当镇静,灌洗液预热,避免咳嗽,增加回收量。②回收液体过程中吸引负压过大可能导致远端气道塌陷或气道黏膜损伤,降低回吸收率或改变 BALF 的组分。③注意注入灌洗液注入的速度。④重症感染患者,要保证其通气与氧合。

mNGS 有助于肺部感染的精准诊断,但仍需结合临床。有时候需与培养和 PCR 技术相结合。为了提高阳性率,也可取活检组织进行 mNGS 检测,意义可能会更大。

二、支气管镜在肺部感染中的鉴别诊断价值

肺部感染性疾病需要与非感染性疾病相鉴别。发热伴肺部阴影常见的非感染性疾病包括:肺癌、血液系统疾病、结缔组织疾病、间质性肺疾病、血管炎、过敏性肺炎、放射学肺炎、肺水肿、肺栓塞等。其中良性疾病主要包括支气管异物合并感染、肺隔离症、肺动脉栓塞、放射性肺炎、肺出血、COP 等;恶性疾病包括肺炎型肺癌、肺淋巴瘤、肺转移瘤等。这些疾病均存在与感染性疾病类似的临床或影像表现。

支气管镜在此类疾病的鉴别诊断中起到了举足轻重的作用。尤其是支气管异物合并感染、COP、肺炎型肺癌、肺淋巴瘤、肺转移瘤等疾病的鉴别。采用目前常规的 TBLB、TBNA、EBUS-TBNA、GS 等支气管镜操作技术,往往能取得明确的病理诊断。

三、支气管镜在肺部感染中的治疗价值

支气管镜在肺部感染中的治疗作用主要包括吸痰、痰痂祛除、支气管冲洗、支气管镜药物灌注治疗及炎性气道狭窄的治疗。

支气管镜药物灌注治疗目前尚不成熟。两性霉素 B 静脉应用有较为严重的毒副作用,限制了其在临床上的应用。但是两性霉素 B 在临床是可以雾化吸入的。

局部应用两性霉素 B 可能避免静脉应用所引起的肝肾功能损伤,可能减少患者经济费用及缩短住院天数。经支气管镜支气管肺泡灌洗术已成为治疗重症肺部感染的重要手段,与传统治疗手段比较,支气管镜肺泡灌洗可以冲洗阻塞支气管的黏稠分泌物,保持气道通畅;将药物直接送入肺部感染组织,保证局部药物浓度处于有效杀菌范围。

我科在部分慢性肺真菌病患者中应用两性霉素 B 注射液进行支气管内注射治疗,获得一定疗效。但截至目前,尚没有相关数据支持,仍需大规模的对照试验证实。

吸入用乙酰半胱氨酸溶液支气管灌洗治疗,可以使乙酰半胱氨酸直接到达支气管内炎症部位,并保留一定时间,可提高局部药物浓度。支气管镜反复灌洗,可清除炎

症病灶的分泌物、病原体、痰液,改善气道阻塞症状。对于大量脓性痰或痰栓形成的肺部感染患者,吸入用乙酰半胱氨酸溶液支气管灌洗治疗有良好的疗效。但目前也缺乏循证医学证据支持。

参 考 文 献

[1] Henan Li. Detection of Pulmonary Infectious Pathogens From Lung Biopsy Tissues by Metagenomic Next-Generation Sequencing. Frontiers in Cellular and Infection Microbiology, 2018,8:205.

[2] Next-Generation Sequencing in Clinical Microbiology. Stephanie L. Gu W, Miller S, Chiu CY. Clinical metagenomic next-generation sequencing for pathogen detection. Annu Rev Pathol,2019,14:319-338.

[3] Tamma PD, Fan Y, Bergman Y, et al. Applying rapid whole-genome sequencing to predict phenotypic antimicrobial susceptibility testing results among carbapenem-resistant Klebsiella pneumoniae clinical isolates. Antimicrob Agents Chemother,2019,63(1).

[4] Langelier C, Kalantar KL, Moazed F, et al. Integrating host response and unbiased microbe detection for lower respiratory tract infection diagnosis in critically ill adults. Proc Natl Acad Sci USA,2018,115(52):E12353-12362.

[5] 卢鑫,孙文逵,高伟,等.雾化吸入两性霉素 B 对侵袭性肺曲霉病预防效果的 Meta 分析.中国呼吸与危重症监护杂志,2012,11(1):28-36.

[6] 隋玲玲,路丽红,孟昭斌.抗菌药物降阶梯疗法联合支气管肺泡灌洗术治疗急性脑梗死患者肺部感染的临床疗效.中华医院感染学杂志,2015,25(20):4679-4681.

[7] 张海英.支气管肺泡灌洗对老年肺部感染性疾病的诊断运用评价.实用临床医药杂志,2015,19(17):82-83.

[8] 杨永.经纤维支气管镜支气管肺泡灌洗抗真菌药治疗肺部真菌感染临床观察.中国实用医刊,2015,42(18):30-31.

[9] 乙酰半胱氨酸溶液联合纤维支气管镜肺泡灌洗方案治疗重症肺炎患者的临床效果.国际感染病学(电子版),2020,9(1):65.

[10] 电子纤维支气管镜保留灌注乙酰半胱氨酸及布地奈德治疗儿童难治性支原体肺炎的临床效果观察.中国医药,2020,15(3)369-373.

6 重症甲流的肺外损伤机制

范红 童翔

一、概论

甲型流感病毒感染（简称甲流）是由流感A病毒感染导致的急性呼吸道疾病，既可引起零星感染，也可导致人群大流行。甲型流感病毒感染的临床表现可以从无症状感染到暴发性起病，症状可表现为发热、寒战、头痛、肌痛、全身乏力和厌食等，常伴有呼吸道症状，如咳嗽、流涕和咽痛等。尽管它在一般人群中常是一种自限性感染疾病（无并发症的流感），但在高风险人群（如结构性肺病、免疫低下宿主、老年人、婴幼儿）中可发展成重症，通常还容易合并一系列全身并发症，致死亡率增加。但是，甲流合并肺外脏器损伤致病机制具体尚不清楚，值得深入探索。此外，通过对甲流合并肺外脏器损伤机制的探讨也将对新冠病毒的致病机制提供重要的借鉴和提示。本文通过文献回顾将重症甲流合并肺外损伤时可能的病理机制简单总结如下。

二、重症甲流肺损伤机制

甲流主要并发症是肺炎，在慢性疾病患者和免疫低下人群中最常见，包括原发性病毒性肺炎，继发性细菌性肺炎或两者混合。甲型流感病毒感染可以分为三个阶段，首先是病毒侵入感染呼吸道和肺泡上皮，并在这些细胞中的复制。第二阶段是对病毒的适应性免疫反应，对病毒的清除具有重要作用，但也会对肺泡上皮和内皮细胞造成损害。第三阶段是对感染病毒株的长期免疫的发展伴随着受损肺组织的浸润和再生，在此期间容易继发性细菌感染。

在上述阶段中，多种信号通路和炎症介质包括Toll样受体（TLR）、NF-κB、白介素、维甲酸诱导基因-1（RIG-1）蛋白质和炎症小体等参与其中，这些免疫相关的应答反应既能促进病毒清除，但也可能导致组织损伤。其中，流感病毒感染导致上、下呼吸道基底膜大面积剥落、肺泡毛细血管屏障被破坏，肺上皮细胞肿胀与坏死、肺泡内纤维蛋白积聚和氧化磷脂（OxPLs）的生成，肺精细微结构丧失，致肺塌陷和不张。大量炎性介质释放还进一步导致免疫损伤的激活和恶化。肺泡内，双潜能肺泡上皮细胞的祖细胞和肺泡Ⅱ型细胞被认为是修复过程中的干/祖细胞，固有淋巴细胞在黏膜表面的维持和再生也具有重要作用。如何快速有效地控制病毒复制并减轻宿主的过度免疫反应是呼吸界的难题，值得未来不断探索。

三、重症甲流肾脏损伤机制

甲型流感病毒感染相关的肾脏并发症并不罕见，其可导致死亡风险增加、住院时间延长及慢性肾脏疾病的发生。研究报道，因感染H1N1入院的患者中急性肾损伤的发病率约为33%。甲型流感病毒感染相关肾损伤主要包括横纹肌溶解综合征、溶血性尿毒症综合征、弥散性血管内凝血、Goodpasture综合征、急性肾小球肾炎、急性肾小管坏死，以及重症患者的急性肾损伤（acute kidney injury, AKI）。重症甲型流感病毒感染患者肾脏并发症以AKI多见。在接受机械通气、入住重症监护室的甲流感染患者中，AKI发生率高达50%，AKI的发生与甲型流感患者死亡率增加密切相关。

重症甲型流感病毒感染患者并发AKI的易感因素包括多个方面。与AKI相关的患者基础条件包括：患者年龄、糖尿病史、肥胖、哮喘病史、慢性肾脏病史、妊娠、吸烟史；与AKI相关的器官功能障碍包括：需要机械通气或呼吸功能障碍、使用血管升压药或心血管功能障碍、休克、血液功能障碍、较高的急性生理和慢性健康Ⅱ评分、较高的器官功能衰竭评分、较高的Murray评分；与AKI相关的实验室检查包括：肌酸激酶水平升高、严重酸中毒、C反应蛋白水平升高、乳酸脱氢酶水平升高、血小板减少。

虽然重症甲型流感病毒引起AKI的发病机制尚未完全阐明，但以下因素被认为参与了AKI的发生发展：急性肾小管坏死、弥散性血管内凝血导致的肾小球微血栓形成及病毒对肾脏的直接损害。其中，多个尸检结果表明，急性肾小管坏死可能是导致甲型流感病毒感染相关AKI的最重要机制。在甲型流感病毒感染导致严重的全身性炎症反应伴细胞因子级联的情况下，肾脏灌注不足、肾血管收缩和横纹肌溶解可能同时但不同程度地发生，其均可导致肾脏急性肾小管坏死。此外，在部分患者肾脏中，也呈现出弥散性血管内凝血和病毒的复制，但目前尚无证据表明病毒对肾脏的直接损伤。

目前重症甲型流感病毒感染导致的AKI的治疗主要以抗病毒治疗、维持内环境稳定、营养支持、防治并发症和肾脏替代治疗为主，尽早纠正病因即抗病毒治疗是促进肾功能恢复的前提条件。此外（美国）免疫实践咨询委员会（the Advisory Committee on Immunization Practices, ACIP）建议,年龄6个月以上且无禁忌证的人群每年常规接种流感疫苗,其可降低接种者罹患流感和发生严重并发症的风险。同时对有流感高危因素的密切接触者(并且未接种疫苗或接种疫苗后尚未获得免疫力)可进行暴露后药物预防。除疫苗和药物外,保持良好的个人卫生也是预防流感的重要手段,主要措施包括:勤洗手,保持室内通风,在流感流行季节尽量减少到人群密集场所活动,咳嗽或打喷嚏时用纸巾遮住口鼻,咳嗽或打喷嚏后及时洗手,出现流感样症状应注意自我隔离,及时就医。

四、重症甲流心血管损伤机制

甲流感染时可通过病毒对心肌的直接影响或导致现有心血管疾病的加重而造成心脏损伤。流感流行与心血管死亡率之间存在关联,而接种流感疫苗后,高风险患者的心血管死亡率有所下降,且流感是公认的心肌炎的重要原因,可导致严重的心脏功能损害和死亡。

心血管损伤是流感过程中的较常见的并发症事件,发病率可高达10%。在一项英国的研究中,152名具有血清学证据的流感染的患者,发现18名患者的CK水平升高(12%)。另一项研究显示30名既往健康、没有已知心血管疾病的年轻人,流感抗原试验阳性,在发病后第1天、第4天、第11天和第28天,分别有53%、33%、27%和23%患者的心电图出现异常。在41例血清学确认为甲型流感的患者中,有6例患者出现急性心肌炎和异常心电图,超声心动图显示这6例患者均有局部心肌功能障碍,且其中3例患者CK-MB同工酶升高。因此,与流感相关的心电图改变通常提示心肌受累,但常是轻症。另一研究显示624例急性病毒性心肌炎患者中,对心脏样本进行PCR检测,鉴定出238名(38%)患者的病毒基因组,发现其中有5个样本(2%)属于甲流。我国的一项回顾性研究发现,2009年甲型H1N1流感危重症患者中CK、CK-MB、hs-CRP及心胸比均较轻症组和重症组高,早期进行分子生物学检测和X线胸片检查有助于发现患者早期的心肌损害。

目前流感引起心肌疾病的具体机制尚未完全阐明,普遍认为心肌损伤过程主要与免疫应答过度维持有关。研究表明,$CD4^+$淋巴细胞亚群(辅助性T细胞1型和2型)的平衡决定了心肌炎的免疫应答特征,这种平衡在免疫初期是重要的,而细胞毒性$CD8^+$淋巴细胞直接参与心肌损伤。活化淋巴细胞克隆清除障碍与心功能不全程度相关,可能是心肌炎进展的机制之一,调节性细胞因子网络系统的失衡或缺陷也可能导致潜在的自身反应性T淋巴细胞的激活。促炎细胞因子,包括肿瘤坏死因子-α(TNF-α),也被认为是炎症性心肌病发生和延续的重要生理致病因子,并可能影响心功能不全的严重程度。此外,向动脉粥样硬化小鼠模型[(apoE(-/-),载脂蛋白E缺陷小鼠]注射甲型流感病毒可导致小鼠动脉粥样硬化斑块中明显的炎症、平滑肌细胞增殖、浅表血小板聚集和偶发的血栓下纤维蛋白血栓,表明流感可以促进了动脉粥样硬化斑块的炎症、平滑肌细胞增殖和纤维蛋白沉积,从而导致心血管损伤。也有个案报道显示流感病毒可以直接造成了心肌细胞的损伤。目前少有关流感并发心血管损伤时治疗的系统研究,其中很大程度主要是支持性治疗为主,包括循环稳定、病毒清除、抗感染治疗等。

五、重症甲流肝损伤机制

甲型流感病毒可以侵犯呼吸道、胃肠道、胰腺等黏膜组织和器官,然而部分患者诊治过程中可出现非黏膜脏器受累并造成肝肾等器官损伤,累及肝脏多是短暂、自限的,主要表现为血清转氨酶和(或)总胆红素水平升高,重症患者则可能出现凝血异常、血氨升高等肝衰竭表现。甲流合并肝损伤的发病情况尚缺乏大规模的流行病学数据,有研究报道,国内甲流合并肝损伤的发生率为12.2%~43.8%,而重症甲流患者中肝损伤的发生率可能更高。

关于重症甲流导致肝损伤的具体机制尚不明确,可能与病毒的直接侵犯或者系统性炎性反应的激活有关。重症甲流往往伴随高水平的鼻咽部病毒载量和持续的病毒血症,一方面,病毒随血液循环进入肝脏,直接造成细胞损伤。一项重症甲流患者的多脏器病理研究发现,病毒主要分布于坏死和损伤区域的肝细胞、血管内皮细胞、肝窦上皮细胞及巨噬细胞内,而损伤轻微和结构完整的细胞中病毒较少。另一项研究结果显示,小鼠肝内流感病毒载量与肝脏组织学损伤的严重程度呈正相关,提示我们病毒在肝脏的复制可能是肝损伤的原因之一。另一方面,病毒的持续存在激活细胞免疫。有研究发现,在流感相关性肝炎的发病过程中,凋亡的肝细胞、流感特异性$CD8^+$T淋巴细胞和Kupffer细胞参与了肝内病灶形成和肝细胞破坏。流感病毒再次感染时,肝脏损伤与Kupffer细胞耗竭及免疫反应过程中产生的流感特异性T细胞的动力学和数量有关,肝炎是活化的$CD8^+$T淋巴细胞扩散和肝内滞留的直接后果,活化的$CD8^+$T淋巴细胞和Kupffer细胞相互作用进一步加重了肝细胞损伤。此外,Papic等发现,甲型流感感染期间血清肝酶的异常与低氧血症有关。重症甲流感染会导致呼吸衰竭和细胞因子风暴,进而导致肝脏供氧突然减少,出现缺氧性肝炎,表现为继发于缺氧性小叶中心性坏死的肝转氨酶突然急剧升高。最后,甲流患者中细菌共感染并不少见,并且与肝功能损害相关,然而目前缺乏足够研究,上述机制可能在细菌共感染的过程中得到进一步加强从而加重甲流患者的肝功能损害。综上,甲型流感病毒不仅能够直接感染肺组织,引起病毒性肺炎,而且可以影响肝脏功能,造成肝细胞损伤和功能衰竭,导致患者病情加重和死亡。

六、重症甲流脑损伤机制

流感感染可以伴随一些中枢神经系统疾病,包括瑞氏综合征(Reye's syndrome),流感相关脑炎/脑病(influenza-associated encephalitis/encephalopathy,IAE),发热性癫痫,脊髓炎和吉兰-巴雷综合征等,以儿童常见,主要表现为意思障碍、抽搐、呕吐、头痛、运动麻痹及感觉丧失等。

Reye综合征,是与流感流行相关的最著名的脑病之一,以服用水杨酸类药物(如阿司匹林)为重要病因,经典的Reye综合征通常与B型流感有关。广泛的线粒体受损为其病理基础。Reye综合征会影响身体的所有器官,但对肝脏和大脑带来的危害最大,患者常出现低血糖和(或)高氨血症。但应注意的是,一些非水杨酸解热药,如双氯芬酸钠和美芬那酯,可能与流感相关脑炎/脑病的发生有关,或影响疾病的严重程度。

IAE是一种快速进行性脑病,出现在流感感染的早期阶段。由于中枢神经系统缺乏炎症,IAE一直被称为流感相关性急性脑病,包括急性坏死性脑病(acute necrotizing encephalitis,ANE)。1995年Mizuguchi等发现,流感患儿,尤其是小于5岁的流感患儿,常合并脑炎,首先描述了急性坏死性脑炎。在随后的流感暴发和大流行期间,ANE在儿科人群中反复出现。相比之下,成人发病少见。流感相关脑炎/脑病的发病机制尚不清楚,可能的机制如下:①流感病毒直接入侵脑实质。Fujimoto等用RT-PCR方法检测了7个流感患者,其中有5人脑脊液中检测到了病毒RNA。然而,更多的报告显示,在大多数流感相关脑炎/脑病患者的脑脊液中未检测到病毒RNA。病理显示,在脑组织中缺乏可检测的病毒抗原,也表明病毒的直接侵袭和炎症不太可能是本病的病因。疾病进展似乎太快,病毒无法直接侵入中枢神经系统,并在中枢神经系统组织中复制,造成脑损伤。所以,这仍是一个有争议的问题。②细胞因子风暴(cytokine storm)是IAE最为可能的发病机制。人体免疫系统过度激活导致的"细胞因子风暴"学说常在IAE的文献中提出。细胞因子风暴是指机体感染微生物后引起体液中多种细胞因子迅速大量的产生,如TNF-α、IL-1、IL-6、IL-12、IFN-α、IFN-β、IFN-γ、MCP-1和IL-8等,标志着一种不受控制和功能失调的免疫反应,涉及淋巴细胞和巨噬细胞的持续激活和扩增。细胞因子通过改变血管通透性导致脑损伤,导致肝脏和肾脏等多个器官损伤,发生弥散性血管内凝血。转氨酶和乳酸脱氢酶水平升高,全身血管损伤且进展迅速,多器官衰竭提示高细胞因子血症对血管或血管内皮的损伤可能在流感相关脑炎/脑病发病机制中起重要作用。这些特征通常见于病毒相关性噬血细胞综合征或全身性炎症反应综合征。流式细胞仪分析发现,在ANE恢复期患者外周血淋巴细胞中,CD56$^+$自然杀伤(NK)细胞比例增加,这些细胞产生高水平的细胞因子。在流感相关脑炎/脑病中,几种细胞因子,如可溶性TNF受体-1、IL-1β和IL-6在流感患者血清和脑脊液升高。许多促炎细胞因子,如IL-6,与IAE严重程度正相关。IL-6和TNF-α,可以诱导血管内皮细胞、胶质细胞、神经元凋亡,损伤血脑屏障,增加血脑屏障通透性从而引起脑水肿和损伤、中枢神经系统紊乱和(或)全身性症状。③遗传背景可能有一定的相关性。IAE首先被学者在日本发现提出。IAE和川崎病有类似的地方,如炎症反应和心血管损伤,所以有学者提出,日本人可能有促进全身炎症反应或高细胞因子血症的遗传背景,因此,更容易患流感相关性脑炎的倾向/脑病。一位母亲和她的女儿在患甲型H1N1流感后都出现急性脑病,表明IAE可能存在遗传易感性。目前尚不清楚是否有某些遗传背景的患者对IAE更敏感。Ran结合基因2(RANBP2)的突变表现为家族性或复发性病毒性ANE。人类白细胞抗原(HLA)DRB/HLADQB基因可能参与了ANE的发病机制。④其他可能的机制。有些IAE患者出现肝和(或)肾功能不全,例如血清肌酐和天冬氨酸转氨酶升高,血尿或蛋白尿;在某些病例中,还报告了低血红素血症、弥散性血管内凝血(DIC)和血清CD40配体降低,因此,代谢紊乱和凝血障碍也可能参与IAE的发病机制。

重症甲流合并脑损伤治疗方面,尚不明确。首先,因为IAE是由流感病毒感染引起的,抗病毒奥司他韦磷酸盐治疗必要的,有学者推荐对于重症IAE给药高剂量奥司他韦治疗。其次,亚低温治疗和抗细胞因子药物可能对重度IAE治疗有效。最后,应对重症甲流合并脑损伤患者进行必要的支持治疗。

七、小 结

综上所述,目前重症甲流肺外损伤机制不完全清楚,可能主要聚焦于以下几方面:第一,病毒直接损伤靶器官,造成结构破坏及功能丧失;第二,流感引发的宿主免疫应答并过度反应或持续存在,造成组织免疫损伤;第三,流感继发的细菌感染、凝血功能障碍等异常病理生理过程可以对已损伤的组织造成进一步打击,导致损伤恶化。针对重症甲流肺外损伤治疗,主要以抗病毒、脏器支持、抗炎、免疫调节等为主,此外接种流感疫苗可能是预防重症甲流及肺外损伤最有效的手段。

参 考 文 献

[1] Iwasaki A, Pillai PS. Innate immunity to influenza virus infection. Nat Rev Immunol, 2014, 14: 315-328.

[2] Thomas PG, Dash P, Aldridge JR, et al. The intracellular sensor NLRP3 mediates key innate and healing responses to influenza A virus via the regulation of caspase-1. Immunity, 2009, 30: 566-575.

[3] Leeman KT, Fillmore CM, Kim CF. Lung stem and progenitor cells in tissue homeostasis and disease. Curr Top Dev Biol, 2014, 107: 207-233.

[4] Desai TJ, Brownfield DG, Krasnow MA. Alveolar progenitor and stem cells in lung development, renewal and cancer. Nature, 2014, 507: 190-194.

[5] Asaka M, Ishikawa I, Nakazawa T, Tomosugi N, Yuri T, Suzuki K. Hemolytic uremic syndrome associated with influenza A virus infection in an adult renal allograft recipient: case report and review of the literature. Nephron, 2000, 84(3): 258-266.

[6] Koegelenberg CF, Irusen EM, Cooper R, et al. High mortality from respiratory failure secondary to swine-origin influenza A (H1N1) in South Africa. QJM: monthly journal of the Asso-

ciation of Physicians,2010,103(5):319-325.
[7] Watanabe T. Renal complications of seasonal and pandemic influenza A virus infections. Eur J Pediatr, 2013, 172(1): 15-22.
[8] Bal A,Suri V,Mishra B,et al. Pathology and virology findings in cases of fatal influenza A H1N1 virus infection in 2009-2010. Histopathology,2012,60(2):326-335.
[9] Ayala E, Kagawa FT, Wehner JH, Tam J, Upadhyay D. Rhabdomyolysis associated with 2009 influenza A(H1N1). JAMA,2009,302(17):1863-1864.
[10] Greaves K,Oxford JS,Price CP,et al. The prevalence of myocarditis and skeletal muscle injury during acute viral infection in adults: measurement of cardiac troponins I and T in 152 patients with acute influenza infection. Arch Intern Med, 2003,163(2):165-168.
[11] Ison MG,Campbell V,Rembold C,Dent J,Hayden FG. Cardiac findings during uncomplicated acute influenza in ambulatory adults. Clin Infect Dis,2005,40:415-422.
[12] Karjalainen J, Nieminen MS, Heikkila J. Influenza A1 myocarditis in conscripts. Acta Med Scand, 1980, 207 (1-2): 27-30.
[13] Bowles NE,N Ji,Kearney DL,et al. Detection of viruses in myocardialtissues by polymerase chain reaction: evidence of adenovirus as a common cause of myocarditis in children and adults. JACC,2003,42(3):466-472.
[14] 张天奇,王齐齐,吴涛,等.甲型H1N1流感患者心肌损害的研究.心脑血管病防治,2014,2:135-136.
[15] Calabrese F,Carturan E,Chimenti C,et al. Overexpression of tumor necrosis factor(TNF)alpha and TNFalpha receptor I in human viral myocarditis: clinicopathologic correlations. Mod Pathol,2004,17(9):1108-1118.
[16] Naghavi, M. Influenza Infection Exerts Prominent Inflammatory and Thrombotic Effects on the Atherosclerotic Plaques of Apolipoprotein E-Deficient Mice. Circulation, 2003, 107 (5):762-768.
[17] Whitworth JR,Mack CL,O"Connor JA,et al. Acute hepatitis and liver failure associated with influenza A infection in children. J Pediatr Gastroenterol Nutr,2006,43(4):536-538.
[18] 周大明,姜继军,宗文宏,等,甲型H1N1流感合并肝损害的临床特点分析,中华肝脏病杂志,2010,18(12):940-941.
[19] Zhang Y M,Liu J M,Yu L,et al. Prevalence and characteristics of hypoxic hepatitis in the largest singlecentre cohort of avian influenza A(H7N9)virus-infected patients with severe liver impairment in the intensive care unit. Emerging Microbes & Infections,2016,5(1):e1.
[20] Zhang S,Hu B,Xu J,et al. Influenza A virus infection induces liver injury in mice. Microbial Pathogenesis,2019,137:103736.
[21] Polakos NK,Cornejo JC,Murray DA,et al. Kupffer cell-dependent hepatitis occurs during influenza infection. Am J Pathol,2006,168(4):1169-1405.
[22] Waseem N, Chen P H. Hypoxic Hepatitis: A Review and Clinical Update. Journal of Clinical & Translational Hepatology,2016,4(003):263-268.
[23] Stephen Toovey. Influenza-associated central nervous system dysfunction: A literature review. Travel Medicine & Infectious Disease,2008,6(3):114-124.
[24] Fujimoto S,Kobayashi M,Uemura O,et al. PCR on cerebrospinal fluid to show influenza-associated acute encephalopathy or encephalitis. Lancet,1998,352(9131):873-875.
[25] Kansagra SM,Gallentine WB. Cytokine storm of acute necrotizing encephalopathy. Pediatr Neurol,2011,45(6):400-402.
[26] Lee N,Wong CK,Chan PK,et al. Acute encephalopathy associated with influenza A infection in adults. Emerg Infect Dis,2010,16(1):139-142.
[27] Morishima T,Togashi T,Yokota S,et al. Encephalitis and encephalopathy associated with an influenza epidemic inJapan. Clin Infect Dis,2002,35(5):512-517.
[28] Yao D,Kuwajima M,Chen Y,et al. Impaired long-chain fatty acid metabolism in mitochondria causes brain vascular invasion by a non-neurotropic epidemic influenza A virus in the newborn/suckling period: implications for influenza-associated encephalopathy. Mol Cell Biochem,2007,299(1-2):85-92.

7 脑卒中相关性肺炎诊治中国专家共识解读

黄 怡

脑卒中相关性肺炎(stroke-associated pneumonia,SAP)的概念由 Hilker 于 2003 年首先提出,是卒中后致死的重要危险因素之一,并且增加住院时间及医疗费用,给家庭和社会带来沉重的负担。我国神经内科、急诊科、呼吸科、感染科及重症医学科等多学科专家,对 2010 版进行更新和修订,以适应 SAP 临床防治工作的需要。

SAP 定义为非机械通气的卒中患者在发病 7 d 内新出现的肺炎。其发病群体为脑卒中后患者,SAP 最主要的发病机制是脑卒中后意识障碍、吞咽功能障碍造成的误吸,以及卒中引起的免疫抑制。国外流行病学数据显示,SAP 发病率为 7%~38%。我国国家脑卒中登记中心的资料统计缺血性脑卒中患者 SAP 发病率为 11.4%,出血性脑卒中患者为 16.9%。有研究显示 SAP 的发病率为 35.97%,远高于通常意义上的院内获得性下呼吸道感染的发病率 1.76%~1.94%。SAP 增加卒中患者的 30d 病死率达 3 倍,同时 1 年和 3 年死亡风险均上升。

SAP 病原菌尚缺乏大规模多中心的流行病学调查数据,通常认为以 G⁻ 杆菌为主,多种细菌及厌氧菌混合感染多见,而且疾病过程中病原体往往多变,病原学检查难度较大,易出现多耐药菌。El-Solh 等应用保护性肺泡灌洗研究发现,最多见的病原体是 G⁻ 杆菌(49%)如肺炎克雷伯杆菌、大肠埃希菌等,厌氧菌(16%)及金黄色葡萄球菌(12%),最多见的厌氧菌是普雷沃菌和梭状杆菌,22% 为混合感染,20% 是 2 种病原体混合感染,2% 为 3 种病原体。

1. SAP 的诊断标准
(1)至少符合下列标准中任意 1 项:
①无其他明确原因出现发热(体温≥38℃)。
②白细胞减少(≤4×10⁹/L)或白细胞增多(≥10×10⁹/L)。
③年龄≥70 岁老年人,无其他明确原因出现意识状态改变。

(2)并且至少符合下列标准中任意 2 项:①新出现的脓痰,或 24 h 内出现痰液性状改变或呼吸道分泌物增加或需吸痰次数增加。②新出现或加重的咳嗽或呼吸困难或呼吸急促(呼吸频率>25 次/min)。③肺部听诊发现啰音或爆裂音或支气管呼吸音。④气体交换障碍[如低氧血症(PaO_2/FiO_2≤300),需氧量增加]。

(3)胸部影像检查至少具有下列表现中任意 1 项:新出现或进展性的浸润影、实变影或磨玻璃影。

SAP 需要与医院获得性肺炎(hospital-acquired pneumonia,HAP)、社区获得性肺炎(community-acquired pneumonia,CAP)、呼吸机相关性肺炎(ventilator-associated pneumonia,VAP)及吸入性化学性肺炎(chemical pneumonitis)相鉴别。

2. 卒中相关性肺炎的治疗与管理 应积极治疗原发病;加强口腔护理及综合管理,可以减少或预防肺部感染的发生。早期营养支持:发病 24~48 h 尽量让脑卒中患者口服食物;若患者不能经口进食,推荐应用持续肠内营养,能肠内营养者尽量不采用静脉营养的方式。存在经口进食或肠内营养禁忌证者,需要在 3~7 d 启动肠外营养。

SAP 抗感染的治疗原则是经验性治疗与目标抗感染治疗有机结合,初始方案的选择应该综合考虑宿主因素、病原菌特点、药物的抗菌谱、抗菌活性、药动学/药效学特征及当地病原流行病学特点,兼顾厌氧菌的混合感染治疗等因素,选择起效迅速、神经毒性和肝肾毒性较低的抗感染药物,必要时联合用药。通常推荐选用静脉制剂,期间应在疗效反应和病原学资料的基础上及时调整用药。根据 CURB-65 或 PSI 量表评估,轻中度 SAP 患者首选 β-内酰胺类/酶抑制剂的复合制剂(如阿莫西林/克拉维酸、哌拉西林/他唑巴坦、头孢哌酮/舒巴坦等)或头霉素类(头孢西丁、头孢美唑等)或氧头孢烯类抗感染药物(拉氧头孢或氟氧头孢),疗程一般 5~7 d;评估为中重症者首选厄他培南,或者美罗培南、亚胺培南、比阿培南等,平均疗程 7~10 d。抗厌氧菌的治疗可以首选硝基咪唑类药物(如左旋奥硝唑、甲硝唑、替硝唑等)。根据耐药菌危险因素评估或者微生物培养证实为耐甲氧西林的金黄色葡萄球菌(methicillin-resistant Staphylococcus aureus,MRSA)、铜绿假单胞菌、鲍曼不动杆菌和碳青霉烯耐药肠杆菌(carbapenem-resistant Enterobacter,CRE)感染,应适当延长疗程至 10~21 d。MRSA 感染时可应用万古霉素、去甲万古霉素、利奈唑胺或者替考拉宁;铜绿假单胞菌感染时建议应用抗假单胞菌的 β-内酰胺类抗菌药物(哌拉西林/他唑巴坦、头孢哌酮/舒巴坦、头孢他啶、头孢吡肟、亚胺培南或美罗培南等)治疗,必要时联合应用喹诺酮类(环丙沙星或左氧氟沙星等)或氨基糖苷类药物;鲍曼不动杆菌的耐药率普遍很高,可以应用舒巴坦制剂(如头孢哌酮/舒巴坦、氨苄西林/舒巴坦)或碳青霉烯类、替加环素、多黏菌素治疗,甚至可前述药物联合应用;CRE 感染的患者应用头孢他啶/阿维巴坦、多黏菌素或替加环素。注意喹诺酮类药物会导致中枢神经系统不良反应的问题,特别是对于本次脑卒中较严重、病变邻近皮质或既往有癫痫史者。

患者床头抬高30°～45°是预防SAP的有效措施。对卒中患者早期吞咽功能评估和训练可减少SAP发生。应加强气道管理和喂养管理，存在幽门梗阻、胃瘫、食管反流或误吸的患者，采用幽门后置管喂养的方式可以减少肺炎的发生。

参 考 文 献

[1] Li J, Zhang P, Wu S, et al. Stroke-related complications in largehemisphere infarction: incidence and influence on unfavorableoutcome. Ther Adv Neurol Disord, 2019, 12: 1-10.

[2] De Montmollin E, Ruckly S, Schwebel C, et al. Pneumonia in acuteischemic stroke patients requiring invasive ventilation: mpact on short and long-term outcomes. J Infect, 2019, 79(3): 220-227.

[3] Wilson RD. Mortality and cost of pneumonia after stroke for differentrisk groups. J Stroke Cerebrovasc Dis, 2012, 21(1): 61-67.

[4] Hannawi Y, Hannawi B, Rao CP, et al. Stroke-associated pneumonia: major advances and obstacles. Cerebrovasc Dis, 2013, 35(5): 430-443.

[5] Ji R, Wang D, Shen H, et al. Interrelationship among common medical complications after acute stroke: pneumonia plays an important role. Stroke, 2013, 44(12): 3436-3444.

[6] Smith CJ, Bray BD, Hoffman A, et al. Can a novel clinical risk score improve pneumonia prediction in acute stroke care? A UK multicenter cohort study. J Am Heart Assoc, 2015, 4(1): e001307.

[7] Teh WH, Smith CJ, Barlas RS, et al. Impact of stroke-associated pneumonia on mortality, length of hospitalization, and functional outcome. Acta Neurol Scand, 2018, 138(4): 293-300.

[8] Yu YJ, Weng WC, Su FC, et al. Association between pneumonia in acute stroke stage and 3-year mortality in patients with acute first-ever ischemic stroke. J Clin Neurosci, 2016, 33: 124-128.

[9] Ji R, Shen H, Pan Y, et al. Novel risk score to predict pneumonia after acute ischemic stroke. Stroke, 2013, 44(5): 1303-1309.

[10] Ji R, Shen H, Pan Y, et al. Risk score to predict hospital-acquired pneumonia after spontaneous intracerebral hemorrhage. Stroke, 2014, 45(9): 2620-2628.

[11] 吴安华, 文细毛, 李春辉, 等. 2012年全国医院感染现患率与横断面抗菌药物使用率调查报告. 中国感染控制杂志, 2014, 13(1): 8-15.

[12] Jin JF, Guo ZT, Zhang YP, et al. Prediction of motor recovery after ischemic stroke using diffusion tensor imaging: A meta-analysis. World J Emerg Med, 2017, 8(2): 99-105.

[13] El-Solh AA, Pietrantoni C, Bhat A, et al. Microbiology of severe aspiration pneumonia in institutionalized elderly. Am J Respir Crit Care Med, 2003, 167(12): 1650-1654.

[14] 卒中相关性肺炎诊治中国专家共识组. 卒中相关性肺炎诊治中国专家共识. 中华内科杂志, 2010, 49(12): 1075-1078.

8 肺炎影像学复查的争议与探讨

沈 宁

胸部影像学在社区获得性肺炎（community acquired pneumonia，CAP）诊断中占有核心地位。在治疗随访过程中，由于胸部恶性肿瘤、特殊感染及其他非恶性肺部疾病影像表现可以与肺炎类似，因此，多数临床呼吸科和影像科医生都建议治疗后应进行影像学复查以保证CAP影像吸收，从而可以确认患者的症状和影像学改变确实由CAP所致而非其他原因。临床工作中，对于CAP影像学复查的问题仍存在很多问题，如，是否所有的CAP治疗后都需要复查胸部影像学？如果复查，应该选择胸部X线还是胸部CT？应该随访多长时间复查？本文就上述问题结合相关文献进行阐述。

一、各国指南对肺炎影像学复查的要求

在我国2016年CAP指南中，关于影像学提出：大多数CAP患者在初始治疗后72h临床症状改善，但影像学改善滞后于临床症状。应在初始治疗后72h对病情进行评价，部分患者对治疗的反应相对较慢，只要临床表现无恶化，可以继续观察。初始治疗后评价的内容包括临床表现、生命体征、一般实验室检查、微生物学指标和胸部影像学。对于胸部影像学，临床症状明显改善的患者不推荐常规复查胸部影像；症状或体征持续存在或恶化时，应复查X线胸片或胸部CT确定肺部病灶变化。

美国IDSA/ATS2019年CAP指南中，第16问提出成人CAP治疗有改善，是否需要随访胸部影像学？推荐意见是成人CAP症状在5~7d缓解，建议不需要常规复查胸部影像学（有条件推荐，低证据级别）。

英国胸科协会指南对影像学复查的建议：CAP患者临床治疗满意不需要在出院前复查胸部影像学；无论是否收入院治疗，对于有持续存在症状或体征、或有潜在恶性肿瘤风险（特别是吸烟和年龄50岁以上的患者）应该在6周时进行胸部影像学复查；对于完成治疗后6周持续有症状体征、影像学异常的患者应该考虑进行进一步包括支气管镜在内的检查；医院内治疗团队有责任和患者，以及家庭医生一起对于收住院的CAP患者制订随访计划。

瑞典2017年CAP指南提出：临床过程复杂、仍有症状的患者随访是应该进行胸部X线片复查，还包括反复发作肺炎、免疫抑制人群或潜在恶性肿瘤风险高的患者。推荐对于40岁以上现在吸烟者和50岁以上既往吸烟者CAP随访时复查X线胸片。仍有持续症状或胸片仍有异常的患者应该进行胸部CT，必要时进行支气管镜检查以明确有无其他需要鉴别的疾病。

二、影像学复查的意义

各国指南对于CAP影像学复查都认为不是必须的，大多数建议有肺癌高危因素和临床持续不缓解的患者应该进行影像学检查，对于复查的时间也没有明确界定。但实际临床工作中，绝大多数临床和放射科医生都建议CAP患者应该进行影像学复查，甚至很多患者进行反复多次复查。

CAP诊断标准中，胸部影像学检查显示新出现的斑片状浸润影、叶或段实变影、磨玻璃影或间质性改变是必备条件，同时明确提出"除外肺结核、肺部肿瘤、非感染性肺间质性疾病、肺水肿、肺不张、肺栓塞、肺嗜酸性粒细胞浸润症及肺血管炎等后，可建立临床诊断"。在疾病诊断初期很多临床情况并不典型，可能不容易确定诊断，但随访的影像学检查可以提供很多有用的信息。例如合并阻塞性肺炎的肺癌，抗感染治疗后复查影像学阻塞性肺炎吸收后可能发现肿瘤的影像。由于恶性肿瘤和其他非恶性肺部疾病可以表现为类似肺炎的影像，因此，对于疑诊肺炎的患者，应该进行影像学复查以除外这些疾病，特别是肺癌。

1. 排除胸部恶性肿瘤 肺炎后复查胸部影像学主要的目的是为了排除潜在的胸部恶性肿瘤，主要是肺癌。既往研究显示诊断肺炎患者随访发现肺癌发生率为0.4%~9.2%。Tang KL等进行了一项队列研究，入组了从2000—2002年影像诊断确诊肺炎的3398名患者，随访5年，结果发现肺炎后发现肺癌的比例很低，90d复查有约1%，1年1.7%，随访5年仅有2.3%。新发现癌的危险因素是50岁以上，男性和吸烟。没有在40岁以下的肺炎患者发现肺癌，仅有3例50岁以下的患者发现肺癌。因此肺炎后常规复查胸部影像学检查以发现有无肺癌并不是很必要，研究建议对50岁以上人群，特别是男性吸烟人群进行影像学复查随访。Little BP等研究805名可疑CAP患者，年龄20~98岁，其中618名（77%）患者进行了影像学随访，其中胸片53.6%，胸片和CT17.5%，CT5.6%。共有15名患者诊断恶性肿瘤，9例影像学复查发现，8例为新诊断或非小细胞肺癌复发，1例为大B细胞淋巴瘤。胸片仅1例表现为结节影，其他都表现为渗出或实变。CT显示7例有结节，2例有肿块但没有导致叶或段不张，2例有实变，1例肿物导致右中叶和下叶不张。9例患者平均年龄68.4岁，5例有恶性肿瘤病史，3例有COPD，2例吸烟。随访发现肺癌比例最

高的是美国的一项研究,9.2%初步诊断肺炎的患者随访发现诊断为肺部肿瘤,这项研究是在退伍军人医院进行的,均为65岁以上老年住院患者,且男性为主。提示这类人群患肺炎后应该复查胸部影像学检查。

2. 鉴别其他非肿瘤性疾病　很多肺部疾病不是由感染造成但是能表现出炎症的病理状态,例如BOOP、嗜酸细胞性肺炎、狼疮性肺炎、结节病等,这种情况应引起临床医师的重视并建立完善的鉴别诊断思路。Little BP等研究还发现23例患者复查影像学诊断为非肿瘤肺部疾病,其中肺结核或非结核分枝杆菌6例,真菌感染5例,机化或嗜酸性粒细胞肺炎5例,球形肺不张3例,肺泡出血1例,肺脓肿1例,肺孢子虫病1例,脓毒性肺栓塞1例。平均第1次复查影像学的时间为80d,恶性肿瘤的患者复查时间为17.9d。

三、胸片和胸部CT在复查中的作用和优劣

X线胸片因其低辐射、价廉、普及率高成为肺部感染初步筛查及治疗后随访的首选方法,而CT检查的敏感性及特异性明显优于X线胸片,但存在射线量大、费用较高的缺点。

1. X线胸片和CT在CAP诊断中的应用　X线胸片是CAP诊断首选的方法,但由于X线胸片的敏感性、特异性差,容易造成CAP的漏诊和误诊。研究显示,和胸片相比,胸部CT修正了8%~18%的肺炎诊断。Claessens YE等研究发现,在急诊就诊的疑诊CAP的患者,早期胸部CT检查可以明显改变胸片的诊断进而影响临床治疗。319名患者在4h内进行了胸部CT检查,结果发现188名患者胸片提示肺部渗出影,其中143名(44.8%)诊断为CAP,172名(55.8%)疑诊CAP,排除了4名(1.2%)。CT在胸片阴性的患者中发现40名(33%)有肺部渗出影,在188名胸片有渗出影的患者中56名(29.8%)排除了CAP的诊断。由于进行了CT扫描,启动了51名患者的抗菌药物治疗,停用了29名患者的抗菌药物,72患者收入院,23名患者出院。由于CT检查的敏感性及特异性明显优于X线胸片,对于临床高度怀疑肺部感染而胸片正常者,可以选择CT扫描。

2. X线胸片和CT在CAP随访复查中的应用　对于有随访指征的CAP患者,选择胸片或胸部CT复查需要取决于复查的时间、CT的可及性、费用及是否需要频繁复查等因素。胸片仍然是复查的首选方法,但对于初始胸部CT发现的影像改变,特别是影像特点不典型的患者,可以考虑行胸部CT检查,也可以结合医院和患者的情况选择低剂量CT进行复查和随访。

四、个体化制订影像学复查的方案

影像学检查能实时监测肺部感染治疗后病灶的消散吸收过程,但是否所有肺部感染患者都需要影像学随访目前存在争议,有些通过患者临床病程的好转反映治疗的有效性,反复进行影像学检查可能有辐射过多和增加治疗成本的问题。因此临床医师应充分把握进行影像学随访的指征及原则。总体来说,大部分肺部感染的浸润灶在发病10~21d逐渐消散,2/3的CAP患者肺部病灶在3个月内完全消失,而对于老年人,有肺部基础疾病或免疫抑制患者,肺部病灶的完全消失需要6个月或者更长时间。因此,对于有明确指征需要复查肺部影像学检查的患者应该根据个体差异的不同制订个体化随访的方案。

1. 建议复查胸部影像学的人群　目前公认需要复查胸部影像学的CAP患者主要是有肺癌高危因素的患者(吸烟和年龄50岁以上的患者)、有持续临床症状的患者。对于一些影像学不典型的患者,如以团块、多发结节、合并纵隔肺门淋巴结肿大、游走性改变、空洞样病变等为特点的CAP患者,也应特别注意临床改善的情况,必要时应该复查胸部影像学检查。

2. 复查胸部影像学的时间　复查影像学的时间应该依据患者年龄、病情严重程度、临床症状改善情况等综合判断。2005年ACCP建议诊断后8周复查以保证影像吸收,BTS2009年建议对于临床症状持续或有肿瘤高危因素的患者6周时复查。由于肺部影像学改善滞后于临床症状,对于病情平稳的患者,不建议过早复查胸部影像学。我国的小样本研究显示12.5%患者第1周复查时临床症状好转,而影像学表现有所进展,特别是在老年患者中更为明显。因此建议第2周后复查为宜。目前关于复查胸部影像学的时间尚无明确的界定,但我国普遍存在过早、过多复查胸部CT的现状,应加以适当限制和引导,并根据患者特点进行治疗随访。

3. 加强临床-影像学科沟通　放射科专家对于复查推荐意见不一致,研究显示42%的放射科医生对于新出现的肺内渗出影怀疑CAP的都建议复查,55%建议根据影像特点、患者年龄、临床症状的不同有时需要复查。临床医生在开具影像检查申请时,应该写清症状改善情况、基本药物治疗情况、吸烟史等临床信息,给放射科医生足够的信息进行病情判断。同时新旧影像学的对比至关重要。尽管对于呼吸科医生来说,胸部影像学是必修的知识,但遇到影像学异常与临床情况不符时,也应积极和影像科专家进行沟通,采用多学科合作的门诊-病房-社区联动机制,才能获得最佳效果。

总之,对于CAP的影像复查是临床医生经常进行的工作,但目前的研究显示如果症状短时间内缓解,不需要进行影像学复查。由于目前对于可能类似肺炎表现的肺部肿瘤、其他非感染性肺部疾病的担忧,在我国无论是临床医生还是放射科医生对于CAP影像学复查相对更积极,同时由于CT的普及性和检查费用逐渐降低,使得胸部CT诊断和随访的比例越来越高,但仍然应该以科学审慎地态度对CAP患者进行影像学复查和随访。特别是新冠肺炎疫情来袭后,胸部CT受到高度重视,使患者短时间内复查影像学成为很多医院的临床流程,但作为一种病毒性肺炎,其诊治流程仍应遵循CAP常规,在保证临床有效性安全性的同时,减少射线损害及降低医疗费用。

参 考 文 献

[1] 中华医学会呼吸病学分会.中国成人社区获得性肺炎诊断和治疗指南(2016版).中华结核和呼吸杂志,2016,39:253-279.

[2] Metlay JP,Waterer GW,Long AC,et al. Diagnosis and treatment of adults with community-acquired pneumonia. An official clinical practice guideline of the American Thoracic Society and Infectious Diseases Society of America. Am J Respir Crit Care Med,2019,200: e45-e67.

[3] Lim WS,Baudouin SV,George RC,et al. Pneumonia Guidelines Committee of the BTS Standards of Care Committee. BTS guidelines for the management of community acquired pneumonia in adults: update 2009. Thorax,2009,64(Suppl 3):1-55.

[4] Athlin S,Lidman C,Lundqvist A,et al. Management of community-acquired pneumonia in immunocompetent adults: updated Swedish guidelines 2017. Infectious Disease,2018,50:247-272.

[5] Holmberg H,Kragsbjerg P. Association of pneumonia and lung cancer: the value of convalescent chest radiography and follow-up. Scand J Infect Dis,1993,25:93-100.

[6] Bochud PY,Moser F,Erard P,et al. Communityacquired pneumonia: a prospective outpatient study. Medicine(Baltimore),2001,80:75-87.

[7] Marrie TJ. Pneumonia and carcinoma of the lung. J Infect,1994,29:45-52.

[8] Woodhead MA,Macfarlane JT,McCracken JS,et al. Prospective study of the aetiology and outcome of pneumonia in the community. Lancet,1987,329:671-674.

[9] Tang KL,Eurich DT,Minhas-Sandhu JK,et al. Incidence,correlates,and chest radiographic yield of new lung cancer diagnosis in 3398 patients with pneumonia. Arch Intern Med,2011,171:1193-1198.

[10] Mortensen EM,Copeland LA,Pugh MJ,et al. Diagnosis of pulmonary malignancy after hospitalization for pneumonia. Am J Med,2010,123:66-71.

[11] Little BP,Gilman MD,Humphrey KL,et al. Outcome of Recommendations for Radiographic Follow-Up of Pneumonia on Outpatient Chest Radiography. AJR,2014,202:54-59.

[12] Garin N,Marti C,Scheffler M,et al. Computed tomography scan contribution to the diagnosis of community-acquired pneumonia. Curr Opin Pulm Med,2019,25:242-248.

[13] Claessens YE,Debray MP,Tubach F,et al. Early chest computed tomography scan to assist diagnosis and guide treatment decision for suspected community-acquired pneumonia. Am J Respir Crit Care Med,2015,192:974-982.

[14] 余业洲,赵红,邹立巍,等.社区获得性肺炎治疗前后的影像学表现.中国医学影像学杂志,2019,27:674-676.

9 新型冠状病毒的实验室检测

叶 枫

随着新型冠状病毒性肺炎(coronavirus disease 2019,COVID-19)的暴发和广泛扩散,对全球公共卫生造成了巨大威胁。随着对该疾病认识的不断深入,发现部分无症状感染者有较强的传染性。高效、敏感、精准的实验室检测对于诊断新型冠状病毒(severe acute respiratory syndrom coronavirus 2,SARS-CoV-2)感染至关重要。目前实验室检测技术主要包括病原体检测、血清免疫学检测技术和常规的实验室检查。

一、病原体检测

(一)病毒分离与鉴定

从人呼吸道样本中分离出新型冠状病毒并加以鉴定是实验室诊断病毒感染的"金标准"。目前不但从患者的口/鼻咽拭子、嗽口液、鼻咽抽取物或抽取气管和支气管分泌物、肺组织样本,还从尿液和粪便中成功分离出了新型冠状病毒。此过程需在生物安全三级实验室中进行,且耗时较长,不作为常规诊断方法。但COVID-19作为一种新型的传染病,其病毒的分离与培养对病毒来源、疫苗研发及致病机制等研究均具有重要意义。

(二)病原体核酸检测

1. 实时荧光PCR(reverse transcription-polymerase chain reaction,RT-PCR) 是将RNA的反转录(RT)和cDNA的聚合酶链式扩增(PCR)相结合的技术。自SARS-CoV-2基因序列被公布后,Corman等针对*RdRp*基因设计了2种探针,既可特异性识别SARS-CoV-2的*RdRp*基因,又可鉴别SARS-CoV-2与其外的其他冠状病毒,具有很强的特异性和相对较高的灵敏性。机体被病毒感染后,病毒通过鼻腔和口腔进入到咽喉部,再到气管和支气管,进而到达肺泡。相关研究发现下呼吸道的病毒量会明显高于上呼吸道,其中肺泡灌洗液中最容易检出病毒核酸,其次是痰液、咽漱液,再次是鼻咽拭子、咽拭子。病程不同阶段及机体不同部位的病毒载量会有所不同。患者病毒载量低、病毒出现了变异、标本采集不当或深度不够、样本未能及时送检等因素均可能导致假阴性的结果,不同试剂盒的敏感性和特异性也存在差异。因此当核酸检测结果为阴性时,并不能排除SARS-CoV-2感染,建议采用同一患者多部位标本检测来提高阳性率,选用引物不同的试剂盒对可疑结果进行复核验证。由于RT-qPCR具有较高的临床检测普及率,目前仍作为SARS-CoV-2感染确诊的金标准。

2. 反转录数字PCR(RT-dPCR) 反转录数字PCR(reverse transcription digital PCR,RT-dPCR)主要采用微流控或微滴化方法,将大量核酸分子通过一系列手段制备成单个DNA分子,并转移到独立的反应室后进行扩增检测,甚至可检测出单个拷贝的病毒样本的方法。前期对于HBV和HIV的检测发现RT-dPCR比传统的RT-qPCR具有更高的灵敏性和准确性。现有研究表明RT-dPCR较RT-PCR检测SARS-CoV-2更敏感,更适用于检测病毒载量低的标本,对降低假阴性率更有优势,提示RT-dPCR可作为COVID-19诊断的补充检测。但是SARS-CoV-2基因组中引物与其他病毒或细菌共同感染产生的核酸交叉反应可产生假阳性结果,引物和探针靶区的突变则会导致假阴性结果,应该用不同的引物对同一基因靶标的结果进行验证,进一步提高检测准确率。

3. 反转录环介导等温扩增(RT-LAMP) 反转录环介导等温扩增(reverse transcriptional loop-mediated isothermal amplification,RT-LAMP)是在恒温条件下将RNA反转录进行核酸扩增的方法。与普通PCR相比,RT-LAMP具有4~6个引物,能够针对性地识别ORF1ab靶区的8个不同区域,敏感性与RT-PCR相当,不但可鉴别出其他冠状病毒,还能够检测出更低拷贝的SARS-CoV-2。Lu R等发现这种新型的RT-LAMP与商业化的RT-qPCR具有很高的一致性(92.9%),并且能将检测SARS-CoV-2时间缩短到10~40 min,但有产生气溶胶的风险。由于LAMP技术具有高灵敏度、操作简单、扩增时间短、可视化等优点,这将更有益于发展中国家的基层医院进行现场快速检测。

4. 纳米孔测序(NTS) 纳米孔测序(nanopore target sequencing,NTS)是借助电泳驱动单链DNA/RNA分子序列逐一通过纳米孔来实现测序,即将核酸化学信号转变为计算机可处理的数字信号的一个过程。目前基因测序技术已从第一代发展到第四代。我国科学家采用宏基因组学二代测序技术在短时间内从患者呼吸道样本鉴定了新型病原体SARS-COV-2,而后快速对病毒培养物进行了基因组测序,并与世界卫生组织分享了新型冠状病毒的基因序列信息,为其他国家开发特定诊断工具提供了便利。传统的高通量测序成本较高,对样本制备及场地要求高,且耗时较长,难以用于大量COVID-19疑似患者的快速诊断。NTS文库构建相对简单,可在6~10 h高灵敏地监测突变的核酸序列并对SARS-CoV-2的类型进行分类测序,能准确地检测出完整的病毒基因组并同时检测出其他呼吸道病毒。NTS通过对内标基因的分析,排除了核酸提取及反转录的影响,对全基因组的测序有效避免了病毒突变而产生的漏检情况,不但可以实现新冠病毒和基因突变的检测,还可以监控病毒变异引起的毒性和传播能力改变的情况,但对操作要求更高。对于流行病学史、临床特征、影像学特征高度疑似 COVID-19,但常规 RT-PCR 检测阴性的患者,纳米孔测序技术可作为补充诊断,有望在未来得到更广泛的应用。

5. CRISPR 基因编辑系统　CRISPR(clustered regularly interspaced short palindromic repeat)系统可高精度编辑靶基因,使基因组更有效地产生变化或突变,可用于控制各种类型的遗传疾病。由于该系统具有靶向 RNA 的特性,因此可以鉴定出样本中是否存在特定的序列,从而达到检测病原体的目的。目前主要有 2 种 CRISPR 系统用于核酸特定序列的检测,分别是 CRISPR/Cas13a 和 CRISPR/Cas12a 系统。有学者发现当 SARS-CoV-2 核酸存在时,只需 40min 即被 Cas12a 裂解发出视觉可见的绿色荧光,并且 CRISPR 可检测出单个病毒拷贝,与 RT-PCR 相比具有 95.8% 的一致性。但如果核酸靶序列发生了突变,基于 CRISPR 的诊断也可能发生错误。这一简单快捷的现场诊断方法,仍需大量临床样本来进一步验证其敏感性和特异性。

此外,还有一些新兴的分子诊断技术被研发用于呼吸道病原体诊断,例如核酸质谱技术和生物基因芯片技术等,但由于检测设备和技术难度较高,因此目前并不适合用于 COVID-19 临床大样本诊断。各种常见核酸检测技术比较见表 4-9-1。

表 4-9-1　各种常见新型冠状病毒核酸检测技术比较

检测技术	灵敏度	检测时间	检测范围	操作程序	检测成本	报告方式	临床应用
实时荧光 PCR(RT-PCR)	较高	4~6 h	单一病原体	一般	一般	定性	快速筛查及确诊
反转录数字 PCR(RT-dPCR)	高	8~10 h	单一病原体	复杂	高	绝对定量	量化核酸水平,为病程和疗效提供依据
反转录环介导等温扩增(RT-LAMP)	较高	10~40 min	多种病原体	简便	较低	定性	快速确诊并排除疑似病例
纳米孔测序(NTS)	高	6~8 h	多种病原体	复杂	高	半定量	确诊及监测病毒变异
CRISPR 基因编辑系统	高	约 40 min	多种病原体	简便	高	定性	快速筛查及确诊

二、血清免疫学检测

机体感染 SARS-CoV-2 后,大多数患者可在 7 d 内检测到 IgM 抗体,14 d 左右达到高峰,随后开始下降,IgM 升高提示患者新近发生感染。IgG 抗体出现的时间稍晚于 IgM 抗体,在发病后 10 d 内可检测到,21 d 左右达高峰,并维持在一个较高的水平,通常提示病情进入恢复期或存在既往感染。血清新型冠状病毒特异性 IgM 抗体和 IgG 抗体阳性;特异性 IgG 抗体由阴性转为阳性或恢复期较急性期 4 倍及以上升高,可作为 COVID-19 疑似病例的确诊条件之一。对于已确诊患者,可通过动态监测新型冠状病毒抗原与抗体的滴度变化以评估疗效和疾病转归。IgM 和 IgG 联合检测较单一的 IgM 或 IgG 检测具有更高的敏感性和临床价值,且末梢血、静脉血和血浆的检测结果具有较高的一致性。新型冠状病毒特异性抗体检测可用于回顾性诊断及对核酸检测结果存疑时的辅助诊断,但不能用于新型冠状病毒肺炎的确诊和排除。迄今为止,新型冠状病毒血清学检测常用的方法包括酶联免疫吸附测定(ELISA)、免疫层析法(ICA)和化学发光免疫测定(CLIA)技术。血清学检测常用方法比较见表 4-9-2。

表 4-9-2　新型冠状病毒血清学检测常用方法比较

项目	胶体金免疫层析	酶联免疫吸附	化学发光法
敏感性	低	中	高
检测时间	10~20 min	2~3 h	0.5~1 h
检测通量	低	高	高
操作步骤	简便	复杂	较简便
检测设备	无须	酶标仪、洗板仪	化学发光仪
判读方式	人眼	仪器	仪器
报告形式	定性/半定量	定性/定量	定量

(一)酶联免疫吸附测定

酶联免疫吸附测定(enzyme linked immunosorben tassay, ELISA)是将已知的抗原或抗体吸附在固相载体(聚苯乙烯微量反应板)表面,使酶标记的抗原抗体反应在固相表面进行,利用酶与底物的显色反应对待测物进行定性和定量检测方法。有学者开发了针对 IgM 和 IgG 的 ELISA 检测方法,多次采样发现其阳性率随着病程的延长而增高。该法特异性较强且检测成本低,可定性或半定量检测,但是操作步骤烦琐,耗时较长,因此 ELISA 可能比较适合基层医疗机构的筛查。

(二)免疫层析法

免疫层析(immu-nochromatography assay, ICA)是出现于 20 世纪 80 年代初期的一种新型的免疫分析方式,是在免疫渗滤(immunofiltration asay, IFA)的基础上建立的一种简单快速的免疫学检测技术。现应用于临床的主要是胶体金免疫层析法(GICA),能在 15 min 内同时检测新型冠状病毒特异性的 IgM 和 IgG 抗体,敏感率和特异性较高;但目前胶体金免疫层析法尚不能进行定量检测,而不同冠状病毒 N 蛋白或 S 蛋白可能存在免疫交叉反应从而导致假阳性结果。由于其操作简单、检测速度快、成本低等优点,可作为新型冠状病毒肺炎核酸检测前的分诊方法。主要应用于以下几种情况:SARS-CoV-2 传播地区门诊发热不明患者的诊断;密切接触疫区的疑似病例的管理;无症状感染患者的筛查。

(三)化学发光免疫分析

化学发光免疫分析(chemiluminescent immunoassay, CLIA)是将具有高灵敏度的化学发光测定技术与高特异性的免疫反应相结合,用于各种抗原抗体等的检测分析技术,是继放射免疫技术、酶联免疫技术、荧光免疫技术和时间分辨荧光免疫技术之后发展起来的一项新型免疫测定技术。该法特异性高,检测速度快,可广泛应用于临床样本的检测。相关研究发现化学发光免疫分析技术对 COVID-19 患者血清中的 IgM 和 IgG 检测具有较高的敏感性和特异性,对 COVID-19 早期诊断、流行病学筛查、病程预测及转归方面具有重要意义。但其依赖大型仪器设备支持,难以实现现场筛查。

血清免疫学检测的方法相较于核酸检测更易操作且快捷,对临床实验室的专业设备及专业人员的操作要求相对较低。许多医院已将免疫学检测作为核酸检测的补充手段。值得注意的是,基于抗原抗体接合的免疫学方法的局限性,标本中会存在干扰物质(如类风湿因子、嗜异性抗体、补体、溶菌酶等),标本溶血,标本被细菌污染,标本凝固不全残留有纤维蛋白原,以及与其他类型冠状病毒的抗原交叉反应等因素影响而出现"假阳性"结果。在疾病感染早期,抗体尚未产生或病毒滴度很低,抗体检测试剂盒灵敏度的差异,患者免疫功能受损,标本采集后未在 2 h 内送检或待检测的标本未置于 2~8℃保存等处理不当可导致"假阴性"结果。抗体检测必须采用 IgM 和 IgG 同时检测且通常需多次(2 次以上)动态检测确认,其敏感性、临床应用效率还需要进一步大样本的验证和评估。因此,血清学检测结果不能作为新型冠状病毒感染的独立确诊依据,需结合患者流行病学史、临床表现、其他实验室检查结果即影像学进行综合判断。核酸和抗体联合检测的结果解读见表 4-9-3。

表 4-9-3 核酸和抗体联合检测的结果解读

序号	核酸	IgM	IgG	解读
1	+	−	−	可能为感染"窗口期",一般为 1~2 周
2	+	+	−	可能为感染早期机体已产生 IgM,暂未产生 IgG 或或 IgG 含量未达到诊断试剂的检测下限
3	+	−	+	可能为感染中晚期或复发感染
4	+	+	+	可能为感染活跃期,但人体已产生一定免疫能力
5	−	+	+	核酸假阴性,患者处于感染活跃期。或近期曾感染并处于恢复期,体内病毒被清除,IgM 尚未降至检测下限
6	−	+	−	疑似急性感染,可能为疾病的早期,尚未产生 IgG,需反复取样复查;或因抗体交叉反应等引起的 IgM 假阳性
7	−	±	−	初次感染早期,病毒载量低于核酸检测下限,机体产生少量 IgM,尚未产生 IgG;或由于抗体交叉反应等引起的 IgM 假阳性
8	−	−	+	既往感染或 IgG 结果假阳性,现处于恢复期或体内病毒被清除
9	−	−	−	处于感染潜伏期或为健康人群

三、实验室多指标联合检查

COVID-19 患者血常规、血生化、免疫检查等多项指标均存在着规律性的变化。发病早期常规实验室检查发现外周血白细胞计数一般正常或减少,淋巴细胞计数通常减少(严重者呈现进行性淋巴细胞减少),多数患者 C 反应蛋白(CRP)和红细胞沉降率(ESR)正常或升高,降钙素原(PCT)正常。部分患者可出现乳酸脱氢酶、谷丙转氨酶、谷草转氨酶、肌酸激酶、肌红蛋白升高,严重者肌钙蛋白、D-二聚体升高。而重型、危重型患者常有 IL-6、IL-10 等炎症因子升高。

总之,关于新型冠状病毒的实验室检测技术各有优缺点,应根据实际情况合理选择检测方法。多方法相结合的实验室检测技术将更有益于未来新型冠状病毒肺炎的快速确诊。

参 考 文 献

[1] SUN J,ZHU A,LI H,et al. Isolation of infectious SARS-CoV-2 from urine of a COVID-19 patient. Emerging microbes & infections,2020,9(1):991-993.

[2] XIAO F,SUN J,XU Y,et al. Infectious SARS-CoV-2 in Feces of Patient with Severe COVID-19. Emerging infectious diseases,2020,26(8):1920-1922.

[3] CORMAN V M,LANDT O,KAISER M,et al. Detection of 2019 novel coronavirus(2019-nCoV)by real-time RT-PCR. Euro Surveill,2020,25(3):2000045.

[4] GUO WL,JIANG Q,YE F,et al. Effect of throat washings on detection of 2019 novel coronavirus. Clinical infectious diseases,2020,71(8):1980-1981.

[5] HUANG J T,LIU Y J,WANG J,et al. Next generation digital PCR measurement of hepatitis B virus copy number in formalin-fixed paraffin-embedded hepatocellular carcinoma tissue. Clinical chemistry,2015,61(1):290-296.

[6] YU F,YAN L,WANG N,et al. Quantitative Detection and Viral Load Analysis of SARS-CoV-2 in Infected Patients. Clinical infectious diseases,2020.

[7] SUO T,LIU X,FENG J,et al. ddPCR:a more accurate tool for SARS-CoV-2 detection in low viral load specimens. Emerging microbes & infections,2020,9(1):1259-1268.

[8] LI J,MACDONALD J. Advances in isothermal amplification:novel strategies inspired by biological processes. Biosensors & bioelectronics,2015,64:196-211.

[9] YU L,WU S,HAO X,et al. Rapid Detection of COVID-19 Coronavirus Using a Reverse Transcriptional Loop-Mediated Isothermal Amplification(RT-LAMP)Diagnostic Platform. Clinical chemistry,2020,66(7):975-977.

[10] LU R,WU X,WAN Z,et al. A Novel Reverse Transcription Loop-Mediated Isothermal Amplification Method for Rapid Detection of SARS-CoV-2. International journal of molecular sciences,2020,21(8):2826.

[11] LEE S H,BAEK Y H,KIM Y H,et al. One-Pot Reverse Transcriptional Loop-Mediated Isothermal Amplification(RT-LAMP)for Detecting MERS-CoV. Frontiers in microbiology,2016,7:2166.

[12] BAYLEY H. Nanopore sequencing:from imagination to reality. Clinical chemistry,2015,61(1):25-31.

[13] HUI D S,E I A,MADANI T A,et al. The continuing 2019-nCoV epidemic threat of novel coronaviruses to global health-The latest 2019 novel coronavirus outbreak in Wuhan,China. Int J Infect Dis,2020,91:264-266.

[14] WANG M,FU A,HU B,et al. Nanopore Targeted Sequencing for the Accurate and Comprehensive Detection of SARS-CoV-2 and Other Respiratory Viruses. Small(Weinheim an der Bergstrasse,Germany),2020,e2002169.

[15] CHAN W M,IP J D,CHU A W,et al. Identification of nsp1 gene as the target of SARS-CoV-2 real-time RT-PCR using nanopore whole-genome sequencing. Journal of medical virology,2020.

[16] LI Z,LI Y,CHEN L,et al. A Confirmed Case of SARS-CoV-2 Pneumonia with Routine RT-PCR Negative and Virus Variation in Guangzhou,China. Clinical infectious diseases:an official publication of the Infectious Diseases Society of America,2020.

[17] HSU P D,LANDER E S,ZHANG F. Development and applications of CRISPR-Cas9 for genome engineering. Cell,2014,157(6):1262-1278.

[18] BROUGHTON J,DENG X,YU G,et al. CRISPR-Cas12-based detection of SARS-CoV-2. 2020,38(7):870-874.

[19] HOU T,ZENG W,YANG M,et al. Development and Evaluation of A CRISPR-based Diagnostic For 2019-novel Coronavirus. 2020,36:100713.

[20] 国家卫生健康委员会.新型冠状病毒肺炎诊疗方案(试行第七版). http://www. nhc. gov. cn/yzygj/s7653p/202003/46c9294a7fdc4cef80dc7f5912eb1989. shtml? spm=C73544894212. P59511941341.0.0):

[21] Z L,Y Y,X L,et al. Development and clinical application of a rapid IgM-IgG combined antibody test for SARS-CoV-2 infection diagnosis. 2020.

[22] IHA K,INADA M,KAWADA N,et al. Ultrasensitive ELISA Developed for Diagnosis. Diagnostics(Basel),2019,9(3):78.

[23] ZHANG W,DU R H,LI B,et al. Molecular and serological investigation of 2019-nCoV infected patients:implication of multiple shedding routes. Emerging microbes & infections,2020,9(1):386-389.

[24] CHOE J Y,KIM J W,KWON H H,et al. Diagnostic performance of immunochromatography assay for rapid detection of IgM and IgG in coronavirus disease 2019. Journal of medical virology,2020.

[25] LI H,LIU Z,HE Y,et al. A new and rapid approach for detecting COVID-19 based on S1 protein fragments. Clinical and translational medicine,2020.

[26] LI Z,YI Y,LUO X,et al. Development and clinical application of a rapid IgM-IgG combined antibody test for SARS-CoV-2 infection diagnosis. Journal of medical virology,2020.

[27] WANG Q,DU Q,GUO B,et al. A Method To Prevent SARS-CoV-2 IgM False Positives in Gold Immunochromatography and Enzyme-Linked Immunosorbent Assays. Journal of clinical microbiology,2020,58(6):e00375.

[28] PAN Y,LI X,YANG G,et al. Serological immunochromatographic approach in diagnosis with SARS-CoV-2 infected COVID-19 patients. The Journal of infection,2020,81(1):e28-e32.

[29] 李振甲,应希堂,马世俊.化学发光免疫分析技术的研究现状与展望.国际检验医学杂志,2006,01:95-97.

[30] XF C,J C,J L H,et al. A Peptide-Based Magnetic Chemiluminescence Enzyme Immunoassay for Serological Diagnosis

of Coronavirus Disease 2019. The Journal of infectious diseases,2020,222(2):189-193.

[31] 邹明园,吴国球.抗原交叉反应对新型冠状病毒血清特异性抗体检测的影响.临床检验杂志,2020,38(03):161-163.

[32] CHEN Z M,FU J F,SHU Q,et al. Diagnosis and treatment recommendations for pediatric respiratory infection caused by the 2019 novel coronavirus. World journal of pediatrics:WJP,2020,16(3):240-246.

10 糖皮质激素在COVID-19及其他病毒性肺炎的应用及潜在机制

徐金富

【摘要】

糖皮质激素因其抗炎作用常被用作急性呼吸窘迫综合征的辅助治疗。然而，其在病毒性肺炎中的应用却极具争议。本文旨在系统评价糖皮质激素在流行性病毒性肺炎中的应用及潜在机制。我们从PubMed、EMBASE、Cochrane数据库中全面检索了关于糖皮质激素治疗流感、严重急性呼吸综合征(SARS)、中东呼吸综合征(MERS)和新型冠状病毒性肺炎(COVID-19)的文献。研究表明糖皮质激素治疗与流感肺炎患者的死亡率和院内感染率增加相关。并且糖皮质激素应用与SARS、MERS患者病毒清除延迟相关。综述目前已发表的关于糖皮质激素治疗COVID-19相关研究，表明接受糖皮质激素治疗组患者病死率明显高于非激素治疗组（69/443, 15.6% vs. 56/1310, 4.3%）。与非重症患者相比，重症患者更有可能接受糖皮质激素治疗（201/382, 52.6% vs. 201/1310, 15.3%）。尽管目前没有循证医学证据表明糖皮质激素治疗能降低COVID-19患者的死亡率，但在一些临床观察性研究中显示，糖皮质激素治疗可改善重症COVID-19患者的临床症状和氧合功能。过度的炎症反应和淋巴细胞减少与COVID-19的严重程度和死亡相关。

自2019年12月下旬以来，随着新型冠状病毒性肺炎的暴发流行，截至2020年6月30日全球确诊病例已达1 019 422例，其中死亡病例503 907。目前关于COVID-19的发病机制及临床过程还有待于充分研究，也没有具体的药物治疗被证明是有效的。对于严重的COVID-19患者短期内发展为急性呼吸衰竭、肺水肿和急性呼吸窘迫综合征(ARDS)，伴大量炎性因子释放。因此，对其的治疗显得尤为重要。先前的随机对照临床试验表明糖皮质激素可以调节炎症反应，减少社区获得性肺炎患者治疗失败发生率，缩短到临床稳定的时间，且无明显不良事件发生。此外，Villar等通过一项随机对照临床试验证实早期给予地塞米松治疗可减少中重度ARDS患者的机械通气持续时间和死亡率。尽管糖皮质激素在病毒性肺炎的应用存在很大争议，但在流感病毒暴发流行期间，它们仍被广泛用作流行性病毒性肺炎的辅助治疗。然而，在过去的20年中，几乎没有临床研究的数据表明糖皮质激素治疗使病毒性肺炎患者获益，甚至与患者的不良预后相关。Russell等认为，基于以前发表的关于糖皮质激素在流感、SARS、MERS病毒性肺炎中应用的研究，支持糖皮质激素治疗COVID-19所致肺损伤的临床证据尚不确定。然而我们中国专家组有不同的观点，他们认为对患有COVID-19的危重症患者，可短期谨慎使用低至中等剂量糖皮质激素治疗。这促使我们进一步寻找糖皮质激素在COVID-19中应用的依据和潜在机制。

我们进行了一项全面的搜索，检索了以往所有关于糖皮质激素治疗流感、SARS、MERS肺炎和COVID-19的文献。并从原始研究中提取有用的信息和数据，进行统计分析。我们试图探讨皮糖皮质激素在病毒性肺炎中的应用及潜在作用机制，以便将来在病毒性肺炎患者的治疗中更合理地使用糖皮质激素。

一、糖皮质激素在流感肺炎中的应用

多项研究报道了糖皮质激素治疗与流感肺炎患者死亡率和医院感染率的增加相关。一项对2008年至2011年来自三个亚洲队列（香港、新加坡和北京）的2649名实验室确诊的流感肺炎患者的研究发现糖皮质激素治疗增加流感肺炎患者二重感染率（9.7% vs. 2.7%）和死亡风险（adjusted HR 1.73, 95% CI 1.14~2.62）。另一项研究纳入了2009年6月至2014年4月来自西班牙148个ICU的1846名流感肺炎患者，该研究显示Cox回归分析（HR 1.32, 95% CI 1.08~1.60）和竞争风险分析（SHR 1.37, 95 CI 1.12~1.68）均表明糖皮质激素应用与流感肺炎患者的ICU死亡率相关。此外，还有相关研究显示早期使用糖皮质激素治疗严重的H1N1感染，延长患者的机械通气时间和ICU住院时间。我们对目前已发表的关于糖皮质激素治疗流感肺炎的系统综述和荟萃分析的结果进行了汇总，结果均显示糖皮质激素治疗与流感肺炎患者死亡率（图4-11-1a）和医院感染率（图4-11-1b）显著相关。

因此，对流感肺炎患者不推荐使用糖皮质激素治疗。然而这些结果主要来自观察性研究，尽管一些统计模型被用来调整混杂因素，未来仍需要足够有力的随机对照临床试验来验证这一结论。

二、糖皮质激素在SARS中的应用

在SARS暴发流行期间，糖皮质激素被广泛用于治疗重症SARS患者。然而关于糖皮质激素应用与SARS患者病死率之间的关系的报道不尽相同。陈荣昌教授团队发

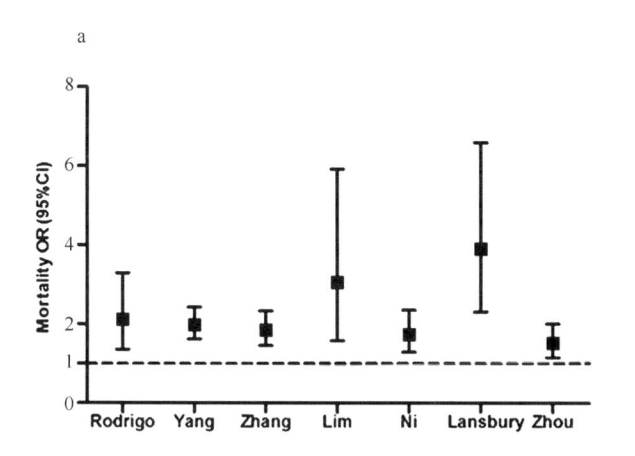

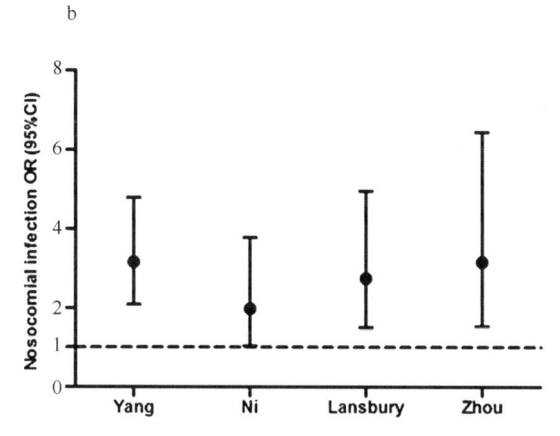

图 4-11-1 糖皮质激素治疗增加流感肺炎患者死亡率(a)和院内感染率(b)

表在 Chest 上的一项研究显示,对于重症 SARS 患者,适当应用糖皮质激素治疗可降低患者病死率,缩短住院时间,且与继发性下呼吸道感染和其他并发症无显著相关性。而 Auyeung 等发现,接受糖皮质激素治疗的 SARS 患者,其入住重症监护室或死亡的风险更高。另一项来自中国香港的回顾性研究共纳入 1287 名重症 SARS 患者,报道称接受糖皮质激素治疗组的患者死亡率高于未接受糖皮质激素治疗组(28.3% vs. 17%)。此外,Lee 等研究发现,对重症 SARS 患者进行早期糖皮质激素治疗与随后较高的血病毒载量相关,糖皮质类激素的应用延迟 SARS 冠状病毒的清除。据报道,重症 SARS 患者在接受糖皮质激素治疗后可出现侵袭性真菌感染、骨坏死等情况。因此,根据目前已发表的研究,对于 SARS 患者接受糖皮质激素治疗的有效性和安全性,我们无法得出明确的结论。

三、糖皮质激素在 MERS 中的应用

关于糖皮质激素治疗 MERS 的研究相对较少。Arabi 等报道了一项多中心、回顾性队列研究,研究对象为 2012 年 9 月至 2015 年 10 月,14 家沙特阿拉伯三级保健医院收治的 309 例 MERS 患者。其中 151 名患者接受了糖皮质激素治疗。研究结果显示接受糖皮质激素治疗的患者更有可能接受有创机械通气治疗(141/151,93.4% vs. 121/158,76.6%,$P<0.0001$),90 d 死亡率更高(112/151,74.2% vs. 91/158,57.6%,$P<0.002$)。然而在矫正了混杂因素后,回归分析结果显示糖皮质激素治疗与 MERS 患者 90 d 死亡率无显著相关性(adjusted OR 0.75,95% CI 0.52~1.07,$P=0.12$),但与 MERS-RNA 病毒清除延迟相关(adjusted HR 0.35,95% CI 0.17~0.72,$P=0.005$)。因此,对于 MERS 患者接受糖皮质激素治疗可能会延迟 MERS-RNA 病毒的清除。

四、糖皮质激素在 COVID-19 中的应用

目前,关于糖皮质激素在 COVID-19 中应用的有效性和安全性尚未确定,研究报道较少,专家意见不一。Russell 等认为先前发表的研究显示糖皮质激素应用与流感肺炎患者死亡率和继发感染风险增加相关,并且延迟 SARS、MERS 冠状病毒的清除,暂无支持糖皮质激素治疗 COVID-19 所致肺损伤的临床依据。然而中国专家组通过对新冠肺炎的救治及相关研究,认为对重症 COVID-19 患者可短期谨慎使用低至中等剂量的糖皮质激素治疗。

我们回顾了从开始到 2020 年 4 月 30 日所有关于激素治疗 COVID-19 的研究。系统分析发现糖皮质激素在新冠肺炎中的应用率为 22.4%(670/2995)。这些患者总体病死率为 4.2%(127/2995),糖皮质激素治疗组患者的病死率明显高于非糖皮质激素治疗组(69/443,15.6% vs. 56/1310,4.3%)。这可能与重症患者更倾向使用糖皮质激素组治疗相关。重症组激素使用率明显高于非重症组(201/382,52.6% vs. 301/1310,23.0%)。在临床实践中,一些小样本的观察性研究报道了糖皮质激素应用可改善严重的 COVID-19 患者的临床症状、氧合功能、减少住院时间和 ICU 入住时间。此外,宋元林教授团队的研究显示甲泼尼龙治疗可降低 COVID-19 合并 ARDS 患者的死亡风险(HR 0.38,95% CI 0.20~0.72)。然而这些研究均为样本量有限的单中心观察性研究,存在潜在偏倚和混杂因素,这些结果应谨慎解释。

总之,目前虽然没有循证医学证据支持糖皮质激素治疗降低 COVID-19 患者的死亡率,但一些临床观察研究显示糖皮质激素治疗可改善新冠肺炎患者的临床症状和氧合功能。尤其对有 ARDS 的新冠肺炎患者可能从糖皮质激素治疗中获益。甲泼尼龙是目前报道最多的治疗 COVID-19 的糖皮质激素,其他类型的糖皮质激素是否在 COVID-19 中起作用尚不确定。就剂量和持续时间而言,根据我们救治 COVID-19 的经验和中国专家共识,认为短期疗程的低至中等剂量的甲泼尼龙[0.5~1mg/(kg·d)]可能是合理的。因此,对于炎症反应剧烈的重症 COVID-19 患者,可以考虑及时、适当地使用糖皮质激素治疗,以防止发生急性呼吸窘迫综合征。遗憾的是,目前没有已证实的生物标记物来指导糖皮质激素在 COVID-19 中的应用。

五、糖皮质激素在 COVID-19 中的潜在作用机制

对于重症 COVID-19 患者在发病 1 周左右的时间内科出现严重的呼吸困难、急性呼吸窘迫综合征、多器官功能障碍，甚至死亡，并且重症患者血清中细胞因子和趋化因子浓度明显升高。我们知道，当病毒侵入呼吸道上皮细胞和肺泡上皮细胞时，刺激特异性免疫细胞(包括单核细胞、T 细胞、B 细胞、自然杀伤细胞)迅速产生大量细胞因子和趋化因子，如 TNF-α、IL-1、IL-6、IL-12、IFN-α、IFN-β、IFN-γ、MCP-1、IP10 和 IL-8。它们反过来促进炎性细胞浸润，从而产生更多细胞因子，这一过程被称为"细胞因子风暴"，在抗病毒的同时也会对肺部造成损害。先前的研究表明，过多的促炎细胞因子的释放，例如 IL-1β、IL-6、IFN-γ 的释放促进 SARS、MERS 患者发生 ARDS、MODS，甚至死亡。而 COVID-19 患者有同样现象。有研究报道 IL-1β、IFN-γ、IP10、MCP1、GSCF、IP10、MCP1、MIP1A 在重症 COVID-19 患者血清中显著增加，表明"细胞因子风暴"与 COVID-19 的严重程度相关。

而淋巴细胞减少可能是与 COVID-19 严重程度和死亡率相关的另一关键因素。先前的研究表明在病毒性肺炎中，死亡患者的 CD3$^+$ T 细胞、CD3$^+$ CD4$^+$ T 细胞和 CD3$^+$ CD8$^+$ T 细胞的绝对计数明显低于存活者，这表明重症病毒性肺炎患者的细胞免疫功能明显受到抑制。T 细胞免疫可能是一种重要的抗病毒机制，特别是关于 CD4$^+$ T 细胞的作用。

我们推测当 SARS-CoV-2 侵入肺泡上皮细胞时，病毒在早期阶段会强烈复制，激活淋巴细胞、巨噬细胞、自然杀伤细胞等。产生大量的细胞因子和趋化因子，它们反过来促进炎症细胞大量迁移到肺部。适度的免疫反应可及时清除病毒，而过度的免疫反应则导致大量炎症因子释放，形成炎症因子风暴，导致 ALI/ARDS。糖皮质激素治疗是一把双刃剑，可能会抑制过度的免疫反应，抑制炎症因子风暴，减轻肺损伤，也可能会抑制 T 淋巴细胞免疫反应，导致持续的病毒复制和随后的清除延迟(作用机制见图 4-11-2)。基于此，临床医师应谨慎合理使用糖皮质激素治疗病毒性肺炎。

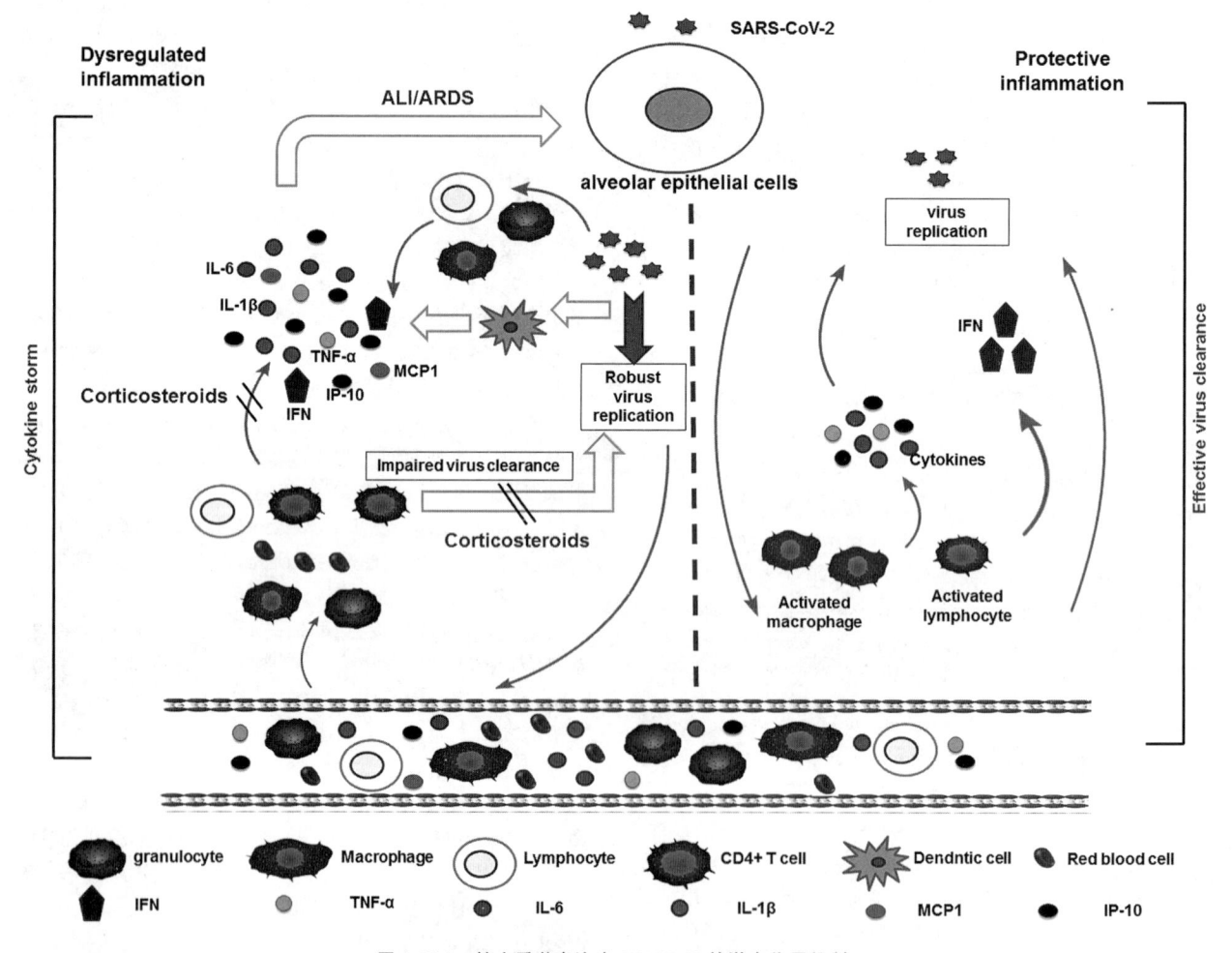

图 4-11-2 糖皮质激素治疗 COVID-19 的潜在作用机制

六、结论和未来展望

总之,对于糖皮质激素在病毒性肺炎中的应用仍然是一个具有挑战性的临床难题。尽管目前没有循证医学证据表明糖皮质激素治疗能降低 COVID-19 患者的病死率,但一些临床观察性研究显示,糖皮质激素治疗可以改善 COVID-19 患者的临床症状和氧合功能。细胞因子风暴和 T 细胞免疫的抑制和缺乏可能是重症 COVID-19 的主要潜在机制。因此,对于炎症反应剧烈的 ARDS 患者早期合理应用糖皮质激素治疗可能使其获益。未来需要对有 ARDS 的病毒性肺炎患者早期给予低至中等剂量甲泼尼龙进行随机对照临床试验,以确认糖皮质激素治疗的有效性和安全性,并进一步探索糖皮质激素治疗对病毒性肺炎患者的长期影响。

参 考 文 献

[1] WHO. Coronavirus disease (COVID-19) outbreak situation. June 30, 2020. http://covid19.who.int.

[2] Torres A, Sibila O, Ferrer M, et al. Effect of corticosteroids on treatment failure among hospitalized patients with severe community-acquired pneumonia and high inflammatory response: a randomized clinical trial. JAMA, 2015, 313: 677-686.

[3] Blum CA, Nigro N, Briel M, et al. Adjunct prednisone therapy for patients with community-acquired pneumonia: a multicentre, double-blind, randomised, placebo-controlled trial. Lancet, 2015, 385: 1511-1518.

[4] Villar J, Ferrando C, Martinez D, et al. Dexamethasone treatment for the acute respiratory distress syndrome: a multicentre, randomised controlled trial. Lancet Respir Med, 2020, 8: 267-276.

[5] Russell CD, Millar JE, Baillie JK. Clinical evidence does not support corticosteroid treatment for 2019-nCoV lung injury. Lancet, 2020, 395: 473-475.

[6] Shang L, Zhao J, Hu Y, Du R, Cao B. On the use of corticosteroids for 2019-nCoV pneumonia. Lancet, 2020, 39: 683-684.

[7] Lee N, Leo YS, Cao B, et al. Neuraminidase inhibitors, superinfection and corticosteroids affect survival of influenza patients. Eur Respir J, 2015, 45: 1642-1652.

[8] Moreno G, Rodríguez A, Reyes LF, et al. Corticosteroid treatment in critically ill patients with severe influenza pneumonia: a propensity score matching study. Intensive Care Med, 2018, 44: 1470-1482.

[9] Yang JW, Yang L, Luo RG, et al. Corticosteroid administration for viral pneumonia: COVID-19 and beyond. Clin Microbiol Infect, 2020.

[10] Chen RC, Tang XP, Tan SY, et al. Treatment of severe acute respiratory syndrome with glucosteroids. Chest, 2006, 129: 1441-1452.

[11] Auyeung TW, Lee JS, Lai WK, et al. The use of corticosteroid as treatment in SARS was associated with adverse outcomes: a retrospective cohort study. J Infect, 2005, 51: 98-102.

[12] Yam LY, Lau AC, Lai FY, et al. Corticosteroid treatment of severe acute respiratory syndrome in Hong Kong. J Infect, 2007, 54: 28-39.

[13] Lee N, Allen Chan KC, Hui DS, et al. Effects of early corticosteroid treatment on plasma SARS-associated Coronavirus RNA concentrations in adult patients. J Clin Virol, 2004, 31: 304-309.

[14] Arabi YM, Mandourah Y, Al-Hameed F, et al. Corticosteroid therapy for critically ill patients with the Middle East respiratory syndrome: a multicenter retrospective cohort study. Am J Respir Crit Care Med, 2018, 197: 757-767.

[15] Zhou W, Liu Y, Tian D, et al. Potential benefits of precise corticosteroids therapy for severe 2019-nCoV pneumonia. Signal Transduct Target Ther, 2020, 5: 18.

[16] Wang Y, Jiang W, He Q, et al. A retrospective cohort study of methylprednisolone therapy in severe patients with COVID-19 pneumonia. Signal Transduct Target Ther, 2020, 5: 57.

[17] Li R, Tian J, Yang F, et al. Clinical characteristics of 225 patients with COVID-19 in a tertiary Hospital near Wuhan, China. J Clin Virol, 2020, 127: 104363.

[18] Wu C, Chen X, Cai Y, et al. Risk factors associated with acute respiratory distress syndrome and death in patients with coronavirus disease 2019 pneumonia in Wuhan, China. JAMA Intern Med, 2020.

[19] Huang C, Wang Y, Li X, et al. Clinical features of patients infected with 2019 novel coronavirus in Wuhan, China. Lancet, 2020, 395: 497-506.

[20] Guo L, Wei D, Zhang X, et al. Clinical features predicting mortality risk in patients with viral pneumonia: The MuLBSTA Score. Front Microbiol, 2019, 10: 2752.

第五部分

间质性肺疾病

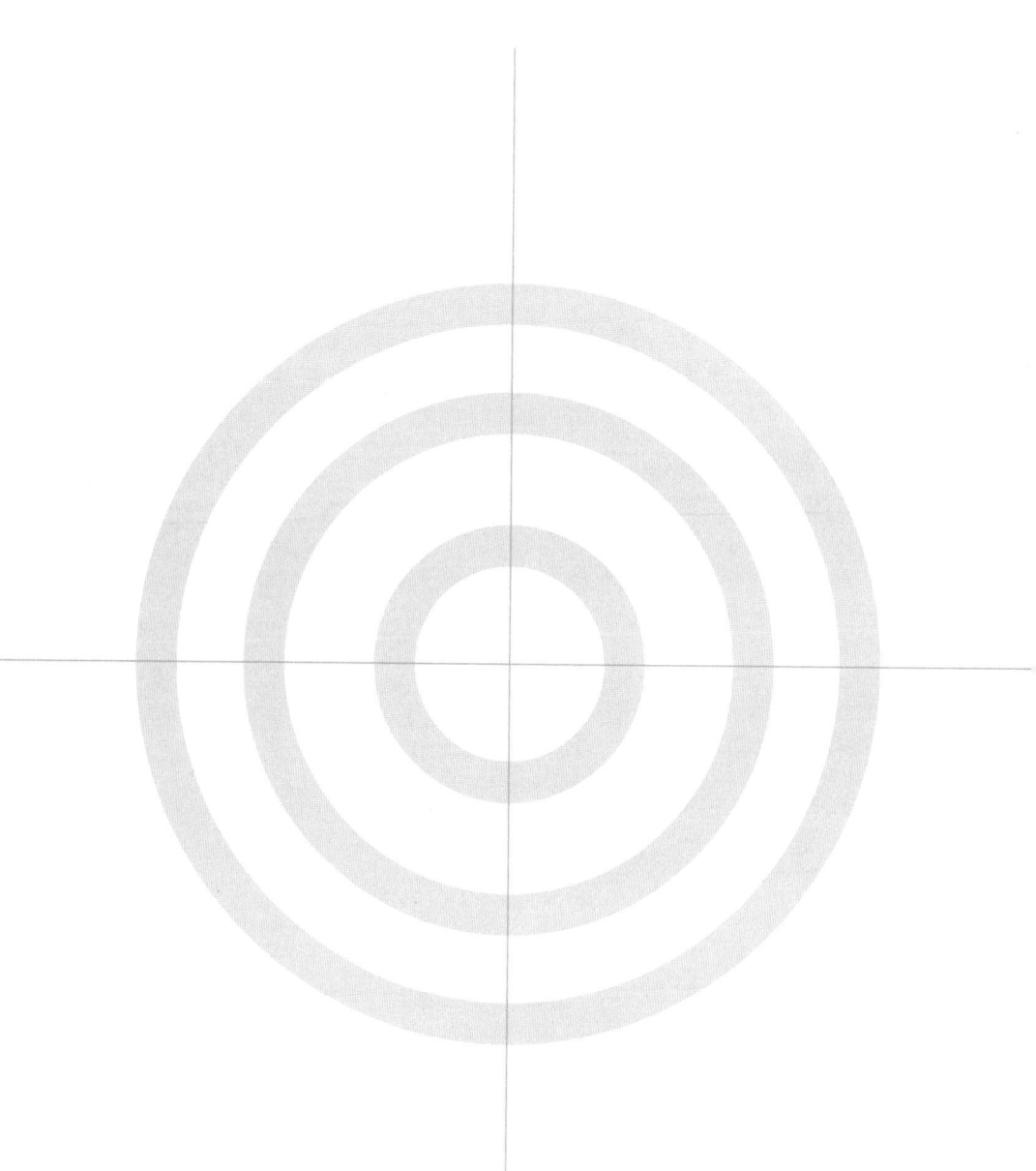

1 间质性肺疾病的影像学新进展：多模态成像定量影像学研究进展与临床应用

于 楠 郭佑民

间质性肺疾病（interstitial lung diseases，ILD）是一组具有高度异质性的疾病，从发病原因、病理特点，到影像学表现都具有相当的复杂性。对临床的诊断、治疗、评估造成困难。影像学是诊断及评估 ILD 的常用方法，然而大多为定性诊断，存在相当的主观性。随着近年来兴起的计算机辅助诊断（computer aided diagnosis，CAD），纹理分析、影像组学为基于 CT 图像的近一步特征提取和分析提供技术手段，能够区分肺实质不同病变的特点，发现支气管、肺血管的改变等。除此之外，新型的影像学成像技术也为形态学和功能学的结合提供信息，例如超极化气体 MRI 及正电子发射断层扫描（positron emission tomography，PET）。而基于多模态的 ILD 评价方法和技术探索是近年来影像学对 ILD 诊疗的最大贡献。

一、概 述

根据美国胸科学会（ATS）和欧洲胸科协会（ERS）的分类标准，ILD 的亚型主要包括以下几类：环境暴露有关的 ILD、继发于结缔组织疾病的 ILD、结节病和特发性间质性肺炎（idiopathic interstitial pneumonias，IIPs），例如特发性肺纤维化（idiopathic pulmonary fibrosis，IPF）、非特异性间质性肺炎。其中 IPF 是主要的亚型（图 5-1-1）。

ILD 患者早期症状并不典型，常被按照肺部感染或者肺水肿进行诊断和治疗。因此，多学科团队（a multidisciplinary team，MDT）需要结合患者的病史、临床表现、实验室检测、影像学表现及病理结果做出正确的诊断。此外，年龄也是 ILD 亚型判断的一个依据，IPF 患者年龄常介于 60～70 岁，而结缔组织相关性肺疾病（CTD-ILD）年龄多小于 50 岁。

影像学检查在 ILD 的诊断和评估中起着关键作用。仰卧位的深吸气扫描胸部 CT 是最常用的方法，薄层的胸部 CT 能够发现有无纤维化的发生、病变范围及病变的特点。俯卧位的扫描方式更有利于发现或鉴别两下肺胸膜下的细微的纤维化改变（图 5-1-2）。

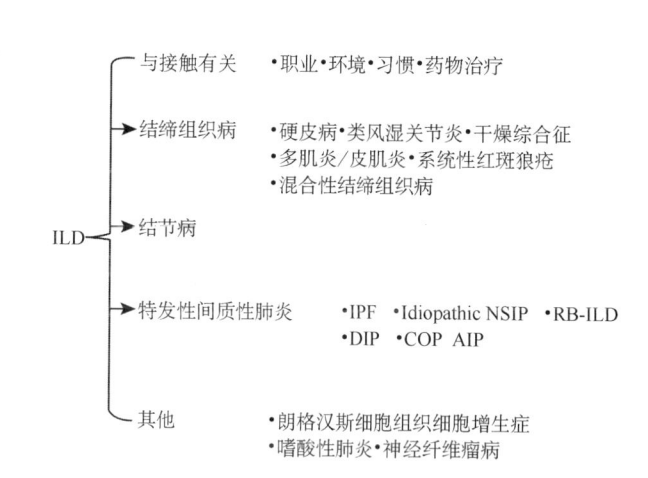

图 5-1-1 ILD 的分类

ILD. 间质性肺疾病；AIP. 急性间质性肺炎；COP. 隐源性组织性肺炎；DIP. 脱屑性间质性肺炎；IPF. 特发性肺纤维化；NSIP. 非特异性间质性肺炎；RB-ILD. 呼吸细支气管炎相关间质性肺病

胸部 CT 可发现病变以双下肺胸膜下、基底部分布为著，可表现为：①蜂窝影：表现为胸膜下簇状分布的囊状影，边界清楚，直径为 3～10mm。②不规则线影：为增厚的小叶间隔、小叶内间隔及蜂窝影的壁形成。③由于邻近纤维组织增生及肺结构破坏所致的牵拉性支气管不规则管腔扩张。④磨玻璃影：表现为肺密度的增加，但是仍不掩盖肺血管（图 5-1-3）。如出现下面任何一项则不考虑 ILD 诊断：病灶以中上肺为主，病灶以支气管周围为主，广泛的磨玻璃影（程度超过网状影）；多量的小结节（两侧分布，上肺占优势）；不连续的囊腔（两侧多发，远离蜂窝肺区域）；弥漫性马赛克密度/空气潴留（两侧分布，3 个或更多肺叶受累），支气管肺段/叶实变。

然而胸部 CT 对病变特点、范围的评估往往是主观的，而缺乏量化的手段，随着定量影像学及其他影像学成像手段的应用，为全面评估 ILD 病变发生与变化提供技术手段。

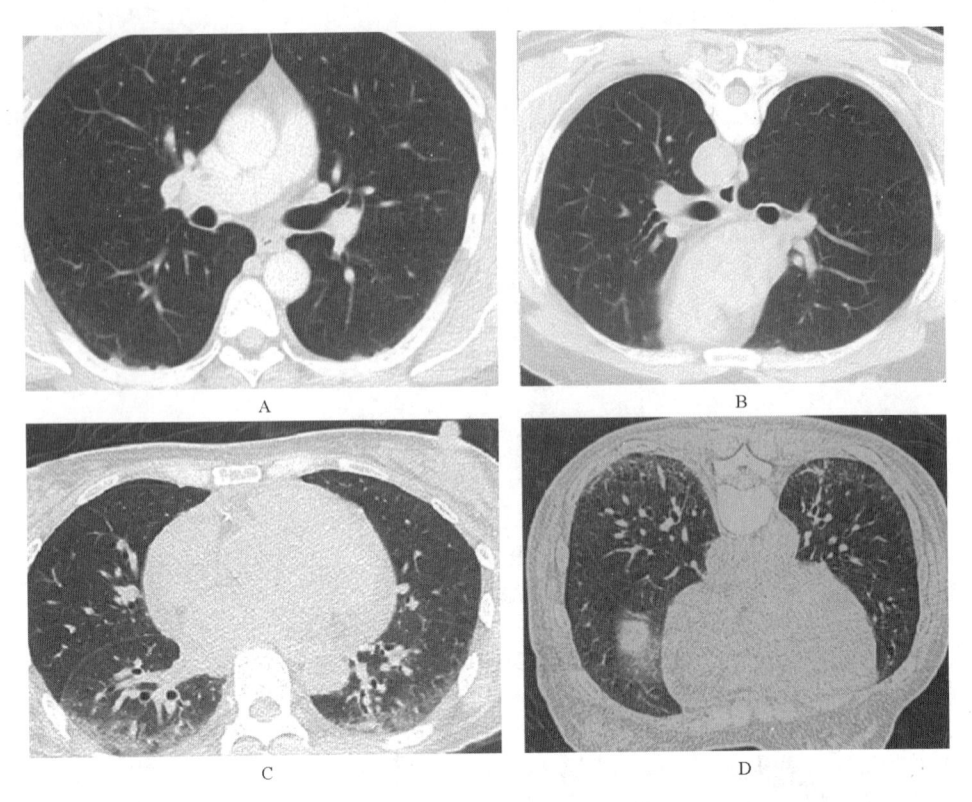

图 5-1-2 仰卧位和俯卧位 CT 的比较

A、B. 乳腺癌患者胸部 CT 轴位图像仰卧位显示两下肺胸膜下不规则影,俯卧位显示胸膜下无异常密度影;C、D. 系统性红斑狼疮患者,仰卧位胸部 CT 显示两下肺胸膜下磨玻璃影,俯卧位显示原先磨玻璃影为不规则线影,边界清楚(引自 Thoracic Imaging,2019:361-423.)

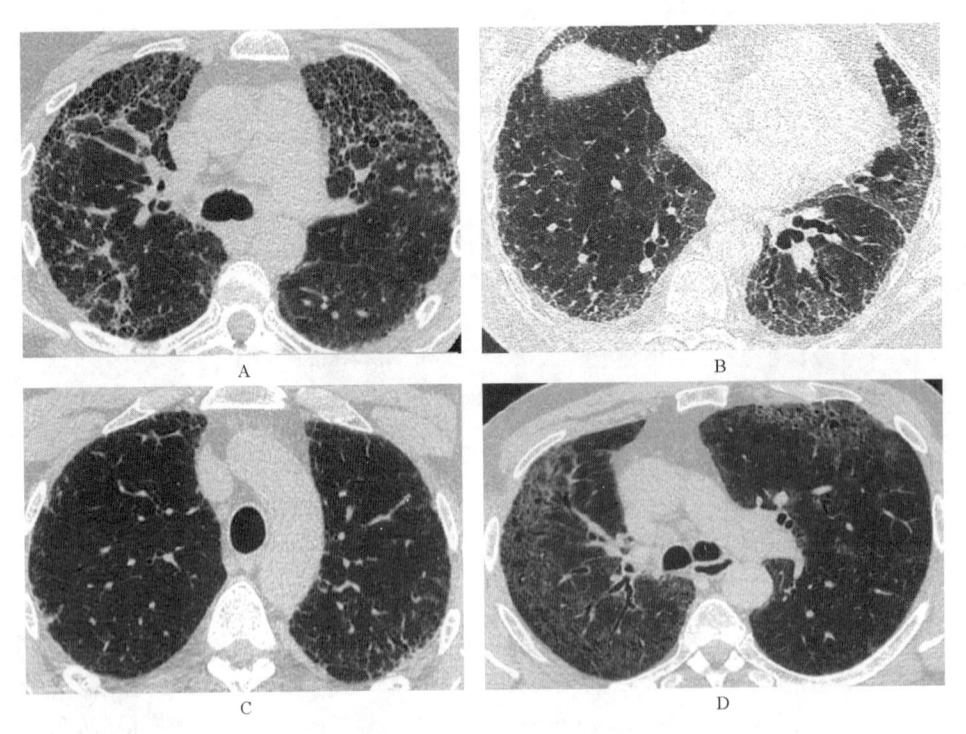

图 5-1-3 ILD 的胸部 CT 表现

A. 两肺上叶腹侧为主的蜂窝征;B. 左肺下叶胸膜下可见牵拉性支气管扩张;C. 左肺上叶胸膜下可见不规则线影;D. 两上肺胸膜下广泛分布的磨玻璃影,其内可见扩张支气管影[引自 J Comput Assist Tomogr,2019,43(6):898-905.]

二、定量 CT 分析

(一) 半定量分析

CT 半定量分析方法是影像学医生根据 ILD 的各影像学特点在各肺叶中累及百分比来计算的方法。需要影像科医生的主观判断，但是在一定程度上引入了定量的概念，并且经过量化的病变范围能够用来随访病变进展、对患者预后做出判断。Nurmi 等采用 CT 半定量手段也证实网格影、牵拉支气管扩张及肺结构变形的范围与类风湿关节炎患者预后不良有关。Moore 等对系统性硬化症肺损伤情况进行评价发现，使用半定量 CT 评价肺病变范围对患者死亡率具有预测作用。然而半定量手段的缺点在于，仍然依赖医生的主管判断。观察者的内部与外部异质性都较差。

(二) 肺密度与体积的定量分析

目前使用的 CT 定量分析对 ILD 的评估主要通过两个方面：肺密度（图 5-1-4，图 5-1-5）和肺体积（图 5-1-6）。正

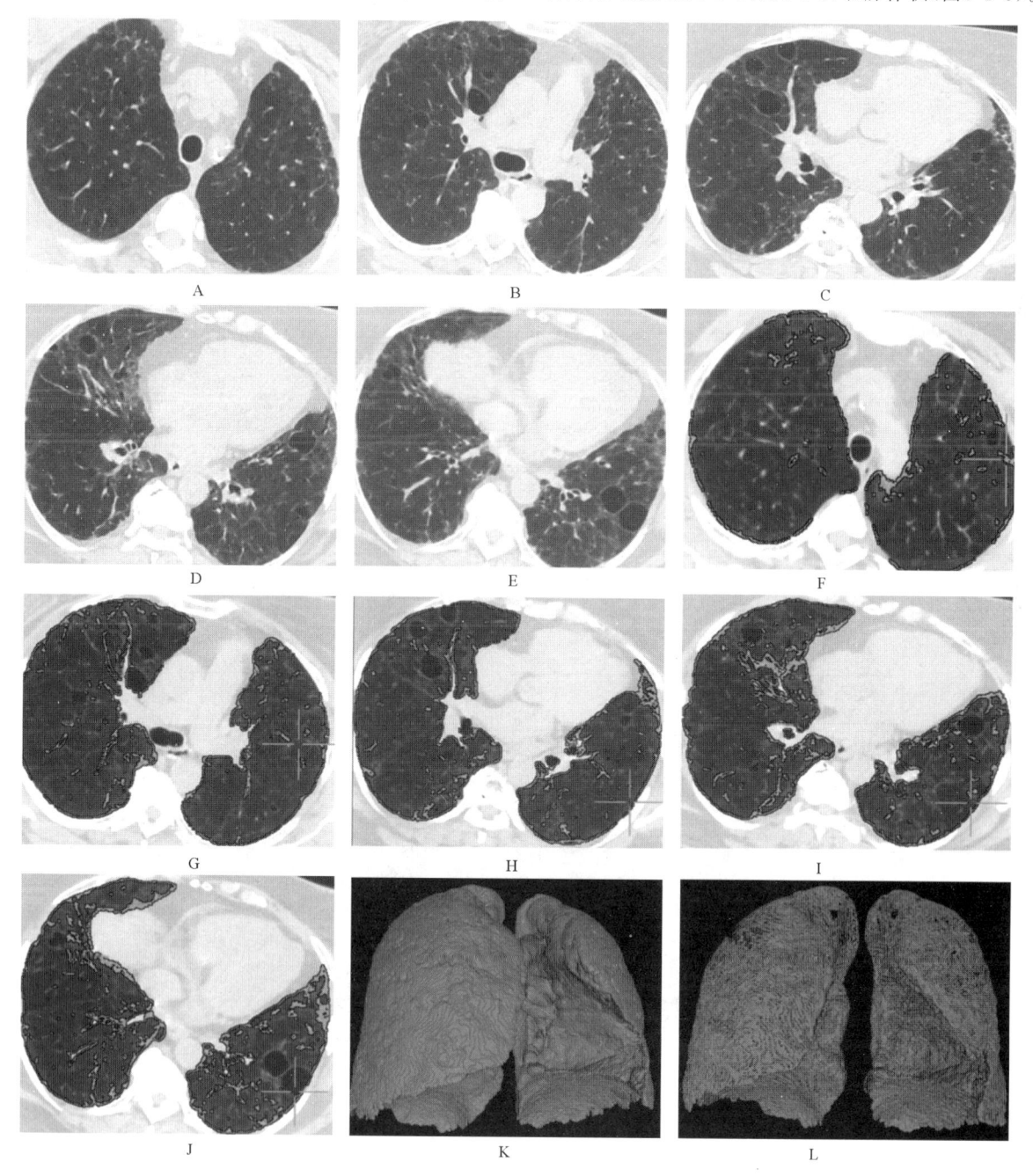

图 5-1-4 56 岁女性，干燥综合征相关性间质性肺病，诊断为淋巴细胞性间质性肺炎

A~E. 轴位高分辨率 CT 原始图像的不同层面显示双侧间质增厚，斑片状磨玻璃和散在的薄壁圆形气囊，主要分布胸膜下；F~J. 对同一患者的肺定量评价图像。在 -200 HU 和 -950 HU 之间的所有体素提取作为总肺容积（TLV）TLV 计算为 3602 cm³（K.）。在 -200 和 -700 HU 之间的所有体素显示了 ILD 的体积，发现为 404 cm³（L.）。ILD 指数 =（ILD 体积/TLV）×100
[引自 European Journal of Radiology,2020,7(1):109030.]

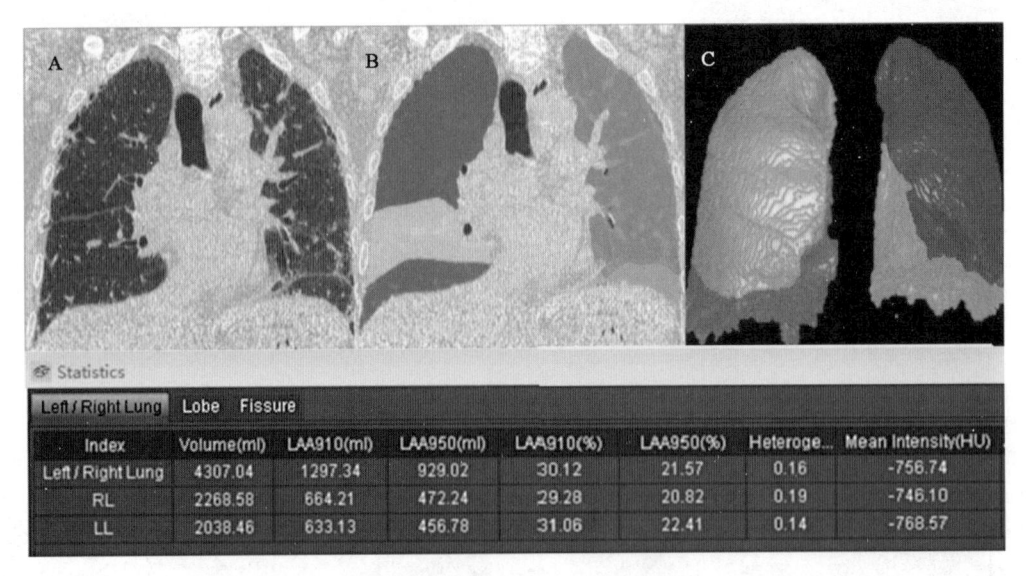

图 5-1-5 全肺及各肺叶的分割及提取

A~C. 分别为 CT 冠状位、肺叶二维分割结果和三维分割结果,能够计算全肺及各肺叶的体积、平均密度等指标[引自 Journal of X-Ray Science and Technology,2019,27(4):591-603.]

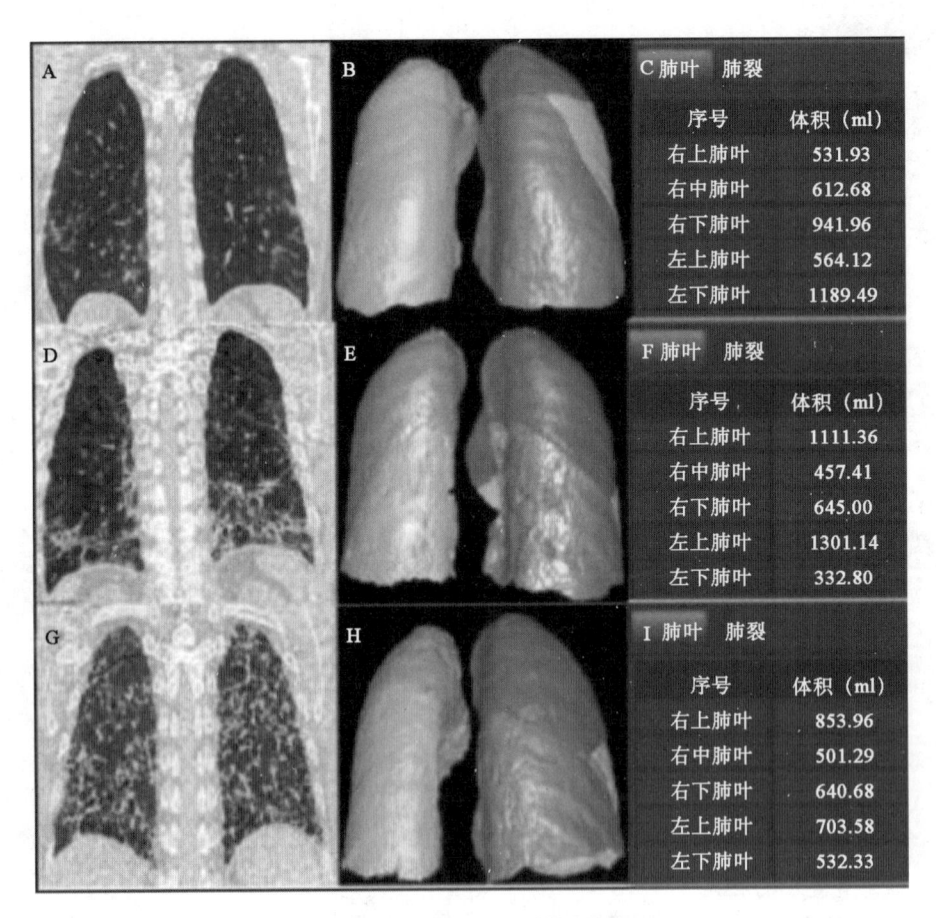

图 5-1-6 不同程度 ILD 肺体积比较

A~C. 男性,40 岁,结缔组织相关性间质性肺疾病,按照 Ashcroft 8 级及 Jacob 4 级评分法肺间隔中等程度纤维化,肺泡结构无明显破坏,为 3 分,轻度病变。全肺容积 3840.19ml,全肺容积未明显缩小,肺密度改变不显著,全肺肺气肿容积及占比明显增大。D~F. 62 岁,UIP。按照 Ashcroft 8 级及 Jacob 4 级评分法肺组织结构破坏,明显纤维化,纤维团灶状增生,为 5 分,中度病变。病变累及 1/3~2/3 肺泡间隔和细小支气管周围肺间质,双肺下叶体积缩小 20%~40%,双肺上叶容积代偿性增 20%~30%。G~I. 65 岁,IPF。按照 Ashcroft 8 级及 Jacob 4 级评分法肺间隔严重破坏,伴蜂窝肺形成,为 7 分,重度病变。病变累及>2/3 的肺泡间隔和细小支气管周围肺间质,双肺下叶体积缩小 30%~50%,全肺容积缩小约 38%。全肺密度升高,双肺下叶明显,全肺肺气肿容积及占比增大,双肺上叶明显(郭佑民团队研究结论)

常肺密度CT值的峰值在-800HU,并且左偏。当发生纤维化时,平均肺密度(mean lung density,MLD)增加,密度直方图显示肺密度分布的峰度和偏度减低。有研究证明MLD的增加与ILD疾病严重程度有关。

然而,MLD是基于全肺的测量,肺内局部发生的空气潴留、肺气肿的低密度区域都可能会影响MLD的测量值,使得全肺的MLD值减低,影响对整体肺实质病变的判断。除此之外,对于ILD的不同病理特点的区别,依靠肺密度的区分仍然是有争议的。有研究认为依靠MLD和肺密度峰度和偏度能够区分NSIP和UIP,而有些研究不能发现两者差异。肺体积的测量是通过对全肺进行分割后对整体肺体积进行定量测量。ILD后期多伴有肺体积缩小,然而肺外围病变可能会影响整体肺的分割,且患者扫描时的呼吸配合也会影响到肺体积的测量。

(三)肺纹理分析与机器学习

基于CT的纹理分析能够通过对肺组织每个像素密度和形态的特点提取和分析获得整个及局部肺实质的纹理特征。基于这些纹理学信息可以用来描述及区别ILD的不同影像学特征,例如区分肺气肿、蜂窝征,在纤维化组织中发现磨玻璃影,在肺气肿中提取纤维化组织。例如自适应多特征方法(adaptive multiple feature method,AMFM)肺纹理分析软件,三维的AMFM软件能够区分肺气肿、肺实变和蜂窝征,敏感性和特异性均在95%以上。在一项关于IPF的大型临床研究中,使用AMFM软件进行定量分析,发现磨玻璃影的范围为IPF进展密切相关。

关于肺实质纹理分析的机器学习有两种类型:监督型和无监督型。非监督的数据驱动的组织纹理分析(data-driven textural analysis,DTA)软件机器被赋予没有任何预标记的数据,并且必须独立地确定如何对数据进行分组。DTA能够从CT原始数据中获得组织纹理信息。通过相同像素纹理的聚类从正常组织中分离出纤维组织,并且对其定量,获得纤维化程度值。有研究对280例IPF患者肺纤维化定量值与肺功能相关性做出分析,发现二者相关性好,且在随访过程中,肺功能的下降伴随着肺纤维化值的增加。

另一种监督型的机器学习模型为用于病理评估和分型的计算机辅助肺信息学模型(computer aided lung informatics for pathology evaluation,CALIPER,图 5-1-7),这种分析方法利用肺组织研究联盟(Lung Tissue Research Consortium)数据库中病理证实的14例ILD患者的薄层CT图像,将肺实质分为感兴趣容积区(volumes of interest,VOIs)。再随机选择的VOIs由4位胸部放射专家分为以下五类:正常、磨玻璃影、不规则网格影、蜂窝影、低密度衰减区和(或)肺气肿(图 5-1-8)。使用CALIPER分析55例IPF患者发现,ILD的总体积、不规则网格影的总体积都和患者的生存率有关(图 5-1-9)。

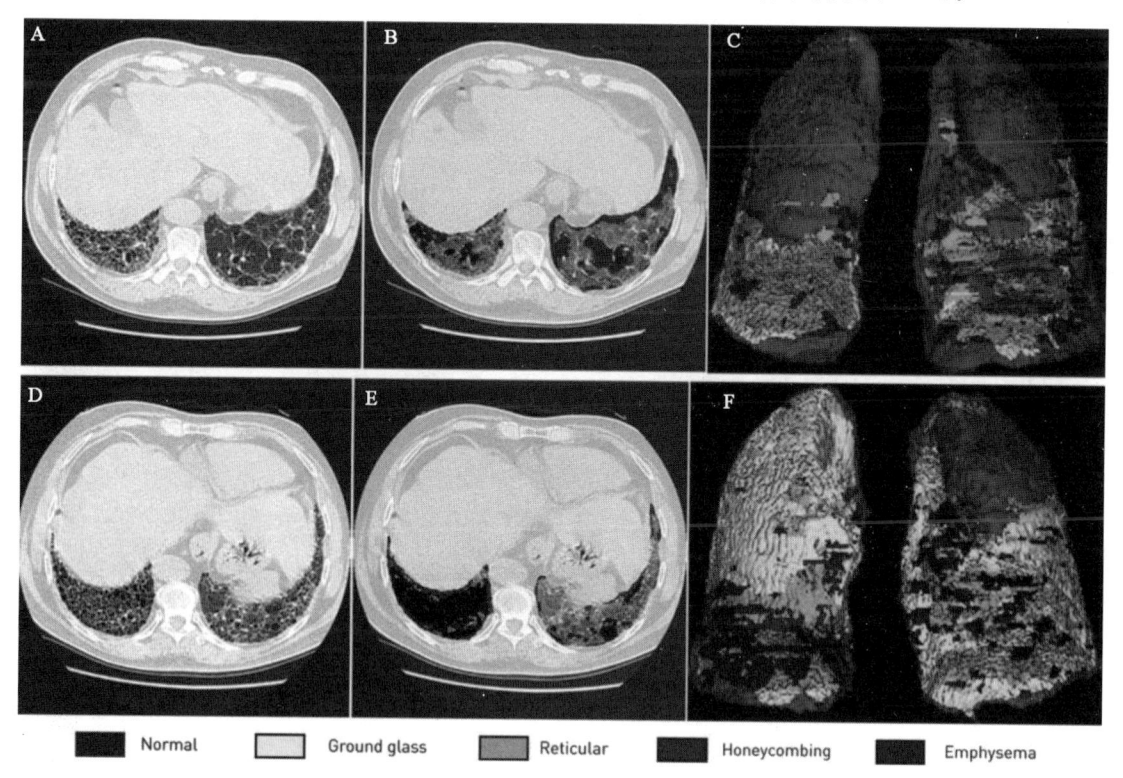

图 5-1-7 CALIPER 的定量分析结果展示

A~C和D~F分别是同一患者不同时间的2次影像学分析结果。三维定量结果在D和F中呈现。不同颜色分别代表正常肺组织、磨玻璃影、不规则线影、蜂窝征和肺气肿[引自 Eur Respir J,2014,43(1):204-212.]

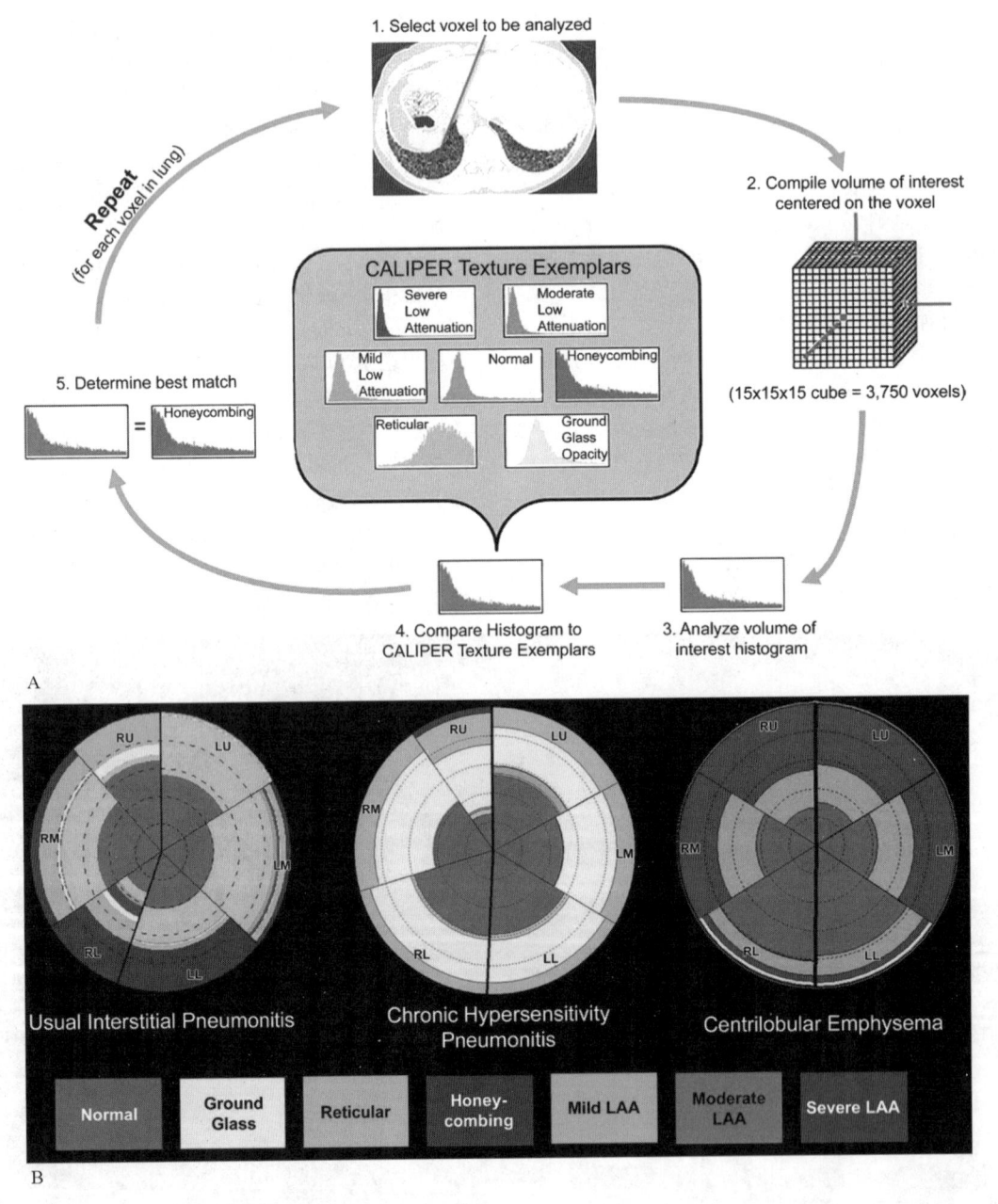

图 5-1-8　基于 CALIPER 纹理分析的流程

A. 流程图显示了 CALIPER 测量肺实质的过程。对于每个 15×15×15 大小的体素，计算基于直方图的特征，然后与已经标记并训练获得的组学特征比对，然后进行分类。B. 图中显示了纹理特征输出。整个圆形代表整个肺容积，并按肺解剖结构划分，同心圆中扇形虚线内代表该肺叶的 20%。肺实质异常的分布和模式表明疾病过程，如 UIP 的双基底层蜂窝状改变（左），慢性过敏性肺炎（CHP）的磨玻璃改变（中），或小叶中心性肺气肿（右）以上肺为主的低密度区（LAA）[引自 RadioGraphics,2020,40(1):28-43.]

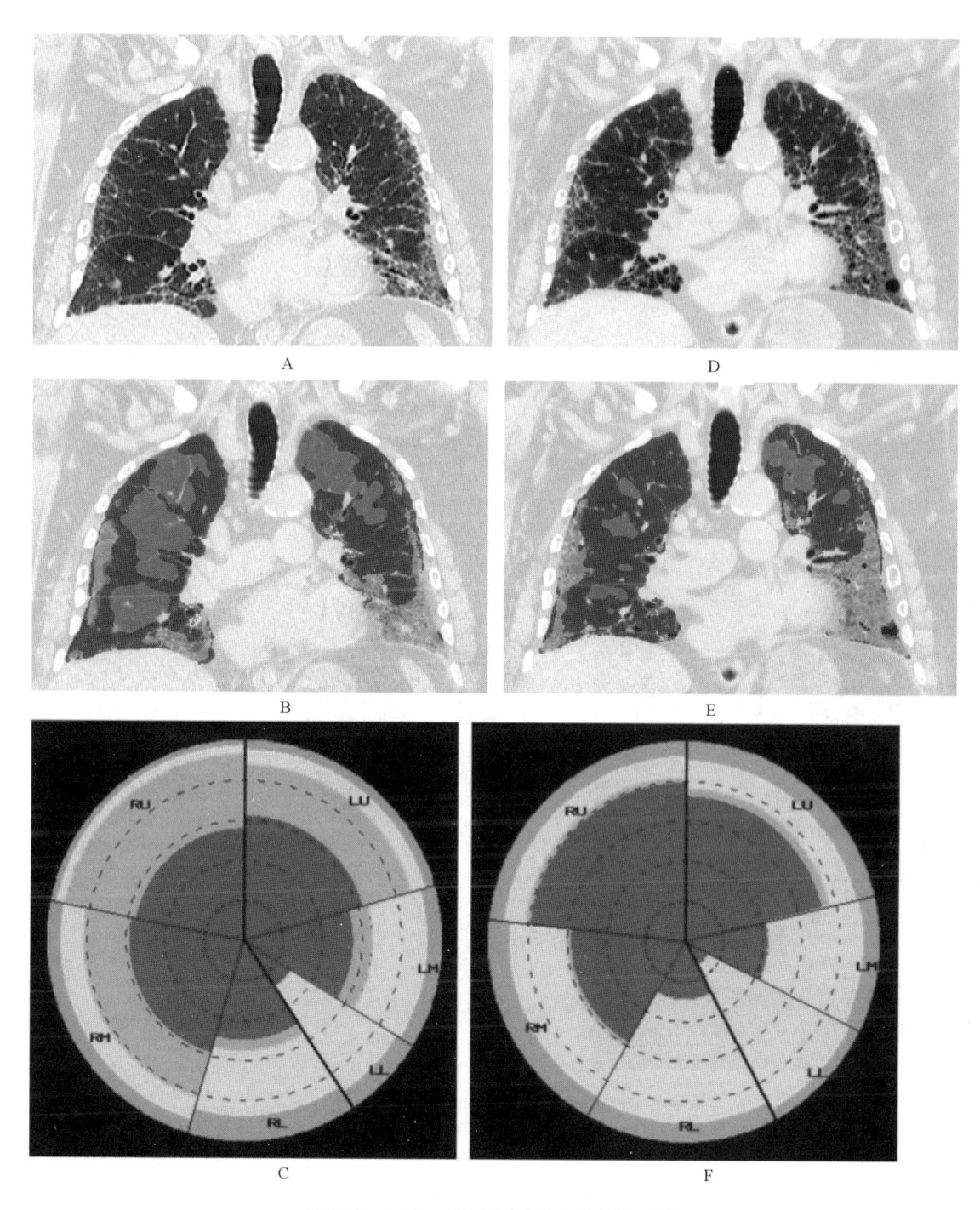

图 5-1-9　CALIPER 纹理分析量化患者的纵向变化

IPF 患者基线 CT 冠状位（A～C）和 2 年随访（D～F）图像,原始图像对病变范围评估较为困难,病变范围没有明显变化。而通过定量分析发现磨玻璃影、网状变化和蜂窝状影在随访中范围扩大。其他区域为正常肺实质[引自 RadioGraphics,2020,40(1):28-43.]

(四) 肺血管分析

肺间质病疾病常常累及肺血管,因此对肺血管病变的分割和定量是评价也是需要研究的。通过对全肺血管体积(pulmonary vessel volume,PVV)的提取和定量不仅与 ILD 病变范围有关,并且当结合 PPV 与 CALIPER 指标后(图 5-1-10),对 ILD 预后评价更好。目前使用的 PVV 分割方法有基于 CT 的血管横截面积定量法。然而关于肺血管的分割(图 5-1-11)、定量及对血管分支的形态测量仍然是分割的难点,需要进一步的人工智能模型进行分析。

总之,CT 定量分析是 ILD 定量分析的主要手段,但目前 CT 定量分析仍然存在以下问题:①CT 扫描数据的同质化问题,多中心研究所面临的扫描设备、扫描参数、重建参数的方式不同可能会影响定量分析结果,因此需要对不同

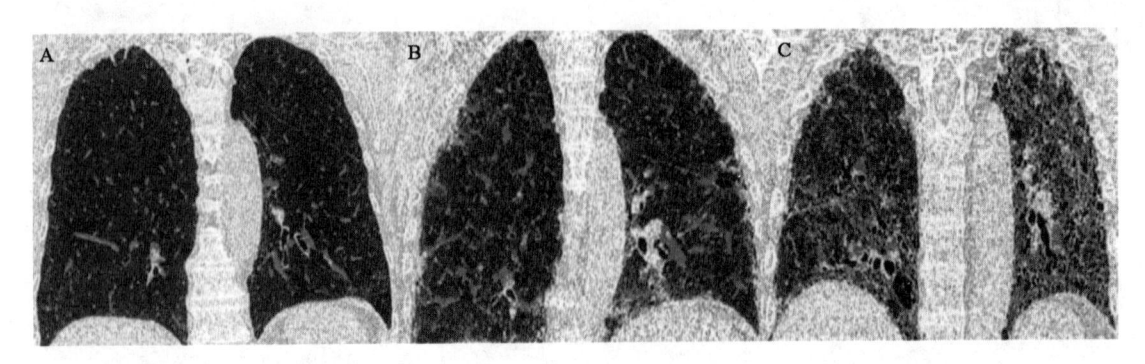

图 5-1-10 肺血管测量的方法

肺动脉和静脉分割的结果(红色)以肺血管容积(PVV)描述及与 CALIPER 定量结果的关系。图 A 病例 1:62 岁女性戒烟者,有 15 包/年的吸烟史,CALIPER 肺的总 ILD 范围为 2%(磨玻璃影 0.7% 和网状型 0.9%),PVV 占肺容积的 2%。图 B 病例 2:61 岁的女性,既往吸烟,有 25 包/年的吸烟史,CALIPER 检查显示 ILD 的总范围为 27%(磨玻璃影 15.2%,网格影 11.4%)。PVV 占肺容积的 6%。图 C 病例 3:64 岁,男性、戒烟者,有 40 包/年的吸烟史,CALIPER 确定的 ILD 总范围为 55%(磨玻璃影 41.1%,网格影 12%,蜂窝影 1.3%)。PVV 占肺容积的 9%[引自 Eur Respir J,2017,49(1):16.]

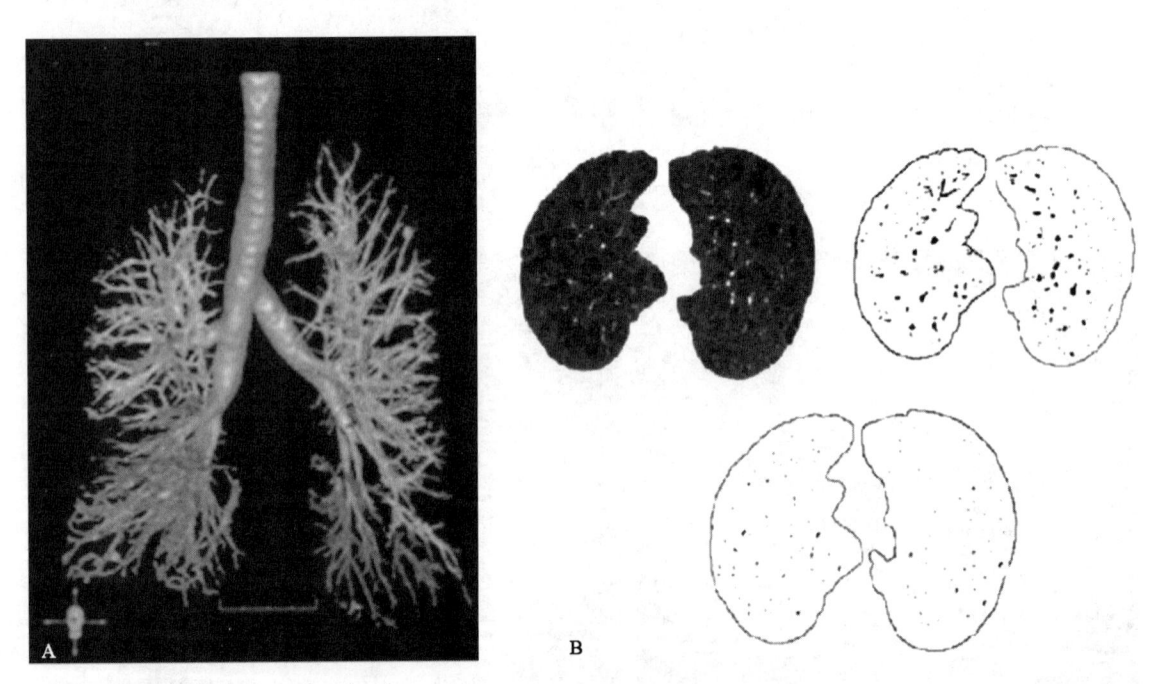

图 5-1-11 肺血管的分割和定量测量的两种方法

A~B 分别表示肺血管的两种定量测量方法。A. 肺血管三维结构的提取和显示,通过对全肺血管的提取,获得全肺血管的总体积;B 肺血管二维提取和定量,通过对 CT 断面的肺血管横断面(黑点、线)的分离,对垂直走形的肺血管进行提取(黑点),最后进行定量测量,获得肺血管断面的总体横截面积[引自 J Xray Sci Technol,2017,25(3):391-402.]

数据来源进行标准化。②患者扫描时的呼吸配合问题,对于深吸气扫描的训练、患者配合都可能影响肺密度,因此需要对数据进行校正。③定量分析反映的主要是肺结构的改变,但不能完全反映肺功能改变。因此,在有解剖成像的同时,需要进一步采用影像学多模态的技术方法,从功能方面对肺间质纤维化进行评估。

三、磁共振成像功能评价

近年来的磁共振成像(magnetic resonance imaging,MRI)新的序列,例如超短回波时间序列(ultrashort echo time,UTE,图 5-1-12)为 ILD 结构评价提供可能性。尤其是 3D 自由呼吸序列,在自由呼吸模式下采用较长的采集时间能够获得高质量的图像,有研究证明 UTE MRI 能够获得和 CT 类似的图像效果。也有研究证明 T_1 和 T_2 弛豫时间能够显示 ILD 的肺实质特征。发生纤维化的肺组织较肺气肿 T_1 弛豫时间更长,也有研究证明磨玻璃影、不规则线状影及蜂窝征之间 T_2 弛豫时间有差异。当 ILP 伴发感染时,T_2 弛豫时间增加。

(一)磁共振弹性成像

磁共振弹性成像(MR elastography,MRE)是测量组织硬度的一种方法(图 5-1-13)。通过评价机械波在组织中的

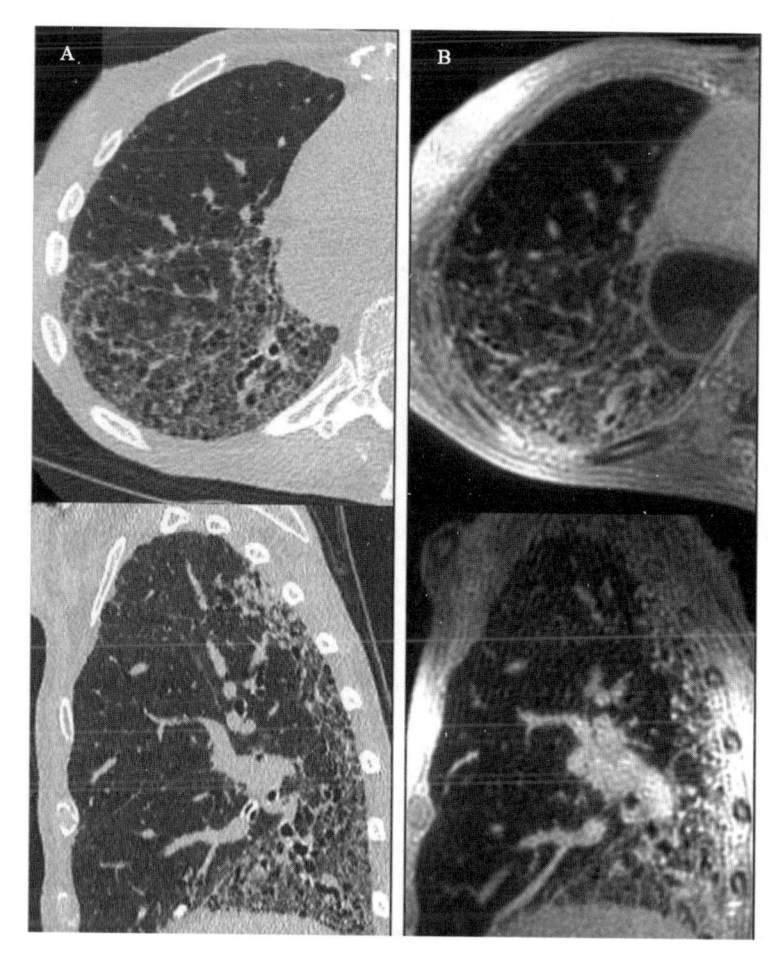

图 5-1-12 轴位和矢状位 CT 和相应的 3D-UTE 图像
A、B. 3D-UTE 与 CT 同样能够发现胸膜下的蜂窝征,但 CT 图像分辨率仍然好于 3D-UTE(引自 Magn Reson Med(2013),70:1241-1250.)

传播,从而提供关于组织弹性的信息。MRE 已经在临床上被用来评价慢性肝病患者的情况,是一种安全的、可靠的、无创的、可以代替肝脏活检用来对肝脏纤维化进行分期的新型技术。有研究使用 MRE 技术对 ILD 患者和正常对照组之间进行比较发现两者差异,因此 MRE 是否可用来进行 ILD 进展的评价仍需要进一步研究的积累。

轴位 CT 和 MRI 与弹性成像的融合图像,观察残余容积(RV)和总肺容量(TLC)轴向 CT 图像对应于 MR 融合图的大致解剖位置。

(二)超极化气体 MRI

超极化气体 MRI(MR Imaging with hyperpolarized gas)是指患者吸入氦(^{3}He)或氙气(^{129}Xe)提高肺部的磁性的 MR 肺成像方法。超极化气体是在纯气体制备,或与氮气或氧气混合。患者吸入后屏住呼吸数秒钟进行图像采集。

吸入 ^{129}Xe 不局限在气道内,而是穿过肺泡间质进入毛细血管血液。利用氙气 ^{129}Xe 在气相和水相[组织和血浆,tissue and plasma,(TP)]和红细胞(red blood cell,RBC)中的化学位移,使用光谱技术能够发现肺泡到毛细血管之间的扩散受限(图 5-1-14)。在 IPF 患者中,RBC 信号峰值较 TP 信号峰值相对减低(图 5-1-15)。且有研究证明信号峰度的改变与 IPF 和 CTD-ILD 患者的一氧化碳弥散(diffusing capacity of the lungs for carbon monoxide,DLCO)值相关。

(三)动态增强 MRI

MRI 肺功能成像除上述的技术以外,还有动态增强显像。动态增强磁共振成像(dynamic contrast-enhanced MRI,DCE)为肺血流动力学评估提供了一种手段。与一组没有肺部疾病的志愿者相比,ILD 患者的肺动脉流量较慢(图 5-1-16)。然而,肺动脉流量作为一种单一的测量方法并没有显示出与疾病严重程度的相关性。

总之,MRI 作为肺功能的评价是一种无辐射的检测手段,且新的检查序列还需要不断的探索对 ILD 的评价。

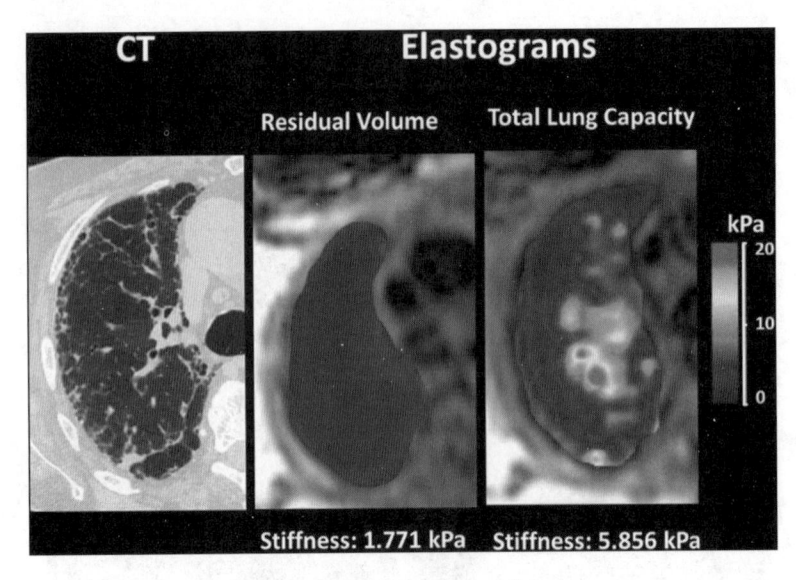

图 5-1-13　男性,76 岁,ILD 患者

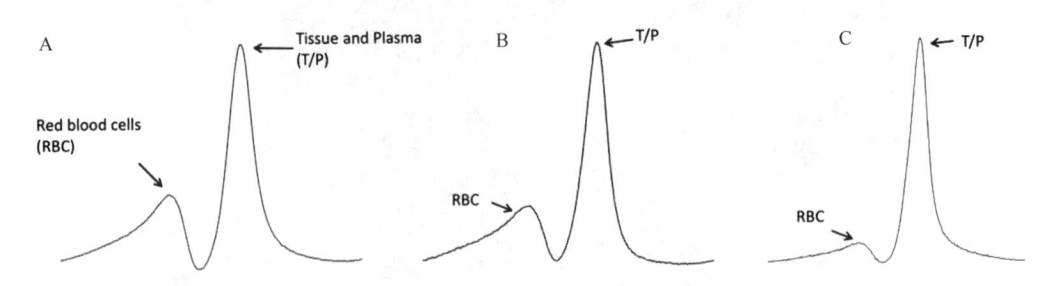

图 5-1-14　超极化气体 MRI 的谱峰
A. 正常志愿者 RBC 和 TP 峰值;B. 轻度 IPF;C. 重度 IPF 显示 RBC 谱峰相对 TP 峰减低(引自 Thorax,2019,0:1-9.)

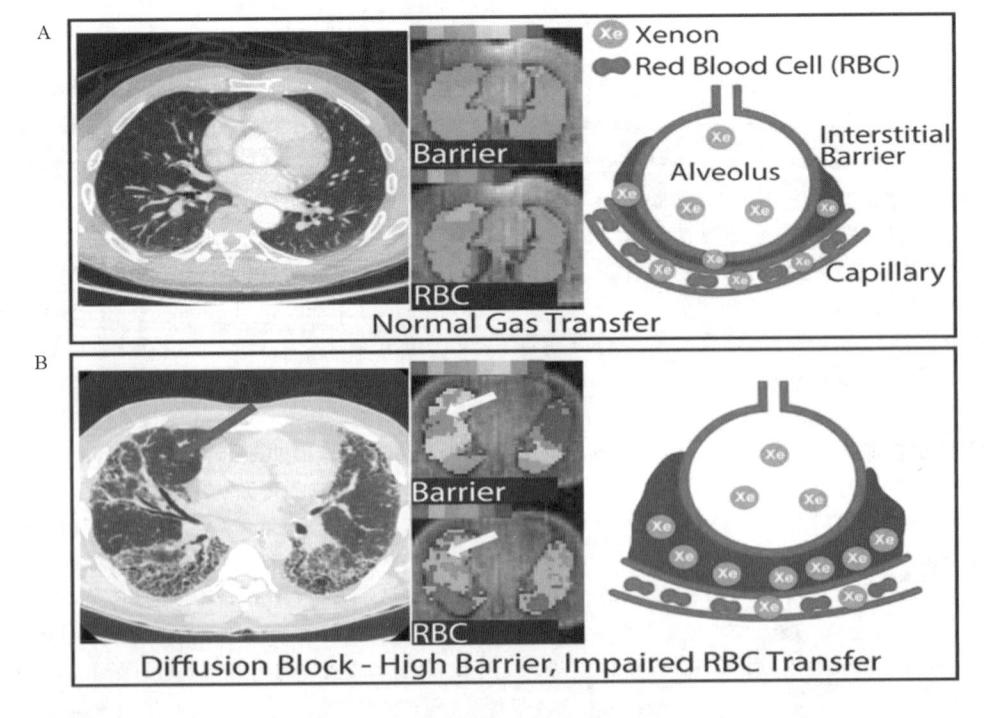

图 5-1-15　超极化气体 MRI 的扩散示意图
在健康肺(图 A)中,氙气有效地穿过肺泡膜扩散到红细胞中(红细胞),信号强度在 2 个腔隙的信号都正常;在 IPF 中,间质增厚,增加组织中氙的摄取。在某些区域(图 B,箭头),扩散速度减慢,导致红细胞转移减少

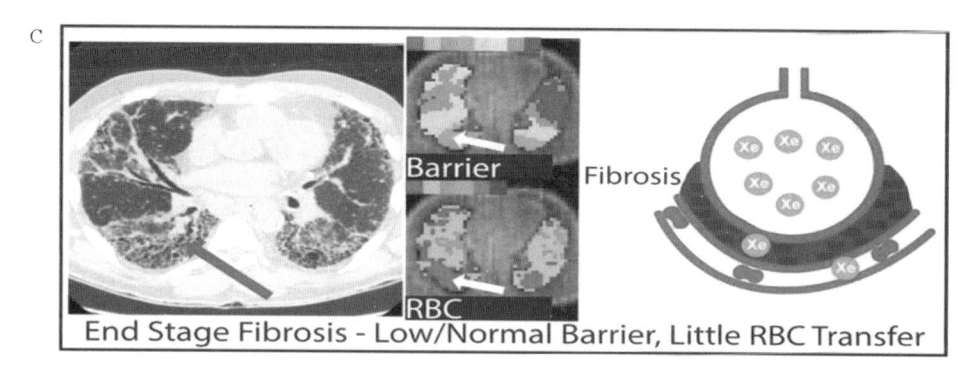

图 5-1-15(续)

随着疾病的进展(图C),间质增厚更加严重^{129}Xe不再扩散到或通过屏障(引自 Thorax,2018,73:21-28.)

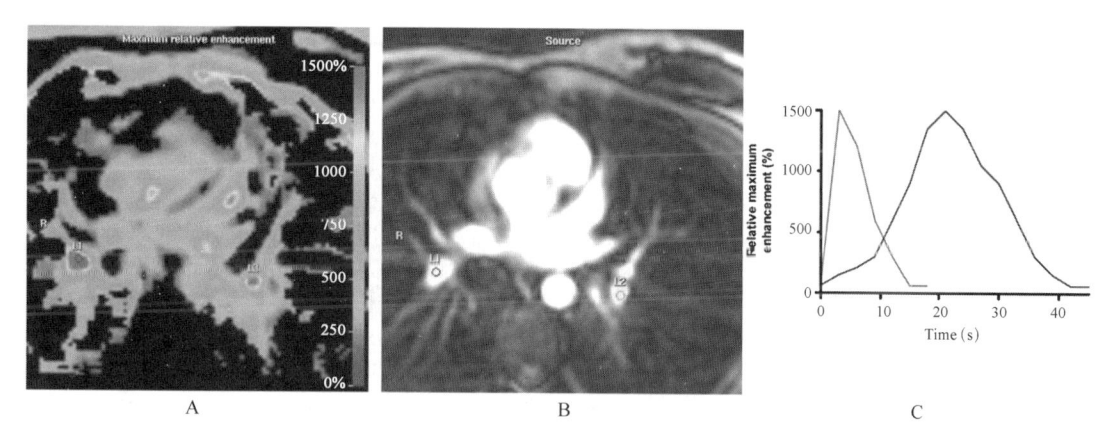

图 5-1-16 男性,58岁,肺纤维化肺气肿综合征

在肺血管区域的彩色编码图上手动绘制ROI(A),显示最高信号强度投影值(红色)。然后在解剖对比增强图像上自动叠加ROI(B)。在一个心动周期内生成的时间-信号强度曲线。绿色代表50岁男性对照组的曲线。红色代表肺纤维化肺气肿综合征患者曲线(C)(引自 Radiology,2010;254:601-608.)

四、正电子发射断层扫描

正电子发射断层扫描(positron emission tomography,PET)在ILD的评估中很少使用。FDG的标准化摄取值(SUV)与22例机化性肺炎患者的淋巴细胞活性有关。PET在纤维占优势的ILD中的作用不太直观。但在ILD患者中正常肺组织的SUV值较高。因此多时间点的数据有利于评估SUV值与ILD病变进展的关系。此外,新的PET示踪剂的研发也是PET在ILD评估的另一个趋势。

五、小 结

多模态成像的定量分析在ILD评估中发挥越来越大的作用。虽然这些方法需要进一步的外部验证,尚未在临床实践中常规使用,但它们有望成为ILD评估的辅助工具,并可能在诊断和评估治疗反应中发挥重要作用。量化肺血管变化可能被证明是ILD评估中一个全新的指标。纹理分析、聚类技术和机器学习可以使自动分层疾病的图像,并提供决策支持。MRI和PET仍然是ILD中的探索性技术,但可能提供疾病的功能和解剖元素之间的联系。

参 考 文 献

[1] American Thoracic Society. Idiopathic pulmonary fibrosis:diagnosis and treatment. International consensus statement. American Thoracic Society(ATS),and the European Respiratory Society(ERS). Am J Respir Crit Care Med,2000,161(2 pt 1):646-664.

[2] Raghu G,Remy-Jardin M,Myers JL,et al. Diagnosis of idiopathic pulmonary fibrosis. AN official ATS/ERS/JRS/ALAT clinical practice guideline. Am J Respir Crit Care Med,2018,198:e44-e68.

[3] Raghu G,Collard HR,Egan JJ,et al. An official ATS/ERS/JRS/ALAT statement: idiopathic pulmonary fibrosis: evidence based guidelines for diagnosis and management. Am J Respir Crit Care Med,2011,183:788-824.

[4] 中国医师协会风湿免疫科医师分会风湿病相关肺血管/间质

病学组国家风湿病数据中心. 2018 中国结缔组织病相关间质性肺病诊断和治疗专家共识. 中华内科杂志, 2018, 57(8): 558-565.

[5] Kim M, Lee SM, Song JW, et al. Added value of prone CT in the assessment of honeycombing and classification of usual interstitial pneumonia pattern. Eur J Radiol, 2017, 91: 66-70.

[6] Ashish Chawla Tze Chwan Lim Vijay Krishnan Chai Gin Tsen. Imaging of Interstitial Lung Diseases. Thoracic Imaging, 2019: 361-423.

[7] 中华医学会病理学分会胸部疾病学组. 中国特发性肺纤维化临床-影像-病理诊断规范. 中华病理学杂志, 2018, 47(2): 81-86.

[8] Lucia Chen, Varsha Halai, Andreea Leandru, and Adam Wallis. Interstitial Lung Disease: Update on the Role of Computed Tomography in the Diagnosis of Idiopathic Pulmonary Fibrosis. J Comput Assist Tomogr, 2019, 43(6): 898-904.

[9] Alicia Chen, Ronald A. Karwoski, BA, David S. Gierada, Brian J. Bartholmai, Chi Wan Koo, Quantitative CT Analysis of Diffuse Lung Disease. 2020, RadioGraphics, 2020, 40(1): 28-43.

[10] Nurmi HM, Kettunen HP, Suoranta SK, et al. Several high-resolution computed tomography findings associate with survival and clinical features in rheumatoid arthritis-associated interstitial lung disease. Respir Med, 2018, 134: 24-30.

[11] oore OA, Goh N, Corte T, et al. Extent of disease on high-resolution computed tomography lung is a predictor of decline and mortality in systemic sclerosis-related interstitial lung disease. Rheumatology, 2013, 52(1): 155-160.

[12] Colombi D, Dinkel J, Weinheimer O, et al. Visual vs Fully Automatic Histogram Based Assessment of Idiopathic Pulmonary Fibrosis (IPF) Progression Using Sequential Multidetector Computed Tomography (MDCT). PLoS One, 2015, 10: e0130653.

[13] Ash SY, Harmouche R, Vallejo DL, et al. Densitometric and local histogram based analysis of computed tomography images in patients with idiopathic pulmonary fibrosis. Respir Res, 2017, 18: 45.

[14] urkan Ufuka, Mahmut Demircia, Goksel Altinisikb, Ugur Karasuc. Quantitative analysis of Sjogren's syndrome related interstitial lung disease with different methods. European Journal of Radiology, 2020, 7(1): 109030.

[15] Do KH, Lee JS, Colby TV, et al. Nonspecific interstitial pneumonia versus usual interstitial pneumonia: differences in the density histogram of high-resolution CT. J Comput Assist Tomogr, 2005, 29: 544-548.

[16] Sverzellati N, Calabrò E, Chetta A, et al. Visual score and quantitative CT indices in pulmonary fibrosis: Relationship with physiologic impairment. Radiol Med, 2007, 112: 1160-1172.

[17] Nan Yin, Cong Shen, Fuwen Dong, Jun Wang, Youmin Guo, Lu Bai. Computer-aided identification of interstitial lung disease based on computed tomography. Journal of X-Ray Science and Technology, 2019, 27(4): 591-603.

[18] Salisbury ML, Lynch DA, van Beek EJ, et al. Idiopathic Pulmonary Fibrosis: The Association between the Adaptive Multiple Features Method and Fibrosis Outcomes. Am J Respir Crit Care Med, 2017, 195: 921-929.

[19] Humphries SM, Yagihashi K, Huckleberry J, et al. Idiopathic pulmonary fibrosis: data-driven textural analysis of extent of fibrosis at baseline and 15-month follow-up. Radiology, 2017, 285: 270-278.

[20] Salisbury ML, Lynch DA, van Beek EJ, et al. Idiopathic Pulmonary Fibrosis: The Association between the Adaptive Multiple Features Method and Fibrosis Outcomes. Am J Respir Crit Care Med, 2017, 195: 921-929.

[21] Humphries SM, Yagihashi K, Huckleberry J, et al. Idiopathic pulmonary fibrosis: data-driven textural analysis of extent of fibrosis at baseline and 15-month follow-up. Radiology, 2017, 285: 270-278.

[22] Erickson BJ, Korfiatis P, Akkus Z, Kline TL. Machine Learning for Medical Imaging. RadioGraphics, 2017, 37(2): 505-515.

[23] Bartholmai BJ, Raghunath S, Karwoski RA, et al. Quantitative computed tomography imaging of interstitial lung diseases. J Thorac Imaging, 2013, 28(5): 298-307.

[24] Maldonado F, Moua T, Rajagopalan S, et al. Automated quantification of radiological patterns predicts survival in idiopathic pulmonary fibrosis. Eur Respir J, 2014, 43(1): 204-212.

[25] Jacob J, Bartholmai BJ, Rajagopalan S, et al. Mortality prediction in idiopathic pulmonary fibrosis: evaluation of computer-based CT analysis with conventional severity measures. Eur Respir J, 2017, 49(1): 16.

[26] Jacob J, Bartholmai BJ, Rajagopalan S, et al. Predicting outcomes in idiopathic pulmonary fibrosis using automated computed tomographic analysis. Am J Respir Crit Care Med, 2018, 198: 767-776.

[27] Pinal-Fernandez I, Pineda-Sanchez V, Pallisa-Nuñez E, et al. Fast 1.5 T chest MRI for the assessment of interstitial lung disease extent secondary to systemic sclerosis. Clin Rheumatol, 2016, 35: 2339-2345.

[28] Johnson KM, Fain SB, Schiebler ML, et al. Optimized 3D ultrashort echo time pulmonary MRI. Magn Reson Med, 2013, 70: 1241-1250.

[29] Buzan MTA, Wetscherek A, Heussel CP, et al. Texture analysis using proton density and T2 relaxation in patients with histological usual interstitial pneumonia (UIP) or nonspecific interstitial pneumonia (NSIP). PLoS One, 2017, 12: e0177689.

[30] Marinelli JP, Levin DL, Vassallo R, et al. Quantitative assessment of lung stiffness in patients with interstitial lung disease using MR elastography. J Magn Reson Imaging, 2017, 46: 365-374.

[31] Wang Z, Robertson SH, Wang J, et al. Quantitative analysis of hyperpolarized 129 Xe gas transfer MRI. Med Phys, 2017, 44: 2415-2428.

[32] Wang JM, Robertson SH, Wang Z, et al. Using hyperpolarized 129Xe MRI to quantify regional gas transfer in idiopathic pulmonary fibrosis. Thorax, 2018, 73: 21-28.

[33] Weatherley ND, Stewart NJ, Chan HF, et al. Hyperpolarised xenon magnetic resonance spectroscopy for the longitudinal

assessment of changes in gas diffusion in IPF. Thorax,2019,74:500-502.
[34] Tsuchiya N,Ayukawa Y,Murayama S. Evaluation of hemodynamic changes by use of phase-contrast MRI for patients with interstitial pneumonia,with special focus on blood flow reduction after breath-holding and bronchopulmonary shunt flow. Jpn J Radiol,2013,31:197-203.
[35] Gianluigi Sergiacomi,Francesca Bolacchi,Marcello Cadioli. Combined pulmonary fibrosis and emphysema:3D time-resolved MR angiographic evaluation of pulmonary arterial mean transit time and time to peak enhancement. Radiology,2010,254(2):601-608.
[36] Mostard RL,Verschakelen JA,van Kroonenburgh MJ,et al. Severity of pulmonary involvement and(18)F-FDG PET activity in sarcoidosis. Respir Med,2013,107:439-447.
[37] Jacquelin V,Mekinian A,Brillet PY,et al. FDG-PET/CT in the prediction of pulmonary function improvement in nonspecific interstitial pneumonia. A Pilot Study. Eur J Radiol,2016,85:2200-2205.

2 间质性肺疾病药物治疗进展

郭 建 徐作军

间质性肺疾病(ILD)是一组可以累及肺间质、肺实质、小气道、肺血管和淋巴管的异源性疾病,不同的原因,治疗的方法和预后各不相同。虽然 ILD 的病因多样,但从临床治疗角度来说,可以将 ILD 大致分为非致纤维化性间质性肺病和致纤维化性间质性肺病两大类,对于前者治疗方案主要针对不同的原因和(或)辅以糖皮质激素和免疫抑制剂治疗,预后往往相对较好;而对于致纤维化性间质性肺病,治疗方案除了针对不同的原因和(或)辅以糖皮质激素和免疫抑制剂治疗外,还需要考虑给予抗纤维化治疗,预后相对较差,是临床治疗的难点。本文就临床常见的几种致纤维化性间质性肺病的抗纤维化治疗进展做一简要介绍。

一、特发性肺纤维化(IPF)的药物治疗

(一)吡非尼酮和尼达尼布

抗纤维化一直是 IPF 治疗研究的热点,自 2014 年美国 FDA 批准吡非尼酮和尼达尼布用于治疗 IPF 以来,先后多个版本的指南都对这两种药物进行了酌情推荐,其有效性和安全性一直也是关注的焦点。

2019 年,Bargagli 等报道了分别使用吡非尼酮和尼达尼布治疗 82 位 IPF 患者,发现予抗纤维化治疗后,两组患者 FVC、FEV1 和 TLC 与基线相比均未见明显下降,而对照组下降明显,提示两种抗纤维化药物效果确切,但这两种药物之间未见明显差异。

TOMORROW 和 INPULSIS 研究事后分析了尼达尼布在 52 周治疗+7d 期间进展事件的发生情况。进展事件定义为 FVC%预计值下降≥10%,急性加重,IPF 相关住院和死亡。结果显示在尼达尼布组($n=723$)和安慰剂组($n=508$),分别有 36.4% 和 53.5% 发生≥1 次进展事件($P<0.001$);有 32.5% 和 49.0% 患者发生≥1 次的 FVC%预计值相对下降≥10%($P<0.001$),4.4% 和 6.9% 的患者发生≥1 次急性加重($P=0.061$),5.0% 和 7.1% 的患者发生≥1 次 IPF 相关住院($P=0.121$),5.8% 和 8.3% 的患者死亡($P=0.092$)。在尼达尼布组和安慰剂组中,分别有 27.0% 和 39.2% 的患者发生 1 次进展事件,6.4% 和 9.3% 的患者发生 2 次进展事件,2.9% 和 3.3% 的患者发生 3 次进展事件,0.1% 和 1.8% 的患者发生≥4 次进展事件。与安慰剂相比,尼达尼布显著降低了发生首次进展事件(HR 0.62 [95%CI:0.53,0.74];$P<0.0001$)和第二次进展事件(HR 0.63 [95%CI:0.45,0.88];$P=0.0098$)的风险。

目前临床上大多是应用尼达尼布或吡非尼酮的单药治疗,两药联合是否可以让患者获益更大尚无定论,近年来也有学者进行尝试。2017 年,Vancheri 在先给予尼达尼布治疗 4~5 周后的患者中加用吡非尼酮,对比单用尼达尼布发现两药联合安全性和耐受性良好,效果确切。2018 年,Kevin R.F 一项纳入 89 名 IPF 患者,持续 24 周的 4 期临床研究揭示对比单药吡非尼酮,加用尼达尼布两药联用,安全性尚可,大多数患者可耐受。2019 年,Luca Richeldi 发现在单用或联用吡非尼酮或尼达尼布,两种药物不存在药代动力学的相互影响。虽然上述研究展示出两药联用治疗 IPF 的新前景,但尚不能根据这些结果推荐在 IPF 治疗过程中联合应用吡非尼酮和尼达尼布。

(二)新型抗纤维化药物

1. 自溶素-卵磷脂酸通路抑制剂(Autotaxin lysophosphatidic acid,LPA) LPA 参与多种器官的纤维化过程,通过靶向阻断自溶素或 LPA 受体抗纤维化是目前研究热点内容之一。2018 年发表的 FLORA 研究,发现自溶素阻滞剂 GLPG1690 可以延缓治疗组 FVC 下降速度,治疗后 FVC 与基线水平基本平行,甚至略有提高,但对照组下降明显,提示 GLPG1690 有望成为 IPF 治疗的新干预靶点,目前已获批进入 3 期临床试验。在另一项研究中,BMS-986020(LPA 受体阻滞剂),可以明显延缓治疗组 FVC 下降,并呈现剂量相关性,但由于 BMS-986020 可导致肝酶升高和胆囊炎,目前实验已停止。以上两项实验展现出 LPA 通路在抗 IPF 的治疗中的新希望,但是其安全性还需进一步评价。

2. 抗结缔组织生长因子抗体 结缔组织生长因子(connective tissue growth factor,CTGF)参与介导了多种器官纤维化过程,包括 IPF。研究发现,约 1/3 的 IPF 患者在应用 Pamrevlumab(FG-3019,抗 CTGF 抗体)后,可稳定或改善 FVC 和 HRCT 下肺纤维化的程度。基于此,一项 2 期实验 PRAISE(NCT01890265)获批进行,现有的数据表明,相对于安慰剂,Pamrevlumab 治疗可以显著延缓 FVC 下降,改善 IPF 患者症状,但更全面的资料有待于更新公布。

3. 正五聚蛋白-2(血清淀粉样蛋白 P,SAP) 动物实验揭示 SAP 可以抑制小鼠博来霉素诱导的肺纤维化,抑制中性粒细胞黏附细胞外基质蛋白。一项应用 PRM-151(重组人正五聚蛋白-2)治疗 IPF 的研究发现 FVC 预测值在治

疗组和对照组分别下降2.5%和4.8%($P<0.05$),且患者安全性和耐受性良好,提示PRM-151可以减缓IPF患者肺功能下降。

除上述所述,还有许多治疗IPF的新型药物目前尚处于临床试验阶段,其有效性和安全性还需进一步评价。比如GPR40激动剂/GPR84拮抗剂,PBI-4050通过调节巨噬细胞、成纤维细胞和上皮细胞等多种细胞抑制博来霉素诱导的小鼠肺纤维化。NCT02538536研究者发现PBI-4050可以和吡非尼酮或尼达尼布联用,且安全性、耐受性良好。抗αvβ6整合蛋白抗体BG00011可以抑制IPF患者肺泡上皮细胞TGF-β信号表达从而抑制IPF纤维化过程。

(三)其他治疗相关进展

1. 抗酸治疗 2015年,IPF指南对抗酸治疗做出了弱推荐,随后不断有学者对抗酸治疗的有效性及安全性提出质疑。Michael Kreuter在对623例患者的研究中发现,服用抗酸药物+吡非尼酮与单用吡非尼酮在延缓FVC下降等关键指标上未见差异。相似的一项IPF患者外科胃底折叠术(WRAP-IPF)抑酸治疗亦抑酸治疗对改善IPF预后的作用。

2. 抗生素治疗 不断有研究发现,IPF患者和健康群体间存在菌群差异,提示在抗IPF时可加入抗生素,相关治疗方案目前已取得一定进展。目前,两项磺胺甲噁唑和多西环素的研究正在进行,相关结果尚未公布。

二、结缔组织病相关的间质性肺病(CTD-ILD)

多种结缔组织病均可累及肺脏,表现为间质性肺病(ILD),CTD-ILD在ILD中占据着相当的比例。以系统性硬化症(SSc)为例,ILD是SSc的一种常见表现(16%~91%),也是导致SSc死亡的首要原因(30%~35%)。目前SSc的治疗有多种药物可选,但患者是需要初始治疗还是强化治疗应综合考虑疾病进展速度、并发症、药物毒性等多方面因素。

(一)SSc的免疫抑制治疗

硬皮病-肺-研究Ⅰ发现(环磷酰胺口服1年,最大剂量2mg/kg)对比安慰剂组,治疗组FVC改善2.5%($P<0.05$),且这种改善效应停药后消失。硬皮病-肺-研究Ⅱ发现[比较口服环磷酰胺2mg/(kg·d)×1年和吗替麦考酚酯1.5g bid×2年]发现口服吗替麦考酚酯与环磷酰胺效果相当,且更为安全。

(二)SSc的生物制剂治疗

Khanna D等研究者托珠单抗的3期临床试验显示出其稳定FVC的效果优于对照组。最近日本一项对比利妥昔单抗和环磷酰胺的研究显示接受利妥昔单抗治疗的患者FVC和DLCO变化情况均明显好于环磷酰胺组(20.6%±8.8% vs 1.1%±3.9% $P<0.05$;34.0%±6.0% vs -1.5%±2.8%,$P<0.01$)。

(三)SSc的抗纤维化治疗

SSc-ILD和IPF在成纤维细胞增殖、迁移和分化等病理机制上有相似之处。尼达尼布作为一种细胞内酪氨酸激酶抑制剂,在SSC-ILD的临床前模型中,显示出了良好的抗纤维化和抗炎作用。

2020年ATS发布了SENSCIS研究中SSc-ILD接受尼达尼布治疗的情况。SENSCIS是一项多中心、随机、双盲、安慰剂对照的Ⅲ期临床试验,旨在探究尼达尼布治疗系统性硬化病相关间质性肺疾病(SSc-ILD)患者52周的疗效及安全性。共有576例患者接受了至少一剂尼达尼布或安慰剂治疗;51.9%的患者存在弥漫性皮肤型系统性硬化病,48.4%的患者在基线时接受麦考酚酯治疗。在主要终点分析中,尼达尼布组的调整后FVC年下降率为-52.4 ml/年,安慰剂组为-93.3 ml/年[组间差异为41.0 ml/年;95%置信区间(CI):2.9~79.0;$P=0.04$],展现出良好的改善SSc-ILD FVC的作用。

三、进行性纤维化性间质性肺疾病(PF-ILD)

PF-ILD是近年来提出的概念,指对治疗无反应,HRCT持续纤维化,肺功能进行性下降,症状逐渐加重的一组ILD。PF-ILD治疗相对困难,但近2年抗纤维化治疗取得一些进展。

2019年,新英格兰发表了一项关于尼达尼布治疗PF-ILD的研究。该研究是在15个国家开展的双盲、安慰剂对照的Ⅲ期临床试验。随机分配患者至尼达尼布150 mg每日2次治疗组和安慰剂组。主要终点是52周内评估的FVC年下降率。结果在总人群中,尼达尼布组的调整后FVC下降率为-80.8 ml/年,安慰剂组的下降率为-187.8 ml/年,组间差异为107.0 ml/年(95% CI:65.4~148.5;$P<0.001$)。在UIP样纤维化类型患者中,尼达尼布组的调整后FVC下降率为-82.9 ml/年,安慰剂组的下降率为 211.1 ml/年,组间差异128.2 ml/年(95% CI:70.8~185.6;$P<0.001$)。腹泻是最常见的不良事件。后续对该研究的亚组分析发现,慢性过敏性肺炎173例(26%),CTD-ILD 170例(26%),NSIP 125例(19%),不能分类的IIP 114例(17%),其他ILD 81例(12%)。与对照组相比,尼达尼布在延缓FVC下降速度(ml/年)方面的作用是一致($P=0.41$)。

四、IPF急性加重期的治疗(AE-IPF)

AE-IPF是IPF患者死亡的首要原因。目前尚无循证医学证据支持的AE-IPF的治疗方案。临床实践中,除改善氧供、减轻症状等支持治疗法外,2018版日本AE-IPF指南,建议糖皮质激素冲击疗法3 d,后续根据患者情况,决定是否重复用药。

尽管抗纤维化药物吡非尼酮和尼达尼布在IPF治疗中发挥了重要作用,但对于AE-IPF的治疗,目前作用仍比较局限。不过有学者发现抗纤维化药物可以通过减缓IPF的进程,减少AE-IPF发作频率。2019年日本一篇个案还曾报道了一位75岁老年男性AE-ILD发作时单用尼达尼布治疗后症状、影像学、血氧情况明显改善的病例。

此外,近2年有学者发现重组人可溶性血栓调节蛋白(rhTM),可用于AE-IPF的治疗,静脉给药连续6 d,可以有效改善AE-IPF患者的生存率。另外一些小样本观察性研究提示,激素联合其他免疫抑制剂如环磷酰胺、他克莫司或环孢素可能会使患者部分获益,但这些结果的可信度和安全性还需进一步评估。

参 考 文 献

[1] Saito S, Alkhatib A, Kolls JK, et al. Pharmacotherapy and adjunctive treatment for idiopathic pulmonary fibrosis(IPF). Journal of thoracic disease, 2019, 11(Suppl 14): 1740-1754.

[2] Bargagli E, Piccioli C, Rosi E, et al. Pirfenidone and Nintedanib in idiopathic pulmonary fibrosis: Real-life experience in an Italian referral centre. Pulmonology, 2019, 25(3): 149-153.

[3] Vancheri C, Kreuter M, Richeldi L, et al. Nintedanib with Add-on Pirfenidone in Idiopathic Pulmonary Fibrosis. Results of the INJOURNEY Trial. Am J Respir Crit Care Med, 2018, 197(3): 356-363.

[4] Flaherty KR, Fell CD, Huggins JT, et al. Safety of nintedanib added to pirfenidone treatment for idiopathic pulmonary fibrosis. Eur Respir J, 2018, 52(2).

[5] Richeldi L, Fletcher S, Adamali H, et al. No relevant pharmacokinetic drug-drug interaction between nintedanib and pirfenidone. Eur Respir J, 2019, 53(1).

[6] Maher TM, van der Aar EM, Van de Steen O, et al. Safety, tolerability, pharmacokinetics, and pharmacodynamics of GLPG1690, a novel autotaxin inhibitor, to treat idiopathic pulmonary fibrosis(FLORA): a phase 2a randomised placebo-controlled trial. The Lancet. Respiratory medicine, 2018, 6(8): 627-635.

[7] Palmer SM, Snyder L, Todd JL, et al. Randomized, Double-Blind, Placebo-Controlled, Phase 2 Trial of BMS-986020, a Lysophosphatidic Acid Receptor Antagonist for the Treatment of Idiopathic Pulmonary Fibrosis. Chest, 2018, 154(5): 1061-1069.

[8] Raghu G, Scholand MB, de Andrade J, et al. FG-3019 anti-connective tissue growth factor monoclonal antibody: results of an open-label clinical trial in idiopathic pulmonary fibrosis. Eur Respir J, 2016, 47(5): 1481-1491.

[9] Pilling D, Gomer RH. The Development of Serum Amyloid P as a Possible Therapeutic. Frontiers in immunology, 2018, 9: 2328.

[10] Raghu G, van den Blink B, Hamblin MJ, et al. Effect of Recombinant Human Pentraxin 2 vs Placebo on Change in Forced Vital Capacity in Patients With Idiopathic Pulmonary Fibrosis: A Randomized Clinical Trial. Jama, 2018, 319(22): 2299-2307.

[11] Khalil N, Manganas H, Ryerson CJ, et al. Phase 2 clinical trial of PBI-4050 in patients with idiopathic pulmonary fibrosis. Eur Respir J, 2019, 53(3).

[12] Kreuter M, Spagnolo P, Wuyts W, et al. Antacid Therapy and Disease Progression in Patients with Idiopathic Pulmonary Fibrosis Who Received Pirfenidone. Respiration; international review of thoracic diseases, 2017, 93(6): 415-423.

[13] Raghu G, Pellegrini CA, Yow E, et al. Laparoscopic anti-reflux surgery for the treatment of idiopathic pulmonary fibrosis(WRAP-IPF): a multicentre, randomised, controlled phase 2 trial. The Lancet. Respiratory medicine, 2018, 6(9): 707-714.

[14] Shulgina L, Cahn AP, Chilvers ER, et al. Treating idiopathic pulmonary fibrosis with the addition of co-trimoxazole: a randomised controlled trial. Thorax, 2013, 68(2): 155-162.

[15] Brownell R, Kaminski N, Woodruff PG, et al. Precision Medicine: The New Frontier in Idiopathic Pulmonary Fibrosis. Am J Respir Crit Care Med, 2016, 193(11): 1213-1218.

[16] Roofeh D, Jaafar S, Vummidi D, Khanna D. Management of systemic sclerosis-associated interstitial lung disease. Current opinion in rheumatology, 2019, 31(3): 241-249.

[17] Khanna D, Denton CP, Jahreis A, et al. Safety and efficacy of subcutaneous tocilizumab in adults with systemic sclerosis(faSScinate): a phase 2, randomised, controlled trial. Lancet(London, England), 2016, 387(10038): 2630-2640.

[18] Ebata S, Yoshizaki A, Fukasawa T, et al. Rituximab therapy is more effective than cyclophosphamide therapy for Japanese patients with anti-topoisomerase I-positive systemic sclerosis-associated interstitial lung disease. J Dermatol, 2019, 46(11): 1006-1013.

[19] Wong AW, Ryerson CJ, Guler SA. Progression of fibrosing interstitial lung disease. Respir Res, 2020, 21(1): 32.

[20] Flaherty KR, Wells AU, Cottin V, et al. Nintedanib in Progressive Fibrosing Interstitial Lung Diseases. N Engl J Med, 2019, 381(18): 1718-1727.

[21] Wells AU, Flaherty KR, Brown KK, et al. Nintedanib in patients with progressive fibrosing interstitial lung diseases-subgroup analyses by interstitial lung disease diagnosis in the INBUILD trial: a randomised, double-blind, placebo-controlled, parallel-group trial. The Lancet. Respiratory medicine, 2020, 8(5): 453-460.

[22] Homma S, Bando M, Azuma A, et al. Japanese guideline for the treatment of idiopathic pulmonary fibrosis. Respiratory investigation, 2018, 56(4): 268-291.

[23] Crestani B, Huggins JT, Kaye M, et al. Long-term safety and tolerability of nintedanib in patients with idiopathic pulmonary fibrosis: results from the open-label extension study, INPULSIS-ON. The Lancet. Respiratory medicine, 2019, 7(1): 60-68.

[24] Ito Y, Tazaki G, Kondo Y, Takahashi G, Sakamaki F. Therapeutic effect of nintedanib on acute exacerbation of interstitial lung diseases. Respiratory medicine case reports, 2019, 26: 317-320.

[25] Hayakawa S, Matsuzawa Y, Irie T, Rikitake H, Okada N, Su-

zuki Y. Efficacy of recombinant human soluble thrombomodulin for the treatment of acute exacerbation of idiopathic pulmonary fibrosis: a single arm, non-randomized prospective clinical trial. Multidisciplinary respiratory medicine, 2016, 11: 38.

[26] Leuschner G, Behr J. Acute Exacerbation in Interstitial Lung Disease. Frontiers in medicine, 2017, 4: 176.

3 尘肺中的免疫防御机制研究进展:2019—2020年

罗 娅 王 婧

一、概 述

尘肺是由于长期暴露于职业性粉尘(如石英、煤矿和石棉纤维等)而导致的致命性肺部疾病,是我国最严重的职业病。其中,最常见的尘肺类型包括硅沉着病(又称矽肺)、煤工尘肺和石棉肺。近年来,尘肺呈现出新暴发和年轻化趋势,其发病率仍居高不下,考虑主要与一些新兴产业、新型材料的使用增加相关,如牛仔布喷砂和珠宝抛光等。尘肺虽可预防,但是目前尚无有效治疗药物,死亡率仍较高,严重威胁着全球公共健康,带来了沉重的医疗负担。对于晚期尘肺患者,肺移植仍是延长患者生存期的唯一方法。目前尘肺患者的治疗选择受限,主要是由于对尘肺的关键致病机制认识不足,缺乏有效的治疗靶点。因此,加深对尘肺致病机制的认识对于减轻全球尘肺疾病负担至关重要。

尘肺主要的病理特征表现为肺部慢性炎症和进行性加重的肺纤维化,同时伴随肺泡结构破坏和肺泡重塑。尘肺致病机制复杂,涉及多种免疫炎症细胞异常活化和募集、肺上皮损伤和修复异常、肺干(祖)细胞再生异常、上皮间质转化、多种促纤维通路如转化生长因子(TGF)-β、WNT/β-catenin等异常激活、胶原及细胞外基质沉积,以及纤维化形成等。历经多年对尘肺的机制研究,目前我们对尘肺致病的关键通路和分子靶点的认识取得了一定的进展。值得一提的是,肺部免疫(包括先天性和适应性免疫)防御机制在尘肺的机制研究中越来越受重视。起初,肺部的正常防御机制如黏液纤毛清除系统和肺上皮屏障可清除各种职业性粉尘和帮助修复肺部损伤。然而,若长期吸入各种粉尘,一旦超过可调控的临界范围,这些防御机制失衡,将不能再维持肺部微环境的稳态,造成呼吸系统的毒性、损伤,可导致肺泡上皮细胞损伤、凋亡,过度激活肺泡巨噬细胞和促进中性粒细胞募集;同时,也可激活T或B淋巴细胞等免疫细胞,这些对于启动和维持肺部炎症反应和纤维化过程都至关重要。

本文主要就尘肺的先天性免疫(黏液纤毛清除系统、肺上皮细胞、巨噬细胞)和适应性免疫(Th1,Th2,Th17,Treg和Breg)防御机制相关的研究进展进行综述,以加深对尘肺潜在致病机制的认识和促进尘肺关键靶点的临床转化,从而加速尘肺"精准医疗"进程。

二、尘肺中的先天性免疫防御机制

肺部先天性免疫防御机制主要包括黏液纤毛清除系统、肺上皮屏障、先天性免疫细胞(如巨噬细胞、中性粒细胞、肥大细胞等),以及体液因子(如溶菌酶和表面活性剂蛋白)等。当前研究表明,二氧化硅(silica)暴露可诱导巨噬细胞和肥大细胞产生白三烯B4(LTB4),LTB4作为中性粒细胞趋化因子,可促进中性粒细胞募集,是引起矽肺中性粒细胞浸润和肺部炎症的重要趋化因子。目前,黏液纤毛清除系统、肺上皮细胞及巨噬细胞是尘肺先天性防御机制的研究重点,因此我们主要就这三方面进行详细论述。

(一)黏液纤毛清除系统

黏液纤毛清除(mucociliary clearance,MCC)系统是分布于传导性气道,由黏液毯(黏液层和浆液层)、运输黏液的纤毛柱状上皮细胞及纤毛、形成黏液毯的杯状细胞和浆液分泌腺组成的复合系统,可清除鼻腔后部2/3、咽、喉到终末细支气管之间的所有吸入性颗粒及外来微生物,是机体防御外部异物侵入的重要屏障之一。黏液纤毛清除功能取决于黏液毯与纤毛间的互动平衡,可发挥运输、湿润、屏障、免疫等作用。若黏液纤毛清除受损或发生功能障碍,则可引起多种肺部疾病,如肺部阻塞性疾病[慢性阻塞性肺病(COPD)和哮喘]、遗传性疾病(原发性纤毛运动障碍和囊性纤维化),以及纤维性间质性肺病[特发性肺纤维化(IPF)、尘肺等],且被认为是以上疾病发生发展的重要环节之一。

既往研究发现,矽肺、煤工尘肺和石棉肺患者可出现黏液纤毛清除受损。随着研究不断深入,目前我们对尘肺患者黏液纤毛清除受损潜在的分子机制有了一定的认识。黏液是由杯状细胞和黏膜下浆液分泌腺合成的黏蛋白,以及水、电解质、代谢物等组成的复杂混合物。其中,MUC5B(最重要)和MUC5AC是最主要的黏蛋白组成成分。*MUC5B*和*MUC5AC*基因正常表达对于维持正常的黏液纤毛清除功能至关重要。Platenburg等的研究证实,*MUC5B* rs35705950等位基因与石棉肺发生风险相关。最新一项研究在Silica诱导的矽肺小鼠黏膜下腺观察到*MUC5B*表达明显增加及伴有黏液纤毛结构受损,该研究提示MUC5B黏蛋白分泌增加可能参与了矽肺的发生发展。此外,既往研究显示*MUC5B*基因表达与金属蛋白酶 MMP7 的浓度相关。然而,Grubb 等人的研究提示,老年小鼠的 MCC 功能降低可能与 MUC5B 黏蛋白分泌减少有关。与此同时,在 MUC5B 缺陷型小鼠中也发现 MCC 功能障碍。因此,MUC5B 过度分泌常见于尘肺在内的多种肺部疾病,而分泌不足可见于老年人群。MUC5B 分泌或许与年龄相关,且无论 MUC5B 过多或过少分泌,都可能引起 MCC 受损。关于 MUC5AC,目前暂缺乏与尘肺致病机制相关的直接研究。先前 Koeppen 等的研究表明,MUC5AC 缺陷型小鼠伴有黏液纤毛清除功能严重受损和急性肺损伤。同时,气道上皮细胞中 MUC5AC 分泌增加对流感引起的肺损伤具有保护作用,且并不会引起气道阻塞。这些研究提示过表达 MUC5AC 在小鼠肺中可发挥保护作用,且提示 MUC5AC 与 MUC5B 在肺中发挥的效应并不完全相同。综上,目前关于 MUC5B、MUC5AC 与尘肺之间的关系仍有待进一步探索。

气道纤毛可到达黏液毯的凝胶层,发挥"刷子"样运输功能,确保黏液毯的持续流动,纤毛与黏液毯之间保持互动平衡对于有效清除体内异物至关重要。既往研究发现,纤毛相关的编码基因众多,如 DNAH5、DNAH12、DNAH1、DNAH11、CCDC151、CCDC14、CCDC114、FOXJ1、CFAP206 等,这些基因编码的蛋白对于维持纤毛的正常功能至关重要。当机体暴露于各种粉尘时,可引起纤毛结构损伤及数量减少,使得纤毛的摆动频率、幅度及协调性降低,从而导致 MCC 能力下降,并进一步减弱其先天性免疫防御功能,同时可增加尘肺患者肺部感染风险。Li 等的最新研究,在矽肺患者及矽肺大鼠中发现 Silica 可干扰原发性纤毛功能,并参与矽肺纤维化的发生发展。整体而言,尚缺乏纤毛在尘肺中具体致病机制的研究,目前结果表明纤毛功能障碍可能是尘肺加重的重要诱因之一,而改善纤毛功能可能是缓解尘肺的有效方法。

(二)肺上皮细胞

肺上皮细胞以多种方式参与机体固有免疫防御,除了通过上皮细胞间紧密连接形成致密的屏障,也通过其表面受体(如 Toll 样受体和糖基化终末产物受体)和分泌肺表面活性物质蛋白(SP),以及与多种免疫细胞相互作用来维持肺部稳态。肺上皮细胞的异常损伤、过度修复和细胞衰老、凋亡与多种肺部疾病密切相关,如急性肺损伤、IPF、COPD 及尘肺等。当粉尘沉积在肺内,可引起肺上皮细胞损伤,引起细胞肿胀、脱落及细胞间的连接缺失。同时,目前研究表明肺上皮细胞损伤是粉尘在肺内沉积后的早期事件,可通过多种信号因子和途径促进肺纤维化,包括:①激活凝血级联反应,活化的血小板可释放促纤维化因子如血小板衍生长因子(PDGF)和 TGF-β1。②释放多种趋化因子,如粒细胞巨噬细胞集落刺激因子(GM-CSF)、单核细胞趋化蛋白-1(MCP-1)等,可将单核细胞和中性粒细胞募集到损伤部位,可进一步产生活性氧(ROS)加重肺纤维化。③引起肺泡上皮细胞发生上皮-间质转化(EMT)表型改变,活跃的 EMT 事件可导致大量的成纤维细胞/肌成纤维细胞活化、增殖,以及其他促纤维化因子生成。

Silica 对肺具有非常强的毒性,矽肺也被认为是一种持续的 Silica 损伤后过度的肺间质重塑疾病。Peeters 等的研究表明,二氧化硅可诱导人肺上皮细胞中的 NLRP3 炎性小体和 caspase-1 的激活,增加 IL-1β、高迁移率组族蛋白 1(HMGB1)、碱性成纤维细胞生长因子(bFGF)等炎症因子分泌,以及成纤维细胞的增殖,从而促进肺纤维化和矽肺疾病进展。最近的一项研究,在暴露于二氧化硅的矽肺小鼠模型中观察到明显的 DNA 双链断裂和细胞凋亡,该研究证实了 N-乙酰基-丝氨酰-天冬氨酰-赖氨酰脯氨酸(Ac-SDKP),一种抗纤维化的四肽,可抑制二氧化硅诱导的上皮细胞凋亡,并抑制纤维化反应。因此,Ac-SDKP 可能对矽肺患者具有潜在的抗纤维化效果。线粒体功能障碍和线粒体缺陷引起的肺泡上皮细胞(AEC)凋亡在促进肺纤维化中起关键作用。Kim 等的研究团队,首次在过表达线粒体 8-氧鸟嘌呤 DNA 糖基化酶(mtOGG1)的转基因小鼠中证实了 mtOGG1 可减轻肺泡上皮细胞假定激酶1(PINK1)缺乏、线粒体 DNA 损伤及细胞凋亡,同时减轻石棉和博来霉素诱导的肺纤维化。该研究提示增加 mtOGG1 表达可能有助于改善石棉肺纤维化。

(三)巨噬细胞

参与肺部先天性免疫的巨噬细胞包括气道巨噬细胞、肺泡巨噬细胞、间质巨噬细胞及外周募集浸润于肺部的巨噬细胞等,是肺部抵御各种职业性粉尘的重要细胞成分,也是尘肺组织及肺泡灌洗液中数量最多的一类炎症细胞。巨噬细胞对异物的识别、吞噬及巨噬细胞的凋亡、自噬,可引起炎性细胞的募集和促进炎症因子释放,在尘肺的发生发展中发挥至关重要的作用。

1. 巨噬细胞的识别与吞噬　肺泡中的巨噬细胞在执行固有免疫时,第一步就是对抗原进行识别。研究发现巨噬细胞上的清道夫受体(SR)是巨噬细胞识别粉尘(如二氧化硅颗粒、石棉纤维、二氧化钛颗粒等)的重要受体。Murthy 等人的研究发现,SR-A 家族 MARCO 敲除的原代肺泡巨噬细胞,在给予石棉纤维刺激后,TGF-β 产生减少为原来的 1/7。同时,Thakur 等发现,在二氧化硅诱导的矽肺小鼠中,MARCO 阳性的巨噬细胞明显增加,然而在 MARCO 敲除的小鼠肺部炎症反应更显著,这提示除了 MARCO 可能还有其他受体参与到巨噬细胞的识别。随后,Tsugita 等发现,SR-B 家族的 SR-B1 通过胞外 α-螺旋结构,可特异识别二氧化硅,但对其他形式的粉尘不具有识别作用。二氧化硅刺激 BMDM 原代巨噬细胞后,发现 SR-B1 敲除小鼠对粉尘的吞噬作用减弱,炎症因子 IL-1α 和 IL-β 释放明显减少,以及细胞死亡减少。并进一步通过体内试验验证,给予 SR-B1 中和抗体的小鼠在 Silica 刺激下肺部的炎症浸润和纤维化程度明显改善。

2. 巨噬细胞的凋亡与自噬　巨噬细胞吞噬二氧化硅颗粒后,吞噬泡与溶酶体结合。由于巨噬细胞溶酶体内不产生能分解二氧化硅的酶,并且二氧化硅等颗粒可破坏溶酶体膜,从而使巨噬细胞溶酶体崩解,溶酶体内各种酶类(如组织蛋白酶)和酸性物质释放到细胞质,导致细胞损伤,细胞则会根据细胞自身状态选择不同方式的死亡,主要包括凋亡与自噬。普遍认为,巨噬细胞受损后凋亡是巨噬细胞死亡的主要方式之一。Joshi 等通过 time-lapse imaging 方法发现,在给予二氧化硅刺激后,80% 的细胞死于凋亡,

20%的细胞死于坏死。该研究发现,在吞噬二氧化硅后的3~6 h,巨噬细胞可出现以caspase3和caspase9激活、线粒体超极化、细胞膜肿胀为特征的凋亡表型,只有少部分巨噬细胞不表现为caspase活化的坏死死亡。

近年来的研究发现,职业性粉尘的暴露可增加巨噬细胞的自噬活性。

虽然当前研究提示巨噬细胞自噬与尘肺的发生发展密切相关,但目前对于巨噬细胞自噬与尘肺的致病关系仍无定论。一方面,既往研究指出巨噬细胞的自噬活性增加对矽肺具有保护作用。Xi等的研究发现,在巨噬细胞中使用自噬激活剂后可明显抑制二氧化硅刺激巨噬细胞所引起的IL-1β、TNF-α的释放,以及抑制巨噬细胞中NF-κB通路激活。Jessop等用自噬功能缺陷小鼠Atg5(fl/fl)LysM-Cre(+)构建矽肺动物模型,发现敲除鼠NLRP3炎性小体激活增加,导致炎症因子IL-18等的释放明显增加,从而加重了肺部炎症和纤维化。另一方面,也有研究指出巨噬细胞的自噬增加可能促进矽肺疾病进展。Liu等的研究发现,暴露于二氧化硅的巨噬细胞自噬活性增加,可能是通过巨噬细胞中的BCL2结合成分3(BBC3)诱导自噬活性增加从而促进矽肺肺纤维化。同时,最近的一项研究表明巨噬细胞衍生的单核细胞趋化蛋白1诱导蛋白1(MCPIP1)通过增加巨噬细胞自噬介导了二氧化硅诱导的肺纤维化,该研究也提示MCPIP1可能是矽肺的潜在治疗靶点。综上,巨噬细胞自噬与尘肺之间的相关性尚未明确,仍需深入研究明确巨噬细胞自噬对尘肺的影响。

三、尘肺中的适应性免疫防御机制

目前,T淋巴细胞(如Th1、Th2、Th17和Treg)和B淋巴细胞(如Breg)的免疫调节作用是尘肺适应性防御机制的研究重点,现就这两方面在尘肺中的作用进行阐述。

(一)T淋巴细胞

T淋巴细胞在尘肺早期的致病过程中发挥了重要作用。CD4[+]T细胞在不同因子的诱导下可分化成Th1型、Th2型、Th17型和Treg细胞。其中Th1/Th2型细胞失衡和Th17/Treg失衡在尘肺致病过程中至关重要。尘肺发生过程中促炎型Th1细胞数量增加,Th2型细胞数量减少,可产生大量的炎性因子。CD4[+]T细胞在TGFβ的刺激下可分化成Th17和Treg两种细胞,而IL-6决定了具体的分化方向。TGF-β和IL-6的共同作用可使T细胞分化成Th17细胞,反之则分化为Treg细胞。Th17细胞可释放IL-17,IL-17具有强大的中性粒细胞募集作用。因此,Th17/Treg细胞失衡(Th17>Treg)通过促进IL-17释放,也可增加中性粒细胞的募集。改善Th1/Th2和Th17/Treg细胞比例失衡,以及抑制炎性因子如IL-1、IL-6、IL1-7等的释放,将有助于改善尘肺的肺部炎症。

Liu等用anti-CD25 mAbs PC61构建Treg细胞耗竭的小鼠模型,研究早期可观察到Treg缺陷的矽肺小鼠肺部炎症反应明显,中性粒细胞浸润增加,Th1型细胞因子IL-2和IFNγ明显升高,这些提示Treg细胞在限制尘肺早期炎症中发挥重要作用。同样的,Song等用anti-CD25 mAbs PC61构建TregTreg免疫缺陷小鼠,也发现Treg缺陷的矽肺小鼠肺组织中中性粒细胞浸润明显增加,同时调节Th17分化的转录因子RORγt和Th17细胞分泌的IL-17A明显减少,说明Treg可促进Th17细胞的分化成熟。此外,对二氧化硅诱导的矽肺小鼠肺泡灌洗液中的巨噬细胞和淋巴细胞进行体外细胞实验,发现IL-17A mAb和IL-1Ra抗体处理淋巴细胞后,可抑制Th1型而促进Th2型细胞分化,并且增强了Treg细胞的分泌功能。在矽肺动物模型中,通过给予IL-17A中和抗体,可观察到中性粒细胞浸润明显减少,减弱Th1/Th2型细胞的免疫反应,而增强Treg细胞反应,以及减轻了矽肺早期阶段肺部炎症。Mi等发现,IL-17A除了可以趋化中性粒细胞外,还可以促进小鼠肺泡上皮细胞系MLE12的上皮间质转化,并且可以促进MLE12细胞系分泌胶原纤维。尽管很多研究表明拮抗Th17型细胞因子IL-17A可减缓炎症反应,但研究也表明IL-17A的拮抗并不能直接影响最终的纤维化程度。Liu等用anti-CD25 mAbs PC61 Treg细胞耗竭的小鼠模型,发现虽然加重了肺部炎症,但改善了肺纤维化程度。此外,Lo等发现,在炎症依赖的肺纤维化产生过程中,效应性T细胞(Teff)产生的一些细胞因子会促进成纤维细胞产生胶原沉积,而在炎症抑制的情况下,Treg则可以通过分泌PDGF-B和TGFb来刺激成纤维细胞产生胶原,促进肺纤维化。

(二)B淋巴细胞

T淋巴细胞在肺纤维化产生过程中发挥重要作用,而B淋巴细胞与尘肺间的相关研究较少。现对于B淋巴细胞的研究主要集中在分泌IL-10的调节性B细胞(Breg)。研究发现,在小鼠尘肺模型中,小鼠肺淋巴结和脾脏中B10细胞浸润明显增加,并且B10细胞可以通过调节T细胞平衡,减少Th1型细胞比例,减少肺部炎症反应,进而缓解肺纤维化。

四、展 望

尽管目前仍无有效缓解尘肺疾病进展的治疗药物,但随着研究的不断深入,使我们对尘肺的致病机制有了更深刻的认识。免疫防御机制在尘肺的致病过程中发挥着举足轻重的作用,本文通过对既往尘肺免疫相关研究进行综述,使我们认识到除了适应性免疫防御机制,先天性免疫在尘肺致病过程中的作用也是不可忽视的。然而,这些免疫防御机制在尘肺中具体的致病机制仍不完全清楚,且部分具有争议,如巨噬细胞自噬与尘肺的关系,因此仍有待进一步深入研究。此外,除了通过传统的研究方法,利用组学方法包括基因组学、转录组学、表观遗传组学、蛋白质组学、代谢组学等有助于揭示尘肺疾病过程中的全面分子改变和关键分子靶点,尤其是单细胞组学可在单个细胞层面通过联合多种组学技术,探究与疾病发生发展的关系。但遗憾的是,目前尘肺组学研究主要是在动物模型和细胞系(如巨噬细胞和肺上皮细胞)中进行的,仍缺乏尘肺患者样本(如肺组织、肺泡灌洗液、血尿标本等)的组学研究。未来,对尘肺患者进行组学研究是非常有必要的,这将有助于揭示参与尘肺发病的重要分子靶点和潜在生物标志物,同时加强对关键致病分子的临床转化,可促进尘肺"个体化治疗"的发展。

参 考 文 献

[1] Cullinan P, Reid P. Pneumoconiosis. Prim Care Respir J, 2013,22(2):249-252.

[2] Hoy RF, Chambers DC. Silica-related diseases in the modern world. Allergy,2020.

[3] Rose C, Heinzerling A, Patel K, et al. Severe Silicosis in Engineered Stone Fabrication Workers-California, Colorado, Texas, and Washington,2017-2019. MMWR Morb Mortal Wkly Rep,2019,68(38):813-818.

[4] Satpathy SR, Jala VR, Bodduluri SR, et al. Crystalline silica-induced leukotriene B4-dependent inflammation promotes lung tumour growth. Nat Commun,2015,6:7064.

[5] Bustamante-Marin XM, Ostrowski LE. Cilia and Mucociliary Clearance. Cold Spring Harb Perspect Biol,2017,9(4).

[6] Yoruk O, Ates O, Araz O, et al. The effects of silica exposure on upper airways and eyes in denim sandblasters. Rhinology, 2008,46(4):328-333.

[7] Peksoy I, Ugur MB, Altin R, et al. Evaluation of nasal mucociliary functions with rhinoscintigraphy in coal workers' pneumoconiosis. ORL J Otorhinolaryngol Relat Spec,2005, 67(3):163-167.

[8] Abú-Shams K, Pascal I. Asbestos: characteristics, properties, pathogenesis and sources of. exposure. An Sist Sanit Navar, 2005,28(Suppl 1):7-11.

[9] Whitsett JA. Airway Epithelial Differentiation and Mucociliary Clearance. Ann Am Thorac Soc,2018,15(Suppl 3):S143-S148.

[10] Roy MG, Livraghi-Butrico A, Fletcher AA, et al. Muc5b is required for airway defence. Nature, 2014, 505 (7483): 412-416.

[11] Koeppen M, McNamee EN, Brodsky KS, et al. Detrimental role of the airway mucin Muc5ac during ventilator-induced lung injury. Mucosal Immunol,2013,6(4):762-775.

[12] Platenburg M, Wiertz IA, van der Vis JJ, et al. The MUC5B promoter risk allele for idiopathic pulmonary fibrosis predisposes to asbestosis. Eur Respir J,2020,55(4).

[13] Yu Q, Fu G, Lin H, et al. Influence of silica particles on mucociliary structure and MUC5B expression in airways of C57BL/6 mice. Exp Lung Res,2020,46(7):217-225.

[14] Gharib SA, Altemeier WA, Van Winkle LS, et al. Matrix metalloproteinase-7 coordinates airway epithelial injury response and differentiation of ciliated cells. Am J Respir Cell Mol Biol,2013,48(3):390-396.

[15] Grubb BR, Livraghi-Butrico A, Rogers TD, Yin W, Button B, Ostrowski LE. Reduced mucociliary clearance in old mice is associated with a decrease in Muc5b mucin. Am J Physiol Lung Cell Mol Physiol,2016,310(9):860-867.

[16] Ehre C, Worthington EN, Liesman RM, et al. Overexpressing mouse model demonstrates the protective role of Muc5ac in the lungs. Proc Natl Acad Sci U S A, 2012, 109 (41): 16528-16533.

[17] Beckers A, Adis C, Schuster-Gossler K, et al. The FOXJ1 target Cfap206 is required for sperm motility, mucociliary clearance of the airways and brain development. Development,2020,147(21).

[18] Li S, Wei Z, Li G, et al. Silica Perturbs Primary Cilia and Causes Myofibroblast Differentiation during Silicosis by Reduction of the KIF3A-Repressor GLI3 Complex. Theranostics,2020,10(4):1719-1732.

[19] Peeters PM, Perkins TN, Wouters EF, Mossman BT, Reynaert NL. Silica induces NLRP3 inflammasome activation in human lung epithelial cells. Part Fibre Toxicol,2013,10:3.

[20] Shifeng L, Hong X, Xue Y, et al. Ac-SDKP increases α-TAT 1 and promotes the apoptosis in lung fibroblasts and epithelial cells double-stimulated with TGF-β1 and silica. Toxicol Appl Pharmacol,2019,369:17-29.

[21] Kim SJ, Cheresh P, Jablonski RP, et al. Mitochondrial 8-oxoguanine DNA glycosylase mitigates alveolar epithelial cell PINK1 deficiency, mitochondrial DNA damage, apoptosis, and lung fibrosis. Am J Physiol Lung Cell Mol Physiol,2020, 318(5):L1084-L1096.

[22] Murthy S, Larson-Casey JL, Ryan AJ, et al. Alternative activation of macrophages and pulmonary fibrosis are modulated by scavenger receptor, macrophage receptor with collagenous structure. FASEB J,2015,29(8):3527-3536.

[23] Thakur SA, Beamer CA, Migliaccio CT, Holian A. Critical role of MARCO in crystalline silica-induced pulmonary inflammation. Toxicol Sci,2009,108(2):462-471.

[24] Tsugita M, Morimoto N, Tashiro M, et al. SR-B1 Is a Silica Receptor that Mediates Canonical Inflammasome Activation. Cell Rep,2017,18(5):1298-1311.

[25] Joshi GN, Knecht DA. Silica phagocytosis causes apoptosis and necrosis by different temporal and molecular pathways in alveolar macrophages. Apoptosis,2013,18(3):271-285.

[26] Chen S, Yuan J, Yao S, et al. Lipopolysaccharides may aggravate apoptosis through accumulation of autophagosomes in alveolar macrophages of human silicosis. Autophagy,2015,11 (12):2346-2357.

[27] Zhu HX, Gao JL, Zhao MM, et al. Effects of bone marrow-derived mesenchymal stem cells on the autophagic activity of alveolar macrophages in a rat model of silicosis. Exp Ther Med,2016,11(6):2577-2582.

[28] Xi C, Zhou J, Du S, Peng S. Autophagy upregulation promotes macrophages to escape mesoporous silica nanoparticle(MSN)-induced NF-κB-dependent inflammation. Inflamm Res, 2016, 65 (4): 325-341.

[29] Jessop F, Hamilton RF, Rhoderick JF, Shaw PK, Holian A. Autophagy deficiency in macrophages enhances NLRP3 inflammasome activity and chronic lung disease following silica exposure. Toxicol Appl Pharmacol,2016,309:101-110.

[30] Liu H, Cheng Y, Yang J, et al. BBC3 in macrophages promo-

ted pulmonary fibrosis development through inducing autophagy during silicosis. Cell Death Dis,2017,8(3):e2657.

[31] Liu H,Fang S,Wang W,et al. Macrophage-derived MCPIP1 mediates silica-induced pulmonary fibrosis via autophagy. Part Fibre Toxicol,2016,13(1):55.

[32] Liu F,Liu J,Weng D,et al. CD4+CD25+Foxp3+ regulatory T cells depletion may attenuate the development of silica-induced lung fibrosis in mice. PLoS One,2010,5(11):e15404.

[33] Song L,Weng D,Liu F,et al. Tregs promote the differentiation of Th17 cells in silica-induced lung fibrosis in mice. PLoS One,2012,7(5):e37286.

[34] Tang W,Liu F,Chen Y,et al. Reduction of IL-17A might suppress the Th1 response and promote the Th2 response by boosting the function of Treg cells during silica-induced inflammatory response in vitro. Mediators Inflamm, 2014, 2014:570894.

[35] Chen Y,Li C,Weng D,et al. Neutralization of interleukin-17A delays progression of silica-induced lung inflammation and fibrosis in C57BL/6 mice. Toxicol Appl Pharmacol, 2014,275(1):62-72.

[36] Mi S,Li Z,Yang HZ,et al. Blocking IL-17A promotes the resolution of pulmonary inflammation and fibrosis via TGF-beta1-dependent and-independent mechanisms. J Immunol, 2011,187(6):3003-3014.

[37] Lo Re S,Lecocq M,Uwambayinema F,et al. Platelet-derived growth factor-producing CD4+ Foxp3+ regulatory T lymphocytes promote lung fibrosis. Am J Respir Crit Care Med, 2011,184(11):1270-1281.

[38] Liu F,Dai W,Li C,et al. Role of IL-10-producing regulatory B cells in modulating T-helper cell immune responses during silica-induced lung inflammation and fibrosis. Sci Rep,2016, 6:28911.

[39] Lu Y,Liu F,Li C,Chen Y,Weng D,Chen J. IL-10-Producing B Cells Suppress Effector T Cells Activation and Promote Regulatory T Cells in Crystalline Silica-Induced Inflammatory Response In Vitro. Mediators Inflamm,2017,2017:8415094.

4 肺纤维化诊断与预测的生物标志物

范亚丽 叶俏

肺纤维化是由多种不同致病因素导致的间质性肺部疾病的共同结局，病因复杂，发病机制尚未完全阐明，临床特征经常重叠，但病程进展生存预后表现出明显的异质性。肺功能、影像学对早期诊断、治疗效果的评价和预后的判断方面还是存在明显的局限性。因此，发现可以指导疾病诊断、治疗和预后管理的生物标志物，对肺纤维化患者具有重大意义。近年来，学者们致力于探寻和研究各种肺纤维化相关的生物标志物（表 5-4-1）。

表 5-4-1 肺纤维化相关生物标志物

	生物标志物	诊断/疾病易感性标志物	疾病进展/活动性标志物	预后标志物	治疗标志物
基因标志物	端粒长度	√	√	√	
	TERT	√		√	
	TERC	√		√	
	RTEL1	√		√	
	PARN	√		√	
	MUC5B	√		√	
	TOLLIP	√		√	√
	TLR3		√	√	
	SFTPA₂	√			
	SFTPC	√			
蛋白标志物	SP-A	√		√	√
	SP-D	√	√	√	√
	KL-6	√	√	√	√
	MMP-1	√			
	MMP-7	√		√	
	MMP-3			√	
	CA125		√	√	
	CA19-9	√	√	√	
	CCK18	√			
	CXCL13		√	√	
	CCL18	√	√	√	
	MCP-1	√		√	
	Periostin			√	
	Osteopontin	√		√	
循环细胞标志物	Circulating fibrocytes		√	√	
	CD28% CD4⁺ T cells		√	√	
	Semaphorin 7a+ Tregs		√	√	

一、基因标志物

(一)端粒长度及相关基因

1. 端粒长度 端粒是细胞染色体末端的帽状结构,其主要作用是在细胞分裂及DNA复制期保护染色体的完整性和稳定性。当端粒长度低于临界阈值时,细胞就会发生衰老或凋亡。由于端粒酶活性的存在,使端粒长度处于竞争性平衡状态,延缓由于染色体复制、环境损伤等引起的缩短。

(1)疾病诊断:不同肺纤维化患者的外周血端粒长度均明显短于健康人的,端粒长度依次为结节病＞吸烟相关肺纤维化＞隐源性机化性肺炎(COP)＞特发性非特异性间质性肺炎(iNSIP)＞过敏性肺炎(HP)＞结缔组织病(CTD)相关性肺纤维化＞特发性肺纤维化(IPF),且携带端粒酶反转录酶(TERT)基因突变的IPF的端粒长度最短。这表明端粒变异对IPF的影响最大,对纤维化性肺疾病易感性起着重要作用,同时提示端粒长度可能是IPF潜在的诊断标志物,是否有助于与其他纤维化性肺疾病相鉴别还需进一步研究。

(2)风险预测:端粒长度与IPF疾病进展及无肺移植生存率有关,可能是IPF预后的潜在生物标志物,但端粒长度缩短与其他纤维化性肺疾病预后的关系尚未完全阐明。在IPF和具有自身免疫特征的间质性肺炎(IPAF)患者中,外周血细胞端粒长度＜第10百分位数者比≥第10百分位数者肺功能下降更快,是无移植生存期的危险因素。同时,外周血细胞端粒缩短与CHP死亡风险增加有关,但与其他包括CTD相关性肺纤维化、结节病、药物或放射相关的肺纤维化患者无肺移植生存期不具有相关性。这可能受研究样本量小的影响,端粒长度能否用于评估其他肺纤维化的预后,有待大样本研究进一步证实。

2. 端粒酶反转录酶(telomerase reverse transcriptase, TERT)和端粒酶RNA组分(telomerase RNA component, TR/TERC) TERT是一种由TERT基因编码的RNA依赖的DNA聚合酶,在合成、延伸端粒DNA序列中起催化作用。TERC中包含与端粒互补的序列,是端粒酶延长端粒DNA的模板。TERT和TERC是端粒酶恢复端粒长度的重要组成部分。TERT/TERC基因突变是肺纤维化潜在的易感性标志物。

(1)疾病诊断:在多种纤维化性肺疾病患者外周血中检测到TERT/TERC基因突变,包括IPF、CTD相关肺纤维化、HP、iNSIP、脱屑性间质性肺炎等。与非肺纤维化人群相比,肺纤维化患者TERT/TERC基因突变频率显著增加,在散发性IPF中为1%~6%,在FPF中高达8%~18%,在类风湿关节炎相关纤维化性肺疾病中为5.9%。

(2)风险预测:TERT/TERC基因突变与肺纤维化患者预后差相关。携带TERT/TERC基因突变的肺纤维化患者无肺移植生存率明显低于无TERC/TERC突变患者。端粒相关基因突变还可以预测肺纤维化患者肺移植后的临床转归。一项研究纳入262例因肺纤维化接受肺移植术患者(213例IPF,30例CTD相关肺纤维化,19例NSIP),经检测TERT、RTRL1、PARN基因突变频率分别为5%、3.8%和3%;携带TERT、RTEL1或PARN基因突变的肺纤维化接受肺移植术患者的死亡风险升高(HR 1.82),慢性肺移植排斥反应发生率明显增加(HR 2.88)。这表明端粒相关基因突变与肺纤维化患者肺移植后预后不良有关。

(二)黏蛋白5B(mucin 5B,MUC5B)

MUC5B基因编码高度糖基化的前体蛋白即MUC5B蛋白,MUC5B蛋白主要由黏膜下腺体分泌,分布在传导性支气管,是呼吸道黏液的主要成分,在保护呼吸道上皮细胞和呼吸道免疫防御中发挥重要作用。在肺间质改变特别是IPF时,肺组织结构破坏,蜂窝样改变,引起MUC5B异常分泌。蜂窝样改变周围远端气道含有一层假复层黏膜纤毛上皮,由高表达MUC5B的基底上皮细胞和黏液细胞组成,而正常情况下在终末细支气管及肺泡并无MUC5B分泌。

(1)疾病诊断:Seibold等采用全基因组连锁扫描83例家族性间质性肺炎、492例散发性IPF患者和322例对照人群肺组织的MUC5B基因启动子区多态性,发现rs35705950最小等位基因频率(MAF)分别为34%、38%和9%,携带突变T基因(TT型和GT型)者与无T基因者相比,其家族性间质性肺炎(OR 6.8和20.8)与IPF(OR 9.0和21.8)的患病风险显著增加,该结果在不同队列中得到验证。在非西班牙裔白种人患者中CHP的MUC5B启动子rs35705950的MAF与IPF相似,MUC5B启动子rs35705950多态性也是CHP的患病危险因素(OR 1.91),但与CTD相关肺纤维化、肌炎相关肺纤维化、系统性硬化症(SSc)相关纤维化及结节病无关。此外,MUC5B rs357057950多态性可能增加肺间质异常(ILA)易感性,携带rs357057950-T基因型ILA患者影像表现为可能UIP型和UIP型的可能性大,表明MUC5B启动子多态性对早期肺间质改变具有提示作用。

(2)风险预测:MUC5B基因突变可能对评估疾病的预后具有一定价值。以美国非西班牙裔白种人群为主分两个队列研究均发现MUC5B rs35705950-T基因型使CHP和IPAF死亡风险增加,可改善IPF患者的生存率,与CTD相关肺纤维化无相关性。而在中国人群MUC5B rs35705950和rs868903基因多态性是IPF生存率降低的危险因素,这可能与种族异质性有关。针对上述研究结果不一致,Dudbridge F等重新分析了612例IPF和3366例对照者的MUC5B启动子多态性与IPF患者生存率之间的关系,经调整全基因组关联研究中的指数事件偏倚,逆转了易感基因MUC5B与增加生存率的矛盾关联,发现MUC5B启动子多态性与IPF生存率降低有关。将MUC5B rs35705950加入IPF病死率预测模型中,能提高模型的预测效能(ROC曲线下面积可从0.68~0.69提高到0.71~0.73),表明MUC5B基因多态性可能是一种预后标志物。

(三)Toll样作用蛋白(Toll-interacting protein,TOLLIP)

TOLLIP是一种可与泛素相结合的接头蛋白,它广泛表达于体内各组织,参与Toll样受体、IL-1及转化生长因子β(TGF-β)信号转导通路,在炎症反应的负调控中发挥重要作用。

(1) 疾病诊断与风险预测:TOLLIP 基因不仅可作为 IPF 易感性标志物,也可以反映 IPF 的预后。三阶段全基因组关联研究发现欧裔美国人群中 TOLLIP 多态性 (rs111521887,rs5743894,rs5743890)是 IPF 患病危险因素,可作为 IPF 疾病易感性标志物;生存分析发现,TOLLIP rs5743890-G 基因型增加 IPF 的死亡风险。

(2) 治疗反应评估:TOLLIP 基因多态性还影响 IPF 的治疗效果。一项事后研究发现携带 rs3750920-TT 基因型的 IPF 患者可以在 N-乙酰半胱氨酸(NAC)治疗中获益(HR 0.14);而 NAC 对 CC 基因型 rs3750920 患者具有潜在的危害(HR 3.23),其机制尚不清楚。建议 IPF 患者在选择 NAC 治疗时应进行 TOLLIP 基因多态性检测。

(四)表面活性物质蛋白(surfactant proteins,SP)

表面活性物质由脂质(主要是磷脂酰胆碱)、2 个低分子疏水蛋白 SP-B 和 SP-C,以及 2 个高分析亲水寡聚蛋白 SP-A 和 SP-D 组成;几乎全部由 Ⅱ 型肺泡上皮细胞分泌,具有维持肺泡表面活性膜的稳定,调节肺组织免疫的功能。SP-A₂ 和 SP-C 基因变异会导致内质网应激,肺泡上皮细胞分泌 TGF-β₁ 增加,及 TGF 活化,进而促进肺纤维化发生发展。

疾病诊断:SP-A₂ 和 SP-C 基因突变与 FIP 易感性相关,但在散发性 IPF 中属于罕见突变。此外,通过对 81 例类风湿关节炎(RA)相关肺纤维化与 1010 例对照者进行全外显子组测序,发现 TERT、RTEL1、PARN 和 SP-C 基因突变可能导致 RA 相关肺纤维化发病风险增加(OR 3.17)。SP-C 基因突变也是儿童间质性肺疾病发生的重要原因。

二、蛋白标志物

(一)表面活性物质蛋白

1. SP-A 和 SP-D

(1) 疾病诊断:SP-A 和 SP-D 是辅助肺纤维化诊断的潜在生物标志物。研究通过检测 33 例肺纤维化患者(IPF 21 例,CTD 相关肺纤维化 12 例)和 82 例对照组(细菌性肺炎 12 例,健康志愿者 70 例)的血清 SP-A 和 SP-D 水平,分析发现肺纤维化患者 SP-A 和 SP-D 水平显著高于对照组,SP-A 和 SP-D 诊断准确率最高的临界值分别为 48.2 ng/ml 和 116 ng/ml,敏感性、特异性和诊断准确率分别为 81.8%、86.6% 和 85.2%,69.7%、95.1% 和 87.8%。血清 SP-A 和 SP-D 还有助于将 IPF 和其他肺纤维化区分开,且对 IPF 的诊断准确率 SP-D 优于基质金属蛋白酶-7(MMP-7)和 MMP-1。IPF 患者在急性加重(AE)时较稳定期 SP-A 和 SP-D 水平显著升高,两者联合还可提高 AE-IPF 的诊断准确率。此外,血清 SP-A 水平可作为鉴别 UIP 和 NSIP 的潜在生物标志物。血清 SP-D 有助于从 SSc 患者中筛查肺纤维化患者,SP-D 与抗拓扑异构酶 I 抗体组合,诊断 SSc 相关肺纤维化的敏感性和特异性分别为 97% 和 69%。

(2) 风险预测:血清 SP-A 和 SP-D 可提高对肺纤维化预后的评估。血清 SP-A 和 SP-D 升高均是 IPF 患者预后的独立危险因素,血清 SP-A 基线水平每增加 49 ng/ml,患者 1 年内死亡的风险增加 3.27 倍,将 SP-A 和 SP-D 放入临床预测模型,对 IPF 患者 1 年死亡率预测效能显著提高。日本一项研究分析了 10 例 AE-IPF 患者基线血清 Ⅱ 型肺泡细胞表面抗原(krebs von den lungen-6/mucin 1,KL-6)和 SP-D 水平与 AE-IPF 预后的关系,随访 180 d 后 6 例患者死于 AE,死亡组基线 KL-6 和 SP-D 水平显著高于存活组,血清 KL-6 和 SP-D 升高可作为 AE-IPF 预后不良的生物指标。PROFILE 研究对 IPF 患者血清中的 123 个生物标志物进行评估,证实血清 SP-D 高水平与 IPF 疾病进展和死亡率增加密切相关。

(3) 治疗反应评估:SP-A 和 SP-D 还可作为预测 IPF 患者抗纤维化药物治疗效果的生物标志物。研究纳入 49 例患者(吡非尼酮 23 例,尼达尼布 26 例),监测肺功能和血清 SP-A、SP-D、KL-6 水平从基线到 3 个月、6 个月的变化,将 6 个月内用力肺活量(FVC)下降 10% 或一氧化碳弥散量(DLCO)下降 15% 分为进展组(17 例),其余为稳定组(32 例),6 个月时,血清 SP-A 的变化与 FVC 及 DLCO 的变化呈负相关,SP-A 的在 3 个月、6 个月变化识别疾病进展的灵敏度和特异度分别为 93% 和 75%、81% 和 81%。SP-D 在接受吡非尼酮治疗的 IPF 队列中起到提示疾病进展和生存预后的作用。

2. 前 SP-B 疾病诊断:通常血液中很少检测到 SP-B,与 SP-B 相比,前 SP-B 水平在急性肺损伤患者血液中含量高且持续时间长。研究纳入包含纤维化性肺疾病、慢性阻塞性肺疾病(COPD)、哮喘、肺癌、肺动脉高压、炎症、需要呼吸机支持在内的 283 例慢性肺部疾病患者,通过检测血清前 SP-B(C-proSP-B)水平,发现 C-proSP-B 水平在 IPF 患者中最高,可以将 IPF 与其他肺部疾病区分开。

(二)KL-6

KL-6 是黏蛋白家族中的一组附膜糖蛋白,主要由肺泡 Ⅱ 型上皮细胞和支气管上皮细胞表达。在正常情况下血清 KL-6 分泌较少,当肺组织受损,KL-6 分泌增加,进入血液循环,反映肺部 KL-6 的产生情况,故检测其水平有助于判断肺泡损伤、Ⅱ 型肺泡细胞再生和多种肺部疾病的活动情况。

1. 疾病诊断 KL-6 是肺纤维化的潜在诊断标志物。KL-6 在多种间质性肺疾病(ILD)患者血清中均明显升高,包括 IPF、CTD-ILD、HP、放射性肺炎、药物诱导性 ILD、结节病、急性呼吸窘迫综合征及肺泡蛋白沉积症等。国内多中心大样本研究证实 KL-6 能将 ILD 从其他良性肺部疾病中区别开来,当临界线为 500U/ml 时,其诊断 ILD 敏感性和特异性分别为 77.75% 和 94.51%;而且血清 KL-6 对肺纤维化的诊断识别力优于 CCL18、单核细胞趋化蛋白-1(MCP-1)、SP-A 和 SP-D。血清 KL-6 同样有助于识别 CTD 患者是否合并肺纤维化,为 CTD 相关肺纤维化的筛查和管理提供依据。

2. 风险预测 血清 KL-6 水平同样有助于评估疾病的活动情况及生存预后。血清 KL-6 是 IPF 发生 AE 的独立预测因子,发生 AE 的 IPF 患者基线血清 KL-6 水平显著高于稳定期患者,且 KL-6 水平≥1300U/ml 的患者发生 AE 的时间较早。动态监测血清 KL-6 有助于评估 IPF 疾病状态及预后,对 66 例 IPF 患者进行回顾性分析,发现随访期间血清 KL-6 水平升高的患者 FVC 下降幅度明显大于无 KL-6 升高的患者,基线血清 KL-6＜1000U/ml 且 KL-6 无连续升高者预后优于基线 KL-6≥1000U/ml 且连续升高者,KL-6 连续变化＜51.8U/ml/年患者的生存率明显高于 KL-6 连续变化≥51.8U/ml/年患者的。KL-6 水平与 CTD 相关肺纤维化患者(包括 RA-ILD、SSc、炎性肌炎)的 CT 半定量分级呈正相关,与 FVC、DLCO 呈负相关,血清 KL-6 水平可反映 CTD 相关肺纤维化的严重程度。高水平的 KL-6 与非 IPAF 的特发性纤维化性-NSIP 的疾病进展相关,是判断 RA 相关肺纤维化患者是否为 UIP 型(≥640U/ml)和预后差的潜在生物标志物(≥685U/ml);也是 SSc 相关肺纤维化疾病严重程度、活动性及预后的潜在标志物。正常参考界限值有待进一步确定。

3. 治疗反应评估　为评估血清 KL-6 在肺纤维化治疗中的预测价值,Hu Y 等比较了多种肺纤维化患者接受相应治疗前后总体血清 KL-6 水平,发现治疗后病情改善组 KL-6 水平显著降低,而加重组 KL-6 水平显著升高,KL-6 水平起到提示病情变化的作用,但该研究并没有对 KL-6 预测单一疾病的某种药物的治疗效果进行评估。另外两项研究评估抗氧化、抗纤维化药物治疗 IPF 对 KL-6 的影响,发现 NAC 治疗可能抑制了血清 KL-6 的升高,尼达尼布对 KL-6 水平无调节作用。KL-6 是否可作为药效评价的生物标志物,其结果的临床意义还需要多中心、大样本的队列研究证实。

(三)基质金属蛋白酶(matrix metalloproteinase,MMPs)

MMPs 是一类结构中含有锌离子和钙离子的蛋白水解酶类,由体内多种组织和肿瘤细胞产生,能降解多种细胞外基质成分,促进细胞迁移、增殖,在组织重塑及创伤修复中发挥作用。

1. 疾病诊断　MMPs 是肺纤维化潜在的诊断生物标志物。一项研究通过检测 74 例 IPF 患者和 53 例正常对照者中 49 种血浆蛋白的浓度,发现 5 种蛋白(MMP-7、MMP-1、MMP-8、IGFBP1 和 TNFRSF1A)组合可以准确区分 IPF 组和对照组,其敏感性为 98.6%,特异性为 98.1%,MMP-7 和 MMP-1 组合稍逊与上述 5 种组合,单一蛋白以 MMP-7 诊断准确率最高。血清 MMP-1,尤其 MMP-7 还有助于将 IPF 与其他肺纤维化区分开(曲线下面积分别为 0.63 和 0.73,两者结合为 0.74),MMP-7 截点为 3.91 ng/ml 时,其敏感性和特异性最高。MMP-7 和 MMP-1 组合还可以将 IPF 和 COPD、HP、结节病区分开来,将 IPF 和 HP 区分的敏感性为 96.3%,特异性为 87.2%。血清 MMP-2 也可辅助用于石棉肺和矽肺的诊断。

2. 病情评估　血清 MMP-7 水平与疾病的严重程度有关,血清 MMP-7 每增加 1 ng/ml,IPF 及亚临床 ILD 患者的 FVC% 下降 4.0%、DLCO% 下降 4.1%,而血清 MMP-1 水平与肺功能不具有相关性;并且亚临床 ILD 患者的 MMP-7 显著低于已确诊 IPF 患者的,提示血清 MMP7 水平可反映疾病的严重程度。

3. 风险预测　MMP-7 可能是评估 IPF 患者的预后生物标志物。通过检测 IPF 患者从基线到 3 个月血清 MMP-7 水平的变化,发现无论在稳定组还是进展组,MMP-7 水平没有随时间而变化,不能预测 IPF 进展,但基线高水平的 MMP-7 的 IPF 患者死亡风险增加。长期随访发现,以 4.3 ng/ml 为 MMP-7 的临界线,血清 MMP-7＞4.3 ng/ml 的 IPF 患者中位生存期仅 2 年,MMP-7＜4.3 ng/ml 的中位生存期为 4.6 年。另外,研究还发现血浆 MMP-7 的水平与 GAP 评分呈正相关,当血浆 MMP-7＞12.1 ng/ml 时,能够独立预测 IPF 患者的全因死亡率及无肺移植生存率。综上,血液中 MMP-7 升高预示 IPF 患者的生存预后较差。

(四)骨桥蛋白(osteopontin,OPN)

OPN 是一种参与免疫反应和组织修复的糖蛋白,在人体内合成 OPN 最多的组织是骨组织和上皮组织;在 IPF 肺组织中,骨桥蛋白与 MMP-7 共定位于肺泡上皮细胞,可诱导成纤维细胞和上皮细胞迁移和增殖,促进细胞外基质沉积。

疾病诊断与风险预测　OPN 可能是 IPF 潜在诊断生物标志物。从 35 种生物标志物中筛选有助于区分 IPF 和其他纤维化性肺疾病的生物标志物,发现 OPN＞6 ng/ml、SP-D＞31 ng/ml、MMP-7＞1.75 ng/ml,无论是单独 OPN 还是其联合 SP-D 或 MMP-7,均能显著区分 IPF 和其他纤维化性肺疾病。此外,研究发现血清 OPN 和 KL-6 水平升高预示 IPF 发生 AE 和死亡的风险显著增加,为 AE-IPF 的发生及预后评价提供依据。

(五)细胞角蛋白 18 片段(cleaved cytokeratin 18,CCK18)

CCK18 是一种细胞骨架蛋白,通过凋亡蛋白酶分解成片段而形成,存在于包含肺泡上皮细胞在内的多种细胞。CCK18 是肺泡上皮细胞凋亡和未折叠蛋白反应激活有关标志物。

疾病诊断:通过对 84 例 IPF、24 例 HP、22 例 NSIP、33 例正常对照血清 CCK-18 水平分析,发现 IPF 患者的血浆 CCK-18 水平较非 IPF 组明显升高,CCK-18 可作为 IPF 潜在的诊断性生物标志物(ROC 曲线下面积 0.76)但血清 CCK-18 与疾病严重程度及预后无关。

(六)趋化因子

1. 趋化因子 13(CXCL13)　是基质细胞所产生的一种趋化因子,介导 B 淋巴细胞向炎症病灶迁移,参与许多免疫性疾病的发生发展。

疾病评估与风险预测:CXCL13 与 IPF 患者的病情严重程度和生存率相关。研究报道 IPF 患者肺组织中 CXCL13 mRNA 表达水平及血浆 CXCL13 水平均显著高于 COPD 患者和健康对照,尤其在 IPF 伴肺动脉高压或 AE 时血浆 CXCL13 水平升高更明显;将 CXCL13 浓度随时间变化的幅度分层,当 CXCL13 的增加超过 50% 时,预示着患者将出现呼吸衰竭,预后不良。此外,CXCL13 与 SSc 并发肺纤维化及疾病严重程度有关,SSc 并发肺纤维化的血清 CXCL13 水平显著高于 SSc 患者和健康对照者,CXCL13 与肺功能(VC% 和 DLCO%)呈负相关,与皮肤评分呈正相关;在血清 CXCL13 升高组肺纤维化、肺动脉高压、雷诺现象、指端溃疡等发生率较高，表明血清 CXCL13 水平有助于 SSc 患者肺纤维化的筛查及疾病严重的评估。

2. CC-趋化因子配体 18（CC-chemokine Ligand 18，CCL18） 是一种主要由单核细胞、巨噬细胞、树突状细胞等抗原呈递细胞分泌的 CC 趋化因子，对 T 淋巴细胞具有趋化作用。CCL18 在体外可刺激正常肺成纤维细胞分化产生胶原增加。

（1）疾病诊断：在多种纤维化性肺疾病中血清 CCL18 水平均高于正常对照组，包括 IPF、HP、iNSIP、COP、结节病和 SSc 相关纤维化性肺疾病，其中 HP 的 CCL18 水平最高，支持 CCL18 参与机体免疫炎症反应。最近研究证实 KL-6、SP-D 和 CCL18 可有助于从 SSc 患者中识别并发肺纤维化患者，诊断能力依次为 SP-D、KL-6、CCL18。

（2）病情评估：CCL18 可作预测肺纤维化疾病活动性的潜在生物标志物。对 40 例不同肺纤维患者的血清 CCL18 水平动态检测至少 6 个月，发现血清 CCL18 的变化与总肺活量的变化呈负相关；与 6 个月内病情稳定者相比，病情好转者 CCL18 显著降低，病情恶化者 CCL18 显著升高，血清 CCL18 水平反映了肺纤维化的活动性。但是基线 CCL18 不能用于预测 IPF 患者 AE 的发生。

（3）风险预测：CCL18 可能是疾病进展及生存预后的潜在生物标志物。血清 CCL18 基线水平与 6 个月内 IPF 患者肺功能的下降程度呈正相关，以 150 ng/ml 作为 CCL18 的临界值，CCL18＞150 ng/ml 组较 CCL18 低水平组 IPF 疾病进展发生率及死亡风险明显增高。血清 CCL18 还可以预测 SSc 相关肺纤维化的疾病进展及死亡风险。一项前瞻性研究发现基线 CCL18、性别和免疫抑制剂使用情况是随访期间 SSc 相关肺纤维化患者 FVC＞下降 10% 的独立预测因子；根据基线 CCL18 水平、性别及免疫抑制剂使用情况建立模型，预测随访期间患者肺纤维化进展风险：CCL18＜40pg/ml，使用免疫抑制剂治疗的女性患者肺纤维化进展风险为 0，CCL18＞84pg/ml，未使用免疫抑制剂治疗的男性患者肺纤维化进展风险最大，为 44%。此外，当血清 CCL18＞187 ng/ml 时，其疾病进展发生率及死亡风险均明显增高。

（4）治疗反应评估：血清 CCL18 不能作为药效评价的生物标志。对吡非尼酮治疗 IPF 的 3 个临床研究的所有数据进行事后分析，发现在试验队列的安慰剂组基线血浆 CCL13、CCL18、COMP、CXCL13、CXCL14、骨膜蛋白、YKL40 水平可用于预测疾病进展，但在验证队列只有 CCL18 能标准可靠地预测 FVC%pred 的绝对变化，是预测 IPF 疾病进展的良好标志物；但无论基线生物标志物浓度如何，吡非尼酮治疗效果一致，吡非尼酮并不能调节生物标志物的纵向浓度。

三、循环细胞标志物

（一）循环纤维细胞（circulating fibrocytes CF）

CF 是一类存在于外周血中骨髓来源的间充质祖细胞，在 TNF-$β_1$ 或内皮素-1 刺激下可分化为肌成纤维细胞，分泌细胞外基质。在肺纤维化疾病中，CF 分化为参与胶原生成的细胞达所有成纤维细胞/肌成纤维细胞的 25%。

1. 病情评估与风险预测　IPF 患者 CF 数量较健康对照显著增加，尤其在 AE 期间，CF 计数比疾病稳定时增加 10 倍，可作为 IPF 疾病活动性的指标；COX 回归显示 CF 数量是 IPF 死亡率的独立预测因子，CF 占白细胞总数＞5% 的患者平均生存期为 7.5 个月，＜5% 的患者平均生存期为 27 个月，表明对 CF 进行定量可以预测 IPF 患者的死亡率。另外，IPF 患者接受尼达尼布（8 例）或吡非尼酮（4 例）治疗 6 个月后，CF 百分比较基线水平显著降低，但由于该研究例数较少，不能与临床指标进行统计分析。

2. 病情评估　为研究 CF 与其他肺纤维化性疾病的关系，对包括特发性间质性肺炎（IIP）、结节病、CTD 相关肺纤维化在内的 41 例 ILD 患者外周血 CF 数量进行分析，发现 ILD 患者 CF 数量均明显高于正常对照组，尤以 IIP 和 CTD 相关肺纤维化患者更显著，按病理分类以 UIP 和 NSIP 型更显著；相关性分析显示 CF 细胞数与 VC% 和 DLCO% 呈负相关，与 KL-6 呈正相关；对 2 名患者的 CF 数量和 KL-6 随病情变化进行了评估，发现只有 CF 变化与病情变化平行；提示 CF 数量与疾病严重及活动性有关。

（二）T 淋巴细胞亚群

T 淋巴细胞作免疫系统的重要组成部分，在细胞免疫中发挥核心作用，其水平能反映机体的免疫状态。多项研究发现 T 细胞介导的免疫抑制与 IPF 患者的预后不良有关。

1. 病情评估与风险预测　外周血活化的调节性 T 淋巴细胞（aTreg）百分比与 IPF 患者 DLCO 呈负相关，与 GAP 评分呈正相关。循环 $CD4^+ CD28^+$ T 细胞百分比 FVC% pred 和 DLCO% pred 呈正相关，当 $CD4^+ CD28^+/CD4_总 ≥ 82\%$ 和 $CD4^+ CD28^+/CD4_总 < 82\%$ 时，IPF 患者 1 年内无死亡或者肺移植比率分别 $(56±6)\%$ 和 $(9±9)\%$，$CD4^+ CD28^+$ T 细胞百分比下降提示 IPF 生存预后较差。另一项研究证实 $CD4^+$ T 细胞表面 ICOS 和 CD28 表达下调预示 IPF 死亡风险增加，按照 ICOS 和 CD28 表达量将死亡风险进行分级：低 ICOS 和低 CD28＞低 ICOS 和高 CD28＞高 ICOS。上述结果强调了患者免疫状态对其 IPF 生存预后的影响。

综上，多种生物标志物可以在临床、影像、病理基础上，对肺纤维化的疾病诊断、病情评估、治疗反应和风险预测起到辅助作用，几种生物标志物的组合有可能提高肺纤维化诊断、病情评估和预后判断的准确性。目前，大部分生物标志物缺乏特异性，仍然需要更多的研究，更新的技术，继续寻找敏感度和特异长高、可重复性好的肺纤维化生物标志物，为早期诊断和指导个性化治疗提供依据。

致谢：本文得到国家自然科学基金上项目（81970061）和首都临床特色应用研究项目（Z181100001718118）的资助。

参 考 文 献

[1] Snetselaar R, van Moorsel C, Kazemier K M, et al. Telomere length in interstitial lung diseases. Chest, 2015, 148(4):1011-1018.

[2] Newton C A, Oldham J M, Ley B, et al. Telomere Length and Genetic Variant Associations with Interstitial Lung Disease Progression and Survival. Eur Respir J, 2019.

[3] Adegunsoye A, Vij R, Noth I. Integrating Genomics Into Management of Fibrotic Interstitial Lung Disease. Chest, 2019, 155(5):1026-1040.

[4] Swaminathan A C, Neely M L, Frankel C W, et al. Lung Transplant Outcomes in Pulmonary Fibrosis Patients with Telomere-Related Gene Variants. Chest, 2019.

[5] Seibold M A, Wise A L, Speer M C, et al. A common MUC5B promoter polymorphism and pulmonary fibrosis. N Engl J Med, 2011, 364(16):1503-1512.

[6] Ley B, Newton C A, Arnould I, et al. The MUC5B promoter polymorphism and telomere length in patients with chronic hypersensitivity pneumonitis: an observational cohort-control study. Lancet Respir Med, 2017, 5(8):639-647.

[7] Putman R K, Gudmundsson G, Araki T, et al. The MUC5B promoter polymorphism is associated with specific interstitial lung abnormality subtypes. Eur Respir J, 2017, 50(3).

[8] Newton C A, Oldham J M, Ley B, et al. Telomere length and genetic variant associations with interstitial lung disease progression and survival. Eur Respir J, 2019, 53(4).

[9] Jiang H, Hu Y, Shang L, et al. Association between MUC5B polymorphism and susceptibility and severity of idiopathic pulmonary fibrosis. Int J Clin Exp Pathol, 2015, 8(11):14953-14958.

[10] Wang H, Zhuang Y, Peng H, et al. The relationship between MUC5B promoter, TERT polymorphisms and telomere lengths with radiographic extent and survival in a Chinese IPF cohort. Sci Rep, 2019, 9(1):15307.

[11] Dudbridge F, Allen R J, Sheehan N A, et al. Adjustment for index event bias in genome-wide association studies of subsequent events. Nat Commun, 2019, 10(1):1561.

[12] Noth I, Zhang Y, Ma S F, et al. Genetic variants associated with idiopathic pulmonary fibrosis susceptibility and mortality: a genome-wide association study. Lancet Respir Med, 2013, 1(4):309-317.

[13] Oldham J M, Ma S F, Martinez F J, et al. TOLLIP, MUC5B, and the Response to N-Acetylcysteine among Individuals with Idiopathic Pulmonary Fibrosis. Am J Respir Crit Care Med, 2015, 192(12):1475-1482.

[14] Juge P A, Borie R, Kannengiesser C, et al. Shared genetic predisposition in rheumatoid arthritis-interstitial lung disease and familial pulmonary fibrosis. Eur Respir J, 2017, 49(5).

[15] Hong D, Dai D, Liu J, et al. Clinical and genetic spectrum of interstitial lung disease in Chinese children associated with surfactant protein C mutations. Ital J Pediatr, 2019, 45(1):117.

[16] Ohnishi H, Yokoyama A, Kondo K, et al. Comparative study of KL-6, surfactant protein-A, surfactant protein-D, and monocyte chemoattractant protein-1 as serum markers for interstitial lung diseases. Am J Respir Crit Care Med, 2002, 165(3):378-381.

[17] Elhai M, Hoffmann-Vold A M, Avouac J, et al. Performance of Candidate Serum Biomarkers for Systemic Sclerosis-Associated Interstitial Lung Disease. Arthritis Rheumatol, 2019, 71(6):972-982.

[18] Kinder B W, Brown K K, Mccormack F X, et al. Serum surfactant protein-A is a strong predictor of early mortality in idiopathic pulmonary fibrosis. Chest, 2009, 135(6):1557-1563.

[19] Nakamura M, Ogura T, Miyazawa N, et al. Outcome of patients with acute exacerbation of idiopathic interstitial fibrosis (IPF) treated with sivelestat and the prognostic value of serum KL-6 and surfactant protein. Nihon Kokyuki Gakkai Zasshi, 2007, 45(6):455-459.

[20] Maher T M, Oballa E, Simpson J K, et al. An epithelial biomarker signature for idiopathic pulmonary fibrosis: an analysis from the multicentre PROFILE cohort study. Lancet Respir Med, 2017, 5(12):946-955.

[21] Ikeda K, Shiratori M, Chiba H, et al. Serum surfactant protein D predicts the outcome of patients with idiopathic pulmonary fibrosis treated with pirfenidone. Respir Med, 2017, 131:184-191.

[22] Kahn N, Rossler A K, Hornemann K, et al. C-proSP-B: A Possible Biomarker for Pulmonary Diseases?. Respiration, 2018, 96(2):117-126.

[23] Hamai K, Iwamoto H, Ishikawa N, et al. Comparative Study of Circulating MMP-7, CCL18, KL-6, SP-A, and SP-D as Disease Markers of Idiopathic Pulmonary Fibrosis. Dis Markers, 2016, 2016:4759040.

[24] Wakamatsu K, Nagata N, Kumazoe H, et al. Prognostic value of serial serum KL-6 measurements in patients with idiopathic pulmonary fibrosis. Respir Investig, 2017, 55(1):16-23.

[25] Hu Y, Wang L S, Jin Y P, et al. Serum Krebs von den Lungen-6 level as a diagnostic biomarker for interstitial lung disease in Chinese patients. Clin Respir J, 2017, 11(3):337-345.

[26] Tomioka H, Kuwata Y, Imanaka K, et al. A pilot study of aerosolized N-acetylcysteine for idiopathic pulmonary fibrosis. Respirology, 2005, 10(4):449-455.

[27] Bergantini L, Bargagli E, Cameli P, et al. Serial KL-6 analysis in patients with idiopathic pulmonary fibrosis treated with nintedanib. Respir Investig, 2019, 57(3):290-291.

[28] Rosas I O, Richards T J, Konishi K, et al. MMP1 and MMP7 as potential peripheral blood biomarkers in idiopathic pulmonary fibrosis. PLoS Med, 2008, 5(4):e93.

[29] Morais A, Beltrao M, Sokhatska O, et al. Serum metalloproteinases 1 and 7 in the diagnosis of idiopathic pulmonary fibrosis and other interstitial pneumonias. Respir Med, 2015, 109(8):1063-1068.

[30] Xue C, Wu N, Li X, et al. Serum concentrations of Krebs von den Lungen-6, surfactant protein D, and matrix metallopro-

teinase-2 as diagnostic biomarkers in patients with asbestosis and silicosis: a case-control study. BMC Pulm Med, 2017, 17 (1):144.

[31] Richards T J, Kaminski N, Baribaud F, et al. Peripheral blood proteins predict mortality in idiopathic pulmonary fibrosis. Am J Respir Crit Care Med, 2012, 185(1):67-76.

[32] Tzouvelekis A, Herazo-Maya J D, Slade M, et al. Validation of the prognostic value of MMP-7 in idiopathic pulmonary fibrosis. Respirology, 2017, 22(3):486-493.

[33] White E S, Xia M, Murray S, et al. Plasma Surfactant Protein-D, Matrix Metalloproteinase-7, and Osteopontin Index Distinguishes Idiopathic Pulmonary Fibrosis from Other Idiopathic Interstitial Pneumonias. Am J Respir Crit Care Med, 2016, 194(10):1242-1251.

[34] Gui X, Qiu X, Xie M, et al. Prognostic Value of Serum Osteopontin in Acute Exacerbation of Idiopathic Pulmonary Fibrosis. Biomed Res Int, 2020, 2020:3424208.

[35] Cha S I, Ryerson C J, Lee J S, et al. Cleaved cytokeratin-18 is a mechanistically informative biomarker in idiopathic pulmonary fibrosis. Respir Res, 2012, 13:105.

[36] Vuga L J, Tedrow J R, Pandit K V, et al. C-X-C motif chemokine 13(CXCL13) is a prognostic biomarker of idiopathic pulmonary fibrosis. Am J Respir Crit Care Med, 2014, 189(8):966-974.

[37] Prasse A, Pechkovsky D V, Toews G B, et al. CCL18 as an indicator of pulmonary fibrotic activity in idiopathic interstitial pneumonias and systemic sclerosis. Arthritis Rheum, 2007, 56(5):1685-1693.

[38] Schupp J, Becker M, Gunther J, et al. Serum CCL18 is predictive for lung disease progression and mortality in systemic sclerosis. Eur Respir J, 2014, 43(5):1530-1532.

[39] Neighbors M, Cabanski CR, Ramalingam TR, et al. Prognostic and predictive biomarkers for patients with idiopathic pulmonary fibrosis treated with pirfenidone: post-hoc assessment of the CAPACITY and ASCEND trials. Lancet Respir Med, 2018, 6(8):615-626.

[40] Moeller A, Gilpin SE, Ask K, et al. Circulating fibrocytes are an indicator of poor prognosis in idiopathic pulmonary fibrosis. Am J Respir Crit Care Med, 2009, 179(7):588-594.

[41] De Biasi S, Cerri S, Bianchini E, et al. Levels of circulating endothelial cells are low in idiopathic pulmonary fibrosis and are further reduced by anti-fibrotic treatments. BMC Med, 2015, 13:277.

[42] Fujiwara A, Kobayashi H, Masuya M, et al. Correlation between circulating fibrocytes, and activity and progression of interstitial lung diseases. Respirology, 2012, 17(4):693-698.

[43] Hou Z, Ye Q, Qiu M, et al. Increased activated regulatory T cells proportion correlate with the severity of idiopathic pulmonary fibrosis. Respir Res, 2017, 18(1):170.

[44] Gilani S R, Vuga L J, Lindell K O, et al. CD28 down-regulation on circulating CD4 T-cells is associated with poor prognoses of patients with idiopathic pulmonary fibrosis. PLoS One, 2010, 5(1):e8959.

[45] Bonham C A, Hrusch C L, Blaine K M, et al. T cell Co-Stimulatory molecules ICOS and CD28 stratify idiopathic pulmonary fibrosis survival. Respir Med X, 2019, 1:100002.

5 经支气管冷冻肺活检术诊断间质性肺疾病的临床应用进展

周国武　任雁宏　李　俊　耿　菁　代华平

间质性肺疾病(interstitial lung disease,ILD)是呼吸系统的常见病,它是一组复杂的异质性疾病,诊断分类较难,往往需要综合临床表现、血清学检查结果、高分辨率CT (high-resolution CT,HRCT)等特征进行多学科诊断(multidisciplinary discussion,MDD),而对于上述方法仍无法诊断的患者,则需要采用侵入性诊断方法获取组织标本进行病理评估,以提高ILD诊断效率。

一、间质性肺疾病诊治方法概述

既往获取ILD组织标本的方法包括经支气管肺活检术(transbronchial lung biopsy,TBLB)和外科肺活检术(surgical lung biopsy,SLB)。由于TBLB获取的组织标本量较小,平均约4mm²,其病理诊断率较低,仅约64.3%,因此目前诸多指南均未推荐TBLB作为ILD的常规活检方法。与之相反,SLB可获得大组织标本,新近一项meta分析显示,SLB的平均病理诊断率高达91.1%,高于其他侵入性诊断方法,因此截至目前SLB仍是指南中唯一获得推荐的侵入性诊断方法。而另一方面,虽然SLB具有较高的诊断率,但临床实际工作中普及难度大,患者接受度不高,主要原因是较高的术后严重并发症和医疗费用。Hutchinson等先后分别总结了英国1997—2008年、美国2000—2011年接受SLB的ILD患者,发现SLB术后并发症分别高达13.9%和30%,约8.4%的ICU入住率,住院期间死亡率均达1.7%,而对于非选择性手术患者,住院期间死亡率分别高达4.6%和16%。新近Meta分析显示,SLB平均并发症发生率约12.9%,死亡率约2.3%(表5-5-1)。因此,有必要寻求一种诊断率较高、安全性更好的活检方法。

经支气管冷冻肺活检术(transbronchial lung cryobiopsy,TBLC)是近年来兴起的一项新技术,它是利用冷冻探头在冷冻过程中的黏附性,将经支气管进入的探头周围的组织暴力撕裂,获得组织学标本的一项技术。研究显示,TBLC获取的标本量显著大于TBLB(20mm² vs 4mm²)。而一项Meta分析显示TBLC的诊断率和安全性均介于TBLB和SLB之间,那么TBLC是否有可能替代SLB成为ILD活检的主要方法呢?

表 5-5-1　ILD不同活检方法的诊断率与安全性

活检方法	研究数	病例数	诊断率(%)	死亡率(%)	并发症(%)
TBLC	11	704	84.4(75.9~91.4)	0.5	气胸:10(5.3~16.1) 中重度出血:20.99(5.6~42.8)
TBLB	11	1214	64.3(52.6~75.1)	0	气胸:6.0(3.2~9.6) 出血:10.1(4.4~17.8)
SLB	24	2665	91.1(86.9~93.2)	2.3(1.3~3.6)	总体并发症:12.9(9.3~16.9)

二、冷冻肺活检术的适应证和禁忌证

2018年欧洲冷冻协作组专家共识认为TBLC的适应证整体与SLB一致,即结合临床表现、实验室检查、HRCT特征等仍无法诊断的ILD,但鉴于TBLC在安全性方面的优势,该专家共识认为只要临床有理由需要组织病理学评估,HRCT表现典型的UIP并不是TBLC的绝对禁忌证。此外,对于IPF急性加重低风险、未急速进展的急性、亚急性ILD患者,TBLC亦是适用的。整体而言,TBLC的适应证比SLB更为宽泛,而且越来越多的研究亦在不断尝试拓展TBLC的应用范畴。Yarmus等率先使用TBLC进行肺移植术后评估;中日友好医院周国武等报道了使用TBLC诊断病情无缓解ARDS患者,并系统综述了文献报道的病例,结果发现TBLC能有效诊断病情无缓解ARDS,对改变临床决策具有指导意义,而且并发症是可接受的。但是,TBLC的拓展应用在普及之前还需更多高证据等级的循证医学研究加以验证。

另一方面关于TBLC禁忌证,2018年欧洲冷冻协作组专家共识认为若患者存在以下情况,应视为相对禁忌证:出血倾向、抗凝/抗血小板治疗中、血小板$<50\times10^9$/L、肺

动脉高压,以及肺功能 FVC<50%、DLCO<35%,而年龄不是 TBLC 的禁忌证。

三、冷冻肺活检诊断 ILD 的效能评价

2015 年,Tomassetti 等发表在《美国呼吸与危重症医学杂志》上的一项横断面研究纳入 117 位患者,其中 58 位患者接受了 TBLC,59 位接受了 SLB,结果显示,TBLC 和 SLB 均能显著增加 MDD 诊断率,且两者间 MDD 诊断率相当。遗憾的是,由于缺少更多循证医学证据,2018 年 ATS/ERS 等联合发布的 IPF 指南亦未对冷冻肺活检作出推荐意见。

2019 年,Romagnoli 等发表在《美国呼吸与危重症医学杂志》的一项前瞻性自身对照研究,共纳入 21 位 ILD 患者,每位患者依次行 TBLC 和 SLB 手术,结果显示:TBLC 的病理诊断率较 SLB 低,且两者一致性差,相符率仅为 38%;而且 TBLC 病理诊断与 MDD 诊断相符率亦显著低于 SLB,分别为 48% 和 62%。因此,研究者认为 TBLC 不能替代 SLB。本项研究发表后引起了激烈的争论,一方面样本量太小,不能有效排除选择偏倚,另一方面,病理判读过程中盲法不够严谨。不久之后,Troy 等在《柳叶刀:呼吸医学》杂志上发表了另一项前瞻性自身对照研究,共纳入 65 位 ILD 患者,依次行 TBLC 和 SLB,结果显示,两者病理诊断率没有显著差别,且一致性好,两者相符率达 70.8%(κ 值 0.70),而分别基于两者病理诊断的 MDD 诊断相符率亦达 76.9%(κ 值 0.62)。令人鼓舞的是,2020 年 ATS/JRS/ALAT 等发布的成人过敏性肺炎诊治指南明确推荐了 TBLC 作为纤维化型过敏性肺炎的活检手段之一。笔者相信随着越来越多正面循证医学证据的出现,TBLC 将来有望取代 SLB 作为 ILD 的首选活检方法。

四、冷冻肺活检技术的安全性

如上所述,冷冻肺活检技术的安全性介于 TBLB 和 SLB 之间,仍然有着较高的手术并发症,尤其是操作相关的显量出血(中大量)和气胸,发生率分别达 20.99% 和 10%,此外还有术后 ILD 急性加重、术后发热等并发症,亦有个别致死病例的报道。TBLC 安全性可能最主要取决于活检位置,一般认为过于接近胸膜(<1cm)容易引起气胸,过于远离胸膜又容易引起显量出血,因此,多部 TBLC 专家共识或指南均推荐在距离胸膜 1~2cm 处行 TBLC。

TBLC 除了可导致上述急性并发症之外,能否引起远期并发症也值得关注。Aburto 等回顾性分析了 257 例接受了 TBLC 的患者,长期随访后发现 30 d 和 90 d 再入院率分别为 1.3% 和 3.5%,再入院原因包括肺部感染、原发病加重等,30 d 和 90 d 死亡率分别为 0.38% 和 0.78%。遗憾的是,该研究无法回答 TBLC 与上述远期事件的关联性,亦未能与 SLB 进行对照分析。

五、如何提高冷冻肺活检的诊断率和手术安全性

虽然 Troy 等的研究显示,TBLC 和 SLB 的病理诊断率(含确定 UIP 和可能 UIP)相当,但是 SLB 的确定 UIP 占比显著高于 TBLC,因此仍需通过改进 TBLC 来提高其诊断效能。TBLC 操作方法可能对其诊断率具有显著影响,Ravaglia 等回顾性分析了 699 例接受了 TBLC 的 ILD 患者,结果显示标本数量和活检位置数与 TBLC 的病理诊断率和 MDD 诊断率密切相关。两块标本的病理和 MDD 诊断率分别为 91.0% 和 87.0%,仅一块标本的病理诊断率和 MDD 诊断均为 67.6%(P<0.05);而两个肺段活检的病理诊断和 MDD 诊断率分别为 92.5% 和 92.9%,一个肺段活检分别为 84.8% 和 88.4%(P<0.05);冷冻探头类型和多肺叶活检与诊断率无显著相关性。此外,联合其他诊断方法也可能是提高 TBLC 诊断率的重要策略,有研究者探索了 TBLC 联合基因组分析诊断 ILD 的效能,结果显示,联合 TBLC 病理诊断和基因分析后,可显著增加 MDD 诊断信度。

至于如何提高安全性,患者选择是提高 TBLC 安全性的首要措施,这其中最需要我们关注的是患者肺功能,欧洲冷冻肺协作组专家共识建议将 FVC<50%、DLCO<35% 视为 TBLC 禁忌证,Aburto 的研究亦提示 MRC 气促评分≥2、FVC<50% 是术后再入院的预测因素,Ravaglia 的研究提示患者基础肺功能与气胸发生率成负相关。另一方面,HRCT 表型亦可能与 TBLC 并发症密切相关,我们课题组的一项前瞻性队列研究显示,HRCT 为纤维化表型(蜂窝影、细网格影和牵拉性支扩等)的显量出血风险明显高于非纤维化型。

其次,TBLC 操作方法是影响其安全性的另一重要因素,CHEST 冷冻肺活检指南及其他专家共识均提出了相应推荐意见。如前所述,冷冻活检位置是 TBLC 的关键技术要点,寻求一种精准的冷冻探头放置引导技术有望显著降低操作相关并发症,既往指南/共识推荐术中透视引导 TBLC,但由于透视是二维重叠图像,尤其是当探头走行方向与透视方向平行时,透视是无法精准评估探头-胸膜距离的。Ravaglia 大宗回顾性研究显示,透视引导下 TBLC 的气胸发生率仍高达 19.2%,其中 70% 的患者需要引流,一项 Meta 分析亦提示透视引导 TBLC 的气胸发生率平均约为 9.4%。因此,有必要寻找一种更为精准的引导方法。我们课题组前期一项纳入 155 例 ILD 患者的前瞻性队列研究,通过术中使用锥形束 CT(cone-beam CT,CBCT)三维图像进行探头定位,其气胸发生率仅为 1.9%。此外,还有数位学者初步探索了径向超声支气管镜(radial probe endobronchial ultrasound, RP-EBUS)引导 TBLC 的可能性,通过不同组织结构的不同超声表现来辨认间质性肺病变、周围血管等,从而进行定位,初步结果显示这种方式也可能是可行的,但目前尚缺少大样本研究加以验证。

冷冻探头类型、活检数量、活检位置、位置数等技术

要点也可能是影响TBLC安全性的重要因素。Ravaglia的研究显示，2.4mm冷冻探头的气胸发生率显著高于1.9mm探头（21.2% vs 2.7%），因此，众多指南/共识均推荐使用1.9mm冷冻探头；此外，多位置活检、下肺活检、3块以上标本等均可能是增加气胸发生率的原因。Hagmeyer等的研究通过改变冷冻肺活检操作模式，即预置球囊、缩短冷冻时间、减少活检数量可显著减少操作并发症，并发症总体发生率从84%降至14%。然而，总体而言目前尚缺少更多、尤其是高证据等级的临床研究加以证实，仍需后续更多研究探索提高TBLC安全性的操作方法，并通过制定标准化操作规程，更加规范地普及该项技术。

六、发展前景

TBLC由于能够获取相对较大的组织标本，显著提高了支气管镜技术诊断ILD的效能，并有望替代SLB成为ILD的首选侵入性诊断方法。随着临床实践的不断探索，TBLC的应用范畴也越来越广泛，具有乐观的临床应用前景。但我们还需认识到，TBLC的诊断效能和安全性受较多因素影响，在更大范围普及该技术之前，仍亟需基于更多高质量临床研究结果来制定规范的TBLC操作规程，从而最终提升临床医生诊治ILD的水平。

参 考 文 献

[1] Sharp C, McCabe M, Adamali H, Medford AR. Use of transbronchial cryobiopsy in the diagnosis of interstitial lung disease-a systematic review and cost analysis. QJM, 2017 Apr 1, 110(4): 207-214.

[2] Raghu G, Remy-Jardin M, Myers JL, et al. Diagnosis of Idiopathic Pulmonary Fibrosis. An Official ATS/ERS/JRS/ALAT Clinical Practice Guideline. Am J Respir Crit Care Med, 2018, 198(5): e44-e68.

[3] Hutchinson JP, McKeever TM, Fogarty AW, Navaratnam V, Hubbard RB. Surgical lung biopsy for the diagnosis of interstitial lung disease in England: 1997-2008. Eur Respir J, 2016, 48(5): 1453-1461.

[4] Hutchinson JP, Fogarty AW, McKeever TM, Hubbard RB. In-Hospital Mortality after Surgical Lung Biopsy for Interstitial Lung Disease in the United States. 2000 to 2011. Am J Respir Crit Care Med, 2016, 193(10): 1161-1167.

[5] Babiak A, Hetzel J, Krishna G, Fritz P, Moeller P, Balli T, Hetzel M. Transbronchial cryobiopsy: a new tool for lung biopsies. Respiration, 2009, 78(2): 203-208.

[6] Hetzel J, Maldonado F, Ravaglia C, et al. Transbronchial Cryobiopsies for the Diagnosis of Diffuse Parenchymal Lung Diseases: Expert Statement from the Cryobiopsy Working Group on Safety and Utility and a Call for Standardization of the Procedure. Respiration, 2018, 95(3): 188-200.

[7] Yarmus L, Akulian J, Gilbert C, et al. Cryoprobe transbronchial lung biopsy in patients after lung transplantation: a pilot safety study. Chest, 2013, 143(3): 621-626.

[8] Zhou G, Feng Y, Wang S, et al. Transbronchial lung cryobiopsy may be of value for nonresolving acute respiratory distress syndrome: case series and systematic literature review. BMC Pulm Med, 2020, 20(1): 183.

[9] Tomassetti S, Wells AU, Costabel U, et al. Bronchoscopic Lung Cryobiopsy Increases Diagnostic Confidence in the Multidisciplinary Diagnosis of Idiopathic Pulmonary Fibrosis. Am J Respir Crit Care Med, 2016, 193(7): 745-752.

[10] Romagnoli M, Colby TV, Berthet JP, et al. Poor Concordance between Sequential Transbronchial Lung Cryobiopsy and Surgical Lung Biopsy in the Diagnosis of Diffuse Interstitial Lung Diseases. Am J Respir Crit Care Med, 2019, 199(10): 1249-1256.

[11] Troy LK, Grainge C, Corte TJ, et al. Diagnostic accuracy of transbronchial lung cryobiopsy for interstitial lung disease diagnosis (COLDICE): a prospective, comparative study. Lancet Respir Med, 2020, 8(2): 171-181.

[12] Raghu G, Remy-Jardin M, Ryerson CJ, et al. Diagnosis of Hypersensitivity Pneumonitis in Adults. An Official ATS/JRS/ALAT Clinical Practice Guideline. Am J Respir Crit Care Med, 2020, 202(3): e36-e69.

[13] Maldonado F, Danoff SK, Wells AU, et al. Transbronchial Cryobiopsy for the Diagnosis of Interstitial Lung Diseases: CHEST Guideline and Expert Panel Report. Chest, 2020, 157(4): 1030-1042.

[14] 中华医学会呼吸病学分会介入呼吸病学学组、中国医师协会呼吸医师分会介入呼吸病学工作委员会，经支气管冷冻活检技术临床应用专家共识，中华结核和呼吸杂志，2019，42(6): 405-412.

[15] Aburto M, Pérez-Izquierdo J, Agirre U, et al. Complications and hospital admission in the following 90 days after lung cryobiopsy performed in interstitial lung disease. Respir Med, 2020, 165: 105934.

[16] Ravaglia C, Wells AU, Tomassetti S, et al. Diagnostic yield and risk/benefit analysis of trans-bronchial lung cryobiopsy in diffuse parenchymal lung diseases: a large cohort of 699 patients. BMC Pulm Med, 2019, 19(1): 16.

[17] Kheir F, Alkhatib A, Berry GJ, et al. Using Bronchoscopic Lung Cryobiopsy and a Genomic Classifier in the Multidisciplinary Diagnosis of Diffuse Interstitial Lung Diseases. Chest, 2020, 158(5): 2015-2025.

[18] Zhou G, Ren Y, Li J, et al. Safety and diagnostic efficacy of cone beam computed tomography-guided transbronchial cryobiopsy for interstitial lung disease: a cohort study. Eur Respir J, 2020, 56(2): 2000724.

[19] Sethi J, Ali MS, Mohananey D, Nanchal R, Maldonado F, Musani A. Are Transbronchial Cryobiopsies Ready for Prime Time?: A Systematic Review and Meta-Analysis. J Bronchology Interv Pulmonol, 2019, 26(1): 22-32.

[20] Gnass M, Filarecka A, Pankowski J, et al. Transbronchial lung cryobiopsy guided by endobronchial ultrasound radial

miniprobe in interstitial lung diseases: preliminary results of a prospective study. Pol Arch Intern Med, 2018, 128 (4): 259-262.

[21] Chang CH, Lee CS, Li SH, et al. Feasibility of Radial Endobronchial Ultrasound-Guided Bronchoscopic Cryobiopsy without Fluoroscopy for Lung Parenchymal Lesions. Can Respir J, 2017, 2017: 7170687.

[22] Hagmeyer L, Theegarten D, Wohlschläger J, et al. Transbronchial cryobiopsy in fibrosing interstitial lung disease: modifications of the procedure lead to risk reduction. Thorax, 2019, 74(7): 711-714.

6 特发性肺纤维化的随访和管理

赵亚滨

特发性肺纤维化(idiopathic pulmonary fibrosis,IPF)是一种病因不清、慢性、进行性、纤维化性间质性肺疾病,病变局限在肺脏。好发于中老年人群,其肺组织学和(或)胸部高分辨率CT(HRCT)特征性表现为普通型间质性肺炎(UIP),平均生存期为2.5~3.5年。IPF的自然病程各异,每个个体的病程差异很大,难以预测。一些IPF患者表现相对的稳定,肺功能缓慢下降,伴随着一次或多次的急性恶化;一些患者经历肺功能快速下降,疾病迅速进展。大多数IPF患者直接死于急性加重或肺功能恶化引起的呼吸衰竭。如何能够准确预测患者的生存期是目前研究者需关注的课题。因此IPF的随访中需关注肺功能、影像学、生物学标志物及临床指标等多维参数进行评估,这些参数可以帮助确定疾病在诊断时的初始严重程度,提供基线预后评估,并随着时间的推移来评估疾病进展的速度。

一、评估指标

(一)肺功能

Collard等采用的肺功能(PFTs)标准来定义疾病的进展、稳定性或改善,被认为是经典的标准。用力肺活量(FVC)和一氧化碳弥散量(DLCO)占预计值的百分比、静息时的脉搏血氧饱和度测定是用于监测和评估IPF疾病的重要肺功能参数。基线PFTs与生存有一定的相关性,Nathan等对446名IPF患者进行回顾性分析,按FVC占预计值的百分比(FVC%pre)预测轻度、中度和重度(FVC%pre≥70%,55%~69%和<55%)患者的中位生存期分别为55.6个月、38.7个月和27.4个月;按DLCO占预计值的百分比(DLCO%pre)预测轻度、中度和重度(DLCO%pre≤50%,35%~49%和<35%)患者中位生存期分别为67.3个月、47.8个月和31.3个月。不同的预测结果可能存在影响PFTs的共同条件例如检测条件、肺气肿、肥胖等。

FVC%pre的下降是预测死亡率的最佳肺功能参数。目前普遍采用6个月或12个月内FVC或DLCO百分比的变化来确定IPF的恶化、稳定或改善:FVC的下降≥10%或DLCO的下降≥15%定义为恶化,是预后不良因素。2个临床试验共计1156例IPF患者的研究表明,24周内FVC%pre绝对下降≥10%的患者中1年的死亡率与比FVC%pre下降<5%的患者几乎高5倍(*HR*4.78;95%*CI* 3.12~7.33),比FVC绝对下降5%~10%者增高2倍以上(*HR*2.14;95%*CI* 1.43~3.20)。

尽管某些患者疾病早期肺功能是正常的,即使年度变异度较低,较少的FVC变化也意味着疾病的恶化或进展。目前FVC或DLCO下降5%~10%被认为是恶化的指征,意味着患者预后更差和生存更短。需要注意的是在IPF合并肺气肿患者中,肺容量可能是正常的或轻度下降,此时FVC下降不能很准确的预测生存;尤其是肺气肿程度超过15%时FVC的下降毫无价值的。已证明使用FVC评估预后优于DLCO。12个月内肺泡-动脉氧分压差下降>15 mmHg也可以预测死亡。

(二)6min步行距离测试

在运动测试中,6 min步行距离测试(6MWD)是目前使用最多的公认的工具,它能够确定IPF的初始严重程度,并评估其演变和预测预后。还可用于心脏疾病、慢性阻塞性肺疾病(COPD)和肺动脉高压的评估。主要指标为步行开始和结束时的脉搏血氧饱和度测定(SpO_2),6 min内连续步行距离,以及连续记录SpO_2及步行距离的变化。6 min结束时的SpO_2<88%提示预后不良。748名IPF患者6MWD数据分析表明基线6MWD<250 m和24周6MWD下降>50 m是独立的死亡预测因子。

(三)肺HRCT

胸部HRCT是评估ILD纤维化和蜂窝肺程度的标准方法,能够提供详细的信息,缩小ILD的诊断范围,甚至能够直接确诊不需要外科肺活检。2018年,ATS/ERS/JRS/ALAT发布的IPF诊断指南中明确指出对于HRCT为确定UIP者,除外其他原因可直接确诊为IPF,不需进行外科肺活检。HRCT对判断预后也有着重要的意义。HRCT纤维化与蜂窝范围可以预测死亡率,并FVC%和DLCO%预测相一致。

初始HRCT不仅要描述纤维化及蜂窝肺,而且要对其进行量化。尤其是对于某些患者因临床和功能恶化使其无法进行肺功能等参数测试的严重病例,HRCT能够反映病变进展及严重程度。因此量化的HRCT将是可以客观地评价IPF纤维化程度和进展的工具。一些研究表明,在HRCT中肺功能与IPF的程度之间存在良好的相关性,既往文献大多采用半定量方法,目前一种新的自动分析系统称为CALIPER(计算机辅助肺脏病理评估和评级信息系统)能够测量新的改变,如肺血管的大小,有助于IPF纤维化及蜂窝肺半定量的评估。不建议IPF患者的随访中常规 HRCT 检查,除非怀疑出现特定情况,如疾病的进展,急性加重,合并肺肿瘤,肺栓塞,肺气肿或肺动脉高压。

(四)生物学标志物

生物学标志物一般被用于疾病诊断及分类,评估病情严重程度及疾病进展,预测及评价疗效,预测急性加重,预估发生疾病的风险。理想的生物学标志物在非目标疾病中正常表达;在目标疾病中表达异常,并在治疗后可恢复正常;要准确、无创。尽管目前没有一个对IPF的监测、随访和判断预后有着重要的意义。

1. 反映肺泡上皮细胞损伤的标志物

(1)涎液化糖链抗原-6(Krebs Von den Lungen-6, KL-6):是一种高分子量糖蛋白,属于上皮黏蛋白(MUC)1;在各种上皮细胞表面表达,并通过再生或受损的Ⅱ型肺泡上皮高度表达;在正常组织和细支气管上皮细胞中极少量表达。在中国 ILD 患者中以500U/ml作为诊断的cut-off 值,KL-6的灵敏度和特异性达到77.75%和94.51%。KL-6 可用于 IPF 诊断、病情活动性、治疗效果和预后的评估。KL-6 增高意味着IPF病情进展及预后不佳,经过吡非尼酮治疗后血清 KL-6 水平可显著降低。

(2)表面活性蛋白(surfactant protein,SP)A 和 D:SP-A、SP-D 为亲水肺表面活性蛋白。由于肺泡-毛细血管膜的存在,SP一般不能释放入血。研究发现当呼吸膜受损时,SP-A 和 SP-D 在血清中的浓度显著增加。有研究表明 SP-D 在 UIP 晚期水平增高;IPF 不同血清 SP-A 水平预后有显著的差异,SP-A 升高者死亡率增高达3.3倍。

(3)CC16(Club cell protein 16)为Clara细胞分泌蛋白,在抗炎、抗氧化、抗纤维化、免疫调节方面具有强大的生物学活性。CC16为组织特异性蛋白,主要在肺组织中表达。血中的 CC16 几乎全部来自肺组织, Buendia-Roldán I 等报道 IPF 患者血清及 BALF 中 CC16 水平显著高于非IPF ILD 及对照组。

2. 反映间质修复及纤维增殖的标志物 包括基质金属蛋白酶-7(MMP-7)、骨膜蛋白(periostin)、循环成纤维细胞、赖氨酰氧化酶样蛋白2(LOXL2)、HSP47、Ospeopontin、Fibulin-1、胰岛素样生长因子结合蛋白(IGFBPs)等。MMP-7在IPF中显著增高,且与FVC% pre, DLCO%pre 呈负相关,与GAP评分呈正相关,并有助于判断预后,基线高水平 MMP-7 可早于FVC 4个月预测IPF进展。

3. 免疫及炎症标志物 包括CCL18、YKL-40、Anti-HSP70、ICAM、IL-6 等。CCL18(CC-chemokine ligand 18)由树突细胞和单核-巨噬细胞释放的炎症趋化因子;具有激活多个信号转导途径;具有介导免疫反应,激发炎症反应,活化淋巴细胞、单核-巨噬细胞、成纤维细胞等作用;IPF患者基线血清CCL18增高预示着随访6个月后TLC和FVC的下降,死亡风险增高。HSP70 具有抗炎、抗氧化、抗凋亡的作用,可减少肺损伤及纤维化。IPF 患者肺成纤维细胞HSP70 表达减少,Anti-HSP70 表达与肺功能呈负相关,且 Anti-HSP70 阳性者1年生存率显著降低。

4. 分子生物学标志物 近年来,分子生物学标志物越来越多的用于IPF的评估。端粒的缩短影响上皮再生,其在白细胞中的缩短与IPF的预后不良有关。多项临床试验中发现MUC5B基因多态性是预后良好的标志。另外不典型患者如同时出现*MUC5B*基因及端粒的缩短可能意味着更高风险发展为IPF。更有学者提出利用分子内型(molecular endotypes)来分层患者,预测患者未来风险及治疗反应

(五)临床指标及共病

IPF 临床表现的异质性使得临床指标与预后的相关性更加复杂。男性、<70岁、基线呼吸困难低评分常常意味着预后不佳,随诊6个月及12个月呼吸困难评分下降均预示着生存期的缩短。因此,应每3个月或6个月对病情进行评估,使用包括呼吸困难问卷,mMRC 评分、Borg 量表等工具评估患者呼吸困难症状及生活质量的改变。在疾病快速进展的情况下,随访应该更频繁,可每3个月或更短时间进行。

此外,共同疾病和并发症的存在,如肺气肿、肺动脉高压、心血管疾病和支气管肺癌等与IPF的更快进展有关。部分吸烟患者影像学上表现为同时存在肺气肿与纤维化,称为肺纤维化合并肺气肿(CPFE),其中位生存期为2.1~8.5年,目前尚不确定是否较单纯IPF预后会更差。有8.1%~86.4%的IPF存在肺动脉高压,在诊断或随访中发现肺动脉高压常是预后不良的因素。心脏彩超无创而且安全,是发现肺动脉高压的重要手段,建议IPF患者至少每年进行心脏彩超的检查及早发现肺动脉高压。在诊断明确的IPF患者中,仅在以下情况下使用右心导管:①肺移植前。②临床恶化、运动能力受限、DLCO下降(特别是DLCO<40%预计值)或严重低氧血症伴限制性通气障碍,特别是在合并肺气肿的情况下。③如果认为对严格评估预后至关重要。④如果超声心动图诊断为严重的前负荷性高压,评估治疗肺动脉高压的可能性。⑤怀疑有收缩功能正常的左心室功能障碍。IPF 合并肺癌的发生率4.8%~8.0%,较正常人明显增高。Ozawa 等报道IPF随访1年、5年、10年合并肺癌的累计发生率分别为3.3%、15.4%和54.7%,高龄和吸烟与肺癌的发生显著相关。IPF合并肺癌的病理类型和普通人群患肺癌的病理类型相似,男性中鳞状细胞癌最多见,占47%;女性中腺癌最多见,占64%,其他如小细胞癌、支气管肺泡癌等也可以见到。

二、多维评估体系

目前通常使用"轻度、中度、重度""早期、进展期"等描述IPF的不同状态,但尚没有指南性的文献来明确定义IPF的分期。临床试验大多采用FVC% pred 为50%~55%、DLco 占预计值百分比(DLco% pre)为35%~40%作为轻-中度的标准。由于IPF的自然病程异质性较大,某个单一的指标并不能完全反映IPF的状态,比如单纯的肺功能指标与IPF的预后不完全呈线性关系。临床需要更好的方法评估IPF个体的疾病走向和死亡风险。同其他慢性进展性肺疾病如支气管哮喘、慢性阻塞性肺疾

病等一样,IPF 也需要综合性的指标来预估风险和指导治疗。

Ley 等提出采用多变量的 GAP 模型评价 IPF。GAP 模型(表 5-6-1,表 5-6-2)包括 4 个变量:性别(G)、年龄(A)及生理性指标(P)——两项肺功能指标(FVC、DLco),根据不同得分将 IPF 分为 Ⅰ 期、Ⅱ 期和 Ⅲ 期。GAP 分期与预后相关,GAP Ⅰ、GAP Ⅱ、GAP Ⅲ 期患者的 1 年病死率分别为 5.6%、16.2% 及 39.2%,2 年病死率分别为 10.9%、29.9% 及 62.1%,3 年病死率分别为 16.3%、42.1% 及 76.8%。GAP 分期能够简捷分析 IPF 患者的风险和预测预后。

原始的 GAP 分级没有包括肺 HRCT 评分及病情变化对预后的影响,HRCT 纤维化或蜂窝范围的增加、患者肺功能下降的速度、急性加重或住院都会影响患者的预后。因此,Ley 等又提出纵向 GAP 的概念,即在最初的 GAP 变量基础上添加了由于呼吸原因住院和 24 周 FVC% 的变化这 2 项变量。

Du Bois 团队也做了一个死亡风险评估系统(表 5-6-3),该系统包括了 FVC 下降及住院对死亡风险的影响。这个评分系统略显复杂,限制了其在临床的应用。

表 5-6-1　ILD 中 GAP 评分模型

	预测指标	评分
ILD 亚型	IPF	0
	未分类 ILD	0
	CTD-ILD,iNSIP	-2
	慢性 HP	-2
G 性别	男	1
	女	0
A 年龄	≤60 岁	0
	61~65 岁	1
	>65 岁	2
P 生理学指标		
FVC%pre	>75%	0
	51%~75%	1
	≤50%	2
DLCO%pre	>50%	0
	36%~50%	1
	≤35%	2
	未实施	3
	最高总得分	8

表 5-6-2　IPF GAP 分期与预后

GAP 分期	Ⅰ 期	Ⅱ 期	Ⅲ 期
总得分	0~3	4~5	6~8
死亡率			
1 年	5.6%	16.2%	39.2%
2 年	10.9%	29.9%	62.1%
3 年	16.3%	42.1%	76.8%

表 5-6-3　Du Bois 死亡风险预测系统

风险评分		预期死亡风险	
风险因素	评分	总危险评分	预期 1 年死亡风险
年龄			
≥70	8		
60~69	4	0~4	<2%
<60	0	8~14	2%~5%
呼吸疾病住院史		16~21	5%~10%
有	14	22~29	10%~20%
无	0	30~33	20%~30%
FVC%pre		34~37	30%~40%
≤50	18	38~40	40%~50%
51~65	13	41~43	50%~60%
66~79	8	44~46	60%~70%
≥80	0	47~49	70%~80%
24 周 FVC%pre 变化		>50	>80%
≤-10	21		
-5~-9.9	10		
>-4.9	0		

两种评分系统都有其局限性,试验设计、纳入的病例数、采用的参数、随访时限等均不尽相同,临床尚需更多的研究建立适合 IPF 的评估系统。

三、随　访

IPF 是慢性进行性纤维化性肺疾病,病程中涉及评估病情进展、评估治疗疗效、调整治疗方案、预防急性加重、预测死亡风险等方面,需要对患者进行系统性的随访,取得相关资料。通常每 3~6 个月进行评估,内容包括呼吸困难评分、生活质量评分、FVC、DLCO、6 min 步行距离、脉搏血氧饱和度(SpO_2);至少每年进行肺 HRCT、心电图、心脏超声检查。病情进展迅速时可增加随访的频次。

四、IPF 的管理

IPF 病情发展缓慢,常伴有不可预测的病情恶化、急性加重,病情的异质性需要对每一个个体进行评估和管理,全面的管理包括药物治疗和非药物治疗、姑息治疗、共病的控制、患者教育和支持疗法,达到控制疾病进展,减少急性加重,减轻症状,减少经济及精神负担,提高生活质量的目的。

(一)药物治疗

1. 早期的抗纤维化治疗　临床实践中,由于技术要求高、移植后生存率不确定、供体肺稀缺、费用昂贵等多种因素客观上限制了肺移植的实施,抗纤维化治疗是普遍可行的治疗方案。尼达尼布是一种多靶点酪氨酸激酶抑制剂,能够抑制成纤维细胞生长因子受体(FGFR)、血小板衍化生长因子受体(PDGFR),以及血管内皮生长因子受体(VEGFR),发挥抗炎、抗纤维化作用。吡非尼酮是一种多效性的吡啶化合物,具有抗炎、抗氧化与抗纤维化特性。研究显示以尼达尼布和吡非尼酮为代表的抗纤维化药物能有效延缓各个严重度和GAP分期患者的FVC下降速率，降低急性加重风险和死亡风险，改善疾病预后。INPULSIS研究汇总数据的事后亚组分析显示，无论是基线FVC%pre>90%或≤90%及DLco%pre>40%或≤40%的患者，应用尼达尼布治疗一年后均较安慰剂显著延缓FVC下降速率约50%、改善圣乔治呼吸问卷（SGRQ）评分、延长距发生首次急性加重的时间，显著延长无进展生存期，降低疾病进展风险约40%，并降低相关病死率。INPULSIS-ON延长研究显示，接受尼达尼布治疗48周，FVC%pred≤50%患者和>50%患者的FVC较基线的下降值相仿。CAPACITY和ASCEND研究汇总数据分析显示，对于肺功能较好的早期患者（FVC%pre≥80%或GAP Ⅰ期）和肺功能相对差的中晚期患者（FVC%pre<80%或GAP Ⅱ～Ⅲ期），吡非尼酮延缓FVC下降速率、改善6min步行距离和呼吸困难的疗效相仿。因此，对各个阶段的IPF患者均应尽早干预以改善预后。

抗纤维化药物的安全性和耐受性在大型RCT临床试验中和真实世界的报道是相似的。TOMORROW（NCT00514683）研究和phase 3 INPULSIS-1和-2报道尼达尼布的主要不良事件是腹泻（61.5%）和恶心（24.3%）。吡非尼酮常见不良反应是恶心（35.5%）、皮疹（29.2%）、腹泻（24.6%）和乏力（23.016.8%）。光过敏是吡非尼酮特有的不良反应，尼达尼布的特有不良反应为出血（10%）和心脏事件（2.5%）。不良事件可能导致治疗的中断，预防和控制不良事件的发生十分必要。建议吡非尼酮饭中或饭后服用，减缓增量的速度，可在4周内增加到治疗剂量，保护好皮肤避免阳光直射，定期复查肝脏功能，及时处理等；尼达尼布可在饭后服用，根据腹泻的次数给予加用止泻药物、停药后调整药物剂量等处理。

2. 抗酸治疗　胃食管反流（GERD）在IPF患者中发生率较高，且有25%～50%的患者无症状。继发于GERD的慢性微吸入可能在IPF的发生进展中起一定的作用，并可能继发肺脏炎症或急性加重。应用抗酸治疗包括质子泵抑制剂（PPIs），或组胺2阻断受体激动剂（H2RAs），可能降低微吸入相关性肺损伤的风险。但是目前没有足够的证据证实抗酸药物治疗能够延缓IPF肺功能的下降，也不能降低IPF患者的全因死亡率或住院率。2015年，ATS/ERS/JRS/ALAT IPF治疗指南的更新中，将抗酸治疗作为弱推荐药物列入IPF治疗方案中。

3. N-乙酰半胱氨酸　高剂量N-乙酰半胱氨酸（1800mg/d）起到抗氧化作用。N-乙酰半胱氨酸单药治疗，不能延缓IPF患者FVC的下降，不能改善生活质量，也不能降低IPF急性加重频率和病死率。因此，2015年对ATS/ERS/JRS/ALAT治疗指南的更新中不推荐应用N-乙酰半胱氨酸单药治疗IPF。对于已经应用N-乙酰半胱氨酸单药治疗的IPF患者，可以维持治疗。作为传统的治疗药物N-乙酰半胱氨酸在IPF治疗中的地位受到挑战，直至Oldham等再次分析了Panther研究的结果，根据TOLLIP基因（约25%IPF患者有此基因）中RS3750920位点的基因型进行分层，与安慰剂相比，N-乙酰半胱氨酸治疗可以显著改善TT基因型IPF患者的生存率，这个结果解释了部分患者对N-乙酰半胱氨酸的良好治疗反应。

（二）非药物治疗

1. 氧疗　2011年及2015年ATS/ERS/JRS/ALAT IPF治疗指南中均强烈推荐氧疗。调整吸氧浓度使得患者SpO$_2$保持在休息时92%～95%，或运动时≥88%；每60～90 d（或者更短时间）复查。

2. 机械通气　对于预后不良的终末期肺纤维化患者，一般不主张气管插管机械通气治疗。机械通气可能是极少数IPF患者与肺移植之间的过渡方式。无创正压通气可能改善部分IPF患者的缺氧，延长生存时间。

3. 肺移植　肺移植技术已经成为各种终末期肺疾病的主要治疗手段。2011年及2015年ATS/ERS/JRS/ALAT IPF治疗指南均强烈推荐肺移植技术。考虑到IPF高度异质、整体预后差、疾病进展难于预测，肺移植患者通常需要长时间等待合适供体等情况，肺移植候选患者的国际共识推荐对符合指征的IPF患者在确诊后立即进入等候名单。IPF患者接受肺移植可以提高生存率，改善生活质量，5年生存率达50%～56%。由于缺乏RCT研究，目前尚不能确定单肺移植还是双肺移植使IPF患者获益更多。

4. 肺康复训练　2011年ATS/ERS/JRS/ALAT治疗指南建议鼓励IPF患者诊断后立即进行肺康复训练，在病情恶化之前多数患者均可应用。对于改善呼吸困难、减轻抑郁、焦虑和疲劳，增强运动能力、提高生活质量和认知功能均有益处。

（三）姑息治疗

姑息治疗的目的是减轻患者的症状，安慰患者，而不是治疗疾病本身。有学者建议成立由多学科的团队包括ILD专家、肺姑息治疗专家、护士、呼吸治疗师、理疗师和营养师共同帮助患者。工作目标包括①建立定期监测和优化症状管理。②推荐适当的药物，如阿片类药物，密切监测和管理剂量。③协助患者了解疾病的发展轨迹。④参与关于护理目标的讨论，包括长期目标和进一步的护理规划。⑤酌情从门诊和（或）医院护理过渡到家庭护理或临终关怀。⑥与患者和家属讨论临终关怀的期望，并调动离家近的资源支持临终关怀。⑦如果患者家中无法提供最佳护理，则安排转移到其他地点。⑧尽可能的提高生活质量。

（四）其他

由于IPF发病率不高，很多患者对IPF没有正确认识，部分患者对疾病的严重程度没有足够的认识，部分患者高度紧张，影响休息和睡眠。应进行患者教育，充分告知患者IPF的临床发展特点和恶化的特征表现，治疗的方法及药物不良反应控制方法；劝诫和帮助吸烟的患者戒烟；评估患者焦虑和抑郁的程度，必要时给予药物干预，如甲基苯甲酸酯、血清素和去甲肾上腺素再摄取抑制剂、选择性去甲肾上腺素再摄取抑制剂等。由于疾病影响或抗纤维化治疗带来的不良反应可能导致患者营养不良，应注意加强患者蛋白及脂肪的补充。呼吸道感染常引发IPF急性加重，应指导患者减少感染机会，根据当地情况给予疫苗增强抗感染能力。

(五)急性加重的处理

IPF急性加重定义为已诊断或同期诊断为IPF,1个月内发生的呼吸困难急性加重;影像学在原有IPF表现的基础上,新出现两侧的磨玻璃影和(或)实变影,不能完全用心衰或液体过多解释,其组织病理学通常表现为UIP和弥漫性肺泡损伤(DAD)同时存在,可以出现机化性肺炎和显著的成纤维细胞灶。目前临床治疗缺乏有效的治疗方法,氧疗及对症支持治疗是IPF急性加重的主要治疗方法;糖皮质激素、机械通气、抗生素治疗、免疫抑制剂、血浆置换、免疫球蛋白、抗酸治疗等措施疗效均不肯定。TOMORROW和INPULSIS汇总分析提示尼达尼布能够显著降低研究者评估的IPF急性加重发生率,2017专家观点推出预防和治疗的意见(表5-6-4),推荐尼达尼布作为预防IPF急性加重的药物。

表 5-6-4 预防和治疗IPF急性加重的可能措施

预防	推荐	治疗	推荐
流感和肺炎疫苗	+	机械通气	
手卫生,避免与病患接触	+	低潮气量通气	+
控制胃食管反流	+/-	无创通气	+
避免气道刺激及空气污染	+	高流量鼻导管氧疗	+/-
如必须机械通气要采取最小肺脏损伤策略	+/-	药物	
低潮气量通气		糖皮质激素	+
无创通气		经验性抗菌药物	+/-
高流量鼻导管氧疗		免疫抑制剂	-/+
尼达尼布	+/-	血栓调节素	-/+
吡非尼酮	-/+	肺移植	+/-
避免使用泼尼松和硫唑嘌呤	+	其他	
		体外膜肺	-
		多黏菌素B血液灌流	-/+
		利妥昔单抗、血浆置换、静脉免疫球蛋白	-
		非类固醇类治疗	-

注:+:潜在的益处似乎大于潜在的伤害,会考虑在大多数患者中使用;+/-:利益和风险因临床而异,将考虑在选定的患者中使用;-/+:利益和风险因临床而异,不考虑在大多数患者中使用;-:因为缺乏证据来支持临床获益,不会考虑在大多数患者中使用

总而言之,IPF病情复杂多变,异质性强,需要多个指标、多维度评价患者状态和预后。定期随访十分重要,随访中不仅要注意功能性指标的变化,还应注意发现及处理共病,调整药物,给予恰当的心理支持,共同做好预防ILD急性加重的工作。

参 考 文 献

[1] Raghu G, Collard HR, Egan JJ, et al. An Official ATS/ERS/JRS/ALAT Statement: Idiopathic Pulmonary Fibrosis: Evidence-based Guidelines for Diagnosis and Management. Am J Respir Crit Care Med, 2011, 183: 788-824.

[2] American Thoracic Society/European Respiratory Society. International Multidiscipline Consensus Classification of the Idiopathic Interstitial Pneumonias. Am J Respir Crit Care Med, 2002, 165: 277-304.

[3] Kim DS, Collard HR, King Jr TE. Classification and natural history of the idiopathic interstitial pneumonias. Proc Am Thorac Soc, 2006, 3: 285-292.

[4] Nathan SD, Shlobin OA, Weir N, et al. Long-term course and prognosis of idiopathic pulmonary fibrosis in the new millennium. Chest, 2011, 140: 221-229.

[5] Ley B, Collard HR, King Jr TE. Clinical course and prediction of survival in idiopathic pulmonary fibrosis. Am J Respir Crit Care Med, 2011, 183: 431-440.

[6] Collard HR, King TE Jr, Bartelson BB, et al. Changes in clinical and physiologic variables predict survival in idiopathic pulmonary fibrosis. Am. J. Respir. Crit. Care Med, 2003, 168: 538-542.

[7] American Thoracic Society. Idiopathic pulmonary fibrosis: Diagnosis and treatment. International consensus statement. Am. J. Respir. Crit. Care Med, 2000, 161: 646-666.

[8] DuBois RM, Weycker D, Albera C, et al. Forced vital capacity in patients with idiopathic pulmonary fibrosis: test properties and minimal clinically important difference. Am J Respir Crit Care Med, 2011, 184: 1382-1389.

[9] Cottin V, Hansell DM, Sverzellati N, et al. Effect of emphysema extent on serial lung function in patients with idiopathic

pulmonary fibrosis. Am. J. Respir. Crit. Care Med, 2017, 196:1162-1171.

[10] Flaherty KR, Andrei AC, Murray, S, et al. Idiopathic pulmonary fibrosis: Prognostic value of changes in physiology and six-minute-walk-test. Am. J. Respir. Crit. Care Med, 2006, 174:803-809.

[11] Du Bois RM, Weycker D, Albera C, et al. Six Minute Walk Test in Idiopathic Pulmonary Fibrosis. Test Validation and Minimal Clinically Important Difference. Am. J. Respir. Crit. Care Med, 2011, 183:1231-1237.

[12] Eaton T, Young P, Milne D, Wells AU. Six-minute-walk, maximal exercise tests: Reproducibility in fibrotic interstitial pneumonia. Am. J. Respir. Crit. Care Med, 2005, 171: 1150-1157.

[13] Lama VN, Flaherty KR, Toews GB, et al. Prognostic value of desaturation during a 6-minute walk test in idiopathic interstitial pneumonia. Am. J. Respir. Crit. Care Med, 2003, 168: 1084-1090.

[14] Du Bois RM, Albera C, Bradford WZ, et al. 6-minute walk distance is an independent predictor of mortality in patients with idiopathic pulmonary fibrosis. Eur. Respir. J, 2014, 43, 1421-1429.

[15] Du Bois RM, Albera C, Bradford WZ, et al. A novel clinical prediction model for near term mortality in patients with idiopathic pulmonary fibrosis (IPF). Am J Respir Crit Care Med, 2013, 187:A2357.

[16] Raghu G, Remy-Jardin M, Myers J, et al. Diagnosis of Idiopathic Pulmonary Fibrosis An Official ATS/ERS/JRS/ALAT Clinical Practice Guideline. Am J Respir Crit Care Med, 2018, 198(5):e44-e68.

[17] Sumikawa H, Johkoh T, Colby TV, et al. Computed tomography findings in pathological usual interstitial pneumonia: relationship to survival. Am J Respir Crit Care Med, 2008, 177:433e9.

[18] Lynch DA, Godwin JD, Safrin S, et al. High-resolution computed tomography in idiopathic pulmonary fibrosis: diagnosis and prognosis. Am J Respir Crit Care Med, 2005, 172: 488-493.

[19] Xaubet A, Agusti C, Luburich P, et al. Pulmonary Function Tests and CT Scan in the management of Idiopathic Pulmonary Fibrosis. Am. J. Respir. Crit. Care Med, 1998, 158: 431-436.

[20] Hu Y, Wang LS, Jin YP, et al. Serum Krebs Von Den Lungen-6 Level as a Diagnostic Biomarker for Interstitial Lung Disease in Chinese Patients. Clin Respir J, 2017, 11: 337-345.

[21] Kinder BW, Brown KK, McCormack FX, et al. Serum surfactant protein-A is a strong predictor of early mortality in idiopathic pulmonary fibrosis. Chest, 2009, 135:1557-1563.

[22] Buendia-Roldán I, Ruiz V, Sierra P, et al. Increased Expression of CC16 in Patients with Idiopathic Pulmonary Fibrosis. PLoS One, 2016, 11:e0168552.

[23] Tzouvelekis A, Herazo-Maya JD, Slade M, et al. Validation of the prognostic value of MMP-7 in Idiopathic Pulmonary Fibrosis. Respirology, 2017, 22:486-493.

[24] Bauer Y, White ES, Bernard S, et al. MMP-7 is a predictive biomarker of disease progression in patients with idiopathic pulmonary fibrosis. ERJ Open Res, 2017, 3:1-10.

[25] Prasse A, Probst C, Bargagli E, et al. Serum CC-chemokine ligand 18 concentration predicts outcome in idiopathic pulmonary fibrosis. Am. J. Respir. Crit. Care Med, 2009, 179, 717-723.

[26] Sellare J, Veraldi KL, Thiel KJ, et al. Intracellular heat shock protein 70 deficiency in pulmonary fibrosis. Am J Respir Cell Mol Biol, 2019, 60:629-636.

[27] Kahloon RA, Xue J, Bhargava A, et al. Patients with idiopathic pulmonary fibrosis with antibodies to heat shock protein 70 have poor prognoses. Am J Respir Crit Care Med, 2013, 187:768.

[28] Kropski JA, Blackwell TS, Lloyd JE. The genetic basis of idiopathic pulmonary fibrosis. Eur. Respir. J, 2015, 45: 1717-1727.

[29] Seibold MA, Wise AL, Speer MC, et al. A common MUC5B promoter polymorphism and pulmonary fibrosis. N. Engl. J. Med, 2011, 364:1503-1512.

[30] Goodwin AT, MBChB, Jenkins G. Molecular Endotyping of Pulmonary Fibrosis. Chest, 2016, 149:228-237.

[31] Collard HR, King Jr TE, Bartelson BB, et al. Changes in Clinical and Physiologic Variables Predict Survival in Idiopathic Pulmonary Fibrosis. Am J Respir Crit Care Med, 2003, 168: 538-542.

[32] Jankowich MD, Rounds SIS. Combined pulmonary fibrosis and emphysema syndrome: a review. Chest, 2012, 141: 222-223.

[33] Nadrous HF, Pellikka PA, Krowka MJ, et al. H. Pulmonary hypertension in patients with idiopathic pulmonary fibrosis. Chest, 2005, 128:2393-2399.

[34] Nathan SD, Shlobin OA, Barnett SD, et al. Right ventricular systolic pressure by echocardiography as a predictor of pulmonary hypertension in idiopathic pulmonary fibrosis. Respir. Med, 2008, 102:1305-1310.

[35] Ozawa Y, Suda T, Naito T, et al. Cumulative incidence of and predictive factors for lung cancer in IPF. Respirology, 2009, 14:723-728.

[36] King TE Jr, Behr J, Brown KK, et al. BUILD-1: a randomized placebo controlled trial of bosentan in idiopathic pulmonary fibrosis. Am J Respir Crit Care Med, 2008, 177:75-81.

[37] Noble PW, Albera C, Bradford WZ, et al. Pirfenidone in patients with idiopathic pulmonary fibrosis (CAPACITY): two randomised trials. Lancet, 2011, 377(9779):1760-1769.

[38] Idiopathic Pulmonary Fibrosis Clinical Research N, Raghu G, Anstrom KJ, et al. Prednisone, azathioprine, and N-acetylcysteine for pulmonary fibrosis. N Engl J Med, 2012, 366: 1968-1977.

[39] Ley B, Ryerson CJ, Vittinghoff E, et al. A multidimensional index and staging system for idiopathic pulmonary fibrosis. Ann Intern Med, 2012, 156:684-691.

[40] Ley B, Bradford WZ, Weycker D, et al. Unified baseline and longitudinal mortality prediction in idiopathic pulmonary fibrosis. Eur. Respir. J, 2015, 45:1374-1381.

[41] DuBois RM, Weycker D, Albera C, et al. Ascertainment of individual risk of mortality for patients with idiopathic pulmonary fibrosis. Am. J. Respir. Crit. Care Med, 2011, 184: 459-466.

[42] Albera C, Costabel U, Fagan EA, et al. Efficacy of pirfenidone in patients with idiopathic pulmonary fibrosis with more preserved lung function. Eur Respir J, 2016, 48: 843.

[43] Kolb M, Richeldi L, Behr J, et al. Nintedanib in patients with idiopathic pulmonary fibrosis and preserved lung volume. Thorax, 2016, 72: 340-346.

[44] Robalo-Cordeiro C, Campos P, Carvalho L, et al. Idiopathic pulmonary fibrosis in the era of antifibrotic therapy: Searching for new opportunities grounded in evidence. Rev Port Pneumol, 2017, 23: 287-293.

[45] Wuyts WA, Kolb M, Stowasser S, et al. First data on efficacy and safety of nintedanib in patients with idiopathic pulmonary fibrosis and forced vital capacity of ≤50% of predicted value. Lung, 2016, 194: 739-743.

[46] Richeldi L, Cottin V, Du Bois RM, et al. Nintedanib in patients with idiopathic pulmonary fibrosis: combined evidence from the TOMORROW and INPULSIS® trials. Respir Med, 2016, 113: 74-79.

[47] Noble PW, Albera C, Bradford WZ, et al. Pirfenidone for idiopathic pulmonary fibrosis: analysis of pooled data from three multinational phase 3 trials. Eur Respir J, 2016, 47: 243-253.

[48] Raghu G, Freudenberger TD, Yang S, et al. High prevalence of abnormal acid gastro-oesophageal reflux in idiopathic pulmonary fibrosis. Eur Respir J, 2006, 27: 136-142.

[49] Tobin RW, Pope CE, Pellegrini CA, et al. Increased prevalence of gastroesophageal reflux in patients with idiopathic pulmonary fibrosis. Am J Respir Crit Care Med, 1998, 158: 1804-1808.

[50] Lee JS, Collard HR, Anstrom KJ, et al. IPF net Investigators. Anti-acid treatment and disease progression in idiopathic pulmonary fibrosis: an analysis of data from three randomized controlled trials. Lancet Repir Med, 2013, 1: 369-376.

[51] Raghu G, Rochwerg B, Zhang Y, et al. An official ATS/ERS/JRS/ALAT clinical practice guideline: treatment of idiopathic pulmonary fibrosis. an update of the 2011 clinical practice guideline. Am J Respir Crit Care Med, 2015, 192: e3-e19.

[52] Oldham JM, Ma SF, Martinez FZ, et al. TOLLIP, MUC5B, and the Response to N-Acetylcysteine among Individuals with Idiopathic Pulmonary Fibrosis. Am J Respir Crit Care Med, 2015, 192: 1475-1482.

[53] Mallick S. Outcome of patients with idiopathic pulmonary fibrosis (IPF) ventilated in intensive care unit. Respir Med, 2008, 102: 1355-1359.

[54] 中华医学会呼吸病学分会肺间质病学组 特发性肺纤维化诊断和治疗中国专家共识. 中华结核和呼吸杂志, 2016, 39: 427-432.

[55] Keating D, Levvey B, Kotsimbos T, et al. Lung transplantation in pulmonary fibrosis: challenging early outcomes counterbalanced by surprisingly good outcomes beyond 15 years. Transplant Proc, 2009, 41: 289-291.

[56] Kalluri M, Claveria F, Ainsley E, et al. Beyond idiopathic pulmonary fibrosis diagnosis: multidisciplinary care with an early integrated palliative approach is associated with a decrease in acute care utilization and hospital deaths. J Pain Symptom Manage, 2018, 55(2): 420-426.

[57] Lanken PN, Terry PB, Delisser HM, et al. An official American Thoracic Society clinical policy statement: palliative care for patients with respiratory diseases and critical illnesses. Am J Respir Crit Care Med, 2008, 177: 912-927.

[58] Collard HR, Ryerson CJ, Corte TJ, et al. Acute exacerbation of idiopathic pulmonary fibrosis. an international working group report. Am J Respir Crit Care Med, 2016, 194: 265-275.

[59] Kondoh Y, Cottin V, Brown KK. Recent lessons learned in the management of acute exacerbation of idiopathic pulmonary fibrosis. Eur Respir Rev, 2017, 26: 170050.

7 特异性肺纤维化的全新发病机制

汤 楠

特发性肺纤维化(idiopathic pulmonary fibrosis, IPF)是一种常见的肺泡疾病,肺健康组织被过量的间质细胞和细胞外基质逐渐取代,导致肺泡结构被破坏、肺泡区域逐渐致密化,最终导致呼吸衰竭和死亡。IPF 患者诊断的中位生存时间为 2~4 年,约 80% 的患者从确诊到死亡不超过 5 年,5 年生存率仅高于胰腺癌和肺癌,因而被无奈地称为"不是癌症的癌症"。因为 IPF 发病年龄大多在 50~70 岁,随着人口的老龄化,在全球范围内,该疾病的发病率越来越高,世界 IPF 联合协会统计,约有 320 万人患 IPF,每年新增 122 万病例。

一、特发性肺纤维化的主要临床症状

IPF 的主要临床症状及常见体征:①患者多呈现进行性肺功能衰竭,尤其以发病后期及剧烈运动时表现最为明显。②患者早期少见咳嗽,随着病程进行,会出现轻咳及少量痰液,直至后期出现继发性感染等肺炎症状。③患者多见消瘦、乏力及杵状指(趾)等长期缺氧的表征。

IPF 发病率较高,具体到性别和年龄段,该调查显示:男性较女性更易罹患 IPF,而随着年龄的增长,不管是男性还是女性,罹患 IPF 的概率都大大增加。

IPF 治愈率和预后极差,约有 80% 的患者从最初确诊到死亡不超过 5 年时间,该死亡率甚至超过大多数肺部癌症的死亡率。匮乏的治疗手段和药物很大程度上源于 IPF 发病机制探究的滞后。

特发性肺纤维化(IPF)是一种致命的疾病,由于缺乏有效的治疗药物和手段,患者在诊断后的存活率很低,其恶化程度堪比恶性癌症。

二、特发性肺纤维化的主要病理特征

IPF 是多种肺间质疾病中的一种,与其他多种间质疾病在一些特征上具有共性,如何对 IPF 患者进行确切的诊断在过去的很长一段时间比较模糊和经验主义。随着肺活检技术和肺移植手术的成熟,以及追踪患者系统的完善,目前初步得出了两个极为重要的诊断特征:进行性恶化趋势及病变部位结构异质性。

IPF 的进行性恶化趋势是患者致死的主要原因:在患者发病初期,纤维化病变区域往往只出现在肺泡的很小一部分区域,很难在肺功能上得到察觉。而且,这样的区域一般首先出现在肺叶边缘。在后续的时间内,病变区域逐步蔓延,直到整个肺叶均呈现致密状。这个过程一般需要 2~4 年的时间,但在极少数有其他诱发因素的存在下,这样的过程可能只发生在短短的几个月。经过大范围的临床统计,医学工作者发现,大部分的 IPF 患者均具有这样的特质:起始于肺叶边缘的纤维化小块,后逐渐进行,直到整个肺部变得致密。因此,这个特质被称为进行性,而 IPF 也被称为进行性肺纤维化。这样的特质也是 IPF 临床诊断的主要标准之一。但为什么患者的纤维化发生于肺叶边缘,又是什么样的驱动因素促使了纤维化的进行性,这些问题却没有答案。究其原因,主要有两个。首先,因为在正常呼吸状态下,我们人体的肺部的很多肺泡区域并不会完全被利用,而是有很大的富裕,因此,在 IPF 患者肺部刚开始发生纤维化的时候,患者并不能够有很直接的呼吸困难等反应。如果这个时候不去做 CT 扫描的检测,就很难捕捉到早期发病可能的触发因素,也很难及时做出治疗干预,因此,IPF 的进行性也被认为是最为致命的特征。其次,目前存在的肺纤维化的小鼠模型的表型并不能够模拟 IPF 的边缘起始性和进行性,那么揭示这样的特质背后的机制便更加困难。

在临床研究中,医生们通过影像学扫描观测到 IPF 患者纤维化的发病模式是从肺叶边缘到中心,并把该特征作为 IPF 的关键诊断标准。这个过程一般需要 3~5 年,但有时,会因为一些未知的原因进入急剧恶化期,只需要数月便出现急剧的扩散。

特发性肺纤维化(IPF)患者呈现进行性病程进展。这也是该疾病最为致命的特征,即使一开始病程进展缓慢的患者,如果肺部遭遇二次伤害,也会出现急剧的恶化。

结构异质性是 IPF 的另外一个特有的主要特征,这也是肺活检技术鉴定的依据之一。具体而言,结构异质性是指在 IPF 患者的肺部,同一时间可见多种程度不一的纤维化区域,包括蜂窝状结构(honeycombing),致密纤维化区域(dense fibrosis),纤维化早期区域(fibroblastic foci),以及严重的病变区域和相对正常的肺泡的过渡区域(transition)。这 4 种结构源于大量 IPF 患者的肺部活检结果,之后便作为确诊 IPF 的主要依据之一。其中,纤维化早期区域(fibroblastic foci)同时也是纤维化过程最活跃的区域,在这个区域，可以看到活跃的细胞外基质的沉积，同时伴随着间质细胞，尤其以 α-SMA 标记的肌成纤维细胞为主要类型，这些间质细胞呈现高比例的 Ki-67 细胞复制标志物的表达。同时，在这样的小块区域中，可以看到典型的有规律的结构：紧邻活跃的间质区，但位于这样的间质区的内表面，是一些呈异常聚集状的 AT2 细胞，而 AT1 细胞却消失了。这些聚集的 AT2 细胞呈现微弱升高的细胞复制标志物 Ki-67 的表达。更加值得注意的是，这个典型的区域多数位于 IPF 肺组织的过渡区。结合 IPF 的进行性和边缘起始性，纤维化早期区域（fibroblastic foci）被认为是 IPF 中高度活跃和病变的区域。因此，围绕这个区域展开研究，可能有助于我们找到早期的真正驱动不变的机制。

在特发性肺纤维化的患者肺部，可以发现一个标志性的区域：纤维细胞病灶（fibroblatic foci），在这个区域可以看到肌成纤维细胞的生成及胶原的大量沉积。同时，可以看到被激活的缓慢增殖的 AT2 细胞。这样的区域被认为是纤维化病变的的积极活跃区，这样的区域的数目被临床上作为预测患者病程进展快慢的参考指标。

病理结构的背后是错综复杂的致病机制。而每一种细微的结构必然对应其特别的发病机制，因此，对于病理结构的细致描述和对比，必然会对我们阐明机制提供方向和思路。

三、特发性肺纤维化发病机制的多种假说

关于 IPF 的发病机制一直以来是困扰肺部基础研究和疾病领域的难题之一，原因有以下几点：首先，IPF 是一种慢性进行性疾病，患者在发病初期往往不易察觉，因而错失了研究和发现起始发病因素的机会；其次，IPF 的病程往往伴随着多种肺泡细胞的参与，包括肺泡上皮细胞，肺泡间质细胞，免疫细胞等细胞类群，复杂的关系网给基础探究带来一定的阻力。

虽然精确的诱发 IPF 的机制尚未完全阐明，但目前相关研究工作者对其发病机制提出了一些假说，依据这些假说，一些针对 IPF 的药物也被开发出来，但目前这些药物都未能起到彻底的治愈效果。这些假说及其相关药物主要有以下两个方面。

1. 损伤导致的免疫异常 在疾病的早期阶段，由于一些未知的原因导致的细胞死亡等过程会促进肺部细胞分泌 TGFβ，IL-1β 及 CXCL 等分子，这些过度的持续高表达的细胞因子会再次刺激肺泡间质细胞，如成纤维细胞和周皮细胞的复制和分化，同时激活的间质细胞开始大量地分泌细胞外基质如胶原蛋白、弹性纤维等。过多的纤维化细胞，以及细胞外基质造成肺部不可逆转的纤维化改变。依据这样的假说，一些干预免疫的药物被开发出来，但是，治疗效果却并不理想，因此，科学家开始反思这个假说，又提出了另外一种对 IPF 的解释。

2. AT2 细胞可能是 IPF 起始的关键分子 当重新审视表皮细胞在 IPF 中的作用时，研究领域认为 IPF 的起始者很有可能是受伤失控的表皮细胞。通过对家族性肺纤维化患者的肺组织进行外显子测序，科学家发现了多个和肺泡上皮干细胞（AT2 细胞）相关的基因突变，例如 *Sftpc*、*Sftpa* 和 *Muc5b* 等基因，这更加将起始细胞类型锁定在了 AT2 细胞上。

基于组织病理学的观察，IPF 的肺组织中，尤其是间质细胞高度活跃致密的地方，经常可以观察到聚集的 AT2 细胞，这不禁让人猜想是否 AT2 细胞会直接转变为间质细胞，参与纤维化发生过程中。为了探究这个问题，研究团队使用谱系追踪的手段，特异性地在博来霉素诱导的小鼠纤维化模型中追踪了 AT2 细胞的行为特征，结果表明 AT2 细胞并不会向间质细胞转变，而是一部分分化为肺泡一型细胞，一部分继续保持 AT2 细胞的性质。这个发现否定了 AT2 细胞通过转变为间质细胞参与到纤维化病变的可能性。那么，AT2 细胞是否是特发性肺纤维化发病的源头，如果确实如此，AT2 细胞本质的异常主要在哪里？它又究竟是如何导致了纤维化的发生呢？

通过对家族性肺纤维化患者的肺组织进行外显子测序，发现了多个和肺泡上皮干细胞（AT2 细胞）相关的基因的突变，例如 *SPC*、*SPA* 和 *MUC5B* 等，这指示 AT2 细胞在 IPF 中的异常。

为了回答这个问题，研究团队继续回到了 IPF 患者的组织中寻找答案。同时得益于单细胞 RNA 测序技术的发展，通过对多个 IPF 的患者组织中的细胞进行单细胞 RNA 测序分析，进一步对比正常供体患者中的单个细胞的基因表达谱发现：相较于其他细胞类群，IPF 患者中的 AT2 细胞的基因录表达谱的变化是最显著也是最大的；同时，可以看到这些细胞呈现高度活跃状态，也高度富集了 Hippo 信号通路和 TGFβ 信号通路。其中，Hippo 信号通路被多个团队证明对上皮的损伤应激响应具有关键作用，而 TGFβ 信号通路被认为是器官纤维化病变的关键，以及普适性的信号通路，这主要由于其激活状态在多种纤维化病变组织中被检测和捕捉到。虽然看到了这些促纤维化信号通路在 AT2 细胞中的富集，但是关于 AT2 细胞的细胞行为，TGFβ 等促纤维化信号通路以及纤维化改变之间具体的连接依然未被阐明。

通过对多个 IPF 的患者组织中的细胞进行单细胞 RNA 测序分析，进一步对比正常供体患者中的单个细胞的基因表达谱发现：IPF 患者中的 AT2 细胞的基因录表达谱与对照 AT2 细胞的基因表达谱差别很显著。

四、肺纤维化发病的全新机制

之前由于缺乏有效的动物模型，肺特发性肺纤维化确切的病理生理学仍不清楚，但是大量的研究暗示了上皮细胞和间质细胞都有参与这一过程。例如，对 AT2 细胞的反复损伤导致间质细胞不受控制的激活，从而引起自己瘢痕，即纤维化的形成和细胞外基质的沉积，因此，了解肺泡上皮细胞损伤后再生和修复，以及错误的再生和修复是如何影响间质细胞最终导致纤维化的发生具有重要意义。

北京生命科学研究所汤楠团队一直致力于探究肺损伤后肺泡再生的调控机制。团队前期建立了左肺切除

(pneumonectomy,PNX)诱导肺泡再生的小鼠模型。通过研究发现,左肺切除手术后剩余肺泡(右肺)被暴露于升高的呼吸张力下,因此激活了肺泡干细胞的增殖和分化,最终新肺泡的建立,呼吸功能的恢复,肺泡区域的呼吸张力恢复到正常生理水平。

进一步,团队的研究人员发现细胞周期调控蛋白Cdc42在肺泡再生过程中发挥了重要的作用。Cdc42基因缺失的肺泡干细胞在肺损伤后无法建立新的肺泡,导致了升高的肺泡张力无法恢复到正常生理水平。当研究人员继续追踪该肺泡再生障碍小鼠(Cdc42肺泡干细胞null小鼠)时,发现小鼠的肺部发生纤维化病变,同时病程模拟了IPF的疾病发展。具体表现如下:①小鼠肺纤维化进展从肺叶边缘起始并不断向肺叶中心进行。②肺泡逐步被过度增殖的成纤维细胞和增加的细胞外基质所替代。③小鼠肺活量和肺顺应性进行性下降,小鼠最终死于呼吸功能衰竭。同时,在老年Cdc42 null小鼠里,研究人员也能观察到同样的病理改变。

通过单细胞测序分析,研究人员发现肺纤维化的小鼠肺部富集了一群肺泡干细胞亚群。进一步的生物信息分析表明,该干细胞亚群是肺泡干细胞分化过程中的一种中间态。通过和IPF患者肺泡干细胞单细胞测序数据库的比较,研究人员发现①小鼠模型中激活的肺泡干细胞亚群里上调的基因与IPF患者的肺泡干细胞中上调的基因有高度重叠。②小鼠肺泡干细胞亚群和IPF患者肺泡干细胞中都有显著升高的机械张力相关信号通路和TGFbeta信号通路。

与IPF相似的发病模式及高度重叠的上调基因让研究人员猜想:机械张力相关的信号通路和TGFbeta信号通路可能共同参与了IPF发病。为了探究这个猜想,研究人员首先将假体置于左肺切除手术(PNX)后的Cdc42 null小鼠胸腔内,进而缓解了PNX诱导的肺泡呼吸张力的增加,结果发现假体的植入可以显著抑制肺纤维化的进展。另一方面,研究人员在Cdc42缺失的肺泡干细胞中,通过对TGFbeta信号通路进行干扰(分别干扰配体和受体),发现在Cdc42 null的再生障碍的小鼠中,阻断AT2细胞中的TGFbeta信号通路可以显著阻止肺纤维化的进展。

在临床研究中,医生们通过影像学扫描观测到IPF患者纤维化的发病模式是从肺叶边缘到中心,并把该特征作为IPF的关键诊断标准。但是,为什么肺纤维化会起始于肺边缘和为什么纤维化是进行性,相关的发病机制却完全不清楚,这也是在本研究之前没有一个真实模仿IPF小鼠模型的关键。基于此,研究人员采用机械通气手段对小鼠进行不同程度从低到高的呼吸机械张力模拟,同时结合数学模型运算和拟合,证明了随着呼吸运动机械张力的增加,位于肺叶边缘的肺泡首先承受高的机械张力,高的机械张力进一步激活肺泡干细胞中不断级联放大的TGFbeta信号通路,从而诱导肺泡周围间质细胞的响应和激活。

综上,汤楠实验室的研究人员在本文中首次建立了高度模拟IPF发病特征的小鼠疾病模型,并进一步发现Cdc42缺失的肺泡干细胞由于无法分化和建立新肺泡,导致肺泡干细胞被持续暴露于升高的肺泡机械张力下,从而持续激活肺泡干细胞里TGFbeta信号通路,最终导致从边缘到中心的肺纤维化病变。该研究从细胞行为和分子机理双重层面阐述了进行性肺纤维化的发生和发展,为肺纤维化的研究和治疗提供了思路。

参考文献

[1] Wynn TA. Cellular and molecular mechanisms of fibrosis. The Journal of pathology,2008,214:199-210.

[2] Wynn TA, Ramalingam TR. Mechanisms of fibrosis: therapeutic translation for fibrotic disease. Nature medicine,2012, 18:1028-1040.

[3] Bongartz T, et al. Incidence and mortality of interstitial lung disease in rheumatoid arthritis: a population-based study. Arthritis & Rheumatism,2010,62:1583-1591.

[4] King Jr TE, Pardo A, Selman M. Idiopathic pulmonary fibrosis. The Lancet,2011,378:1949-1961.

[5] Raghu G, Weycker D, Edelsberg J, et al. Incidence and prevalence of idiopathic pulmonary fibrosis. American journal of respiratory and critical care medicine,2006,174:810-816.

[6] Bjoraker JA, et al. Prognostic significance of histopathologic subsets in idiopathic pulmonary fibrosis. American journal of respiratory and critical care medicine,1998,157:199-203.

[7] Selman M, King TE, Pardo A. Idiopathic pulmonary fibrosis: prevailing and evolving hypotheses about its pathogenesis and implications for therapy. Annals of internal medicine, 2001,134:136-151.

[8] Meltzer EB, et al. Bayesian probit regression model for the diagnosis of pulmonary fibrosis: proof-of-principle. BMC medical genomics,2011,4:1-13.

[9] Kim DS, Collard HR, King Jr TE. Classification and natural history of the idiopathic interstitial pneumonias. Proceedings of the American Thoracic Society,2006,3:285-292.

[10] Noble PW, Barkauskas CE, Jiang D. Pulmonary fibrosis: patterns and perpetrators. The Journal of clinical investigation, 2012,122:2756-2762.

[11] Lynch DA, et al. Diagnostic criteria for idiopathic pulmonary fibrosis: a Fleischner Society White Paper. The Lancet Respiratory Medicine,2018,6:138-153.

[12] Chapman HA. Epithelial-mesenchymal interactions in pulmonary fibrosis. Annual review of physiology, 2011, 73: 413-435.

[13] Tolle LB, Southern BD, Culver DA. et al. Idiopathic pulmonary fibrosis: What primary care physicians need to know. Cleve Clin J Med,2018,85:377-386.

[14] Kropski JA, Blackwell TS, Loyd JE. The genetic basis of idiopathic pulmonary fibrosis. European Respiratory Journal, 2015,45:1717-1727.

[15] Goodwin AT, Jenkins G. Molecular endotyping of pulmonary fibrosis. Chest,2016,149:228-237.

[16] Wang Y, et al. Genetic defects in surfactant protein A2 are

associated with pulmonary fibrosis and lung cancer. American journal of human genetics,2008,84:52-59.

[17] Seibold MA, et al. A common MUC5B promoter polymorphism and pulmonary fibrosis. The New England journal of medicine,2011,364:1503-1512.

[18] Nogee LM, et al. A mutation in the surfactant protein C gene associated with familial interstitial lung disease. The New England journal of medicine,2001,344:573-579.

[19] Rock JR, et al. Multiple stromal populations contribute to pulmonary fibrosis without evidence for epithelial to mesenchymal transition. Proceedings of the National Academy of Sciences of the United States of America,2011,108:1475-1483.

[20] Xu Y, et al. Single-cell RNA sequencing identifies diverse roles of epithelial cells in idiopathic pulmonary fibrosis. JCI Insight,2016,1(20):e90558.

[21] Liu Z, et al. MAPK-Mediated YAP Activation Controls Mechanical-Tension-Induced Pulmonary Alveolar Regeneration. Cell reports,2016,16:1810-1819.

[22] Wu H, et al. Progressive pulmonary fibrosis is caused by elevated mechanical tension on alveolar stem cells. Cell,2020,180:107-121.

[23] Gross TJ, Hunninghake GW. Idiopathic pulmonary fibrosis. New England Journal of Medicine,2001,345:517-525.

8 肺纤维化动物模型的制备与评价

崔 烨

一、前言

肺纤维化可以由遗传缺陷、职业暴露、环境因素或药物引起,也可以是特发性的。各种类型肺纤维化的发病机制目前还不完全清楚。随着纤维化严重程度的进展,肺顺应性逐渐丧失,气体交换受损,最终可导致呼吸衰竭。为了更好地了解肺纤维化的发病机制,在过去的几十年里,研究者已制备出多种肺纤维化的动物模型。

动物模型在疾病的研究中扮演着重要的角色,它们可以帮助我们理解疾病在体内形成的病理生理机制。一种理想的动物模型应该是最能模拟人类疾病的模型,具有高度的可复制性和一致性,易于实施,可广泛使用,且不太昂贵。建立任何一种人类慢性疾病的动物模型都具有很大的难度。毋庸置疑,动物模型对于加深我们对肺纤维化的认识和药物研发都是必不可少的,但肺纤维化的年龄相关性及病理的高度复杂性,给动物模型的制备和评估都带来了极大的挑战。遗憾的是,目前还没有任何一种动物模型能够从各个方面都完全复制人类肺纤维化的发生和进展。

正是因为如此,虽然许多化合物在体外能有效地限制成纤维细胞/肌成纤维细胞的激活,也在动物模型上显示了减轻肺纤维化的功效,但只有极少数化合物在临床试验中能够控制或减缓患者肺纤维化的逐渐恶化,而绝大多数化合物最终无法成功地转化为肺纤维化有效的治疗方式。诸多不成功的临床试验在一定程度上浪费了宝贵的患者资源和经济资源。因此,我们迫切需要增强临床前肺纤维化动物模型的成功转化,以便更好地识别和选择临床上有意义的干预靶点,帮助制药企业决定哪些药物值得研究开发,并有效促进候选药物早日进入临床试验。

本文旨在总结常用肺纤维化模型的研究现状,并提出未来的发展前景。

二、实验动物的选择

一些家畜(比如马和狗)已经被证明可以自发出现肺纤维化病理改变。此外,在体型较大的动物中,还可以使用纤维支气管镜在选定的节段诱导严重的纤维化病变,并开展临床相关的检测,比如重复测量肺功能和肺活检。尽管对这些家畜模型的研究有助于探究肺纤维化的发病机制,但较为高昂的购买费用和饲养成本使得我们很难广泛采用这些物种开展临床前研究。目前,研究肺纤维化发病机制和临床前治疗评估最不可或缺的模型仍然是啮齿类动物模型。诸多传统的和新型的啮齿类动物模型为我们深入了解肺纤维化的发病机制提供了宝贵的资源。

由于高龄实验动物的饲养耗时较长且价格不菲,大多数研究选用的仍是低龄实验动物,这与临床上肺纤维化多在中老年阶段发病是不符的。目前尚无确切证据表明高龄与低龄动物中实验性肺纤维化发病机制的区别,但有研究报道称,在高龄小鼠中,博来霉素可诱导更为严重的肺纤维化病理改变,且高龄小鼠肺组织的损伤修复机能严重受损。随着我国人口老龄化进程的持续发展,肺纤维化在未来十几年中的发病率也将会逐渐上升。因此,有必要探索肺纤维化与衰老的相关性,并研究在高龄实验动物中衰老相关靶点在肺纤维化发病及进展中作用和变化。

三、肺纤维化动物模型的种类

用于肺纤维化模型制备的诱导因素很多,如博来霉素、二氧化硅、放射线等。此外,通过病毒载体过度表达致纤维化细胞因子也可以导致肺纤维化。

(一)博来霉素肺纤维化模型

目前,博来霉素模型已成为国际上最常用的实验性肺纤维化动物模型。因此,在本文中,我们将对该模型进行详细的阐述。博来霉素是一种临床上常用的广谱抗肿瘤药物。博来霉素进入肿瘤细胞后,可与铁离子和氧结合反应,产生活性氧类(reactive oxygen species, ROS),如 O_2^- 和 ·OH,这些自由基可直接攻击 DNA,引起 DNA 断裂,最终导致肿瘤细胞的凋亡,这是博来霉素抗肿瘤的作用机制之一。然而,肺组织中博来霉素水解酶含量较低,因此,摄入博来霉素后,肺组织中的博来霉素不能被及时有效地降解,同时博来霉素所介导的 DNA 断链过程中涉及到 ROS 的大量生成,这可引起肺部的急性损伤,并可发展成肺纤维化,博来霉素诱导的肺纤维化模型也正是利用了博来霉素的肺毒性。建立模型时,博来霉素可通过静脉、腹腔注射或气道多种途径单次或多次给药。在动物模型中无论采用哪种给药途径,博来霉素均会导致肺纤维化。但是,损伤的最初部位取决于暴露的方式,比如系统性给药会导致内皮损伤,而经气管给药则会引起上皮的损伤。另外,值得注意的是,博来霉素模型中纤维化的发展取决于小鼠的品系,相对于BALB/C小鼠而言,C57BL/6小鼠对博来霉素更敏感,肺纤维化病变也更加明显,因此更适合用作制备肺纤维化模型。

在经气道给药的动物模型制备过程中,可以采用经气管注射、经鼻或经口气管滴注给予博来霉素。气管内注射需要在实验动物的颈部中线切口,注射博来霉素后立即缝合切口。此外,还可将动物固定在倾斜操作台上,利用喉镜暴露声门,将带有气溶胶雾化喷射头的雾化针插入气管后,使用相连的高压注射器将博来霉素喷射入气管。这种无创气管插管造模的优点在于其对动物的伤害较小,同时采用喷雾给药比传统滴注法给药使博来霉素在肺部的分布更加均一。这种给药途径不仅适用于博来霉素模型,也适用于气管内给药诱发肺纤维化的其它动物模型。

博来霉素诱导的实验性肺纤维化动物模型可被称之为"损伤-修复"模型,其病程进展可分为两个阶段:首先,博来霉素气管滴注后会造成急性肺损伤期(第0～7d),此阶段的主要病理表现为肺内大量炎性细胞的浸润。在急性期后,第二阶段的主要病理表现为细胞外基质的重塑和胶原的大量沉积。需要注意的是,博来霉素模型后期肺纤维化的形成完全依赖于起始阶段肺组织所受到的损伤,且肺纤维化病变呈自限性,持续时间仅在4个月左右,此后纤维化会随着时间的推移而逐渐消失,这与临床上特发性肺纤维化持续进展性和不可逆性是有巨大差别的。另外,小鼠博来霉素模型也缺乏人类疾病的关键病理学表现,如成纤维细胞灶的形成。目前,我们对实验性肺纤维化的认识大多是建立在这种动物模型的基础上,同时,也有大量药物都被证明可以缓解博来霉素导致的急性肺部炎症和继发的肺纤维化。遗憾的是,多数药物在临床特发性肺纤维化的治疗中并没有表现出与基础研究相似的有效作用。因此,学术界现已对基于博来霉素模型药物研发的应用价值产生了一些质疑。

临床上,肺纤维化往往起病隐匿,随着疾病的进展,肺功能逐渐恶化,出现明显症状后,患者才会来医院就诊。这就意味着在动物实验中,只观察药物对肺纤维化的预防作用是远远不够的。为了评估药物真正的抗肺纤维化功效,在使用博来霉素动物模型时,我们首先应精准把握治疗时机,以保证干预措施抑制的是纤维化病理改变而不影响早期炎症。一项有关博来霉素动物模型的回顾性研究表明,在2008—2019年发表的976篇文献中,干预措施开始于博来霉素造模后七d之内的研究高达60%以上。博来霉素造模后七天内给予药物治疗即使减轻了肺部炎症,也减少了继发的纤维化病变,但药物干预的可能仅仅是肺部的炎症反应,而不是持续性的肺纤维化过程。因此,美国胸科学会官方报告建议在博来霉素模型动物中,治疗干预时间应在纤维化出现后,即不早于造模后第7～10d。

(二)二氧化硅肺纤维化模型

矽肺是由于长期吸入大量游离二氧化硅引起的肺进行性纤维化疾病,是尘肺中的一个重要类型。动物实验中可将二氧化硅悬液通过雾化吸入或气管滴注方式建立这种肺纤维化模型。肺泡巨噬细胞吞噬二氧化硅后,发生呼吸爆发,激活电子传递系统,产生大量ROS。此外,还有研究表明石英可不依赖肺泡巨噬细胞产生ROS。通过对新研磨的石英尘采用电子自旋共振波谱技术,检测到每克石英尘在空气中研磨30min后可产生约10^{18}个硅载自由基,硅载自由基与水反应生成·OH。这些ROS可引起细胞膜脂质过氧化,最终导致细胞损伤并释放多种致纤维化性细胞因子,参与肺部纤维化形成和进展。

二氧化硅肺纤维化模型的优势在于吸入的二氧化硅不容易从肺中被清除,因此体内存在持久的纤维化刺激。另外,这种动物模型的一个特征为肺巨噬细胞NALP3炎性小体的激活,这对研究肺纤维化的固有免疫调节作用具有重要意义。

(三)放射性肺纤维化模型

放射性肺纤维化是临床上胸部恶性肿瘤放疗和骨髓移植预处理后常见的并发症,放射疗法在杀伤肿瘤细胞或抑制肿瘤细胞生长的同时,也对健康组织产生有害作用,即放射性损伤。因此,建立放射性肺纤维化动物模型对研究放射性肺损伤的机制和防治手段十分有利。实验证明,ROS在射线诱发的组织损伤中起重要作用,电离辐射可通过产生ROS引起细胞DNA损坏,此外,ROS还会攻击和破坏生物膜脂质成分和其他生物大分子,形成氧化损伤,最终可诱导肺纤维化的形成。

在模型制备过程中,可以通过实验动物胸部局部暴露单剂量辐射诱导纤维化的产生。需要注意的是,肺纤维化的产生取决于辐射剂量和实验动物的品系。另外,放射性肺纤维化模型的制备是一个相对缓慢的过程,需要至少16周的时间才会出现明显的纤维化病变,这在一定程度上限制了它的广泛应用。

(四)病毒载体介导过度表达致纤维化细胞因子诱导的肺纤维化模型

腺病毒和慢病毒载体已被用来在实验动物的肺组织中过度表达多种致纤维化细胞因子诱导肺纤维化。其中,利用腺病毒载体介导的转化生长因子(TGF)-β1所诱导的肺纤维化动物模型应用最为广泛。TGF-β1是一种多功能的细胞因子,对细胞的增殖、分化、凋亡及细胞外基质的合成等起重要的调节作用。国内外研究表明TGF-β1在炎症性疾病、脏器纤维化、创伤修复、肿瘤及免疫性疾病的发生发展中都具有重要意义。在众多与肺纤维化有关的细胞因子中,以TGF-β1研究的最为透彻。大量人体及动物研究均表明TGF-β1在肺纤维化过程中起着举足轻重的作用,它是目前公认的致肺纤维化细胞因子网络的枢纽。TGF-β1可促使激活的炎性细胞聚集和上皮细胞向间充细胞转化,并可诱导成纤维细胞分化为肌成纤维细胞分泌大量细胞外基质,此外,TGF-β1还通过对基质降解酶和降解酶抑制剂的调控促进细胞外基质沉积。

腺病毒载体所介导的基因转移具有高效性,与慢病毒载体不同,腺病毒载体在感染细胞后并不整合入宿主基因组,是目前公认的最有效的基因转移载体之一。在大鼠接受TGF-β1腺病毒气管滴注后,外源性活化的TGF-β1在大鼠肺中过度表达的持续时间为7～10d,在此同时,外源性活化的TGF-β1会诱导内源性TGF-β1的表达和激活,从而形成正反馈调节。这种在大鼠肺中过度表达TGF-β1

的方法可诱导大鼠形成严重而持续性的肺纤维化,病变持续时间长达8个月以上。与传统的博来霉素模型相比而言,这种腺病毒介导单基因过度表达动物模型中的肺纤维化病变完全是由肺中过度表达的活化TGF-β1造成的,而并不是由炎症反应驱动的。

病毒载体介导过度表达致纤维化细胞因子诱导的肺纤维化模型也存在着一些缺点:人类肺纤维化涉及到诸多致纤维化细胞因子,但这些模型只局限于单基因过度表达所引起的肺纤维化;转基因在动物模型肺组织中的过度表达高于正常的生理水平;实验动物对病毒载体会产生免疫应答,这会严重影响病毒载体的重复干预。

四、小结与展望

综上所述,尽管目前的肺纤维化动物模型具有一定的局限性,还不能全面地反映出肺纤维化患者体内复杂的病理改变,但以上这些动物模型为我们研究肺纤维化的病因、发病机制及防治提供了必不可少的实验手段。在严格控制各种条件下,我们可以观察肺纤维化的发生、发展和疾病转归及这些不同改变在形态学、影像学和分子生物学上的表现等规律。

肺纤维化动物模型可分为炎症驱动和非炎症驱动两类,其中,博来霉素、二氧化硅和放射性肺纤维化模型中纤维化的发生是炎症反应驱动的,而TGF-β1过度表达动物模型中炎症程度相对轻微,且其纤维化的发展不依赖炎症驱动。因此,在评估药物潜在的抗纤维化作用时,使用不同类别的动物模型有助于确定药物的抗纤维化作用是否独立于其抗炎作用。有趣的是,吡非尼酮(pirfenidone)和尼达尼布(nintedanib)这两种临床上用于肺纤维化治疗的药物在多种肺纤维化动物模型中都显示出了疗效。这就说明多种肺纤维化动物模型的联合使用可能有助于提高我们对纤维化形成过程的理解,并促进新一代抗纤维化药物的研发。

参 考 文 献

[1] Lederer DJ, Martinez FJ. Idiopathic Pulmonary Fibrosis. N Engl J Med, 2018, 378(19):1811-1823.

[2] Tashiro J, Rubio GA, Limper AH, et al. Exploring Animal Models That Resemble Idiopathic Pulmonary Fibrosis. Front Med (Lausanne), 2017, 4:118.

[3] Ochi A, Sekiguchi M, Tsujimura K, et al. Two Cases of Equine Multinodular Pulmonary Fibrosis in Japan. J Comp Pathol, 2019, 170:46-52.

[4] Piras IS, Bleul C, Siniard A, et al. Association of Common Genetic Variants in the CPSF7 and SDHAF2 Genes with Canine Idiopathic Pulmonary Fibrosis in the West Highland White Terrier. Genes (Basel), 2020, 11(6).

[5] Redente EF, Jacobsen KM, Solomon JJ, et al. Age and sex dimorphisms contribute to the severity of bleomycin-induced lung injury and fibrosis. Am J Physiol Lung Cell Mol Physiol, 2011, 301(4):510-518.

[6] Hecker L, Logsdon NJ, Kurundkar D, et al. Reversal of persistent fibrosis in aging by targeting Nox4-Nrf2 redox imbalance. Sci Transl Med, 2014, 6(231):231-247.

[7] Fyfe AJ, McKay P. Toxicities associated with bleomycin. J R Coll Physicians Edinb, 2010, 40(3):213-215.

[8] Lazo JS, Humphreys CJ. Lack of metabolism as the biochemical basis of bleomycin-induced pulmonary toxicity. Proc Natl Acad Sci USA, 1983, 80(10):3064-3068.

[9] Chaudhary NI, Schnapp A, Park JE. Pharmacologic differentiation of inflammation and fibrosis in the rat bleomycin model. Am J Respir Crit Care Med, 2006, 173(7):769-776.

[10] Chua F, Gauldie J, Laurent GJ. Pulmonary fibrosis: searching for model answers. Am J Respir Cell Mol Biol, 2005, 33(1):9-13.

[11] Yang J, Cui Y, Kolb M. How useful is traditional herbal medicine for pulmonary fibrosis? Respirology, 2009, 14(8):1082-1091.

[12] Moeller A, Ask K, Warburton D, et al. The bleomycin animal model: a useful tool to investigate treatment options for idiopathic pulmonary fibrosis? Int J Biochem Cell Biol, 2008, 40(3):362-382.

[13] Gauldie J, Kolb M. Animal models of pulmonary fibrosis: how far from effective reality? Am J Physiol Lung Cell Mol Physiol, 2008, 294(2):L151.

[14] Kolb P, Upagupta C, Vierhout M, et al. The importance of interventional timing in the bleomycin model of pulmonary fibrosis. Eur Respir J, 2020, 55(6).

[15] Jenkins RG, Moore BB, Chambers RC, et al. An Official American Thoracic Society Workshop Report: Use of Animal Models for the Preclinical Assessment of Potential Therapies for Pulmonary Fibrosis. Am J Respir Cell Mol Biol, 2017, 56(5):667-679.

[16] Brown T. Silica exposure, smoking, silicosis and lung cancer--complex interactions. Occup Med (Lond), 2009, 59(2):89-95.

[17] Hamilton RF, Jr, Thakur SA, Holian A. Silica binding and toxicity in alveolar macrophages. Free Radic Biol Med, 2008, 44(7):1246-1258.

[18] Vallyathan V, Shi XL, Dalal NS, et al. Generation of free radicals from freshly fractured silica dust. Potential role in acute silica-induced lung injury. Am Rev Respir Dis, 1988, 138(5):1213-1219.

[19] Cassel SL, Eisenbarth SC, Iyer SS, et al. The Nalp3 inflammasome is essential for the development of silicosis. Proc Natl Acad Sci USA, 2008, 105(26):9035-9040.

[20] Hanania AN, Mainwaring W, Ghebre YT, et al Radiation-Induced Lung Injury: Assessment and Management. Chest, 2019, 156(1):150-162.

[21] Tominaga H, Kodama S, Matsuda N, et al. Involvement of reactive oxygen species (ROS) in the induction of genetic instability by radiation. J Radiat Res (Tokyo), 2004, 45(2):181-188.

[22] Satterwhite DJ, Moses HL. Mechanisms of transforming growth factor-beta 1-induced cell cycle arrest. Invasion Metastasis, 1994, 14(1-6):309-318.

[23] Lee CG, Kang HR, Homer RJ, et al. Transgenic modeling of transforming growth factor-beta(1): role of apoptosis in fibrosis and alveolar remodeling. Proc Am Thorac Soc, 2006, 3(5):418-423.

[24] Yoshimura A, Wakabayashi Y, Mori T. Cellular and molecular basis for the regulation of inflammation by TGF-beta. J Biochem, 2010, 147(6):781-792.

[25] Lijnen PJ, Petrov VV, Fagard RH. Induction of cardiac fibrosis by transforming growth factor-beta(1). Mol Genet Metab, 2000, 71(1-2):418-435.

[26] Brunner G, Blakytny R. Extracellular regulation of TGF-beta activity in wound repair: growth factor latency as a sensor mechanism for injury. Thromb Haemost, 2004, 92(2):253-261.

[27] Li AG, Lu SL, Han G, et al. Current view of the role of transforming growth factor beta 1 in skin carcinogenesis. J Investig Dermatol Symp Proc, 2005, 10(2):110-117.

[28] Rico MC, Rough JJ, Del Carpio-Cano FE, et al. The axis of thrombospondin-1, transforming growth factor beta and connective tissue growth factor: an emerging therapeutic target in rheumatoid arthritis. Curr Vasc Pharmacol, 2010, 8(3):338-343.

[29] Prud'homme GJ, Piccirillo CA. The inhibitory effects of transforming growth factor-beta-1 (TGF-beta1) in autoimmune diseases. J Autoimmun, 2000, 14(1):23-42.

[30] Strieter RM. What differentiates normal lung repair and fibrosis? Inflammation, resolution of repair, and fibrosis. Proc Am Thorac Soc, 2008, 5(3):305-310.

[31] Wahl SM, Hunt DA, Wakefield LM, et al. Transforming growth factor type beta induces monocyte chemotaxis and growth factor production. Proc Natl Acad Sci USA, 1987, 84(16):5788-5792.

[32] Reibman J, Meixler S, Lee TC, et al. Transforming growth factor beta 1, a potent chemoattractant for human neutrophils, bypasses classic signal-transduction pathways. Proc Natl Acad Sci USA, 1991, 88(15):6805-6809.

[33] Doerner AM, Zuraw BL. TGF-beta1 induced epithelial to mesenchymal transition (EMT) in human bronchial epithelial cells is enhanced by IL-1beta but not abrogated by corticosteroids. Respir Res, 2009, 10:100.

[34] Zavadil J. New TGF-beta and Ras crosstalk in EMT. Cell Cycle, 2009, 8(2):184.

[35] Guo W, Shan B, Klingsberg RC, et al. Abrogation of TGF-beta1-induced fibroblast-myofibroblast differentiation by histone deacetylase inhibition. Am J Physiol Lung Cell Mol Physiol, 2009, 297(5):864-870.

[36] Eickelberg O, Kohler E, Reichenberger F, et al. Extracellular matrix deposition by primary human lung fibroblasts in response to TGF-beta1 and TGF-beta3. Am J Physiol, 1999, 276(5 Pt 1):814-824.

[37] Heilbronn R, Weger S. Viral vectors for gene transfer: current status of gene therapeutics. Handb Exp Pharmacol, 2010(197):143-170.

[38] Sime PJ, Xing Z, Graham FL, et al. Adenovector-mediated gene transfer of active transforming growth factor-beta1 induces prolonged severe fibrosis in rat lung. J Clin Invest, 1997, 100(4):768-776.

[39] Ask K, Labiris R, Farkas L, et al. Comparison between conventional and "clinical" assessment of experimental lung fibrosis. J Transl Med, 2008, 6:16.

第六部分

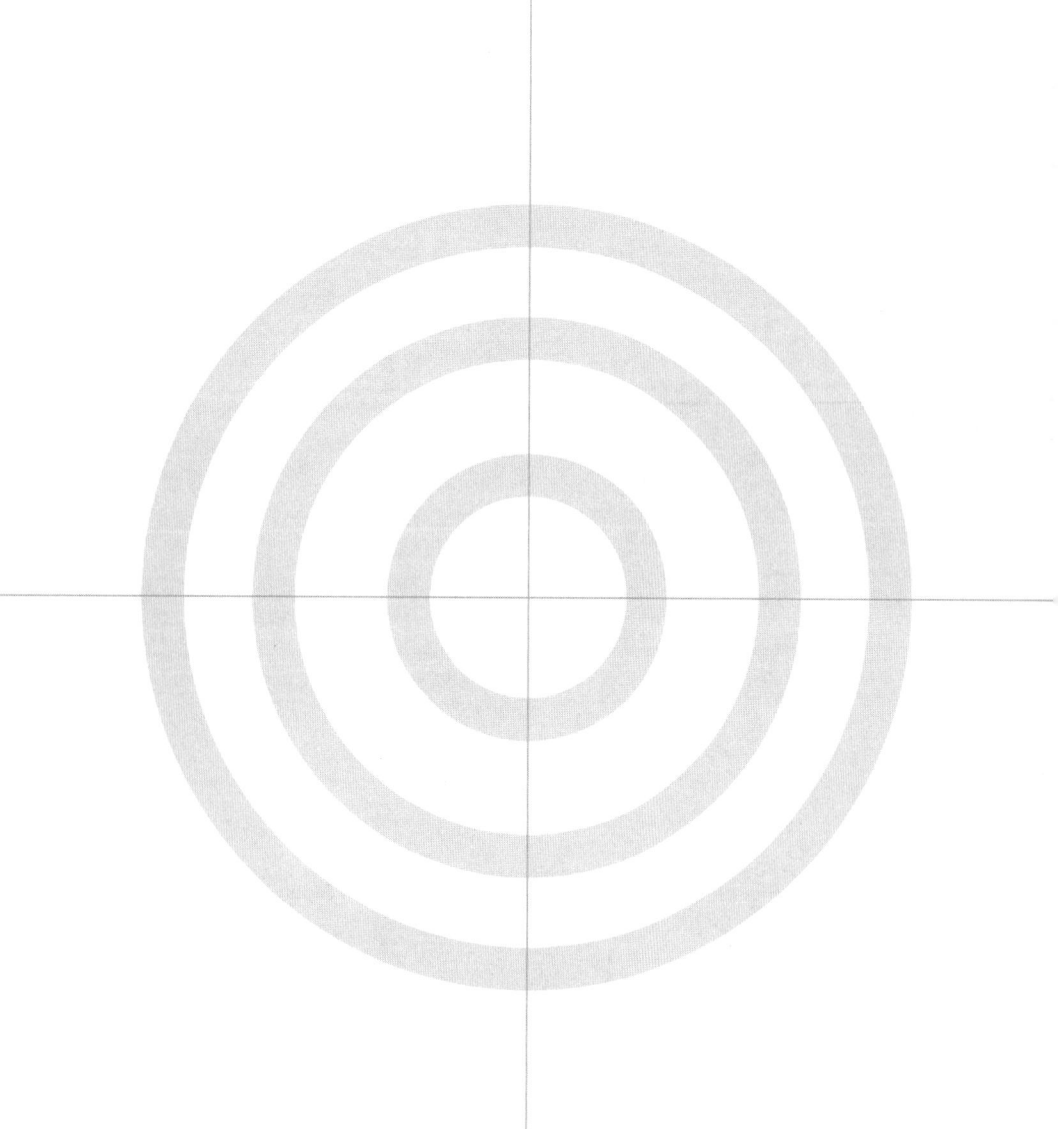

肺　癌

1 ALK阳性非小细胞肺癌的治疗进展

陈 茜 周建英

近10多年来,随着分子生物学的进展和靶向药物的不断涌现,非小细胞肺癌(non-small cell lung cancer, NSCLC)的治疗已进入了个体化分子靶向治疗时代。目前临床应用的个体化分子靶向治疗主要针对表皮生长因子受体(epithelial growth factor receptor,EGFR)突变型、间变淋巴瘤激酶(anaplastic lymphoma kinase,ALK)融合基因型和c-ros肉瘤致癌因子-受体酪氨酸激酶(ROS proto-oncogene 1,receptor tyrosine kinase)融合基因型肺癌。这3种基因变异型的靶向药物显著提高了晚期NSCLC的临床疗效。

2007年,日本学者Soda等首次报道从1例62岁吸烟的肺腺癌患者肿瘤组织中扩增出由3926bp组成的DNA片段,编码1059个氨基酸组成的蛋白质,即融合蛋白EML4-ALK,即棘皮动物微管结合蛋白4(echinoderm microtubule associated protein-like 4,EML4)与ALK的融合基因(*EML4-ALK*)蛋白,并明确了*EML4-ALK*融合基因具有致癌性,是肺癌的驱动基因之一。

*EML4*和*ALK*两个基因分别位于人类2号染色体的p21和p23带,相隔约10Mb距离。这2个基因片段的倒位融合能够使组织表达新的融合蛋白EML4-ALK,含EML4的氨基端和ALK的胞内酪氨酸激酶。迄今,已经发现了多种融合类型,在所有的类型中均为相同的ALK断裂位点与不同EML4断裂位点之间的融合,其中最常见的融合类型为E13:A20和E6a/b:A20,即变体1和3a/b,在NSCLC患者融合类型中分别占33.0%和29.0%。除了*EML4*外,肺癌中与*ALK*基因融合的其他基因还包括*TFG*、*KIF5B*、*KLC1*、*STRN*等。国内外大量的研究数据显示,发生ALK重排的NSCLC患者占3%~7%。

一、第一代ALK-TKI

克唑替尼(crizotinib)是一种小分子ATP竞争性抑制剂,对ALK、c-MET和ROS1驱动的肿瘤具有选择性抑制作用。2011年8月26日,美国食品药品监督管理局(Food and Drug Administration,FDA)批准了克唑替尼用于ALK FISH阳性的局部晚期或转移性NSCLC患者的治疗。2013年6月,克唑替尼在中国上市。

PROFILE1007为评估克唑替尼对比培美曲塞或多西他赛二线治疗晚期ALK重排NSCLC患者的Ⅲ期临床试验。研究共入组347例患者,接受克唑替尼和接受化疗患者的客观缓解率(objective response rate,ORR)分别为65%和20%($P<0.001$),克唑替尼组的无进展生存时间(progression-free survival,PFS)也显著优于化疗组(7.7个月 vs. 3.0个月)($P<0.01$)。该研究结果奠定了克唑替尼用于晚期ALK阳性NSCLC患者二线治疗的地位。

PROFILE1014为评估一线克唑替尼对比标准化疗治疗晚期ALK重排NSCLC患者的Ⅲ期临床试验。研究共入组343例患者,结果提示克唑替尼组的ORR显著优于化疗组(74% vs. 45%)($P<0.001$)。同时,克唑替尼组的PFS也显著优于化疗组(10.9个月 vs. 7.0个月)。该研究结果奠定了克唑替尼作为晚期ALK阳性NSCLC患者的一线治疗地位。

克唑替尼最常见的不良反应(≥25%)为视觉异常、腹泻、恶心、呕吐、食欲缺乏、水肿、转氨酶升高及疲劳。但通常这些反应的级别为1或2级。PROFILE 1014研究中3/4级不良反应中发生率较高的为转氨酶升高(14%)及中性粒细胞减少(11%),临床应用中需关注肝功能及血常规的检测。严重不良反应为间质性肺炎,但发生概率低,PROFILE 1014研究中其发生概率约为1%,在临床中应用中一旦发现间质性肺炎,须永久停药。克唑替尼推荐起始治疗剂量为250mg,每日2次口服。治疗过程中,如果出现3或4级不良反应,须一次或多次减少剂量。中国临床肿瘤学会(Chinese Society of Clinical Oncology,CSCO)推荐第1次减少剂量:200mg,每日2次;第2次减少剂量:250mg,每日1次;如果每日1次250mg仍不能耐受,则永久停药。

二、第二代ALK-TKI

(一)艾乐替尼

艾乐替尼(alectinib)是第二代ALK抑制剂,是一种强效的选择性ALK抑制剂,其效力比克唑替尼强10倍。P-糖蛋白在血脑屏障上有典型表达,与克唑替尼和色瑞替尼比较,艾乐替尼不是P-糖蛋白的底物,它能够很好地通过血脑屏障。

FDA已批准艾乐替尼作为ALK阳性晚期NSCLC患者的一线治疗。ALEX研究是一项比较艾乐替尼与克唑替尼一线治疗303例ALK阳性晚期NSCLC的Ⅲ期临床试验。结果提示艾乐替尼的研究者评估的中位PFS为34.8个月(17.7-未达到),显著优于克唑替尼的10.9个月

(9.1～12.9)(HR=0.43)。对于基线存在脑转移的患者，艾乐替尼的中位PFS为27.7个月(9.2-未达到)，克唑替尼为7.4个月(6.6～9.6)(HR=0.35)。相较于克唑替尼，艾乐替尼发生率更高的不良反应包括贫血(22.4% vs.7.3%)、血胆红素升高(19.1% vs.1.3%)、肌肉痛(16.4% vs.2.0%)、体重增加(9.2% vs.0%)、光敏反应(5.9% vs.0%)。而克唑替尼组发生率更高的不良反应包括恶心(49.7% vs.15.8%)、腹泻(6.45% vs.13.2%)和呕吐(41.1% vs.9.2%)。艾乐替尼组3～5级不良反应发生率为44.7%，而克唑替尼组为51.0%，其中最常见的为实验室指标异常包括谷丙转氨酶升高、谷草转氨酶升高、肌酸激酶升高、QT间期延长和血胆红素升高等。

此外，艾乐替尼已获美国FDA批准用于克唑替尼治疗进展的ALK阳性晚期NSCLC患者的治疗。艾乐替尼对L1196M、C1156Y、G1269A、S1206Y、L1152R、F1174L、1151Tins等ALK激酶区突变引起的克唑替尼耐药有效，对G1202R、I1171N、I1171S等效果不佳。两项单臂Ⅱ期临床试验(NCT01871805和NCT01801111)提示艾乐替尼治疗克唑替尼进展的ALK阳性患者，ORR分别为38%和44%，中位缓解时间分别为7.5个月和11.2个月。对该两项试验颅内转移患者的数据进行Pooled分析，基础有可测量颅内病灶的患者，艾乐替尼的颅内客观缓解率为64.0%，颅内疾病控制率为90.0%，中位缓解时间为10.8个月。可见，艾乐替尼对有无颅内转移的克唑替尼治疗失败的ALK阳性NSCLC患者均有较好的疗效。

(二)色瑞替尼

FDA已批准第二代ALK抑制剂色瑞替尼作为ALK阳性晚期NSCLC患者的一线治疗。色瑞替尼(ceritinib, LDK378)是一种二氨基嘧啶化合物，对ALK酪氨酸激酶的抑制活性是克唑替尼的20倍，同时可抑制胰岛素样生长因子1受体(insulin-like growth factor1 receptor, IGF-1R)，但对其抑制活性低于ALK激酶的1/50，对c-MET无抑制活性。

ASCEND-4是一项对比色瑞替尼和化疗一线治疗晚期ALK阳性NSCLC的Ⅲ期临床试验。共入组376例患者，接受色瑞替尼治疗189例，化疗187例。色瑞替尼对比化疗显著延长患者PFS，分别为16.6个月和8.1个月($P<0.00001$)。色瑞替尼组的2年生存率为70.6%，化疗组为58.2%，其中有72%的患者在化疗进展后接受ALK抑制剂的治疗。色瑞替尼的总缓解率也显著高于化疗组(72.5% vs.26.7%)。平均应答时间色瑞替尼为6.1周，化疗组为13.4周。对于脑转移患者，色瑞替尼同样有效。色瑞替尼治疗脑转移的PFS为10.7个月，化疗组为6.7个月。

此外，色瑞替尼已获美国FDA批准用于克唑替尼治疗进展的ALK阳性NSCLC患者的治疗。体外实验显示，色瑞替尼对L1196M、G1269A、S1206Y、11171T等ALK激酶区突变引起的耐药具有显著活性，但对C1156Y、G1202R、1151Tins、L1152R、F1174C等引起的耐药活性差。ASCEND-5是一项全球、多中心的色瑞替尼对比二线化疗治疗既往化疗和克唑替尼进展的ALK阳性NSCLC患者。色瑞替尼治疗的PFS显著长于化疗(5.4个月 vs.1.6个月，P<0.0001)，两者的总缓解率分别为39.1%和6.9%，疾病控制率分别为76.5%和36.2%。对于基础有脑转移的患者，色瑞替尼PFS为4.4个月，化疗为1.5个月。因此，色瑞替尼治疗克唑替尼进展的ALK阳性NSCLC患者优于二线化疗，颅内转移患者也能从色瑞替尼治疗中获益。

(三)Brigatinib(AP26113)

Brigatinib是一种二氨基嘧啶类化合物，可有效抑制ALK、ROS1、IGF-1R、FLT-3及EGFR的活性。ALTA-1L是一项对比Brigatinib和克唑替尼一线治疗晚期ALK阳性NSCLC的Ⅲ期临床试验。研究共入组275例ALK阳性NSCLC患者，Brigatinib组预估的12个月无进展生存率为67%，显著优于克唑替尼的43%($P<0.001$)。Brigatinib组和克唑替尼组的ORR分别为71%和60%。对颅内有可测量病灶的患者，两组的颅内客观缓解率分别为78%和29%。因此，该研究提示Brigatinib一线治疗晚期ALK阳性NSCLC的疗效优于克唑替尼，且对脑转移患者有较好的疗效。

2017年4月28日FDA批准Brigatinib用于对克唑替尼不耐受或用药后疾病进展的ALK阳性的转移性NSCLC患者。Brigatinib对G1123，T1151，L1152，C1156，I1171，F1174，L1196，G1202，D1203，S1206和G1269等ALK激酶区突变引起的耐药具有显著活性。一项Ⅱ期临床试验(ALTA)入组克唑替尼治疗进展的ALK阳性NSCLC患者，分成A组(112例，口服Brigatinib 90mg，1次/d)和B组(110例，Brigatinib前7d 90 mg，1次/d，此后180 mg，1次/d)。两组中基线有颅内可测量病灶患者的颅内病灶的客观缓解率分别为50%和67%；基线有任何脑转移的患者，两组的中位颅内PFS为12.8个月和18.4个月。

(四)Ensartinib(X-396)

Ensartinib是一种氨基哒嗪类ALK抑制剂，和克唑替尼一样有一个共同的疏水性2,6-二氯-3-氟-苯乙氧基团和一个激酶铰链结合基团，不同的是Ensartinib有一个氨基哒嗪基，对EML4-ALK融合和ALK点突变如L1196M、C1156Y、T1151M等均有效。此外，Ensartinib还能抑制MET、ABL、Axl、EPHA2、LTK、ROS1和SLK。目前，Ensartinib还未获得FDA批准用于晚期ALK阳性NSCLC患者的治疗。

Ⅱ期临床试验研究入组了160例克唑替尼治疗进展的ALK阳性NSCLC患者，研究表明ORR为52%，中位PFS为9.6个月(95% CI 7.4～11.6个月)，颅内有可测量病灶患者的颅内客观缓解率为70%。91%的患者至少发生1种治疗相关不良反应，而多数为1～2级。最常见的不良反应包括皮疹(56%)、ALT升高(46%)、AST升高(41%)、血清肌酐升高(19%)、便秘(18%)。23%的患者发生3级治疗相关不良反应，无4级治疗相关不良反应。且该研究中，未发现间质性肺炎和QT间期延长。后续的Ensartinib一线治疗的Ⅲ期临床试验(NCT02767804)正在进行中，期待其结果。

三、第三代 ALK-TKI

Lorlatinib 是一种高颅内穿透力、高效、高选择性 ALK/ROS1 抑制剂。对野生型 ALK，Lorlatinib 平均 Ki 值<0.07nM，而对 L1196M、G1269A、1151Tins、F1174L、C1156Y、L1152R 和 S1206Y 等克唑替尼耐药突变，平均 Ki 值<0.1~0.9nM。在体外细胞和体内小鼠临床前研究中，Lorlatinib 显著抑制肿瘤细胞的生长。

Ⅱ期临床试验入组 276 例晚期 ALK 阳性 NSCLC 患者。其中，30 例既往未接受治疗的患者中，Lorlatinib 的 ORR 为 90%，颅内客观缓解率为 66.7%。在 198 例既往接受至少一种 ALK-TKI 治疗的患者中，Lorlatinib 治疗的 ORR 为 47%，81 例颅内有可测量病灶的患者中，颅内客观缓解率为 63%。而仅接受克唑替尼治疗的患者中，客观缓解率为 69.5%，仅接受一种非克唑替尼 ALK-TKI 治疗的患者的 ORR 为 32.1%，两种或两种以上 ALK-TKI 治疗的 ORR 为 38.1%。最常见的治疗相关不良反应包括高胆固醇血症(81%，其中 3~4 级占 16%)、高三酰甘油血症(60%，其中 3-4 级占 16%)。

同时，该Ⅱ期临床试验获取患者的基础血浆和肿瘤组织标本进行二代测序，研究发现克唑替尼耐药的患者中，血浆或组织中 ALK 突变阳性和阴性患者 Lorlatinib 治疗的疗效无明显差异。既往一种或两种以上第二代 ALK-TKI 治疗失败的患者中，血浆或组织中 ALK 突变阳性的患者的 ORR 显著优于血浆阴性的患者(62% vs. 32%)或组织阴性的患者(69% vs. 27%)。而血浆 ALK 突变阴性和阳性患者的中位 PFS 无明显差异(7.3 个月 vs. 5.5 个月，HR=0.81)。但是，组织 ALK 突变阳性患者的 PFS 显著优于阴性患者(11.0 个月 vs. 5.4 个月，HR=0.47)。因此，对于既往一种或两种以上第二代 ALK-TKI 治疗失败的患者，组织的 ALK 突变检测可能作为预测疗效的有效指标。

四、ALK-TKI 联合免疫治疗

CheckMate 370 研究是一项Ⅰ/Ⅱ期评估克唑替尼联合 nivolumab 一线治疗晚期 ALK 阳性 NSCLC 的安全性和耐受性的研究，研究发现克唑替尼 250mg，2 次/d，口服联合 nivolumab 240mg 每 2 周 1 次，5/13(38%)因严重肝脏毒性而停止联合治疗，其中，有 2 例患者可能因严重肝脏毒性而死亡。因此，该研究结果不支持该剂量的克唑替尼联合 nivolumab 作为晚期 ALK 阳性 NSCLC 的一线治疗。

另一项ⅠB期临床试验入组了 9 例患者，2 例患者接受克唑替尼 250mg，2 次/d 联合 pembrolizumab 200mg，每 3 周 1 次治疗(DL0)，因出现剂量限制性毒性，后续 7 例患者接受 3 周的克唑替尼 2 次/d 单药治疗，3 周后联合 pembrolizumab 200mg 3 周 1 次治疗(DL1)。结果表明 4 例患者出现剂量限制性毒性，包括 3 级的 ALT 和 AST 升高和 3 级的疲乏。因此，关于克唑替尼联合 pembrolizumab 的安全剂量有待进一步的研究。

此外，一项多中心的开放性ⅠB期临床试验入组了 36 例患者，其中，14 例患者接受 450mg/d 色瑞替尼口服联合 nivolumab 3mg/kg 每 2 周静脉注射，22 例患者接受 300mg/d 色瑞替尼口服联合 nivolumab 3mg/kg 每 2 周静脉注射，研究表明，450mg 组中，4 例患者发生剂量限制性毒性，而 300mg 组中，2 例患者发生剂量限制性毒性。既往未接受 ALK-TKI 治疗的患者中，450mg 组的 ORR 为 83%，300mg 组为 60%。而曾接受 ALK-TKI 治疗的患者中，450mg 组的 ORR 为 50%，300mg 组为 25%。同时，研究发现 PD-L1 表达阳性的患者的 ORR(64%)大于表达阴性的患者(31%)。最常见的 3~4 级不良反应包括 ALT 升高(25%)、γ-GT 升高(22%)、淀粉酶升高(14%)、脂肪酶升高(11%)和丘疹(11%)。因此，该研究表明色瑞替尼联合 nivolumab 有较好的疗效，且疗效与 PD-L1 的表达相关，但同时，不良反应有增加。

五、其他

第一代 ALK-TKI 的继发耐药机制除了 ALK 的耐药突变，还包括 ALK 基因拷贝数的增加，旁路途径的激活如 EGFR、HER2、KIT、IGF-1R 通路激活等，上皮间质转化，小细胞癌转化等。因此，如出现以上继发耐药机制后，联合其他通路抑制剂或针对小细胞肺癌的化疗方案可能取得临床获益。

六、总结

晚期 ALK 阳性 NSCLC 患者一线首选 ALK-TKI 治疗，目前国内 CFDA 批准的一线治疗药物为克唑替尼，二代或三代药物作为一线治疗还未获批，故首选克唑替尼治疗，进展后推荐二次活检，根据耐药机制选择后续精准治疗，包括二代、三代药物或者化学治疗，旨在延长患者的总生存时间。

参考文献

[1] Shackelford RE, Vora M, Mayhall K, et al. ALK-rearrangements and testing methods in non-small cell lung cancer: a review. Genes Cancer, 2014, 5(1-2):1-14.

[2] Pan Y, Zhang Y, Li Y, et al. ALK, ROS1 and RET fusions in 1139 lung adenocarcinomas: a comprehensive study of common and fusion pattern-specific clinicopathologic, histologic and cytologic features. Lung Cancer, 2014, 84(2):121-126.

[3] 张绪超, 陆舜, 张力, 等. 中国间变性淋巴瘤激酶(ALK)阳性非小细胞肺癌诊疗指南. 中华病理学杂志, 2015, 44(10):696-703.

[4] Katayama R, Sakashita T, Yanagitani N, et al. P-glycoprotein mediates ceritinib resistance in anaplastic lymphoma kinase-rearranged non-small cell lung cancer. E Bio Medicine, 2015, 3: 54-66.

[5] Camidge DR, Dziadziuszko R, Peters S, et al. Updated Efficacy and Safety Data and Impact of the EML4-ALK Fusion Variant on the Efficacy of Alectinib in Untreated ALK-Positive Advanced Non-Small Cell Lung Cancer in the Global Phase III ALEX Study. J Thorac Oncol, 2019, 14(7): 1233-1243.

[6] Gainor JF, Dardaei L, Yoda S, et al. Molecular mechanisms of resistance to first-and second-generation ALK inhibitors in ALK-rearranged lung cancer. Cancer Discov, 2016, 6 (10): 1118-1133.

[7] Gadgee SM, Shaw AT, Govindan R, et al. Pooled analysis of CNS response to Alectinib in two studies of pretreated patients With ALK-positive non-small-cell lung cancer. J Clin Oncol, 2016, 34(34): 4079-4085.

[8] Soria JC, Tan DSW, Chiari R, et al. First-line ceritinib versus platinum-based chemotherapy in advanced ALK-rearranged non-small-cell-lung cancer(ASCEND-4): a randomized, open-label, phase 3 study. Lancet, 2017, 389(10072): 917-929.

[9] Shaw AT, Kim TM, Crinò L, et al. Ceritinib versus chemotherapy in patients with ALK-rearranged non-small-cell lung cancer previously given chemotherapy and crizotinib (ASCEND-5): a randomised, controlled, open-label, phase 3 trial. Lancet Oncol, 2017, 18(7): 874-886.

[10] Camidge DR, Kim HR, Ahn MJ, et al. Brigatinib versus crizotinib in ALK-Positive non-small-cell lung cancer. N Engl J Med, 2018, 379(21): 2027-2039.

[11] Zhang S, Anjum R, Squillace R, et al. The potent ALK inhibitor brigatinib(AP26113)overcomes mechanisms of resistance to first-and second-generation ALK inhibitors in preclinical models. Clin Cancer Res, 2016, 22(22): 5527-5538.

[12] Huber RM, Kim DW, Ahn WJ, et al. Brigatinib(BRG) in crizotinib(CRZ)-refractory ALK＋ non-small cell lung cancer (NSCLC): efficacy updates and exploratory analysis of CNS ORR and overall ORR by baseline(BL) brain lesion status. J Clin Oncol, 2018, 36(15).

[13] Yang Y, Zhou J, Zhou J, et al. Efficacy, safety, and biomarker analysis of ensartinib in crizotinib-resistant, ALK-positive non-small-cell lung cancer: a multicentre, phase 2 trial. Lancet Respir Med, 2020, 8(1): 45-53.

[14] Solomon BJ, Besse B, Bauer TM, et al. Lorlatinib in patients with ALK-positive non-small-cell lung cancer: results from a global phase 2 study. Lancet Oncol, 2018, 19 (12): 1654-1667.

[15] Shaw AT, Solomon BJ, Besse B, et al. ALK resistance mutations and efficacy of lorlatinib in advanced anaplastic lymphoma kinase-positive non-small-cell lung cancer. J Clin Oncol, 2019, 1802236.

[16] Spigel DR, Reynolds C, Waterhouse D, et al. Phase 1/2 Study of the Safety and Tolerability of Nivolumab Plus Crizotinib for the First-Line Treatment of Anaplastic Lymphoma Kinase Translocation-Positive Advanced Non-Small Cell Lung Cancer (CheckMate 370). J Thorac Oncol, 2018, 13 (5): 682-688.

[17] Patel SP, Pakkala S, Pennell NA, et al. Phase Ib Study of Crizotinib Plus Pembrolizumab in Patients with Previously Untreated Advanced Non-Small Cell Lung Cancer with ALK Translocation. Oncologist, 2020, 25(7): 562-e1012.

[18] Felip E, Braud FG, Maur M, et al. Ceritinib plus Nivolumab in Patients with Advanced ALK-Rearranged Non-Small Cell Lung Cancer: Results of an Open-Label, Multicenter, Phase 1B Study. J Thorac Oncol, 2020, 15(3): 392-403.

[19] Rothenstein JM, Chooback N. ALK inhibitors, resistance development, clinical trials. Curr Oncol, 2018, 25 (Suppl 1): S59-S67.

2 晚期非小细胞肺癌分子靶向治疗现状与进展

张文静 徐瑜 白莉

肺癌是我国及全球范围内发病率、死亡率最高的恶性肿瘤,其中80%~85%的患者为非小细胞肺腺癌(NSCLC),大部分患者就诊时已为晚期,失去手术机会。近20年来,随着二代测序技术(next generation sequencing,NGS)、肿瘤相关信号通路的研究及相应酪氨酸激酶抑制剂的研发不断深入,越来越多的NSCLC已经被证实存在驱动基因突变导致肿瘤的发生发展,包括表皮生长因子受体(epithelial growth factor receptor,EGFR)、间变性淋巴瘤激酶(anaplastic lymphoma kinase,ALK)、ROS1、KRAS、NRAS、c-MET、HER2、RET、NTRK、PIK3A等,晚期NSCLC患者的治疗模式已经从基于组织病理分型的传统化疗、放疗模式,发展到基于分子病理分型、个体化的分子靶向治疗。本文主要阐述晚期NSCLC驱动基因和分子靶向治疗药物的研究现状及未来发展方向。

一、NSCLC中常见驱动基因突变和分子靶向治疗药物研究进展

(一) EGFR

EGFR突变是NSCLC中最常见的驱动基因,30%~50%的亚裔NSCLC患者存在EGFR基因突变,EGFR在不吸烟腺癌患者中发生率较高,最常见的EGFR突变类型是19外显子缺失和21外显子L858R点突变,占EGFR突变类型80%~90%。目前已经获批上市的EGFR小分子酪氨酸激酶抑制剂(tyrosine kinase inhibitor,TKI)包括一、二、三代药物,均被NCCN指南推荐用于EGFR敏感突变晚期NSCLC的一线治疗。不同EGFR TKI与EGFR靶点细胞内区酪氨酸激酶结合的位点、可逆程度、是否具有高选择性及疗效有所不同。第一代EGFR-TKI是可逆的、非选择性的酪氨酸激酶抑制剂,包括吉非替尼、厄洛替尼或埃克替尼,一代EGFR TKIs与经典含铂双药方案相比,显示出更高的客观缓解率(objective response rate,ORR)和无进展生存期(progression free survival,PFS)第二代EGFR TKI的作用特点为不可逆、非选择性、为ErbB受体家族阻断剂(泛-HER抑制剂),包括阿法替尼和达克替尼。Lux-lung3、Lux-lung6研究证实,阿法替尼一线用于EGFR敏感突变晚期NSCLC患者,较标准含铂双药化疗能显著延长无进展生存期。ARCHER1050研究显示,与标准的一代EGFR TKI吉非替尼相比,达克替尼显示出更高的PFS。第三代EGFR TKI如奥西替尼,选择性地抑制EGFR敏感突变和T790M突变,对野生型EGFR亲和力很低,不良反应小。颅内AURA3研究显示,奥希替尼二线治疗一代、二代EGFR TKI耐药后T790MT突变的患者优于化疗(PFS 10.1个月 vs. 4.4个月)。FLAURA研究探讨奥希替尼对比一代EGFR-TKI一线治疗EGFR敏感突变晚期NSCLC患者的疗效,奥希替尼组较对照组显著延长患者PFS(18.9个月 vs.10.2个月)和OS(38.6个月 vs.31.8个月)。此外,奥希替尼可以有效穿透血脑屏障,更好地发挥颅内疗效,奥希替尼组脑转移患者客观缓解率(objective response rate,ORR)优于对照组(66% vs. 43%),显著降低脑转移进展和死亡风险(HR=0.48;95% CI:0.26~0.86)。

EGFR 20外显子插入突变是EGFR少见突变中最常见的突变类型,占EGFR所有突变4%,除了一种EGFR 20外显子插入类型A763_Y764insFQEA对EGFR TKI敏感外,大多数EGFR20外显子插入类型使用EGFR TKI疗效差,中位PFS仅约2个月。针对EGFR外显子20插入突变这种突变类型至今尚无获批的靶向治疗药物。TAK-788(AP32788)是一种选择性的针对EGFR/HER2抑制剂,临床前研究显示,TAK-788对EGFR外显子20插入突变活性比野生型更好,I/II期临床研究结果显示(n=28),在各种EGFR外显子20插入突变的NSCLC患者中,TAK-788 ORR为43%,mPFS为7.3个月。波齐替尼(poziotinib)治疗EGFR外显子20插入ORR为55%,mPFS为5.5个月。

(二) ALK

NSCLC患者中ALK基因重排的发生率3%~7%,其中最常见的是棘皮动物微管相关蛋白样基因(EML4-ALK)。不同种族ALK重排发生率无明显差异,临床上常见于从未吸烟(少量吸烟)、50岁左右的腺癌患者。第一代ALK TKI克唑替尼(crizotinib)改善了该类型患者的ORR和PFS。基于PROFILE1014研究,对比传统化疗,克唑替尼组显示出更好的ORR(74% vs.45%)和PFS(10.9个月 vs. 7.0个月)。阿来替尼(alectinib)作为国内第一个上市的第二代ALK-TKI,对大多数的ALK激酶区突变有效。ALEX研究对比阿来替尼和克唑替尼一线治疗ALK阳性晚期NSCLC患者的Ⅲ期临床研究,结果显示阿来替尼组较对照组显著延长患者PFS(34.8个月 vs 10.9个月)。第二代ALK-TKI还有色瑞替尼(ceritinib)、布加替尼(Brigatinib)。色瑞替尼对 ALK 阳性 C1156Y 突变的肿瘤细胞具有良好的抗肿瘤活性。在 ASCEND-4 研究中，色瑞替尼一线治疗 ALK 阳性 NSCLC 对比化疗获得了很好的疗效，其 PFS 显著优于化疗对照组（16.6 个月 vs. 8.1 个月）。ALTA-1L 研究比较一线使用布加替尼对比克唑替尼治疗 ALK 阳性患者，BIRC 评估的中位 mPFS 克唑替尼组为 9.8 个月，而布加替尼组尚未达到，1 年 PFS 率两组分别为 67% 和 43%（HR=0.49，P=0.0007）。既往克唑替尼治疗后耐药进展的患者大多数能从第二代 ALK 抑制剂包括阿来替尼，色瑞替尼，布加替尼中获益。劳拉替尼（lorlatinib）作为第三代 ALK-TKI，可以克服目前大多数临床观察到单一 ALK 耐药突变，尤其是对于第一、二代 ALK-TKI 易发生耐药的位点 G1202R 突变疗效显著。2018 年底 FDA 批准劳拉替尼用于治疗 ALK 阳性晚期 NSCLC 的二线或三线治疗。

二、NSCLC 少见驱动基因突变及分子靶向治疗药物研究进展

（一）ROS 1

ROS1 重排在 NSCLC 发生频率约为 1%~2%，多发生在年轻、不吸烟的肺腺癌患者，最常见的是与 CD74 基因融合。由于 ROS1 与 ALK 的酪氨酸激酶区域有高度同源性，ALK-TKI 包括克唑替尼、色瑞替尼、劳拉替尼在 ROS1 阳性的肿瘤中显示出抗肿瘤活性。PROFILE 1001 临床研究发现克唑替尼治疗 ROS1 重排 NSCLC 的 ORR 分别于 72%，疾病控制率（DCR）为 90%，mPFS 为 19.3 个月。基于此研究结果，2016 年 FDA 批准克唑替尼用于 ROS1 阳性晚期 NSCLC 患者的一线治疗。一项韩国 II 期临床研究在评估色瑞替尼治疗 ROS1 阳性晚期 NSCLC 疗效中，ORR 达到 67%，既往未使用克唑替尼的患者 PFS 为 19.3 个月，全部患者为 9.3 个月。Entrectinib 是具有抑制 ALK、ROS1 和 NTRK 活性的多靶点靶向药，STARTRK-2 的 II 期临床研究中，BICR 评估的 Entrectinib 治疗 ROS1 阳性患者的 ORR 77.4%，对脑转移患者缓解率达 55%，中位 PFS 达 19 个月。目前克唑替尼治疗 ROS1 阳性 NSCLC 患者的耐药最常见的机制是酪氨酸激酶区的继发突变（约 53%）及旁路激活途径，耐药突变常见位点分别为 G2032R（41%）、D2033N（6%）、S19886F（6%）。劳拉替尼是一种覆盖突变位点较为广泛的三代 ALK/ROS1 TKI，可更好地通过血脑屏障，ESMO 2017 年会上报道了劳拉替尼治疗 ROS1 阳性 NSCLC 的 II 期临床试验部分数据：47 例 ROS1 阳性 NSCLC 患者接受劳拉替尼治疗，其中 25 例患者合并脑有转移，34 例既往接受过克唑替尼治疗，总有效率为 36%，一年无进展生存概率 48%，有效缓解的 17 例患者中有 71% 患者 PFS 大于 6 个月，颅内有效率为 56%。因此对于 ROS1 阳性晚期 NSCLC 患者接受克唑替尼进展后、出现脑转移的患者可以选择劳拉替尼和色瑞替尼。

（二）c-MET

c-MET 激活方式包括 MET 突变以 14 外显子跳跃突变（MET ex14）为主，MET 扩增（包括整体染色体重复和局部基因重复）、MET 蛋白过表达。c-MET 下游通路的激活也是造成 EGFR 抑制剂原发和获得性耐药的主要原因之一。针对 MET 通路异常激活的策略包括靶向 MET 基因的小分子 TKI 包括多靶点激酶抑制剂克唑替尼，卡博替尼，以及选择性 MET 抑制剂如竞争性 ATP 抑制剂 Capmatinib（INC280）等。MET ex14 是 NSCLC 中一种独立的分子亚型，在肺腺癌中的发生率为 3%~4%。2019ASCO 大会报道的高选择性 MET 抑制剂 Capmatinib（INC280）和 Tepotinib 在一线和二线治疗 MET ex14 的 NSCLC 患者中显示了较好的疗效。基于 II 期 GEOMETRY 临床研究，Capmatinib 在初治的 28 例 MET ex14 跳跃突变 NSCLC 患者中，ORR 为 67.9%，疾病控制率（DCR）为 96.4%，中位缓解持续时间（DOR）为 11.14 个月，中位无进展生存期为 9.69 个月。另外在经治的 69 例患者 ORR 约为 40.6%，疾病控制率（DCR）为 78.3%，中位缓解持续时间 DOR 为 9.72 个月，中位无进展生存期为 5.42 个月，并且合并脑转移 13 例，7 例患者对 capmatinib 应答（54%），4 例患者脑部病变消退（31%），颅内疾病控制率 DCR 为 92.3%。2020 年 5 月，美国 FDA 加速批准 MET 抑制剂 Capmatinib 用于治疗携带 MET ex14 的晚期 NSCLC。在 Tepotinib 治疗 MET ex14 跳跃突变晚期 NSCLC 患者的 II 期单臂 VISION 研究中，显示一线 ORR 为 58.8%，二线 ORR 为 53.3%。在二线及以上，ORR 为 45.2%；液体活检确定的 MET ex14 跳跃突变患者的 ORR 为 50%，DOR 中位数为 12.4 个月，DCR 为 66.7%。对于通过组织活检确定的患者，ORR 为 45.1%，中位 DOR 为 15.7 个月，DCR 为 72.5%。脑转移患者可获得同样疗效。FDA 已授予 Tepotinib 突破性药物资格（BTD），用于治疗接受含铂化疗后病情进展、携带 MET 基因第 14 号外显子跳跃突变的转移性 NSCLC 患者。

（三）BRAF

NSCLC 中发生率约有 3%~5%。其中主要针对 BRAF V600E 突变位点的临床研究，BRAF V600E 在肺腺癌中最常见，占 NSCLC 患者的 1%~2%。一项 II 期临床研究表明达拉菲尼（dabrafenib）联合曲美替尼（frametinib）治疗 BRAF 阳性患者，ORR 可达 63%，中位 PFS 达 9.7 个月；既往未治疗的患者中，ORR 达到 64%，中位 PFS 达 10.4 个月。NCCN 指南推荐针对 BRAF V600E 突变 NSCLC 患者，一线可选化疗或达拉菲尼联合曲美替尼治疗。

（四）RET 重排

NSCLC 中发生率约有 12%。最常见的是和 KIF5B 基因融合（占 72%），其次 CCDC6（23%），NCOA4（2%）、EPHA5（1%）和 PICALM（1%）。众多已经上市的多靶点酪氨酸激酶抑制剂包括卡博替尼（cabozantinib）、凡德替尼（vandetanib）、乐伐替尼（lenvatinib）、舒尼替尼（sunitinib）等均能抑制 RET 活性。一项 II 期临床研究显示，卡博替尼治疗 25 例可评估疗效的 RET 重排患者中，有 7 例局部缓解 ORR 达 28%，中位 PFS 为 5.5 个月，中位 OS 为 9.9 个月。日本一项 II 期临床研究研究显示，凡德替尼治疗 17 例可

评估疗效的 RET 重排患者中，ORR 为 53%，中位 PFS 为 4.7 个月，中位 OS 为 11.1 个月。一项韩国的 II 期临床试验评估了 17 例 RET 重排的 NSCLC 患者中接受凡德替尼的疗效，ORR 为 18%（部分缓解 3 例），mPFS 为 4.5 个月，mOS 为 11.6 个月，1 年 OS 率为 33%。其他抑制剂 RX-DX-105，BLU-667 和 LOXO-292，也对 RET 重排患者显示出较好的临床疗效。

（五）NTRK 融合

NTRK 融合在 NSCLC 检出率为 13%。3 项 I/II 期临床研究显示拉罗替尼（larotrectinib）用于 NTRK 融合阳性患者，ORR 可达 80%（95%CI，67%～90%），Entrectinib 在 NTRK 阳性患者中可达到 100% 有效率。2018 年 11 月，FDA 批准拉罗替尼用于治疗携带 NTRK 基因融合的局部晚期或转移性实体瘤成人和儿童。目前正在研发的其他 NTRK 抑制剂包括 entrectinib，repotrectinib（tpx-0005）和 DS-6051b。

（六）HER2

NSCLC 的患者中发生率为 2%～4%，包括过表达、扩增以及突变。20 外显子的插入突变是最常见的突变类型。波齐替尼针对 HER2 20 外显子插入，ORR 可达 55%。TAK788 的 ORR 可达 30%，疾病稳定患者约 66%（Presented at 2018 WCLC，2019 ASCO）。另有抗体偶联药物、吡咯替尼等对抗 HER2 效果值得期待。

（七）KRAS

KRAS 突变在亚裔 NSCLC 患者中发生率约为 13%，KRAS 突变中 G12C 最常见（39%），G12D（17%），G12V（21%）。一直以来缺乏直接针对 KRAS 突变靶向药物。在一项多中心、开放性的 I 期实验（NCT03600883）首次评估了新型 KRAS G 12C 小分子抑制剂 AMG 510 在治疗局部晚期或转移性 KRAS 突变实体瘤的安全性、耐受性、药代动力学和疗效的临床研究，总共入组 10 例患者，其中 5 例患者部分缓解，4 例患者稳定，DCR 达 90%，ORR 达 50%，随后在 2019WCLC 会上报道了扩大样本至 23 例的数据，临床数据显示 ORR 达 48%。其他 KRAS 抑制剂 MRTX849、BI 1701963 及其联合 MEK 抑制剂曲美替尼、针对 KRAS 下游信号 BRAF、MEK、PI3K/AKT 通路抑制剂对 KRAS 突变的疗效仍在探索中。

三、小结和展望

随着对 NSCLC 中驱动基因认识的深入，以及可靶向药物的相继获批上市，大大改善了晚期 NSCLC 患者的临床疗效和预后。但同时，我们必须认识到相当一部分驱动基因如 EGFR20 外显子插入、HER2 扩增、KRAS 突变等仍然缺乏有效的靶向治疗药物，对于上述靶点的新药研发迫在眉睫。即使对于已有可靶向治疗药物的驱动基因类型，不同的突变类型、是否伴随突变对靶向药物的疗效反应性存在明显差异，面对诸多可选择的靶向药物，如何进行选择及如何选择靶向治疗最佳联合治疗策略从而使患者获得最佳临床疗效，是靶向治疗急需探索的领域。针对靶向药物耐药问题，如何排兵布阵延缓或克服耐药及耐药后最佳治疗策略的选择也是亟待解决和探索的难题。

参考文献

[1] Siegel RL, Miller KD. Cancer statistics, 2019, 69(1): 7-34.

[2] Mitsudomi T. Driver gene mutation and targeted therapy of lung cancer. Gan to kagaku ryoho Cancer & chemotherapy, 2013, 40(3): 285-290.

[3] Paez JG, Janne PA, Lee JC, et al. EGFR mutations in lung cancer: correlation with clinical response to gefitinib therapy. Science (New York, NY), 2004, 304(5676): 1497-1500.

[4] Han JY, Park K, Kim SW, et al. First-SIGNAL: first-line single-agent iressa versus gemcitabine and cisplatin trial in never-smokers with adenocarcinoma of the lung. Journal of clinical oncology, 2012, 30(10): 1122-1128.

[5] Maemondo M, Inoue A, Kobayashi K, et al. Gefitinib or chemotherapy for non-small-cell lung cancer with mutated EGFR. The New England journal of medicine, 2010, 362(25): 2380-2388.

[6] Mok TS, Wu YL, Thongprasert S, et al. Gefitinib or carboplatin-paclitaxel in pulmonary adenocarcinoma. The New England journal of medicine, 2009, 361(10): 947-957.

[7] Mitsudomi T, Morita S, Yatabe Y, et al. Gefitinib versus cisplatin plus docetaxel in patients with non-small-cell lung cancer harbouring mutations of the epidermal growth factor receptor (WJTOG3405): an open label, randomised phase 3 trial. The Lancet Oncology, 2010, 11(2): 121-128.

[8] Rosell R, Carcereny E, Gervais R, et al. Erlotinib versus standard chemotherapy as first-line treatment for European patients with advanced EGFR mutation-positive non-small-cell lung cancer (EURTAC): a multicentre, open-label, randomised phase 3 trial. The Lancet Oncology, 2012, 13(3): 239-246.

[9] Sequist LV, Yang JC, Yamamoto N, et al. Phase III study of afatinib or cisplatin plus pemetrexed in patients with metastatic lung adenocarcinoma with EGFR mutations. Journal of clinical oncology, 2013, 31(27): 3327-3334.

[10] Wu YL, Zhou C, Hu CP, et al. Afatinib versus cisplatin plus gemcitabine for first-line treatment of Asian patients with advanced non-small-cell lung cancer harbouring EGFR mutations (LUX-Lung 6): an open-label, randomised phase 3 trial. The Lancet Oncology, 2014, 15(2): 213-222.

[11] Wu YL, Cheng Y, Zhou X, et al. Dacomitinib versus gefitinib as first-line treatment for patients with EGFR-mutation-positive non-small-cell lung cancer (ARCHER 1050): a randomised, open-label, phase 3 trial. The Lancet Oncology, 2017, 18(11): 1454-1466.

[12] Mok TS, Wu YL, Ahn MJ, et al. Osimertinib or Platinum-Pemetrexed in EGFR T790M-Positive Lung Cancer. The New England journal of medicine, 2017, 376(7): 629-640.

[13] Soria JC, Ohe Y, Vansteenkiste J, et al. Osimertinib in Untreated EGFR-Mutated Advanced Non-Small-Cell Lung Cancer. The New England journal of medicine, 2018, 378(2): 113-125.

[14] Yasuda H, Kobayashi S, Costa DB. EGFR exon 20 insertion mutations in non-small-cell lung cancer: preclinical data and clinical implications. The Lancet Oncology, 2012, 13(1): e23-31.

[15] Arcila ME, Nafa K, Chaft JE, et al. EGFR exon 20 insertion mutations in lung adenocarcinomas: prevalence, molecular heterogeneity, and clinicopathologic characteristics. Molecular cancer therapeutics, 2013, 12(2): 220-229.

[16] Doebele R, Riely G, Spira A, et al. First report of safety, PK, and preliminary antitumor activity of the oral EGFR/HER2 exon 20 inhibitor TAK-788 (AP32788) in non-small cell lung cancer (NSCLC). Journal of Clinical Oncology, 2018, 36: 9015-9015.

[17] Shaw AT, Engelman JA. ALK in lung cancer: past, present, and future. Journal of clinical oncology, 2013, 31(8): 1105-1111.

[18] Solomon BJ, Mok T, Kim DW, et al. First-line crizotinib versus chemotherapy in ALK-positive lung cancer. The New England journal of medicine, 2014, 371(23): 2167-2177.

[19] Hida T, Nokihara H, Kondo M, et al. Alectinib versus crizotinib in patients with ALK-positive non-small-cell lung cancer (J-ALEX): an open-label, randomised phase 3 trial. Lancet (London, England), 2017, 390(10089): 29-39.

[20] Soria JC, Tan DSW, Chiari R, et al. First-line ceritinib versus platinum-based chemotherapy in advanced ALK-rearranged non-small-cell lung cancer (ASCEND-4): a randomised, open-label, phase 3 study. Lancet (London, England), 2017, 389(10072): 917-929.

[21] Camidge DR, Kim HR, Ahn MJ, et al. Brigatinib versus Crizotinib in ALK-Positive Non-Small-Cell Lung Cancer. The New England journal of medicine, 2018, 379(21): 2027-2039.

[22] Waqar SN, Morgensztern D. Lorlatinib: a new-generation drug for ALK-positive NSCLC. The Lancet Oncology, 2018, 19(12): 1555-1557.

[23] Takeuchi K, Soda M, Togashi Y, et al. RET, ROS1 and ALK fusions in lung cancer. Nature medicine, 2012, 18(3): 378-381.

[24] Shaw AT, Riely GJ, Bang YJ, et al. Crizotinib in ROS1-rearranged advanced non-small-cell lung cancer (NSCLC): updated results, including overall survival, from PROFILE 1001. Annals of oncology, 2019, 30(7): 1121-1126.

[25] Lim SM, Kim HR, Lee JS, et al. Open-Label, Multicenter, Phase II Study of Ceritinib in Patients With Non-Small-Cell Lung Cancer Harboring ROS1 Rearrangement. Journal of clinical oncology, 2017, 35(23): 2613-2618.

[26] Drilon A, Siena S, Ou SI, et al. Safety and Antitumor Activity of the Multitargeted Pan-TRK, ROS1, and ALK Inhibitor Entrectinib: Combined Results from Two Phase I Trials (ALKA-372-001 and STARTRK-1). Cancer discovery, 2017, 7(4): 400-409.

[27] Shaw AT, Felip E, Bauer T M, et al. Lorlatinib in non-small-cell lung cancer with ALK or ROS1 rearrangement: an international, multicentre, open-label, single-arm first-in-man phase 1 trial. The Lancet Oncology, 2017.

[28] Reungwetwattana T, Liang Y, Zhu V, et al. The race to target MET exon 14 skipping alterations in non-small cell lung cancer: The Why, the How, the Who, the Unknown, and the Inevitable. Lung cancer (Amsterdam, Netherlands), 2017, 103: 27-37.

[29] Vansteenkiste JF, Van De Kerkhove C, Wauters E, et al. Capmatinib for the treatment of non-small cell lung cancer. Expert review of anticancer therapy, 2019, 19(8): 659-671.

[30] Johne A, Scheible H, Becker A, et al. Open-label, single-center, phase I trial to investigate the mass balance and absolute bioavailability of the highly selective oral MET inhibitor tepotinib in healthy volunteers. Investigational New Drugs, 2020.

[31] Planchard D, Kim TM, Mazieres J, et al. Dabrafenib in patients with BRAF(V600E)-positive advanced non-small-cell lung cancer: a single-arm, multicentre, open-label, phase 2 trial. The Lancet Oncology, 2016, 17(5): 642-650.

[32] Drilon AE, Liu S, Doebele R, et al. LBA19A phase 1b study of RXDX-105, a VEGFR-sparing potent RET inhibitor, in RETi-naïve patients with RET fusion-positive NSCLC. Annals of Oncology, 2017, 28.

[33] Subbiah V, Gainor JF, Rahal R. Precision Targeted Therapy with BLU-667 for RET-Driven Cancers, 2018, 8(7): 836-849.

[34] Drilon A, Subbiah V, Oxnard G, et al. A phase 1 study of LOXO-292, a potent and highly selective RET inhibitor, in patients with RET-altered cancers. Journal of Clinical Oncology, 2018, 36: 102-102.

[35] Mendoza L. Clinical development of RET inhibitors in RET-rearranged non-small cell lung cancer: Update. Oncology reviews, 2018, 12(2): 352.

[36] Farago AF, Azzoli CG. Beyond ALK and ROS1: RET, NTRK, EGFR and BRAF gene rearrangements in non-small cell lung cancer. Translational Lung Cancer Research, 2017, 6(5): 550-559.

[37] Laetsch, TW, et al. Larotrectinib for paediatric solid tumours harbouring NTRK gene fusions: phase 1 results from a multicentre, open-label, phase 1/2 study. Lancet Oncology, 2018, 19: 705.

[38] Canon J, Rex K, Saiki AY, et al. The clinical KRAS(G12C) inhibitor AMG 510 drives anti-tumour immunity. Nature, 2019, 575(7781): 217-223.

3 肺癌免疫治疗现在与展望

陈良安

一、肺癌免疫治疗概述

肺癌是常见的恶性肿瘤之一,对人类健康和生命产生严重危害。尽管近些年,手术、化疗、放疗、靶向治疗及综合治疗取得了一定成效,肺癌的死亡率仍呈现攀升趋势。我国卫健委公布的调查结果显示,中国肺癌死亡率已达30.83/10万,比30年前上升了465%,成为我国恶性肿瘤死亡的首位病因。近年来,肺癌治疗取得了重要进展。免疫治疗作为肺癌综合治疗的重要手段,走过了一段曲折的历程。

(一)免疫治疗的历程

人类对肿瘤免疫治疗的研究已逾百年。早在1893年,美国医生William Col-ey意外发现,术后化脓性链球菌感染使肉瘤消退,开始尝试使用灭活的菌毒素治疗肉瘤,揭开了肿瘤免疫治疗的序幕。近百年来,肿瘤免疫治疗进展缓慢,直到20世纪90年代,Weissman首次报道了CIK细胞抗肿瘤有较好疗效,再次引起人们对肿瘤免疫治疗的关注。近年来,肿瘤免疫学技术日益发展,抗PD-1抗体/PD-L1抗体和CTLA-4抗体等免疫检查点抑制剂陆续问世,开启了肺癌免疫治疗新篇章。

(二)免疫检查点抑制剂治疗肺癌的机制

在肺癌免疫应答的过程中,T细胞属于主要效应细胞,T细胞在受到抗原呈递细胞激活后,大量聚集并攻击表达相关抗原的肿瘤细胞。同时,T细胞表面有功能抑制性蛋白表达,也就是所谓的免疫检查点如程序死亡分子1(PD-1)。肿瘤细胞表面表达相应配体,比如PD-L1和PD-L2,在和T细胞表面的PD1结合后,可以促进机体的T细胞发生凋亡,从而实现肿瘤免疫逃逸。免疫检查点抑制剂如PD-1/PD-L1单克隆抗体,可以阻断PD-1/PD-L1通路,重新激活T细胞,恢复其对肿瘤的免疫应答,达到杀伤肿瘤的效果。目前常见的免疫检查点抑制剂主要有以Nivolumab和Pembrolizumab为代表的PD-1抑制剂,以Atezolizumab和Durvalumab为代表的PD-L1抑制剂,以Ipilimumab和Tremelimumab为代表的CTLA-4抑制剂。

二、肺癌免疫治疗的现状

(一)从二线治疗到一线治疗

针对阻断PD-1/PD-L1通路的免疫检查点抑制剂在肺癌中的研究,近几年出现突破性进展。非小细胞肺癌二线治疗的几大经典研究KEYNOTE-010、Checkmate-017、Checkmate-057及OAK实验均证实,与化疗组相比,PD1/PD-L1抑制剂组患者的疾病无进展生存期(PFS)、客观缓解率(ORR)及总生存期(OS)都有不同程度的改善,由此奠定了PD1/PD-L1抑制剂作为非小细胞肺癌二线标准治疗的地位。目前PD1抑制剂nivolumab和pembrolizumad及PD-L1抑制剂atezolizumb和durvalumab获得美国食品药物管理局(food and drug administration,FDA)批准应用于晚期非小细胞肺癌二线治疗。

免疫检查点抑制剂并未止步二线,其在肺癌一线治疗的研究迅速推进。KEYNOTE-024临床试验纳入驱动基因无突变的晚期NSCLC患者,患者肺癌PD-L1高表达(TPS≥50%),研究显示与一线含铂双药化疗相比,一线使用pembrolizumab治疗患者的PFS及ORR优于化疗组,且缓解持续时间更长。美国FDA批准pembrolizumab用于一线治疗EGFR及ALK无敏感突变且PD-L1高表达的转移性非小细胞肺癌患者,免疫检查点抑制剂正式进军肺癌的一线治疗领域。

(二)从单药治疗到联合治疗

免疫检查点抑制剂单药治疗取得突破性进展后,为进一步提高其在肺癌治疗中的疗效,研究者开始探索免疫联合用药的可行性。目前常见的方案主要有免疫检查点抑制剂联合化疗、放疗、抗肿瘤血管生成靶向治疗及两种免疫药物联合等。

化疗既可以减轻肿瘤瘤体负荷,又可以促进肿瘤抗原释放,同时还可以诱导肿瘤微环境趋化因子的释放,与免疫治疗起到协同作用,从而提高肺癌免疫疗效。在免疫检查点抑制剂联合化疗的KEYNOTE-021临床试验中,Pembrolizumab联合化疗组ORR(55%)是单纯化疗组(29%)的近2倍,PFS也显著延长(13个月 vs. 8.9个月,$P=0.010$)。免疫治疗与化疗联用发挥协同功效,使肺癌治疗的疗效得到提升。

放疗作为另一种传统肿瘤治疗手段,可以促进肿瘤抗原释放、提高免疫应答、改善效应T细胞的启动和激活,以及放疗对肿瘤免疫周期的影响,为免疫治疗联合放疗提供基础。免疫联合放疗中适合患者的选择至关重要,主要取决于肿瘤位置、患者临床分期和肺癌组织学类型等。此外还要把握免疫治疗联合放疗的最佳时机及联合用药的顺序。

不同免疫检查点抑制剂具有不同的作用机制,两种免疫检查点抑制剂的联合应用也可提升疗效。除PD-1外，CTLA-4也是另一种免疫检查点，主要表达于机体活化的T细胞表面。CTLA-4与PD-1可通过互补的机制来调节效应T细胞的活化及功能。研究表明CTLA-4与PD-L1抑制剂联合应用可以提高肺癌治疗疗效，但同时毒性也明显增加。

抗血管生成靶向药可抑制肿瘤组织生长，有研究报道VEGF/VEGFR通路与免疫系统之间能够相互促进，为抗血管生成靶向药物与免疫治疗的联合提供了理论依据。Checkmate-012临床试验中PD1抑制剂nivolumab单药治疗或联合贝伐珠单抗治疗结果显示，联合用药组患者的无进展生存期较单药组延长，同时联合用药没有明显增加不良反应的发生。抗血管生成靶向药与肿瘤免疫治疗联合可能是一种相互增益的治疗策略。

为进一步扩大获益人群及提高抗肿瘤疗效，免疫联合治疗是未来研究的热点与重点之一。随着肺癌治疗模式的不断丰富，以及免疫联合治疗研究的不断深入，免疫联合治疗模式也逐渐被接受，联合治疗是免疫治疗的出路，强强联合也是肿瘤治疗的大势所趋。

(三)免疫治疗逐步精准化

免疫检查点抑制剂的研发也推动了精准医疗的发展。在免疫治疗中寻找可以预测免疫疗效的生物标志物，筛选免疫治疗获益人群，最终实现肺癌免疫治疗的精准化尤为重要。PD-L1表达是临床研究中运用最早，也是应用最广泛的PD-1/PD-L1抑制剂疗效预测指标之一。多个临床试验显示，PD-L1的表达水平与免疫治疗的疗效相关。NCCN指南也提出，患者PD-L1表达阳性（尤其PD-L1≥50%）可以作为肺癌免疫治疗患者选择的重要依据之一。

随着全基因组测序技术突飞猛进的发展，多个研究提出肿瘤突变负荷(tumor mutation burden,TMB)可以作为免疫检查点抑制剂疗效的预测指标之一。CheckMate 026、POPLAR、OAK等研究均证实了免疫治疗疗效和TMB具有一定相关性，在TMB高的患者中免疫治疗的客观缓解率及PFS显著优于化疗，TMB作为疗效预测标志物可能有助于筛选出免疫获益人群。

随着免疫检查点抑制剂研究的不断深入，有临床试验发现错配修复基因缺陷(dMMR)及微卫星不稳定性(MSI)、肿瘤微环境、肠道菌群的构成等也会影响免疫检查点抑制剂的疗效，可能成为筛选免疫治疗标志物的突破口。多种潜在免疫疗效预测指标的发现，推动着肺癌免疫治疗精准化及个体化的发展。

三、肺癌免疫治疗需解决的问题与思考启示

近年来，以免疫检查点抑制剂为代表的肺癌免疫治疗获得较好的疗效。但肺癌免疫治疗还存在许多需要解决及思考的问题，例如如何选择肺癌免疫治疗的获益人群、如何筛选免疫治疗的分子标记物，如何确定免疫治疗的最佳时机，如何优化免疫治疗的方案，如何规定免疫治疗的疗程，如何评估免疫治疗的疗效，如何监测管理免疫相关的不良反应，以及如何克服免疫治疗的耐药等诸多问题尚需进一步探索。

(一)免疫治疗疗效预测

PD-L1作为PD1/PD-L1单克隆抗体直接作用的靶点，其表达水平和肺癌免疫治疗的效果存在一定相关性，但将PD-L1作为肺癌免疫疗效的预测指标还存在一定争议。主要原因：①既往的临床研究结果并不统一。PD-L1表达阳性的部分患者的免疫治疗疗效欠佳，同时部分PD-L1表达阴性的患者可以通过免疫治疗获益，使得PD-L1的预测价值受到争议。②PD-L1截断值选择不统一，所规定的PD-L1阳性定义标准也不相同。③PD-L1表达一般是通过免疫组化(IHC)检测，但IHC作为主观的检测手段，有时检验结果的判读因人而异。④此外，PD-L1检测试剂盒及抗体不同，试剂盒之间的检测结果不完全一致。如何使PD-L1检测更加规范化、使不同检测方法之间具有可比性，是我们面临的问题。目前TMB、MSI/MMR、肿瘤微环境及肠道菌群等作为生物标志物尚存在局限性，探索新的免疫治疗生物标志物是目前研究的热点。由于免疫治疗具有复杂性，在筛选更优的免疫治疗分子标记物的基础上，更需要建立多种生物标志物组成的联合评分模型，对免疫疗效开展综合评估，最终实现肺癌免疫治疗的精准化。

(二)免疫治疗疗程

对于免疫检查点抑制剂治疗疗程的规定是需要思考的又一问题。目前尚未界定免疫治疗的持续时间，对于免疫检查点抑制剂治疗获益的人群，临床实验多以2年期作为治疗疗程。有研究显示，用药时间长是良好的预后因素，但免疫治疗的疗效具有相对持久性，是否需要长期使用免疫检查点抑制剂，如何确定最佳治疗持续时间及规定免疫治疗疗程，尚需进一步探索。

(三)免疫治疗疗效评估

免疫检查点抑制剂通过调节机体免疫发挥抗肿瘤作用，同时可能会产生一些非常规的缓解模式，如延迟吸收和假性进展。应用传统的RECIST标准进行疗效评估会存在偏差，这给传统疗效评估模式带来了巨大挑战。免疫治疗疗效评价标准(immune-related response criteria,irRC)及修改版免疫相关缓解标准(immune-related RECIST,irRECIST)的制订与发布，使得免疫治疗评估更具体、更全面、更特异，新的评估标准可以更科学地指导免疫检查点抑制剂的临床应用。

(四)免疫治疗的耐药问题

与其他抗肿瘤药物一样，免疫治疗也存在耐药问题。免疫治疗耐药模式包括原发性耐药、适应性耐药及获得性耐药。原发性耐药是指患者从初始即对肿瘤免疫治疗无应答；适应性耐药是指肿瘤虽可被免疫系统识别，但其对免疫杀伤产生适应性，导致肿瘤细胞可以逃避T细胞攻击；获得性耐药是指患者初始的肿瘤免疫治疗有效，但在治疗一段时间后出现疾病进展。肿瘤免疫耐药可能与肿瘤抗原的表达缺失，肿瘤抗原的呈递缺陷，肿瘤细胞的信号通路异常，T细胞的功能缺陷，靶抗原表达的逐渐减少，肿瘤新突变的产生，免疫细胞对抗原识别被破坏等相关。

目前针对肿瘤免疫耐药的机制尚未完全阐明,但肿瘤免疫治疗耐药与肿瘤细胞、免疫细胞及肿瘤微环境三方面密切相关,机制复杂且涉及多个环节,如何解决肿瘤免疫治疗耐药问题,如何针对不同的耐药机制制订个体化的免疫治疗方案,最终使患者获益是需要思考及解决的问题。

(五)免疫治疗相关不良反应

随着免疫检查点抑制剂在肺癌中的广泛应用,免疫相关不良反应(immune-related adverse events,irAEs)逐渐引起医生的关注与重视。免疫检测点抑制剂可以激活非特异免疫反应,导致免疫相关不良反应的发生。免疫相关不良反应最常累及患者的皮肤、胃肠道、肺、骨骼肌及内分系统。大部分irAEs为轻中度,可被患者耐受,并通过暂时停药或皮质类固醇激素治疗得以控制。但随着研究的不断深入,出现了诸如免疫相关性肺炎、免疫间质性肾炎、免疫性心肌炎等一系列严重危及患者生命的不良反应,亟须引起临床医生的高度重视。由于免疫反应具有滞后性及持续性,一些免疫相关不良反应可能会出现较晚,有时甚至停药后一段时间才出现,故临床上对irAEs的预防、识别、治疗和随访监测应贯穿整个免疫治疗过程。此外免疫治疗与化疗、放疗、双免疫药物等联合应用,增加了药物使用的不良反应,联合用药的安全性、最优治疗方案的选择、最佳剂量的探索、不良反应的监控等一系列问题亟待解决。

四、肺癌免疫治疗的展望

目前免疫检查点抑制剂已成为化疗失败的晚期非小细胞肺癌患者的二线标准治疗方案,其一线治疗的适应证在迅速推进中,联合治疗研究也在不断开展。目前肺癌的免疫治疗正向着新辅助治疗及辅助治疗推进,免疫检查点抑制剂在肺癌维持治疗中的研究也在进行中,肺癌的免疫治疗正在改变肺癌的治疗策略,最终可能使各个阶段和各个分期的肺癌患者得到益处。目前我国研发的免疫检查点单抗也在临床研究和审批中,相信随着研究的逐步深入,肺癌免疫治疗将会给中国肺癌患者带去更多的福音。

参 考 文 献

[1] McCarthy EF. The toxins of William B. Coley and the treatment of bone and soft tissue sarcomas. Iowa Orthop J,2006, 26:154-158.

[2] Postow MA,Callahan MK,Wolchok JD. Immune checkpoint blockade in cancer therapy. J Clin Oncol,2015,33(17):1974-1982.

[3] Topalian SL,Taube JM,Anders RA,et al. Mechanism-driven biomarkers to guide immune checkpoint blockade in cancer therapy. Nat Rev Cancer,2016,16(5):275-287.

[4] Borghaei H,Paz-Ares L,Horn L,et al. Nivolumab versus docetaxel in advanced nonsquamous non-small-cell lung cancer. N Engl J Med,2015,373(17):1627-1639.

[5] Brahmer J,Reckamp KL,Baas P,et al. Nivolumab versus docetaxel in advanced squamous-cell non-small-cell lung cancer. N Engl J Med,2015,373(2):123-135.

[6] Herbst RS,Baas P,Kim DW,et al. Pembrolizumab versus docetaxel for previously treated, PD-L1-positive, advanced non-small-cell lung cancer (KEYNOTE-010):a randomised controlled trial. Lancet,2016,387(127):1540-1550.

[7] Rittmeyer A,Barlesi F,Waterkamp D,et al. Atezolizumab versus docetaxel in patients with previously treated non-small-cell lung cancer(OAK):a phase 3,open-label,multicentre randomised controlled trial. Lancet, 2017, 389 (10066):255-265.

[8] Reck M,Rodriguez-Abreu D,Robinson AG,et al. Pembrolizumab versus chemotherapy for PD-L1-positive non-small-cell lung cancer. N Engl J Med,2016,375(19):1823-1833.

[9] Langer CJ,Gadgeel SM,Borghaei H,et al. Carboplatin and pemetrexed with or without pembrolizumab for advanced, non-squamous nonsmall-cell lung cancer:a randomised, phase 2 cohort of the open-label KEYNOTE-021 study. Lancet Oncol,2016,17(11):1497-1508.

[10] Carbone DP,Reck M,Paz-Ares L,et al. First-Line Nivolumab in Stage IV or Recurrent Non-Small-Cell Lung Cancer. N Engl J Med,2017,376(25):2415-2426.

[11] Gopalakrishnan V,Spencer C,Reuben A,et al. Abstract 2672:response to anti-PD-1 based therapy in metastatic melanoma patients is associated with the diversity and composition of the gut microbiome. Cancer Res, 2017, 77 (13 Suppl):2672.

[12] Nishino M,Giobbie-Hurder A,Gargano M,et al. Developing a common language for tumor response to immunotherapy: immune-related response criteria using unidimensional measurements. Clin Cancer Res,2013,19(14):3936-3943.

[13] Sharma P, Hu-Lieskovan S, Wargo JA. Primary, adaptive, and acquired resistance to cancer immunotherapy. Cell,2017, 168(4):707-723.

[14] Weber JS,Dummer R,de Pril V,et al. Patterns of onset and resolution of immune-related adverse events of special interest with ipilimumab. Cancer,2013,119(9):1675-1682.

[15] Costa R,Carneiro BA,Agulnik M,et al. Toxicity profile of approved anti-PD-1 monoclonal antibodies in solid tumors:a systematic review and meta-analysis of randomized clinical trials. Oncotarget,2017,8(5):8910-8920.

[16] Brahmer J,Reckamp KL,Baas P,et al. Nivolumab versus docetaxel in advanced squamous-cell non-small-cell lung cancer. N Engl J Med,2015,373(2):123-135.

[17] Motzer RJ,Escudier B,McDermott DF,et al. Nivolumab versus everolimus in advanced renal-cell carcinoma. N Engl J Med,2015,373(19):1803-1813.

[18] Rizvi NA,Mazières J,Planchard D,et al. Activity and safety of nivolumab,an anti-PD-1 immune checkpoint inhibitor, for patients withadvanced, refractory squamous non-small-cell lung cancer (CheckMate 063):a phase 2,single-arm trial. Lancet Oncol,2015,16(3):257-265.

4 液体活检在肺癌诊治中的应用和挑战

吴 珍 赵 微 戴 钰 陈良安

肺癌是全球发病率和死亡率均居首位的恶性肿瘤之一。由于早期断不足使得80%的肺癌患者确诊时已处于晚期,而晚期肺癌患者又由于无法耐受组织病理活检而失去精准治疗的机会,极大地影响了肺癌患者的生存期。以安全微创和可重复动态检测为特点的液体活检在肺癌患者的早期诊断、靶点检测、耐药监测和预后评估中均发挥了重要作用。同样,液体活检在肺癌诊疗中也面临一系列的挑战:如何挑选合适的样本类型,如何利用液体活检的多种检测成分,如何选择有效的检测方法,以及如何提高液体活检在免疫治疗中的应用价值等。本文就液体活检在肺癌诊治中的相关应用进展和目前临床应用中面临的相关挑战作一综述。

一、液体活检的发展史

液体活检指的是应用来源于人体循环的体液样本进行疾病相关分子的检测来指导疾病的诊疗,其不仅用于肿瘤疾病的辅助诊疗,还在产前诊断、心血管疾病、慢性肾病、脑卒中等疾病的诊治中发挥重要作用。在肿瘤的液体活检中应用最广泛的为循环游离DNA(cell free DNA,cfDNA)。循环游离DNA首先由Mandel和Metais于1948年发现并报道,是一种存在于人体体液中且游离于细胞之外的核酸,主要由凋亡或坏死细胞释放而成。而后,肿瘤患者外周血中被证实含有更多的cfDNA。1994年,Anker等在肿瘤患者cfDNA中发现了肿瘤相关的RAS基因突变。这部分含有肿瘤相关突变的cfDNA称为循环肿瘤DNA(circulating tumor DNA,ctDNA),来源于凋亡或坏死的肿瘤细胞释放、循环肿瘤细胞(circulating tumor cell,CTC)或外泌体等。随后更多的研究发现,ctDNA可反映肿瘤组织基因组变异和表观遗传学等改变,进一步提升了液体活检在肿瘤诊疗领域的应用与进展。

CTC是另一种常见的液体活检技术,最初在1869年由Ashworth发现。肿瘤患者外周血中存在与肿瘤细胞相似的细胞,首次提出了CTC的概念。直到2003年,CTC才被完全定义:一方面为来源于原发灶或转移灶的肿瘤细胞通过毛细血管入侵血液循环系统形成,另一方面为肿瘤细胞获得间质上皮转化使得细胞的侵袭能力增强入侵基底膜而形成。随着单细胞测序技术的发展,CTC所具有的基因组信息被深入挖掘,证实与肿瘤原发灶和转移灶存在相似的基因谱,其在肿瘤疾病诊治中的作用越来越突出,有望成为补充和替代肿瘤组织的体液样本。并且CTC获取方便,可实现动态监测,有助于肿瘤诊疗过程中的个体化动态指导。

二、液体活检在肺癌诊治中的应用

液体活检以其安全、无创和可重复检测的优势广泛应用于肺癌临床诊疗,为肺癌的早期诊断提供了安全有效的方法,给不能耐受组织活检的患者提供了靶点检测的机会,给治疗过程中的随访和监测也提供了一定的便利,并且减少了耐药后不必要的再活检,贯穿于肺癌患者的全程诊疗过程。

(一)肺癌患者的早期诊断

大多数肺癌患者早期时无明显症状,且目前缺乏有效的早期诊断方法,使得多数患者确诊时已处于晚期。尽管美国NIH于2011年发表研究结果证实,低剂量CT筛查可以降低20%的肺癌病死率及6.7%的总病死率,但是低剂量CT中高达96.4%的假阳性率导致不必要的过度医疗和辐射暴露。液体活检技术通过对其中cfDNA,微小RNA(miRNA),CTC和肿瘤血小板(tumor educated platelet)进行检测可实现肺癌的早期诊断,有望成为将来肺癌早期诊断的又一大策略。早在20世纪,研究发现肿瘤患者外周血中的cfDNA含量比普通健康者更多。Diehn等利用深度测序的方法,再结合机器学习,将早期肺癌患者血浆中的cfDNA与风险匹配对照组血浆中的cfDNA进行差异分析,前瞻性地建立并验证了一种称为"血浆中肺癌可能性"(Lung-CLiP)的机器学习方法用于早期肺癌的筛查。研究者们从TCGA数据库中筛选出3个与肺癌相关性高的miRNA:miR-21-5p,miR-103-3p,miR-126-3p,联合这3个miRNA在肺结节患者中进行肺癌筛查的灵敏度可达到81.2%,而与肺部CT联合诊断可使得肺癌早期诊断的灵敏度上升到89.9%。对miRNA的联合应用还可进一步区分早期肺癌的病理分型,Lu等研究表明应用三个miRNA分子(miR-17,miR-190b和miR-375)可区分小细胞肺癌与非小细胞肺癌,灵敏度和特异度可分别达到82%和84%。肺癌特异性抗体联合肺部CT进行肺癌早期筛查的阳性预测值可达95%,高于单独应用肺部CT(69%)或特异性抗体(85.2%)的阳性预测值。借助于液体活检,能够以更加安全、易于接受的方法提高肺癌早期诊断的普及性，并且与目前已有的影像学筛查结合具有更高的敏感性，可进一步提高肺癌早期诊断的阳性率，做到早发现、早治疗，进而改善肺癌患者的整体生存质量，并延长生存期。

(二)肺癌患者的靶点检测

目前指南推荐非小细胞肺癌患者确诊后应首先进行驱动基因检测以明确下一步治疗方案。尽管靶点检测的金标准仍是组织分子检测，但由于患者身体的耐受性及肿瘤异质性导致的单次活检的局限性使得组织活检在临床的应用受限。采用全身外周体液中的cfDNA、CTC、外泌体、TEP等进行分子靶点的检测，以安全简便、易于动态监测的特点广泛应用于临床以指导个体化精准诊疗。从最初王洁等应用高性能液相质谱检测外周血ctDNA中 *EGFR* 突变到后来实时荧光定量PCR的应用，液体活检在非小细胞肺癌患者靶点检测中的应用越来越广泛。而基于荧光定量PCR平台的Cobas检测技术首先被FDA批准用于液体活检检测EGFR已知突变位点(19外显子缺失、L858R点突变和T790M突变)。随着检测技术的不断发展，使得液体活检在分子检测中的灵敏性能够进一步提升，更好地满足临床诊疗需求。目前二代测序进行液体活检在驱动基因检测中的一致性可以达到90%以上，且转移灶数目越多的患者血浆检测驱动基因的灵敏性和一致性越高。目前液体活检所覆盖的分子谱也越来越广泛，既满足了非小细胞肺癌临床诊疗中的常见分子靶点-EGFR和 *ALK* 等基因的检出，也能发现更多驱动基因的未知位点，还能进一步进行耐药机制的深入探讨。

(三)肺癌患者的耐药监测

耐药是肺癌患者治疗过程中不可避免的结局。耐药后的分子检测仍然以组织。

检测为金标准。由于多数患者耐药后身体状况无法耐受有创的耐药后再活检，使得多数患者在耐药后失去进行分子检测的机会。安全微创的液体活检再次解决了这一难题。研究发现，与组织样本相比，耐药患者血浆样本检出T790M的一致性可达70%以上，且胸腔外转移患者血浆检出T790M突变的阳性率更高。一代EGFR-TKI耐药患者的血浆中能够早于影像学进展2个月检出T790M的存在，有助于患者的耐药监测以便尽早发现耐药。由于肿瘤的异质性导致单次组织活检检出的耐药基因谱不全，而来自外周循环的体液样本同时包含了肿瘤原发灶和转移灶的肿瘤分子背景，能够较全面地检出耐药基因谱。Jeffrey等研究表明耐约患者外周血能检测到肿瘤组织无法检出的T790M耐药突变，进一步为耐药患者提供有效的治疗方案。液体活检，再次为耐药患者提供了安全便利的分子检测方法，不仅有助于检出耐药基因，还能早于临床影像学评估就监测到耐药的出现，并且还能弥补肿瘤组织异质性导致的肿瘤耐药谱不全，更好地指导耐药患者的后续治疗。

(四)肺癌患者的预后评估

越来越多的研究还证实利用液体活检进行疾病监测，可以评估和预测患者的预后。早期肺癌患者术后，外周血中检测ctDNA或CTC阳性组的患者术后1年复发率和术后2年复发率均高于阴性组。TRACERx研究纳入了100例早期肺癌术后的患者通过ctDNA来监测驱动基因数目的变化，结果表明，以ctDNA监测驱动基因数目≥2作为复发的标志，其灵敏度和特异度可达到93%和90%，并且可早于影像学进展之前预测复发的出现。液体活检对靶向治疗的预后同样具有一定作用，BENEFIT研究证实血浆检测 *EGFR* 突变阳性患者接受一代EGFR-TKI的客观缓解率为72.1%，中位无进展生存期(progress free survival, PFS)为9.5个月。同时在接受治疗后的第8周，血浆EGFR转阴的患者可获得更长的PFS。初治时 *EGFR* 突变的频率也被认为与一代EGFR-TKI治疗的预后相关：突变频率大于5.15%的患者接受一代EGFR-TKI治疗获得的PFS长于 *EGFR* 突变频率<5.15%的患者(15.4个月 *vs.* 11.1个月)。血浆中 *ALK* 突变频率的动态变化同样可以评估ALK抑制剂的疗效，动态监测 *BRAF* 突变频率的降低也可提示相关的靶向治疗有效。

三、液体活检在肺癌诊治中的挑战

(一)检测样本的选择

作为临床检测最常见的标本之一，外周血样本是最早应用于肺癌患者液体活检的样本，其获取方便，检测灵敏性高，在肺癌诊疗中的应用也最为广泛。但是，研究者发现，来自于多数肺癌患者外周血中的ctDNA量占总体cfDNA的比值<1%，且受肿瘤分期、患者病灶部位、肿瘤负荷等因素影响而使外周血ctDNA检测存在一定的局限性。近些年来，除外周血以外的其他样本也逐渐被用于肺癌患者的液体活检。痰液样本作为呼吸系统疾病最常见的标本之一，其中含有大量的cfDNA。研究证实，肺癌患者cfDNA可以用于驱动基因检测，尽管驱动基因检测的一致性不如外周血，但是其可以检测到外周血无法检测到的基因突变，两者联合可以检测到更多的肿瘤分子靶点，且吸烟患者的痰液cfDNA检测驱动基因的一致性高于非吸烟患者。基于尿液样本的液体活检也被证实与组织样本一样具有较好的一致性，与血液样本的联合可以检出更多的驱动基因变异。尿液样本cfDNA进行T790M的动态监测还可以评估奥希替尼的早期疗效。胸腔积液作为肺癌患者的常见标本之一，在检测驱动基因中的价值较外周血更胜一筹。胸腔积液上清液中的cfDNA检测到的肿瘤突变负荷(TMB)与肿瘤组织中检测到的TMB相似，高于外周血cfDNA检测到的TMB。在检出的EGFR突变频率比较中胸腔积液cfDNA，也高于外周血cfDNA。而脑脊液在肺癌脑转移患者驱动基因检测中的灵敏性和一致性也要高于外周血样本，并且脑脊液cfDNA能够检出更多的驱动基因拷贝数变异。越来越多的体液样本用于液体活检，在样本选择中我们应该根据患者临床特点和疾病特征，结合标本获取的可行性来有针对性地选择最适合的样本，提高液体活检在肺癌诊疗中的应用价值。

(二)检测成分的取舍

大量研究表明 cfDNA 是液体活检中应用最多的生物标志物,其次是 CTC。CTC 来源于原发或转移灶并具有通过循环系统传播到远处形成转移灶的潜能,携带肿瘤相关分子谱,可以用于肿瘤诊断和评估预后。与健康对照组相比,早期肺癌患者外周血中检测到一定数目的 CTC。利用二代测序技术可以进行 CTC 全基因组扩增测序或单细胞全外显子测序,了解肿瘤特异性的分子变异,评估耐药和分析表型转化。另外,CTC 在融合基因检测中更具优势。利用 CTC 中的 RNA 测序进行 ALK 等融合基因变异检测,与组织分子检测相比具有较高的一致性,并且能够根据其动态变化预测 ALK 抑制剂的疗效。但 CTC 由于其在外周血中的稀缺性、CTC 表型的变异性及单个 CTC 下游分子分析的局限性,使其在临床中的应用有待进一步加强和改善。外泌体是一种具有脂质双层膜结构的微小囊泡,其在肿瘤患者外周体液中含量丰富,其内含有大量的核酸分子,由于外泌体表层的脂膜结构使得包含其中的 DNA 和 RNA 较 cfDNA 更加稳定,且外泌体由活细胞分泌,具有很好的肿瘤特征代表性。二代测序检测外泌体 DNA 中的驱动基因变异,可达到 95% 的灵敏度,并且外泌体 DNA 中所检测的驱动基因频率还可进一步指导肺癌患者的预后。应用外泌体中的 DNA 和 RNA 分子进行 T790M 耐药检测,可获得 92% 的灵敏度,而传统的液体活检应用 ctDNA 检测 T790M 突变的灵敏度仅为 58%。应用外泌体核酸可以使得一代 EGFR-TKI 耐药患者不必要的再活检率从 42% 下降至 8%。但目前外泌体的获取和鉴定方法尚无统一标准,其临床应用有待进一步验证和推广。除此之外,循环 RNA 和肿瘤教育血小板在肺癌早期诊断中也有一定的价值,为肺癌患者的液体活检提供了更多的选择方式。

(三)检测方法的权衡

目前多种方法用于液体活检,基于荧光定量 PCR 平台的 Cobas 方法,数字 PCR 方法和二代测序方法是常见的 3 种检测方法。Cobas 方法是目前 FDA 批准用于临床患者液体活检的检测方法,其检测周期短,成本低,覆盖 EGFR 基因的临床常见和已知位点,但是多中心的研究显示其灵敏度只有 72.1%。数字 PCR 是一种绝对定量方法,其灵敏度高于普通 PCR,且检测阈值能覆盖低频突变位点,对于肺癌患者治疗过程中已知靶点的动态监测意义显著,有助于治疗过程中的疗效预测和耐药监测。二代测序是一种高通量测序方法,可一次检测包括点突变、缺失、融合、拷贝数变异等多个基因的多种已知和未知变异类型,节约样本,一次检测覆盖所有待检测的基因,尤其对耐药基因的探索有重要意义,且具有较高的灵敏,但检测周期往往需要 1~2 周,价格成本较昂贵。针对不同患者的临床需求,选择不同的检测方法使液体活检更好地服务临床,指导患者的精准诊疗。

(四)免疫治疗中的应用价值

免疫治疗是肺癌诊治领域继靶向治疗后又一里程碑式的进展,给许多肺癌患者带来新的希望。在免疫治疗获益人群的挑选上,2020 年 NCCN 指南依然推荐对 PD-L1 阳性且 EGFR,ALK,ROS1 和 BRAF 阴性或突变状态未知的晚期非小细胞肺癌患者使用免疫治疗。PD-L1 表达以组织检测为金标准,但部分晚期患者由于不能耐受组织活检而无法进行 PD-L1 表达的检测。研究者发现外周血 CTC 同样可以用于 PD-L1 表达的检测,并且能够进行免疫治疗的疗效预测,但是其与组织 PD-L1 表达的一致性有待进一步提高。除 PD-L1 表达以外,肿瘤突变负荷(tumor mutation burden,TMB)是免疫治疗另一热门标志物,利用外周血进行 TMB 检测可以通过界定阈值实现免疫治疗的疗效评估。但无论是组织活检出还是液体活检,目前对于 TMB 的检测标准仍然没有统一定论。微卫星不稳定性(microsatellite instability,MSI)检测也为实体瘤免疫治疗的疗效评估提供了一定的依据,液体活检同样为其检测带来了新的途径,并且经外周血检测的 MSI 与组织相比具有 98.4% 的一致性。

四、小 结

毫无疑问,液体活检为肺癌患者的诊治提供了有力帮助,让更多的患者从中获益。基于检测技术的不断进展,液体活检在靶点检测中已经与组织分子检测有很好的一致性,为后续治疗过程中的动态监测和耐药检测打下了坚实的基础。作为一项新兴技术,液体活检仍然存在一定的挑战。外周循环中 ctDNA、CTC 等物质的量和稳定性受肿瘤分期和肿瘤负荷的影响,会影响液体活检在临床应用中的敏感性。CTC 和外泌体的分离和获取也是限制其临床应用的重要因素。另外,如何更好地利用液体活检辅助免疫治疗也是其未来的发展方向。借助于科学技术的不断进展,未来液体活检必将以其安全、便捷的优势更好地应用于肺癌患者的临床诊疗实践。

参 考 文 献

[1] Howlader N NA, Krapcho M, Miller D, et al. SEER Cancer Statistics Review, 1975-2014, National Cancer Institute. Bethesda, MD, 2017.

[2] Ferrari M, Carrera P, Lampasona V, et al. New trend in non-invasive prenatal diagnosis. Clin Chim Acta, 2015, 451: 9-13.

[3] Nascimento da Silva M, Sicchieri LB, de Oliveira Silva FR, et al. Liquid biopsy of atherosclerosis using protoporphyrin IX as a biomarker. Analyst, 2014, 139: 1383-1388.

[4] Diaz LA, Jr, Bardelli A. Liquid biopsies: genotyping circulating tumor DNA. J Clin Oncol, 2014, 32: 579-586.

[5] Korabecna M, Opatrna S, Wirth J, et al. Cell-free plasma DNA during peritoneal dialysis and hemodialysis and in patients with chronic kidney disease. Ann N Y Acad Sci, 2008, 1137: 296-301.

[6] Mandel P, Metais P. Les acides nucleiques du plasma sanguin chez l'homme. C R Seances Soc Biol Fil, 1948, 142: 241-243.

[7] Vasioukhin V, Anker P, Maurice P, et al. Point mutations of the N-ras gene in the blood plasma DNA of patients with myelodysplastic syndrome or acute myelogenous leukaemia. Br J Haematol, 1994, 86: 774-779.

[8] Anker P, Mulcahy H, Chen XQ, et al. Detection of circulating tumour DNA in the blood (plasma/serum) of cancer patients. Cancer Metastasis Rev, 1999, 18: 65-73.

[9] Mulcahy HE, Lyautey J, Lederrey C, et al. Plasma DNA K-ras mutations in patients with gastrointestinal malignancies. Ann N Y Acad Sci, 2000, 906: 25-28.

[10] Xu RH, Wei W, Krawczyk M, et al. Circulating tumour DNA methylation markers for diagnosis and prognosis of hepatocellular carcinoma. Nat Mater, 2017, 16: 1155-1161.

[11] Dianat Moghadam H, Azizi M, Eslami SZ, et al. The Role of Circulating Tumor Cells in the Metastatic Cascade: Biology, Technical Challenges, and Clinical Relevance. Cancers (Basel), 2020, 12.

[12] Shook D, Keller R. Mechanisms, mechanics and function of epithelial-mesenchymal transitions in early development. Mech Dev, 2003, 120: 1351-1383.

[13] Ni X, Zhuo M, Su Z, et al. Reproducible copy number variation patterns among single circulating tumor cells of lung cancer patients. Proc Natl Acad Sci USA, 2013, 110: 21083-21088.

[14] Auer M, Heitzer E, Ulz P, et al. Single circulating tumor cell sequencing for monitoring. Oncotarget, 2013, 4: 812-813.

[15] Aberle DR, Adams AM, Berg CD, et al. Reduced lung-cancer mortality with low-dose computed tomographic screening. N Engl J Med, 2011, 365: 395-409.

[16] Leon SA, Shapiro B, Sklaroff DM, et al. Free DNA in the serum of cancer patients and the effect of therapy. Cancer Res, 1977, 37: 646-650.

[17] Chabon JJ, Hamilton EG, Kurtz DM, et al. Integrating genomic features for non-invasive early lung cancer detection. Nature, 2020, 580: 245-251.

[18] Lin Y, Leng Q, Jiang Z, et al. A classifier integrating plasma biomarkers and radiological characteristics for distinguishing malignant from benign pulmonary nodules. Int J Cancer, 2017, 141: 1240-1248.

[19] Lu S, Kong H, Hou Y, et al. Two plasma microRNA panels for diagnosis and subtype discrimination of lung cancer. Lung Cancer, 2018, 123: 44-51.

[20] Ren S, Zhang S, Jiang T, et al. Early detection of lung cancer by using an autoantibody panel in Chinese population. Oncoimmunology, 2018, 7: e1384108.

[21] Mao C, Yuan JQ, Yang ZY, et al. Blood as a Substitute for Tumor Tissue in Detecting EGFR Mutations for Guiding EGFR TKIs Treatment of Nonsmall Cell Lung Cancer: A Systematic Review and Meta-Analysis. Medicine (Baltimore), 2015, 94: e775.

[22] Coghlin CL, Smith LJ, Bakar S, et al. Quantitative analysis of tumor in bronchial biopsy specimens. J Thorac Oncol, 2010, 5: 448-452.

[23] Bai H, Mao L, Wang HS, et al. Epidermal growth factor receptor mutations in plasma DNA samples predict tumor response in Chinese patients with stages IIIB to IV non-small-cell lung cancer. J Clin Oncol, 2009, 27: 2653-2659.

[24] G. A, Sacher, Kimberly M. Komatsubara, et al. Application of Plasma Genotyping Technologies in Non-Small Cell Lung Cancer: A Practical Review. Journal of Thoracic Oncology, 2017, 12.

[25] Mohrmann L, Huang HJ, Hong DS, et al. Liquid Biopsies Using Plasma Exosomal Nucleic Acids and Plasma Cell-Free DNA Compared with Clinical Outcomes of Patients with Advanced Cancers. Clin Cancer Res, 2018, 24: 181-188.

[26] Jovelet C, Ileana E, Le Deley MC, et al. Circulating Cell-Free Tumor DNA Analysis of 50 Genes by Next-Generation Sequencing in the Prospective MOSCATO Trial. Clin Cancer Res, 2016, 22: 2960-2968.

[27] Wang Y, Tian PW, Wang WY, et al. Noninvasive genotyping and monitoring of anaplastic lymphoma kinase (ALK) rearranged non-small cell lung cancer by capture-based next-generation sequencing. Oncotarget, 2016.

[28] Cui S, Zhang W, Xiong L, et al. Use of capture-based next-generation sequencing to detect ALK fusion in plasma cell-free DNA of patients with non-small-cell lung cancer. Oncotarget, 2017, 8: 2771-2780.

[29] Aguado C, Gimenez-Capitan A, Karachaliou N, et al. Fusion gene and splice variant analyses in liquid biopsies of lung cancer patients. Transl Lung Cancer Res, 2016, 5: 525-531.

[30] Minari R, Mazzaschi G, Bordi P, et al. Detection of EGFR-Activating and T790M Mutations Using Liquid Biopsy in Patients With EGFR-Mutated Non-Small-Cell Lung Cancer Whose Disease Has Progressed During Treatment With First-and Second-Generation Tyrosine Kinase Inhibitors: A Multicenter Real-Life Retrospective Study. Clin Lung Cancer, 2020.

[31] Su KY, Tseng JS, Liao KM, et al. Mutational monitoring of EGFR T790M in cfDNA for clinical outcome prediction in EGFR-mutant lung adenocarcinoma. PLoS One, 2018, 13: e0207001.

[32] Lee JY, Qing X, Xiumin W, et al. Longitudinal monitoring of EGFR mutations in plasma predicts outcomes of NSCLC patients treated with EGFR TKIs: Korean Lung Cancer Consortium (KLCC-12-02). Oncotarget, 2016, 7: 6984-6993.

[33] Parikh AR, Leshchiner I, Elagina L, et al. Liquid versus tissue biopsy for detecting acquired resistance and tumor heterogeneity in gastrointestinal cancers. Nat Med, 2019, 25: 1415-1421.

[34] Thompson JC, Yee SS, Troxel AB, et al. Detection of Therapeutically Targetable Driver and Resistance Mutations in Lung Cancer Patients by Next-Generation Sequencing of Cell-Free Circulating Tumor DNA. Clin Cancer Res, 2016, 22: 5772-5782.

[35] Liang H, Huang J, Wang B, et al. The role of liquid biopsy in predicting post-operative recurrence of non-small cell lung cancer. J Thorac Dis, 2018, 10: 838-845.

[36] Jamal-Hanjani M, Wilson GA, McGranahan N, et al. Tracking the Evolution of Non-Small-Cell Lung Cancer. N Engl J Med, 2017, 376: 2109-2121.

[37] Abbosh C, Birkbak NJ, Wilson GA, et al. Phylogenetic ctDNA analysis depicts early-stage lung cancer evolution. Nature, 2017, 545: 446-451.

[38] Jamal-Hanjani M, Hackshaw A, Ngai Y, et al. Tracking genomic cancer evolution for precision medicine: the lung TRACERx study. PLoS Biol, 2014, 12: e1001906.

[39] Wang Z, Cheng Y, An T, et al. Detection of EGFR mutations in plasma circulating tumour DNA as a selection criterion for first-line gefitinib treatment in patients with advanced lung adenocarcinoma (BENEFIT): a phase 2, single-arm, multicentre clinical trial. Lancet Respir Med, 2018, 6: 681-690.

[40] Yang X, Zhuo M, Ye X, et al. Quantification of mutant alleles in circulating tumor DNA can predict survival in lung cancer. Oncotarget, 2016, 7: 20810-20824.

[41] Mau-Soerensen M, Ahlborn LB, Joenson L, et al. Dynamics of mutant BRAF V600E in free circulating DNA (fcDNA) of non-melanoma cancer patients (pts) in response to treatment with BRAF and MEK/EGFR inhibitors. Journal of Clinical Oncology, 2016, 34.

[42] Zhao X, Han RB, Zhao J, et al. Comparison of epidermal growth factor receptor mutation statuses in tissue and plasma in stage I-IV non-small cell lung cancer patients. Respiration, 2013, 85: 119-125.

[43] Nygaard AD, Holdgaard PC, Spindler KL, et al. The correlation between cell-free DNA and tumour burden was estimated by PET/CT in patients with advanced NSCLC. Br J Cancer, 2014, 110: 363-368.

[44] De Mattos-Arruda L, Mayor R, Ng CKY, et al. Cerebrospinal fluid-derived circulating tumour DNA better represents the genomic alterations of brain tumours than plasma. Nat Commun, 2015, 6: 8839.

[45] van der Drift MA, Prinsen CF, Hol BE, et al. Can free DNA be detected in sputum of lung cancer patients? Lung Cancer, 2008, 61: 385-390.

[46] Wu Z, Yang Z, Li CS, et al. Differences in the genomic profiles of cell-free DNA between plasma, sputum, urine, and tumor tissue in advanced NSCLC. Cancer Med, 2019, 8: 910-919.

[47] Franovic A, Raymond VM, Erlander MG, et al. Urine test for EGFR analysis in patients with non-small cell lung cancer. J Thorac Dis, 2017, 9: 1323-1331.

[48] Reckamp KL, Melnikova VO, Karlovich C, et al. A Highly Sensitive and Quantitative Test Platform for Detection of NSCLC EGFR Mutations in Urine and Plasma. J Thorac Oncol, 2016, 11: 1690-1700.

[49] Husain H, Melnikova VO, Kosco K, et al. Monitoring Daily Dynamics of Early Tumor Response to Targeted Therapy by Detecting Circulating Tumor DNA in Urine. Clin Cancer Res, 2017.

[50] Tong. L, Ding. N, Li. J, et al. etDNA: Tumor-Derived DNA from Pleural Effusion Supernatant as a Promising Source for NGS Based Mutation Profiling in Lung Cancer. Journal of Thoracic Oncology, 2017, 12: S1891.

[51] Li YS, Jiang BY, Yang JJ, et al. Unique genetic profiles from cerebrospinal fluid cell-free DNA in leptomeningeal metastases of EGFR-mutant non-small-cell lung cancer: a new medium of liquid biopsy. Ann Oncol, 2018, 29: 945-952.

[52] He Y, Shi J, Schmidt B, et al. Circulating Tumor Cells as a Biomarker to Assist Molecular Diagnosis for Early Stage Non-Small Cell Lung Cancer. Cancer Manag Res, 2020, 12: 841-854.

[53] Pailler E, Adam J, Barthelemy A, et al. Detection of circulating tumor cells harboring a unique ALK rearrangement in ALK-positive non-small-cell lung cancer. J Clin Oncol, 2013, 31: 2273-2281.

[54] Chemi F, Mohan S, Brady G. Circulating Tumour Cells in Lung Cancer. Recent Results Cancer Res, 2020, 215: 105-125.

[55] van Niel G, D'Angelo G, Raposo G. Shedding light on the cell biology of extracellular vesicles. Nat Rev Mol Cell Biol, 2018, 19: 213-228.

[56] Castellanos-Rizaldos E, Grimm DG, Tadigotla V, et al. Exosome-Based Detection of EGFR T790M in Plasma from Non-Small Cell Lung Cancer Patients. Clin Cancer Res, 2018, 24: 2944-2950.

[57] 张灏,赵立波,叶国栋. 外泌体研究、转化和临床应用专家共识. 转化医学杂志, 2018, 7: 321-325.

[58] Su K, Zhang T, Wang Y, et al. Diagnostic and prognostic value of plasma microRNA-195 in patients with non-small cell lung cancer. World J Surg Oncol, 2016, 14: 224.

[59] Best MG, Sol N, In't Veld S, et al. Swarm Intelligence-Enhanced Detection of Non-Small-Cell Lung Cancer Using Tumor-Educated Platelets. Cancer Cell, 2017, 32: 238-252.e239.

[60] Wu YL, Lee V, Liam CK, et al. Clinical utility of a blood-based EGFR mutation test in patients receiving first-line erlotinib therapy in the ENSURE, FASTACT-2, and ASPIRATION studies. Lung Cancer, 2018, 126: 1-8.

[61] Hindson CM, Chevillet JR, Briggs HA, et al. Absolute quantification by droplet digital PCR versus analog real-time PCR. Nat Methods, 2013, 10: 1003-1005.

[62] Heeke S, Hofman V, Ilie M, et al. Prospective evaluation of NGS-based liquid biopsy in untreated late stage non-squamous lung carcinoma in a single institution. J Transl Med, 2020, 18: 87.

[63] Thress KS, Paweletz CP, Felip E, et al. Acquired EGFR C797S mutation mediates resistance to AZD9291 in non-small cell lung cancer harboring EGFR T790M. Nat Med, 2015, 21: 560-562.

[64] Guibert N, Delaunay M, Lusque A, et al. PD-L1 expression in circulating tumor cells of advanced non-small cell lung cancer patients treated with nivolumab. Lung Cancer, 2018, 120: 108-112.

[65] Yarchoan M, Hopkins A, Jaffee EM. Tumor Mutational Burden and Response Rate to PD-1 Inhibition. N Engl J Med, 2017, 377: 2500-2501.

[66] Gandara DR, Paul SM, Kowanetz M, et al. Blood-based tumor mutational burden as a predictor of clinical benefit in non-small-cell lung cancer patients treated with atezolizumab. Nat Med, 2018, 24: 1441-1448.

[67] Le DT, Durham JN, Smith KN, et al. Mismatch repair deficiency predicts response of solid tumors to PD-1 blockade. Science, 2017, 357: 409-413.

[68] Willis J, Lefterova MI, Artyomenko A, et al. Validation of Microsatellite Instability Detection Using a Comprehensive Plasma-Based Genotyping Panel. Clin Cancer Res, 2019, 25: 7035-7045.

5 肿瘤新抗原预测程序

梁红阁

因肿瘤抗原在肿瘤诊断、预后和靶向治疗中有着至关重要的作用,癌症疫苗和过继T细胞治疗等免疫治疗的个性化也依赖于特异性新表位的识别。然而,确定免疫治疗靶点,以及最可能受益于免疫治疗患者人群的可靠的生物标志物,仍是一个关键的、尚未解决的问题。大量的平行序列分析表明突变负荷和免疫治疗预后之间存在联系,但还需要可靠的方法确定哪些肿瘤特异性突变肽(新抗原)可诱发抗肿瘤T细胞免疫,以提高对免疫检查点抑制剂(immune checkpoint nhibitors, ICIs)治疗反应的预测,确定疫苗和过继T细胞治疗的靶点。随着肿瘤基因组学的发展,肿瘤特异性新抗原的鉴定成为可能。本文综述了目前已报道的基于基因检测的新抗原预测方法、在肿瘤治疗中的验证及其所面临的挑战。

一、引 言

癌症免疫治疗的方法利用了人类免疫系统的监测能力,它能够通过识别肿瘤相关抗原,消除癌细胞。癌症免疫系统相互作用的特征可以识别潜在的生物标志物,包括MHC表达、IFN敏感性、淋巴细胞计数(包括效应细胞和调节性T细胞计数)、肿瘤T细胞、新抗原、Interleukin-6(IL-6)表达、programmed cell death-Ligand 1(PD-L1)表达或肿瘤突变负荷(tumor mutation burden, TMB)。呈递肿瘤特异性新抗原主要组织相容性复合体(MHC)分子,以供T细胞识别。除了表达模式异常外,肿瘤细胞还包含一系列癌症体细胞突变和蛋白编码区突变,这可能产生肿瘤特异性突变蛋白,肿瘤相关的表位可能来源于异常蛋白表达或非同义基因改变,从而产生新的肽序列。肿瘤新抗原作为识别肿瘤细胞的重要的生物标志物和潜在的治疗靶点,在肿瘤诊断、预后和靶向治疗等方面发挥着重要作用。研究发现,突变负荷和预测的新表位数目与肿瘤对免疫检查点抑制剂的临床反应密切相关,包括非小细胞肺癌(non-small cell lung cancer, NSCLC)和黑色素瘤。新抗原负荷与programmed cell death protein-1(PD-1)和cytotoxic T-lymphocyte antigen 4(CTLA-4)治疗效果相关,这表明新抗原负荷不但是肿瘤免疫治疗非常重要的生物标志物,还是肿瘤治疗的强有力的靶点。

使用新抗原的主要问题之一是新抗原的鉴定,虽然基因组学和生物信息学的技术进步为有效地从肿瘤的体细胞突变谱中选择最强的免疫原性新抗原奠定了基础,然而潜在的抗原库是巨大的,并存在很大的特异性。因此在不同的研究中,识别新抗原的标准与其疗效预测相关性并不一致。目前所报道的预测方法主要是全外显子组测序、结合质谱或计算预测模型(主要是human leukocyte antigen(HLA)-I结合亲和力)及体外验证。从概念上讲,基于NGS数据的新表位预测可以分为三个步骤:首先,识别非同义突变,并保留所有可能含有适当长度(一般为8~11mer)的突变所致的新肽;其次,预测与患者特异性MHC等位基因的结合亲和力;最后,根据前两步结果,结合MHC提呈、T细胞识别、与未突变蛋白序列相似性等特征,评估每个肽的免疫原性。新抗原预测软件的最终目标之一是对将受益于免疫治疗的患者进行分类,或设计一种个性化的癌症疫苗。本文综述了目前已报道的基于基因检测的新抗原预测方法及其在肿瘤中的验证,包括pVAC-Seq、MuPeXI、TSNAD、Neopepsee和pTuneos。

二、pVAC-Seq

pVAC-Seq程序是一种自动化新抗原预测程序,可利用DNA和RNA序列数据,从肿瘤突变库中系统地识别出候选新抗原表位。需要输入的信息包括已被"翻译"成氨基酸变化的非同义突变,以及患者特异性的HLA等位基因,之后pVAC-Seq开始运行以最终识别出候选新抗原表位,步骤如下:①表位预测,pVAC-Seq通过计算其与HLA I类分子的结合亲和力来预测突变导致的表位。首先,生成肽序列的FASTA文件;氨基酸FASTA序列是由突变氨基酸每侧8~10个氨基酸组成的;如果突变分别发生在转录本的末端或开始附近,则取前面或后面16~20氨基酸构建FASTA序列。然后运行表位预测软件:根据选择的k-mer窗口大小从表位预测软件(NetMHC v3.4软件)中预测所有候选肽。继而进行解析、筛选和输出:只有突变体(MT)结合分数<500 nM、包含突变氨基酸的特定肽才与相应的野生型进行对比。最后,从所有指定的k-mers和输入的所有独立HLA等位基因类型中选择每个突变的最佳候选(最低的MT结合分数)。②序列信息整合,输入肿瘤DNA序列和RNA序列、正常组织DNA序列信息,利用bam-readcount软件,输出基因表达,是以每千碱基外显子每百万读数的片段数(fragments per kilobase of exon per million reads mapped, FPKM)衡量。③筛选候选新抗原:首先,通过基于测序深度的筛选器(depth based filters)筛选出以下表位:正常组织覆盖率≥5×(最高20×);正常组织VAF≤2%(可以根据正常样本中肿瘤细胞的污染程度

来增加）；肿瘤覆盖率（DNA 和 RNA）≥10×；肿瘤 VAF（DNA 和 RNA）≥40%；其次，通过基于表达的筛选器（expression based filters）筛选出 FPKM>1 的表位。通过这一程序，在所有新表位中快速筛选和识别少量潜在免疫原性的新表位。

为了验证 pVAC-Seq，将其应用于 4 例转移性黑色素瘤患者的分析，所有 4 名患者都参加了树突状细胞疫苗的 I 期临床试验（NCT00683670，BB-IND 13590）。首先由 NetMHC v3.4 预测原始候选抗原的数量，随后通过 pVAC-Seq 程序的解析和筛选确定更合理的高 HLA-I 亲和力的最终候选抗原，并将对最终筛选的抗原进行免疫原性检测和疫苗的设计。其中 3 例患者的临床结果表明，疫苗的免疫接种可扩大抗肿瘤免疫的抗原宽度和克隆多样性。提示 pVAC-Seq 可识别用于树突状细胞个性化疫苗的新抗原肽。

这一程序的优点是可以在较短的时间内评估肿瘤特异性新表位，还提供了除 MHC 结合亲和力之外的预测信息，包括相似性、表达情况等。缺点是①该程序只关注了单纯的体细胞点突变，而未扩展到其他的基因改变，如插入、删失、基因融合等，对评估新抗原负荷本身是否可以作为 ICIs 疗效的生物标志物有一定的限制。②Pvac-Seq 使用默认的筛选值标识零免疫原性肽，说明在确定适当的表位标识阈值方面还存在挑战。③该程序仅预测了可被 T 细胞识别的 I 类 MHC 分子所呈递的新抗原，并未考虑可被突变特异性抗体识别的膜蛋白胞外区域的突变。因此，Pvac-Seq 用户需对所分析的数据有深入的了解，并且需要知道哪些筛选标准适用于来自特定样本的数据，才能找到最优的筛选值并获得相关肽的列表。

三、MuPeXI

MuPeXI 是一个识别肿瘤特异性肽段并评估其成为新表位潜力的程序。程序输入是一个包含体细胞突变、HLA 类型列表和可选的基因表达谱的文件。随后 MuPeXI 对原始的测序数据（WXS/WGS 和 RNA-seq）进行预处理，产生识别变异体的 VCF 文件和表达值，然后进行新抗原的预测。具体步骤如下：①效应预测，通过 Ensembl 变异效应预测器（Ensembls variant effect predictor，VEP）预测突变（SNVs 和插入缺失）对 cDNA 和蛋白序列的影响。②新表位提取：利用来自 VEP 文件中体细胞的突变位置信息来识别新肽。对于框内突变，突变蛋白序列可以直接从 Ensembl 蛋白库中推断出来。对于移码突变，通过翻译突变 cDNA 来推断突变蛋白。③与正常肽段的相似性：整个蛋白质组被切割成自定义的长度，从未突变的氨基酸序列中识别出与新肽最相似的正常肽（对于 SNVs），或者通过蛋白库寻找最多 4 个不匹配的相似肽（对于插入缺失），相似性越高，新表位的优先排序越低。④预测 MHC 结合亲和力：用 NetMHCpan 3.0 检测肽和 HLA 表型的结合能力，并对亲和力及等级评分进行注释。⑤基因表达：提供基因水平或转录水平的表达数据，并对所有转录产物进行注释。⑥注释：对每对突变和正常肽的所有相关信息进行注释。⑦优先级评分排序：根据 MHC-肽结合亲和力、相应基因表达水平和相似性对肽段进行优先级评分和排序，最终程序以表格的形式输出，表中包含了所有来源于单核苷酸变异（single nucleotide variants，SNVs）、插入和缺失的肿瘤特异性肽段以及完整的注释、HLA 结合力、与正常肽段的相似性。并根据这些信息对肽段进行优先排序，粗略预测免疫原性。

MuPeXI 对 3 例 NSCLC 患者（L011，L012，L013）预测的新肽 T 细胞反应活性进行了分析。共鉴定出了 995 个 9～11mer 特定的新肽，在原研究中鉴定的 322 个独特的 9mer 多肽中，只有 190 个被 MuPeXI 鉴定出来，这很可能是由于 NGS 分析的差异，尤其是识别变异体的差异所引起。随后使用荧光素或 DNA 标记的 MHC 多聚物筛选 T 细胞反应活性。最终 11 个预测的新肽在相应的患者样本中得到了 T 细胞识别，为了评估 MuPeXI 优先级评分是否可以区分引起 T 细胞反应的新肽和未引起 T 细胞反应的新肽，构建了基于 MuPeXI 优先级评分的 ROC 曲线。结果显示 ROC 曲线下面积为 0.635，表明 MuPeXI 能够优先选择免疫原性肽。

MuPeXI 对肽段的优先级评分旨在根据引起 T 细胞反应的可能性对肽进行排序。其优点是该程序不仅关注点突变，还可以对插入缺失的相似非突变肽进行搜索。缺点是该程序仅预测了可被 T 细胞识别的 I 类 MHC 分子所呈递的新抗原，并未考虑可被突变特异性抗体识别的膜蛋白胞外区域的突变；且对优先级评分的分析是基于非常少的可用数据，因此是否能准确筛选出具有免疫原性的肽段还需进一步验证。

四、TSNAD

肿瘤特异性新抗原检测（tumour-specific neoantigen detector，TSNAD）由突变检测和新抗原预测两部分组成，可以从肿瘤组织-正常组织配对的基因组/外显子组测序数据中识别出肿瘤体细胞突变。然后，采用两种策略来预测新抗原。首先，根据人类蛋白图谱，有 5462 个预测的膜蛋白，该程序使用 TMHMM 鉴定这些蛋白的跨膜拓扑结构和胞外区域。将筛选的肿瘤错义突变定位到膜蛋白的胞外区域，以鉴定膜蛋白的胞外突变。其次，除了膜蛋白外，由于由 MHC 分子介导的抗原呈递系统，多肽也可在细胞表面出现。使用 SOAP-HLA（v.2.2）对每个样本进行 HLA 分型，然后利用 NETMHCPAN（v.2.8）预测 I 类 MHC 与野生型/突变型多肽的结合亲和力。在不影响正常组织的情况下，HLA 蛋白与突变肽的特异性结合可能成为药物靶点，故该程序还进一步比较了 HLA 分子与野生型和突变型多肽的结合信息，以提取能结合 HLA-A/B/C 分子的突变肽进行进一步分析。

TSNAD 对来自国际癌症基因组协会（ICGC）数据库的 9155 个样本的癌症体细胞突变进行了潜在新抗原的预测。首先，将所有的错义突变定位到膜蛋白的胞外区域，获得 88354 个细胞外突变。其次，基于错义突变提取了 21 个氨基酸长度，突变位点上游有 10 个氨基酸，下游有 10

个氨基酸。通过这些方法预测了包括I类MHC分子所表达的膜蛋白和多肽的胞外突变的大量的新抗原。其中有65个潜在的常见新抗原,它们的相应突变至少出现在20个供体中,且IC50小于500nM。这65个新抗原与12个基因的23个体细胞突变有关。其中KRAS、PIK3CA和TP53比其他基因占据更多的潜在新抗原,最常见的潜在新抗原是由基因KRAS编码的,提示这些基因在肿瘤免疫治疗中发挥更重要的作用。

TSNAD可以预测潜在的新抗原,包括膜蛋白的胞外突变和由MHC I类分子提呈的新抗原。该程序的优点为TSNAD不仅考虑了I类MHC分子所呈递的新抗原,还考虑了膜蛋白的突变;缺点是该程序主要关注MHC-I的结合亲和力,在不确定优先级评分的情况下获得最终的新肽,这阻碍了其进一步的临床应用。

五、Neopepsee

Neopepsee是一个基于机器学习的用于二代测序数据的新抗原预测程序,这一程序利用原始的RNA测序数据和体细胞突变,通过利用免疫原性特征构建的机器学习分类器预测免疫原性,并将其分为高、中、低三类,同时可提供候选肽包括IC50、新肽和免疫调节基因(如PD1、PD-L1)的表达水平、匹配的表位序列等在内的87个免疫原性相关值。

该程序最初收集了13个已被报道用于预测免疫原性的潜在特征,并根据其代表的潜在生物学意义,将13个潜在特征其分为三组。① MHC-I结合和表达:包括基于IC50和百分位等级的MHC-I结合亲和力预测值、基于NetCTLpan的MHC-I结合评分、蛋白裂解、与抗原提呈相关的转运蛋白(transporter associated with antigen processing, TAP)的转运效率及其综合评分、pMHC-I分子的T细胞识别评分;②氨基酸特征:包括T细胞受体(T cell receptor, TCR)接触残基处氨基酸的疏水性;位于2、3、5、6位氨基酸的"极性和荷电值"、分子大小和"肽的熵";③复杂性评分:包括MHC与野生型和相应突变肽结合亲和力之间的差异(differential agretopicity index, DAI)和氨基酸配对的接触电位(amino acid pairwise contact potentials, AAPPs);④此外,还根据之前关于相似性和免疫原性的假设,定义了一个新的评分标准,即"与已知表位的序列相似性"。在以上4个因素中,根据之前研究报道的一致性、每个因素的信息含量和各因素之间的相关性对冗余因素进行了排除,最后,9个因素用于构建机器学习分类器:包括基于IC50和百分位等级的MHC-I结合亲和力预测值、pMHC结合评分、T细胞识别评分、TCR接触残基处氨基酸的疏水性、氨基酸的极性和荷电值、DAI、AAPPs及与已知表位序列相似性。基于对免疫原性特征的选择机器分类器构造了4个学习模型,并在构建的数据集上使用了500次的10次交叉验证,并测量了性能。在训练步骤中,计算出数据集的免疫原性特征被输入到4个分类器中。然后,验证了4种训练好的分类器和传统方法在独立数据集上的性能。

Neopepsee对224例胃腺癌样品进行了分析,共鉴定出3760个预测的新抗原,其中在多个肿瘤样本只发现了16个(0.42%)新抗原。体细胞单核苷酸变异(somatic single-nucleotide variants, SNV)的中位数为49,推测的新抗原中位数为7。微卫星不稳定性(microsatellite instability, MSI)状态的不同导致体细胞SNVs的数量有很大差异[MSI-高的中位SNVs为452, MSI-低的中位SNVs为56,微卫星稳定(microsatellite stable, MSS)肿瘤的中位SNVs为40]。MSI-高的肿瘤中新抗原的数量(中位数为68)高于MSI-低的肿瘤(中位数为10)及MSS肿瘤(中位数为5)。与无新抗原的肿瘤相比,有新抗原的肿瘤预后更好(29.1个月 vs. 14.1个月;log-rank $P=0.024$)。然而,MSI状态与总生存率没有显著的相关性(29.4月 vs. 26.7月,log-rank $P=0.616$)。在cox回归分析中,缺乏新抗原和晚期肿瘤(Ⅲ期和Ⅳ期)是总体生存独立的预后不良因素。无论在单变量分析(风险比 hazard ratio, HR=3.1; $P=0.022$),还是在多变量分析(HR=2.2; $P=0.040$)中,新抗原阳性均与整体生存的改善相关。我们的数据表明,微卫星不稳定灶所引起的新抗原负荷的增加可能是一个有利的预后因素,而非MSI状态本身。

Neopepsee构建了一个基于肽的免疫原性特征的机器学习模型来优化候选新表位。该方法的优点是与IC50为500 nM,百分位等级为2.4的传统免疫原性阈值的预测方法相比,灵敏性和特异性提高了2~3倍,并可用于判断患者的预后。缺点是纳入机器学习模型的9个因素还需进一步验证其生物学特性;此外,由于肽来自通用的抗原而不是通过实验验证的真正的新抗原,故Neopepsee使用的训练数据缺乏特异性。

六、pTuneos

pTuneos基于通过肽-MHC结合的高亲和力预测新抗原,并采用两步筛选和排序策略对新抗原进行优先排序。总体来说,pTuneos预测新抗原包括四个步骤,①数据预处理:对原始测序数据(WGS/WES和/或RNA-seq)进行分析,以识别VCF文件和表达谱中的体细胞突变(SNVs和插入缺失)。②候选新抗原标识:对于单核苷酸变异,将核苷酸的变化转化为相应的氨基酸的变化,然后应用到蛋白质组库;对于核苷酸插入和缺失改变,直接从cDNA翻译成相应的包含基因改变位点的21聚体肽,再将长肽切成9~11肽,然后用NetMHCpan 4.0测定突变肽和正常肽的MHC结合亲和力。③基于模型的筛选:构建一个随机森林模型(forest model),即Pre&RecNeo,根据5个相关特征预测新肽的MHC提呈和T细胞识别率,包括突变肽-MHC亲和力百分位排名、正常肽-MHC亲和力百分位排名、正常肽段与突变肽段序列相似性、肽段疏水性评分和T细胞对肽段-MHC复合物的识别。④筛选新表位:pTuneos开发了一个评分模型RefinedNeo,以细化新表位免疫原性的等级,新表位免疫原性的评估因素包括了新肽的自然处理、MHC提呈和T细胞识别的概率,以及新肽在临床肿瘤治疗中的实际免疫效果。

pTuneos 对一组接受 pembrolizumab(队列 Rizvi)治疗的 IV 期 NSCLC 患者和两组接受抗 CTLA-4 免疫治疗的晚期黑色素瘤患者(队列 Snyder 和队列 Van Allen)进行了分析,以评估识别的新抗原与患者生存之间的关系。在 31 例接受 pembrolizumab 治疗的肺癌患者(队列 Rizvi)中,有 14 例患者获得了持久的临床疗效(durable clinical benefit,DCB),17 例患者没有获得持久的临床疗效(non-durable clinical benefit,NDB)。pTuneos 发现每个肿瘤中候选新抗原的中位数为 41 个(范围为 1~417),整体新抗原免疫原性评分范围为 0~1.93 分。在 59 例接受 ipilimumab 或 tremelimumab(队列 Snyder)治疗的黑色素瘤患者中,有 36 例患者 DCB,23 例患者 NDB。pTuneos 发现每个肿瘤中候选新抗原中位数为 384 个(范围为 0~3299),整体新抗原免疫原性评分范围为 0~8.6 分。在 103 例接受 ipilimumab(队列 Van Allen)治疗的黑色素瘤患者中,21 例为 DCB,72 例为 NDB。pTuneos 在每个肿瘤中鉴定的候选新抗原的中位数为 74 个(范围为 0~2537),整体新抗原免疫原性评分范围为 0~12.07 分。在所有三个队列中,与新抗原负荷相比,新抗原免疫原性评分能更好地区分出长期受益组和无长期受益组的患者。

接下来,对新抗原负荷、新抗原整体免疫原性评分和微卫星不稳定状态对生存的不同预测能力进行了评估。对于队列 Rizvi 和 Snyder,高新抗原负荷(>中位数)与改善无进展生存(PFS)或总体生存(OS)相关(队列 Rizvi:危险比 $HR=0.32,95\%\ CI\ 0.13\sim0.78,P=0.01$;队列 Snyder: $HR=0.38,95\%\ CI\ 0.17\sim0.85,P=0.01$)。而在队列 Van Allen 中,新抗原负荷与总生存(OS)的改善无关($HR=0.72,95\%\ CI\ 0.48\sim1.08$,logrank $P=0.1$)。在所有三个队列中,与新抗原负荷相比,整体新抗原免疫原性评分显示,患者无进展生存期(PFS)及总体生存期(OS)的曲线分离更为显著(队列 Rizvi: $HR=0.27,95\%\ CI\ 0.11\sim0.69,P=0.006$;队列 Snyder: $HR=0.22,95\%\ CI\ 0.09\sim0.52,P=0.0006$;队列 Van Allen: $HR=0.55,95\%\ CI\ 0.36\sim0.84,P=0.006$)。在包括年龄、性别、总体新抗原负荷、总体新抗原免疫原性评分和微卫星不稳定状态的单变量 Cox 回归和多变量 Cox 回归分析显示,只有整体新抗原免疫原性评分与改善的无进展生存(PFS)或整体生存(OS)相关。提示整体新抗原免疫原性评分可能是更好地预测 ICIs 免疫治疗疗效的生物标志物。

pTuneos 还对 TCGA 癌症组 III/IV 期胃腺癌(STAD; $n=166/441$),III/IV 期肺腺癌(LUAD; $n=101/569$)和 III/IV 期皮肤黑色素瘤(SKCM; $n=191/470$)进行了分析,以探讨整体新抗原免疫原性评分、新抗原负荷、微卫星不稳定性状态(microsatellite instability status,MSI)和若干免疫浸润因素之间的关系。还比较了这些因素的总体生存(Overall Survival,OS)预测能力。结果表明,pTuneos 计算的整体新抗原免疫原性评分可以预测所有三组 TCGA 癌症队列的生存,提示整体新抗原免疫原性评分在各种癌症的生存预测方面有一定的潜力。

pTuneos 通过基于高肽-MHC 结合亲和力获得的推测性新抗原,采用两步筛选和排序策略对新抗原进行优先排序。优点为对对免疫原性进行了评分,这一评分结果被证明可以更好地预测各种肿瘤的生存;缺点是只考虑了基于 SNVs 的新抗原,而未纳入其他类型新抗原的鉴定,如基于基因融合的、RNA 选择性剪接的和 RNA 编辑的新抗原;此外,未考虑 MHC-II 类-肽复合物和膜蛋白的突变。

七、挑 战

从 NGS 数据中预测新表位是一项复杂的任务,这其中涉及到数据解析和生物信息学的许多重要步骤。目前主要是基于肽-MHC 的结合亲和力预测新抗原,但这只是部分地描述了潜在的免疫原性,其他预测免疫原性的参数如相似性、MHC 提呈和 T 细胞识别等,在新抗原预测方面也至关重要。虽然目前开发了许多程序用于新抗原的预测,但还有许多问题需要考虑:①目前所有的预测工具都没有考虑 MHC-II 类分析提呈的新抗原的评估,而这些抗原可能是在肿瘤免疫过程中占据更加重要的地位;②我们使用各种工具预测的新抗原是选择合适药物靶点的重要来源,但还需通过更多的体外实验验证,来判断这些工具的预测能力,并筛选出成为 T 细胞或抗体免疫治疗的药物靶点;③将质谱数据运用到新抗原预测的工具中,以提高可识别出刺激 T 细胞反应的候选新抗原的能力,是重要的研究方向。

参 考 文 献

[1] Lundegaard C, Lund O, Buus S, et al. Major histocompatibility complex class I binding predictions as a tool in epitope discovery. Immunology, 2010, 130(3):309-318.

[2] Lin HH, Ray S, Tongchusak S, et al. Evaluation of MHC class I peptide binding prediction servers: Applications for vaccine research. Bmc Immunol, 2008, 9.

[3] Stratton MR, Campbell PJ, Futreal PA. The cancer genome. Nature, 2009, 458(7239):719-724.

[4] Alexandrov LB, Nik-Zainal S, Wedge DC, et al. Signatures of mutational processes in human cancer. Nature, 2013, 500(7463):415-416.

[5] Schumacher TN, Schreiber RD. Neoantigens in cancer immunotherapy. Science, 2015, 348(6230):69-74.

[6] Vormehr M, Diken M, Boegel S, et al. Mutanome directed cancer immunotherapy. Curr Opin Immunol, 2016, 39:14-22.

[7] Rizvi NA, Hellmann MD, Snyder A, et al. Mutational landscape determines sensitivity to PD-1 blockade in non-small cell lung cancer. Science, 2015, 348(6230):124-128.

[8] McGranahan N, Furness AJS, Rosenthal R, et al. Clonal neoantigens elicit T cell immunoreactivity and sensitivity to immune checkpoint blockade. Science, 2016, 351(6280):1463-1469.

[9] Snyder A, Makarov V, Merghoub T, et al. Genetic Basis for

Clinical Response to CTLA-4 Blockade in Melanoma. New Engl J Med,2014,371(23):2189-2199.
[10] Hugo W,Zaretsky JM,Sun L,et al. Genomic and Transcriptomic Features of Response to Anti-PD-1 Therapy in Metastatic Melanoma. Cell,2016,165(1):35-44.
[11] Sharma P,Allison JP. The future of immune checkpoint therapy. Science,2015,348(6230):56-61.
[12] Van Allen EM,Miao D,Schilling B,et al. Genomic correlates of response to CTLA-4 blockade in metastatic melanoma. Science,2015,350(6257):207-211.
[13] Hundal J,Carreno BM,Petti AA,et al. pVAC-Seq:A genome-guided in silico approach to identify tumor neoantigens for personalized immunotherapy. Cancer Research,2016,76.
[14] Bjerregaard AM,Nielsen M,Hadrup SR,et al. MuPeXI:prediction of neo-epitopes from tumor sequencing data. Cancer Immunol Immun,2017,66(9):1123-1130.
[15] Zhou Z,Lyu XZ,Wu JC,et al. TSNAD:an integrated software for cancer somatic mutation and tumour-specific neoantigen detection. Roy Soc Open Sci,2017,4(4).
[16] Kim S,Kim HS,Kim E,et al. Neopepsee:accurate genome-level prediction of neoantigens by harnessing sequence and amino acid immunogenicity information. Annals of Oncology,2018,29(4):1030-1036.
[17] Zhou C,Wei ZT,Zhang ZB,et al. pTuneos:prioritizing tumor neoantigens from next-generation sequencing data. Genome Med,2019,11(1).
[18] Carreno BM,Magrini V,Becker-Hapak M,et al. Cancer immunotherapy. A dendritic cell vaccine increases the breadth and diversity of melanoma neoantigen-specific T cells. Science,2015,348(6236):803-808.
[19] Nielsen M,Andreatta M. NetMHCpan-3.0:improved prediction of binding to MHC class I molecules integrating information from multiple receptor and peptide length datasets. Genome Med,2016,8(1):33.
[20] McGranahan N,Furness AJ,Rosenthal R,et al. Clonal neoantigens elicit T cell immunoreactivity and sensitivity to immune checkpoint blockade. Science,2016,351(6280):1463-1469.
[21] Bentzen AK,Marquard AM,Lyngaa R,et al. Large-scale detection of antigen-specific T cells using peptide-MHC-I multimers labeled with DNA barcodes. Nat Biotechnol,2016,34(10):1037-1045.
[22] Ilyas S,Yang JC. Landscape of Tumor Antigens in T Cell Immunotherapy. J Immunol,2015,195(11):5117-5122.
[23] Robbins PF,Lu YC,El-Gamil M,et al. Mining exomic sequencing data to identify mutated antigens recognized by adoptively transferred tumor-reactive T cells. Nat Med,2013,19(6):747-748.
[24] Uhlen M,Fagerberg L,Hallstrom BM,et al. Tissue-based map of the human proteome. Science,2015,347(6220).
[25] Sonnhammer EL,von Heijne G,Krogh A. A hidden Markov model for predicting transmembrane helices in protein sequences. Proceedings. International Conference on Intelligent Systems for Molecular Biology,1998,6:175-182.
[26] Li RQ,Yu C,Li YR,et al. SOAP2:an improved ultrafast tool for short read alignment. Bioinformatics,2009,25(15):1966-1967.
[27] Hoof I,Peters B,Sidney J,et al. NetMHCpan,a method for MHC class I binding prediction beyond humans. Immunogenetics,2009,61(1):1-13.
[28] Stranzl T,Larsen MV,Lundegaard C,et al. NetCTLpan:pan-specific MHC class I pathway epitope predictions. Immunogenetics,2010,62(6):357-368.
[29] Calis JJA,Maybeno M,Greenbaum JA,et al. Properties of MHC Class I Presented Peptides That Enhance Immunogenicity. Plos Comput Biol,2013,9(10).
[30] Chowell D,Krishna S,Becker PD,et al. TCR contact residue hydrophobicity is a hallmark of immunogenic CD8(+) T cell epitopes. P Natl Acad Sci USA,2015,112(14):E1754-E1762.
[31] Patronov A,Doytchinova I. T-cell epitope vaccine design by immunoinformatics. Open Biol,2013,3.
[32] Dintzis HM,Dintzis RZ,Vogelstein B. Molecular determinants of immunogenicity:the immunon model of immune response. Proc Natl Acad Sci USA,1976,73(10):3671-3675.
[33] Liu MKP,Hawkins N,Ritchie AJ,et al. Vertical T cell immunodominance and epitope entropy determine HIV-1 escape. J Clin Invest,2013,123(1):380-393.
[34] Duan F,Duitama J,Al Seesi S,et al. Genomic and bioinformatic profiling of mutational neoepitopes reveals new rules to predict anticancer immunogenicity. J Exp Med,2014,211(11):2231-2248.
[35] Saethang T,Hirose O,Kimkong I,et al. PAAQD:Predicting immunogenicity of MHC class I binding peptides using amino acid pairwise contact potentials and quantum topological molecular similarity descriptors. J Immunol Methods,2013,387(1-2):293-302.
[36] Hoof I,Perez CL,Buggert M,et al. Interdisciplinary Analysis of HIV-Specific CD8(+) T Cell Responses against Variant Epitopes Reveals Restricted TCR Promiscuity. J Immunol,2010,184(9):5383-5391.
[37] Brown SD,Warren RL,Gibb EA,et al. Neo-antigens predicted by tumor genome meta-analysis correlate with increased patient survival. Genome research,2014,24(5):743-750.
[38] Rizvi NA,Hellmann MD,Snyder A,et al. Cancer immunology. Mutational landscape determines sensitivity to PD-1 blockade in non-small cell lung cancer. Science,2015,348(6230):124-128.
[39] Gao QS,Liang WW,Foltz SM,et al. Driver Fusions and Their Implications in the Development and Treatment of Human Cancers. Cell Rep,2018,23(1):227-228.
[40] Hoyos LE,Abdel-Wahab O. Cancer-Specific Splicing Changes and the Potential for Splicing-Derived Neoantigens. Cancer Cell,2018,34(2):181-183.
[41] Han L,Diao LX,Yu SX,et al. The Genomic Landscape and Clinical Relevance of A-to-I RNA Editing in Human Cancers. Cancer Cell,2015,28(4).
[42] Peng XX,Xu XY,Wang YM,et al. A-to-I RNA Editing Contributes to Proteomic Diversity in Cancer. Cancer Cell,2018,33(5):817-818.
[43] Karosiene E,Lundegaard C,Lund O,et al. NetMHCcons:a

consensus method for the major histocompatibility complex class I predictions. Immunogenetics,2012,64(3):177-186.

[44] Linnemann C,van Buuren MM,Bies L,et al. High-throughput epitope discovery reveals frequent recognition of neo-antigens by CD4 + T cells in human melanoma. Nat Med, 2015,21(1):81-85.

[45] Kreiter S,Vormehr M,van de Roemer N,et al. Mutant MHC class II epitopes drive therapeutic immune responses to cancer. Nature,2015,520(7549):692.

[46] Bassani-Sternberg M,Braunlein E,Klar R,et al. Direct identification of clinically relevant neoepitopes presented on native human melanoma tissue by mass spectrometry. Nat Commun,2016,7.

[47] Abelin JG,Keskin DB,Sarkizova S,et al. Mass Spectrometry Profiling of HLA-Associated Peptidomes in Mono-allelic Cells Enables More Accurate Epitope Prediction. Immunity, 2017,46(2):315-326.

[48] Malaker SA,Ferracane MJ,Depontieu FR,et al. Identification and Characterization of Complex Glycosylated Peptides Presented by the MHC Class II Processing Pathway in Melanoma. J Proteome Res,2017,16(1):228-237.

6 中国肿瘤专科护士在免疫治疗中的角色功能及作用

潘瑞丽

随着对肿瘤免疫学认识的不断深入,肿瘤免疫治疗在临床应用中取得了飞速发展,尤其是对各种实体瘤的治疗,使晚期肿瘤患者的生存率得到极大提高。护理人员在肿瘤免疫治疗的具体实践中发挥着不可或缺的作用,本文着重阐述了肿瘤专科护士在患者的健康评估、宣教指导、症状管理、随访咨询、心理支持乃至在 MDT 团队中发挥的重要作用,并为肿瘤专科护士在专业领域发展上提出展望和建议。

一、免疫治疗及其临床应用现状

肿瘤免疫治疗是一种旨在激活人体免疫系统,依靠自身免疫功能杀灭癌细胞和肿瘤组织的抗癌疗法,与以往的手术、化疗、放疗、靶向治疗不同,该方法针对的靶标不是肿瘤细胞和组织,而是人体自身的免疫系统。肿瘤免疫治疗分为主动免疫治疗、被动免疫治疗。主动免疫治疗主要包括治疗性肿瘤疫苗,被动免疫治疗包括抗体药物治疗、过继性免疫细胞治疗、细胞因子治疗等。在抗体药物治疗中,目前最受关注且应用最广泛的是免疫检查点抑制剂(immune checkpoint inhibitor,ICI)治疗。免疫检查点本是人体免疫系统中起保护作用的分子,可防止 T 细胞过度激活导致的炎症损伤等。而肿瘤细胞利用人体免疫系统这一特性,通过过度表达免疫检查点分子,抑制人体免疫系统反应,逃脱人体免疫监视与杀伤,从而促进肿瘤细胞的生长。

近10年来肿瘤免疫治疗飞速发展,为肿瘤治疗带来了翻天覆地的变革。2011 年,美国食品药物监督管理局(FDA)批准了免疫调节剂 ipilimumab 用于黑色素瘤的治疗。此后一系列 PD-1(PD-L1)抑制剂,如 nivolumab、pembrolizumab、atezolizumab 获得各国管理机构批准用于黑色素瘤、肾癌、肺癌、淋巴瘤、尿路上皮肿瘤、肝癌等多种实体瘤的治疗,肿瘤免疫治疗进入全面发展时期。

大量的基础研究和临床研究证实,免疫检查点抑制剂对于多种实体瘤有效,相比于化疗和靶向治疗,免疫治疗虽然起效相对缓慢,但可以长期维持有效,明显延长患者生存期,提高患者生活质量。随着研究的不断深入,免疫治疗的应用从初始的 IV 期肿瘤的后线治疗逐渐成为一线治疗,并且近年来逐渐走向局部晚期及早期肿瘤的治疗,在新辅助治疗中,也初步显现了令人鼓舞的效果。

二、免疫治疗应用于临床后对护理需求日益增长

近年来,全球癌症发病率和死亡率不断上升,癌症已成为威胁人类健康的重大疾病之一。据 GLOBOCAN 2018 数据显示:世界癌症标化发病率为 197.9/10 万,标化死亡率为 101.1/10 万,中国癌症标化发病率为 201.7/10 万,标化死亡率为 130.1/10 万。根据中国肿瘤登记最新估计结果显示,2015 年中国新发癌症病例数约 392.91 万,全国平均每天 19770 人,每分钟有 7 人被诊断为癌症。癌症不仅使患者及其家庭承担极重的经济与心理负担,更对政府的医疗体制以及公众的健康带来巨大的挑战,公众对癌症医疗与护理的需求日渐增强。

三、护士在免疫治疗中的作用

肿瘤免疫治疗已经成为继手术治疗、放射治疗和化学药物治疗之后的第四大肿瘤治疗疗法,也是目前最热门的肿瘤治疗手段。在实施免疫治疗的过程中,需要护士对患者进行严格的管理,以提高患者的治疗依从率,延长患者生存期。目前肿瘤患者对免疫治疗尚缺乏了解,鉴于免疫治疗带来的明显疗效,以及其潜在的不良反应和巨大经济负担,对接受免疫治疗的肿瘤患者需要给予极大关注,护士作为肿瘤免疫治疗团队的一员,在免疫治疗全程管理中的作用日益突出。

(一)收集患者资料,评估健康状况

以护理程序为指导的整体护理已在国内广泛开展,而健康评估是护理程序中最重要和最基本的一步。健康评估的内容包括常见症状评估、身体评估、心理评估、社会评估、检查化验结果的评估及对特殊人群的评估。肿瘤专科护士在免疫治疗开始前对患者实施规范化的护理评估和预见性护理干预可有针对性地提供护理措施,满足患者需求。美国肿瘤护理学会(ONS)对于管理和护理化疗和生物治疗的护士的要求是,掌握药物制剂的基本知识,包括作用机制、药理学、管理原则、治疗适应证、预期毒性和不良事件、评估和管理建议等。随着越来越多的免疫治疗药物应用于临床,免疫治疗相关不良反应(Immune-related adverse events,irAEs)的发生引起了人们的重视。它们可

能涉及所有器官系统,胃肠道、皮肤、肝脏和内分泌器官毒性占主导地位。进行免疫治疗前,肿瘤专科护士应首先做好患者病史和基本信息的采集,了解患者在开始免疫治疗之前的基线状态,包括基线体格检查、基本实验室检测结果(如血常规、转氨酶、胆红素、血肌酐、尿素氮、空腹血糖、心肌酶、胰酶、甲状腺功能、肾上腺皮质功能等)、影像学结果(如肿瘤原发灶和转移灶部位等)。了解并熟悉患者基线状态将有助于对比患者免疫治疗开始后的变化,便于在治疗实施的过程中重点观察,Suzanne 在文章中强调,基线健康状况的任何变化,无论多么微妙或看似微不足道,都可能是不良反应的征兆,应立即报告给医生。关注患者的既往史(如是否曾患有自身免疫性疾病、间质性肺病等),及时与主管医生进行沟通,确认免疫治疗能否顺利开始。倾听患者的主诉,了解患者在治疗前的不适症状,询问患者的护理需求,教会患者自我观察,及早发现问题,及时处理,最大限度地降低免疫相关不良反应的发生概率减轻其严重程度。

(二)专科领域的健康教育

健康教育可定义为对患者的培训和咨询。对患者进行健康宣教是护士最重要的能力之一。在肿瘤专科领域,基于化疗教育的健康宣教经验表明,在初始治疗前对患者进行健康宣教,向患者交代治疗的选择和相关的的处理,可以减轻其焦虑情绪。充分的宣教可以使护患之间彼此充分信任,增加患者依从性,有助于患者开诚布公的跟医护人员交流,及时汇报治疗早期出现的不适。大量研究证实,在初始诊断和治疗过程中进行有效的患者教育可以增加自我护理决策,减少不良反应,提高生活质量。对于接受免疫治疗的患者,护士通过对患者持续进行宣教,协助患者及时了解疾病进展情况及治疗效果和可能出现的不良反应,使 irAEs 在早期被识别出来,并得到诊断和处理。

肿瘤专科护士对患者进行知识评估,了解患者的学习程度,识别个别患者的学习障碍,这些将直接影响肿瘤患者毒性管理的成功与否。因此,在进行健康宣教时护士需要考虑到患者的基础知识水平、受教育程度及年龄,了解不同类型患者在学习过程中存在的困难,以此对患者进行分组,进而因材施教,设计不同的方案对患者进行宣教。

(三)治疗实施,及症状管理

多模式治疗计划在临床实践中越来越受欢迎,其中包括免疫治疗、化疗、放疗和(或)其他免疫肿瘤药物。随着免疫治疗药物在单药和多药治疗方案中的应用增加,肿瘤专科护士承担了越来越多的接受免疫治疗患者的护理及管理工作,包括治疗过程中疗效的观察和不良事件的管理和监测。美国肿瘤护理学会(ONS)(2015)建议对免疫治疗药物的使用保持与其他抗肿瘤药物相同的护理和警惕性。

在免疫治疗过程中,护士需要对患者病情进行持续密切地观察。这样可以协助患者及时了解治疗效果、可能出现的不良反应以及疾病进展情况。研究证实如果早期治疗,irAEs 大多是可以控制的,并且不需要停止 ICIs 治疗。根据不良反应的严重程度,患者可能会接受类固醇类药物治疗或暂停 ICIs 治疗,直至症状改善。及时报告潜在的不良反应是有效管理和完成 ICIs 治疗的关键。此外,需要注意的是,护士应了解常见的 irAEs 进行有针对性的症状管理,斑丘疹和瘙痒是与 PD-1 抑制剂治疗相关的最常见的 irAEs,通常最先出现。腹泻和结肠炎是 PD-1 抑制剂治疗中第二常见的 irAEs。在临床试验中,腹泻和结肠炎的发作时间分别为 pembrolizumab3.4 个月,nivolumab5.6 个月。在临床实践中,护士与患者接触最为密切,是发现早期症状的第一人。护士对患者病情的观察主要从以下几个方面着手:①患者的主诉。比如患者在治疗过程中出现胸闷、憋气的主诉,需要警惕 irAEs 的肺和心脏毒性;患者出现腹泻,需要想到 irAEs 累及肠道的可能。②患者的体征。关注患者新发的皮疹、皮肤黏膜的出血点、眼睑脚踝的水肿、呼吸音的改变等等,这些异常体征都可能是 irAEs 早期的线索。③关注患者生化检查的异常,辅助检查的异常可能早于症状的发生,所以需密切关注患者化验检查结果的异常。

(四)心理支持,情感疏导

肿瘤疾病的特殊性及治疗方案的复杂性会在许多方面影响患者及家属,恶性肿瘤患者良好的情绪、面对治疗和生活积极的态度,对疾病转归以及身体康复起着至关重要的作用。肿瘤专科护士具备更专业的知识和技能以更综合、全面的视角来评估和管理患者的身心健康,为患者及家属提供心理支持。美国肿瘤护理协会一直提倡癌症患者的整体护理,其中包括社会心理问题的评估。肿瘤相关心理困扰主要表现为焦虑和抑郁,进而严重影响患者的生存质量,有研究显示,对患者实施个体化心理干预,可以改善肿瘤患者的焦虑和抑郁状态,王培红等报道,心理护理可提高患者的生活质量,因此关注患者的不良情绪,加强心理护理,是提升护理工作水平的重要手段。随访咨询、联络沟通。

肿瘤的治疗是一个长期的过程,护士对肿瘤患者的管理不仅包括院内的护理,更包括其出院后的连续性照护。近年来,护士随访的患者数目不断增多,研究指出,患者更愿意接受护士的随访,他们认为护士比起医生更容易亲近和沟通,愿意倾诉更多情绪问题。现有研究证实,以护士为主导的电话随访能显著提高患者的服药依从率、提高治疗依从性,帮助患者解决实际存在的问题,Carper 等研究发现,肿瘤专科护士在随访中可以承担着评估治疗的远期疗效和随访获取肿瘤复发信息等工作。随着经济水平的不断提高,近年来出现了多种新型的随访方式如 QQ、微信的随访、信息平台的随访以及随访 APP 等,与传统的随访方式相比,上述形式增加了交流的丰富性,降低了经济成本,提高了患者随访的依从性,以及治疗的满意度。对于接受肿瘤免疫治疗的患者,护士的随访内容应涉及提醒服药、自身锻炼、心理辅导、生活方式指导、复诊提醒。护士应密切关注出院后患者出现的症状及体征。Champiat 等研究发现,irAEs 可发生在免疫治疗过程的各个时间点,甚至可能在停药后出现。如使用 ipilimumab 治疗黑色素瘤的患者中,免疫相关性肝炎的发生时间在 1~23 周不等。此外,肿瘤专科护士应了解免疫治疗不良反应的分级,有助于决定何时通知临床医生,共同决策是否需要进行不良反应的干预,根据严重程度告知患者是否及时返院接受治疗以及是否停止免疫治疗。

(五)多学科协作团队中的协调枢纽

多学科协作团队(muli-disciplinary team,MDT)是以患者为中心,依托团队成员紧密协作,制订规范化、个体化、连续性的综合治疗方案。由于接受免疫治疗的肿瘤患者常涉及多学科的问题,单一学科治疗无法满足患者阶段性治疗的需求,单纯的治疗手段也无法给患者提供全方位的治疗策略。MDT可以最大限度发挥多学科的优势,为肿瘤患者提供合理优化的治疗方案,有利于提高治疗规范率及患者的依从性和满意率,使患者得到最适宜的治疗。在这个包括不同专科的临床医生、护士、心理治疗师、物理治疗师、职业治疗师、营养师、药剂师、社工和义工等人的团队中,护士是重要的组成部分,负责为团队中其他成员提供患者及其家属的新动态,协助患者决策,计划与安排多学科综合小组的会议,共同以循证原则进行证据的探索与使用等,在MDT综合医疗模式中发挥着协调枢纽的作用。

(六)开展科学研究,推动专科发展

专业学科的发展离不开科研创新及临床实践,护士作为肿瘤免疫治疗团队的一员,与患者接触最为紧密,可根据接受治疗的患者在治疗及随访过程中需要解决的问题及需求展开科学研究,为肿瘤患者提供最佳循证实践。护理科研来源于临床,又可将科研成果应用于临床,促进肿瘤专科护理的发展。

四、展望和建议

近年来,当护理工作中出现障碍如健康指导的困难、交流不良、误导、担忧、焦虑及资源缺乏时,肿瘤导航护士(ONN)应运而生,美国医疗体系内就提出了护士领航员的概念,扩大了肿瘤专科护士的工作范畴并开发了新的服务。肿瘤导航护士在对患者进行身体和心理护理的基础上,帮助面对大量的临床信息和数据资料的患者及家属,对检查和治疗的复杂情况做出决定。护士通过协调服务,为患者和家属提供指导和支持,患者满意度得到提高。随着免疫治疗应用于临床,越来越多的研究着眼于免疫联合治疗方案,使得肿瘤治疗变得越来越复杂,我国的免疫治疗还处于起步阶段,在肿瘤免疫治疗的发展道路上,需要增强我国护理人员特别是肿瘤专科护士在免疫治疗护理及免疫相关不良反应的管理能力,可引入护士领航员的角色,以满足不同医疗服务的需求。

2017年Cancer Support Community(CSC)对95名接受ICIs治疗的患者及其45名护理人员进行了需求评估。大多数患者(55%)和护理人员(85%)认为了解如何应对ICI症状和不良反应非常重要,而许多患者(50%)和护理人员(73%)报告难以获得这些信息。鉴于护理人员在肿瘤免疫治疗专业领域中的重要角色和职能,其专业能力及素养的培养应引起护理管理者的重视。护士要为免疫治疗患者提供最佳的护理,需要不断进行相关知识的更新、补充、拓展和提高。相对于学校系统性的学习课程,继续教育项目可根据目前政策导向、社会需求、学员需求及服务对象需求制定针对性、系统性的培训课程,并邀请国内外专家授课,达到传播新理论、新知识、新技术、新方法的目的,是一种护理人员终身教育的形式,可使护理人员在整个职业生涯中,不断提高专业工作能力和业务水平,提高专科护理服务质量。

五、小 结

随着免疫治疗的不断普及,肿瘤专科护士在接受免疫治疗患者的长期管理过程中的作用日趋重要。在我国,肿瘤专科护士的工作已具备良好的基础,在患者的健康评估、宣教指导、症状管理、随访咨询,以及整个MDT团队中都发挥着重要作用,但未来专科发展之路任重道远,需要医务人员共同努力。作为护理人员,应不断完善自身在肿瘤免疫治疗中的作用和职能,使广大肿瘤患者及家属受益,逐步推动专科领域的发展。

参 考 文 献

[1] Oiseth S J,Aziz M S. Cancer immunotherapy: a brief review of the history, possibilities, and challenges ahead Journal of Cancer Metastasis and Treatment,2017,3(10): 250-261.

[2] Park J,Kwon M,Shin E. Immune checkpoint inhibitors for cancer treatment,2016,39,1577-1587.

[3] Patel SP,Woodman SE. Profile of ipilimumab and its role in the treatment of metastatic melanoma. Drug Des Devel Ther, 2011,5: 489-495.

[4] Park J,Kwon M,Shin E. Immune checkpoint inhibitors for cancer treatment, 2016,39,1577-1587.

[5] Gobbini E,Giaj LM. Is there a room for immune checkpoint inhibitors in early stage non-small cell lung cancer?. J Thorac Dis,2018,10(Suppl 13): S1427-S1437.

[6] Bray F,Ferlay J,Soerjomataram I,et al. Global cancer statistics 2018: GLOBOCAN estimates of incidence and mortality worldwide for 36 cancers in 185 countries. CA Cancer J Clin, 2018,68(6): 394-424.

[7] 孙可欣,郑荣寿,张思维,等.2015年中国分地区恶性肿瘤发病和死亡分析.中国肿瘤,2019,28(01): 1-11.

[8] 郑荣寿,孙可欣,张思维,等.2015年中国恶性肿瘤流行情况分析.中华肿瘤杂志,2019(01): 19-28.

[9] Ledezma B,Heng A. Real-world impact of education: treating patients with ipilimumab in a community practice setting. Cancer Manag Res,2013,6: 5-14.

[10] Madden K M,Hoffner B. Ipilimumab-Based Therapy: Consensus Statement From the Faculty of the Melanoma Nursing Initiative on Managing Adverse Events With Ipilimumab Monotherapy and Combination Therapy With Nivolumab.

Clin J Oncol Nurs,2017,21(4 Suppl):30-41.

[11] Mcgettigan S,Rubin KM. PD-1 Inhibitor Therapy: Consensus Statement From the Faculty of the Melanoma Nursing Initiative on Managing Adverse Events. Clin J Oncol Nurs,2017,21(4 Suppl): 42-51.

[12] Strupeit S,Buss A,Dassen T. Effectiveness of nurse-delivered patient education interventions on quality of life in outpatients: a systematic review. Appl Nurs Res,2013,26(4): 232-238.

[13] Lambert K. Art and science of designing patient education material for the 21st century. Nutr Diet,2019,76(4): 493-495.

[14] Valenti RB. Chemotherapy education for patients with cancer: a literature review. Clin J Oncol Nurs,2014,18(6): 637-640.

[15] Shahsavari H,Matory P,Zare Z,et al. Effect of self-care education on the quality of life in patients with breast cancer. J Educ Health Promot,2015,4: 70.

[16] Tian J,Jia LN,Cheng ZC. Relationships between patient knowledge and the severity of side effects,daily nutrient intake,psychological status,and performance status in lung cancer patients. Curr Oncol,2015,22(4): e254-e258.

[17] Wood LS,Moldawer NP,Lewis C. Immune Checkpoint Inhibitor Therapy: Key Principles When Educating Patients. 2019,23,271-280.

[18] Drake CG. Combination immunotherapy approaches. Ann Oncol,2012,23 Suppl 8: i41-i46.

[19] Programmed Death-1 Inhibition in Cancer With a Focus on Non-Small Cell Lung Cancer: Rationale, Nursing Implications, and Patient Management Strategies. Clin J Oncol Nurs,2016,20(3): 319-326.

[20] Dadu R,Zobniw C,Diab A. Managing Adverse Events With Immune Checkpoint Agents. Cancer J,2016,22(2): 121-129.

[21] Friedman CF,Proverbs-Singh TA,Postow MA. Treatment of the Immune-Related Adverse Effects of Immune Checkpoint Inhibitors: A Review. JAMA Oncol,2016,2(10): 1346-1353.

[22] Larkin J,Chiarion-Sileni V,Gonzalez R,et al. Combined Nivolumab and Ipilimumab or Monotherapy in Untreated Melanoma. N Engl J Med,2015,373(1): 23-34.

[23] Robert C,Long GV,Brady B,et al. Nivolumab in previously untreated melanoma without BRAF mutation. N Engl J Med,2015,372(4): 320-330.

[24] Sheldon LK,Harris D,Arcieri C. Psychosocial concerns in cancer care: the role of the oncology nurse. Clin J Oncol Nurs,2012,16(3): 316-319.

[25] 崔桂琴,潘骥群.个体化心理干预结合姑息护理对晚期肿瘤患者心理状态和生活质量的影响.解放军护理杂志,2017,34(20): 16-20.

[26] 王培红,姚玲,吴五矛.护理干预对妇科肿瘤患者生活质量的影响.解放军护理杂志,2007(02): 74-75.

[27] 商丽艳.肿瘤专科护士角色与工作内容的研究.第二军医大学,2014.

[28] Lewis R,Neal RD,Williams NH,et al. Nurse-led vs. conventional physician-led follow-up for patients with cancer: systematic review. J Adv Nurs,2009,65(4): 706-723.

[29] 朱叶卉,胡雁,吴密彬,等.电话随访对乳腺癌患者服药依从性和生活质量的影响.中华护理杂志,2015,50(01): 69-73.

[30] 孟晓静,丰荣.电话随访专科化管理在肿瘤患者化疗间歇期中的应用与效果分析.中国实用护理杂志,2016,32(26): 2049-2053.

[31] Carper E,Haas M. Advanced practice nursing in radiation oncology. Semin Oncol Nurs,2006,22(4): 203-211.

[32] 张京慧,李靖宇,胡僖苹,等.肺癌出院患者QQ群随访模式的建立与评价.中国现代医学杂志,2012,22(34): 106-108.

[33] 杨晓晴,张兰凤,岳增军,等.肿瘤患者出院延续性护理信息平台的构建与应用.中国护理管理,2014,14(12): 1324-1326.

[34] 金爱山,韩爽,申展.肿瘤患者随访信息平台建设与应用.医学信息学杂志,2012,33(03): 25-27.

[35] 陈海珍,陈建国,张兰凤,等.肿瘤随访现状与进展.中华疾病控制杂志,2015,19(05): 517-523.

[36] Champiat S,Lambotte O,Barreau E,et al. Management of immune checkpoint blockade dysimmune toxicities: a collaborative position paper. Ann Oncol,2016,27(4): 559-574.

[37] Eigentler TK,Hassel JC,Berking C,et al. Diagnosis,monitoring and management of immune-related adverse drug reactions of anti-PD-1 antibody therapy. Cancer Treat Rev,2016,45: 7-18.

[38] Rubin KM,Hoffner B,Bullock AC. Caring for Patients Treated With Checkpoint Inhibitors for the Treatment of Metastatic Merkel Cell Carcinoma[J]. Semin Oncol Nurs,2019,35(5): 150924.

[39] 沈鸣雁,卢芳燕,王仁芳,等.针对胰腺癌患者的多学科专业化护理实践与成效.中华护理杂志,2016,51(05): 542-546.

[40] 闫虹,姜燕平,刘建琴,等.专科护士参与"肿瘤多学科联合会诊"的管理探讨.标记免疫分析与临床,2014,21(5): 618-620.

[41] Sheldon LK,Harris D,Arcieri C. Psychosocial concerns in cancer care: the role of the oncology nurse. Clin J Oncol Nurs,2012,16(3): 316-319.

[42] Brown CG,Cantril C,Mcmullen L,et al. Oncology nurse navigator role delineation study: an oncology nursing society report. Clin J Oncol Nurs,2012,16(6): 581-585.

[43] Wood LS,Moldawer NP,Lewis C. Immune Checkpoint Inhibitor Therapy: Key Principles When Educating Patients. Clin J Oncol Nurs,2019,23(3): 271-280.

[44] 鲍银月,樊洁,王亚军,等.重视继续医学教育、规范继续教育项目管理模式.中国医刊,2015,50(8): 18-20.

7 人工智能病理诊断系统在肺癌诊断及预后判断中的应用

王华南　崔节伟　王　娟　梁志欣

肺癌是目前世界上发病率和死亡率最高的恶性肿瘤，严重危害人类身心健康。目前，肺癌的病理诊断主要依赖于人工病理切片分析，人工阅片效率低且具有一定的主观性，会导致一定的误诊率和漏诊率。近年来，随着人工智能和数字病理学的发展，人工智能在肺癌病理诊断中的巨大应用前景逐渐显现，人工智能可以在短时间内整合大量信息并进行分析，有效提高肺癌的诊断效率，在预测肺癌的突变基因方面也有相关研究报道，从而成为病理学家的有力辅助诊断工具。本文主要针对人工智能病理诊断系统在肺癌的细胞病理诊断、组织病理诊断及突变基因预测中的应用进展进行综述。

2018年全球癌症统计结果显示，肺癌患者占恶性肿瘤总人数的11.6%，死亡人数占所有恶性肿瘤致死人数的18.4%。诊断恶性肿瘤的金标准是病理诊断，传统病理诊断需要病理医师在显微镜下逐个分析病理切片，其诊断结果具有一定的主观性，诊断准确性与病理医师的水平直接相关；同时由于环境污染、人口老龄化等多种因素的影响，肿瘤患者日益增多，病理医师的负担越来越重，疲劳阅片现象经常发生，导致一定的误诊率和漏诊率。如何及时、高效、准确地诊断肺癌，是关乎肺癌患者下一步治疗及预后判断的关键一步。近年来，随着人工智能和数字病理学的发展，医学界越来越认识到人工智能在辅助病理诊断中具有的重大临床及科研价值。人工智能在肺癌病理诊断的应用已成为当前研究热点。本文主要对人工智能在肺癌病理诊断中的应用进展进行综述。

一、人工智能病理诊断系统概述

2016年"阿尔法狗（AlphaGo）"以4:1击败职业围棋九段选手李世石（Lee Sedol），引起人们对人工智能（artificial intelligence，AI）的广泛关注。人工智能是研发用于模拟人类大脑学习并延伸人类能力的新型智能技术。人工智能的核心是机器学习，而深度学习（deep learning，DL）是机器学习的一个分支。深度学习技术目前被认为是用于图像分析的最先进技术。最常用的深度学习模型是卷积神经网络（convolutional neural network，CNN），CNN从90年代开始应用于图像分析，是一种特别适用于解决图像分类问题的监督学习算法。

近年来兴起的数字病理学（digital pathology，DP），旨在用全切片扫描仪对病理切片进行数字化，以及对这些数字化的全切片图像进行分析，其核心技术是全切片成像（whole slide imaging，WSI）技术。2017年FDA批准飞利浦全切片扫描仪进入市场用于病理切片的数字化，标志着迈向真正数字化病理道路上的一个重大转折点。随着大数据技术、数字病理学的发展，以深度学习技术为代表的人工智能，已成功应用于病理图像识别，以辅助医学诊断，并表现出巨大的发展潜力。人工智能和数字病理学的组合，称为人工智能病理诊断系统，国内有人将其称为"病理狗"，它将改变病理诊断专家的工作方式，使广大患者受益，成为"病理学的第三次革命"。在某些情况下，基于深度学习的人工智能在病理学图像的识别方面已经超过了经验丰富的病理学家。人工智能病理诊断系统的应用，已经有了许多成功的案例。例如，Xu等开发了一个深层卷积神经网络（deep convolutional neural network，DCNN），对乳腺癌及大肠癌组织病理学图像中的上皮和间质区域进行分割和分类。Litjens等研究了组织病理学检查的深度学习效果，并验证了其在前列腺癌识别和乳腺癌转移检测中的出色表现。Ertosun和Rubin提出了一种使用深度学习的自动分级胶质瘤系统。

二、人工智能病理诊断系统在肺癌诊断中的应用进展

病理诊断分为细胞病理诊断和组织病理诊断，人工智能病理诊断系统在肺癌的细胞病理及组织病理诊断中均有应用的研究报道。

（一）人工智能细胞病理诊断系统在肺癌诊断中的应用

细胞病理学是研究组织碎片、细胞群团、单个细胞的形态和结构及细胞间比邻关系并探讨组织来源的一门科学。在肺癌诊断中，细胞病理学取材简便、快速，可用于肺癌的筛查或普查，在痰液、支气管刷片及冲洗液中可以查找到肺部病变的癌前病变细胞或者癌细胞，为肺癌的早期诊断和早期治疗提供有力的依据。目前，已有人工智能细胞病理诊断系统应用于肺癌分类诊断的研究。

Teramoto等使用深层卷积神经网络（DCNN）开发了微观图像中的肺癌细胞病理自动分类模型，这是一种主要的深度学习技术。用于分类的DCNN由3个卷积层、3个池化层和2个全连接层组成。在进行的评估实验中，研究者使用原始数据库和图形处理单元对DCNN进行了训练。

他们首先将显微图像裁剪并重新采样,获得分辨率为256×256像素的图像,为了防止过度拟合,又通过旋转、翻转和过滤对收集的图像进行增强,并利用三重交叉验证评估了其分类准确性。在获得的结果中,腺癌、鳞状细胞癌和小细胞癌的分类诊断准确率分别为89.0%、60.0%和70.3%,总准确率为71.1%,这与病理学家的诊断准确率相当。因此,作者表示,他们的方法有助于辅助细胞学检查在肺癌诊断中的应用。另一项研究,Teramoto等开发了一种使用生成对抗网络(generative adversarial networks,GAN)自动生成细胞学图像的方法,目标是通过使用实际的和合成的细胞学图像及生成对抗网络来提高DCNN的分类准确率。该研究从原始显微图像中分割出补丁图像,并使用GAN及渐进生长的GANs(PGGAN)生成高分辨率图像,研究者用这些图像预先训练一个DCNN,并利用训练过的DCNN对良、恶性细胞的分类性能进行了评估。结果显示,他们对肺细胞的总体分类准确率为85.3%,与之前未使用GAN生成的图像进行预训练的研究相比,准确率提高了约4.3%。这些结果证实他们提出的方法在仅获得有限数据的情况下对于细胞学图像的分类是有效的。Zhang等在"肺癌早期诊断立体定位仪"的基础上,研制了基于图像处理和人工神经网络的"肺癌早期细胞病理电脑诊断系统"(lung cancer diagnosing system,LCDS)。该研究选取512例经皮肺穿刺标本涂片,经LCDS检测判定为肺癌者389例,判定为正常细胞者36例,判定为核异型细胞者87例,该系统与病理专家的细胞病理诊断结果相比,470例符合,诊断总符合率达91.8%。接受手术治疗的362例中有307例术后病理确诊为肺癌,以术后组织病理诊断为标准,LCDS对肺癌检测诊断的敏感度为94.79%(291/307例),特异度为90.91%(50/55例),诊断准确性达94.20%(341/362例)。

以上研究表明,人工智能细胞病理诊断系统可以对肺癌细胞进行分类,且其诊断准确率与病理学家的诊断准确率相当,这将大大节约病理学家的时间,减轻病理医师工作负担,有效提高肺癌细胞病理学诊断效率,使病理学家集中精力研究疑难病例。

(二)人工智能组织病理诊断系统在肺癌诊断中的应用

组织病理学检查即活体组织检查,简称活检,是指用局部切取、钳取、穿刺、搔刮和摘取等手术方法,从活体内获取病理组织进行病理检测的诊断方法。组织病理学检查是目前广为采用的诊断方法,对肿瘤良、恶性的鉴别具有确诊价值。腺癌和鳞状细胞癌是肺癌最常见的亚型,病理学切片的目测检查是目前病理学家评估肺部肿瘤分期和亚型的主要方法之一,人工阅片效率低,易出现疲劳阅片现象,人工智能组织病理诊断系统的应用,大大提升了肺癌的诊断效率。

在肺癌组织病理诊断中,已经证明人工智能可以对肺癌亚型准确分类,并能预测非小细胞肺癌患者的生存预后。Kun-Hsing Yu及其同事使用了来自癌症基因组图谱(the cancer genome atlas,TCGA)的2 186张肺腺癌和鳞状细胞癌患者的组织切片的全扫描图像和来自斯坦福组织芯片(tissue microarray,TMA)数据库的294张图像进行验证。他们使用图像分析软件提取了9 879个用于预测结果的形态学图像特征,用机器学习软件评估了这些图像,并开发了可以识别肿瘤细胞的分类器,以区分腺癌和鳞状细胞癌,并预测生存期。结果显示,分类器能够有效地区分恶性肿瘤和相邻健康组织(AUC=0.81),并且能够区分两种不同类型的非小细胞肺癌(non-small cell lung cancer,NSCLC)(AUC>0.75)。此外,它也能准确预测Ⅰ期腺癌(log-rank检验,$P=0.0023$)和鳞状细胞癌(log-rank检验,$P=0.023$)的长期生存。目前,传统的病理方法尚无法确定哪些Ⅰ期NSCLC患者在手术后可能复发,而人工智能机器学习模型可以成功辅助预测。Luo等基于形态学特征开发了一个统计模型来预测肺癌患者的生存,他们从癌症基因组图谱数据集中下载523例肺腺癌和511例鳞状细胞癌患者的病理图像,提取了943个特征,运用此模型进行分析。预测模型是从训练集开发的,并分别在独立的肺腺癌和鳞状细胞癌的测试集中进行了验证。结果表明,基于数字病理成像的人工智能可以预测肺癌患者的预后。Coudray等对从癌症基因组图谱获得的全部切片图像训练出了一个深层卷积神经网络,该网络可以准确自动地将肺组织病理图像分类为腺癌、鳞状细胞癌和正常肺组织,其结果与病理学家的分析结果一致,平均曲线下面积(AUC)为0.97。他们的模型在冷冻组织、福尔马林固定石蜡包埋组织和活检组织的独立数据集上得到了验证。以上研究显示,人工智能通过对数字病理组织切片的分析,可以帮助病理学家迅速判断肺癌类型,并预测患者的预后,显著提高了肺癌的诊断效率,明显减少了误诊率及漏诊率,大幅减轻了病理工作者的工作负担。

(三)人工智能组织病理诊断系统在预测肺癌突变基因中的应用

目前,用于疾病诊断的基因突变检测较少。2015年美国甲状腺协会发布的关于甲状腺结节分子谱在外科手术中的应用的声明指出,BRAF-V600E突变对于甲状腺乳头状癌的诊断具有关键作用,术前细针穿刺细胞学标本进行基因诊断可用于甲状腺结节良恶性的鉴别,有研究报道,BRAF-V600E基因检测判断甲状腺良、恶性结节的敏感度和特异度分别为72.6%和100%。而对于包括肺癌的大多数癌症,基因检测目前大多仍限于疾病的靶向治疗或预后判断。

目前,已有针对肺癌特定基因突变的多种靶向药物问世,对于伴有基因突变的肺癌患者,可以使用具有针对性的靶向药物对基因进行阻断,以控制肿瘤继续增长,因此基因突变的检测是当今肺癌常规且重要的治疗及判断预后的方法之一。已有研究证明,人工智能可以帮助检测肺癌突变基因。Coudray等推测某些基因突变会改变全切片图像上肺癌肿瘤细胞的排布,因而他们对腺癌中最常见的10个突变基因通过训练神经网络进行了预测,结果发现其中的6个(STK11、EGFR、FAT1、SETBP1、KRAS、TP53)可以通过病理图像进行预测,其准确率为73.3%~85.6%。该发现表明深度学习模型可以帮助病理学家快速检测肺癌突变基因。另外一项研究,Wang等选取南京军区总医院病理科50例肺腺癌病理切片,其中包含表皮生长因子受体(epidermal growth factor receptor,EGFR)基因突变21例和EGFR基因未突变29例,运用条件生成对抗网络(conditional generative adversarial networks,CGAN)分割癌变上皮组织内的细胞核,构建有效的病理组学特征以描述肺部肿瘤,从而运用支持向量机(support vector machine,SVM)分类器构建EGFR基因突变风险预测模型。实验结果表明,他们构建的EGFR基因突变风险预测模型的曲线下面积(AUC)在测试集上可达72.4%,准确率为70.8%,提示EGFR基因突变与肺腺癌全扫描组织病理图像中的组织形态学特征密切相关,证明了从全扫描组织病理图像中预测EGFR基因突变的可行性。这些研究说明,人工智能组织病理诊断系统有可能帮助病理学家快速检测肺癌突变基因,便于指导患者尽早开始靶向药物治疗,以提高治疗效果,改善患者预后。

目前,指导肺癌靶向治疗的基因检测大多依赖于组织活检标本,相对于传统组织病理学,液体活检是一类新兴的病理检测技术。液体活检以血液、尿液、痰液等液体样本中的肿瘤循环细胞(circulating tumor cell,CTC)、肿瘤循环DNA(circulating tumor DNA,ctDNA)、小RNA(microRNA,miRNA)以及外泌体(exosome)等为检测目标,通过荧光原位杂交(fluorescence in situ hybridization,FISH)、二代测序(next generation sequencing,NGS)等技术获取肿瘤基因突变等相关信息,以指导临床治疗和预后判断,液体活检技术由于其无创、取材方便、操作风险低及避免局部取样偏差从而获取肿瘤组织的全面信息等优势成为当前研究热点。随着人工智能的发展及拉曼光谱等新兴检测技术的进步,人工智能病理诊断系统在液体活检中的应用将会大大提高肺癌基因检测的准确率和效率。

三、人工智能在肺癌病理诊断的局限性和未来展望

人工智能病理诊断系统在肺癌中的应用,不但提高了病理工作者的工作效率,且具有良好的稳定性,能发现人肉眼、镜下不易察觉的细节,有效降低了漏诊率及误诊率。然而现阶段人工智能病理诊断进展大多还停留在实验室研究阶段,未能真正进入临床,其局限性表现在:①数据质量问题。目前,标本处理、切片染色及图像标注尚未形成标准化流程,用于人工智能训练的数据量不足,影响诊断的可靠性;②数据整合问题。目前,人工智能模型的数据主要来源于病理切片,而没有结合患者的症状、体征及其他检查化验结果等信息,削弱了诊断的准确性;③法律责任界定问题。单独应用人工智能发生医疗错误时责任的界定亟待相关法律法规的出台。

目前,虽然大多数人工智能在肺癌病理学方面的研究仍然集中在肿瘤的检测和分级上。然而,随着人工智能及数字病理技术的进步,人工智能在肺癌病理诊断领域中的应用,正逐步扩展至与临床特征密切结合的疾病严重程度评估和预后预测方面,同时在新兴的液体活检相关技术领域也具有巨大发展前景。而且随着越来越多的经验丰富的病理学家们参与到人工智能的肺癌病理图像标注工作中,我们相信,整合临床数据、遗传数据和形态数据的人工智能病理诊断系统在肺癌的精准病理诊断中将发挥更大的应用价值。

参 考 文 献

[1] Bray F, Ferlay J, Soerjomataram I, et al. Global cancer statistics 2018: GLOBOCAN estimates of incidence and mortality worldwide for 36 cancers in 185 countries. CA Cancer J Clin, 2018, 68(6): 394-424.

[2] Gurcan MN, Boucheron LE, Can A, et al. Histopathological image analysis: a review. IEEE Rev Biomed Eng, 2009, 2: 147-171.

[3] WebsterJD, DunstanRW. Whole-slide imaging and automated image analysis: considerations and opportunities in the practice of pathology. Vet Pathol, 2014, 51(1): 211-223.

[4] Silver D, Huang A, Maddison CJ, et al. Mastering the game of go with deep neural networks and tree search. Nature, 2016, 529(7587): 484-489.

[5] Russakovsky O, Deng J, Su H, et al. Imagenet large scale visual recognition challenge. Int J Comput Vis, 2015, 115(3): 211-252.

[6] FDA. Press Announcements-FDA allows marketing of first whole slide imaging system for digital pathology. 2017. https://www.fda.gov/news-events/press-announcements/fda-allows-marketing-first-whole-slide-imaging-system-digital-pathology.

[7] Hamilton PW, Bankhead P, Wang Y, et al. Digital pathology and image analysis in tissue biomarker research. Methods, 2014, 70(1): 59-73.

[8] 许燕,汤烨,闫雯,等.病理人工智能的现状和展望.中华病理学杂志,2017,46(9):593-595.

[9] Salto-Tellez M, Maxwell P, Hamilton P. Artificial intelligence-The third revolution in pathology. Histopathology, 2019, 74(3): 372-376.

[10] Xu J, Luo X, Wang G, et al. A Deep Convolutional Neural Network forsegmenting and classifying epithelial and stromal regions in histopathological images. Neurocomputing, 2016, 191: 214-223.

[11] Litjens G, Sanchez C I, Timofeeva N, et al. Deep learning as a tool for increased accuracy and efficiency of histopathological diagnosis. Scientific Reports, 2016, 6: 26286.

[12] Ertosun MG, Rubin DL. Automated grading of gliomas using deep learning in digital pathology images: A modular approach with ensemble of convolutional neural networks. AMIA AnnuSymp proc, 2015, 2015: 1899-1908.

[13] Teramoto A, Tsukamoto T, Kiriyama Y, et al. Automated classification of lung cancer types from cytological images using deep convolutional neural networks. BioMed Res Int, 2017, 2017: 4067832.

[14] Teramoto A, Tsukamoto T, Yamada A, et al. Deep learning approach to classification of lung cytological images: Two-step training using actual and synthesized images by progressive growing of generative adversarial networks. PLoS ONE, 2020, 15(3): e0229951.

[15] 张缨, 叶玉坤, 汪栋, 等. 图像处理和人工神经网络在肺癌细胞病理诊断中的应用. 中华胸心血管外科杂志, 2005, 21(4): 238-240.

[16] Yu KH, Zhang C, Berry GJ, et al. Predicting non-small cell lung cancer prognosis by fully automated microscopic pathology image features. Nat Commun, 2016, 7: 12474.

[17] Luo X, Zang X, Yang L, et al. Comprehensive computational pathological image analysis predicts lung cancer prognosis. J Thorac Oncol, 2017, 12(3): 501-509.

[18] Coudray N, Ocampo PS, Sakellaropoulos T, et al. Classification and mutation prediction from non-small cell lung cancer histopathology images using deep learning. Nat Med, 2018, 24(10): 1559-1567.

[19] Ferris R L, Baloch Z, Bernet V, et al. American Thyroid Association statement on surgical application of molecular profiling for thyroid nodules: current impact on perioperative decision making. Thyroid, 2015, 25(7): 760-768.

[20] 李晓锋, 刘希, 汪园园, 等. BRAF-V600E 突变检测在 B 超引导下甲状腺细针穿刺标本中的应用及意义. 临床与病理杂志, 2020, 40(2): 381-387.

[21] Chan BA, Hughes BG. Targeted therapy for non-small cell lung cancer: current standards and the promise of the future. Transl Lung Cancer Res, 2015, 4(1): 36-54.

[22] Junttila MR, de Sauvage FJ. Influence of tumourmicroenvironment heterogeneity on therapeutic response. Nature, 2013, 501(7467): 346-354.

[23] 王荃, 沈勤, 张泽林, 等. 基于深度学习和组织形态分析的肺癌基因突变预测. 生物医学工程学杂志, 2020, 37(1): 10-18.

[24] Isola P, Zhu J, Zhou T, et al. Image-to-image translation with conditional adversarial networks. IEEE Conference on Computer Vision and Pattern Recognition (CVPR 2017), 2017: 5967-5976.

[25] Furey TS, Cristianini N, Duffy N, et al. Support vector machine classification and validation of cancer tissue samples using microarray expression data. Bioinformatics, 2000, 16(10): 906-914.

8 雾霾与肺癌

王 平

雾霾与肺癌的关系已被广泛关注与讨论。肺癌的发生是环境因素与宿主因素共同作用的结果，虽然目前尚没有明确的证据证明雾霾与肺癌的因果关系，但从目前现有的研究结果看雾霾可能作为一个重要的环境因素与肺癌的发生发展关系密切。

一、雾霾与全球疾病负担

2017年全球疾病负担调查显示：肺癌死亡人数为188万人，相比于2007年增加了29.6%。肺癌死亡人群中有18.6%，约35万人死于环境与职业暴露因素中空气污染所致的肺癌。

二、雾霾的定义

雾霾是一种自然现象，是人为因素与自然因素共同作用的结果。雾霾的成因既包括扬尘、海盐、植物花粉、火山爆发引起的火山灰等因素，也包括工业污染与生活污染形成的人为因素，特别需要注意的是各种污染物间接通过核反应、凝聚而成的二次污染物对人体健康的危害更大。

污染物颗粒根据大小不同而命名。PM10是指环境空气中，空气动力学当量直径≤$10\mu m$的颗粒物，也称为可吸入颗粒物。PM2.5是指环境空气中空气动力学当量直径≤$2.5\mu m$的颗粒物，也称为可入肺颗粒物。各级颗粒物成分复杂，既有细菌、真菌，也包括烟草成分，灰尘等。

三、雾霾与肺癌的关系

一项前瞻性研究评价了空气污染中PM10的增加与患者入院的相关关系，研究结果显示：当PM10增加到$150\mu g/m^3$时，儿童住院率增加300%，成人住院率增加了44%。另外一项ESCAPE研究，评价了欧洲国家PM2.5与肺癌的相关关系，平均观察12.8年后，共有2095例患者发生了肺癌，研究结果显示：PM10每增加$10\mu g/m^3$，患者发生肺癌的相对危险度（HR）为1.22（95% CI 1.03～1.45）。ESCAPE的后续研究中继续评价了空气污染物成分（铜、铁、锌、硫、镍、钒、硅、钾）与肺癌发生的相关关系，研究结果显示：PM2.5-铜/PM10-铜，PM2.5-铁/PM10-铁，PM2.5-硫和PM10-镍与肺癌的发生呈正相关。AH-SMOG-2研究中评价了不吸烟患者中PM2.5与肺癌的相关关系，在80285例不吸烟或已经戒烟的患者中，平均观察7.5年后，共有250例患者发生了肺癌，在不吸烟/已戒烟的患者中发生肺癌的风险因素不仅与患者的年龄、既往吸烟史、戒烟时间、既往吸烟量有关，同时还与患者的每日户外暴露时间，以及在当地的居住时间显著相关。Johanna等研究评价了哈佛地区6城市空气污染与疾病的相关关系，随访35年后，结果显示：PM2.5每增加$10\mu g/m^3$，全因死亡风险增加14%（95% CI：7%～22%），心血管疾病死亡风险增加26%（95% CI：14%～40%），肺癌死亡风险增加37%（95% CI：7%～75%）。

2017年全球健康数据统计中，我国女性寿命约为79.9岁，男性约为74.5岁，导致我国患者死亡最多的疾病是脑卒中，而肺癌所致的死亡已经从2007年的第五位上升为第三位，死亡人数增加了约50%。我国患者死亡相关的危险因素分析中，空气污染仍是重要的危险因素，2017年与2007年相比，空气污染所致死亡人数增加了1.7%。

全国各地雾霾来源不同。全国各地雾霾成因的分析中，京津冀地区雾霾构成中二次气溶胶贡献显著，而二次气溶胶的形成对于机体危害更大。北京某一周内空气质量监控结果显示，O_3，NO_2相比其他污染物对于PM2.5的影响更为显著。

随着《大气污染防治行动计划》的实施，京津冀地区2013-2017年PM2.5相关疾病死亡减少了102,133人，肺癌相关死亡减少了约7800人，PM2.5相关的肺癌死亡率下降了11.5%。

四、雾霾致肺癌的分子机制

多种机制可能参与了空气污染物导致的细胞损伤过程。小鼠吸入雾霾后24h，肺组织表现为间质性炎症改变，140d后肺组织损伤更加明显。在细胞水平，无论急性暴露还是慢性暴露，PM2.5均可以增加A549细胞的迁徙能力及上皮-间质分化能力。

多种机制参与了肺癌的发生、发展，目前的研究证实空气污染物在肺癌的发生中也扮演了重要的角色，有效控制空气污染物的水平与肺癌发生率的下降有显著相关关系。但目前分子机制的研究仍不充分，有待于进一步的研究证实。

参 考 文 献

[1] GBD 2017 Mortality Collaborators. Global, regional, and national age-sex-specific mortality and life expectancy, 1950-2017: a systematic analysis for the Global Burden of Disease Study 2017. Lancet, 2018, 392(10159): 1684-1735.

[2] GBD 2017 Risk Factor Collaborators. Global, regional, and national comparative risk assessment of 84 behavioural, environmental and occupational, and metabolic risks or clusters of risks for 195 countries and territories, 1990-2017: a systematic analysis for the Global Burden of Disease Study 2017. Lancet, 2018, 392(10159): 1923-1994.

[3] Schulze F, Gao X, Virzonis D, et al. Air Quality Effects on Human Health and Approaches for Its Assessment through Microfluidic Chips. Genes (Basel), 2017, 8(10): 244.

[4] Pope CA 3rd. Respiratory disease associated with community air pollution and a steel mill, Utah Valley. Am J Public Health, 1989, 79(5): 623-628.

[5] Raaschou-Nielsen O, Andersen ZJ, Beelen R, et al. Air pollution and lung cancer incidence in 17 European cohorts: prospective analyses from the European Study of Cohorts for Air Pollution Effects (ESCAPE). Lancet Oncol, 2013, 14(9): 813-822.

[6] Gharibvand L, Shavlik D, Ghamsary M, et al. The Association between Ambient Fine Particulate Air Pollution and Lung Cancer Incidence: Results from the AHSMOG-2 Study. Environ Health Perspect, 2017, 125(3): 378-384.

[7] Lepeule J, Laden F, Dockery D, et al. Chronic exposure to fine particles and mortality: an extended follow-up of the Harvard Six Cities study from 1974 to 2009. Environ Health Perspect, 2012, 120(7): 965-970.

[8] http://www.healthdata.org/china.

[9] Bi W, Chen K, Xiao Z, et al. Health Benefit Assessment of China's National Action Plan on Air Pollution in the Beijing-Tianjin-Hebei Area. Aerosol Air Qual, 2019, 19: 383-389.

9 导航支气管镜新技术在肺癌诊断的应用进展

杨 震 梁志欣 陈良安

肺癌诊断的金标准是病理诊断,其前提是获得足量的活检组织样本。传统呼吸镜诊断技术主要采用可弯曲支气管镜(broncoscopy)和超声支气管镜(endobronchial ultrasound)用于中央型肺癌和纵隔/肺门淋巴结的活检诊断。在周围型肺癌,传统呼吸内镜因到达困难而应用受限,临床多采用CT引导经皮肺穿刺活检。但近年来新型导航支气管镜技术快速发展,大幅提升了呼吸内镜在周围型肺癌的诊断能力,本文就相关新技术进展进行文献回顾。

一、小探头超声(radical endobronchial ultrasound,REBUS)

REBUS是一种纤细而柔软的超声探头,可通过几乎所有支气管镜的工作通道,也可以与引导鞘管(guided-sheaths,GS)配合在具有更大工作孔道的治疗性支气管镜上使用。REBUS提供了一个从设备头端旋转探头向外发散的二维平面内的360°超声视图,可以实时定位支气管镜所能触及的远端病变,以及支气管镜视野下不可见的更远端的病变。在REBUS图像中,实性病变通常表现为一个完全围绕中心探头的圆形(同心视野,当REBUS探头进入气道,直接进入周围病变时,如图6-9-1A所示)或仅在屏幕部分可见的半圆(偏心视野,当REBUS探头被引导到只与病灶周围接触的气道时,如图6-9-1B)。有时可以通过"暴风雪征"检测到磨玻璃病灶(ground glass opacity,GGO)(图6-9-1C)。

1项关于REBUS用于周围型肺癌诊断的meta分析纳入了16项研究,包含至少6个月随访数据的1420名患者,结果显示REBUS用于周围型肺癌诊断的总体诊断率为73%,气胸的发生率为1%,其中0.4%需要放置胸导管。与偏心视野相比,同心视野的病灶诊断率更高,>20mm病灶比≤20mm病灶的诊断率更高。

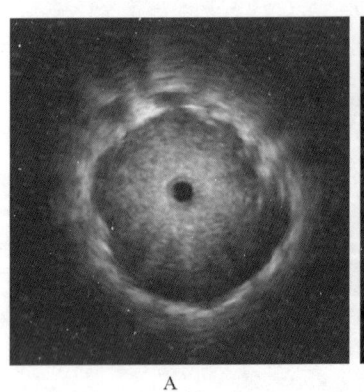

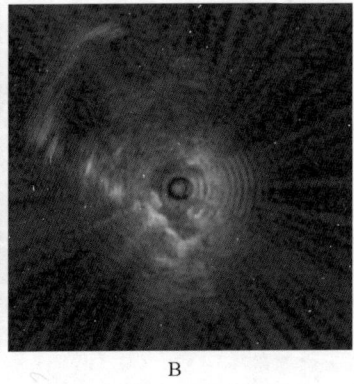

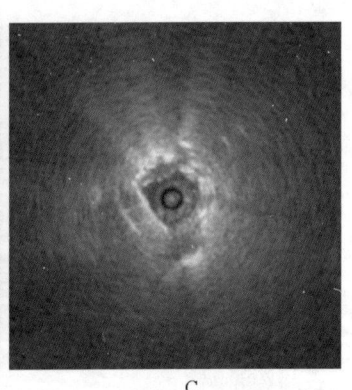

图 6-9-1 小探头超声图像

虽然REBUS可以让术者观察病灶并进行活检,但它仍有局限性。GGO病灶虽然可通过"暴风雪征"来识别,但在临床实践中准确识别这种征象通常很难,特别是对于小的GGO病灶。肺不张常常被错误的识别为病灶而导致诊断结果不准确。此外,偏心视野病灶的REBUS图像无法告诉术者病灶相对于探头所在气道的具体空间方位,病灶距离支气管镜末端所在位置太远导致探头无法定位到病灶,此时术者往往须借助C形臂X光机来调整支气管镜或引导鞘管的方向,努力使探头进入病灶。

二、细支气管镜和超细支气管镜(thin and ultrathin bronchoscopy,TB和UTB)

细支气管镜和超细支气管镜的定义尚无共识,现有文献中通常是指外径小于4mm或3mm的支气管镜(图6-9-2)。细支气管镜和超细支气管镜更小的外径允许其更好地进入亚段支气管,并可能到达肺外周病变。标准支气管镜可以到达第3级或第4级支气管,而超细支气管镜据报道可以到达最多至第9级支气管。

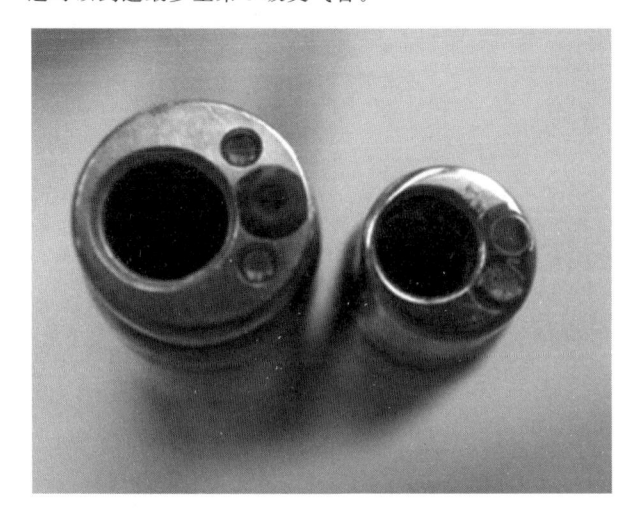

图 6-9-2 细支气管镜(左)和超细支气管镜(右)

1项前瞻性多中心随机对照试验比较了外径4mm的细支气管镜联合引导鞘管与外径3mm的超细支气管镜的诊断价值。该研究招募了310例肺结节患者,其中305例接受了支气管镜检查。术中两组患者也同时联合了X线胸片、虚拟导航和REBUS。尽管两组采用的支气管镜的外径仅相差1mm,但超细支气管镜组的诊断率明显优于细支气管镜组(74% vs. 59%)。近期发表的1项比较细支气管镜和超细支气管镜诊断率的RCT研究显示,356例肺结节患者随机分配接受细支气管镜或超细支气管镜检查,超细支气管镜组的诊断率也明显优于细支气管镜组(70.1% vs. 98.7%)。

总体而言,与互补技术(如X线胸片、REBUS、引导鞘管和导航系统)联合应用更细的支气管镜可提高进入肺外周病变的能力。

三、虚拟导航(virtual bronchoscopic navigation, VBN)

接近肺外周病变需要精确的选择支气管,虚拟导航利用螺旋CT数据重建生成气管-支气管树的三维图像,并在三围支气管树中标记目标病灶并规划出一条经支气管入路到达病灶的气道内导航路径(图6-9-3)。在支气管镜检查期间,术者借助虚拟导航系统生成的气道内图像和导航路径,快速准确地操作支气管镜前行和转向以通过复杂的支气管分支,最终到达目标病灶。

1项多中心前瞻性研究将199例肺结节患者随机分为VBN辅助组(VBNA)和无VBN辅助组(NVBNA),所有操作均联合应用引导鞘管、REBUS探针和X线胸片,VBNA组的诊断率显著高于NVBNA组(80% vs. 67%, P = 0.03)。1项针对VBN的系统评价显示,VBN的总体诊断率为74%,<20mm病灶的诊断率为67%,纳入的这些研究中VBN均联合了其他技术,包括UTB、X线胸片、引导鞘管和REBUS。

VBN通过有效的术前计划辅助术者在术中更高效地选择正确的支气管分支抵达目标病灶。但需要注意的是,VBN不能针对基于术前CT的重建图像与术中实际差异进行实时地匹配和调整,也无法将操作工具头端的具体位置实时反馈给操作者,VBN本身不能确认是否最终到达病灶,术中往往需要借助其他技术。

四、电磁导航(electromagnetic navigation, ENB)

ENB技术的基本原理是术前应用患者胸部的薄层CT数据生成三维支气管树,然后在三维支气管树中标记目标病灶并规划出一条从气管至病灶的导航路径,术中通过一块磁板在患者胸部生成一个磁场,然后利用贴在患者胸部的电磁传感器对电磁导航管或活检工具进行实时的三角定位,引导电磁导航管或活检工具沿预定的行进路线到达病灶。与VBN相似,ENB同样不能针对基于术前CT的重建图像与术中实际差异进行实时的匹配和调整。目前国内可获得的商用电磁导航系统有3种,分别是SuperDimension(Medtronic, Minneapolis, MN, USA)、SPiNDrive(VeranMedical Technologies, St Louis, MO, USA)和朗开医疗的电磁导航系统。

(一)SuperDimension电磁导航系统

该系统将一个钝头的电磁探头附在一根远端带预弯角度(有多个弯曲度可用)的导航鞘管末端用来定位鞘管,并实时引导鞘管沿术前规划的路径行进至目标病灶。到达位置后,将电磁探头撤出,导航鞘管仍保留在原位,作为活检工具进入的通道(图6-9-4)。在活检工具通过鞘管送入病灶进行活检之前,通常还需要采用超声小探头或C形臂X光机的实时影像再次确认导航鞘管已经达到目标病灶,以提高导航和诊断的准确率。

1项纳入15个研究的meta分析显示,1033个肺结节的总体诊断率为64.9%,气胸发生率为3.1%,其中1.6%需要胸腔置管。病灶越大和支气管征阳性的病灶诊断率越高,联合REBUS或X线胸片相比不联合的诊断率更高。1项前瞻性多中心的真实世界Navigate研究显示,1157例患者中94%(1092/1157)导航成功并完成活检,经1年随访确认的诊断准确率为73%。

SuperDimension电磁导航系统在导航过程中受生理运动的影响较大,实时生成的电磁探头在导航路径上的图像可出现较明显的往返漂移,术者需要花一定时间适应这种图像漂移,但并不困难。此外,SuperDimension电磁导航系统在支气管征阳性病灶的诊断准确率更高。因此针对无支气管征病灶,SuperDimension电磁导航系统还提供了一个配套的穿刺打孔装置(crosscountry system),当导航鞘管到达临近病灶的支气管,该装置通过鞘管进入到预定的穿刺点进行穿刺并扩张穿刺点,使导航鞘管通过穿刺点进入肺组织,然后再导航至目标病灶进行活检(图6-9-5)。该装置在国内尚未注册,国内有学者尝试借助通用的穿刺针进行穿刺打孔或直接进行穿刺活检。

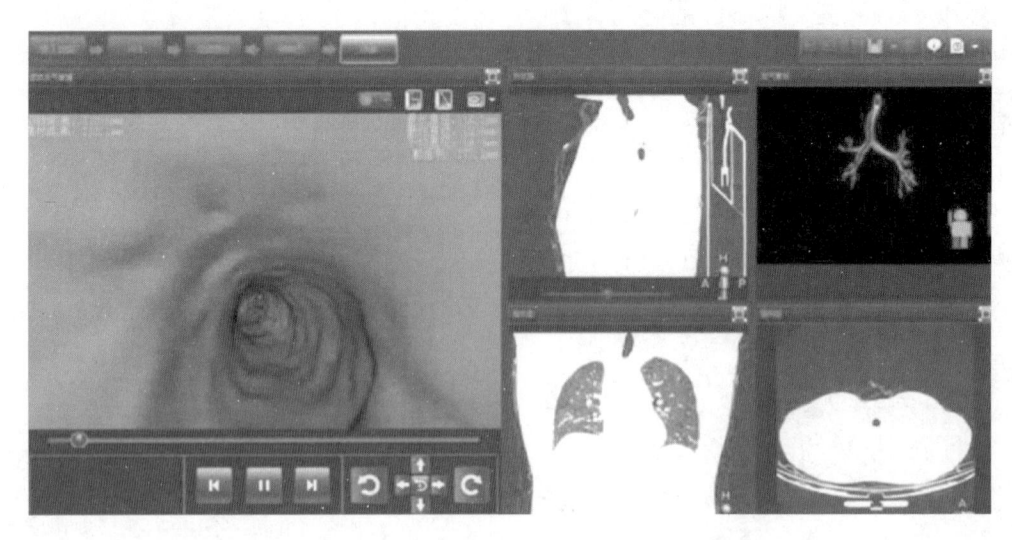

图 6-9-3 虚拟导航图像

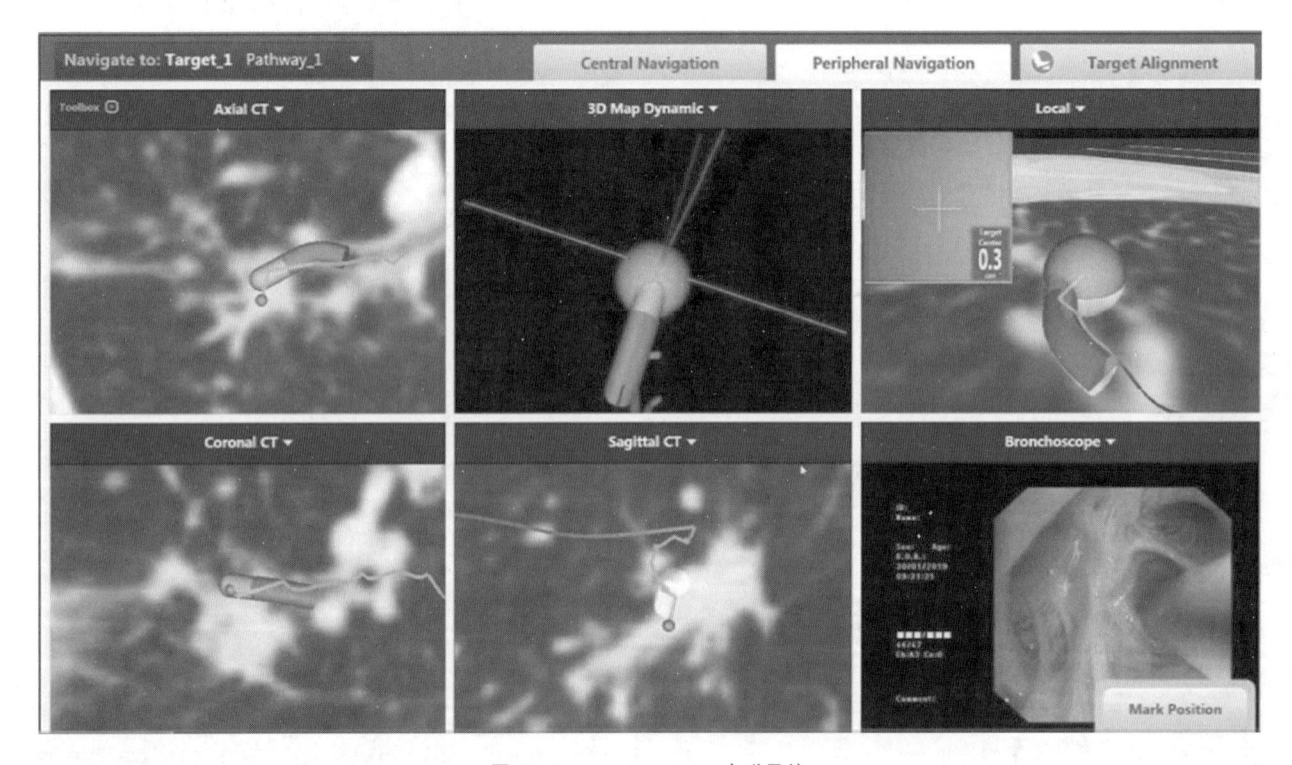

图 6-9-4 SuperDimension 电磁导航

（二）SPiNDrive 电磁导航系统

该系统实时引导带有电磁探头的活检工具沿术前规划的路径行进至目标病灶,可在活检取样时对活检工具的位置进行实时跟踪,还提供带有电磁探头的经皮活检针进行经皮穿刺肺活检。此外,SPiNDrive 电磁导航系统利用深吸气相 CT 数据进行三维重建用于术前规划,术中利用平静呼吸相 CT 数据进行导航,与 SuperDimension 电磁导航相比,SPiNDrive 电磁导航系统术中电磁探头图像漂移的情况大大改善（图 6-9-6）。

1 项回顾性研究发现,SPiNDrive 电磁导航系统用于肺结节患者的诊断率为 83.3%（40/48）,1 例患者发生气胸（2%）。近期发表的一个多中心病例系列报道显示,129 例患者采用 SPiNDrive 电磁导航系统进行经皮肺穿刺的诊断率为 73.7%,当同时进行电磁导航支气管镜检查时,诊断率增加至 81.1%。

（三）朗开电磁导航系统

朗开电磁导航系统是国内自主研发的设备（图 6-9-7）,已开发可适配超细支气管镜电磁探头,以及针对无支气管征病灶的专用穿刺针（ENB-TPNA 穿刺针）,目前处于临床应用初期阶段。

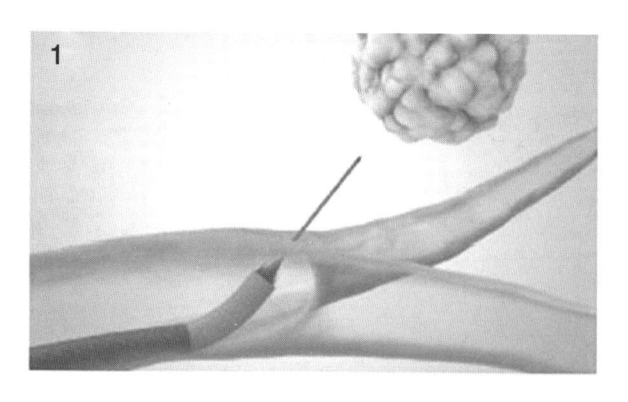

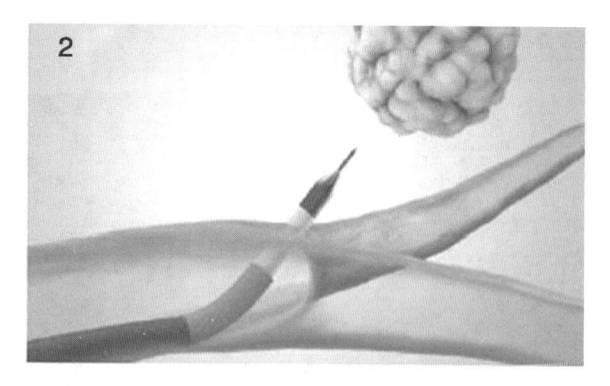

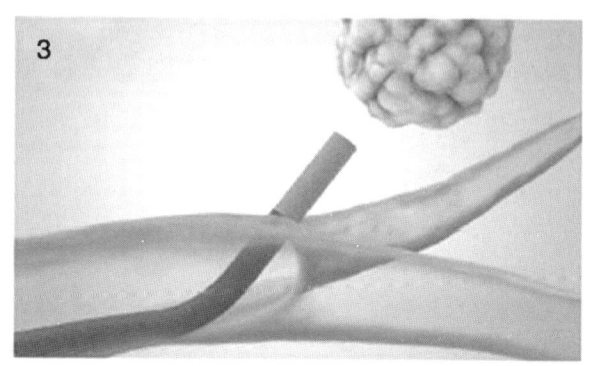

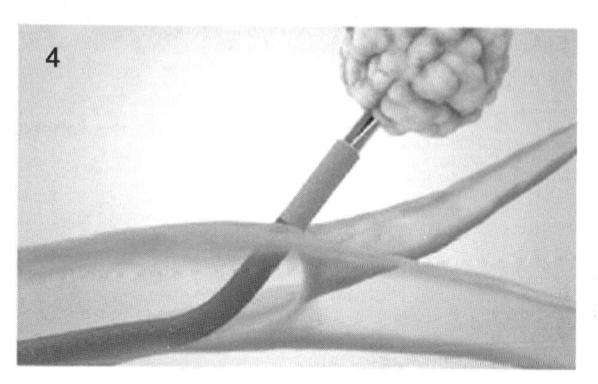

图 6-9-5 穿刺打孔装置

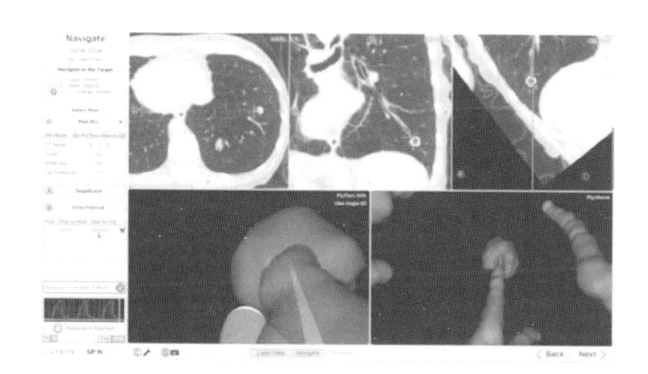

图 6-9-6 SPiNDrive 电磁导航系统

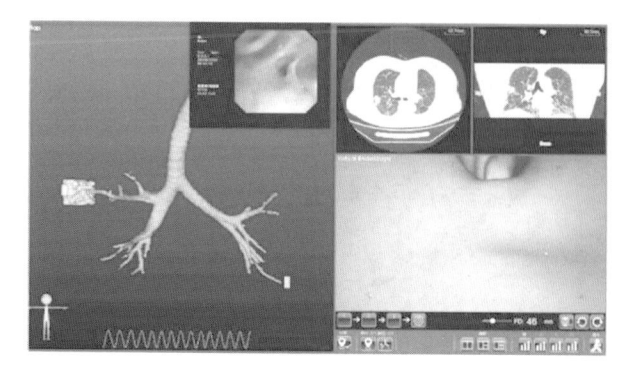

图 6-9-7 朗开电磁导航系统

五、增强现实导航

增强现实导航,同样应用患者胸部 CT 数据生成三维支气管树,一方面可以类似于 VBN 在三维支气管树中标记目标病灶并规划出一条从气管至病灶的导航路径,但较 VBN 的技术优势在于可将 VBN 气道内图像与支气管镜下图像进行实时匹配和关联(图 6-9-8),对有支气管征病灶进行气道内的实时导航活检;另一方面,可提供专用工具对气道进行穿刺打孔,并穿过肺实质建立一条从气道至目标病灶的隧道,用于无支气管征病灶的活检,因此也被称为支气管镜下经肺实质结节抵达术(bronchoscopic trans-parenchymal nodule access,BTPNA)。在建立隧道的过程中,该技术可以将无法在 C 形臂 X 光机下显影的 GGO 病灶和较小的病灶,通过增强现实技术融合至 C 形臂 X 光机

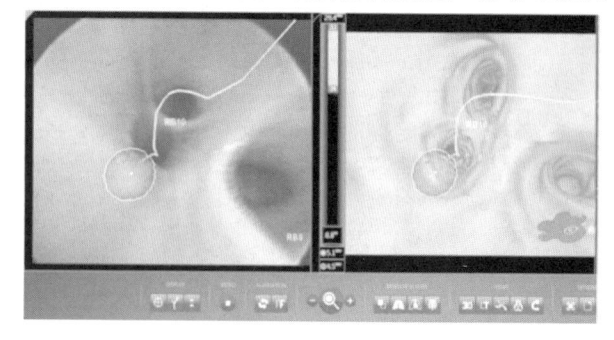

图 6-9-8 增强现实导航的气道内导航部分

的实时影像上,提高对 GGO 病灶和较小的病灶的定位能力(图 6-9-9)。2015 年首份 BTPNA 临床研究报道,12 名肺结节患者经 BTPNA 的诊断率为 83%,没有出现明显的并发症。

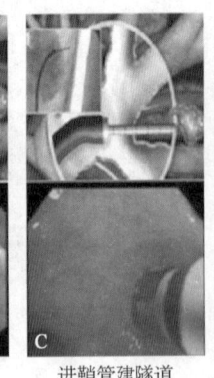

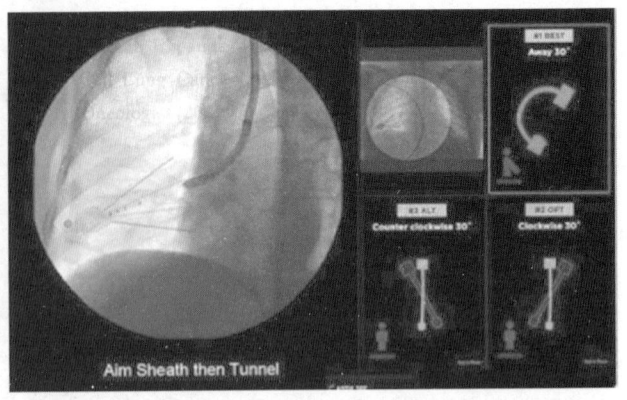

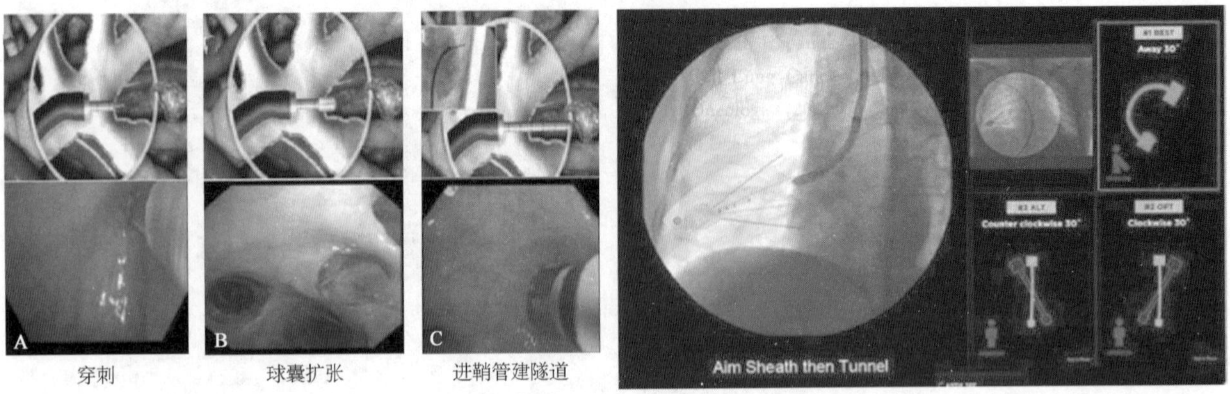

图 6-9-9　增强现实导航的 BTPNA 部分

六、小　结

从目前的研究进展来看,导航支气管镜将成为肺癌特别是早期周围型肺癌的关键诊断工具,其气胸和出血的发生率远低于 CT 引导经皮肺穿刺,诊断率已提升至 80%～90%。未来通过优化患者筛选,将多种导航技术融合建立优化的复合导航支气管镜技术,有望将诊断率提升至更高水平。

参 考 文 献

[1] Steinfort DP, Khor YH, Manser RL, et al. Radial probe endobronchial ultrasound for the diagnosis of peripheral lung cancer: systematic review and meta-analysis. Eur Respir J, 2011, 37: 902-910.

[2] Wang Memoli JS, Nietert PJ, Silvestri GA. Meta-analysis of guided bronchoscopy for the evaluation of the pulmonary nodule. Chest, 2012, 142(2): 385-393.

[3] Ishiwata T, Gregor A, Inage T, et al. Bronchoscopic navigation and tissue diagnosis. Gen Thorac Cardiovasc Surg, 2020, 68(7): 672-678.

[4] Oki M, Saka H, Ando M, et al. Ultrathin bronchoscopy with multimodal devices for peripheral pulmonary lesions. A randomized trial. Am J Respir Crit Care Med, 2015, 192: 468-476.

[5] Asano F, Shinagawa N, Ishida T, et al. Virtual bronchoscopic navigation combined with ultrathin bronchoscopy. A randomized clinical trial. Am J Respir Crit Care Med, 2013, 188: 327-333.

[6] Oki M, Saka H, Asano F, et al. Use of an ultrathin vs thin bronchoscope for peripheral pulmonary lesions: a randomized trial. Chest, 2019, 156: 954-964.

[7] Ishida T, Asano F, Yamazaki K, et al. Virtual bronchoscopic navigation combined with endobronchial ultrasound to diagnose small peripheral pulmonary lesions: a randomized trial. Thorax, 2011, 66: 1072-1077.

[8] Asano F, Eberhardt R, Herth FJ. Virtual bronchoscopic navigation for peripheral pulmonary lesions. Respiration, 2014, 88: 430-440.

[9] Gex G, Pralong JA, Combescure C, et al. Diagnostic yield and safety of electromagnetic navigation bronchoscopy for lung nodules: a systematic review and meta-analysis. Respiration, 2014, 87: 165-176.

[10] Folch EE, Pritchett MA, Nead MA, et al. Electromagnetic Navigation Bronchoscopy for Peripheral Pulmonary Lesions: One-Year Results of the Prospective, Multicenter NAVIGATE Study. J Thorac Oncol, 2019, 14(3): 445-458.

[11] Raval AA, Amir L. Community hospital experience using electromagnetic navigation bronchoscopy system integrating tidal volume computed tomography mapping. Lung Cancer Manag, 2016, 5(1): 9-19.

[12] Mallow C, Lee H, Oberg C, et al. Safety and diagnostic performance of pulmonologists performing electromagnetic guided percutaneous lung biopsy (SPiNperc). Respirology, 2019, 24: 453-458.

[13] Herth FJ, Eberhardt R, Sterman D, et al. Bronchoscopic transparenchymal nodule access (BTPNA): first in humantrial of a novel procedure for sampling solitary pulmonary nodules. Thorax, 2015, 70: 326-332.

10 生物标志物在肺癌免疫治疗中的预测价值

周英 张艰

免疫检查点抑制剂(ICIs)的发展，极大地改变了肺癌治疗的格局，但这一新进治疗模式的局限性及其带来的不良反应仍不容忽视。研究发现多达60%的晚期非小细胞肺癌患者不能从ICIs中获益，甚至出现了严重的免疫毒性，且治疗成本高，严重影响了其在临床治疗晚期非小细胞肺癌中的应用。因此，探索与ICIs预后相关的生物标志物，对提高疗效及预防不良反应具有重要意义。目前肺癌免疫治疗疗效预测生物标志物主要有两大类，肿瘤相关的生物标志物和系统性炎症反应相关的生物标志物。本文系统地回顾了多种生物标志物在肺癌患者免疫治疗后的预测价值。这些结果可用于日常临床实践，并有助于医生在未来的免疫治疗中对肺癌患者进行筛选及分层。同时，为减少免疫治疗不良反应的发生，提高晚期肺癌患者生存率提供理论基础。

一、前言

肺癌在全球的发病率和死亡率均位居癌症榜的首位。肺癌的治疗也经历了细胞毒性化疗药物、靶向治疗、免疫疗法三次革命洗礼，免疫疗法的成功不仅革命性地改变了癌症治疗的格局，而且革命性地改变癌症治疗的理念。它的目标不是肿瘤本身，而是免疫系统，通过刺激免疫系统间接抑制肿瘤细胞的生长。目前正在进行临床试验的免疫疗法有：细胞因子、肿瘤疫苗接种、抗体、过继性细胞转移、免疫检查点抑制剂。在所有的免疫疗法中，临床上最广泛、最成功使用的是免疫检查点抑制剂(immune checkpoint inhibitors, ICIs)，如细胞毒性T淋巴细胞抗原4(cytotoxic T-lymphocyte antigen 4, CTLA-4)和程序性死亡1/配体1(programmed death 1/ligand 1, PD1/PD-L1)。但是伴随这一新进展而来的一些缺陷也不容忽视，研究发现多达60%的晚期NSCLC患者不能从ICIs中获益，出现低应答甚至无应答，甚至有些患者出现了严重的免疫毒性。而且ICIs治疗的成本很高，对卫生医疗系统造成了重大的经济影响。基于此研究者开始对可能与预后相关的各种生物标志物的积极探索，如肿瘤相关和系统性炎症反应相关的生物标志物，筛选最佳应答者规避这种风险。本文就肺癌免疫治疗疗效预测或预后的生物标志物概述如下。

二、肿瘤相关的生物标志物(tumour-related biomarkers)

(一)PD-L1表达

PD-L1表达量是指通过免疫化学方法测定肿瘤细胞和(或)免疫细胞表达PD-L1的比例。目前，已有4个抗体克隆(22C3、28-8、SP263和SP142)被批准用于测定非小细胞肺癌患者的PD-L1表达。大部分研究将PD-L1≥1%定义为阳性，将PD-L1≥50%定义为高表达。研究发现高PD-L1表达与使用PD-1/PD-L1抑制剂治疗的高应答率及临床疗效有关，PD-L1高表达者有更好的OS和PFS。同样，在二线治疗中，在PD-L1高表达的患者中，免疫治疗患者比化疗患者表现出更长的生存期。然而，也有研究结果表明，即使在PD-L1阳性的人群中，免疫治疗的效果也没有在整个人群中体现。另一方面，一些患者无论肿瘤细胞PD-L1表达水平如何甚至是阴性，都表现出临床疗效。

因此，PD-L1表达是免疫治疗反应的一个有争议的生物标志物，其在临床应用过程中的不完美性也逐渐凸显，不同的肿瘤亚型、不同检测平台、不同的截断值和评估方法及时间和空间的异质性均会导致PD-L1表达量不同。

(二)肿瘤突变负荷(tumour mutation burden, TMB)和血TMB(blood-TMB, bTMB)

TMB是指肿瘤细胞基因组编码区每百万碱基发生非同义突变的总数，目前使用Foundation Medicine公司的新一代测序技术(NGS)来测量TMB。大部分研究将TMB≥10mut/Mb定义为高TMB。大量临床研究结果显示，接受ICIs的肺癌患者中，高TMB具有更高的总体应答率(ORR)、无进展生存期(PFS)及持久的临床获益(DCB)，甚至是OS。bTMB是另一个引起人们兴趣的血清标志物，在POPLAR和OAK研究发现，血液TMB与组织TMB呈正相关，bTMB越高，PFS越长，他们的研究建议bTMB≥16muts/Mb定义为高bTMB截断值。

当然(b)TMB作为一种生物标志物也有它的局限性，如基因测序成本高且耗时，需专业人士解读报告，缺乏标准化检测平台，并且目前缺乏统一的TMB阈值。

(三) DNA 错配修复缺陷 (DNA mismatch repair deficiency, dMMR) 和微卫星不稳定性 (microsatellite instability, MSI)

MMR 是一个识别和修复 DNA 复制和重组过程中可能出现突变的系统。许多类型的癌细胞在 MMR 中有缺陷，导致错误基因序列的积累，这些错误序列通常被重复，称为微卫星，呈现微卫星高度不稳定性 (MSI-H)。但研究发现 NSCLC 中 MSI-H 发生率较低 (约 0.6%)。Le 等报道了在接受帕博利珠单抗治疗不同的癌症类型患者，其中 dMMR 或 MSI-H 的患者分别获得 53% 的 ORR 和 64% 的 2 年生存率。因此 FDA 首次批准帕博利珠单抗用于 MSI-H 和 dMMR 的进展期实体肿瘤治疗。然而，本研究未纳入 NSCLC 患者。目前针对肺癌的研究较少，需要更多的大型研究探索其在肺癌中的价值。

还有一些新的肿瘤相关生物标志物如基因表达特征、肿瘤基因型 (如肿瘤驱动突变的存在) 以及肿瘤微环境中肿瘤浸润淋巴细胞的密度似乎会影响免疫治疗的反应，目前正在研究中。

三、系统性炎症反应 (systemic inflammatory response, SIR) 相关的生物标志物

肿瘤微环境 (tumor microenvironment, TME) 是肿瘤细胞与免疫系统细胞相互作用的主要场所，这有助于肿瘤的进展、扩散和转移。对于恶性肿瘤患者，尽管肿瘤的发生、发展与基因遗传相关，但越来越多的研究结果证实 SIR 与肿瘤的发生发展有着千丝万缕的联系，而炎症也会影响宿主癌症的免疫反应，可能会干扰免疫治疗的效果。理解炎症、癌症和免疫反应之间的因果关系很重要。此外，外周促炎状态与癌症患者较差的预后有关。许多血常规参数已被作为癌症患者潜在的炎症生物标志物，如循环白细胞、绝对中性粒细胞计数、绝对血小板计数和乳酸脱氢酶 (LDH) 浓度升高，这些参数与几种癌症的不良预后相关。

(一) 中性粒细胞淋巴细胞比率 (neutrophil to lymphocyte ratio, NLR) 和衍生中性粒细胞淋巴细胞比率 (derived neutrophil-to-lymphocyte ratio, dNLR)

肿瘤相关中性粒细胞 (tumor-associated neutrophils, TANs) 是肿瘤内浸润的中性粒细胞，在肿瘤从恶性转化到肿瘤进展、细胞外基质修饰、血管生成、细胞迁移和免疫抑制等多个方面都有重要的作用。肿瘤区域淋巴细胞浸润增加与实体瘤患者对治疗良好的应答相关。中性粒细胞作为一种炎症反应，通过抑制免疫细胞尤其是活化 T 细胞的细胞毒活性来抑制抗肿瘤免疫反应。因此研究者提出了中性粒细胞淋巴细胞比率 (neutrophil to lymphocyte ratio, NLR) 这个概念，即中性粒细胞绝对值计数 (ANC)/淋巴细胞绝对值计数 (ALC)。新的证据表明，NLR 升高代表了循环淋巴细胞的相对减少和循环炎症细胞因子或介质的升高。循环淋巴细胞的减少会削弱免疫检查点抑制剂的作用，主要释放 T 细胞 (淋巴细胞的主要亚型) 功能的抑制信号。目前研究中缺乏一个统一的截止值 (cut-off)，从 1.9 到 9.21 都有。NLR 的预后价值已在各种癌症类型中得到验证，同样在肺癌免疫治疗，Bagley、Soyano 等团队的研究结果均显示：高 NLR 与 NSCLC 免疫治疗较差的 OS、PFS 相关。有趣的是，除了基线 NLR 水平预后及预测价值外，NLR 在晚期癌症患者后续治疗中也具有预测价值，如在晚期 NSCLC 患者中，接受 ICIs 治疗 6 周后，NLR≥5 与较差的 PFS 和 OS 相关。因 NLR 只涉及到中性粒细胞和淋巴细胞，但未涉及到单核细胞和其他粒细胞亚群，因此研究者提出了 dNLR 这个概念，即 dNRL = ANC/(WBC-ANC)。在接受 ICIs 晚期 NSCLC 患者中，基线 dNLR>3 与较差 OS 相关。但也有研究显示，高 dNLR 与 PFS 及 OS 的相关性无明显统计学意义。

当然 NLR 和 dNLR 也有一定的局限性，目前研究缺乏一个统一的截止值，且迄今为止关于 NLR、dNLR 的研究规模较小，具有回顾性，因此需要进行大量前瞻性研究验证。

(二) 肺癌免疫预后指数 (lung immune prognostic index, LIPI)

为了提高生物标志物的预测价值，研究者发现通过组合不同的指标可以产生预测的相加性或协同作用。研究证实血清乳酸脱氢酶 (LDH) 水平升高与许多实体肿瘤的不良预后有关，因此 Mezquita 和同事将 dNLR 和 LDH 进行组合，在 JAMA 上提出了 LIPI 这一概念，这一综合指标根据 dNLR>3 和 LDH>正常值上限将其分为 3 组，低风险组 LIPI=0 分 (0 因素)、中风险组 LIPI=1 分 (1 因素)、高风险组 LIPI=2 分 (2 因素)。这项研究基于 466 例接受了免疫治疗的 NSCLC 患者，发现低风险 LIPI 与较好的 OS 和 PFS 相关，而在化疗组却没有显著的相关性。但是 2019 年同样发表在 JAMA 上的研究，Kazandjian 等发现，无论 NSCLC 患者采用何种治疗方法，低风险 LIPI 与较长的 OS 和 PFS 相关，认为基线 LIPI 可能是预后的生物标志物。

(三) 格拉斯哥预后评分系统 (Glasgow prognostic score, GPS)

除了 LIPI，还有其他组合指标，如将 C-反应蛋白>10mg/L 和白蛋白<35g/L 纳入到 GPS，即低风险 GPS=0 (0 因素)，中风险 GPS=1 (1 因素)，高风险 GPS=2 (2 因素)。研究发现高风险 GPS 与 NSCLC 治疗的不良预后相关。华西医学院李为民教授团队通过检索数据库的 10 项研究，涉及来自几个地区的 5369 名化疗或手术的肺癌患者，结果发现，在综合数据中高风险 GPS (1~2 分) 与较差的 OS 相关。然而，中高风险 GPS 与 PFS 值之间没有显著的相关性。

最近，Shafique 等发现改良 GPS (mGPS) 优于 GPS，是癌症患者强有力的预后因素，与肿瘤部位无关。定义低风险 mGPS=0 (CRP≤10mg/L)，中风险 GPS=1 (CRP>10mg/L 且 ALB≥35g/L)，高风险 GPS=2 (CRP>10mg/L 且 ALB<35g/L)。同样是华西医学院李为民教授团队分析了来自多个国家的 5817 名肺癌患者 (手术、化疗或放疗) 的 11 项研究，结果显示高 mGPS 与较差的 OS

相关（HR＝1.77；95%CI:1.35~2.31；$P<0.05$），而接受手术的患者中，mGPS与较差OS之间的相关性不显著，这可能归因于较低的肿瘤负荷。但是目前关于GPS及mGPS在肺癌ICIs的预后及预测价值的研究相对较少。

（四）免疫代谢预后指数（immune-metabolic-prognostic index, IMPI）

还有些研究评估了全身炎症相关生物标记物联合代谢指标F-18葡萄糖正电子发射断层扫描/计算机断层扫描（F-18 FDG PET/CT），即使用免疫代谢预后指数（IMPI）对ICIs治疗的NSCLC患者进行预后评估。我们知道F-18 FDG PET检查中肿瘤代谢值的预后价值是公认的，病变总糖酵解（total lesion glycolysis, TLG）＝平均SUV×代谢瘤体积（MTV）。IMPI定义为使用NLR≥4.9联合TLG≥541.5 ml建立了IMPI，将其分为3组：低风险IMPI＝0分（0因素）；中风险IMPI＝1分（1因素）；高风险IMPI＝2分（2因素）。如Castello等研究的多变量分析结果提示，肺癌免疫治疗患者中IMPI与PFS及OS显著相关，低、中、高风险IMPI组PFS中位值分别为7.8个月（95% CI 4.6~11.0）、5.6个月（95% CI 3.8~7.4）和1.8个月（95% CI 1.6~2.0）（$P<0.001$）。中位OS分别为15.2个月（95% CI 10.9~19.6）、13.2个月（95% CI 5.9~20.3）和2.8个月（95% CI 1.4~4.2）（$P<0.001$）。因此IMP也是一种潜在的有预测价值的生物标记物，可用于识别可能从ICI获益的NSCLC患者。

四、结语与展望

推进肺癌患者个体化免疫治疗既能保证患者选择最合适的方案，得到最佳获益避免不必要的不良事件，又能够支付合理的医疗费用。由于免疫系统的复杂性及动态变化的特性，不太可能确定较完美的免疫治疗预测生物标志物，这种生物标志物的临床应用和适用性可能会因治疗的线数、不同的时间点、可替代的治疗方案和关注的健康经济考虑而有所不同。但是尽管如此，一方面，我们可以通过协同或结合不同的生物标志物来进一步提高其预测能力；另一方面我们也可以寻找一个提示免疫治疗预后不良或治疗无反应的标志物（类似于KRAS突变提示EGFR TKIs效果差预后不良）。这种精确的预测生物标志物，会更好地将疾病风险、预后或治疗反应分类，进而引导我们为癌症患者提供更好的医疗保健，同时更好地筛选出无应答者避免不必要的毒性和花费，这仍然是一个持续的挑战。虽然血液相关生物标志物已显示出一定的预测价值，且血液标志物易于获得、成本低、侵入性较小，希望未来可以将这些血液相关生物标志物纳入到肺癌患者免疫治疗前瞻性随机临床试验中。

参 考 文 献

[1] BRAY F, FERLAY J, SOERJOMATARAM I, et al. Global cancer statistics 2018: GLOBOCAN estimates of incidence and mortality worldwide for 36 cancers in 185 countries. CA, 2018, 68(6): 394-424.

[2] COUZIN-FRANKEL J. Breakthrough of the year 2013. Cancer immunotherapy. Science (New York, NY), 2013, 342 (6165): 1432-1433.

[3] CHAE YK, OH MS, GILES FJ. Molecular Biomarkers of Primary and Acquired Resistance to T-Cell-Mediated Immunotherapy in Cancer: Landscape, Clinical Implications, and Future Directions. The oncologist, 2018, 23(4): 410-421.

[4] GALLUZZI L, CHAN TA, KROEMER G, et al. The hallmarks of successful anticancer immunotherapy. Science translational medicine, 2018, 10(459).

[5] RITTMEYER A, BARLESI F, WATERKAMP D, et al. Atezolizumab versus docetaxel in patients with previously treated non-small-cell lung cancer (OAK): a phase 3, open-label, multicentre randomised controlled trial. Lancet (London, England), 2017, 389(10066): 255-265.

[6] RECK M, RODRíGUEZ-ABREU D, ROBINSON AG, et al. Pembrolizumab versus Chemotherapy for PD-L1-Positive Non-Small-Cell Lung Cancer. The New England journal of medicine, 2016, 375(19): 1823-1833.

[7] MOK TSK, WU YL, KUDABA I, et al. Final analysis of the phase III KEYNOTE-042 study: Pembrolizumab (Pembro) versus platinum-based chemotherapy (Chemo) as first-line therapy for patients (Pts) with PD-L1-positive locally advanced/metastatic NSCLC. Annals of oncology, 2019, 30 Suppl 2(i38).

[8] MUKHERJI D, JABBOUR MN, SAROUFIM M, et al. Programmed Death-Ligand 1 Expression in Muscle-Invasive Bladder Cancer Cystectomy Specimens and Lymph Node Metastasis: A Reliable Treatment Selection Biomarker?. Clinical genitourinary cancer, 2016, 14(2): 183-187.

[9] BORGHAEI H, PAZ-ARES L, HORN L, et al. Nivolumab versus Docetaxel in Advanced Nonsquamous Non-Small-Cell Lung Cancer. The New England journal of medicine, 2015, 373(17): 1627-1639.

[10] HERBST RS, BAAS P, KIM DW, et al. Pembrolizumab versus docetaxel for previously treated, PD-L1-positive, advanced non-small-cell lung cancer (KEYNOTE-010): a randomised controlled trial. Lancet (London, England), 2016, 387(10027): 1540-1550.

[11] HELLMANN M D, CIULEANU TE, PLUZANSKI A, et al. Nivolumab plus Ipilimumab in Lung Cancer with a High Tumor Mutational Burden. The New England journal of medicine, 2018, 378(22): 2093-2104.

[12] RIZVI NA, HELLMANN MD, SNYDER A, et al. Cancer immunology. Mutational landscape determines sensitivity to PD-1 blockade in non-small cell lung cancer. Science, 2015, 348(6230): 124-128.

[13] KOWANETZ M, ZOU W, SHAMES DS, et al. Tumor mutation load assessed by FoundationOne (FM1) is associated with improved efficacy of atezolizumab (atezo) in patients

with advanced NSCLC. Ann Oncol,2016,27.

[14] FEHRENBACHER L,SPIRA A,BALLINGER M,et al. Atezolizumab versus docetaxel for patients with previously treated non-small-cell lung cancer (POPLAR): a multicentre, open-label,phase 2 randomised controlled trial. Lancet (London,England),2016,387(10030): 1837-1846.

[15] GANDARA DR,PAUL SM,KOWANETZ M,et al. Blood-based tumor mutational burden as a predictor of clinical benefit in non-small-cell lung cancer patients treated with atezolizumab. Nature medicine,2018,24(9): 1441-1448.

[16] DUDLEY JC,LIN MT,LE DT,et al. Microsatellite Instability as a Biomarker for PD-1 Blockade. Clinical cancer research,2016,22(4): 813-820.

[17] VANDERWALDE A,SPETZLER D,XIAO N,et al. Microsatellite instability status determined by next-generation sequencing and compared with PD-L1 and tumor mutational burden in 11,348 patients. Cancer medicine,2018,7(3): 746-756.

[18] LE DT,DURHAM JN,SMITH KN,et al. Mismatch repair deficiency predicts response of solid tumors to PD-1 blockade. Science,2017,357(6349): 409-413.

[19] CRUSZ SM,BALKWILL FR. Inflammation and cancer: advances and new agents. Nature reviews Clinical oncology, 2015,12(10): 584-596.

[20] LAIRD BJA,FALLON M,HJERMSTAD MJ,et al. Quality of Life in Patients With Advanced Cancer: Differential Association With Performance Status and Systemic Inflammatory Response. Journal of clinical oncology, 2016, 34 (23): 2769-2775.

[21] MCMILLAN DC. The systemic inflammation-based Glasgow Prognostic Score: a decade of experience in patients with cancer. Cancer Treat Rev,2013,39(5): 534-540.

[22] PETRELLI F,CABIDDU M,COINU A,et al. Prognostic role of lactate dehydrogenase in solid tumors: a systematic review and meta-analysis of 76 studies. Acta oncologica (Stockholm,Sweden),2015,54(7): 961-970.

[23] PARAMANATHAN A,SAXENA A,MORRIS DL. A systematic review and meta-analysis on the impact of pre-operative neutrophil lymphocyte ratio on long term outcomes after curative intent resection of solid tumours. Surgical oncology, 2014,23(1): 31-39.

[24] TEMPLETON AJ,ACE O,MCNAMARA MG,et al. Prognostic role of platelet to lymphocyte ratio in solid tumors: a systematic review and meta-analysis. Cancer Epidemiol Biomarkers Prev,2014,23(7): 1204-1212.

[25] SHAVERDIAN N,LISBERG AE,BORNAZYAN K,et al. Previous radiotherapy and the clinical activity and toxicity of pembrolizumab in the treatment of non-small-cell lung cancer: a secondary analysis of the KEYNOTE-001 phase 1 trial. The Lancet Oncology,2017,18(7): 895-903.

[26] NAKAMURA Y,WATANABE R,KATAGIRI M,et al. Neutrophil/lymphocyte ratio has a prognostic value for patients with terminal cancer. World J Surg Oncol,2016,14(148).

[27] BAGLEY SJ,KOTHARI S,AGGARWAL C,et al. Pretreatment neutrophil-to-lymphocyte ratio as a marker of outcomes in nivolumab-treated patients with advanced non-small-cell lung cancer. Lung cancer (Amsterdam, Netherlands),2017, 106(1-7).

[28] SOYANO AE,DHOLARIA B,MARIN-ACEVEDO JA,et al. Peripheral blood biomarkers correlate with outcomes in advanced non-small cell lung Cancer patients treated with anti-PD-1 antibodies. Journal for immunotherapy of cancer, 2018,6(1): 129.

[29] SUH KJ,KIM SH,KIM YJ,et al. Post-treatment neutrophil-to-lymphocyte ratio at week 6 is prognostic in patients with advanced non-small cell lung cancers treated with anti-PD-1 antibody. Cancer immunology,immunotherapy,2018,67(3): 459-470.

[30] MEZQUITA L,AUCLIN E,FERRARA R,et al. Association of the Lung Immune Prognostic Index With Immune Checkpoint Inhibitor Outcomes in Patients With Advanced Non-Small Cell Lung Cancer. JAMA Oncol,2018,4(3): 351-357.

[31] RUSSO A,FRANCHINA T,RICCIARDI GRR,et al. Baseline neutrophilia, derived neutrophil-to-lymphocyte ratio (dNLR), platelet-to-lymphocyte ratio (PLR),and outcome in non small cell lung cancer (NSCLC) treated with Nivolumab or Docetaxel. Journal of cellular physiology, 2018, 233 (10): 6337-6343.

[32] DOLAN RD,LAIRD BJA,HORGAN PG,et al. The prognostic value of the systemic inflammatory response in randomised clinical trials in cancer: A systematic review. Critical reviews in oncology/hematology,2018,132:130-137.

[33] WEIDE B,MARTENS A,HASSEL JC,et al. Baseline Biomarkers for Outcome of Melanoma Patients Treated with Pembrolizumab. Clinical cancer research, 2016, 22 (22): 5487-5496.

[34] KAZANDJIAN D,GONG Y,KEEGAN P,et al. Prognostic Value of the Lung Immune Prognostic Index for Patients Treated for Metastatic Non-Small Cell Lung Cancer. JAMA Oncol,2019.

[35] JIN J,HU K,ZHOU Y,et al. Prognostic value of the Glasgow prognostic score in lung cancer: evidence from 10 studies. The International journal of biological markers,2018,33 (2): 201-207.

[36] SHAFIQUE K,PROCTOR MJ,MCMILLAN DC,et al. The modified Glasgow prognostic score in prostate cancer: results from a retrospective clinical series of 744 patients. BMC cancer,2013,13(292).

[37] JIN J,HU K,ZHOU Y,et al. Clinical utility of the modified Glasgow prognostic score in lung cancer: A meta-analysis. PloS one,2017,12(9): e0184412.

[38] LIU J,DONG M,SUN X,et al. Prognostic Value of 18F-FDG PET/CT in Surgical Non-Small Cell Lung Cancer: A Meta-Analysis. PloS one,2016,11(1): e0146195.

[39] CASTELLO A,TOSCHI L,ROSSI S,et al. The immune-metabolic-prognostic index and clinical outcomes in patients with non-small cell lung carcinoma under checkpoint inhibitors. J Cancer Res Clin Oncol,2020.

11 肺癌免疫治疗相关生物标记物的应用现状

史文佳 赵 微

免疫检查点抑制剂(ICI)具有较好的疗效和安全性,因而被广泛应用于肺癌治疗,并且全面改变了晚期肺癌的治疗格局。但是,只有部分肺癌患者能从免疫治疗中获益,所以我们亟待找出可以预测其疗效的生物标记物。程序性细胞死亡蛋白配体1(PD-L1)可在肿瘤细胞和免疫细胞上表达,并在免疫检查点通路中起关键作用。因此,PD-L1表达是评价程序性细胞死亡蛋白1/程序性细胞死亡蛋白配体1[PD-1(PD-L1)]抑制剂疗效的一种生物标记物。然而,PD-L1表达的预测结果与实际疗效并非完全符合,表明其他因素也参与了免疫反应过程。本文详细介绍了与肿瘤异质性和宿主免疫性相关的生物标记物,包括PD-L1表达、肿瘤突变负荷(TMB)、新抗原、特定突变基因、循环肿瘤DNA(ctDNA)、人类白细胞抗原I(HLA-I)、肿瘤微环境(TME)、外周血炎细胞和肠道微生物等。

一、研究背景

肺癌是我国最常见的恶性肿瘤,占全球癌症相关死亡数的首位。肺癌的5年生存率低于20%,约半数患者确诊时已发生转移,其5年生存率约为5%。晚期肺癌的治疗目前仍以化疗为主,分子靶向治疗只适用于约30%驱动基因阳性的患者,且受到耐药性的制约。近年来,以免疫检查点抑制剂(ICI)为主的免疫治疗实现了肺癌治疗的重大突破,ICI疗效显著、持久,不良反应少,因此用于肺癌的一线、二线和维持治疗。但是,并非所有肺癌患者都能从ICI治疗中获益,部分患者产生耐药性或发生严重的免疫相关不良反应(irAEs),因此需要进一步探索可以预测ICI疗效及预后的生物标记物。

二、免疫检查点抑制剂

(一)免疫检查点机制

免疫检查点的主要作用是调节免疫细胞的功能,在生理条件下保护正常组织和细胞免受免疫系统的攻击,而肿瘤细胞利用此特点来逃避免疫细胞对其识别和清除。免疫检查点主要包括细胞毒性T淋巴细胞抗原4(CTLA-4)和程序性细胞死亡蛋白1(PD-1)(程序性细胞死亡蛋白配体1)(PD-L1)途径。CTLA-4在抗原呈递阶段干扰淋巴细胞的激活,PD-1(PD-L1)则破坏活化T细胞的功能,为肿瘤的生长提供有利的微环境。因此,针对这两种途径的抑制剂可以恢复并强化特异性抗肿瘤免疫反应。近年来,ICI的发现、研究和应用为肺癌的治疗做出了重要贡献。

(二)免疫检查点抑制剂的应用

主要的ICI包括PD-1抑制剂(纳武利尤单抗、帕博利珠单抗和信迪利单抗)、PD-L1抑制剂(阿特珠单抗、德瓦鲁单抗和阿维单抗)和CTLA-4单克隆抗体(ipilimumab和tremelimumab)。纳武利尤单抗被美国食品药物监督管理局(FDA)批准用于治疗转移性非小细胞肺癌(NSCLC),也可用于转移性小细胞肺癌(SCLC)的三线治疗。帕博利珠单抗用于PD-L1评分大于50%的转移性NSCLC患者,帕博利珠单抗联合含铂双药化疗用于晚期患者的一线治疗。另外,帕博利珠单抗单药治疗被批准为SCLC患者的三线治疗。信迪利单抗目前正处于临床试验阶段,并且,已有研究报道其应用于NSCLC患者的新辅助治疗。阿特珠单抗获批为晚期NSCLC患者的二线治疗,有研究报道其疗效与PD-L1的表达水平相关。但是,无论PD-L1的表达水平如何,阿特珠单抗联合化疗对NSCLC患者都具有很好的疗效。研究发现阿特珠单抗联合化疗对晚期SCLC患者有效,但治疗费用与化疗相当。德瓦鲁单抗被批准用于治疗III期不可切除的NSCLC肺癌。关于阿维单抗的多个临床试验也正在进行。此外,多项关于ICI单药治疗及联合免疫、化疗、放疗、靶向治疗等相关临床试验均在开展。

尽管ICI在肺癌治疗方面取得了一定进展,但仅对15%~25%的患者有效。一方面归因于免疫治疗的耐药性,某些癌基因或抑癌基因如EGFR和STK11与ICI耐药有关,也有报道使用抗生素后肠道微生物的多样性变化可能与ICI耐药有关。另一方面,约20%~30%的患者在接受PD-1/PD-L1抑制剂治疗后出现免疫相关不良反应(irAEs),主要由免疫系统的过度激活或自身免疫反应所致,可涉及内分泌系统、皮肤、心血管系统、呼吸道、消化系统等。以上提及的ICI疗效的局限性推动了生物标记物的研究发展,从而有益于肺癌患者的针对性治疗和不良反应的预测。

三、生物标记物

生物标记物可以预测免疫治疗的疗效、预后和不良反应,从而指导其临床应用。PD-1(PD-L1)信号通路是ICI的关键靶点,因此PD-L1可作为PD-1(PD-L1)抑制剂的生物标记物,但也有研究发现其疗效预测作用的缺失。通过针对肿瘤与免疫系统之间相互作用的研究,发现肿瘤突变负荷、新抗原、肿瘤微环境、肠道微生物等复杂因素可作为生物标记物。以下将讨论目前发现的主要生物标记物,部分源于肿瘤的异质性,另一部分与免疫反应相关。

(一)肿瘤异质性相关生物标记物

1. PD-L1 表达 PD-L1 在肿瘤细胞和免疫细胞中均有表达,可以通过免疫组织化学(IHC)方法分析其表达水平。据报道,NSCLC 的 PD-L1 表达水平明显高于肾细胞癌和黑色素瘤。既往研究表明 PD-L1 高表达与 PD-1(PD-L1)抑制剂治疗后的无进展生存期(PFS)和总生存期(OS)呈正相关。然而,另一些研究报道 PD-1(PD-L1)抑制剂对 PD-L1 低表达的患者也有较好的疗效。6 个 III 期临床试验报道了 ICI 治疗对 PD-L1 高表达(≥50%)的 NSCLC 患者疗效显著。相反,1 项荟萃分析报道 PD-1/PD-L1 抑制剂联合化疗在 PD-L1<1% 的 NSCLC 患者中比化疗更有效。此外,多项研究报道 ICI 联合化疗对 NSCLC 患者的效应与 PD-L1 表达水平无关。在 SCLC 患者中,基质 PD-L1 表达与帕博利珠单抗的疗效呈正相关,然而,在纳武利尤单抗治疗后的客观缓解率(ORR)与 PD-L1 表达无关。PD-L1 的以上预测性差异可能源于病理标本的代表性和检测技术的可靠性。首先,PD-L1 在肿瘤组织中的分布不均一,因此组织活检标本或切除组织对 PD-L1 表达水平的判断不准确。1 项研究通过比较 268 例患者的 5 份核心活检标本与完整组织标本的 PD-L1 表达水平来了解其差异。结果,1% 为截断点时有 39% 的样本阳性率相符,50% 为截断点时只有 10% 相符。其次,PD-L1 的表达不具有一贯性,前期治疗会改变其表达水平,从而影响其疗效预测作用。据报道,PD-L1 除了构成性表达外,兼具诱导性表达,在免疫细胞中尤其明显。研究人员对应用阿特珠单抗的 4549 例 NSCLC 患者的 PD-L1 表达谱进行了分析,发现干扰素-γ 可上调 PD-L1 在免疫细胞中的表达,但其在肿瘤细胞中的表达水平与基因功能失调有关,并且 PD-L1 在两种细胞中均有预测作用。第三,目前有 5 种经 FDA 批准的抗体可用于 PD-L1 检测。BluePrint 研究报道了 22C3、28-8 和 SP263 抗体染色结果的一致性,但是在肿瘤细胞中,SP142 的敏感性较低,73-10 的敏感性较高,而在免疫细胞中各个抗体的评分有较大差异。除了抗体间的不一致,病理医师对 PD-L1 表达水平的评估也可能导致结果的差异。另外,目前的研究并没有确切定义 PD-L1 表达的截断点,以指导 ICI 的临床应用。

PD-L1 作为有效的生物标记物,其应用有待进一步优化。PD-L1 可与其他因素结合来指导 ICI 治疗。有研究探讨了 PD-L1 表达联合 CD8$^+$ 肿瘤浸润淋巴细胞(TILs)密度对 NSCLC 患者的预测价值,得出 PD-L1$^+$(CD8^{low})组与肿瘤的高分级和晚分期相关,而 PD-L1$^-$(CD8^{low})组与较好的 OS 和 PFS 相关。但是研究样本量较小(55 例),其临床意义有待证实。另外,除了组织学标本,也有研究探索了肺癌患者外周血免疫细胞中 PD-L1 的表达水平与缓解率之间的关系,报道了治疗前 PD-L1$^+$CD11b$^+$ 细胞≥30% 的患者可达到 50% 的缓解率。甚至有研究发现正电子发射断层扫描-计算机断层摄影(PET-CT)可反映 NSCLC 患者 PD-1(PD-L1)的表达水平,并证实了肿瘤示踪剂摄取和 ICI 疗效之间的相关性。

2. 肿瘤突变负荷(TMB) TMB 指肿瘤中非同义突变的总数,可以用每兆(Mb)的体细胞突变数来表示。应用下一代测序(NGS)技术于肺组织标本可测定 TMB。TMB 作为 ICI 治疗的生物标志物主要是由于高水平的基因突变可导致新抗原增加,进而激活特异性免疫功能。1 项回顾性分析显示,在接受纳武利尤单抗治疗的 NSCLC 患者中,高 TMB(全基因组测序结果>243 个突变)的患者有更好的 PFS 和 ORR。在另一项研究中,接受纳武利尤单抗和 ipilimumab 联合治疗的 NSCLC 患者中,高 TMB(≥10 Mut/Mb)者 ORR 或 PFS 也较高。同样的,在接受纳武利尤单抗单药或 ipilimumab 联合治疗的 SCLC 患者中也报道了 TMB 的类似预测结果。

TMB 的疗效预测作用与新抗原产生有关,但两者的关系并非一一对应,某些突变基因更容易形成新抗原。例如,与微卫星不稳定性(MSI)伴随的错配修复缺陷(MMRd)突变与新抗原的相关性更高。与 TMB 相比,MMRd 代表了更多的插入缺失(indel)突变,以及随之出现的框移突变,这些突变能形成更多的新抗原。虽然 MMRd/MSI 只占 NSCLC 突变的一小部分,但其预测价值值得进一步探讨。

TMB 的检测对于时间和标本的要求比较高,为了克服这些缺点,一些研究人员对替代方法进行了探索。有研究利用高敏 NGS 技术检测血液 TMB(bTMB),发现其能有效估计 ICI 治疗的 NSCLC 患者的缓解率和生存率,包括阿特珠单抗单药和德瓦鲁单抗 + tremelimumab。另外,TMB 水平的截断值目前还没有定论,可以通过测序技术和分析方法的改进以及数据规模的扩大来不断克服。

3. 新抗原 如上所述,新抗原可以反映特异性免疫反应的强度,其作为 ICI 治疗生物标记物的作用不仅体现在数量(可通过 TMB 来初步估计),还体现在其质量。首先,克隆突变分布于整个肿瘤,亚克隆突变存在于肿瘤的部分组织,据此可将新抗原分为两类。克隆突变产生的新抗原对免疫细胞的攻击更敏感,而新抗原的瘤内不均一性(ITH)与克隆突变呈负相关,因此,ITH 可作为 ICI 疗效的阴性预测因子。其次,主要组织相容性复合体 I(MHC I)与 T 细胞受体(TCR)的结合是 T 细胞-新抗原反应的一个步骤,MHC I 与 TCR 的结合亲和力也与免疫反应相关,可通过差异性一致性指数(DAI)来衡量。1 项关于帕博利珠单抗的研究报道,DAI 可用于预测 NSCLC 患者的 OS。此外,通过对新抗原表位与已知的免疫源性微生物表位进行相似性分析,可得到序列同源性结果,也可用于评估免疫反应强度。研究人员基于以上三项因素建立新抗原适应度模型,应用于 PD-1 抑制剂治疗的患者,证明了其对肺癌等肿瘤的生存预测作用。

4. 特定突变基因 研究表明,肺癌中一些突变基因,主要是肿瘤驱动基因,与 ICI 的疗效相关。1 项荟萃分析报道,在抗 PD-1(PD-L1)治疗的 NSCLC 患者中,EGFR 突变患者的ORR较低,可能由于EGFR突变患者的TMB水平较低。另一项研究也报道TMB高水平与EGFR野生型肺癌高度相关。但也有研究报道德瓦鲁单抗可改善EGFR/ALK突变、PD-L1表达≥25% NSCLC患者的OR。另外,阿特珠单抗联合酪氨酸激酶抑制剂(TKI)据报道可对TKI无效的患者起效。STK11基因突变也可影响ICI疗效。STK11联合KRAS突变与肺腺癌患者的缓解和生存率降低有关。在非鳞NSCLC队列中,STK11(KRAS)共突变患者在接受帕博利珠单抗＋双药化疗后PSF和OS均较低。相反,基因组分析表明STK11(TP53)野生型NSCLC患者存在更长的OS。大多数突变基因对ICI治疗存在不良影响,但其机制及解决方法仍需进一步研究。

5. 循环肿瘤DNA(ctDNA)　ctDNA检测属于"液体活检",利用NGS技术测试突变基因片段,用于评估实时肿瘤细胞死亡,从而监测免疫治疗效果。1项关于转移性NSCLC患者的小样本研究报告了抗PD-1(PD-L1)治疗下ctDNA变化和放射学表现具有一致性,同时表明低水平的ctDNA是PFS和OS的阳性预测因子。另一个队列研究显示,在PD-1抑制剂治疗的肺癌患者中,ctDNA的疗效预测作用早于CT图像平均8.7周。这一发现为动态监测ICI疗效提供了一种有效的方法,但其准确性还有待进一步验证。

(二)宿主免疫相关生物标记物

1. 人类白细胞抗原I(HLA-I)　人类白细胞抗原基因在体内编码免疫监视功能,HLA-I基因主要与抗原呈递有关。因此HLA-I基因的多样性与多种抗原的识别相关。1项关于1535名接受抗PD-1或抗CTLA-4治疗的癌症患者的研究显示,HLA-I杂合度与更长的生存期呈正相关。相反,HLA-I基因抗原呈递功能受损对肺癌患者的PD-1/PD-L1抑制剂治疗起负性作用。

2. 肿瘤微环境(TME)　TME在肿瘤生长中发挥重要作用,包括肿瘤相关巨噬细胞(TAM)、自然杀伤细胞(NK)、树突状细胞(DC)、淋巴细胞和骨髓来源的抑制细胞(MDSCs)等多种免疫细胞,其中,肿瘤浸润淋巴细胞(TILs)是ICI治疗的抗肿瘤活性的主力军,既往研究报道肿瘤微环境中细胞毒性T细胞、辅助T细胞、记忆T细胞等TILs聚集与ICI治疗NSCLC患者的疾病缓解相关,不同的TILs在肿瘤-免疫相互作用中发挥不同的作用。1项研究运用免疫组化技术分析NSCLC组织样本中CD8和CD4分子的表达,得出较高的$CD8^+$T细胞计数(886～1899/mm^2)和较高的$CD8^+/CD4^+$比值(>2)与抗PD-1治疗的较高缓解率呈正相关。另一项研究表明基质中$CD8^+$和$CD4^+$免疫细胞浸润程度高的NSCLC患者在纳武利尤单抗治疗后表现出更好的OS。也有关于纳武利尤单抗治疗的肺癌患者的研究,分析了基质转化生长因子诱导蛋白(TGFBI)和瘤间$CD8^+$T细胞,结果显示低TGFBI和高CD8表达水平与肿瘤的高缓解率呈正相关。TILs表面的PD-1表达也是一个潜在的预测因子,有研究报道抗PD-1治疗前PD1表达最高($PD1^T$)的$CD8^+$T细胞与较好的药物疗效呈正相关。另一项关于CD3、CD8、CD4、PD1和FoxP3在TILs中的表达的研究表明,高$CD3^+$TILs(>617.5/mm^2)和低$FoxP3^+/CD8^+$T细胞(<25%)是NSCLC患者抗PD1治疗的预后因素。然而在另外的情况下,FoxP3高表达与治疗反应呈正相关。1项针对接受纳武利尤单抗治疗的EGFR突变NSCLC患者的研究报道,$CD4^+$和$FoxP3^+$T细胞是阳性预后因素,而PD-L1的表达不能预测疗效。另外,1项研究发现在根据基因表达分组的某一种NSCLC亚型中,TAM细胞和调节B细胞与ICI的疗效呈负相关。实际上,TME的复杂性决定了其中的少数细胞类型不具有完全代表性,因此有研究设计了免疫图谱,并据此将肺癌患者的TME分为T细胞富集型、T细胞贫乏型和T细胞中等型,此分类不受组织学类型的影响。这种免疫图谱兼具全面性和个性化,可作为较为理想的生物标记物。另一项研究通过比较188例NSCLC患者的mRNA测序,建立了基于转录组的模型,并证实其中一种以高$CD8^+$T细胞和记忆B细胞与低$CD4^+$ Treg和肿瘤相关骨髓细胞为特征的肺腺癌分子亚型是抗PD-1治疗的阳性预测因子。

3. 外周血指标　血液样本中的免疫细胞可作为生物标志物。1项对NSCLC患者抗PD-1(PD-L1)治疗前或刚开始抗PD-1(PD-L1)治疗时外周血T淋巴细胞分布的研究发现,高$PD1^+CD4^+$/总$CD4^+$T细胞比率与长PFS呈正相关。另外,血液中$CD4^+$和$CD8^+$中央记忆T细胞(TM)与效应T细胞(Eff)的高比值与纳武利尤单抗治疗的NSCLC患者的高PD-L1表达水平和PFS呈正相关。此外,对阿特珠单抗治疗的晚期NSCLC患者血液免疫细胞亚型的分析显示,在疾病缓解的患者中,调节性T细胞(Treg)和MDSCs明显减少。除此之外,利用外周免疫细胞可以预测ICI治疗患者的高进展性疾病(HPD)。1项针对263例抗PD-1(PD-L1)治疗的NSCLC患者的前瞻性研究报道,HPD在$CCR7^-CD45RA^-/CD8^+$T细胞比例较低、$TIGIT^+/PD-1^+CD8^+$T细胞比例较高的患者中发生频率较高。

外周炎症细胞水平也可用于评价ICI疗效,其中中性粒细胞与淋巴细胞比值(NLR)与ICI疗效高度相关。既往研究报道了NLR在预测PD-1抑制剂治疗的肺癌患者的PFS和OS中的作用。在接受二线纳武利尤单抗治疗的NSCLC患者中,△NLR>1与肿瘤的进展及短OS相关。1项关于绝对淋巴细胞计数(ALC)的研究报道,基线和治疗后6周的ALC高水平与PD-1抑制剂治疗的NSCLC患者OS升高相关,并且考虑到治疗后ALC水平的下降,建议谨慎联合ICI和放疗。最近的1项研究报道了应用免疫-代谢-预后指数(IMPI)来评价PD-1抑制剂在NSCLC患者中的有效性,研究采用全血细胞计数测定和F-18 FDG PET(CT)检测,发现IPMI两参数低水平(NLR<4.9和病灶糖酵解总量<541.5ml)与患者的PFS和OS呈正相关。其他涉及炎症、代谢和营养因素的评分系统,如肺免疫预后指数(LIPI)、晚期肺癌炎症指数(ALI)、RMH预后评分和MDACC预后评分的研究都已开展。还有研究探索了其他的生物标志物,包括红细胞分布宽度、基线血清钠浓度、血清催乳素(PRL)等。

4. 微生物　临床前和临床研究报道指出,共生菌群特别是肠道微生物的多样性在抗肿瘤免疫反应中起重要作用，因此微生物是肺癌患者 ICI 治疗的潜在生物标志物。通过对肺癌患者粪便标本进行分析，发现肠道菌群多样性与 ICI 治疗效果呈正相关。此外，PD-1 抑制剂治疗过程中抗生素的使用与 ICI 疗效呈负相关，这可能与肠道微生物多样性的变化有关。在非小细胞肺癌患者中，ICI 治疗前服用抗生素与短 PSF 和短 OS 相关。1 项对纳武利尤单抗治疗的 NSCLC 患者和健康人群的研究报道，治疗前微生物组成影响抗 PD-1 反应。微生物多样性受到多种因素的干扰，包括身体状况、饮食模式、烟草吸入和居住环境等。1 项针对国内 NSCLC 患者的研究报道，特定的菌群与 PD-1 抑制剂的反应相关。此外，肠道菌群是 irAEs 的一个潜在预测因子。有关黑色素瘤患者的研究显示特定菌群与 ICI 相关的结肠炎呈正相关，但其在肺癌患者中还未得到研究。

四、小 结

肺癌是发病率、死亡率均很高的恶性肿瘤，ICI 为其治疗开创了新的突破口，但疗效具有局限性。由于肿瘤组织与免疫系统之间的作用是一个多因素的动态过程，为 ICI 的疗效预测带来了困难。任何单一的生物标记物都不足以准确预测缓解率及生存率，因此可将不同因素进行组合建模。目前研究已经探索了不同生物标记物的组合，但大多只涉及少量指标，未来可探索一个涵盖基因测序、细胞染色、分子鉴定和影像学检查等多维指标的综合模型，从而增加 ICI 治疗的选择和预测准确性。另一方面，预测模型可能存在较差的时效性和便捷性，而液体活检操作简便、实施容易，且与其他生物标记物具有相当的一致性，因此受到广泛关注。另外，液体活检可重复操作，能够监测指标的动态变化，有助于更好地检测 ICI 的实时效应。生物标记物的研究在一些领域还没有被充分的研究，例如 ICI 在难治的 SCLC 患者以及联合化疗患者中的疗效预测。此外，目前关于生物标记物的报道大多是基于对现有队列的回顾性分析，可能存在偏倚，因此需要更多的前瞻性研究来进一步验证。

综上所述，肺癌患者 ICI 治疗的生物标记物研究已经取得了一定的成果，PD-L1 表达已被 FDA 批准作为预后性标志物，并且研究报道 TMB 和 TILs 与 ICI 治疗呈高度正相关。通过对治疗反应或耐药性机制的研究，目前已发现很多潜在的生物标记物，包括免疫相关新抗原、特定突变基因和微生物多样性等。但是，由于各个生物标记物的局限性，并没有预测 ICI 疗效的"金标准"，因此，需要进行更多的研究来进一步探索精准预测模型。

参 考 文 献

[1] Siegel RL, Miller KD, Jemal A. Cancer Statistics, 2020. CA Cancer J Clin, 2020, 70: 7-30.

[2] Khaltaev N, Axelrod S. Global Lung Cancer Mortality Trends and Lifestyle Modifications: Preliminary Analysis. Chin Med J (Engl), 2020, 133: 1526-1532.

[3] Arbour KC, Riely GJ. Systemic Therapy for Locally Advanced and Metastatic Non-Small Cell Lung Cancer: A Review. Jama, 2019, 322: 764-774.

[4] Lim SW, Ahn MJ. Current Status of Immune Checkpoint Inhibitors in Treatment of Non-Small Cell Lung Cancer. Korean J Intern Med, 2019, 34: 50-59.

[5] Brahmer J, Reckamp KL, Baas P, et al. Nivolumab Versus Docetaxel in Advanced Squamous-Cell Non-Small-Cell Lung Cancer. N Engl J Med, 2015, 373: 123-135.

[6] Borghaei H, Paz-Ares L, Horn L, et al. Nivolumab Versus Docetaxel in Advanced Nonsquamous Non-Small-Cell Lung Cancer. N Engl J Med, 2015, 373: 1627-1639.

[7] Ready N, Farago AF, De Braud F, et al. Third-Line Nivolumab Monotherapy in Recurrent Sclc: Checkmate 032. J Thorac Oncol, 2019, 14: 237-244.

[8] Herbst RS, Baas P, Kim DW, et al. Pembrolizumab Versus Docetaxel for Previously Treated, Pd-L1-Positive, Advanced Non-Small-Cell Lung Cancer (Keynote-010): A Randomised Controlled Trial. Lancet, 2016, 387: 1540-1550.

[9] Garon EB, Rizvi NA, Hui R, et al. Pembrolizumab for the Treatment of Non-Small-Cell Lung Cancer. N Engl J Med, 2015, 372: 2018-2028.

[10] Reck M, Rodríguez-Abreu D, Robinson AG, et al. Pembrolizumab Versus Chemotherapy for Pd-L1-Positive Non-Small-Cell Lung Cancer. N Engl J Med, 2016, 375: 1823-1833.

[11] Langer CJ, Gadgeel SM, Borghaei H, et al. Carboplatin and Pemetrexed with or without Pembrolizumab for Advanced, Non-Squamous Non-Small-Cell Lung Cancer: A Randomised, Phase 2 Cohort of the Open-Label Keynote-021 Study. Lancet Oncol, 2016, 17: 1497-1508.

[12] Gandhi L, Rodríguez-Abreu D, Gadgeel S, et al. Pembrolizumab Plus Chemotherapy in Metastatic Non-Small-Cell Lung Cancer. N Engl J Med, 2018, 378: 2078-2092.

[13] Paz-Ares L, Luft A, Vicente D, et al. Pembrolizumab Plus Chemotherapy for Squamous Non-Small-Cell Lung Cancer. N Engl J Med, 2018, 379: 2040-2051.

[14] Chung HC, Piha-Paul SA, Lopez-Martin J, et al. Pembrolizumab after Two or More Lines of Previous Therapy in Patients with Recurrent or Metastatic Sclc: Results from the Keynote-028 and Keynote-158 Studies. J Thorac Oncol, 2020, 15: 618-627.

[15] Hoy SM. Sintilimab: First Global Approval. Drugs, 2019, 79: 341-346.

[16] Gao S, Li N, Gao S, et al. Neoadjuvant Pd-1 Inhibitor (Sintilimab) in Nsclc. J Thorac Oncol, 2020, 15: 816-826.

[17] Fehrenbacher L, Spira A, Ballinger M, et al. Atezolizumab Versus Docetaxel for Patients with Previously Treated Non-Small-Cell Lung Cancer (Poplar): A Multicentre, Open-Label, Phase 2 Randomised Controlled Trial. Lancet, 2016, 387:

1837-1846.

[18] Peters S, Gettinger S, Johnson ML, et al. Phase Ii Trial of Atezolizumab as First-Line or Subsequent Therapy for Patients with Programmed Death-Ligand 1-Selected Advanced Non-Small-Cell Lung Cancer (Birch). J Clin Oncol, 2017, 35: 2781-2789.

[19] Spigel DR, Chaft JE, Gettinger S, et al. Fir: Efficacy, Safety, and Biomarker Analysis of a Phase Ii Open-Label Study of Atezolizumab in Pd-L1-Selected Patients with Nsclc. J Thorac Oncol, 2018, 13: 1733-1742.

[20] Rittmeyer A, Barlesi F, Waterkamp D, et al. Atezolizumab Versus Docetaxel in Patients with Previously Treated Non-Small-Cell Lung Cancer (Oak): A Phase 3, Open-Label, Multicentre Randomised Controlled Trial. Lancet, 2017, 389: 255-265.

[21] West H, Mccleod M, Hussein M, et al. Atezolizumab in Combination with Carboplatin Plus Nab-Paclitaxel Chemotherapy Compared with Chemotherapy Alone as First-Line Treatment for Metastatic Non-Squamous Non-Small-Cell Lung Cancer (Impower130): A Multicentre, Randomised, Open-Label, Phase 3 Trial. Lancet Oncol, 2019, 20: 924-937.

[22] Horn L, Mansfield AS, Szczęsna A, et al. First-Line Atezolizumab Plus Chemotherapy in Extensive-Stage Small-Cell Lung Cancer. N Engl J Med, 2018, 379: 2220-2229.

[23] Li L Y, Wang H, Chen X, et al. First-Line Atezolizumab Plus Chemotherapy in Treatment of Extensive Small Cell Lung Cancer: A Cost-Effectiveness Analysis from China. Chin Med J (Engl), 2019, 132: 2790-2794.

[24] Antonia SJ, Villegas A, Daniel D, et al. Overall Survival with Durvalumab after Chemoradiotherapy in Stage Iii Nsclc. N Engl J Med, 2018, 379: 2342-2350.

[25] Gulley JL, Rajan A, Spigel DR, et al. Avelumab for Patients with Previously Treated Metastatic or Recurrent Non-Small-Cell Lung Cancer (Javelin Solid Tumor): Dose-Expansion Cohort of a Multicentre, Open-Label, Phase 1b Trial. Lancet Oncol, 2017, 18: 599-610.

[26] Barlesi F, Vansteenkiste J, Spigel D, et al. Avelumab Versus Docetaxel in Patients with Platinum-Treated Advanced Non-Small-Cell Lung Cancer (Javelin Lung 200): An Open-Label, Randomised, Phase 3 Study. Lancet Oncol, 2018, 19: 1468-1479.

[27] Jenkins RW, Barbie DA, Flaherty KT. Mechanisms of Resistance to Immune Checkpoint Inhibitors. Br J Cancer, 2018, 118: 9-16.

[28] Skoulidis F, Goldberg ME, Greenawalt DM, et al. Stk11/Lkb1 Mutations and Pd-1 Inhibitor Resistance in Kras-Mutant Lung Adenocarcinoma. Cancer Discov, 2018, 8: 822-835.

[29] Lee CK, Man J, Lord S, et al. Checkpoint Inhibitors in Metastatic Egfr-Mutated Non-Small Cell Lung Cancer-a Meta-Analysis. J Thorac Oncol, 2017, 12: 403-407.

[30] Routy B, Le Chatelier E, Derosa L, et al. Gut Microbiome Influences Efficacy of Pd-1-Based Immunotherapy against Epithelial Tumors. Science, 2018, 359: 91-97.

[31] Baraibar I, Melero I, Ponz-Sarvise M, et al. Safety and Tolerability of Immune Checkpoint Inhibitors (Pd-1 and Pd-L1) in Cancer. Drug Saf, 2019, 42: 281-294.

[32] Barroso-Sousa R, Barry WT, Garrido-Castro AC, et al. Incidence of Endocrine Dysfunction Following the Use of Different Immune Checkpoint Inhibitor Regimens: A Systematic Review and Meta-Analysis. JAMA Oncol, 2018, 4: 173-182.

[33] Mekki A, Dercle L, Lichtenstein P, et al. Detection of Immune-Related Adverse Events by Medical Imaging in Patients Treated with Anti-Programmed Cell Death 1. Eur J Cancer, 2018, 96: 91-104.

[34] Kluger HM, Zito CR, Turcu G, et al. Pd-L1 Studies across Tumor Types, Its Differential Expression and Predictive Value in Patients Treated with Immune Checkpoint Inhibitors. Clin Cancer Res, 2017, 23: 4270-4279.

[35] Gibney GT, Weiner LM, Atkins MB. Predictive Biomarkers for Checkpoint Inhibitor-Based Immunotherapy. Lancet Oncol, 2016, 17: e542-e551.

[36] Hersom M, Jørgensen JT. Companion and Complementary Diagnostics-Focus on Pd-L1 Expression Assays for Pd-1/Pd-L1 Checkpoint Inhibitors in Non-Small Cell Lung Cancer. Ther Drug Monit, 2018, 40: 9-16.

[37] Hellmann MD, Paz-Ares L, Bernabe Caro R, et al. Nivolumab Plus Ipilimumab in Advanced Non-Small-Cell Lung Cancer. N Engl J Med, 2019, 381: 2020-2031.

[38] Melosky B, Chu Q, Juergens RA, et al. Breaking the Biomarker Code: Pd-L1 Expression and Checkpoint Inhibition in Advanced Nsclc. Cancer Treat Rev, 2018, 65: 65-77.

[39] Landre T, Des Guetz G, Chouahnia K, et al. First-Line Pd-1/Pd-L1 Inhibitor Plus Chemotherapy Vs Chemotherapy Alone for Negative or<1% Pd-L1-Expressing Metastatic Non-Small-Cell Lung Cancers. J Cancer Res Clin Oncol, 2020, 146: 441-448.

[40] Reck M, Mok TSK, Nishio M, et al. Atezolizumab Plus Bevacizumab and Chemotherapy in Non-Small-Cell Lung Cancer (Impower150): Key Subgroup Analyses of Patients with Egfr Mutations or Baseline Liver Metastases in a Randomised, Open-Label Phase 3 Trial. Lancet Respir Med, 2019, 7: 387-401.

[41] Gadgeel SM, Pennell NA, Fidler MJ, et al. Phase Ii Study of Maintenance Pembrolizumab in Patients with Extensive-Stage Small Cell Lung Cancer (Sclc). J Thorac Oncol, 2018, 13: 1393-1399.

[42] Ready NE, Ott PA, Hellmann MD, et al. Nivolumab Monotherapy and Nivolumab Plus Ipilimumab in Recurrent Small Cell Lung Cancer: Results from the Checkmate 032 Randomized Cohort. J Thorac Oncol, 2020, 15: 426-435.

[43] Munari E, Zamboni G, Lunardi G, et al. Pd-L1 Expression Heterogeneity in Non-Small Cell Lung Cancer: Defining Criteria for Harmonization between Biopsy Specimens and Whole Sections. J Thorac Oncol, 2018, 13: 1113-1120.

[44] Sheng J, Fang W, Yu J, et al. Expression of Programmed Death Ligand-1 on Tumor Cells Varies Pre and Post Chemotherapy in Non-Small Cell Lung Cancer. Sci Rep, 2016, 6: 20090.

[45] Kowanetz M, Zou W, Gettinger SN, et al. Differential Regulation of Pd-L1 Expression by Immune and Tumor Cells in Nsclc and

the Response to Treatment with Atezolizumab (Anti-Pd-L1). Proc Natl Acad Sci USA,2018,115:10119-10126.

[46] Tsao MS, Kerr KM, KockxM, et al. Pd-L1 Immunohistochemistry Comparability Study in Real-Life Clinical Samples: Results of Blueprint Phase 2 Project. J Thorac Oncol,2018, 13: 1302-1311.

[47] El-Guindy DM, Helal DS, Sabry NM, et al. Programmed Cell Death Ligand-1 (Pd-L1) Expression Combined with Cd8 Tumor Infiltrating Lymphocytes Density in Non-Small Cell Lung Cancer Patients. J Egypt Natl Canc Inst,2018,30: 125-131.

[48] Bocanegra A, Fernandez-Hinojal G, Zuazo-Ibarra M, et al. Pd-L1 Expression in Systemic Immune Cell Populations as a Potential Predictive Biomarker of Responses to Pd-L1/Pd-1 Blockade Therapy in Lung Cancer. Int J Mol Sci,2019,20.

[49] Niemeijer AN, Leung D, Huisman MC, et al. Whole Body Pd-1 and Pd-L1 Positron Emission Tomography in Patients with Non-Small-Cell Lung Cancer. Nat Commun,2018,9: 4664.

[50] Peters S, Creelan B, Hellmann MD, et al. Abstract Ct082: Impact of Tumor Mutation Burden on the Efficacy of First-Line Nivolumab in Stage Iv or Recurrent Non-Small Cell Lung Cancer: An Exploratory Analysis of Checkmate 026. Cancer Research,2017,77.

[51] Hellmann MD, Ciuleanu TE, Pluzanski A, et al. Nivolumab Plus Ipilimumab in Lung Cancer with a High Tumor Mutational Burden. N Engl J Med,2018,378: 2093-2104.

[52] Ricciuti B, Kravets S, Dahlberg SE, et al. Use of Targeted Next Generation Sequencing to Characterize Tumor Mutational Burden and Efficacy of Immune Checkpoint Inhibition in Small Cell Lung Cancer. J Immunother Cancer, 2019, 7: 87.

[53] Hellmann MD, Callahan MK, Awad MM, et al. Tumor Mutational Burden and Efficacy of Nivolumab Monotherapy and in Combination with Ipilimumab in Small-Cell Lung Cancer. Cancer Cell,2019,35: 329.

[54] Campbell BB, Light N, Fabrizio D, et al. Comprehensive Analysis of Hypermutation in Human Cancer. Cell,2017,171: 1042-1056.

[55] Gandara DR, Paul SM, Kowanetz M, et al. Blood-Based Tumor Mutational Burden as a Predictor of Clinical Benefit in Non-Small-Cell Lung Cancer Patients Treated with Atezolizumab. Nat Med,2018,24: 1441-1448.

[56] Wang. Z, Duan J, Cai S, et al. Assessment of Blood Tumor Mutational Burden as a Potential Biomarker for Immunotherapy in Patients with Non-Small Cell Lung Cancer with Use of a Next-Generation Sequencing Cancer Gene Panel. JAMA Oncol,2019,5: 696-702.

[57] Ghorani E, Rosenthal R, Mcgranahan N, et al. Differential Binding Affinity of Mutated Peptides for Mhc Class I Is a Predictor of Survival in Advanced Lung Cancer and Melanoma. Ann Oncol,2018,29: 271-279.

[58] Łuksza M, Riaz N, Makarov V, et al. A Neoantigen Fitness Model Predicts Tumour Response to Checkpoint Blockade Immunotherapy. Nature,2017,551: 517-520.

[59] Tsakonas G, Ekman S. Oncogene-Addicted Non-Small Cell Lung Cancer and Immunotherapy. J Thorac Dis, 2018, 10: 1547-1555.

[60] Ozaki Y, Muto S, Takagi H, et al. Tumor Mutation Burden and Immunological, Genomic, and Clinicopathological Factors as Biomarkers for Checkpoint Inhibitor Treatment of Patients with Non-Small-Cell Lung Cancer. Cancer Immunol Immunother,2020,69: 127-134.

[61] Garassino MC, Cho BC, Kim JH, et al. Durvalumab as Third-Line or Later Treatment for Advanced Non-Small-Cell Lung Cancer (Atlantic): An Open-Label, Single-Arm, Phase 2 Study. Lancet Oncol,2018,19: 521-536.

[62] Skoulidis F, Arbour KC, Hellmann MD, et al. Association of Stk11/Lkb1 Genomic Alterations with Lack of Benefit from the Addition of Pembrolizumab to Platinum Doublet Chemotherapy in Non-Squamous Non-Small Cell Lung Cancer. Journal of Clinical Oncology,2019,37: 102.

[63] Willard MD, Smyth ENN, Tiu RV, et al. Genomic Characterization of Lung Tumors and Metastatic (Met) Sites in Advanced (Adv) Nsclc. Journal of Clinical Oncology, 2019, 37: 2014.

[64] Goldberg SB, Narayan A, Kole AJ, et al. Early Assessment of Lung Cancer Immunotherapy Response Via Circulating Tumor DNA. Clin Cancer Res,2018,24: 1872-1880.

[65] Anagnostou V, Forde PM, White JR, et al. Dynamics of Tumor and Immune Responses During Immune Checkpoint Blockade in Non-Small Cell Lung Cancer. Cancer Res,2019, 79: 1214-1225.

[66] Chowell D, Morris LGT, Grigg CM, et al. Patient Hla Class I Genotype Influences Cancer Response to Checkpoint Blockade Immunotherapy. Science,2018,359: 582-587.

[67] Gettinger S, Choi J, Hastings K, et al. Impaired Hla Class I Antigen Processing and Presentation as a Mechanism of Acquired Resistance to Immune Checkpoint Inhibitors in Lung Cancer. Cancer Discov,2017,7: 1420-1435.

[68] Hornyák L, Dobos N, Koncz G, et al. The Role of Indoleamine-2,3-Dioxygenase in Cancer Development, Diagnostics, and Therapy. Front Immunol,2018,9: 151.

[69] Niemeijer AN, Sahba S, Smit EF, et al. Association of Tumour and Stroma Pd-1, Pd-L1, Cd3, Cd4 and Cd8 Expression with Dcb and Os to Nivolumab Treatment in Nsclc Patients Pre-Treated with Chemotherapy. Br J Cancer,2020.

[70] Nakazawa N, Yokobori T, Kaira K, et al. High Stromal Tgfbi in Lung Cancer and Intratumoral Cd8-Positive T Cells Were Associated with Poor Prognosis and Therapeutic Resistance to Immune Checkpoint Inhibitors. Ann Surg Oncol,2020,27: 933-942.

[71] Thommen DS, Koelzer VH, Herzig P, et al. A Transcriptionally and Functionally Distinct Pd-1(+) Cd8(+) T Cell Pool with Predictive Potential in Non-Small-Cell Lung Cancer Treated with Pd-1 Blockade. Nat Med,2018,24: 994-1004.

[72] Cai MC, Zhao X, Cao M, et al. T-Cell Exhaustion Interrelates with Immune Cytolytic Activity to Shape the Inflamed Tumor Microenvironment. J Pathol,2020,251: 147-159.

[73] Sato M, Watanabe S, Tanaka H, et al. Retrospective Analysis of Antitumor Effects and Biomarkers for Nivolumab in Nsclc Pa-

tients with Egfr Mutations. PLoS One,2019,14: e0215292.

[74] Seo JS,Kim A,Shin JY,et al. Comprehensive Analysis of the Tumor Immune Micro-Environment in Non-Small Cell Lung Cancer for Efficacy of Checkpoint Inhibitor. Sci Rep,2018,8: 14576.

[75] Karasaki T,Nagayama K,Kuwano H,et al. An Immunogram for the Cancer-Immunity Cycle: Towards Personalized Immunotherapy of Lung Cancer. J Thorac Oncol,2017,12: 791-803.

[76] Jang HJ,Lee HS,Ramos D,et al. Transcriptome-Based Molecular Subtyping of Non-Small Cell Lung Cancer May Predict Response to Immune Checkpoint Inhibitors. J Thorac Cardiovasc Surg,2020,159: 1598-1610.

[77] Inomata M,Kado T,Okazawa S,et al. Peripheral Pd1-Positive Cd4 T-Lymphocyte Count Can Predict Progression-Free Survival in Patients with Non-Small Cell Lung Cancer Receiving Immune Checkpoint Inhibitor. Anticancer Res,2019, 39: 6887-6893.

[78] Manjarrez-Orduño N,Menard LC,Kansal S,et al. Circulating T Cell Subpopulations Correlate with Immune Responses at the Tumor Site and Clinical Response to Pd1 Inhibition in Non-Small Cell Lung Cancer. Front Immunol,2018,9: 1613.

[79] Zhuo M,Chen H,Zhang T, et al. The Potential Predictive Value of Circulating Immune Cell Ratio and Tumor Marker in Atezolizumab Treated Advanced Non-Small Cell Lung Cancer Patients. Cancer Biomark,2018,22: 467-476.

[80] Kim CG,Kim KH,Pyo KH,et al. Hyperprogressive Disease During Pd-1/Pd-L1 Blockade in Patients with Non-Small-Cell Lung Cancer. Ann Oncol,2019,30: 1104-1113.

[81] Jiang T,Qiao M,Zhao C,et al. Pretreatment Neutrophil-to-Lymphocyte Ratio Is Associated with Outcome of Advanced-Stage Cancer Patients Treated with Immunotherapy: A Meta-Analysis. Cancer Immunol Immunother, 2018, 67: 713-727.

[82] Dusselier M,Deluche E,Delacourt N,et al. Neutrophil-to-Lymphocyte Ratio Evolution Is an Independent Predictor of Early Progression of Second-Line Nivolumab-Treated Patients with Advanced Non-Small-Cell Lung Cancers. PLoS One,2019,14: e0219060.

[83] Karantanos T,Karanika S,Seth B,et al. The Absolute Lymphocyte Count Can Predict the Overall Survival of Patients with Non-Small Cell Lung Cancer on Nivolumab: A Clinical Study. Clin Transl Oncol,2019,21: 206-212.

[84] Castello A,Toschi L,Rossi S,et al. The Immune-Metabolic-Prognostic Index and Clinical Outcomes in Patients with Non-Small Cell Lung Carcinoma under Checkpoint Inhibitors. J Cancer Res Clin Oncol,2020,146: 1235-1243.

[85] Varga A,Bernard-Tessier A,Auclin E,et al. Applicability of the Lung Immune Prognostic Index (Lipi) in Patients with Metastatic Solid Tumors When Treated with Immune Checkpoint Inhibitors (Ici) in Early Clinical Trials. Ann Oncol, 2019,30(Suppl 1): i2.

[86] Shiroyama T,Suzuki H,Tamiya M,et al. Pretreatment Advanced Lung Cancer Inflammation Index (Ali) for Predicting Early Progression in Nivolumab-Treated Patients with Advanced Non-Small Cell Lung Cancer. Cancer Med,2018,7: 13-20.

[87] Maymani H,Hess K,Groisberg R,et al. Predicting Outcomes in Patients with Advanced Non-Small Cell Lung Cancer Enrolled in Early Phase Immunotherapy Trials. Lung Cancer, 2018,120: 137-141.

[88] Kiriu T,Yamamoto M,Nagano T,et al. Prognostic Value of Red Blood Cell Distribution Width in Non-Small Cell Lung Cancer Treated with Anti-Programmed Cell Death-1 Antibody. In Vivo,2019,33: 213-220.

[89] Fucà G,Galli G,Poggi M,et al. Low Baseline Serum Sodium Concentration Is Associated with Poor Clinical Outcomes in Metastatic Non-Small Cell Lung Cancer Patients Treated with Immunotherapy. Target Oncol,2018,13: 795-800.

[90] Caponnetto S,Iannantuono GM,Barchiesi G,et al. Prolactin as a Potential Early Predictive Factor in Metastatic Non-Small Cell Lung Cancer Patients Treated with Nivolumab. Oncology,2017,93: 62-66.

[91] Schett A,Rothschild SI,Curioni-Fontecedro A,et al. Predictive Impact of Antibiotics in Patients with Advanced Non Small-Cell Lung Cancer Receiving Immune Checkpoint Inhibitors: Antibiotics Immune Checkpoint Inhibitors in Advanced Nsclc. Cancer Chemother Pharmacol,2020,85: 121-131.

[92] Botticelli A,Vernocchi P,Marini F,et al. Gut Metabolomics Profiling of Non-Small Cell Lung Cancer (Nsclc) Patients under Immunotherapy Treatment. J Transl Med, 2020, 18: 49.

[93] Jin Y,Dong H,Xia L,et al. The Diversity of Gut Microbiome Is Associated with Favorable Responses to Anti-Programmed Death 1 Immunotherapy in Chinese Patients with Nsclc. J Thorac Oncol,2019,14: 1378-1389.

[94] Chaput N,Lepage P,Coutzac C,et al. Baseline Gut Microbiota Predicts Clinical Response and Colitis in Metastatic Melanoma Patients Treated with Ipilimumab. Ann Oncol,2017, 28: 1368-1379.

12 真实世界肺癌免疫治疗的有关问题和思考

邓海怡 王李强 王 飞 周承志

一、研究背景

肺癌是世界范围内发病率和死亡率最高的恶性肿瘤。据 Globocan 2018 统计,肺癌发病率占癌症总发病人数的 11.6%,死亡率占癌症总死亡人数的 18.4%。近年来,免疫治疗快速发展,尤其是免疫检查点抑制剂（immune checkpoint inhibitors,ICI）取得重大的突破。多项临床研究表明 ICIs 比传统化疗明显延长晚期肺癌患者总生存期。但临床研究入组条件严格,排除了 PS 评分高、高龄、自身免疫疾病、应用激素、有症状的脑转移等患者。真实世界这些特殊人群的免疫治疗是值得探讨的问题。临床研究表示 ICI 无论在一线还是二线,单药还是联合都有显著疗效。在真实世界中何时应用免疫治疗、是单药治疗还是联合治疗是值得思考的问题。本文结合临床研究与真实世界的数据加以分析,以供广大临床工作者参考。

二、肺癌免疫治疗现状

目前,NMPA 批准用于肺癌的有 Nivolumab、Pembrolizumab、Atezolizumab、durvalumab（详见表 6-12-1）,还有不少原研药物正处于临床研究中。如：替雷利珠单抗联合培美曲塞及铂类一线治疗非鳞状非小细胞肺癌（NSCLC）患者的 III 期研究 BGB-A317-307；比较信迪利单抗联合培美曲塞含铂双药（TP）与安慰剂联合 TP III 期临床研究 ORIENT-11；信迪利单抗联合化疗一线治疗鳞状 NSCLC 的 III 期临床研究 ORIENT-12；卡瑞利珠单抗联合化疗一线治疗非鳞 NSCLC 的 III 期临床研究；特瑞普利单抗用于 EGFR-TKI 治疗失败的 EGFR 突变阳性 T790M 阴性晚期 NSCLC 患者的 II 期研究。

表 6-12-1 肺癌免疫治疗的适应证

药物	临床研究	适应证	生物标志物	NMPA	FDA	EMA
Nivolumab	CM-017	2 线鳞癌	None		2015.3.4	2015.7.20
Nivolumab	CM-057	2 线非鳞 NSCLC	None		2015.10.9	2016.4.6
Nivolumab	CM-078	2 线 NSCLC	PD-L1 ≥ 1%, EGFR-/ALK-	2018.6.15		
Nivolumab	CM-032	3 线 SCLC	None		2018.8.17	
Pembrolizumab	KN-001	2 线 NSCLC	PD-L1 ≥ 1%, EGFR-, ALK-		2015.10.2	2016.8.2
Pembrolizumab	KN-024	1 线 NSCLC	PD-L1 ≥ 50%, EGFR-, ALK-		2016.10.24	2017.1.31
Pembrolizumab	KN-042	1 线 NSCLC	PD-L1≥1%	2019.9.29	2019.4.11	
Pembrolizumab+卡铂/培美曲塞	KN-189	1 线非鳞 NSCLC	EGFR-, ALK-	2019.3.28	2018.8.20	2018.9.10
Pembrolizumab+卡铂/紫杉醇(白蛋白紫杉醇)	KN-407	1 线鳞癌	EGFR-, ALK-	2019.11.26	2018.10.30	2019.3.14
Pembrolizumab	KN-028,KN-015	3 线 SCLC	None		2019.6.18	
Atezolizumab	POPLAR OAK	2 线 NSCLC	None		2016.10.18	2017.9.25

(续　表)

药物	临床研究	适应证	生物标志物	获批时间 NMPA	获批时间 FDA	获批时间 EMA
Atezolizumab+贝伐珠单抗/紫杉醇/卡铂	IMpower150	1线非鳞 NSCLC	EGFR-,ALK-		2018.12.6	2019.3.7
Atezolizumab+卡铂/白蛋白紫杉醇	IMpower130	1线非鳞 NSCLC	EGFR-,ALK-		2019.12.3	2019.9.6
Atezolizumab+卡铂/依托泊苷	IMpower133	1线 ES-SCLC	EGFR-,ALK-	2020.2.13	2019.3.18	2019.9.6
Durvalumab	PACIFIC	III期 NSCLC	None	2019.12.9	2018.2.16	2018.9.24
Durvalumab+卡铂/依托泊苷	CASPIAN	1线 ES-SCLC	EGFR-,ALK-		2020.3.30	

注：NSCLC为非小细胞肺癌，ES-SCLC为广泛期小细胞肺癌，CM-为CheckMate，KN-为KEYNOTE

三、免疫治疗的疗效

(一)ICI 单药一线治疗

宜选择 PD-L1 高表达人群，PD-L1≥50% 是目前标准。

KEYNOTE-024 研究显示在 PD-L1 表达≥50% 的晚期 NSCLC，Pembrolizumab 组的总生存期(median overall survival，mOS)和无进展生存期(Median progression-free survival，mPFS)均优于化疗组。KEYNOTE-042 研究显示无论 PD-L1 表达状态如何，晚期 NSCLC 一线治疗 Pembrolizumab 都优于化疗组，亚组分析显示 PD-L1 表达≥50% 是主要获益人群。

日本的 1 项真实世界研究显示 Pembrolizumab 在治疗 PD-L1 表达≥50% 的晚期 NSCLC，mPFS 为 8.3 个月，mOS 为 17.8 个月。法国的 1 项研究也显示 Pembrolizumab 一线治疗 PD-L1 高表达的晚期 NSCLC 患者的优势。两项真实世界研究显示 OS 均能获益，但均短于临床研究。

(二)ICI 二线及以上单药治疗

相对于多西他赛组，疗效和不良反应均有优势。

4 项大型的临床研究表明，ICI 单药二线或以上治疗晚期 NSCLC 的疗效也显著优于化疗组，ICI 组的 mPFS 为 2.3～5.2 个月，mOS 为 9.2～17.3 个月，而多西他赛化疗组的 mPFS 为 2.8～4.0 个月，mOS 为 6.0～9.7 个月。本文总结了 4 项真实世界中 ICI 单药二线及以上治疗晚期 NSCLC 的研究，数据显示 mPFS 为 2.2～5.7 个月，mOS 为 7.9～13.21 个月。真实世界研究的 mOS 均比临床研究稍短。

(三)免疫治疗应用的时机

早用获益更长久，而且不良反应发生率也低。

KEYNOTE-001 显示，Pembrolizumab 一线比二线治疗疗效更显著，mOS 和 5 年生存率分别是 22.1 个月 vs.10.5 个月和 23.2% vs.15.5%。KEYNOTE-024、KEYNOTE-189 研究交叉治疗组分析显示一线免疫治疗较一线化疗后选择免疫治疗明显增加患者生存获益，而且不良反应也低。

1 项真实世界研究显示，pembrolizumab 一线比二线治疗的 mOS 延长 10.4 个月。Afzal 等的研究比较 Pembrolizumab 联合化疗和单纯化疗，化疗组中 45.9% 进展后选择免疫治疗，但也不如一线免疫治疗的疗效显著(ORR：58.3% vs.80%)。因此，无论临床研究还是真实世界均证实早期应用免疫治疗获益更大。

(四)单药还是联合

PD-L1 高表达人群可以单药，低表达人群更倾向联合；联合的方式：化疗为主，抗血管数据少，双免疫有争议。

KEYNOTE-189、KEYNOTE-407 研究分别显示在晚期非鳞癌及肺鳞癌中证实了 Pembrolizumab 联合化疗相对于化疗显著延长 mOS。IMpower150 研究对比 Atezolizumab+贝伐珠单抗+化疗(ABCP组)与贝伐珠单抗+化疗(BCP组)一线治疗转移性非鳞 NSCLC，结果显示：ABCP 组 mPFS 优于 BCP 组，基因野生型患者中 ABCP 组 mOS 较 BCP 组延长。CheckMate227 研究显示在高 TMB 组，Ipilimumab 联合 Nivolumab 组 mPFS 和 ORR 均优于化疗。而 MYSTIC 研究则显示，相比化疗组和 durvalumab 单药组，durvalumab 联合 tremelimumab 组在 PD-L1 表达≥25% 的患者中，PFS 和 OS 均无获益，仅在 bTMB≥20 mut/Mb 的患者中，联合治疗组 OS 延长。

免疫单药治疗比化疗明显改善生存期，但 KEYNOTE-042 研究表明疗效与 PD-L1 表达有关。PD-L1 低表达患者优选联合化疗治疗。KEYNOTE-024、KEYNOTE-042、KEYNOTE-189 研究的数据显示，PD-L1 表达≥50% 的 NSCLC 单药与联合化疗的 2 年生存率相近，但单药 OS 风险比更低，安全性更好。

(五)特殊人群

老年人与 PS 评分年龄不是大问题，PS 评分影响可能更大。1 项汇总了 4 项 NSCLC 的临床试验，对不同年龄进行分析显示：年龄＜65 岁，65～69 岁，70～74 岁和≥75 岁的 OS 的 HR 分别是 0.71、0.66、0.67 和 0.81；≥75 岁患者 3/4 级不良反应发生率比年轻组更低。Checkmate153 和 Checkmate171 研究显示，高龄组与总体人群的 OS 相近，PS 为 2 分的 OS 显著降低。但最近一项 Pembrolizumab 治疗 PS 为 2 分的 NSCLC 单臂 II 期临床研究显示疗效与 PS 为 0～1 分的相似，而且并不增加不良反应的发生。在真实世界中：1 项意大利的研究数据显示年龄对疗效的影响并不显著,而 PS 评分越高疗效越差;加拿大的 1 项研究也显示高龄并不降低疗效,但 PS 评分为 0~1 分比≥2 分的 mOS 延长 9.9 个月。

(六)脑、肝转移患者

脑转移疗效不差,肝转移疗效欠佳。

KEYNOTE-189 研究显示脑转移的 HR 为 0.41,无脑转移患者的 HR 为 0.59。但真实世界的 3 项免疫单药治疗研究都显示有脑转移的疗效比无脑转移差,mOS 分别为 5.09~8.6 个月和 11.4~16.3 个月。另一项非随机Ⅱ期临床研究显示免疫单药用于脑转移的 NSCLC 也有疗效。美国 1 项研究也显示,在脑转移患者中,免疫联合化疗比单纯化疗组的 ORR 升高(80% vs. 41.7%)。可见,脑转移患者也能从免疫治疗中获益。

KEYNOTE-189 研究显示肝转移的 HR 为 0.62,而无肝转移患者的 HR 为 0.58,与单纯化疗相比,mOS 分别是 12.6 个月 vs. 6.6 个月和 23.7 个月 vs. 13.2 个月。而在 1 项真实世界的研究显示,肝转移患者比无肝转移的 mOS 明显缩短,HR 为 2.02。另一项日本的研究显示肝转移影响疗效,HR 为 1.60。可见,肝转移患者免疫治疗获益有限。

(七)激素的使用

影响疗效,尽量不用,实在要用选择短疗程低剂量。

1 项回顾性研究显示在免疫治疗的前 30d 内使用糖皮质激素,mOS 显著下降(4.3 个月 vs. 11 个月)。Fucà 等的研究显示免疫治疗前应用激素组比未使用激素组的疾病控制率更低(34% vs. 62%),mOS 缩短 10.28 个月,但在免疫治疗期间因不良反应使用激素对疗效影响并不显著。另一项研究回顾性分析显示在免疫开始时使用泼尼松≥10mg 患者的 ORR 降低,mPFS 和 mOS 也明显缩短。

(八)合并自身免疫性疾病患者

疗效无差异,但要更加重视不良反应的管理。

1 项真实世界的研究纳入的 751 例患中 11.3% 有自身免疫性疾病,数据显示自身免疫性疾病的病人不良反应明显增加(65.9% vs. 39.9%),但 PFS 和 OS 无显著差异。另一项研究也显示 45 例自身免疫性疾病患者中 2 级及以上的不良反应会增多,但免疫治疗的疗效并无显著差异。

四、疗效标志物的探索

PD-L1 是目前唯一推荐,多维度检测是未来方向。

相关标志物的检测可以评估患者对免疫治疗获益的可能性。目前研究的正性标志物有 PD-L1、TMB、dMMR/MSI-H、TP-53、KRAS、CD8+TIL 等,负性的标志物有 STK11m、KEAP1m、MDM2/4、EGFR 突变、PTEN 缺失等。KEYNOTE-001、KEYNOTE-042 研究证实了 PD-L1 表达水平高的患者疗效更显著。CheckMate227 研究显示 TMB 可作为正性标志物,但 KEYNOTE-189 和 KEYNOTE-021 研究则显示 TMB 无法预测免疫治疗联合化疗的疗效。有文献报道 dMMR/MSI-H 与疗效成正相关,2017 年 FDA 批准了 pembrolizumab 用于治疗 MSI-H/dMMR 变异的任何实体瘤患者。生物标记物的研究不断深入,但目前在肺癌方面指南仅推荐 PD-L1 的检测。

五、疗效评价标准

RECIST 1.1 是目前临床研究的评估标准;iRECIST 循证医学证据尚少,可用于真实世界疗效评估;imRECIST 仅适用于经验丰富的专家和治疗团队。

免疫治疗与传统化疗不同,可出现假性进展和超进展,用传统的疗效评价标准是无法做出准确的评估。随着对免疫治疗的认识,疗效评价标准也在不断完善,2009 年免疫相关反应标准(irRC)、2013 年实体瘤免疫相关疗效评价标准(irRECIST)和 2017 年基于 RECIST 1.1 标准的实体瘤免疫治疗疗效评价标准(iRECIST)。RECIST1.1 标准已评定为进展的患者还不能确认免疫治疗进展,即 iUPD,iUPD 后仍可能出现 iCR/iPR/iSD,需 4~8 周再次评估,若影像学评估证实靶病灶增加至少 5mm,则可评为确认的疾病进展(iCPD)。2018 年 imRECIST 提出疾病进展后可以继续使用免疫治疗,但需结合患者病情及预测获益情况慎重决定。

六、不良反应

不良反应与疗效相关,轻度不良反应有利于长生存,重点关注致死性不良反应。

免疫相关性不良反应(immune-related adverse events,irAEs)可以累及人体的任何器官,大多数 irAEs 为 1~2 级,但仍有部分患者会产生严重的、甚至威胁生命的 3~4 级免疫异常毒性反应。

Wang 等回顾性查询 WHO 药物警戒数据库,报道了 613 例致命性 irAEs,其发生率在 CTLA-4 抑制剂中最高是结肠炎,而抗 PD-1/PD-L1 的是肺炎;心肌炎发生率低,但死亡率最高(39.7%)。在 6 项真实世界的 PD-1/PD-L1 抑制剂研究,≥3 级 irAEs 发生率为 11%~26%,其中发生率最高的也是肺炎。致死性 irAEs 发生率并不高(0.36%~1.23%),但是发展迅速,病死率高,应早期识别,尽早诊断和治疗。

有轻度 irAEs 的患者免疫治疗的疗效反而显著。1 项荟萃分析显示,有 irAE 的癌症患者的 PFS 和 OS 都获益(OS 的 HR 为 0.54,95%CI:0.45~0.65),而轻度 irAE 与 OS 获益相关(HR:0.57),而重度 irAE 与 OS 没有显著相关(HR:0.99)。另一项研究结果显示:首次出现≥2 级 irAE 对 PFS 和 OS 都有积极影响(PFS 的 HR:0.63,OS 的 HR:0.57)。

七、小细胞肺癌的免疫治疗

30 余年不停探索,2 个多月 OS 的突破,未来任重道远。

广泛期小细胞肺癌一线治疗方案 30 多年一直未变,直到 2018 年首个 PD-L1 单抗 Atezolizumab 阳性结果出现,即 IMpower133,Atezolizumab 联合化疗比化疗组疗效更显著(mPFS:5.2个月 vs.4.3个月,mOS:12.3个月 vs.10.3个月)。随后,相似的 CASPIAN 研究对比 Durvalumab 联合化疗与单纯化疗,结果显示:两组的 PFS 并无显著差异,但免疫联合组的中位 OS 明显延长(13个月 vs.10.3个月)。

八、结 语

肺癌已步入免疫治疗时代,ICI 药物相继上市,真实世界中使用免疫治疗的人越来越多。真实世界研究与临床研究结果基本一致:免疫治疗可以明显延长肺癌患者的生存期,而且越早应用免疫治疗获益更大。免疫治疗可以根据患者 PD-L1 的表达情况选择单药还是联合治疗。高龄、PS 评分高、自身免疫疾病等特殊人群并不是免疫治疗的禁忌证。年龄并非影响免疫治疗的重要因素,更需要关注的是患者的 PS 评分情况。PS 评分影响免疫治疗的疗效,积极治疗肺癌的并发症可改善患者 PS 评分。脑转移患者同样能从免疫治疗中获益,自身免疫疾病并不影响免疫治疗的疗效,不良反应的管理是关键所在。激素会降低免疫治疗的疗效,尽量减少不必要的激素使用。目前在肺癌方面指南仅推荐 PD-L1 的检测,多维检测是未来方向。RECIST 1.1 仍然是目前临床研究的评估标准,但在真实世界需要结合临床个体化考虑。免疫治疗耐受性良好,大部分 irAEs 程度较轻,但也存在致命性 irAEs,早期识别、及时治疗是关键。

表 6-12-2 真实世界研究结果

研究者	国家	药物	亚组	线程	mPFS(月)	mOS(月)
Tamiya et al	日本	Pem	NA	1L	8.3	17.8
Amrane et al	法国	Pem	NA	1L	10.1	15.2
Merino et al	西班牙	Niv	NA	2L	5.3	9.7
CRINÒ et al	意大利	Niv	NA	≥2L	4.2	7.9
Weis et al	美国	Niv Ate	NA	≥2L	2.2 vs. 2.0	8.4 vs. 6.5
Figueir et al	葡萄牙	Niv	NA	≥2L	4.91	13.21
Ksienski et al	加拿大	Pem	线程:1/2L	≥1L	3.7	总:13.4;线程:24.3 vs. 13.9
Afzal et al	美国	Pem+AP vs. AP	脑转移(+/−)	1/2L	总:NA vs. 3.55 脑转移:4.1 vs. NA	NA
Galli et al	意大利	ICIs	PS 评分:0,1,≥2;年龄:<70,70~79,≥80	≥1L	总:3.0;PS 评分:5.49 vs. 2.63 vs. 1.88;年龄:2.8 vs. 3.5 vs. 2.6	总:9.93;PS:21.91 vs. 7.57 vs. 2.67;年龄:9.1 vs. 11.3 vs. 9.6
Muchnik et al	加拿大	ICIs	PS 评分:0~1,≥2	≥1L	NA	总:8.2;PS 评分:13.7 vs. 3.8
Ahn et al	韩国	Niv/Pem	脑转移(+/−)肝转移(+/−)	≥1L	总:3.06	总:10.25;脑转移:5.09 vs. 15.08;肝转移:4.93 vs. 13.54
Bjørnhart et al	丹麦	Niv/Pem	脑转移(+/−)	≥1L	总:6.3;脑转移:4.2 vs. 7.1	总:16.1;脑转移 8.2 vs. 16.3
Hendriks et al	法国	ICIs	脑转移(+/−)	≥1L	脑转移:1.7 vs. 2.1	脑转移:8.6 vs. 11.4
Goldberg et al		Pem	NA	≥1L	NA	7.7
Scott et al	美国	Nivo	激素(+/−)	≥1L	NA	4.3 vs.11
Fucà et al	意大利	ICIs	激素(+/−)	≥1L	1.98 vs. 3.94	4.86 vs. 15.14
Arbour et al	美国法国	Anti-PD-(L)1	激素(+/−)	≥1L	激素:MSKCC 1.9 vs. 2.6;GRCC:1.7 vs. 1.8	激素:MSKCC 5.4 vs. 12.1;GRCC 3.3 vs. 9.4

注:Pem 为 Pembrolizumab,Niv 为 Nivolumab,Anti-PD-(L)1 为 PD-(L)1 抑制剂,AP:培美曲塞+卡铂,-L 为-线,mPFS:中位无进展生存期,mOS:中位总生存期,ORR:客观缓解率,NA:文中未提及或未达到

参 考 文 献

[1] Bray F, Ferlay J, Soerjomataram I, et al. Global cancer statistics 2018: GLOBOCAN estimates of incidence and mortality worldwide for 36 cancers in 185 countries. CA Cancer J Clin, 2018, 68(6):394-424.

[2] Zhou C, Chen G, Huang Y, et al. A Randomized Phase 3 Study of Camrelizumab plus Chemotherapy as 1st Line Therapy for Advanced/Metastatic Non-Squamous Non-Small Cell Lung Cancer. J Thorac Oncol, 2019, 14S(10): S215-S216.

[3] Zhang J, Zhou C, Zhao Y, et al. A PII Study of Toripalimab, a PD-1 mAb, in Combination with Chemotherapy in EGFR+ Advanced NSCLC Patients Failed to Prior EGFR TKI Therapies. J Thorac Oncol, 2019, 14(10, Supplement): S292.

[4] Reck M, Rodriguez-Abreu D, Robinson AG, et al. Updated Analysis of KEYNOTE-024: Pembrolizumab Versus Platinum-Based Chemotherapy for Advanced Non-Small-Cell Lung Cancer With PD-L1 Tumor Proportion Score of 50% or Greater. J Clin Oncol, 2019, 37(7):537-546.

[5] Mok T SK, Wu Y, Kudaba I, et al. Pembrolizumab versus chemotherapy for previously untreated, PD-L1-expressing, locally advanced or metastatic non-small-cell lung cancer (KEYNOTE-042): a randomised, open-label, controlled, phase 3 trial. Lancet, 2019, 393(10183):1819-1830.

[6] Tamiya M, Tamiya A, Hosoya K, et al. Efficacy and safety of pembrolizumab as first-line therapy in advanced non-small cell lung cancer with at least 50% PD-L1 positivity: a multicenter retrospective cohort study (HOPE-001). Invest New Drugs, 2019, 37(6):1266-1273.

[7] Amrane K, Geier M, Corre R, et al. First-line pembrolizumab for non-small cell lung cancer patients with PD-L1≥50% in a multicenter real-life cohort: The PEMBREIZH study. Cancer Med, 2020, 9(7):2309-2316.

[8] Brahmer J, Reckamp KL, Baas P, et al. Nivolumab versus Docetaxel in Advanced Squamous-Cell Non-Small-Cell Lung Cancer. N Engl J Med, 2015, 373(2):123-135.

[9] Borghaei H, Paz-Ares L, Horn L, et al. Nivolumab versus Docetaxel in Advanced Nonsquamous Non-Small-Cell Lung Cancer. N Engl J Med, 2015, 373(17):1627-1639.

[10] Wu YL, Lu S, Cheng Y, et al. Nivolumab Versus Docetaxel in a Predominantly Chinese Patient Population With Previously Treated Advanced NSCLC: CheckMate 078 Randomized Phase III Clinical Trial. J Thorac Oncol, 2019, 14(5): 867-875.

[11] Herbst RS, Baas P, Kim DW, et al. Pembrolizumab versus docetaxel for previously treated, PD-L1-positive, advanced non-small-cell lung cancer (KEYNOTE-010): a randomised controlled trial. Lancet, 2016, 387(10027):1540-1550.

[12] Merino Almazán M, Duarte Pérez JM, Marín Pozo JF, et al. A multicentre observational study of the effectiveness, safety and economic impact of nivolumab on non-small-cell lung cancer in real clinical practice. Int J Clin Pharm, 2019, 41(1): 272-279.

[13] Crino L, Bidoli P, Delmonte A, et al. Italian Cohort of Nivolumab Expanded Access Program in Squamous Non-Small Cell Lung Cancer: Results from a Real-World Population. Oncologist, 2019, 24(11):e1165-e1171.

[14] Weis TM, Hough S, Reddy HG, et al. Real-world comparison of immune checkpoint inhibitors in non-small cell lung cancer following platinum-based chemotherapy. J Thorac Oncol, 2020, 26(3):564-571.

[15] Figueiredo A, Almeida MA, Almodovar MT, et al. Real-world data from the Portuguese Nivolumab Expanded Access Program (EAP) in previously treated Non Small Cell Lung Cancer (NSCLC). Pulmonology, 2020, 26(1):10-17.

[16] Garon EB, Hellmann MD, Rizvi NA, et al. Five-Year Overall Survival for Patients With Advanced Non-Small-Cell Lung Cancer Treated With Pembrolizumab: Results From the Phase I KEYNOTE-001Study. J Clin Oncol, 2019 (37): 2518-2527.

[17] Gadgeel S, Rodríguez-Abreu D, Speranza G, et al. Updated Analysis From KEYNOTE-189: Pembrolizumab or Placebo Plus Pemetrexedand Platinum for Previously Untreated Metastatic Nonsquamous Non-Small-Cell Lung Cancer. J Clin Oncol, 2020, 38(14):1505-1517.

[18] Ksienski D, Wai ES, Croteau N, et al. Pembrolizumab for advanced nonsmall cell lung cancer: Efficacy and safety in everyday clinical practice. Lung Cancer, 2019, 133:110-116.

[19] Afzal MZ, Dragnev K, Shirai K. A tertiary care cancer center experience with carboplatin and pemetrexed in combination with pembrolizumab in comparison with carboplatin and pemetrexed alone in non-squamous non-small cell lung cancer. J Thorac Dis, 2018, 10(6):3575-3584.

[20] Paz-Ares L, Luft A, Vicente D, et al. Pembrolizumab plus Chemotherapy for Squamous Non-Small-Cell Lung Cancer. N Engl J Med, 2018, 379(21):2040-2051.

[21] Deng Y, Cappuzzo F, Jotte RM, et al. Atezolizumab for First-Line Treatment of Metastatic Nonsquamous NSCLC. N Engl J Med, 2018, 378(24):2288-2301.

[22] Hellmann MD, Ciuleanu TE, Pluzanski A, et al. Nivolumab plus Ipilimumab in Lung Cancer with a High Tumor Mutational Burden. N Engl J Med, 2018, 378(22):2093-2104.

[23] Rizvi NA, Cho BC, Reinmuth N, et al. Durvalumab With or Without Tremelimumab vs Standard Chemotherapy in First-line Treatment of Metastatic Non-Small Cell Lung Cancer. JAMA Oncol, 2020.

[24] Marur S, Singh H, Mishra-Kalyani P, et al. FDA analyses of survival in older adults with metastatic non-small cell lung cancer in controlled trials of PD-1/PD-L1 blocking antibodies. Semin Oncol, 2018, 45(4):220-225.

[25] Spigel DR, McCleod M, Jotte RM, et al. Safety, Efficacy, and Patient-Reported Health-Related Quality of Life and Symptom Burden with Nivolumab in Patients with Advanced Non-Small Cell Lung Cancer, Including Patients Aged 70 Years or Older or with Poor Performance Status (CheckMate 153). J Thorac Oncol, 2019, 14(9):1628-1639.

[26] Felip E, Ardizzoni A, Ciuleanu T, et al. CheckMate 171: A phase 2 trial of nivolumab in patients with previously treated advanced squamous non-small cell lung cancer, including ECOG PS 2 and elderly populations. Eur J Cancer, 2020, 127: 160-172.

[27] Middleton G, Brock K, Savage J, et al. Pembrolizumab in patients with non-small-cell lung cancer of performance status 2 (PePS2): a single arm, phase 2 trial. Lancet Respir Med. 2020.

[28] Galli G, De Toma A, Pagani F, et al. Efficacy and safety of immunotherapy in elderly patients with non-small cell lung cancer. Lung Cancer, 2019, 137: 38-42.

[29] Muchnik E, Loh KP, Strawderman M, et al. Immune Checkpoint Inhibitors in Real-World Treatment of Older Adults with Non-Small Cell Lung Cancer. J Am Geriatr Soc, 2019, 67(5): 905-912.

[30] Ahn B, Pyo K, Xin C, et al. Comprehensive analysis of the characteristics and treatment outcomes of patients with non-small cell lung cancer treated with anti-PD-1 therapy in real-world practice. J Cancer Res Clin Oncol, 2019, 145(6): 1613-1623.

[31] Bjornhart B, Hansen KH, Jorgensen TL, et al. Efficacy and safety of immune checkpoint inhibitors in a Danish real life non-small cell lung cancer population: a retrospective cohort study. Acta Oncol, 2019, 58(7): 953-961.

[32] Hendriks L, Henon C, Auclin E, et al. Outcome of Patients with Non-Small Cell Lung Cancer and Brain Metastases Treated with Checkpoint Inhibitors. J Thorac Oncol, 2019, 14(7): 1244-1254.

[33] Goldberg SB, Gettinger SN, Mahajan A, et al. Pembrolizumab for patients with melanoma or non-small-cell lung cancer and untreated brain metastases: early analysis of a non-randomised, open-label, phase 2 trial. Lancet Oncol, 2016, 17(7): 976-983.

[34] Morita R, Okishio K, Shimizu J, et al. Real world effectiveness and safety of nivolumab in patients with non-small cell lung cancer: A multicenter retrospective observational study in Japan. Lung Cancer, 2020, 140: 8-18.

[35] Scott SC, Pennell NA. Early Use of Systemic Corticosteroids in Patients with Advanced NSCLC Treated with Nivolumab. J Thorac Oncol, 2018, 13(11): 1771-1775.

[36] Fuca G, Galli G, Poggi M, et al. Modulation of peripheral blood immune cells by early use of steroids and its association with clinical outcomes in patients with metastatic non-small cell lung cancer treated with immune checkpoint inhibitors. ESMO Open, 2019, 4(1): e457.

[37] Arbour KC, Mezquita L, Long N, et al. Impact of Baseline Steroids on Efficacy of Programmed Cell Death-1 and Programmed Death-Ligand 1 Blockade in Patients With Non-Small-Cell Lung Cancer. J Clin Oncol, 2018, 36(28): 2872-2878.

[38] Cortellini A, Buti S, Santini D, et al. Clinical Outcomes of Patients with Advanced Cancer and Pre-Existing Autoimmune Diseases Treated with Anti-Programmed Death-1 Immunotherapy: A Real-World Transverse Study. Oncologist, 2019, 24(6): e327-e337.

[39] Danlos F, Voisin A, Dyevre V, et al. Safety and efficacy of anti-programmed death 1 antibodies in patients with cancer and pre-existing autoimmune or inflammatory disease. Eur J Cancer, 2018, 91: 21-29.

[40] Garassino M, Rodriguez-Abreu D, Gadgeel S, et al. Evaluation of TMB in KEYNOTE-189: Pembrolizumab Plus Chemotherapy vs Placebo Plus Chemotherapy for Nonsquamous NSCLC. J Thorac Oncol, 2019, 14S(10): S216-S217.

[41] Langer C, Gadgeel S, Borghaei H, et al. KEYNOTE-021: TMB and Outcomes for Carboplatin and Pemetrexed With or Without Pembrolizumab for Nonsquamous NSCLC. J Thorac Oncol, 2019, 14S(10): S216.

[42] Le DT, Kim TW, Van Cutsem E, et al. Phase II Open-Label Study of Pembrolizumab in Treatment-Refractory, Microsatellite Instability-High/Mismatch Repair-Deficient Metastatic Colorectal Cancer: KEYNOTE-164. J Clin Oncol, 2020, 38(1): 11-19.

[43] Lemery S, Keegan P, Pazdur R. First FDA Approval Agnostic of Cancer Site-When a Biomarker Defines the Indication. N Engl J Med, 2017, 377(15): 1409-1412.

[44] Wolchok JD, Hoos A, O'Day S, et al. Guidelines for the Evaluation of Immune Therapy Activity in Solid Tumors, Immune-Related Response Criteria. Clin Cancer Res, 2009, 15(23): 7412-7420.

[45] Nishino M, Giobbie-Hurder A, Gargano M, et al. Developing a common language for tumor response to immunotherapy: immune-related response criteria using unidimensional measurements. Clin Cancer Res, 2013, 19(14): 3936-3943.

[46] Seymour L, Bogaerts J, Perrone A, et al. iRECIST: guidelines for response criteria for use in trials testing immunotherapeutics. Lancet Oncol, 2017, 18(3): E143-E152.

[47] Hodi FS, Ballinger M, Lyons B, et al. Immune-Modified Response Evaluation Criteria In Solid Tumors (imRECIST): Refining Guidelines to Assess the Clinical Benefit of Cancer Immunotherapy. J Thorac Oncol, 2018, 36(9): 850.

[48] Wang DY, Salem J, Cohen JV, et al. Fatal Toxic Effects Associated With Immune Checkpoint Inhibitors. JAMA Oncol, 2018, 4(12): 1721.

[49] Zhou X, Yao Z, Yang H, et al. Are immune-related adverse events associated with the efficacy of immune checkpoint inhibitors in patients with cancer? A systematic review and meta-analysis. BMC Med, 2020, 18(1).

[50] Maillet D, Corbaux P, Stelmes JJ, et al. Association between immune-related adverse events and long-term survival outcomes in patients treated with immune checkpoint inhibitors. Eur J Cancer, 2020, 132: 61-70.

[51] Horn L, Mansfield AS, Szczęsna A, et al. First-Line Atezolizumab plus Chemotherapy in Extensive-Stage Small-Cell Lung Cancer. N Engl J Med, 2018, 379(23): 2220-2229.

[52] Paz-Ares L, Dvorkin M, Chen Y, et al. Durvalumab plus platinum-etoposide versus platinum-etoposide in first-line treatment of extensive-stage small-cell lung cancer (CASPIAN): a randomised, controlled, open-label, phase 3 trial. Lancet, 2019, 394(10212): 1929-1939.

第七部分

睡眠呼吸障碍

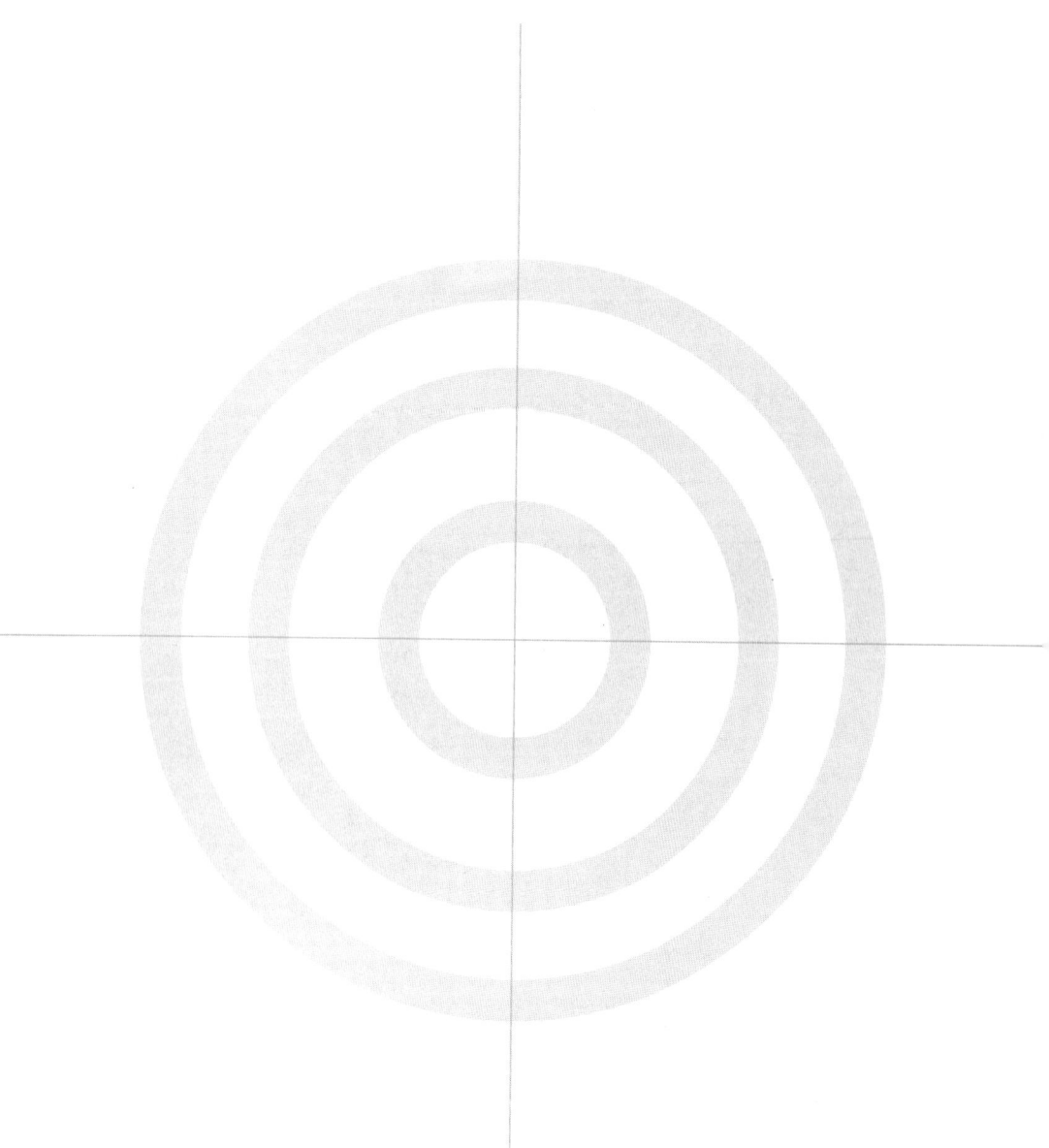

1 阻塞性睡眠呼吸暂停2019年年度进展

王晓娜　肖　毅

阻塞性睡眠呼吸暂停(obstructive sleep apnea，OSA)是一种常见的慢性疾病，以夜间间歇性低氧和睡眠片段化为特征。未治疗的OSA患者生活质量差，交通事故、心血管疾病、代谢性疾病和神经认知障碍的发生率较高，给家庭和社会带来了巨大的经济负担，已成为一个关注度较高的健康问题。近些年在OSA及其并发症方面取得了较多的进展，本文将对过去一年OSA的主要进展进行简要总结。

一、流行病学

根据2012年AASM中成人OSA的诊断标准(apnea hypopnea index，AHI≥5次/h或AHI≥15次/h)，全球30~69岁的人群中有9.36亿人患OSA，4.25亿人患中、重度OSA(AHI≥15次/h)。中国OSA的人数最多，达1.76亿，中、重度OSA人数达6600万。

二、诊　断

OSA是一种复杂异质性的疾病，OSA的诊治也应当实现精准治疗。Santamaria等发现了一组特殊的miRNAs可用来鉴别OSA(AHI≥15次/h)和非OSA患者。Miguel等提出可以从疾病的严重程度、生物活性、患者的主观感受和病理生理特征这4个方面对OSA进行评估和干预。

人工智能技术也越来越多地用于OSA的诊断。利用人工智能图像识别技术分析颅面形态诊断OSA(AHI≥5次/h)的敏感性是74%，特异性是88%，诊断重度OSA(AHI≥30次/h)的敏感性是80%，特异性是91%。Martinot等发现利用计算机算法自动分析下颌运动所得的阻塞性呼吸障碍指数与经多导睡眠图分析所得的阻塞性呼吸障碍指数一致性较高，且能够用于OSA严重程度的分级。

三、疾病负担

(一)OSA和高血压

OSA是高血压的独立危险因素。Esther等的研究发现顽固性高血压患者中OSA的患病率较高，顽固性高血压患者的血压与OSA的严重程度呈剂量-效应关系，尤其是夜间血压。我国一项横断面研究发现在中重度OSA患者中慢波睡眠减少和高血压相关，慢波睡眠减少的比例和血压呈剂量-效应关系。

在血压控制较好的OSA患者中，持续正压通气(continuous positive airway pressure，CPAP)治疗能够降低醒后血压而不是睡前血压，CPAP治疗2个月后醒后收缩压下降最明显。一项随机、双盲、交叉试验发现中重度OSA患者停用CPAP治疗后，吸氧可降低醒后血压和氧减指数(oxygen desaturation index，ODI)，但不影响夜间觉醒和晨起的嗜睡症状。因此，推测间歇性缺氧可能是OSA患者白天血压升高的主要原因。

(二)OSA和心血管疾病

嗜睡症状作为心血管疾病风险评估的新指标。中重度OSA患者(AHI≥15次/h)中，OSA症状亚型(睡眠障碍型、症状轻微型、中度嗜睡型和过度嗜睡型)与心血管疾病的患病率相关，其中过度嗜睡型OSA患者心血管疾病的患病率明显高于其他3个亚型。ISAACC研究发现在无嗜睡症状的急性冠脉综合征患者中，OSA不会导致急性冠脉事件后心血管事件明显增加。

低氧血症与OSA患者心血管疾病关系密切。通过多导睡眠图将OSA患者分为呼吸暂停事件为主的亚型、低通气事件为主的亚型和睡眠相关微觉醒为主的亚型，低通气事件为主的亚型与其他两型相比，高脂血症、心力衰竭和冠心病的发病率更高。也有研究提出，相比AHI，低氧负荷与心血管疾病的死亡率更相关。

睡眠呼吸疾病是缺血性脑卒中可逆的危险因素。美国德克萨斯州Nueces县的一项流行病学调查数据表明，睡眠呼吸疾病(AHI≥10次/h)与脑卒中复发相关，但与死亡率无关，推测睡眠呼吸疾病是脑卒中可逆的危险因素之一。

重叠综合征患者的心脑血管疾病风险更高。57%重叠综合征患者的运动心脏功率(exercise cardiac power，ECP，指心肺运动测试期间最大耗氧量与收缩压峰值的比值)是降低的，提示重叠综合征患者不良冠脉事件的风险高。OSA同时合并COPD、夜间低氧(夜间$SaO_2<90\%$持续时间>10 min)的患者心血管疾病死亡率和全因死亡率高于OSA组、COPD组。通过分析2005-2008年美国NHANES的数据发现重叠综合征患者较COPD或OSA患者的脑卒中风险增加，其中65岁以上的女性重叠综合征患者脑卒中风险更高。

(三)OSA和肺动脉高压

Mehra等发现睡眠呼吸疾病在不同类型肺动脉高压

的特点不同:左心疾病所致的肺动脉高压(第2类)和血液系统疾病/结节病所致的肺高压(第5类)患者中,睡眠呼吸疾病和OSA发病率最高,但未发现合并中枢性睡眠呼吸暂停;动脉性肺动脉高压患者(第1类)和肺血栓栓塞疾病所致的肺动脉高压患者(第4类)中夜间血氧饱和度最高,可能和通气/血流比例失调或生理分流相关。Puri等发现睡眠呼吸疾病会增加动脉性肺动脉高压患者(第1类)的平均肺动脉压和肺血管阻力,对肺毛细血管楔压无影响。

(四)OSA和糖尿病

OSA与糖尿病之间的关系是相互的。OSA所致的间歇性缺氧和觉醒可导致胰岛素敏感性降低、交感神经兴奋和全身性炎症,最终导致糖尿病。同时,血糖水平控制不佳会使颈动脉体和咽扩张肌敏感性降低,从而促进OSA患者的睡眠呼吸事件。肥胖和糖尿病神经病可能会加重OSA疾病的严重程度。糖尿病足、胰岛素治疗是糖尿病者出现OSA的危险因素。通过研究超重/肥胖成人糖尿病前期和近期被诊断但未经治疗的2型糖尿病患者,发现OSA的严重程度和睡眠时间仅与高水平的HbA1c有关,与胰岛素敏感性和β细胞功能无关。

(五)OSA和认知功能

帕金森病(Parkinson disease,PD)患者往往会存在包括OSA在内的睡眠障碍。Kaminska等发现已经诊断为OSA且MoCA分数较低的PD患者呼吸紊乱指数、AHI、呼吸相关的觉醒指数显著升高,总觉醒指数和ODI与MoCA评分正常者无差异。因此认为PD患者的认知功能障碍与OSA相关的睡眠碎片化相关,而不与整夜的睡眠片段化相关。

空间定向障碍是阿尔兹海默病患者认知功能障碍的最早标志之一。认知正常、合并轻度OSA的老年患者和不合并OSA的老年患者相比,睡前完成空间迷宫的时间、早晨的心理运动警觉性测试没有显著差异,但醒后前者在空间迷宫试验中表现明显较差,提示OSA和老年患者的认知功能下降相关。

四、治 疗

(一)CPAP

CPAP治疗是OSA患者的一线治疗,主要适用于中重度OSA患者中,对于轻度OSA的疗效尚不明确。Wimms等研究发现轻度OSA(5≤AHI<15)患者接受3个月CPAP治疗与接受3个月单纯的护理治疗相比,生活质量(SF-36健康调查量表)明显升高。

CPAP治疗能够改善OSA患者的抑郁症状。通过对SAVE研究二次分析和对其他20个研究进行Meta分析发现,CPAP治疗能够改善OSA患者抑郁的情况,在CPAP治疗前抑郁症状明显的患者中效果更明显。通过对RICCADSA研究的二次分析,CPAP治疗能够改善非嗜睡OSA患者的抑郁评分(ZUNG抑郁自评量表)。

CPAP依从性差是影响其疗效的关键因素。Taweesedt等对诊断为OSA的退伍军人进行研究发现,退伍军人对CPAP的整体依从性差,前30 d内鼻罩的依从性高于口鼻罩,但3个月后面罩类型对依从性的影响很小。使用自动调压的CPAP和治疗依从性差有关。

(二)体重管理

2019年美国胸科协会对成人OSA患者的体重管理发布了一项指南。低热量饮食与普通饮食相比,能够有效减轻体重、改善超重/肥胖的OSA的AHI,故推荐超重/肥胖的OSA患者采用低热量饮食。体育锻炼对超重/肥胖的OSA疾病严重程度的影响尚无一致的结论,但能够改善他们心血管疾病的预后,故推荐超重/肥胖的OSA患者加强体育锻炼。低热量饮食、加强体育锻炼和行为指导的综合生活方式管理能有效的减轻体重,且可降低超重/肥胖的OSA的AHI和日间嗜睡症状,故强烈推荐对超重/肥胖的OSA患者进行综合的生活方式干预。

BMI≥27kg/m² 的OSA患者,如不能通过综合生活管理有效减重,且无明确的禁忌证或急性的心血管疾病(指6个月内没有急性心脑血管事件、未控制的高血压、危及生命的心律失常或心力衰竭失代偿),建议使用减肥药物减轻体重。

BMI≥35kg/m² 的OSA患者,如果不能通过综合生活管理有效减重,且没有明显的禁忌,建议行减肥手术。虽然减肥手术不能够改善OSA的严重程度,但减肥手术能够有效的减重,且能够改善患者的生活质量和血糖控制情况。

(三)药物治疗

Solriamfetol是一种选择性的多巴胺和去甲肾上腺素再摄取抑制剂,可有效改善OSA和发作性睡病患者的白天嗜睡症状、延长睡眠潜伏期,目前已被FDA批准用于治疗存在白天嗜睡症状的发作性睡病和OSA患者。

回顾过去1年的进展,OSA的疾病负担依然不容小觑,探究新技术新方法在睡眠呼吸疾病中的应用是非常有意义的。在现有的基础上,我们可以继续探究OSA的临床表型及病理生理机制之间的关系,最终实现OSA的精准医疗。OSA的治疗仍存在挑战,提高CPAP的依从性,发现新的治疗方法将是我们后续努力的方向。

参 考 文 献

[1] Benjafield A V,Ayas N T,Eastwood P R,et al. Estimation of the global prevalence and burden of obstructive sleep apnoea: a literature-based analysis. Lancet Respiratory Medicine, 2019,7(8):687-698.

[2] Santamaria-Martos F,Benitez I,Giron C,et al. Utility of microRNAs for Obstructive Sleep Apnea Identification. American Journal of Respiratory and Critical Care Medicine, 2019,199.

[3] Angel Martinez-Garcia M,Campos-Rodriguez F,Barbe F,et al. Precision medicine in obstructive sleep apnoea. Lancet Re-

spiratory Medicine,2019,7(5):456-464.

[4] Rong Y,Liu Z,Li Z,et al. A Screening Test on the Diagnosis of Obstructive Sleep Apnea Hypopnea Syndrome(OSAHS) Using Facial Recognition Technology. American Journal of Respiratory and Critical Care Medicine,2019,199.

[5] Martinot J,Cuthbert V,Dedave A,et al. Automated Diagnosis of Sleep-Disordered Breathing (SDB) Using Mandibular Movements Analysis and Supervised Machine Learning. American journal of respiratory and critical care medicine, 2019,199.

[6] Sapina-Beltran E,Torres G,Benitez I,et al. Prevalence,Characteristics,and Association of Obstructive Sleep Apnea with Blood Pressure Control in Patients with Resistant Hypertension. Annals of the American Thoracic Society, 2019, 16 (11):1414-1421.

[7] Ren R,Covassin N,Zhang Y,et al. Interaction Between Slow Wave Sleep and Obstructive Sleep Apnea in Prevalent Hypertension. Hypertension,2019:A11913720.

[8] Javaheri S,Gottlieb D J,Quan S F. Effects of continuous positive airway pressure on blood pressure in obstructive sleep apnea patients:The Apnea Positive Pressure Long-term Efficacy Study(APPLES). J Sleep Res,2019:e12943.

[9] Turnbull C D,Sen D,Kohler M,et al. Effect of Supplemental Oxygen on Blood Pressure in Obstructive Sleep Apnea (SOX). A Randomized Continuous Positive Airway Pressure Withdrawal Trial. Am J Respir Crit Care Med,2019,199(2): 211-219.

[10] Mazzotti D R,Keenan B T,Lim D C,et al. Symptom Subtypes of Obstructive Sleep Apnea Predict Incidence of Cardiovascular Outcomes. American Journal of Respiratory and Critical Care Medicine,2019,200(4):493-506.

[11] Sanchez-De-La-Torre M,Sanchez-De-La-Torre A,Bertran S, et al. Effect of obstructive sleep apnoea and its treatment with continuous positive airway pressure on the prevalence of cardiovascular events in patients with acute coronary syndrome(ISAACC study):a randomised controlled trial. Lancet Respir Med,2019.

[12] Kim S,Park S,Shin B,et al. Prevalence and risk factors for cardiovascular diseases according to phenotypes of obstructive sleep apnea syndrome:a retrospective cohort study. SLEEP,2019,421.

[13] Azarbarzin A,Sands S A,Stone K L,et al. The hypoxic burden of sleep apnoea predicts cardiovascular disease-related mortality:the Osteoporotic Fractures in Men Study and the Sleep Heart Health Study. European Heart Journal,2019,40 (14):1149.

[14] Brown D L,Shafie-Khorassani F,Kim S,et al. Sleep-Disordered Breathing Is Associated With Recurrent Ischemic Stroke. Stroke,2019,50(3):571-576.

[15] Macrea M,Zuwallack R L,Martin T J,et al. Exercise Cardiac Power and Coronary Artery Disease Mortality Risk in Patients with Chronic Obstructive Pulmonary Disease(COPD) and Obstructive Sleep Apnea(OSA)Overlap Syndrome(OS). American Journal of Respiratory and Critical Care Medicine, 2019,199.

[16] Kendzerska T,Leung R S,Aaron S D,et al. Cardiovascular Outcomes and All-Cause Mortality in Patients with Obstructive Sleep Apnea and Chronic Obstructive Pulmonary Disease (Overlap Syndrome). Annals of the American Thoracic Society,2019,16(1):71-81.

[17] Olanipekun T,Oni O,Effoe V,et al. Obstructive Sleep Apnea-Chronic Obstructive Pulmonary Disease Overlap Syndrome and the Risk of Stroke:Findings from the 2005-2008 National Health and Nutrition Examination Survey (NHANES). American Journal of Respiratory and Critical Care Medicine, 2019,199.

[18] Mehra R,Wang L,Nawabit R,et al. Sleep Disordered Breathing Phenotype Across Pulmonary Hypertension Group:Insights from the Pulmonary Vascular Disease Phenomics Study. American Journal of Respiratory and Critical Care Medicine,2019,199.

[19] Puri R,Vanderpool R,Airhart S, et al. Additive Effect of Sleep Disordered Breathing on the Severity of Pulmonary Vascular Disease in Patients with Pulmonary Arterial Hypertension. American Journal of Respiratory and Critical Care Medicine,2019,199.

[20] Song S O,He K,Narla R R,et al. Metabolic Consequences of Obstructive Sleep Apnea Especially Pertaining to Diabetes Mellitus and Insulin Sensitivity. Diabetes Metab J,2019,43 (2):144-155.

[21] Subramanian A,Adderley N J,Tracy A,et al. Risk of Incident Obstructive Sleep Apnea Among Patients With Type 2 Diabetes. Diabetes Care,2019,42(5):954-963.

[22] Mokhlesi B,Tjaden A H,Temple K A,et al. Impact of Obstructive Sleep Apnea and Sleep Duration on Glucose Tolerance and Beta-Cell Function in Adults with Prediabetes or Untreated Type 2 Diabetes. American Journal of Respiratory and Critical Care Medicine,2019,199.

[23] Kamınska M,Lafontaine A,Leonard G,et al. Obstructive Sleep Apnea-Related Sleep Fragmentation Is Associated with Cognitive Dysfunction in Parkinson's Disease. American Journal of Respiratory and Critical Care Medicine,2019,199.

[24] Varga A W,Williams M,Mullins A E,et al. Effects of Obstructive Sleep Apnea on Human Spatial Navigational Memory Processing in Cognitively Normal Older Individuals. American Journal of Respiratory and Critical Care Medicine, 2019,199.

[25] Wimms A J,Kelly J L,Turnbull C D,et al. Continuous positive airway pressure versus standard care for the treatment of people with mild obstructive sleep apnoea(MERGE):a multicentre,randomised controlled trial. Lancet Respir Med,2019.

[26] Zheng D,Xu Y,You S,et al. Effects of continuous positive airway pressure on depression and anxiety symptoms in patients with obstructive sleep apnoea:results from the sleep apnoea cardiovascular Endpoint randomised trial and meta-analysis. EClinicalMedicine,2019,11:89-96.

[27] Balcan B,Thunstrom E,Strollo P J,et al. Continuous Positive Airway Pressure Treatment and Depression in Adults with Coronary Artery Disease and Nonsleepy Obstructive Sleep Apnea. A Secondary Analysis of the RICCADSA Trial. Ann

Am Thorac Soc,2019,16(1):62-70.
[28] Taweesedt P T, Herve N N, Kim J W, et al. Comparison of Continuous Positive Airway Pressure Compliance Using a Nasal Vs. Oronasal Mask in Veterans with Obstructive Sleep Apnea. American Journal of Respiratory and Critical Care Medicine,2019,199.
[29] Billings M E, Krishnan V, Su G, et al. Clinical Practice Guideline Summary for Clinicians: The Role of Weight Management in the Treatment of Adult Obstructive Sleep Apnea. Annals of the American Thoracic Society, 2019, 16(4): 405-408.
[30] Schweitzer P K, Rosenberg R, Zammit G K, et al. Solriamfetol for Excessive Sleepiness in Obstructive Sleep Apnea (TONES 3) A Randomized Controlled Trial. American Journal of Respiratory and Critical Care Medicine,2019,199(11): 1421-1431.
[31] Thorpy M J, Shapiro C, Mayer G, et al. A randomized study of solriamfetol for excessive sleepiness in narcolepsy. Annals of Neurology,2019,85(3):359-370.

2 阻塞性睡眠呼吸暂停与免疫功能

黄 红 王 玮

阻塞性睡眠呼吸暂停（obstructive sleep apnea,OSA）是最常见的睡眠相关呼吸疾病，主要特征为睡眠中反复发生上气道塌陷导致慢性间歇低氧伴和反复微觉醒、睡眠片段化，并因此引起系统性炎症、氧化应激、胰岛素抵抗及内皮功能紊乱等一系列病理生理改变，进而导致心脑血管、内分泌系统等全身损害。近期研究表明 OSA 患者发生社区获得性肺炎的风险较未合并 OSA 者明显升高。大型流行病学研究结果亦显示，在校正了包括体重指数（（body mass index,BMI)在内的混杂因素影响后，OSA 患者中各类癌症发生率及死亡率均较普通人群增高，且 OSA 患者肿瘤的发生发展与其免疫功能的失衡相关。现针对 OSA 患者免疫功能失衡表现及可能机制作一综述。

一、OSA 患者的免疫失衡情况

(一) 固有免疫

固有免疫是一切免疫应答的基础，常见的固有免疫细胞包括巨噬细胞、中性粒细胞、自然杀伤细胞和树突状细胞等。Wang 等学者发现，与常氧组相比，慢性间歇低氧组小鼠的皮下脂肪中 M1 型巨噬细胞增多，进而通过分泌多种促炎因子促进机体产生炎症损伤。慢性间歇低氧亦能增加小鼠肿瘤组织中巨噬细胞的浸润，并改变其极性，使 M2 型巨噬细胞明显增多，并通过促进血管形成、基质及骨架重建等功能增加肿瘤的侵袭及转移。Sharma 等的研究表明，与健康对照组相比，肥胖 OSA 患者的肺泡巨噬细胞中过氧化物酶体增殖物激活受体-γ 的 mRNA 水平较对照组减少 2 倍，且其蛋白活性下降 48%，提示 OSA 患者存在肺泡巨噬细胞功能受损，并可能因此增加其肺部疾病的易感性。有趣的是，OSA 患者外周血中性粒细胞计数虽然明显增加，但其吞噬细菌的能力却下降。同样，未经治疗的 OSA 患者外周血中自然杀伤细胞所占比例增加，但其成熟能力及功能却下降，且这一损伤作用由 OSA 患者体内异常向免疫抑制表型转换的单核细胞介导，并可能因此促进肿瘤逃逸，导致 OSA 患者肿瘤发生率增加。Galati 等发现，与健康对照组相比，OSA 患者组所有树突状细胞亚型均明显降低，而树突状细胞是机体中专职的抗原呈递细胞，在免疫应答的启动、调控和维持阶段均至关重要。同时，髓源性抑制细胞——巨噬细胞、树突状细胞、粒细胞的前体计数在重度 OSA 患者外周血中明显升高，并通过增加转化生长因子 β_1 (transforming growth factor-β_1, TGF-β_1)等抑制性细胞因子的分泌，加强对 T 细胞的抑制作用，进而促进肿瘤免疫逃逸。

(二) 细胞免疫

参与细胞介导的免疫反应的细胞主要为辅助性 T ($CD4^+$ T)细胞、抑制/杀伤 T ($CD8^+$ Tc)细胞和自然杀伤 T (NKT)细胞，其中 $CD4^+$ T 细胞又包括 Th1、Th2、调节性 T 细胞(Treg)等。OSA 患儿外周血中 $CD4^+$ T 细胞及 Th1 细胞数量增加，Treg 和 NKT 细胞计数减少；扁桃体中 $CD4^+$ T 细胞增加，FoxP3 $CD8^+$ T 细胞减少，提示 OSA 患者存在 T 细胞免疫失衡。Vicente 等亦发现，OSA 患者鼻咽部灌洗液中 $CD4^+$ T 细胞比例较单纯鼾症组及正常对照组均明显增加，且增加程度与睡眠呼吸暂停低通气指数（apnea hypopnea index,AHI) 呈正相关。Akbarpour 等的研究结果显示，与常氧组小鼠相比，经慢性间歇低氧或者睡眠片段化预处理的小鼠的瘤组织中颗粒酶 B 和穿孔素表达水平明显下降，且颗粒酶 B 水平与肿瘤重量呈负相关，提示 $CD8^+$ T 细胞功能受损。同时，慢性间歇低氧组及睡眠片段化组小鼠肿瘤干细胞中的 $Oct4^+$、$CD44^+$ 及 $CD133^+$ 表达均明显增高，提示慢性间歇低氧和睡眠片段化干预可能通过改变肿瘤免疫微环境促进肿瘤的增长及转移。OSA 患者循环中 $CD8^+$ 细胞/淋巴细胞比值表现为升高，且 $CD8^+$ 细胞对人脐静脉内皮细胞及人慢性髓系白血病细胞的细胞毒性作用增强。Liu 等对 44 例罹患小细胞肺癌的患者进行 2 年随访，发现与未合并 OSA 的肺癌患者相比，合并 OSA 的肺癌患者血中 TGF-β_1、血管内皮生长因子（vascular endothelial growth factor, VEGF）水平及 Foxp3+Treg 细胞数量均升高，而 TGF-β_1 和 VEGF 又分别能促进 Treg 细胞发育、引导 Treg 向肿瘤组织浸润，进而抑制抗肿瘤免疫效应，这与此研究中 VEGF 表达水平同肺癌患者总生存期呈负相关的结果相一致。

(三) 体液免疫

Domagała-Kulawik 等将 48 位重度 OSA 患者（平均 AHI 为 52.92 次/h）外周血淋巴细胞进行流式细胞分型，发现 OSA 患者 B 细胞数量较正常组减少，且 B 细胞所占淋巴细胞比例与 OSA 患者并发症评分呈负相关，提示循环中 B 细胞的耗竭促进了 OSA 患者的全身炎症反应。Korin 等发现，6 h 睡眠剥夺导致小鼠大脑中 B 细胞丰度增加，提示睡眠障碍可能参与中枢神经系统的自身免疫性疾病。健康受试者经 24 h 睡眠剥夺后，血清免疫球蛋白

IgG、IgA、IgM 和补体 C3 及 C4 均较对照组升高，表明睡眠-觉醒活动在体液免疫中有着重要作用。

（四）免疫相关的细胞因子

免疫相关细胞因子多由活化的免疫细胞、血管内皮细胞、肿瘤细胞等分泌，参与免疫调节、炎症反应及抗肿瘤等生物过程。白细胞介素（interleukin，IL）-6 能刺激活化的 B 细胞及 T 细胞增殖，是重要的促炎因子之一。OSA 患者外周血单个核细胞中 IL-6 转录水平明显升高，IL-6 在 OSA 外周血中、鼻咽部灌洗液中以及慢性间歇低氧小鼠鼻部和肺部组织中均表达增高。与正常对照组相比，OSA 患者中 IL-1β、IL-4、IL-8、肿瘤坏死因子 α（tumor necrosis factor alpha，TNF-α）等促炎因子亦明显增加。Tang 等将 OSA 患者进一步依据 BMI 或 AHI 分层分析显示，超重者和重度 OSA 患者 IL-6、IL-1β、TNF-α 均分别较体重正常者及轻度 OSA 患者升高，多元回归分析显示 AHI、氧减指数、觉醒指数、夜间平均血氧饱和度和 BMI 均显著影响上述细胞因子的表达水平，提示 OSA 患者存在全身系统性炎症反应，且这一效应由间歇低氧、睡眠片段化及肥胖等因素介导。相反，有研究显示抑制性免疫细胞因子——IL-10、TGF-β₁ 在 OSA 患者中表达水平较正常者下降，Motamedi 等则发现，与轻度 OSA 患者和正常对照组相比，中重度 OSA 患者血中 IL-10 表达无明显差异。干扰素-γ（interferon-γ，IFN-γ）既是促炎因子又能通过增强细胞毒性 T 细胞及自然杀伤细胞的杀伤功能达到抗肿瘤效应。关于 IFN-γ 变化的研究亦未达成一致结论。Su 等发现肥胖 OSA 患儿外周血中 IFN-γ 水平升高，Said 等的研究结果则显示重度 OSA 患者血中 IFN-γ 表达下降。

以上结果表明 OSA 患者中多种免疫细胞及相关细胞因子的表达水平和生物功能发生变化，提示 OSA 患者存在不同层面的免疫功能紊乱，而具体紊乱情况则可能因患者机体性能、组织特异性、OSA 本身疾病进展程度、合并症等情况不同而不同。

二、OSA 导致免疫失衡的可能机制

（一）内脏脂肪的影响

肥胖是 OSA 的重要致病因素之一，50% 以上的 OSA 患者属于肥胖者，且 OSA 患者系统炎症反应的增加主要源于内脏脂肪的堆积。一方面，肥大的脂肪细胞能通过分泌 TNF-α，刺激前脂肪细胞和周围的内皮细胞分泌单核细胞趋化蛋白-1，促进巨噬细胞富集并向 M1 型巨噬细胞极化，进而增加 TNF-α、IL-1β 和 IL-6 等促炎因子分泌。另一方面，单核巨噬细胞和脂肪细胞中的饱和脂肪酸可通过激活 Toll 样受体 4/核因子-κB（nuclear factor kappa-B，NF-κB）通路促进脂肪细胞中单核细胞趋化蛋白-1 和促炎因子——抵抗素的分泌。

（二）慢性间歇低氧

夜间反复缺氧—复氧所致的氧化应激可导致体内 Toll 样受体-4 依赖的活性氧增多，进而激活 NF-κB、激活蛋白-1 等转录因子，上调 IL-6、IL-8、TNF-α 等细胞因子的表达，最终促进中性粒细胞及单核巨噬细胞的活化及浸润。另一方面，慢性间歇低氧导致缺氧诱导因子-1（hypoxia-inducible factor-1，HIF-1）表达增多，而 HIF-1 可通过与程序性死亡配体 1（programmed death ligand 1，PD-L1）启动子区域的缺氧反应元件结合激活 PD-L1 转录，增加单核细胞表面 PD-L1 的表达，进而通过与 T 细胞表面程序性死亡受体-1 相结合，抑制 T 淋巴细胞的增殖并下调 CD⁺8T 细胞的细胞毒性作用。

（三）睡眠片段化

睡眠片段化一方面可能通过 Toll 样受体-4/NADPH 氧化酶 2/活性氧通路增加巨噬细胞的聚集，并改变其极性；另一方面可通过抑制下丘脑分泌素表达增加集落刺激因子 1 水平，进而增加单核细胞的产生。

三、治疗 OSA 对免疫功能的影响

Halawani 等发现，109 名 OSA 患者经持续正压通气（continuous positive airway pressure，CPAP）治疗后，外周血中中性粒细胞/淋巴细胞比值较前明显下降。Al-Halawani 等的研究结果表明，3 个月的下颌前移矫治器治疗亦显著降低 OSA 患者中性粒细胞/淋巴细胞比值，进一步亚组分析发现这一改善只在 OSA 治疗效果最佳组（治疗后氧减指数<10 次/h，或较基线下降 50% 以上）中有统计学差异，提示中性粒细胞/淋巴细胞比值的降低与氧减指数下降相关。也有学者报道，OSA 患者经悬雍垂腭咽成形术加舌根射频消融联合治疗 4 周后，外周血中 IL-6 及 TNF-α 水平均较术前明显下降。李蔚等发现，每晚 8h 以上、持续 3 个月的 CPAP 治疗能有效降低 OSA 患者 TNF-α、IL-8 及 NF-κB 水平。Perrini 等纳入 31 名合并病态肥胖的 OSA 患者及 15 名无 OSA 的病态肥胖者，两组间 IL-2、IL-4、IL-6、单核细胞趋化蛋白-1、VEGFα 及 BMI 的基线水平无明显差异，分别对两组进行减肥＋CPAP 治疗、单纯减肥治疗 6 个月，发现治疗后两组受试者 BMI 均明显下降，但上述炎症因子血清表达水平只在每天坚持 CPAP 治疗 4 h 以上的 OSA 患者中明显下降，同时此组患者腹部皮下脂肪中 IL-6 及 VEGFα 的 mRNA 水平亦较前明显降低，表明有效的 CPAP 治疗能改善 OSA 患者系统性及肥胖相关性炎症反应。Borges 等则发现 8 周的 CPAP 治疗能提高 18 名中重度 OSA 患者的睡眠质量，却并不能改善其血中 TNF-α、IL-1β、IL-6 和 IL-8 水平，提示 CPAP 治疗的受益与治疗时长及患者依从性相关。

综上所述，OSA 患者存在免疫功能失衡，涉及固有免疫、细胞及体液免疫等多个方面，具体紊乱情况则可能因患者机体性能、组织特异性、OSA 本身疾病进展程度、合并症等情况不同而不同。OSA 患者发生免疫紊乱的原因可能归结于慢性间歇低氧、睡眠片段化所致氧化应激损伤及肥胖的交互影响，有效地针对 OSA 进行治疗可一定程度上改善 OSA 患者紊乱的免疫功能，但未来需要更多的高质量研究进一步探究 OSA 患者免疫损伤的具体机制及相关治疗所带来的长期改善效果。

参 考 文 献

[1] Campos-Rodriguez F, Martinez-Garcia MA, Martines M, et al. Association between obstructive sleep apnea and cancer incidence in a large multicenter Spanish cohort. American Journal of Respiratory and Critical Care medicine, 2013, 187(1):99-105.

[2] Wang Y, Lee MYK, Mak JCW, et al. Low-Frequency Intermittent Hypoxia suppresses subcutaneous adipogenesis and induces macrophage polarization in lean mice. Diabetes & Metabolism Journal, 2019, 43(5):659-674.

[3] Torres M, Martinez-Garcia MÁ, Campos-Rodriguez F, et al. Lung cancer aggressiveness in an intermittent hypoxia murine model of postmenopausal sleep apnea. Menopause, 2020, 27(6):706-713.

[4] Sharma S, Malur A, Marshall I, et al. Alveolar macrophage activation in obese patients with obstructive sleep apnea. Surgery, 2012, 151(1):107-112.

[5] Hernández-Jiménez E, Cubillos-Zapata C, Toledano V, et al. Monocytes inhibit NK activity via TGF-β in patients with obstructive sleep apnoea. European Respiratory Journal, 2017, 49(6):1602456.

[6] Galati D, Zanotta S, Canora A, et al. Severe depletion of peripheral blood dendritic cell subsets in obstructive sleep apnea patients: A new link with cancer?. Cytokine, 2020, 125:154831.

[7] 陈思文, 李洁, 向彬, 等. 阻塞性睡眠呼吸暂停综合征患者髓源性抑制细胞的免疫功能及其机制. 中华医学杂志, 2020, 100(4):295-300.

[8] Su MS, Xu L, Xu K, et al. Association of T lymphocyte immune imbalance and IL-10 gene polymorphism with the risk of obstructive sleep apnea in children with obesity. Sleep and Breathing, 2017, 21(4):929-937.

[9] Anderson ME Jr, Buchwald ZS, Ko J, et al. Patients with pediatric obstructive sleep apnea show altered T-cell populations with a dominant TH17 profile. Otolaryngology--Head and Neck Surgery, 2014, 150(5):880-886.

[10] Vicente E, Marin JM, Carrizo SJ, et al. Upper airway and systemic inflammation in obstructive sleep apnoea. European Respiratory Journal, 2016, 48(4):1108-1117.

[11] Akbarpour M, Khalyfa A, Qiao Z, et al. Altered CD8+ T-cell lymphocyte function and TC1 cell stemness contribute to enhanced malignant tumor properties in murine models of sleep apnea. Sleep, 2017, 40(2).

[12] Domagala-Kulawik J, Osinska I, Piechuta A, et al. T, B, and NKT cells in systemic inflammation in obstructive sleep apnoea. Mediators of inflammation 2015, 2015:161579.

[13] Dyugovskaya L, Lavie P, Hirsh M, et al. Activated CD8+ T-lymphocytes in obstructive sleep apnoea. European Respiratory Journal, 2005, 25(5):820-828.

[14] Liu Y, Lao M, Chen J, et al. Short-term prognostic effects of circulating regulatory T-Cell suppressive function and vascular endothelial growth factor level in patients with non-small cell lung cancer and obstructive sleep apnea. Sleep Medicine, 2020, 70:88-96.

[15] Korin B, Avraham S, Azulay-Debby H, et al. Short-term sleep deprivation in mice induces B cell migration to the brain compartment. Sleep, 2020, 43(2):222.

[16] Tang T, Huang Q, Liu J, et al. Oxidative stress does not contribute to the release of proinflammatory cytokines through activating the nod-like receptor protein 3 inflammasome in patients with obstructive sleep apnoea. Sleep and Breathing, 2019, 23(2):535-542.

[17] Reale M, Velluto L, Nicola MD, et al. Cholinergic markers and cytokines in OSA patients. International Journal of Molecular Sciences, 2020, 21(9):3264.

[18] Said EA, Al-Abri MA, Al-Saidi I, et al. Altered blood cytokines, CD4 T cells, NK and neutrophils in patients with obstructive sleep apnea. Immunology Letters, 2017, 190:272-278.

[19] Lackey DE, Olefsky JM. Regulation of metabolism by the innate immune system. Nat Rev Endocrinol, 2016, 12(1):15-28.

[20] Gill R, Tsung A, Billiar T. Linking oxidative stress to inflammation: Toll-like receptors. Free Radical Biology and Medicine, 2010, 48(9):1121-1132.

[21] Cubillos-Zapata C, Avendaño-Ortiz J, Hernandez-Jimenez E, et al. Hypoxia-induced PD-L1/PD-1 crosstalk impairs T-cell function in sleep apnoea. European Respiratory Journal, 2017, 50(4):1700833.

[22] Mcalpine CS, Kiss MG, Rattik S, et al. Sleep modulates haematopoiesis and protects against atherosclerosis. Nature, 2019, 566(7744):383-387.

[23] Al-Halawani MD, Kyung C, Liang F, et al. Treatment of obstructive sleep apnea with CPAP improves chronic inflammation measured by neutrophil-to-lymphocyte ratio. Journal of Clinical Sleep Medicine, 2020, 16(2):251-257.

[24] Naik S, Chan M, Kreinin I, et al. Neutrophil-to-lymphocyte ratio decreases in obstructive sleep apnea treated with mandibular advancement devices. Sleep and Breathing, 2018, 22(4):989-995.

[25] 李蔚, 江程澄. 阻塞性睡眠呼吸暂停综合征患者持续正压通气治疗后血清细胞因子的变化. 中国老年医学杂志, 2013, 33:1559-1561.

[26] Peerrini S, Cignarelli A, Quaranta VN, et al. Correction of intermittent hypoxia reduces inflammation in obese subjects with obstructive sleep apnea. JCI Insight, 2017, 2(17):e94379.

[27] Borges YG, Cipriano LHC, Aires R, et al. Oxidative stress and inflammatory profiles in obstructive sleep apnea: are short-term CPAP or aerobic exercise therapies effective?. Sleep and Breathing, 2020, 24(2):541-549.

3 抗击新冠肺炎疫情对医务人员睡眠心理状态的影响

张 笋 杨新艳 张挪富

新型冠状病毒肺炎(coronavirus disease 2019, COVID-19)疫情自去年12月在武汉暴发至今已持续超过6个月。截至目前,全球累计确诊病例已超1200万例,累计死亡病例超过56万例。由于新型冠状病毒(severe acute respiratory syndrome coronavirus 2, SARS-CoV-2)具有强烈的传染性,且人群普遍易感,因此在缺乏有效的阻断病毒传播途径的情况下,极易在短时间内出现大量确诊病例,给医务人员造成巨大的生理及心理压力。多项大样本量研究指出,短期内骤增的工作强度和对于COVID-19这种充满未知性疾病的恐惧感,使得医务人员出现睡眠障碍、焦虑及抑郁等情况的风险大幅增加。因此,在抗击新冠疫情的过程中,要时刻关注医务人员的睡眠及心理状态,同时采取必要的手段进行干预,以保障医务人员的身心健康及医疗工作的正常运行。

一、流行病学及临床表现

武汉是国内新冠疫情暴发的起源地,也是最早采取"封城"等强力隔离措施的城市,因此,武汉市及湖北省当地的医务人员在疫情期间的睡眠及心理状态也受到了格外的关注。一项针对医务人员抗疫期间心理健康状况的研究显示,在纳入的1257例医务人员中,760例为武汉当地医务人员,而参与抗疫一线医务人员有522例。在全部受试者中,有抑郁、焦虑、失眠及感到痛苦等症状的比例分别为50.4%、44.6%、34%和71.5%,其中护士、女性、一线抗疫人员及武汉当地的医务人员表现出了更为严重的精神心理异常。而另一项针对武汉一线抗疫儿科医生睡眠障碍的研究结果显示,身为独生子女或曾接触过COVID-19患者的儿科医生更容易出现睡眠障碍。在疫情初期,由于物资短缺、防护意识及措施不到位等诸多原因,导致部分武汉一线医务人员出现了自身感染的情况。一项纳入了70例确诊或疑似COVID-19的医务人员的研究表明,相较于未感染的医护人员,被感染医护人员存在更高的躯体化症状、抑郁症状及创伤后应激障碍(Post-traumatic stress disorder, PTSD)相关症状,且睡眠质量也较未感染者显著下降。该研究结果提示,感染SARS-CoV-2的医务人员可能存在更严重的睡眠及心理障碍。

与此同时,也有多项研究报道了除武汉地区外的国内外医务人员抗疫期间的睡眠及心理状态。有研究人员通过手机问卷的形式调查了包括武汉在内的全国1563例抗疫医务人员的失眠状况,结果显示超过1/3的医务人员伴有失眠症状,且高中或以下文化程度、在COVID-19隔离病房工作、对COVID-19疫情的担忧使得这类医务人员出现失眠症状的风险更高。另一项样本量超过7000例的研究结果显示,年轻人较老年人更容易出现焦虑和抑郁症状;同时,与其他职业(如教师、企业职工)相比,医务人员的睡眠质量最差。在关注疫情暴发当下医务人员心理睡眠状态的同时,也有学者注意到疫情持续一段时间之后医务人员出现的创伤后应激症状(PTSS)。该研究对国内不同省份的377例医务人员进行了调查,结果表明,疫情暴发1个月后,医务人员中PTSS的患病率为3.8%,同时女性医务工作者更容易受到PTSS的影响。值得注意的是,在缺乏必要的心理干预的情况下,急性应激障碍有可能演变为慢性PTSD,而PTSD患者具有较高的自杀风险。因此,在对医务人员进行心理治疗时需特别关注PTSD及其继发效应。

此外,尽管目前尚无抗疫期间睡眠及心理障碍对医务人员日常诊疗工作的影响的相关报道,但根据既往研究提示,当医务人员出现睡眠及心理障碍时,往往更容易出现记忆力减退、注意力不集中、反应时间延长及自信心不足等情况,从而更容易在医疗工作中出现差错。

二、干预手段

由于此次COVID-19疫情具有突发性和紧迫性等特点,因此目前针对医务人员睡眠及心理障碍的临床研究以观察性和回顾性为主。尽管如此,仍有许多学者就如何缓解此次疫情对医务人员造成的睡眠及心理障碍提出了针对性的意见。来自武汉的一项研究结果显示,在被调查的994例参与抗疫的医务人员中,通过阅读心理学书籍、网络及心理咨询等方式寻求心理问题干预的占比分别为36.3%、50.4%和17.5%。尽管该研究未明确上述干预措施对医务人员的心理障碍是否有影响,但至少可以看出,医务人员对于心理干预治疗的需求十分强烈。

就医务人员自身而言,进行科学合理的认知建构是极为重要的。首先,在COVID-19诊疗过程中,许多医务人员为不能挽救重症或危重症患者而感到内疚和自责。但是,SARS-CoV-2对人类而言是全新且未知的,目前尚未发现有治疗COVID-19的特效药,故医务人员无须将全部责任归咎于自己;其次,医务人员应有意识地延长自己的休息及睡眠时间,不应在没有同事协助的情况下独自工作较长时间,而当工作强度太大产生不良情绪时,需要及时向上级或朋友倾诉自己的问题,必要时接受心理干预。除了医务人员的自我调节外,来自家庭的支持也同样重要。医务人员要保持与家人的沟通,这样有利于疏导不良情绪。除了家人之外,并肩工作的同事是另一个支持来源。同事之间要相互鼓励与肯定,客观地面对治疗结果而不要互相指责,应及时分享和讨论诊疗感受、经验和解决问题的方法。此外,当遇到患者或其家属发泄情绪时,要考虑到他们自己也承受着巨大的压力,有时并非针对医务人员。另一项研究指出,合理的夜班轮换制度不仅可以有效保障医务人员的休息时间,也是调整医务人员心理状态的重要手段之一;同时建议一线医务人员进行适度的有氧运动(如瑜伽、太极拳和气功等),一方面可大大减轻心理压力并改善睡眠质量,另一方面可以改善心肺功能,缓解精神压力。

此外,政府及社会的支持也是不可或缺的一部分。有学者建议,政府相关部门要做好以下几点:①与一线抗疫人员保持良好的沟通,及时回应他们对于睡眠及心理障碍干预的关切。②对于非传染病学背景的医务人员,要做好传染病相关的培训及教育。③充分协调各方资源,保障抗疫一线的物资供应和足够的诊疗场所。④引导媒体正面报道,避免对医务人员的污名化。

三、小结与展望

自2019年12月COVID-19疫情暴发以来,作为抗疫战场的主力军,广大医务工作者承受了空前巨大的心理压力。SARS-CoV-2是未知的、无情的,在短时间内面对大量病情复杂凶险的患者却缺乏循证医学证据提供诊疗指导,生理和心理的双重打击导致部分医务人员出现了明显的失眠、梦魇、焦虑和抑郁等睡眠及心理障碍,睡眠和心理两者之间的交互作用往往使患者的症状产生恶性循环。众所周知,正常、有序的医疗环境需要医务人员保持充足的精力和专注力,合并睡眠及心理障碍的医生和护士往往难以胜任高强度的临床工作,无法高质量地完成医疗救治任务;同时,医生的不良情绪也会间接影响到患者,导致医患之间的信任度下降。因此,及时、有效的心理干预对于诊疗工作的正常开展及医务人员的身心健康都是至关重要的。

我国在心理卫生教育方面起步较西方发达国家晚,公民对于自身心理问题的认知及主动寻求心理干预的意识仍有待提高;同时,"集体利益至上"的理念深入人心,医务人员往往为了顾全抗疫大局而刻意忽略自身存在的睡眠及心理问题,不愿主动寻求心理干预,而这样往往会使得心理问题更加严重。因此,要从政府和个人方面积极做好医务人员的心理健康教育工作。在政府方面,国家卫生健康委印发的《新冠肺炎疫情心理疏导工作方案》中指出,各地卫生健康部门要充分利用当地精神卫生、心理健康及社会工作服务资源,为医疗工作者提供心理服务。对一线医务人员加强关心关爱,在轮休期间由精神卫生专业人员组织开展放松训练等活动。对出现明显应激反应的医务人员,要进行针对性的个体心理治疗或适当的药物干预。湖北省、武汉市要充分发挥当地精神卫生医疗机构和援鄂心理救援队的作用,通过讲座、团体辅导、个体咨询、网络平台、心理热线等方式,为医务人员提供心理服务。而在个人层面,出现心理问题后要及时向家人、朋友及同事倾诉,主动寻求心理干预;同时要注意合理安排工作时间,充分保障睡眠质量。

在今后的临床实践中,要依托大数据、人工智能等高科技手段,继续积极探索新的睡眠和心理治疗干预模式,丰富干预形式,同时在符合医学伦理规范的前提下积极开展前瞻性、干预性的临床试验,为解决医务人员的心理健康问题提供坚实的理论依据。

参 考 文 献

[1] World Health Organization. Coronavirus disease 2019(COVID-19): situation report—175. July 13, 2020. Accessed July 14, 2020. https://www.who.int/docs/default-source/coronaviruse/situation-reports/20200713-covid-19-sitrep-175.pdf? sfvrsn=d8acef25_2.

[2] Wang L, Wang Y, Ye D, et al. Review of the 2019 novel coronavirus(SARS-CoV-2)based on current evidence. Int J Antimicrob Agents, 2020, 55(6):105948.

[3] Song X, Fu W, Liu X, et al. Mental health status of medical staff in emergency departments during the Coronavirus disease 2019 epidemic inChina. Brain Behav Immun, 2020.

[4] Lai J, Ma S, Wang Y, et al. Factors Associated With Mental Health Outcomes Among Health Care Workers Exposed to Coronavirus Disease 2019. JAMA Netw Open, 2020, 3(3):e203976.

[5] Huang Y, Zhao N. Generalized anxiety disorder, depressive symptoms and sleep quality during COVID-19 outbreak inChina: a web-based cross-sectional survey. Psychiatry Res, 2020, 288:112954.

[6] Yin Q, Sun Z, Liu T, et al. Posttraumatic stress symptoms of health care workers during the corona virus disease 2019. Clin Psychol Psychother, 2020, 27(3):384-395.

[7] Zhang C, Yang L, Liu S, et al. Survey of Insomnia and Related Social Psychological Factors Among Medical Staff Involved in the 2019 Novel Coronavirus Disease Outbreak. Front Psychiatry, 2020, 11:306.

[8] Lin LY, Wang J, Ou-Yang XY, et al. The immediate impact of the 2019 novel coronavirus(COVID-19) outbreak on subjective sleep status. Sleep Med, 2020.

[9] Chew N, Lee G, Tan B, et al. A multinational, multicentre study on the psychological outcomes and associated physical symptoms amongst healthcare workers during COVID-19 outbreak. Brain Behav Immun, 2020.

[10] Wang S, Xie L, Xu Y, et al. Sleep disturbances among medical

workers during the outbreak of COVID-2019. Occup Med (Lond),2020.
[11] 梅俊华,张琦,龚雪,等. 医护人员感染新型冠状病毒肺炎后心理及睡眠状态分析. 医药导报,2020,39(3):345-349.
[12] Huang Y,Zhao N. Chinese mental health burden during the COVID-19 pandemic. Asian J Psychiatr,2020,51:102052.
[13] Dutheil F,Mondillon L,Navel V. PTSD as the second tsunami of the SARS-Cov-2 pandemic. Psychol Med,2020:1-2.
[14] Johnson AL,Jung L,Song Y,et al. Sleep deprivation and error in nurses who work the night shift. J Nurs Adm,2014,44(1):17-22.
[15] Parry DA,Oeppen RS,Amin M,et al. Sleep:its importance and the effects of deprivation on surgeons and other healthcare professionals. Br J Oral Maxillofac Surg,2018,56(8):663-666.
[16] Belingheri M,Paladino ME,Riva MA. Working schedule, sleep quality and susceptibility to COVID-19 in healthcare workers. Clin Infect Dis,2020.
[17] Whelehan DF,Alexander M,Ridgway PF. Would you allow a sleepy surgeon operate on you? A narrative review. Sleep Med Rev,2020,53:101341.
[18] Church HR,Rumbold JL,Sandars J. Applying sport psychology to improve clinical performance. Med Teach,2017,39(12):1205-1213.
[19] Kang L,Ma S,Chen M,et al. Impact on mental health and perceptions of psychological care among medical and nursing staff in Wuhan during the 2019 novel coronavirus disease outbreak:A cross-sectional study. Brain Behav Immun,2020,87:11-17.
[20] Kisely S,Warren N,McMahon L,et al. Occurrence,prevention,and management of the psychological effects of emerging virus outbreaks on healthcare workers:rapid review and meta-analysis. BMJ,2020,369:m1642.
[21] 国家卫生健康委员会. 关于印发新冠肺炎疫情心理疏导工作方案的通知:联防联控机制发[2020]34号[EB/OL]. (2020-03-18)[2020-07-17]. http://www.nhc.gov.cn/jkj/s3577/202003/0beb22634f8a4a48aecf405c289fc25e.shtml.

4 阻塞性睡眠呼吸暂停与视神经病变的关系

方媛媛　刘辉国

阻塞性睡眠呼吸暂停低通气综合征(obstructive sleep apnea hypopnea syndrome,OSAHS)是一种临床常见病,主要表现为睡眠时打鼾,夜间睡觉时被憋醒且张口呼吸,白天没精神且容易嗜睡、仪器监测血氧饱和度低等,严重扰乱人们的健康、工作和生活,OSAHS患者在我国有4亿人左右,且患者已经向年轻化发展,其对年轻人的危害更大,会导致幼儿的智力发育不完全,影响幼儿的身高发育、对幼儿的心血管系统提前下了隐患。1990—2010年间,阻塞性睡眠呼吸暂停综合征的患病率增加了约30%。OSAHS以慢性间歇性缺氧和睡眠片段化为主要病理特征,出现氧化应激、高碳酸血症、交感神经激活、内皮功能受损等全身病理生理改变,造成神经系统、心血管系统、呼吸系统、内分泌系统、免疫系统、代谢及生长发育等多系统功能损害,严重影响患者的生活质量,甚至会引发车祸等不可挽回的损失。越来越多的研究表明,OSAHS与多种视神经疾病也具有相关性。OSAHS相关视神经病变主要包括原发性开角型青光眼(primary open angle glaucoma,POAG)、非动脉炎性前部缺血性视神经病变(non-arterial anterior ischemic optic neuropathy,NAION)、视盘水肿(papilledema)等,但关于OSAHS引起视神经病变的具体机制目前研究较少。本文就OSAHS相关视神经病变流行病学、发病机制及治疗方案进行回顾。

一、OASHS相关视神经病变现状

(一)非动脉炎性前部缺血性视神经病变

NAION是50岁以上中老年人最常见的急性视神经前部缺血性疾病,以晨起时突发单眼无痛性视力急剧减退,相对性传入性瞳孔障碍、视野缺损及视盘水肿为特征。在美国每年新发病例至少6000例,我国年发病率约1:16000。多种全身疾病均是NAION的高危因素,例如高血压、糖尿病、高脂血症等,还有部分具有争议的危险因素,如夜间血压下降相关的ONH低灌注,血浆同型半胱氨酸升高,吸烟,使用磷酸二酯酶抑制剂(西地那非、他达拉非)治疗,尤其是在出现AHT或心肌梗死的患者及白内障手术者中。而多项研究表明NAION与睡眠呼吸暂停综合征有显著相关性。Aptel对89例非动脉炎性前部缺血性视神经病变患者进行多导睡眠监测(polysomnography,PSG),其中有67例(75%)确诊为OSAHS患者,对其进行为期3年的随访后显示,有15.4%的OSAHS患者累及另一只眼。WU Yong等对4项前瞻性队列研究及一项病例对照研究进行Meta分析后发现,OASHS患者合并或发展为NAION的风险为非OASHS患者的6倍之多。有研究表示,没有NAION的阻塞性睡眠呼吸暂停患者的眼睛表现为视野受累:根据缺血性视神经病变减压试验分类,30%的眼睛表现为视野缺损。单眼伴有NAION的阻塞性睡眠呼吸暂停患者的对侧视野缺损比无NAION的阻塞性睡眠呼吸暂停患者的对侧视野受到的影响更大。目前,睡眠呼吸暂停综合征是非动脉炎性前部缺血性视神经病变的一个独立高危因素已得到广泛认可。

(二)原发性开角型青光眼

青光眼是一种病理性眼压升高性视神经病变,视神经渐进性受损,伴视野缺损,严重者出现失明,是世界上第二大致盲原因。从病因上可分为原发性青光眼或继发性青光眼。原发性开角型青光眼(POAG)是由虹膜和角膜形成的广角,使房水容易进入小梁网。开角型青光眼临床上可分为正常眼压型青光眼(normal tension glaucoma,NTG)和高眼压型青光眼(high tension glaucoma,HTG)。有研究表明,原发性开角型青光眼与睡眠呼吸暂停综合征相关,但结论并不一致。Kremmer S报道了一例正常眼压性青光眼患者随访8年的结果,虽然通过药物及手术将眼压将至正常,但仍发生了进行性青光眼损害,伴有视神经萎缩和视野缺损增加,通过排查可能的心血管相关因素,最后诊断为睡眠呼吸暂停综合征,予以3年的持续正压通气治疗(continue positive airway pressure,CPAP),视神经损伤得到缓解。该报道提出了睡眠呼吸暂停综合征可能与青光眼具有相关性。但是Aptel F对9580例50岁以上的患者进行横断面调查却得出将混杂因素考虑在内,OSAHS患者相较于非OSAHS,青光眼发病率并没有明显增加的结论。Huon分别从青光眼患者中睡眠呼吸暂停综合征的发病率及OSAHS患者青光眼的发病率两个方面进行Meta分析,结果显示青光眼与睡眠呼吸暂停综合征具有显著相关性,睡眠呼吸暂停综合征更容易并发青光眼。眼压升高是目前青光眼发病的唯一明确的病因,OSAHS患者中有50%缺乏昼夜节律,22%表现为倒置节律(昼夜峰相),予以CPAP治疗后使67%出现异常节律的呼吸暂停患者眼压恢复昼夜节律。

(三)视盘水肿

视盘(又称视乳头)水肿特指颅内压增高导致的视盘水肿,表现为短暂性视物模糊,行眼底检查可发现不同程度的双眼视盘水肿、视野缺损,若颅内高压不能解决,则可能出现晚期视力严重受损。有学者认为阻塞性睡眠呼吸暂停综合征可通过多种机制引起颅内高压,如此,我们有理由认为OSAHS与视盘水肿之间存在联系。多篇报道证实了OSAHS与视盘水肿之间的关系,并且提出CPAP治疗可缓解症状。但目前尚缺乏大样本的临床病例对照研究论证其相关性或队列研究说明其因果关系。

(四)睡眠呼吸暂停患者视网膜神经纤维层厚度的变化

视网膜神经纤维层(retinal nerve fiber layer,RNFL)是视网膜神经节细胞轴突汇聚形成的神经纤维,最后形成视神经。RNFL厚度降低间接说明视网膜神经节细胞的丢失,尤其是轴突的萎缩或破坏,即临床前期的视神经疾病的病例表现。临床上,光学相干断层扫描(optical coherence tomography,OCT)是一种最新的非侵入性眼部成像技术,可以灵敏地显示和量化与视杯增大相关的RNFL厚度的减少。因此,研究表明在青光眼出现视野缺陷之前可能已经丢失40%的视网膜神经节细胞。而目前有大量的研究表明,在诊断为视神经病之前OSAHS可导致RNFL厚度降低,且其严重程度与AHI或最低血氧饱和度呈正相关。与阻塞性睡眠呼吸暂停相关的ET-1和氧化应激的增加可能会对视网膜神经节细胞产生影响,尤其是内皮素1通过直接刺激或干扰视神经内的轴突运输来促进星形胶质细胞反应和视网膜神经节细胞死亡,这可能是OSAHS导致RNFL厚度变薄的机制。

(五)继发性视神经病变

OSA是高血压、糖尿病等多种疾病独立为高危因素,并促进疾病的发展,加剧恶化。高血压、糖尿病等代谢性疾病均可引起视网膜病变,导致视神经萎缩变性,甚至失明。同时,OSA与视神经病变也有着千丝万缕的联系,因此,OSA是否也是诱导高血压视网膜病变、糖尿病视网膜病变(DR)等继发性视神经病变的高危因素或者加重病情发展的因素呢?与轻度OSA相比,重度OSA患者与轻度OSA患者相比,视网膜小动脉改变增加,与高血压视网膜病变相似。在一项后续研究中,OSA也与视网膜血管搏动幅度减弱有关。另外,一项前瞻性研究显示,OSA是增殖前/增殖性DR进展的独立预测因子。持续的气道正压治疗与增前/增生DR降低相关。同时一项荟萃分析显示OSA与DR风险增加显著相关($OR=2.01$,95% $CI=1.49\sim2.72$)。糖尿病视网膜病变是糖尿病最常见的微血管并发症之一,血管内皮生长因子(vascular endothelial growth factor,VEGF)的高表达是DR致病机制之一。OSA合并症使糖尿病性视网膜病变患者的血清VEGF水平显著升高,在2型糖尿病(尤其是OSA合并症)的微血管病变严重程度中起重要作用。另外,OSA患者炎症标志物的水平升高,如酰化刺激蛋白、高敏感的CRP和膜攻击复合物(导致补体替代途径的激活)的成分。有研究观察了OSA患者补体激活情况,发现其C3水平升高,IgM和NK细胞百分比降低。因此,补体介导的炎症激活可能导致糖尿病微血管病变加速,进而导致糖尿病视网膜病变的发展和恶化。

二、OSAHS引起视神经病变可能的机制

阻塞性睡眠呼吸暂停综合征以睡眠期间反复上气道完全或部分阻塞,伴有动脉血氧分压($PaCO_2$)下降,这种反复发作的通气量减低或呼吸暂停引起机体出现类似于缺血再灌注的慢性间歇性缺氧,夜间反复胸内负压增大、二氧化碳潴留和低氧血症等病理生理改变,继发交感神经激活,并出现微觉醒。反复夜间低氧诱发氧化应激损伤,继而出现炎症反应,损伤内皮血管系统,造成全身多系统靶器官的功能障碍。视神经病变主要涉及缺血缺氧低灌注、氧化应激及继发神经轴索受损萎缩等病理生理过程。OSAHS可能通过上述过程造成视神经损伤。

(一)低氧直接损伤

视神经为第Ⅱ对脑神经,为中枢感觉神经,需要高能量代谢来维持正常功能,对缺氧极度敏感。OSAHS发作性低氧血症会通过增加线粒体、内质网内活性氧(ROS)的产生直接损伤中枢皮质神经元及海马体,又或者通过氧化应激、炎症反应进一步加重神经元损伤,引起认知障碍、精神异常等症状。Tsang对41例中重度OSAHS患者进行视野检查发现相对35例非OSAHS患者,经多导睡眠监测检测诊断为睡眠呼吸暂停低通气的患者出现视野缺损的风险明显升高,并提出合理假设,即重复呼吸暂停引起视神经缺氧,或间接引起血管病变导致视野缺损。

慢性间歇性缺氧(chronic intermittent hypoxia,CIH)是OSAHS的主要致病机制。CIH主要通过氧化应激及炎症反应对靶器官造成损伤。体外缺氧刺激视网膜神经细胞诱导产生谷氨酸,另外,caspase级联反应也参与诱导视网膜神经细胞凋亡。同时,研究表明线粒体功能障碍也可能与缺氧诱导的RGC凋亡有关。此外,CIH对视网膜组织的损伤还包括抑制小胶质细胞,即Muller细胞产生各种神经营养因子发挥对RGCs的保护作用,并诱导激活TLR4通路激活,产生$TNF-\alpha$、$IL-1\beta$、COX-2等炎症因子,进一步损伤视网膜神经,最终导致视神经功能障碍。

(二)血管因素

1. 神经血管低灌注　视神经分为眼内段、眶内段、管内段及颅内段,其各段血液供应有所不同。眼内段,为视盘表面的神经纤维层,由视网膜中央动脉来的毛细血管供应,而视盘筛板及筛板前的血供,则由来自睫状后动脉的分支供应。二者之间有沟通。Zinn-Haller环,为视盘周围巩膜内睫状后动脉小分支吻合所成。眶内、管内、颅内段则由视神经中的动脉及颅内动脉、软脑膜血管供应。上述血管均为周围小动脉或者末梢微动脉,当夜间睡眠期间反复出现间歇性缺氧时,颈动脉化学感受体感受循环血中氧分压的下降,产生电信号并兴奋交感神经,外周血管阻力增加,血压急剧升高并持续维持较高的水平,超出眼血管自身调节能力,视神经供应血管收缩,血流量下降,视神经灌注减少,长期暴露于缺血缺氧状态,引起神经水肿甚至萎缩。而眶内、颅内视神经血管受脑血管血流及软脑膜血管血流的影响。软脑膜动脉具有稳定脑血流的作用,抵消

血流速度和脑血流收缩压-舒张压振幅的变化，在OSAHS患者中，因动脉二氧化碳分压（$PaCO_2$）升高，脑血管扩张，另外缺氧、氧化应激及炎症反应影响全身脉管系统，使得软脑膜动脉对$PaCO_2$的稳定能力下降，不再补偿脑血流的变化，那么视神经头部的自动调节将会受损，表现为视盘水肿。

2. 神经血管功能障碍

（1）交感神经兴奋性增加：OSAHS以间歇性缺氧及微觉醒为主要特点，反复发作性间歇性低氧导致循环血氧含量下降，激活交感神经系统。同时，当呼吸暂停，由于血气的变化，机体通过一系列激活链来稳定上呼吸道肌肉张力以中止呼吸暂停，这一过程伴有交感神经的兴奋，并继发心动过速和短暂的血压升高，使得患者从呼吸暂停中醒来，恢复气流，血氧饱和度升高。而交感神经的兴奋除了带来心律失常，血管阻力增加，同时伴随缺氧时，血管内皮受损，自我调节功能下降，舒缩失调。

（2）氧化应激、炎症反应：缺氧-复氧的过程类似于缺血再灌注损伤，间歇性缺氧导致大量的活性氧（ROS）产生而不能被线粒体清除，富余的氧自由基破坏细胞结构，导致细胞功能失调甚至凋亡。而ROS不仅直接损伤细胞结构，而且是低氧诱导因子-1（HIF-1）的诱导剂，诱导多种基因的转录表达，包括各种炎症因子、肿瘤坏死因子（TNF-α）、超敏反应蛋白（CRP）等，加重内皮细胞的破坏，影响其正常自我调节功能。血管内皮的破坏是动脉粥样硬化的起点，视神经供应动脉内皮受损后，则不可避免的出现血管硬化，视神经血管多以玻璃样变为主，加重血管的收缩舒张障碍以至于视神经缺血。

（3）血小板聚集、异常活化：阻塞性睡眠呼吸暂停低通气发生时间歇性缺氧、氧化应激、循环炎症细胞因子和脂质浓度升高是导致OSAHS患者血管稳态破坏的因素。与内皮细胞损伤和其他未暴露的分子相平行，血小板也发生了异常活化和聚集。异常活化的血小板进一步释放生物活性物质，通过与LDL受体的相互作用，活化的血小板有助于脂质过氧化，从而反过来加重氧化应激。血小板是动脉粥样硬化的早期效应细胞。持续的血小板活化可能导致严重的血栓并发症，加重视神经微循环障碍。

3. 血管活性物质不平衡 阻塞性睡眠呼吸暂停低通气患者血氧水平下降，低氧诱导血管内皮细胞产生内皮素-1（ET-1，具有收缩血管的功能）；而内皮细胞通过一氧化氮合酶（eNOS）产生NO（具有舒张血管的功能），慢性间歇性缺氧时，NO生物利用度下降，另外ET-1受体表达水平发生变化，ETRB介导的血管舒张功能降低，一氧化氮介导的血管舒张延迟，细胞色素P450产物对血管张力的贡献失衡。当ET-1/NO平衡被打破时，则出现血管收缩舒张障碍，影响是视神经血流动力学，进而促发视神经缺血缺氧损伤。

（三）机械压力

1. 眼内压升高 眼内压（intraocular pressure，IOP）升高一直被认为是视网膜神经纤维层（retinal nerve fiber layer，RNFL）变薄的病理生理基础。眼灌注压取决于全身血压和眼内压，公式为：眼灌注压＝血压－眼内压。在正常人中，视网膜血流量保持恒定，当血压增加高达40％时视盘血流量要确保维持稳定则眼灌注压需要增加34％。因此，当眼内压升高30～45 mmHg时，就可以使眼灌注压降低。OSAHS呼吸暂停期间，体循环动脉血压由于各种机制升高，为了维持视网膜血流量的恒定，即保证眼灌注压的稳定，必须通过升高眼内压来进行自我调节。IOP升高对视神经及视神经血液供应造成压迫，轴浆流中断；眼内压大于靶水平时，引发视神经纤维和视网膜神经节细胞的丢失及凋亡，其结局致使视野缺损和视神经萎缩。Sergi等报道OSAHS患者的IOP明显更大。另外，夜间仰卧位眼内压可升高，肥胖也可能引起眼内压升高，因为眼眶内脂肪组织过多和外周静脉压力增加。阻塞性睡眠呼吸暂停低通气可通过多种机制引起眼内压升高，进而损伤视神经。

2. 颅内压升高 OSAHS与颅内压（intracranial pressure，ICP）变化的关系已得到论证。呼吸暂停事件发生时，胸腔内压升高，回心血量减少，脑静脉回流量下降，血容量升高，ICP升高；其次，间歇性缺氧引起高碳酸血症，$PaCO_2$升高使脑血管扩张，脑含水量增加可能改变颅内容积。有文献表明，阻塞性睡眠呼吸暂停患者在夜间接受氧气治疗后，大脑体积减少了4％。另一个可能引起颅内压升高的原因是OSAHS患者颅内谷氨酸水平的升高。Alperin等的研究提出呼吸暂停可引起谷氨酸升高，引起脑水肿，从而增加ICP。同时视盘低灌注低氧及继发氧化应激均会升高谷氨酸。谷氨酸作为兴奋性神经毒素，可引起脑水肿、高颅内压。OSAHS通过以上机制引起ICP升高，视神经逆行轴突转运因受压而中断，继而引起视盘水肿，长期压力不解除则出现视神经凋亡，纤维萎缩，表现为视野缺损，视神经功能障碍。

三、CPAP治疗对视神经损伤的作用

持续正压通气（continuous positive airway pressure，CPAP）作为OSAHS的标准治疗方案，已在临床诊疗中广泛使用。CPAP治疗可解除OSAHS患者夜间上气道阻塞，改善缺氧，进一步改善由缺氧等引起的一系列病理生理改变。但CPAP治疗对视神经损伤的作用，仍存在争议。有研究者从电生理的角度说明了CPAP对视神经损伤的改善作用。对20例重度OSAHS患者进行视觉诱发电位（visual evoked potential，VEP）检查发现，CPAP治疗对坚持治疗的OSA患者的VEP有显著改善，就此推测CPAP治疗可以通过恢复和保护视神经功能，将OSA的代谢、炎症和缺血后果降到最低，从而使OSA患者VEP反应的改变正常化。但Cohen等发现，经CPAP治疗的OSAHS患者与未行CPAP治疗的OSAHS患者间的夜间平均眼内压差异无统计学意义。因此CPAP对视神经损伤的作用尚不明晰。

四、小　结

关于OSAHS与视神经病变的关系，目前大多数研究为回顾性及横断面研究，仅能说明两者之间的存在联系，

缺乏前瞻性研究以论证因果关系。另外，阻塞性睡眠呼吸暂停综合征患者常伴有许多潜在混杂因素，包括肥胖、高血压和糖尿病等，都会给疾病之间因果关系的论证带来困难。但无论 OSAHS 与视神经病变有无直接病理生理关系，CPAP 治疗都是 OSAHS 患者所必需的。而对于眼科医生及从事睡眠障碍诊疗的医师而言，需考虑 OSAHS 引起视神经病变可能性。对于是否需要对眼科疾病常规进行多导睡眠监测（polysomnography，PSG）仍需要进一步的研究。

参 考 文 献

[1] Jordan AS, Mcsharry DG, Malhotra A. Adult obstructive sleep apnoea. Lancet, 2014, 383(9918): 736-747.

[2] Garg R K, Afifi A M, Garland C B, et al. Pediatric Obstructive Sleep Apnea: Consensus, Controversy, and Craniofacial Considerations. Plast Reconstr Surg, 2017, 140(5): 987-997.

[3] Peppard P E, Young T, Barnet J H, et al. Increased Prevalence of Sleep-Disordered Breathing in Adults. American Journal of Epidemiology, 2013, 177(9): 1006-1014.

[4] Light M, Mccowen K, Malhotra A, et al. Sleep apnea, metabolic disease, and the cutting edge of therapy. Metabolism, 2018, 84: 94-98.

[5] Mentek M, Aptel F, Godin-Ribuot D, et al. Diseases of the retina and the optic nerve associated with obstructive sleep apnea. Sleep Med Rev, 2018, 38: 113-130.

[6] Sun MH, Liao YJ, Lin CC, et al. Association between obstructive sleep apnea and optic neuropathy: a Taiwanese population-based cohort study. Eye (Lond), 2018, 32(8): 1353-1358.

[7] Mcnab AA. The eye and sleep apnea. Sleep Medicine Reviews, 2007, 11(4): 269-276.

[8] Miller NR, Arnold AC. Current concepts in the diagnosis, pathogenesis and management of nonarteritic anterior ischaemic optic neuropathy. Eye(London, England), 2015, 29(1): 65-79.

[9] Xu L, Wang Y, Jonas JB. Incidence of Nonarteritic Anterior Ischemic Optic Neuropathy in Adult Chinese: The Beijing Eye Study. European Journal of Ophthalmology, 2007, 17(3): 459-460.

[10] Aptel F, Khayi H, Pepin JL, et al. Association of Nonarteritic Ischemic Optic Neuropathy With Obstructive Sleep Apnea Syndrome: Consequences for Obstructive Sleep Apnea Screening and Treatment. JAMA Ophthalmol, 2015, 133(7): 797-804.

[11] Wu Y, Zhou LM, Lou H, et al. The Association Between Obstructive Sleep Apnea and Nonarteritic Anterior Ischemic Optic Neuropathy: A Systematic Review and Meta-Analysis. Curr Eye Res, 2016, 41(7): 987-992.

[12] The ischemic optic neuropathy decompression trial (IONDT): design and methods. Control Clin Trials 1998; 19: 276e96.

[13] Kremmer S, Selbach JM, Ayertey HD, et al. Normal tension glaucoma, sleep apnea syndrome and' nasal continuous positive airway pressure therapy-case report with a review of literature. Klin Monbl Augenheilkd, 2001, 218(4): 263-268.

[14] Aptel F, Chiquet C, Tamisier R, et al. Association between glaucoma and sleep apnea in a large French multicenter prospective cohort. Sleep Med, 2014, 15(5): 576-581.

[15] Huon LK, Liu SY, Camacho M, et al. The association between ophthalmologic diseases and obstructive sleep apnea: a systematic review and meta-analysis. Sleep Breath, 2016, 20(4): 1145-1154.

[16] Pepin J-L, Chiquet C, Tamisier R, et al. Frequent loss of nyctohemeral rhythm of intraocular pressure restored by nCPAP treatment in patients with severe apnea. Arch Ophthalmol Chic Ill, 2010, 128: 1257e63.

[17] Wardly DE. Intracranial hypertension associated with obstructive sleep apnea: a discussion of potential etiologic factors. Med Hypotheses, 2014, 83(6): 792-797.

[18] Javaheri S, Qureshi Z, Golnik K. Resolution of papilledema associated with OSA treatment. J Clin Sleep Med, 2011, 7(4): 399-400.

[19] Quigley HA, Dunkelberger GR, Green WR. Retinal ganglion cell atrophy correlated with automated perimetry in human eyes with glaucoma. Am J Ophthalmol, 1989, 107: 453e64.

[20] Lin P-W, Friedman M, Lin H-C, et al. Decreased retinal nerve fiber layer thickness in patients with obstructive sleep apnea/hypopnea syndrome. Graefes Arch Clin Exp Ophthalmol Albr Von Graefes Arch Für Klin Exp Ophthalmol, 2011, 249: 585e93.

[21] Fraser CL, Bliwise DL, Newman NJ, et al. A prospective photographic study of the ocular fundus in obstructive sleep apnea. J Neuroophthalmol, 2013, 33: 241-246.

[22] Tong JY, Golzan M, Georgevsky D, et al. Quantitative retinal vascular changes in obstructive sleep apnea. Am J Ophthalmol, 2017, 182: 72-80.

[23] Altaf QA, Dodson P, Ali A, et al. Obstructive Sleep Apnea and Retinopathy in Patients with Type 2 Diabetes. A Longitudinal Study. Am J Respir Crit Care Med, 2017, 196(7): 892-900.

[24] Zhu Z, Zhang F, Liu Y, et al. Relationship of Obstructive Sleep Apnoea with Diabetic Retinopathy: A Meta-Analysis. Biomed Res Int, 2017, 2017: 4737064.

[25] Li ZG, Li TP, Ye H, et al. Immune function changes in patients with obstructive sleep apnea hypopnea syndrome. Nanfang Yike Daxue Xuebao, 2011, 31: 1003-1005.

[26] Delaey C, Van De Voorde J. Regulatory Mechanisms in the Retinal and Choroidal Circulation. Ophthalmic Research, 2000, 32(6): 249-256.

[27] Carloni S, Riparini G, Buonocore G, et al. Rapid modulation of the silent information regulator 1 by melatonin after hypoxia-ischemia in the neonatal rat brain. J Pineal Res, 2017, 63(3): e12434.

[28] Shan X, Chi L, Ke Y, et al. Manganese superoxide dismutase protects mouse cortical neurons from chronic intermittent hypoxia-mediated oxidative damage. Neurobiology of disease,

2007,28(2):206-215.

[29] Feng J,Wu Q,Zhang D,et al. Hippocampal impairments are associated with intermittent hypoxia of obstructive sleep apnea. Chinese Medical Journal,2012,125(4):696-701.

[30] Tsang CSL,Chong SL,Ho CK,et al. Moderate to severe obstructive sleep apnoea patients is associated with a higher incidence of visual field defect. Eye,2006,20(1):38-42.

[31] Hayreh SS. Blood supply of the optic nerve head and its role in optic atrophy,glaucoma,and oedema of the optic disc. The British journal of ophthalmology,1969,53(11):721-748.

[32] Lévy P,Pépin J-L,Arnaud C,et al. Obstructive Sleep Apnea and Atherosclerosis. Progress in Cardiovascular Diseases, 2009,51(5):400-410.

[33] Ikram MK,De Jong FJ,Vingerling JR,et al. Are Retinal Arteriolar or Venular Diameters Associated with Markers for Cardiovascular Disorders? The Rotterdam Study. Investigative Ophthalmology & Visual Science, 2004, 45 (7): 2129-2134.

[34] Frydrychowski AF,Wszedybyl-Winklewska M,Bandurski T, et al. Flow-induced changes in pial artery compliance registered with a non-invasive method in rabbits. Microvascular Research,2011,82(2):156-162.

[35] Paiva T,Attarian H. Obstructive sleep apnea and other sleep-related syndromes. Handb Clin Neurol,2014,119:251-271.

[36] Belaidi E,Morand J,Gras E,et al. Targeting the ROS-HIF-1-endothelin axis as a therapeutic approach for the treatment of obstructive sleep apnea-related cardiovascular complications. Pharmacology & therapeutics,2016,168:1-11.

[37] Nadeem R,Molnar J,Madbouly EM,et al. Serum inflammatory markers in obstructive sleep apnea: a meta-analysis. Journal of clinical sleep medicine:JCSM:official publication of the American Academy of Sleep Medicine,2013,9(10): 1003-1012.

[38] Atkeson A,Yeh SY,Malhotra A,et al. Endothelial function in obstructive sleep apnea. Progress in cardiovascular diseases,2009,51(5):351-362.

[39] Gabryelska A,Łukasik ZM,Makowska JS,et al. Obstructive Sleep Apnea: From Intermittent Hypoxia to Cardiovascular Complications via Blood Platelets. Frontiers in neurology, 2018,9:635.

[40] Phillips BG,Narkiewicz K,Pesek CA,et al. Effects of obstructive sleep apnea on endothelin-1 and blood pressure. Journal of Hypertension,1999,17(1):61-66.

[41] Lee PJ,Liu CJL,Wojciechowski R,et al. Structure-function correlations using scanning laser polarimetry in primary angle-closure glaucoma and primary open-angle glaucoma. American journal of ophthalmology, 2010, 149 (5): 817-825.e811.

[42] Sergi M,Salerno DE,Rizzi M,et al. Prevalence of Normal Tension Glaucoma in Obstructive Sleep Apnea Syndrome Patients. Journal of Glaucoma,2007,16(1):42-46.

[43] Jennum P,Børgesen SE. Intracranial Pressure and Obstructive Sleep Apnea. Chest,1989,95(2):279-283.

[44] O'donoghue FJ,Briellmann RS,Rochford PD,et al. Cerebral Structural Changes in Severe Obstructive Sleep Apnea. American Journal of Respiratory and Critical Care Medicine, 2005,171(10):1185-1190.

[45] Alperin N,Ranganathan S,Bagci AM,et al. MRI Evidence of Impaired CSF Homeostasis in Obesity-Associated Idiopathic Intracranial Hypertension. American Journal of Neuroradiology,2013,34(1):29.

[46] Liguori C,Placidi F,Palmieri MG,et al. Continuous Positive Airway Pressure Treatment May Improve Optic Nerve Function in Obstructive Sleep Apnea: An Electrophysiological Study. Journal of clinical sleep medicine:JCSM:official publication of the American Academy of Sleep Medicine,2018,14 (6):953-958.

[47] Cohen Y,Ben-Mair E,Rosenzweig E,et al. The effect of nocturnal CPAP therapy on the intraocular pressure of patients with sleep apnea syndrome. Graefes Arch Clin Exp Ophthalmol,2015,253(12):2263-2271.

5 从睡眠呼吸调控辨析呼吸衰竭——临床病例评析

张晓雷

一、通气功能是由通气肌做功能力、中枢通气驱动和通气负荷决定的

通气系统的三个关键要素包括中枢控制器、通气感受器和效应器。

1. 中枢控制器,主要是脑干(延髓、脑桥)的神经元,产生呼吸驱动,主要两组神经元组成,即背侧呼吸组神经元(DRG)和腹侧呼吸组神经元(VRG)。DRG 主要位于孤束核,是心肺感受器传入的神经冲动在中枢整合的重要部位;VRG 主要包括包钦格复合体、前包钦格复合体、疑核和后疑核等神经核团,其中前包钦格复合体是重要的呼吸发生器。

2. 通气的效应器,即呼吸肌,包括上气道肌群、膈肌及肋间肌等辅助呼吸肌。

3. 通气的感受器,包括中枢及外周化学性感受器、机械性、温度、痛觉等感受器。

呼吸系统由高效的前反馈和后反馈(正/负反馈)调控,清醒状态下,多种调控机制参与通气的调控,即使在外环境明显改变(如高原)或重要通气部件受损情况下,仍可代偿维持通气功能和血气的稳定。机体在睡眠状态下,通气调控能力降低,呼吸系统处于潜在的"脆弱"阶段,轻度的通气功能受损即可出现夜间低通气。因此,睡眠呼吸监测是早期通气功能不全及"不明原因"呼吸衰竭的重要的临床诊断工具。

二、化学性调控是睡眠状态下主要的呼吸调控方式,CO_2 是关键调控因子

清醒状态下的呼吸调控主要包括高位呼吸中枢,即大脑皮质对呼吸的自主调控和中枢及外周化学感受器的代谢性调控。四肢肌肉及关节周围的机械性感受器可感受运动而引起呼吸频率和潮气量增加,触觉、痛觉、温度觉感受器受刺激可引起通气量的变化,肺的过度充气或牵张可通过 Hering-Breuer 反射抑制呼吸,情感应激可引起通气量的增加,如高通气综合征的患者。此外,清醒状态本身可作为独立的通气刺激因子。

化学性调控是机体在清醒安静状态下和睡眠状态下主要的通气调控方式。机体在睡眠状态下,除代谢性调控外,其他通气调控机制明显减弱或消失,而对通气的化学性(代谢性)调控成为最主要的通气调控方式。外周化学感受器位于颈动脉体和主动脉体,感受氧、二氧化碳和氢离子浓度的变化,是即时调控的快反应感受器。延髓斜方体后核是重要的中枢性化学感受器,通过感受脑脊液中 pH 的变化,感受 $PaCO_2$ 的变化。CO_2 是睡眠状态下的关键通气调控因子,当 $PaCO_2$ 水平低于导致呼吸暂停的窒息阈值时,即发生中枢性呼吸暂停。与外周快反应化学感受器不同,中枢感受器需要 1 min 的时间对化学性刺激作出反应,这种反应的延迟与心力衰竭等病理情况下周期性呼吸(Cheyne-Stokes 呼吸)的发生密切相关。

三、不同清醒-睡眠阶段低氧及高二氧化碳通气反应性的变化

从清醒状态到非快动眼睡眠(NREM)再到快动眼睡眠(REM),机体对低氧和高碳酸血症的反应性是逐步降低的。通气调定点,即导致通气量增加的 $PaCO_2$ 的节点,由清醒到稳定睡眠到 REM 睡眠是增高的,即在 REM 睡眠状态下需较高的 $PaCO_2$ 水平,才能启动通气量的增加。这是临床上很多睡眠呼吸障碍性疾病,包括阻塞性睡眠呼吸暂停及大多数睡眠低通气疾病,其低氧血症和高碳酸血症在 REM 睡眠期最为突出的原因之一。此外,低氧和高二氧化碳通气反应性与机体的行为状态密切相关,随清醒、睡眠、运动等行为状态的变化而改变。并且,低氧和高二氧化碳的通气反应具有可塑性,如机体反复暴露于低氧环境中,可导致低氧通气反应的敏感性降低,进而导致睡眠状态下通气不稳定的病理状态;同样睡眠呼吸疾病经无创通气治疗后,其通气反应性的降低可随通气的改善而恢复,这就可解释部分肺泡低通气疾病患者,随着治疗时间的延长,其无创通气压力需求可能会降低。

四、睡眠微觉醒是个双刃剑

睡眠呼吸暂停事件终止时,通常伴随微觉醒的发生,微觉醒一方面导致了睡眠稳态的破坏和碎片化的睡眠,但同时微觉醒导致通气量的恢复和增加是对睡眠低通气的重要保护机制,在某些中枢性低通气疾病的患者,可出现

继发于呼吸暂停或低通气事件的微觉醒的明显降低，进而进一步加重了睡眠低通气。

五、不同睡眠清醒时相呼吸神经元电活动及呼吸肌功能的变化

呼吸运动神经元除接收节律性，即与呼吸运动相关的神经冲动（驱动电位）外，还接收紧张性神经冲动，这种紧张性的神经冲动可理解为背景频率。机体从清醒到 NREM 到 REM 睡眠期，紧张性神经冲动的动作电位降低，可导致呼吸肌肌电活动降低，表现为潮气量和分钟通气量的降低。但是在 REM 睡眠期，存在内源性不规律的，与呼吸运动无关的，且不依赖于 $PaCO_2$ 水平（化学性调控）的紧张性神经冲动的动作电位的增加，导致 REM 期中枢性呼吸事件与 NREM 相比，相对减轻，因此中枢性呼吸暂停及中枢性肺泡低通气在 NREM 期通常较 REM 期更常见，程度更为严重。

呼吸肌，包括上气道肌群、肋间肌和腹肌等辅助呼吸肌的肌电活动从清醒到 NREM，再到 REM 睡眠期，是逐渐降低的，尤其是在 REM 睡眠期，除膈肌之外的呼吸肌均处于类似"瘫痪"的状态；而膈肌作为维持机体呼吸运动的重要肌肉，在清醒及不同睡眠时相，其肌电活动无明显变化，是维持机体在睡眠状态下通气稳态的重要动力源。神经肌肉疾病患者如果膈肌受累，其在睡眠状态下尤其是 REM 睡眠期会出现明显的低通气。因此，REM 期低通气通常是神经肌肉疾病呼吸肌受累的最早和最突出的临床表现，具有重要提示及鉴别诊断意义。

六、病例分析

（一）病例 1

1. 病历资料　38 岁，女性，反复呼吸困难伴双下肢水肿 5 年，近 5 年四肢肌力进行性减退，近 2 年出现咳嗽无力、声音改变、进食水呛咳。30 年前罹患脊髓灰质炎。血气分析（FiO_2 0.21）：pH 7.44，PO_2 50mmHg，PCO_2 63mmHg，HCO_3^- 42.8mmol/L，SO_2 86%。胸部 CT 未见异常。心脏超声提示右心增大，肺动脉高压，估测 SPAP 50mmHg。肺功能提示限制性通气功能障碍，无法配合 P0.1 及最大吸气压检测。多导睡眠监测提示：以低通气事件为主，明显的低氧血症，在快动眼睡眠期（R 期）低氧尤为明显。

2. 诊治经过　病房夜班值班医生给予患者吸氧后，发现血氧基线改善，但睡眠期，尤其是 R 期出现持续时间更长、更深的氧降。患者次夜于睡眠室进行无创通气手工压力滴定，通气模式：BPAP(S/T) IPAP 14cmH$_2$O, EPAP 6cmH$_2$O，备用频率 12 次/min，在未吸氧情况下，其夜间低氧血症基本纠正。此患者给予无创通气治疗，但 1 年后因吸入性肺炎去世。

3. 病例评析

（1）此患者以肺动脉高压收入院，病史及血气分析提示为低氧或肺部疾病相关性肺动脉高压，肺功能检查提示限制性通气功能障碍，因无法配合卧位肺功能和最大吸气压检查，未能获得呼吸肌受累证据。但多导睡眠监测表现为 REM 睡眠期相关的显著的低氧血症和低通气，为呼吸肌受累的特征性表现，提示存在神经肌肉疾病导致肺泡低通气和肺动脉高压。

（2）此患者夜间常规氧疗，为何低氧事件加重？据血气公式 $PAO_2 = FiO_2(760-47)-1.25 \times PaCO_2 = 0.21713-1.25 \times PaCO_2 = 150-1.25 \times PaCO_2$，对于无换气功能异常的单纯肺泡低通气疾病患者，其动脉氧分压的降低是由于肺泡低通气造成的肺泡中二氧化碳分压增高，挤占了氧气的空间所致，因此对于此类患者首要的问题是改善通气，如单纯吸氧，化学感受器的反应性降低，可导致睡眠期尤其是 R 期更为严重的低氧。

（3）对于神经肌肉疾病导致肺泡低通气的患者，无创通气需采用 BPAP(S/T) 模式，而不是无备用频率的 S 模式，需设置较高的吸气触发灵敏度，降低因呼吸肌无力造成的无效触发。此类患者通常不需要较高水平的压力支持，并且对高水平的压力支持耐受性较差，可因压力滴定过程中的快速升压导致觉醒，因此此类患者无创通气需在保证氧合的基础上，合理设置呼吸机参数，维持睡眠连续性。

（4）神经肌肉疾病患者，除注意膈肌等呼吸肌受累之外，还需关注上气道肌群，尤其是对于病变较重，受累层面较高的患者，如出现脑神经受累可出现吞咽困难，需注意气道廓清，降低吸入性肺炎的风险。

（二）病例 2

1. 病历资料　患者男性，15 岁，间断呼吸困难、因呼吸衰竭，4 次气管插管病史。患者从 3 岁开始，即在呼吸道感染、发热及局麻后出现呼吸困难、口唇发绀，神志不清，于当地医院先后 4 次入住 ICU，行气管插管，曾诊断为"重症肺炎、呼吸衰竭、急性心力衰竭、中毒性脑病、症状性癫痫"等，给予机械通气、抗感染、解痉、脱水、降颅压等治疗。自诉平素体力活动不受限，喜欢打篮球，BMI：20.7kg/m^2。以下为患者第 4 次发作时气管插管初及治疗 5d 后胸部 CT（图 7-5-1）。

肺功能检查提示立卧位肺通气、肺容量及弥散功能未见异常。清醒状态未吸氧血气：pH 7.40，PCO_2 61cmH$_2$O，PO_2 80cmH$_2$O。肌电图、肌肉活检、头颅 MRI、脑电图、心脏彩超均未见异常。简易精神状态评价量表（MMSE）提示轻度认知功能障碍。多导睡眠监测提示睡眠呼吸事件以低通气为主，NREM 期更为明显，微觉醒减少。全基因组检测：*PHOX2B* 基因突变阳性。患者于睡眠室进行无创通气压力滴定，通气模式：BPAP(S/T) IPAP 15cmH$_2$O，EPAP 6cmH$_2$O，备用频率 12 次/min，在未吸氧情况下，其夜间低氧血症基本纠正。随访 2 年病情稳定。

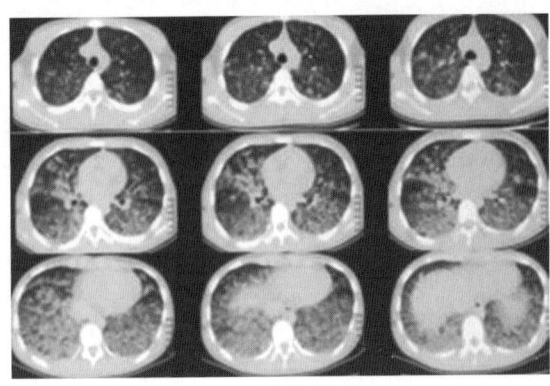

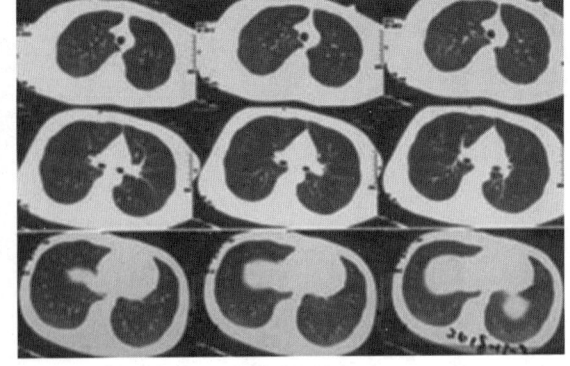

图 7-5-1　患者第 4 次发作时气管插管初及治疗 5d 后胸部 CT

2. 诊断评析

(1)此患者先后 4 次因呼吸道感染、发热或应用局部麻醉药等导致通气需求、氧耗增加或呼吸中枢兴奋性降低的情况下出现呼吸衰竭,辅助检查及病程转归无法用肺实质、气道、肺血管及呼吸肌病变解释。睡眠监测提示主要为 NREM 期的低通气和低氧血症,同时伴微觉醒的减少,提示存在中枢性肺泡低通气,全基因组检查证实为先天性肺泡低通气综合征(CCHS)。

(2)延髓腹外侧区的斜方体后核(RTN)是中枢化学感受器 CO_2/H^+ 依赖信号传输到呼吸中枢控制器的关键位置。CO_2/H^+ 水平升高引起含有 PHOX2B 基因的 RTN 神经元在呼吸中枢控制器前包钦格复合体的轴突终末分泌兴奋性神经递质谷氨酸。而 CCHS 的患者由于相关基因突变导致中枢化学感受器向呼吸中枢控制器神经递质传递障碍。

(3)需注意的是不同于 REM 期存在的内源性兴奋性冲动,NREM 期通气几乎完全依赖于化学性调控,因此中枢性低通气患者的 $PaCO_2$ 水平的增高以 NREM 期更明显,此与神经肌肉疾病导致低通气相鉴别。

七、结　语

睡眠呼吸生理是呼吸与危重症医学科医生知识体系的重要组成部分,了解掌握睡眠呼吸调控的基础知识有助于理清诊断思路,减少临床诊疗的盲点。多导睡眠检测是睡眠状态下睡眠和呼吸最准确和全面的评估方法,是临床上早期发现以及对"unexplained"低通气疾病的重要诊断工具。

6 新型冠状病毒肺炎患者的睡眠呼吸障碍

胡 克

由 SARS-CoV-2 引起的新型冠状病毒肺炎（COVID-19）由于导致大量死亡而对全球健康构成威胁。人群通常容易感染该病毒，特别是患有慢性疾病的中老年人。对1099 例 COVID-19 确诊患者的研究表明，患者的中位年龄为 47.0 岁，其中年龄≥65 岁的占 15.1%，危重患者中年龄≥65 岁的占 27.0%。合并症在 COVID-19 确诊的生存者和死亡者中都非常普遍，主要是高血压、糖尿病、心脑血管疾病等。另一方面，研究表明这些合并疾病也与阻塞性睡眠呼吸暂停密切相关。而且，OSA 也多见于中老年人群，流行病学研究显示，OSA 患者常出现合并症如系统性高血压、心血管疾病、糖尿病和肥胖。因此，包括年龄、性别（男性）、心血管-代谢合并疾病、体型等发生 OSA 的危险因素均与 COVID-19 确诊患者不良预后的危险因素之间，有着很大的重叠，这也表明如果 OSA 患者发生 SARS-CoV-2 感染，则针对 OSA 的有效治疗可使患者受益。虽然一些临床研究表明，在急性期接触 COVID-19 的医护人员和 COVID-19 的患者可能会遭受心理压力和睡眠障碍，例如抑郁、焦虑、失眠等症状，但对于 OSA 是否常见于 COVID-19 患者，以及 OSA 与 COVID-19 的常见合并症之间的关系知之甚少。由于对 COVID-19 大流行期间的感染防护有特殊要求，因此不建议使用多导睡眠图和便携式监测设备来对 COVID-19 患者进行监测，而可穿戴心肺监护装置和基于云平台的系统对于控制和监测 COVID-19 是可行且有效的方法。现有资料表明，超宽带（UWB）雷达睡眠呼吸暂停监测器是一种无线、非接触式监测设备，也是一种便携、方便可靠的用于筛查 OSA 的设备。本研究目的是使用 UWB 雷达监测系统来研究 COVID-19 患者 OSA 的发生状况、临床特征和可能的危险因素。为尽可能避免与急性患者相关的心理压力对睡眠质量的影响，我们探讨了症状消失、但病毒核酸长时间阳性的 COVID-19 康复期患者的 OSA。

一、方 法

1. 研究对象 自 2020 年 3 月 12 日到 2020 年 4 月 23 日，共有 111 例确诊为 COVID-19 的患者连续入组本研究。纳入标准如下：①年龄在 18 岁以上，诊断符合我国指南中 COVID-19 确诊病例诊断标准。②患者为症状消失后的恢复期，但核酸检测持续阳性。③同意进行问卷调查和睡眠监测。排除标准：①重症或危重症患者。②处于急性期。③需要夜间氧疗者。④使用镇静药物如苯二氮䓬类、阿片类、抗精神病药等。⑤拒绝参加本研究者。

收集每位患者的资料，包括人口学资料、实验室检查结果、合并疾病、四份问卷和睡眠监测信息；分析 COVID-19 确诊患者是否存在 OSA 与是否有着合并疾病的相关性。

本研究方案得到我院伦理委员会审查和批准，并获得 COVID-19 患者口头知情同意。在特殊疫情下，本研究申请书面知情同意豁免并获得伦理委员会的同意。

2. 研究方案 COVID-19 确诊患者并曾因病住院，在治疗后达到了临床出院标准（症状消失、胸部 CT 提示肺部急性渗出性病灶基本吸收）、但检测病毒核酸后长时间阳性者，均为本研究的候选者。每位候选者均需都完成包括人口学资料和合并基本等的综合问卷。询问患者此前是否诊断过高血压、糖尿病、心脏病、心绞痛、卒中或其他合并症。然后完成 4 个问卷（ESS、STOP-Bang、ISI、PSQI），在对每位患者安排进行睡眠监测。护士和（或）医生在接诊期间对问卷进行了复核，以确保答案可靠，必要时进行相应的更改。

111 名经实验室确诊断的 COVID-19 患者符合本研究的入、排标准，根据上述原则，有 4 名受试者由于不愿接受睡眠监测（$n=2$）或缺乏足够的睡眠监测记录（$n=2$）而被排除在外，总 107 名患者完成了本研究。

3. 问卷调查 Epworth 嗜睡量表（ESS）用于评价受试者于白天不同情况下的嗜睡程度。在我国，分数≥9 的受试者被认为有白天过度嗜睡的高风险。STOP-Bang 问卷（SBQ）是包括 4 项二分的条目和 4 个临床参数的工具，得分 ≥ 3 被认为具有中度至重度 OSA 风险。失眠严重程度指数（ISI）包括 7 个项目，用于评估失眠症状的严重程度，得分＞15（范围为 0～28）者被认为存在失眠。匹兹堡睡眠质量指数（PSQI）是衡量睡眠质量和睡眠方式的量表，共 7 项，总分 21；得分≥8 被定义为存在失眠的可能，得分越高，睡眠质量越差。

4. 睡眠监测 采用无线、非接触式监测装置进行睡眠监测。所有受试者在单独病房中接受睡眠事件的评估，夜间检测时间不少于 7 h。用于 OSA 筛查的无线非接触式监测系统由中国杭州的兆观公司（Megasens Technology Co. Ltd）提供，该系统包括 UWB 雷达睡眠呼吸暂停监测器（ZG-S01D，图 7-6-1A）和连续血氧监测 Megaring（ZG-P11F，图 7-6-1B）。计算以下睡眠参数：总睡眠时间、睡眠效率、睡眠时间、平均脉搏血氧饱和度(平均SpO_2)、最低脉搏血氧饱和度($Min\ SpO_2$)、氧减指数(ODI)、$SpO_2<90$的睡眠时间所占百分比(T90)、以及呼吸暂停低通气指数(AHI)。AHI≥5次/小时被认为存在OSA。OSA严重程度按照AHI,分为轻度(5~14.9次/h)、中度(15~29.9次/h)和重度(≥30次/h)。

5. COVID-19确诊标准和无症状后病毒携带者 实验室确诊的病例是指符合《新型冠状病毒感染的肺炎诊治指南》中的确诊标准,即该病例具有流行病学史,典型症状和X线影像学表现,通过实时RT-PCR检测SARS-COV-2核酸呈阳性,或血清中具有SARS-COV-2特异性IgM和IgG。对于无症状后的病毒携带者,由于没有标准定义,我们在本文中采用以下定义:即有症状的COVID-19确诊患者,在症状消失后,取鼻咽标本RT-PCR检测核酸持续阳性,时间达2周以上的患者。

6. SARS-CoV-2核酸和血清抗体的检测 收集鼻咽拭子标本,保存在病毒保存培养基中并运输,并由经过培训的技术人员进行检测,通过反转录酶RT-RCR法检测SARS-CoV-2核酸。试剂由中国上海GeneoDx生物技术有限公司提供。通过全自动化学发光免疫分析仪[Uni-Cel DxI800,贝克曼库尔特商业企业(中国)有限公司,上海,中国]检测血清特异性抗SARS-CoV-2的IgG和IgM抗体,试剂盒由中国深圳YHLO Biotech Co.,Ltd提供。

7. 合并疾病诊断 糖尿病的诊断是根据既往的诊断、或空腹血糖≥7.0mmol/L,或随机血糖≥11.1mmol/L,或75g口服葡萄糖耐量试验2h血糖≥11.1mmol/L而做出,使用便携式血糖仪进行测试。高血压定义为收缩压(SBP)≥140 mmHg或舒张压(DBP)≥90 mmHg;在本项研究中,以下三种情况被判定为高血压:①根据临床病史由医生诊断为高血压。②服用过口服降压药。③使用气动微处理器控制的血压测量仪器在傍晚或早晨进行SBP≥140mmHg和(或)DBP≥90mmHg。对心脑血管疾病或其他合并症的判断基于每位患者的既往诊断。心律失常的诊断根据心电图结果而做出。

8. 统计分析 连续描述性统计数据以中位数和四分位间距(IQR)表示,分类变量的统计数据是绝对数和百分比表示。对差异性分析,连续变量以Mann-Whitney U检验,对分类变量进行X^2检验或Fisher精确检验。使用带有Dunn多重比较的Kruskal-Wallis检验来比较各组。单变量和多变量二元逻辑回归分析用于评估COVID-19患者的人口统计学数据、合并疾病、异常实验室发现和OSA因变量之间的相关性,以比值比(OR)和95%置信区间(95%CI)表示。以$P<0.05$被认为具有统计学意义。所有统计分析均使用SPSS 22.0进行。

二、结 果

1. 恢复期COVID-19患者OSA患病率及其特征 在本研究中,所有患者均接受了问卷调查,并使用无线非接触式监测系统进行了整夜睡眠监测。107例恢复期COVID-19患者中,75例(70.1%)合并有OSA。在75例存在OSA的患者中,AHI中位数(IQR)为22.2(12.5~31.0)次/h,其中阻塞性AHI、中枢性呼吸暂停指数和混合性呼吸暂停指数的中位数(IQR)分别为21.7(12.9~32.9)、0.0(0.0~0.1)和0.6(0.3~1.0)次/h。OSA患者的中位数(IQR)ODI为17.7(9.3~30.0)次/h,中位数(IQR)Min SpO_2为72.8(64.1~80.0)%,中位数(IQR)T90为5.4(1.2~16.2)%。

与无OSA的COVID-19患者相比,并存OSA的患者男性更多,颈围和腰围更大,IL-10和干扰素-γ的水平更高,SBQ、ESS和PSQI得分更高。此外,患有OSA的患者的ODI、平均SpO_2、$Min\ SpO_2$和T90与无OSA的患者存在显著差异;但两组患者在年龄、BMI、大多数实验室检查结果、病毒核酸持续时间或住院时间方面差异均无显著性。

2. COVID-19确诊患者的合并疾病 我们分析了COVID-19确诊患者的合并疾病情况。在107例COVID-19确诊病例中,有59例(55.1%)存在合并疾病,48例(44.9%)无合并疾病。合并症的发生顺序为高血压(37.4%)、糖尿病(17.8%)、冠心病(9.3%)、慢性肺病(5.6%)、心律失常(4.7%)、恶性肿瘤(3.7%)、失眠(3.7%)和焦虑症(0.9%)。

3. OSA与合并疾病之间的相关性 在75例存在OSA的COVID-19确诊患者中,34例合并高血压,17例有糖尿病,10有冠心病,2例存在慢性肺病,3例合并心律失常,3例合并恶性肿瘤,2例存在失眠和1例同时有着焦虑。结果发现,高血压(45.3% vs.18.8%,$P=0.009$)、糖尿病(22.7% vs.6.3%,$P=0.042$)和冠心病(13.3% vs.0,$P=0.031$)在存在或不存在OSA的COVID-19患者的组间比较有统计学差异;但两组之间在慢性肺疾病、心律失常、恶性肿瘤、失眠或焦虑的患病率不存在统计学差异。此外,存在与不存在OSA的COVID-19确诊患者合并疾病的总体患病率并无差别(58.7% vs.46.9%,$P=0.261$)。

根据AHI,将COVID-19患者分为4组:非OSA组(AHI 0~4.9),轻度OSA组(AHI 5~14.9)、中度OSA组(AHI 15~29.9)和重度OSA组(AHI≥30)。统计学分析表明,在这4组中,COVID-19患者合并疾病的患病率没有显著性差异,除了慢性肺部疾病的患病率在非OSA患者中略高之外。

4. COVID-19患者OSA的危险因素 单因素分析表明,男性、颈围、腰围、身高、体重和高血压是COVID-19患者发生OSA的危险因素(均$P<0.05$)。多因素Logistic回归显示,COVID-19患者的性别[男性OR 4.352,95% CI 1.642~11.537,$P=0.003$]和高血压(OR 3.133,95% CI 1.111~8.832,$P=0.031$)与OSA显著相关。

三、讨 论

本研究探讨了COVID-19确诊患者OSA的患病率和危险因素,以及OSA与COVID-19患者合并疾病之间的相关性。结果表明,COVID-19确诊患者的OSA和合并疾病均很常见。

已有的研究结果表明，具有任何合并疾病的COVID-19患者的临床结局比没有合并疾病的患者更差，并且合并疾病的数也与临床结局更差有关，但这些合并疾病中，并不包括OSA。在本研究中，我们发现，COVID-19确诊患者的OSA患病率很高（70.1%）；与无OSA的COVID-19患者相比，存在OSA的COVID-19患者中男性更多，颈围和腰围更大，IL-10和干扰素-γ的水平更高，SBQ、ESS和PSQI的得分更高，同时有着更低的夜间氧减；但两组在年龄、BMI、大多数实验室检查结果、病毒核酸持续时间、已经住院时间方面，均无显著性差异。此外我们发现，COVID-19患者的合并疾病患病率很高（55.1%），包括高血压（37.4%），糖尿病（17.8%），冠心病（9.3%），慢性肺病（5.6%），心律失常（4.7%），恶性肿瘤（3.7%），失眠（3.7%）及焦虑症（0.9%）。这些结果说明，高OSA患病率和高合并疾病发生率同时存在于COVID-19患者，表明OSA可能对COVID-19患者的合并症产生影响。

通过单因素逻辑分析确定的OSA危险因素包括男性、颈部和腰围、身高、体重和高血压，这与以往发现的有关晋迪人群OSA危险因素相一致。多因素Logistic回归分析显示，男性和高血压与COVID-19患者的OSA显著相关。我们的结果与既往发现的OSA主要见于男性的流行病学结果相符，但本队列研究并未显示高BMI是COVID-19患者存在OSA的危险因素，这可能与样本量较小有关。

高血压是与COVID-19相关的重要合并症，并严重影响这些患者的预后。最近有报道发现，在对年龄、性别和吸烟状况进行调整之后，高血压被认为是与COVID-19严重程度相关的唯一合并疾病。血管紧张素转换酶受体-2可能是SARS-CoV-2的新型黏附分子，病毒可通过此受体导致COVID-19和肺损伤，而这种受体在高血压和慢性代谢性疾病患者中的表达升高，因此，这可以用来部分解释高血压、糖尿病和其他疾病在COVID-19患者有着高患病率的原因，我们的发现与这些结果一致。

遗憾的是，本研究未能清楚同时存在OSA与心血管代谢合并疾病的COVID-19患者是否具有更高的死亡风险，这主要与数据缺乏有关。因为自2020年3月上旬以来，武汉市新发生的COVID-19病例比1月和2月少得多，而重症和危重症病例就更少，这是我们未能评估OSA对COVID-19患者死亡风险影响的最重要原因。此外，睡眠质量明显受到疾病严重程度和患者心理压力的影响。因此，我们招募了康复期、症状消失后但病毒核酸仍持续阳性而住院的COVID-19患者作为研究对象。

同时应该指出的是，由于在大流行期间对防控SARS-CoV-2感染有特殊的要求，因而我们采用无线非接触式OSA监测系统来进行本项研究。该系统由脉冲无线电超宽带雷达和Megaring（连续脉搏血氧监测指环）组成，雷达监视器放于床头柜上，将脉冲波发射到身体，发射的脉冲被人体反射，然后被接收天线探测到。接收器中配备的软件预设算法可自动对信号进行处理，并且可以连续获取患者的呼吸频率、呼吸幅度、心率和身体运动。该雷达监视系统已被证明可用于对OSA的筛查，是一种便携和可靠的设备，适用于各种紧急情况，尤其是COVID-19大流行期间。本研究所使用的设备见图7-6-1。

本项研究的优势在于，我们不仅针对COVID-19患者的OSA进行了前瞻性分析，而且还避免了与急性期COVID-19相关的心理应压对睡眠质量的影响，这可能更好地反映了COVID-19患者的真实睡眠情况。我们的结果还表明，应更加关注OSA对COVID-19的病程和预后的影响，并且针对OSA的有效治疗可能会使COVID-19患者受益。

我们的研究也存在明显的不足。首先，自2020年3月初以来很少有新发的COVID-19患者，有关睡眠监测和氧合的数据仅是来自恢复期患者而不是急性期患者，这可能会导致评估偏差，并可能降低患者的代表性，因为患者的睡眠条件与急性期不同；其次，OSA的诊断不是基于金标准的客观监测——夜间多导睡眠监测，这可能会影响诊断的准确性。

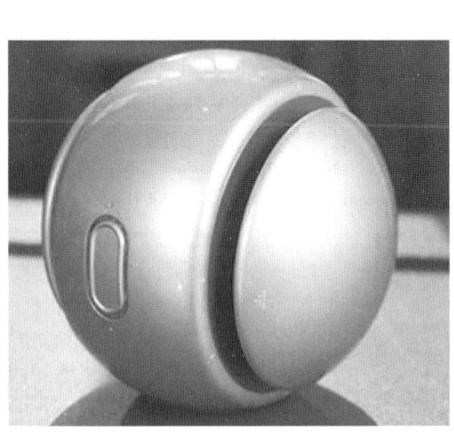

雷达检测装置 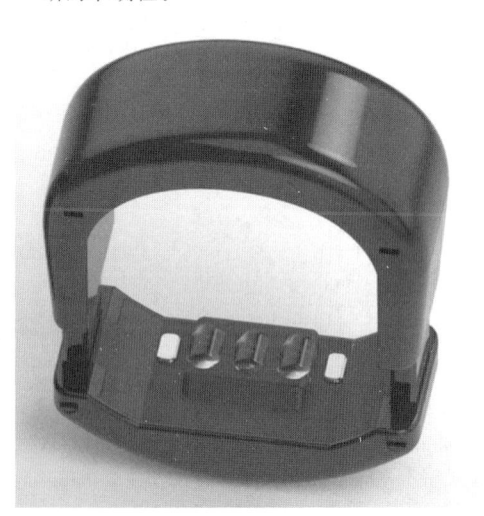　　　　　　指环检测仪

图7-6-1　本研究所使用的设备

总之，本研究结果显示，COVID-19患者OSA和其他合并疾病的患病率均很高，提示OSA可能对COVID-19患者的合并疾病和预后产生影响，需要进一步研究COVID-19所存在OSA是否增加有其他合并疾病的COVID-19患者的死亡风险。

参 考 文 献

[1] Chen N, Zhou M, Dong X, et al. Epidemiological and clinical characteristics of 99 cases of 2019 novel coronavirus pneumonia in Wuhan, China：a descriptive study. Lancet, 2020, 395 (10223)：507-513.

[2] Wang D, Hu B, Hu C, et al. Clinical Characteristics of 138 Hospitalized Patients With 2019 Novel Coronavirus-Infected Pneumonia in Wuhan, China. J Am Med Assoc, 2020, 323 (11)：1061-1069.

[3] Guan WJ, Ni ZY, Hu Y, et al. China Medical Treatment Expert Group for Covid-19. Clinical Characteristics of Coronavirus Disease 2019 in China. N Engl J Med, 2020, 382(18)：1708-1720.

[4] Zhou F, Yu T, Du R, et al. Clinical course and risk factors for mortality of adult in patients with COVID-19 in Wuhan, China：a retrospective cohort study. Lancet, 2020, 395(10229)：1054-1062.

[5] Benjafield AV, Ayas NT, Eastwood PR, et al. Estimation of the global prevalence and burden of obstructive sleep apnoea：a literature-based analysis. Lancet Respir Med, 2019, 7(8)：687-698.

[6] Hedner J, Grote L, Bonsignore M, et al. The European Sleep Apnoea Database(ESADA)：report from 22 European sleep laboratories. Eur Respir J, 2011, 38(3)：635-642.

[7] Chen T, Wu D, Chen H, et al. Clinical characteristics of 113 deceased patients with coronavirus disease 2019：retrospective study. Brit Med J, 2020, 368：m1091.

[8] Baker JG, Sovani M. Case for continuing community NIV and CPAP during the COVID19 epidemic. Thorax, 2020, 75(5)：368.

[9] Liu K, Chen Y, Wu D, et al. Effects of progressive muscle relaxation on anxiety and sleep quality in patients with COVID-19. Complement Ther Clin Pract, 2020, 39：101132.

[10] Lai J, Ma S, Wang Y, et al. Factors associated with mental health outcomes among health care workers exposed to coronavirus disease 2019. J Amer Med Assoc Netw Open, 2020, 3(3)：e203976.

[11] Zhang XL, Xiao Y. Sleep health service in China during the COVID-19 outbreak. J Clin Sleep Med, 2020.

[12] Grote L, McNicholas WT, Hedner J. ESADA collaborators. Sleep apnoea management in Europe during the COVID-19 pandemic：data from the European sleep apnoea database (ESADA). Eur Respir J, 2020, 2001323.

[13] Klum M, Urban M, Tigges T, et al. Wearable cardiorespiratory monitoring employing a multimodal digital patch stethoscope：estimation of ECG, PEP, LVET and respiration using a 55 mm single-lead ECG and phonocardiogram. Sensors(Basel), 2020, 20(7)：E2033.

[14] Gong M, Liu L, Sun X, et al. Cloud-based system for effective surveillance and control of COVID-19：useful experiences from Hubei, China. J Med Internet Res, 2020, 22(4)：e18948.

[15] Zhou Y, Shu D, Xu H, et al. Validation of novel automatic ultra-wide band radar for sleep apnea detection. J Thorac Dis, 2020, 12(4)：1286-1295.

[16] National Health Commission of the People's Republic of China. Diagnosis and treatment of novel coronavirus infected pneumonia（trial 7th edition）[EB/OL]. [2020-03-03]. http：//www. nhc. gov. cn/yzygj/s7653p/202003/46c9294a7dfe4cef80dc7f5912eb1989/files/ce3e6945832a438eaae415350a8ce964. pdf.

[17] Johns MW. A new method for measuring daytime sleepiness：the Epworth sleepiness scale. Sleep, 1991, 14(6)：540-545.

[18] He QY, Chen BY. The interpretation of the guideline of obstructive sleep apnea hypopnea syndrome. Zhonghua Jie He He Hu Xi Za Zhi, 2012, 35(1)：7-8.

[19] Chung F, Yegneswaran B, Liao P, et al. STOP questionnaire：a tool to screen patients for obstructive sleep apnea. Anesthesiology, 2008, 108(5)：812-821.

[20] Yu DS. Insomnia Severity Index：psychometric properties with Chinese community-dwelling older people. J Adv Nurs, 2010, 66(10)：2350-2359.

[21] Liu XC, Tang MQ, Hu L, et al. Reliability and validity of the Pittsburgh sleep quality index. Chin J Psychiatry, 1996, 29(2)：103-107.

[22] Berry RB, Budhiraja R, Gottlieb DJ, et al. Rules for scoring respiratory events in sleep：update of the 2007 AASM Manual for the scoring of sleep and associated events. Deliberations of the sleep apnea definitions task force of the American Academy of Sleep Medicine. J Clin Sleep Med, 2012, 8(5)：597-619.

[23] Standards of medical care in diabetes--2013. Diabetes Care, 2013, 36(Suppl 1)：S11-66.

[24] Pickering TG, Hall JE, Appel LJ, et al. Subcommittee of Professional and Public Education of the American Heart Association Council on High Blood Pressure Research. Recommendations for blood pressure measurement in humans and experimental animals. Part 1：blood pressure measurement in humans：a statement for professionals from the Subcommittee of Professional and Public Education of the American Heart Association Council on High Blood Pressure Research. Hypertension, 2005, 45(1)：142-161.

[25] Guan WJ, Liang WH, Zhao Y, et al. Comorbidity and its impact on 1590 patients with Covid-19 in China：A Nationwide Analysis. Eur Respir J, 2020, 55(5)：2000547.

[26] Franklin KA, Lindberg E. Obstructive sleep apnea is a common disorder in the population-A review on the epidemiology of sleep apnea. J Thorac Dis, 2015, 7：1311-1322.

[27] Li X, Xu S, Yu M, et al. Risk factors for severity and mortality in adult COVID-19 inpatients in Wuhan. J Allergy Clin

Immunol, 2020, 146(1):110-118.
[28] Zhou P, Yang XL, Wang XG, et al. A pneumonia outbreak associated with a new coronavirus of probable bat origin. Nature, 2020, 579(7798):270-273.
[29] Imai Y, Kuba K, Rao S, et al. Angiotensin-converting enzyme 2 protects from severe acute lung failure. Nature, 2005, 436:112-116.
[30] Kuba K, Imai Y, Rao S, et al. A crucial role of angiotensin converting enzyme 2 (ACE2) in SARS coronavirus-induced lung injury. Nat Med, 2005, 11:875-879.
[31] Crackower MA, Sarao R, Oudit GY, et al. Angiotensin-converting enzyme 2 is an essential regulator of heart function. Nature, 2002, 417:822-828.
[32] Danser AHJ, Epstein M, Batlle D. Renin-angiotensin system blockers and the COVID-19 pandemic: at present there is no evidence to abandon renin-angiotensin system blockers. Hypertension, 2020, 75(6):1382-1385.

7 PSG 数据后处理及其临床应用

王 婧 陈 锐

睡眠呼吸障碍包括阻塞性睡眠呼吸暂停(obstructive sleep apnea,OSA)、中枢性睡眠呼吸暂停(central sleep apnea,CSA),伴或不伴陈-施呼吸(Cheyne-Stokes respiration),以及睡眠相关肺泡低通气障碍等,这些疾病各有特征性表现,仅靠病史和体格检查不足以确诊,诊断需要有睡眠技师值守的、在院的整夜多导睡眠图(polysomnography,PSG)监测。PSG 监测的常规记录数据,目前多遵循美国睡眠医师协会(American Academy of Sleep Medicine, AASM)制定的判读标准进行分析,满足常见睡眠障碍性疾病的临床诊断需要。但 PSG 所记录的睡眠中脑电和呼吸的生理信号,后期经软件处理,可用来开展相关的科学研究工作,本文就 PSG 数据后处理方法及临床应用做一总结。

一、PSG 常规记录参数

PSG 监测前 24 h 禁服酒精、咖啡因、镇静药或催眠药,夜间记录时间均在 7 h 以上。PSG 记录的数据主要包括以下部分:①睡眠分期——脑电图(electroencephalogram, EEG)、颏肌电图(electromyography,EMG)和眼电图(electrooculography,EOG)监测用于睡眠分期和识别觉醒,睡眠分期至少需要 3 个 EEG 导联,常规选用在脑部额区、中央区和枕区,但通常会采集双侧电极信号,以便电极失效时有替代,常标记为 F3、F4、C3、C4、O1、O2。②呼吸气流——常使用口鼻热敏电阻和经鼻压力传感器,这两种方法互相补充。③呼吸努力——仅监测气流不足以区分睡眠期间呼吸变化的原因是中枢性还是阻塞性,大多数睡眠实验室会联合使用胸部和腹部呼吸感应体积描记法(respiratory inductance plethysmography,RIP),以准确描记呼吸用力。食管测压是评估呼吸努力的金标准,但考虑患者耐受程度,不常规运用该方法。④脉搏血氧测定——脉搏血氧测定是 PSG 的标准内容,可以连续监测动脉含氧血红蛋白饱和度(SpO_2),要注意收缩性心力衰竭所致循环时间延长的患者中可能会出现较长的信号延迟。⑤通气——成人 PSG 时可选择进行通气评估,无创通气监测技术包括经皮和呼气末二氧化碳监测,以往的设备可能需要夜间多次校准,新一代的经皮监测仪可在整个标准 PSG 中提供可靠的数据。呼气末二氧化碳监测仪不需要频繁的重新校准,但若患者有明显鼻塞或伴有死腔的基础肺部疾病,则可能会低估动脉二氧化碳水平,评估可能不准确。⑥心律——PSG 期间会常规行 ECG 监测,单个导联通常足以识别心律失常,因放置简便,通常使用导联Ⅱ。⑦其他:还有非数值型的参数,包括视频和音频,记录鼾声及体位。

二、PSG 脑电数据后处理及应用

(一) 脑电睡眠微结构改变

1. 循环交替模式 睡眠脑电图不仅提供睡眠宏观结构信息,包括非快速眼动(NREM)睡眠(N1,N2,N3)、快速眼动(REM)睡眠和清醒阶段,还提供了被称为循环交替模式(cyclic alternating pattern,CAP)的微观结构特征。CAP 是一种在非快动眼睡眠期出现的周期性的脑电节律,以一系列突出于背景的短暂性脑事件的发放为特点,且这些事件重复出现,根据其事件数量和持续时间综合判读,提示睡眠不稳定性。Della 等对 17 例短暂性整体失忆患者睡眠微观结构的分析,结果发现,与健康对照者相比,研究组患者的 CAP 时间减少和 CAP 率降低,睡眠效率降低,觉醒指数增加。我们课题组的研究也发现 CAP 可以评估 OSA 患者睡眠紊乱,且较宏观睡眠分期更加敏感。此外,CAP 还与睡眠障碍造成的认知损伤等相关,Bruni 等在对 42 名儿童的睡眠宏观结构和 CAP 进行分析,并采用智力量表和神经心理发育评估对儿童的神经认知进行评估,发现儿童的逻辑推理与 CAP 率相关。我们课题组的研究也发现 CAP 参数的 A3 相指数与 OSA 认知功能呈负相关。

CAP 是涉及皮质的广泛的脑电活动,在 F3、F4、C3、C4、O1 和 O2 脑电电极均可记录到。根据 Terzano 等提供的标准,手工执行 CAP 分析。在 NREM 睡眠中,CAP 出现在整个阶段 N1~N3,其中 A 相由瞬态事件识别,其明显地突出于背景节律即 B 相。CAP 的 A 相可分为 3 种亚型:A1 亚型(EEG 慢节律占主要优势)、A2 亚型(EEG 活动是和快节奏的混合)、A3 亚型(EEG 活动主要为快速低压节律),所有 CAP 序列以 A 相开始,并以 B 相结束。CAP 的每个阶段的持续时间为 2~60 s。当 CAP 不出现超过 60 s 被评为非 CAP,终止 CAP 序列的 A 相被计为非 CAP,即 CAP 序列需要至少 2 个连续的 CAP 循环(图 7-7-1)。CAP 的参数主要包括:CAP 时间、CAP 率(N1、N2、N3 期 CAP 率)、A 相指数(A1、A2、A3 相指数)、A 相平均持续时间和 B 相平均持续时间。

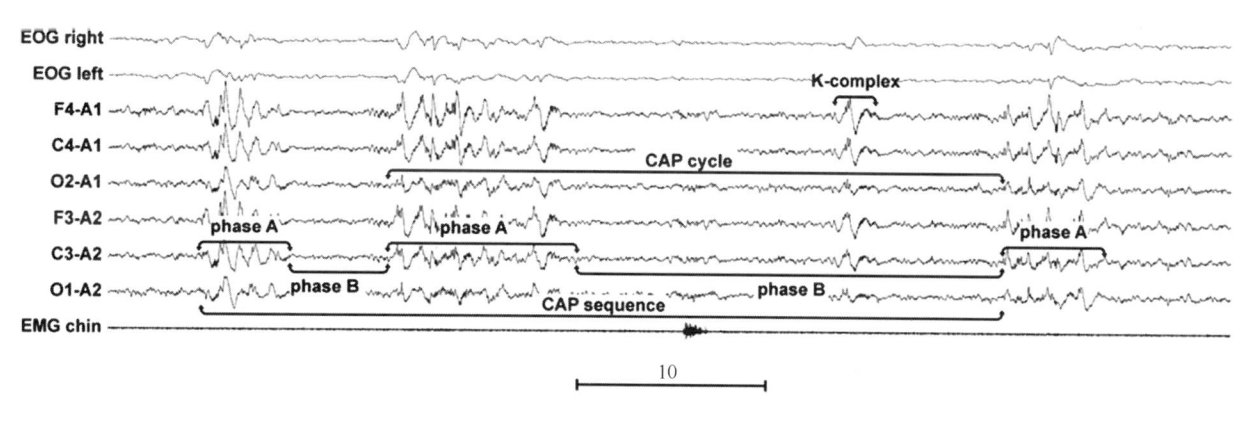

图 7-7-1 CAP 的 EEG 特征

2. Delta/alpha 比值（Delta/alpha ratio，DAR） 脑电的频段一般划分为：delta(1～4 Hz)、theta(4～8 Hz)、alpha(8～13 Hz)、beta(13～30 Hz)、gamma(30～100 Hz)，不同睡眠阶段的特定频段反映了睡眠功能和大脑状态的神经功能，如 delta 活动通常被认为是睡眠深度或睡眠稳态的指标，theta 活性可能参与情绪记忆巩固，alpha 活性反映了皮质抑制的神经元活动等。Delta/alpha 比值（DAR）为 delta 波绝对功率与 alpha 波绝对功率之比，在一定程度上代表脑电图的慢波化程度，其优势在于可以避免由整体的、与频率无关的 EEG 功率增加引起的 delta 增加。DAR 被认为是区分清醒期、1 期和 2 期和慢波睡眠的最佳因子。DAR 可运用 Matlab 软件对患者 PSG 脑电图进行频谱分析获得。

DAR 广泛应用在睡眠领域、神经功能研究等方面，研究表明，DAR 与脑卒中的梗死部位和范围有密切的关系，位于皮质或靠近皮质、病变范围较大的梗死灶，其 DAR 值越大；位于大脑深部靠近底节区，病变范围较小，以及后循环梗死，其 DAR 值偏小，提示 DAR 对前循环较大面积梗死的预测价值。另外，DAR 可反映脑卒中患者的严重程度和预后。有研究显示，亚急性缺血性脑卒中患者的 DAR 比对照组的 DAR 高，且其入院时的 DAR 与入院时的美国国立卫生研究院卒中量表评分（national institutes of health stroke scale，NIHSS，用于评估急性 IS 患者神经功能缺损的严重程度）和卒中 30 d 后的 mRS 评分（改良 Rankin 评分，Modified Rankin Scale，评估脑卒中患者神经功能的恢复状况）正相关。OSA 和肥胖低通气（obesity hypoventilation syndrome，OHS）患者在 NREM 时 DAR 与精神运动警觉测试（PVT）的表现呈负相关，与氧相关指数（如 T90，T80）呈正相关。这突出了脑电图测量得到的 DAR 可作为 OSA 患者嗜睡和认知功能的生物标志物的潜在价值。

（二）脑电频谱分析与脑电连接性分析

脑功能损伤常常出现认知障碍、情绪改变、嗜睡等临床表现，由于传统的将神经症状映射到特定区域的局灶性脑损伤研究具有一定局限性，往往难以找到明确的结构损伤部位，近年来越来越多的研究从功能层面来探究脑功能损伤的病理机制。脑电频谱分析与脑电功能连接性分析提供了一种不同于解剖连接的图谱，可反映大脑区域间更广泛的多突触连接和连接功能关系的影响。分析的具体方法如下。

1. 预处理 利用 Matlab 软件进行数据处理：导入数据、定位电极、剔除无用电极、参考电极的转换（双侧乳突、鼻尖、全脑平均参考）、滤波（高通滤波与低通滤波及 50Hz 干扰）、浏览数据（有无坏电极、去掉漂移很大的时间段数据）、坏电极插补、伪迹的矫正（回归的方法、PCA、ICA）、分段（基线的长度选取）、去掉波幅很大的分段。

2. 频谱分析 在脑电数据进行预处理后，将原本的时域信号经过傅里叶变换得到以频率为横轴，信号幅值为纵轴，且随着频率变化的频域信号。将实验组和对照组分段后 EEG 信号为一个"电极*时间点*分段"的三维矩阵，对所有电极、所有分段的 EEG 信号进行 FFT 变换后，会得到一个"电极*频率点*分段"的三维矩阵存储功率值，进而进行分段间的平均，得到一个"电极*频率点"的二维矩阵。将 delta、theta、alpha、beta、gamma 五个频段相应范围内所有频率点的功率值平均，得到该频段的功率值，每个 EEG 数据集在每个频段的功率均是一个"电极*1"的向量，最终得到一个"N*2*电极"的矩阵存储功率。比较睡眠不同时相和不同频段组合下某些感兴趣的区域，如额叶、顶叶、颞叶、枕叶、中央区的统计学差异。

3. 连接性分析 根据指定的起始和终止结点，分析电极与电极（或脑区与脑区）之间信号的统计学关系。采用相干（coherence）、相位同步（PLV、PLI、wPLI）、格兰杰因果分析（Granger causality）指标构建对应的功能连通性矩阵，绘制功能连接图。为了解决共同源问题，我们将空间滤波后计算功能连接指标。用相干、相位同步、格兰杰因果分析指标等量化脑电连接性，对特定睡眠阶段和波段下额、顶、颞、枕、中央区等区域两两之间的连通性强度进行统计学分析。

4. 脑电频谱分析与连接性分析的临床应用 Musaeus 等利用脑电连接性和与 ApoE 基因相结合的图论分析方法预测轻度认知障碍发展为阿尔茨海默症的风险；Song 等研究发现低频脑电连接性的改变可作为轻度认知障碍临床进展的指标。还有研究发现，阿尔茨海默病脑电连接性下降，且与疾病严重程度相关；脑电频谱及连接性分析在疾病病理生理机制探索、诊断治疗和转归预测等方面都有一定的价值。此外，基于近年来神经影像人脑组学的快速发展，脑电功能连接性研究还可以联合 DTI、fMRI 等影像学技术来实现，为揭示疾病的神经机制提供更加丰富的影像信息。

三、PSG 氧减数据后处理及应用

睡眠呼吸暂停低通气指数（apnea hypopnea index，AHI）是诊断与评估 OSA 严重程度的重要指标，但其对 OSA 多系统合并症发生率的预测价值十分有限，这可能是因为 AHI 仅反映了每小时呼吸事件的发生次数，并不包含 OSA 患者气流受限、缺氧的持续时间和严重程度。一些研究报道指出，PSG 监测中的夜间低氧参数比 AHI 更能反映疾病的转归情况，例如 TS90%（血氧饱和度<90%时间占总监测时间的百分比）等。Gottlieb 等研究发现，心力衰竭时血流动力学的改变与 T90% 有关，而与 AHI 无关；另有研究表明，TS90% 在预测心血管疾病的发病率及预后方面优于 AHI。但 T90% 在合并慢阻肺、肥胖低通气等持续性低氧血症的患者，并不能作为评估间歇缺氧的特异性指标。

最近，Azarbarzin 等提出了一种可以量化 OSA 相关低氧血症的参数——睡眠呼吸暂停特异性低氧负荷（sleep apnea specific hypoxic burden，SASHB），定义为与呼吸事件（暂停或低通气）相关的氧饱和曲线下的面积。SASHB 反映 OSA 的呼吸事件造成低氧血症的频率、持续时间和严重程度，而不反映其他会降低 SpO_2 导致低氧血症的因素。Azarbarzin 等的研究显示，在矫正了心血管疾病的患病率、AHI、TS90%、睡眠时间等因素后，低氧负荷与心血管事件死亡率独立相关；在矫正了人口学特征、吸烟和合并症等因素后，低氧负荷与心力衰竭的患病风险独立相关，与之相比，AHI 并未发现其与心血管不良事件的相关性。研究结果体现了低氧负荷在预测 OSA 导致的心血管不良事件中具有独特的价值，临床上可用于评估 OSA 患者心血管合并症的发病风险。值得一提的是，在低氧负荷计算中，只需要运用气流和 SpO_2 参数，这些信息在 PSG 和便携式睡眠监测设备上均可获得，可应用于多中心、大样本的数据分析。

SASHB 计算方法：在 PSG 记录的通气曲线中，以平静呼吸时的曲线作为基线，曲线下的总面积可量化气道阻塞引起的总通气量缺失。由于不同中心气流测量方法存在差异，故一般使用 SpO_2 曲线替代通气曲线。低氧负荷定义为呼吸事件中 SpO_2 曲线基线下的总面积；对于每一次的呼吸暂停或低通气，基线的 SpO_2 被定义为事件结束前 100s 内 SpO_2 的最高值。这个基线值下的区域是在每个呼吸事件的窗口内计算的。每个部分不饱和的脉氧曲线是通过叠加呼吸事件结束前的 SpO_2 信号来确定的。然后将这些单独的 SpO_2 曲线基线下的面积相加得到总面积，除以睡眠时间，得出低氧负荷的具体数值，单位为（%min）/h（低氧负荷计算示例见图 7-7-2）。例如：SASHB 为 50% min/h 相当于每小时中有 10 min 的时间动脉血氧饱和度比基线低 5%。

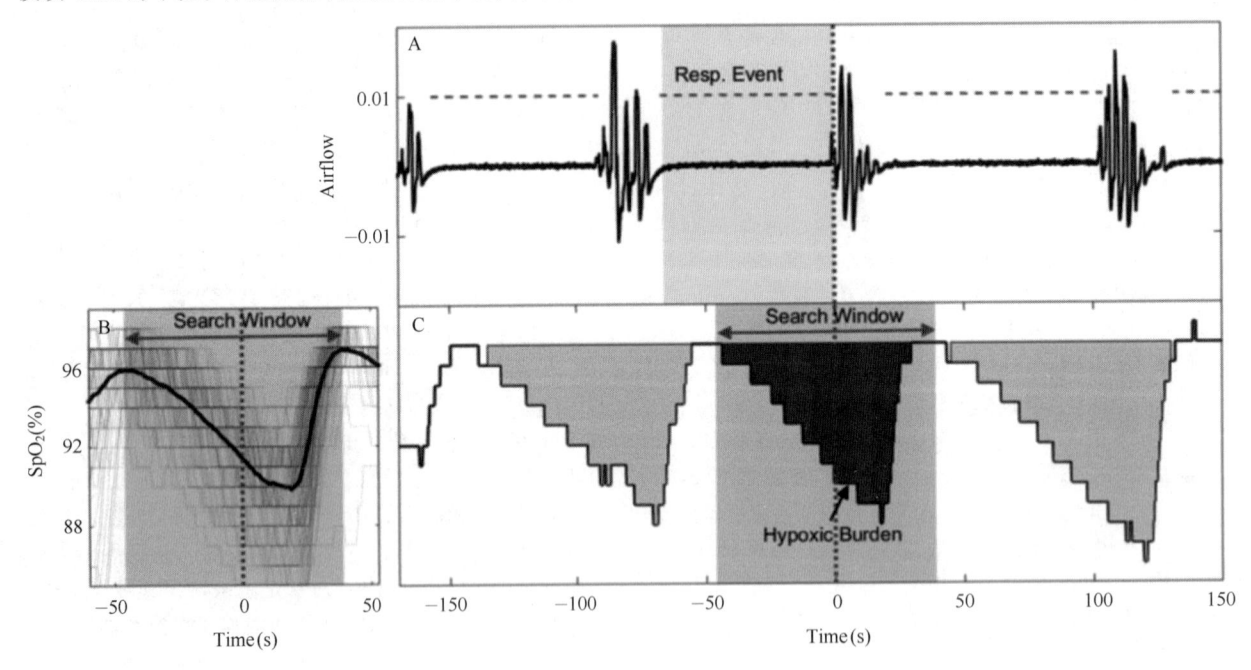

图 7-7-2 低氧负荷计算示例

注：A. 根据鼻导管气流生成的通气曲线和其中的呼吸事件；B. 个体的所有呼吸事件相关的脉搏氧饱和度（SpO_2）信号叠加。信号均在呼吸事件终止时（时间为 0）同步，并计算搜索窗口的时间（2 个峰值之间的时间）。搜索窗口用于计算单次呼吸事件的低氧负荷，即搜索窗口重脉搏氧饱和度曲线基线下的面积。C. 总的低氧负荷定义为单次呼吸事件中脉搏氧饱和度曲线基线下的面积之和除以总睡眠时间

四、PSG 其他相关数据

(一) PSG 下肢肌电数据

睡眠中周期性腿动 (periodic limb movements of sleep, PLMS) 是指在睡眠时出现的周期性、反复发作的、高度刻板的腿部运动。根据 AASM 的判读标准，PSG 记录的下肢肌电数据可判断有意义的腿动事件 (LM)，定义为：①最短持续时间 0.5 s；最长持续时间 10 s；②振幅与静息肌电图相比，肌电图电压增高 8 μV；③起点：以肌电图电压高于基线 8 μV 处作为起点；④终点-肌电图电压并未超过静息肌电图 2 μV，并且持续时间≥0.5 s 的时期的起点处。

周期性腿动序列 (PLMS) 定义为：①LM 事件至少连续出现 4 次才能定义为一组 PLM 序列。②LM 事件之间的周期长期 (连续 LM 事件起始点之前时长) 包括 PLM 事件在内为 5~90s。③左右两腿的腿动，起始点间隔 <5s，计为单次腿动事件。

PLMS 的报告形式：夜间 PLMS 出现的总次数，PLMS 指数 (每小时睡眠发生 PLMS 的次数)，以及与觉醒有关的 PLMS 总次数。

PLMS 的临床意义目前存在争议，有研究发现，伴随每次 PLMs 的发生，平均心率、血压都会出现先增高后降低的变化，增高幅度可达 5%~20%，这种变化在伴有脑电觉醒时交感神经活化程度更加显著。OSA 伴有呼吸事件相关腿动比不伴有患者交感神经活化程度更高，伴随 PLMS 出现的交感神经活化及微觉醒导致的深睡减少，可使夜间血压增高，呈"非杓型"改变，从而影响心脑血管疾病的发生、发展及预后。

(二) 觉醒 (arousal)

睡眠时一系列不同程度的反应，如光、声等外部因素，低氧和胸腔负压等内部刺激，都可以引起觉醒反应。PSG 上表现为脑电图出现稳定睡眠期间脑电频率突然增加，持续 3s 以上。觉醒反应可以分为皮质、皮质下等不同程度的觉醒，在睡眠呼吸障碍中，皮质觉醒最为常见，国人常称之为微觉醒。缺氧、高碳酸血症及呼吸负荷增加是 OSA 患者主要的觉醒刺激因素，其中，呼吸努力/呼吸驱动的增加是觉醒的关键影响因素，也是觉醒阈值常用的测量指标。觉醒阈值用于描述引起微觉醒反应的呼吸刺激大小，通常用测量到的食管压表示。由于食管压的测定通常需要侵入性检查，患者往往不能耐受，寻找非侵入性检查方法十分重要。Edwars 等开发了一种简单的临床筛查方法，定义低觉醒阈值评分标准为：① AHI<30/h。② 最低 SaO_2 > 82.5%。③低通气事件占呼吸事件的百分比 >58.3%；达到 1 条标准计 1 分，总分 2 分或 2 分以上定义为低觉醒阈值。该方法作为无创的觉醒阈值判定方法，期灵敏度为 80.4%，特异性为 88.0%。

五、总 结

PSG 监测记录了整夜睡眠呼吸评估相关的生理信号，包括睡眠分期、呼吸气流、呼吸努力、脉搏血氧饱和度和通气情况等。研究者不仅要掌握常规监测和判定这些信号的技术规范，更要深度挖掘 PSG 数据，进一步进行后处理分析，以期对睡眠相关疾病的诊疗进行更深入的探讨，从 PSG 记录到的众多信号中能筛选出帮助疾病诊疗的标志物参数。本文涉及的脑电微结构、脑电频谱分析与连接性分析、低氧负荷、低觉醒阈值等数据后处理方法是对本课题组长期研究的积累总结及文献阅读的结果，希望能给广大睡眠学工作者带来新的启发与思考。

参 考 文 献

[1] Chervin RD, Aldrich MS. Effects of esophageal pressure monitoring on sleep architecture. Am J Respir Crit Care Med, 1997, 156(3): 881-885.

[2] Caples SM, Rosen CL, Shen WK, et al. The scoring of cardiac events during sleep. J Clin Sleep Med, 2007, 3(2): 147-154.

[3] Manconi M, Ferri R, Miano S, et al. Sleep architecture in insomniacs with severe benzodiazepine abuse. Clin Neurophysiol, 2017, 128(6): 875-881.

[4] Mariani S, Manfredini E, Rosso V, et al. Efficient automatic classifiers for the detection of a phases of the cyclic alternating pattern in sleep. Med Bio Eng Comput, 2012, 50(4): 359-372.

[5] Marca GD, Mazza M, Losurdo A, et al. Sleepmodifications in acute transient global amnesia. J Clin Sleep Med, 2013, 9(9): 921-927.

[6] Li NZ, Wang J, Wang DL, et al. Correlation of sleep microstructure with daytime sleepiness and cognitive function in young and middle-aged adults with obstructive sleep apnea syndrome. Eur Arch Otorhinolaryngol, 2019, 276(12): 3525-3532.

[7] Bruni O, Kohler M, Novelli L, et al. Therole of NREM sleep instability in child cognitive performance. Sleep, 2012, 35(5): 649-656.

[8] Terzano M G, Parrino L, Smerieri A. Atlas, rules, and recording techniques for the scoring of cyclic alternating pattern (CAP) in human sleep. Sleep Med, 2001, 3(2): 187-199.

[9] Parrino L, Ferri R, Bruni O, et al. Cyclic alternating pattern (CAP): The marker of sleep instability. Sleep Med Rev, 2011, 16(1): 27-45.

[10] Knyazev GG. EEG delta oscillations as a correlate of basic homeostatic and motivational processes. Neurosci Biobehav Rev, 2012, 36(1): 677-695.

[11] Neckelmann D, Ursin R. Sleep stages and EEG power spectrum in relation to acoustical stimulus arousal threshold in the rat. Sleep, 1993, 16(5): 467-477.

[12] Nishida M, Pearsall J, Buckner RL, et al. REM sleep, prefrontal theta, and the consolidation of human emotional memory. Cereb Cortex, 2009, 19(5): 1158-1166.

[13] Kraus J, Roman R, Lacinova L, et al. Imagery induced negative affect, social touch and frontal EEG power band activity. Scand J Psychol, 2020, 22.

[14] Hanslmayr S, Volberg G, Wimber M, et al. Prestimulus oscillatory phase at 7 Hz gates cortical information flow and visual perception. Curr Biol, 2013. 23(22):2273-2278.

[15] Weisz N, Hartmann T, et al. Alpha rhythms in audition: Cognitive and clinical perspectives. frontiers in psychology, 2011, 2(73):1-15.

[16] Susmakova K, Krakovska A. Classification of waking, sleep onset and deep sleep by single measures. Meas Sci Rev, 2007, 7:34-38.

[17] Simon P, Michael W, Stephen E, et al. Quantitative EEG indices of sub-acute ischaemic stroke correlate with clinical outcomes. Clin Neurophysiol, 2007, 118(11):2525-2532.

[18] Sheila Sivam1, Joseph Poon, Keith K et al. Slow-frequency electroencephalography activity during wake and sleep in obesity hypoventilation syndrome. Sleep, 2020, 43(2):zsz214.

[19] Musaeus, CS, NielsenMS, Hogh P. Altered low-frequency EEG connectivity in mild cognitive impairment as a sign of clinical progression. J Alzheimers Disease, 2019, 68(3):947-960.

[20] Song, X, Bhaswati Roy, Daniel W, et al. Altered resting-state hippocampal and caudate functional networks in patients with obstructive sleep apnea. Brain and Behavior, 2018, 8(6):e00994.

[21] Kendzerska T, Gershon AS, Hawker G, et al. Obstructive sleep apnea and risk of cardiovascular events and all-cause mortality: a decade long historical cohort study. PLoS Med, 2014, 11(2):e1001599.

[22] Gottlieb J, Schwartz A, Marshall J, et al. Hypoxia, not the frequency of sleep apnea, induces acute hemodynamic stress in patients with chronic heart failure. J Am Coll Cardiol, 2009, 54(18):1706-1712.

[23] Oldenburg O, Wellmann B, Buchholz A, et al. Nocturnal hypoxaemia is associated with increased mortality in stable heart failure patients. Eur Heart J, 2016, 37(21):1695-1703.

[24] Azarbarzin A, Sands SA, Stone KL, et al. The hypoxic burden of sleep apnoea predicts cardiovascular disease-related mortality: theosteoporotic fractures in men study and the sleep heart health study. Eur Heart J, 2019, 40(14):1149-1157.

[25] Azarbarzin A, Sands SA, Taranto ML, et al. The sleep apnea-specific hypoxic burden predicts incident heart failure. Chest, 2020, 158(2):739-750.

[26] Pennestri M H, Montplaisir J, Fradette L, et al. Blood pressure changes associated with periodic leg movements during sleep in healthy subjects. Sleep Med, 2013, 14(6):555-561.

[27] Yang CK, Jordan AS, White DP, et al. Heart rate response to respiratory events with or without leg movements. Sleep, 2006, 29(4):553-556.

[28] Eckert DJ, Younes MK. Arousal from sleep: implications for obstructive sleep apnea pathogenesis and treatment. J Appl Physiolgy(1985), 2014, 116(3):302-313.

[29] Edwards BA, Eckert DJ, McSharry DG, et al. Clinical predictors of the respiratory arousal threshold in patients with obstructive sleep apnea. Am J Respir Crit Care Med, 2014, 190(11):1293-1300.

8 阻塞性睡眠呼吸暂停低通气综合征与肿瘤免疫

刘远灵　高兴林

阻塞性睡眠呼吸暂停低通气综合征（OSAHS）是一种具有潜在危险性的常见及多发病，流行病学调查表明，患有 OSAHS 的患者较普通人而言有更高的癌症风险和癌症相关死亡率。因此，探讨 OSAHS 促发肿瘤发生和进展的机制，对于判断肿瘤合并 OSAHS 患者的预后及指导综合治疗的实施具有重要的意义。

一、肿瘤免疫

肿瘤的特征包括持续增殖，逃避生长抑制因子，抵抗细胞死亡，无限复制，诱导血管生成，侵袭和转移，能量代谢重编程和免疫逃逸。肿瘤免疫学研究的是免疫系统和肿瘤细胞之间的相互作用，其目标是寻找肿瘤免疫诊断的生物标志物和开发新的肿瘤免疫治疗方法。20 世纪初，一名德国医生首次提出了肿瘤免疫的概念。1957 年，第一个以开发肿瘤免疫疗法为目的的纽约癌症研究所成立。如今肿瘤免疫疗法取得了令人鼓舞的成果，尤其是免疫检查点抑制剂的应用大大补充了传统的抗肿瘤治疗方法。

肿瘤细胞与免疫系统之间的相互作用主要包括免疫识别、免疫监视和免疫逃逸三个方面。免疫系统对癌细胞的识别有两种方式：通过对肿瘤特异性抗原（癌细胞特有的分子）或对肿瘤相关抗原（癌细胞与正常细胞表达不同的分子）的辨认。致癌物引起的肿瘤，所产生的肿瘤免疫应答针对的是正常细胞特异基因突变的产物，这些突变蛋白是肿瘤特异性抗原。由病毒引起的肿瘤，病毒抗原作为肿瘤抗原，如人乳头瘤病毒（宫颈癌的病原体）、EB 病毒（鼻咽癌的病原体）等。人体免疫系统通过一系列复杂的过程，对外来细胞，特别是具有高度免疫原性的癌细胞产生内源性免疫反应。免疫系统对肿瘤抗原的识别过程可以描述为：机体免疫系统通过抗原呈递细胞（APC）将肿瘤抗原呈递到 T 细胞，启动和激活淋巴结中的 T 细胞，T 细胞转移和浸润到肿瘤床成为肿瘤浸润淋巴细胞并对癌细胞进行识别，形成抗原特异性效应 T 细胞和记忆 T 细胞，同时启动体液免疫，使效应 T 细胞和其他内源性免疫细胞与肿瘤抗体产生协同作用，以消除肿瘤细胞。主要组织相容性复合体-Ⅰ（MHC-Ⅰ）与 APC 如树突状细胞向分化的 $CD8^+$ T 细胞呈递抗原，产生针对外来抗原的细胞毒性免疫反应，如果这种免疫反应不能提供足够的抗肿瘤免疫，则产生肿瘤免疫逃逸。

免疫监视假说是指机体的免疫系统可以发挥监视作用，识别并消灭任何表达新抗原的"异己"成分或突变细胞，以保持机体内环境的稳定。免疫系统遇到新生肿瘤将启动免疫编辑过程，这一过程可能会带来三种结果：肿瘤消除、肿瘤平衡、肿瘤逃逸。小鼠肿瘤模型可以证实肿瘤免疫编辑的存在，敲除了Ⅰ型干扰素基因的小鼠模型免疫系统肿瘤发生率明显降低。人体免疫监视的证据很难获得，要确定免疫功能是否与癌症发病率相关，需要大量的受试者长期随访，一项研究纳入了 1989－2004 年 905 名接受心脏移植、肺移植或两者皆有的患者，以了解用于防止移植排斥反应的免疫抑制对癌症发病率的影响，在这些患者中，有 102 例新诊断癌症，是普通人群的 7.1 倍，主要类型是白血病和淋巴瘤（一般人群的 26.2 倍）、头颈癌（一般人群的 21 倍）和肺癌（一般人群的 9.3 倍）。

无论免疫原性强弱与否，肿瘤都能产生多种逃避机体免疫系统的策略。这种免疫抑制既可以发生在全身系统中，也可以发生在肿瘤微环境中。下面简要介绍起重要作用的几种免疫细胞和免疫分子。

细胞毒性 T 淋巴细胞相关蛋白 4（CTLA-4）是 T 细胞活化的负调控因子。机体接受抗原刺激后，T 淋巴细胞识别抗原，从而发生活化、增殖、分化，产生效应 T 细胞清除抗原。T 细胞的活化需要第一、第二信号同时存在。T 细胞表面 TCR 识别 APC 提呈的抗原肽-MHC 复合物为活化第一信号，T 细胞表面协同刺激分子 CD28 或者 CTLA-4 与抗原呈递细胞表面的 B7 分子配对结合形成第二信号。共抑制信号分子 CTLA-4 与 CD28 竞争结合 APC 上的 B7 分子，作用于 T 细胞活化的早期，可能是直接通过抑制细胞周期来抑制 T 细胞激活。

抑制性分子程序死亡受体-1（programmed cell death-1，PD-1，也称 CD279）和 CTLA-4 受体有相似的结构，是最热门的肿瘤免疫检查点分子，都可在 T 细胞上表达，但是它们结合的配体不同，PD-1 主要作用于 T 细胞活化晚期，也表达于 B 细胞、NK 细胞和骨髓细胞上。PD-1 的配体是 PD-L1（CD274，也称 B7-H1）和 PD-L2（CD273，也称 B7-DC），在抗原呈递细胞和多种肿瘤细胞均有表达。健康人体中，PD-1（PD-L1）通路主要是防止自身免疫疾病的发生，在肿瘤患者中，该通路促进肿瘤免疫逃逸，降低机体抗肿瘤免疫反应。研究表明肿瘤中 PD-1（PD-L1）通路可诱导 $CD4^+$ T 细胞转化为调节性 T 细胞，间接增强免疫抑制作用。

调节 T 细胞（regulatory T cell，Treg）是具有抑制功能

的 CD4⁺T 细胞亚群,在维持机体免疫耐受及防止自身免疫疾病发生方面有着不可忽视的作用。Treg 来源于天然 CD4 细胞亚群,除表达 CD4、CD25 外,还表达叉头状螺旋转录因子(forkhead helix transcription factor,Foxp3)、CTLA-4、CD127 等。Treg 对肿瘤的影响是复杂的,多种肿瘤患者体内 Treg 表达上调并且被募集到肿瘤组织中。Treg 广泛地抑制多种免疫细胞的增殖,如单核巨噬细胞、树突状细胞、B 细胞、CD4⁺T 细胞、CD8⁺T 细胞等。人体和动物模型研究均表明,肿瘤微环境中 Treg 数量增多是预后不良的象征,Treg 抑制肿瘤免疫,从而阻碍控制癌细胞生长的自身免疫力,针对调节 T 细胞免疫治疗对癌症的治疗可能有帮助。

骨髓来源的抑制细胞(MDSC)是骨髓来源的细胞,在各种病理条件下扩增,如癌症和炎症,它们可以使活性氧和氮的产量增加。单核细胞在骨髓中发育并在进入组织之前转化为巨噬细胞,可以分化为促炎、杀菌(M1)或抗炎(M2)亚型。肿瘤细胞来源的 IL-10 还可诱导单核细胞向 M2 型巨噬细胞极化,从而促进肿瘤相关性巨噬细胞(TAM)的形成,发挥免疫抑制作用。中性粒细胞是循环中最丰富的吞噬细胞,它们是第一批被招募到炎症部位的细胞。然而,中性粒细胞可通过巨噬细胞 1 抗原(MAC1)抑制 T 细胞反应,限制了炎症过程中对宿主组织的损害。因此,增强抗肿瘤免疫反应的总体策略是通过抑制或耗尽特定细胞或细胞类型来中断免疫抑制回路。

新出现的研究表明外泌体可以通过多种机制与肿瘤微环境中的靶细胞相互作用。外泌体存在于各种体液包括外周血中,是由多种类型活细胞分泌到胞外的囊泡小体,含有大量蛋白质、脂质、mRNA、miRNA,具有免疫调节、抗原呈递、细胞间 RNA 和蛋白的交换及信息交流等功能,参与肿瘤发生发展、转移。来自免疫细胞和肿瘤细胞的外泌体具有调节肿瘤免疫的作用。间充质干细胞(MSC)和癌症相关成纤维细胞(CAF)可释放大量的外泌体,破坏间充质肿瘤基质,进入肿瘤实质,并通过特异性相互作用攻击肿瘤细胞。树突状细胞源性外泌体和调节性 T(Treg)细胞源性外泌体分别促进和抑制细胞毒性 T 淋巴细胞(CTL)的产生。

二、OSAHS 与肿瘤

越来越多的证据显示 OSAHS 和肿瘤发生之间密切相关,其中免疫系统被证实参与 OSAHS 促进肿瘤发生的过程。

2012 年,美国 Wisconsin 大型睡眠队列研究对 1522 例患者进行长达 22 年的随访研究,结果显示所有参与者的癌症死亡率为 1.9‰,其中患重度 OSAHS 的肿瘤患者的死亡率是未罹患 OSAHS 对照组患者的 4.8 倍($P<0.01$)。另一项来自西班牙多中心队列研究纳入了 4910 例既往没有肿瘤或呼吸衰竭病史的患者,平均随访时间 4.5 年,该研究以夜间 $SpO_2<90\%$ 占睡眠时间百分比(Tsat90)作为分组标准,研究结果显示随着 Tsat90 增加,肿瘤发生的风险也随之增加;研究还发现与 OSAHS 相关的几种高发的肿瘤类型,包括大肠癌、前列腺癌、肺癌和乳腺癌。在澳大利亚 Brusselton 睡眠队列研究中,中度至重度 OSAHS 患者与未罹患 OSAHS 患者相比,死亡率、肿瘤和脑卒中的风险均升高。但是,另一项来自加拿大队列研究对 10 149 例患者进行平均长达 7.8 年的随访,发现 OSAHS 的严重程度和肿瘤发生率之间并没有独立关联性,该研究是单一中心但样本量大,而西班牙的研究是多中心且入组患者年龄偏小、体重较轻、OSAHS 严重程度偏低。一项荟萃分析结合了已有的研究,发现 OSAHS 与肿瘤发病率和死亡率之间存在相关性。总体而言,目前的研究认为 OSAHS 患者尤其是重度 OSAHS 会增加罹患肿瘤的风险。

近年来,越来越多研究分析了 OSAHS 对肿瘤行为的影响,间歇性低氧(IH)和睡眠片段(SF)是 OSAHS 两个重要的特征。近年来许多体外及动物实验发现 IH 对肺癌的发生和进展起到重要的作用。Almendros 等对 OSAHS 与肿瘤发病机制进行了一系列动物实验研究,发现 IH 能促进黑色素瘤发生和进展,其研究还发现肺泡上皮 TC-1 肿瘤细胞在 IH 条件下生长、增殖速度更快,肿瘤大小和重量达到正常氧浓度条件下培养的 2 倍。Liu 等研究了 IH 条件下缺氧相关的关键基因的表达,经过 IH 条件处理后的两组肺癌细胞(A549 和 H446)增殖能力更强,对放疗的抵抗力更强,且长期处于 IH 暴露下会导致若干个缺氧诱导的基因及其他参与细胞凋亡过程的基因下调。本课题组研究发现 IH 可通过 HIF-1α 介导的途径调控下游基因的表达进而促进肺腺癌细胞的活力,并可通过 RNA 干扰技术沉默 HIF-1α 基因抑制肿瘤细胞生长及转移。SF 是 OSAHS 另一个重要的特征,反复的唤醒干扰了深度睡眠、增加非快速眼动期和快速眼动期的睡眠呼吸暂停总时长进而导致了低质量睡眠,睡眠质量下降可延长睡眠总时间、日间嗜睡,其结局即慢性睡眠剥夺。为进一步证明 SF 影响肿瘤发生,国外学者通过构建动物实验模型证实没有任何缺氧特征的 SF 促进肿瘤的发生。目前,针对 SF 致肿瘤发生的可能免疫机制包括:①通过依赖 TLR-4 信号通路及改变活性氧(ROS)信号募集巨噬细胞、调节性 T 细胞及脂肪干细胞;影响 TAMs 极化和 TLR-4 信号通路进而导致肿瘤的生长速度及侵袭力增加。②睡眠中激素水平的变化可调节多种免疫细胞的功能如巨噬细胞极化等。③SF 可能通过影响 Nox2(NADPH Oxidase2)的活性促进肿瘤的发生。

三、OSAHS 促进肿瘤发生的免疫机制

OSAHS 可影响巨噬细胞表型。巨噬细胞是机体免疫反应中的一种重要细胞,也是肿瘤微环境中最丰富的免疫细胞,参与肿瘤发生发展的若干阶段。肿瘤相关巨噬细胞(tumor associated macrophages,TAMs)主要存在两种表型,M1 表型(产生促进炎症的细胞因子,如肿瘤坏死因子和干扰素-γ,发挥抗肿瘤作用)和 M2 表型(产生抑制炎症的因子,如 IL-10,加速组织修复及促肿瘤发展)。2014 年 Hakim 和 Gozal 首次通过构建动物实验模型证实 SF 通过

TLR-4信号肽、诱导TAMs向M2型巨噬细胞极化促进肿瘤的发生。Almendros等将移植了TC1肺癌细胞的C57(B6)小鼠分别置于常氧及间歇性低氧条件下，发现IH诱导肿瘤周围巨噬细胞的呈M2型改变，且TAM在肿瘤浸润增加约2.2倍，这可能加速IH相关的肿瘤进展。国内学者研究表明间歇性低氧可显著促进Lewis肺癌(LLC)的转移，并伴有原发性肿瘤组织中更多CD209+巨噬细胞浸润，低氧和IL-6协同通过将巨噬细胞从M1向促进肿瘤的M2表型转化，增强体外和体内LLC的转移。此外，该研究还证明，缺氧导致巨噬细胞M2极化主要依赖于ERK信号的激活。

OSAHS影响PD-1(PD-L1)的表达。近年来，免疫治疗是肿瘤治疗的一大热点。PD-1及PD-L1通过相互作用产生免疫耐受防止过度激活免疫系统导致组织损伤及自身免疫疾病。据统计，20%～30%的非小细胞肺癌表达PD-L1，PD-L1阳性的非小细胞肺癌意味着更少的淋巴细胞浸润和更短的无疾病生存期。IH可增强PD-1(PD-L1)相互作用使CD8+细胞毒性T细胞的活化和细胞毒性下降，细胞毒性T细胞可通过释放穿孔素和颗粒酶B直接杀伤肿瘤细胞，颗粒酶B可以抑制肿瘤的生长和扩散。Cubillos-Zapata等研究测定了360例新诊断皮肤黑色素瘤患者血浆可溶性PD-L1的水平后发现，相比于未罹患OSAHS或轻度OSAHS，重度OSA患者血浆可溶性PD-L1水平明显升高，这将作为评估皮肤黑色素瘤侵袭性的一个潜在指标；其另一项研究发现PD-L1在OSAHS患者外周血单核细胞上过表达，PD-1在CD8+T细胞上过表达。在体外间歇性缺氧模型和小鼠模型中或者转染低氧诱导因子-1的情况下，PD-L1和PD-1均被诱导过表达。西班牙的研究团队发现年轻的OSAHS患者PD-L1上调，主要是由于HIF-1α激活。本研究组检测了单纯非小细胞肺癌患者及OSAHS合并非小细胞肺癌患者外周血CD4+T细胞PD-1的表达，发现各组间并无显著差异，OSAHS可能主要影响CD8+T淋巴细胞的功能而影响肿瘤发生发展。在OSAHS间歇性缺氧的条件下，PD-1/PD-L1和HIF表达上调，从而抑制了T细胞的增殖和功能，尤其是CD8+T淋巴细胞；同时增强了骨髓源性抑制细胞(myeloid-derived suppressor sells，MDSCs)的增殖。MDSCs是存在于血液及肿瘤中、由多个分化阶段的髓样细胞组成的异质性群体，通过上调精氨酸酶1(arginase1)、诱导型一氧化氮合酶(iNOS)、ROS和抗炎细胞因子(如IL-10和TGF-b)抑制各类免疫反应。在肿瘤中，缺氧促使MDSCs分化成TAMs，TAMs中的M2型巨噬细胞则发挥免疫抑制及促进肿瘤的生长及转移的作用。

OSAHS影响细胞因子释放：OSAHS患者夜间反复周期性低氧会刺激ROS产生、机体氧化(抗氧化)失衡、上调转录因子NF-κB、AP-1、STAT-3、HIF-1，增加全身炎性因子如TNF-α、IL-1β、IL-6、IL-8及循环中黏附因子如细胞间黏附分子-1(ICAM-1)和血管细胞黏附分子-1(VCAM-1)。炎性因子的增加导致TAMs极化、促进树突细胞转化为肿瘤相关性树突细胞及激活MDSCs的促肿瘤作用。Said等对OSAHS患者血中的细胞因子、CD4+T淋巴细胞等进行测定发现IL-1β、IL-6及CD4+T细胞水平升高，而IFN-γ水平下降，且OSAHS患者的整体免疫反应更倾向表达Th2细胞和调节性T细胞亚群。Th2细胞占主导可能与睡眠障碍或OSAHS患者的儿茶酚胺分泌增加有关，这些介质可以抑制Th1细胞因子的产生。研究证明，恢复足够的氧合可以逆转OSAHS间歇性缺氧环境下的免疫反应障碍。这些数据都与之前的研究相一致，即肿瘤微环境中缺氧恢复后可逆转免疫抑制状态，减少细胞因子如TGF-β，而这些效应可能依赖于调节性T细胞和NK细胞的作用。

OSAHS影响Treg细胞功能。Treg可分泌抑制性细胞因子TGF-β、IL-10，其胞膜上组成性的表达共抑制分子CTLA-4，通过接触抑制的方式与抗原呈递细胞、T细胞表面受体结合，抑制CD4+T细胞作用，参与肿瘤免疫逃逸。多个表明OSAHS患者体内存在Th17/Treg平衡失调。研究发现患有OSAHS或者腺样体肥大的儿童，外周血Th17/Treg比值升高。国内学者发现OSAHS患者外周血Treg细胞数和Foxp3 mRNA水平显著降低了，而OSAHS患者与正常对照组相比，Th17细胞比例明显增高，OSAHS的发展可能与外周血Th17/Treg失衡有关，其特征是促炎细胞因子微环境。在OSAHS患者中，存在致炎因子和抗炎因子的失衡，主要表现为致炎因子表达上调，抗炎因子(如调节T细胞、IL-10、TGF-β)受到抑制，但OSAHS合并肿瘤的患者，Treg的免疫抑制功能却是增强的。本研究组对OSAHS患者，单纯非小细胞肺癌患者，OSAHS合并非小细胞肺癌患者的Treg细胞功能和VEGF水平进行检测，并进行了2年的短期生存率统计，发现OSAHS可能会上调非小细胞肺癌患者TGF-β、VEGF和Foxp3+Tregs表达，Treg数量与ODI呈正相关，而且VEGF水平的升高与非小细胞肺癌合并OSAHS患者短期生存率的降低密切相关。已有研究证明VEGF上调Treg表达，趋化Treg至肿瘤微环境中。因此，OSAHS可能通过调节Treg功能参与肿瘤进展。

间歇缺氧促进外泌体释放，增加肿瘤恶性程度。已有研究表明，缺氧增加了几种类型的肿瘤包括乳腺癌、多发性骨髓瘤、前列腺癌和神经胶质瘤肿瘤细胞中外泌体的分泌。IH促进循环中肿瘤来源外泌体的增加并有选择性地修饰外泌体的内容，使其具备免疫抑制作用。Almendros的研究揭示了间歇性低氧暴露组小鼠来源的循环外泌体可选择性地增强肺癌细胞的增殖、侵袭和迁移能力，同样未治疗的OSAHS患者血清中的外泌体也具有同样的生物学作用。肿瘤来源外泌体通过抑制细胞毒性T细胞、影响抗原呈递、妨碍NK细胞功能和促进免疫抑制性B细胞群的扩增实现肿瘤的免疫逃逸；还可以通过释放血管生长因子如VEGF刺激血管新生及影响细胞间的黏附、细胞外基质重塑，为肿瘤生长及扩散提供了良好的条件。Capello等近期的一项研究表明，外泌体可呈递大量肿瘤相关抗原(tumor-associated antigens，TAAs)，并通过诱导自身抗体发挥对补体介导的细胞毒性的诱饵功能。外泌体作为肿瘤微环境中不同类型细胞交流的重要媒介，是促进肿瘤发生的重要一环，值得更加深入的研究。

总之,目前的流行病学及基于动物实验模型的相关研究表明OSAHS可增加肿瘤发生的风险,免疫细胞、细胞因子、外泌体、PD-1(PD-L1)等介导的免疫反应可能参与了OSAHS致肿瘤发生的过程并扮演重要角色。但目前对于具体的免疫机制、信号通路的认识仍不够深入,仍需要更多的基础和临床研究探索OSAHS、机体免疫、肿瘤三者之间的关系,从而对OSAHS合并肿瘤的患者提供更有效的干预及治疗。

参 考 文 献

[1] Hanahan D, Weinberg RA. Hallmarks of cancer: the next generation. Cell, 2011, 144(5):646-674.

[2] Galluzzi L, Rudqvist NP. Preface: More than two decades of modern tumor immunology. Methods Enzymol, 2019, 629: xxi-xi.

[3] Sukari A, Nagasaka M, Al-Hadidi A, et al. Cancer Immunology and Immunotherapy. Anticancer Res, 2016, 36(11): 5593-5606.

[4] Dunn GP, Old LJ, Schreiber RD. The three Es of cancer immunoediting. Annu Rev Immunol, 2004, 22:329-360.

[5] Roithmaier S, Haydon AM, Loi S, et al. Incidence of malignancies in heart and/or lung transplant recipients: a single-institution experience. J Heart Lung Transplant, 2007, 26(8): 845-849.

[6] Brunner MC, Chambers CA, Chan FK, et al. CTLA-4-Mediated inhibition of early events of T cell proliferation. J Immunol, 1999, 162(10):5813-5820.

[7] Bettelli E, Carrier Y, Gao W, et al. Reciprocal developmental pathways for the generation of pathogenic effector TH17 and regulatory T cells. Nature, 2006, 441(7090):235-238.

[8] Khalyfa A, Almendros I, Gileles-Hillel A, et al. Circulating exosomes potentiate tumor malignant properties in a mouse model of chronic sleep fragmentation. Oncotarget, 2016, 7(34):54676-54690.

[9] Almendros I, Khalyfa A, Trzepizur W, et al. Tumor Cell Malignant Properties Are Enhanced by Circulating Exosomes in Sleep Apnea. Chest, 2016, 150(5):1030-1041.

[10] Seo N, Akiyoshi K, Shiku H. Exosome-mediated regulation of tumor immunology. Cancer Sci, 2018, 109(10):2998-3004.

[11] Gaoatswe G, Kent BD, Corrigan MA, et al. Invariant Natural Killer T Cell Deficiency and Functional Impairment in Sleep Apnea: Links to Cancer Comorbidity. Sleep, 2015, 38(10): 1629-1634.

[12] Almendros I, Wang Y, Becker L, et al. Intermittent hypoxia-induced changes in tumor-associated macrophages and tumor malignancy in a mouse model of sleep apnea. Am J Respir Crit Care Med, 2014, 189(5):593-601.

[13] Nieto FJ, Peppard PE, Young T, et al. Sleep-disordered breathing and cancer mortality: results from the Wisconsin Sleep Cohort Study. Am J Respir Crit Care Med, 2012, 186(2):190-194.

[14] Campos-Rodriguez F, Martinez-Garcia MA, Martinez M, et al. Association between obstructive sleep apnea and cancer incidence in a large multicenter Spanish cohort. Am J Respir Crit Care Med, 2013, 187(1):99-105.

[15] Marshall NS, Wong KK, Cullen SR, et al. Sleep apnea and 20-year follow-up for all-cause mortality, stroke, and cancer incidence and mortality in the Busselton Health Study cohort. J Clin Sleep Med, 2014, 10(4):355-362.

[16] Kendzerska T, Leung RS, Hawker G, et al. Obstructive sleep apnea and the prevalence and incidence of cancer. CMAJ, 2014, 186(13):985-992.

[17] Palamaner Subash Shantha G, Kumar AA, Cheskin LJ, et al. Association between sleep-disordered breathing, obstructive sleep apnea, and cancer incidence: a systematic review and meta-analysis. Sleep Med, 2015, 16(10):1289-1294.

[18] Almendros I, Montserrat JM, Ramirez J, et al R. Intermittent hypoxia enhances cancer progression in a mouse model of sleep apnoea. Eur Respi J, 2012, 39(1):215-217.

[19] Almendros I, Gozal D. Intermittent hypoxia and cancer: Undesirable bed partners? Respir Physiol Neurobiol, 2018, 256: 79-86.

[20] 杨士芳,李晓明,安弘,等. HIF-1α介导了间歇低氧对人肺腺癌A549细胞体外生物学行为的影响. 中国病理生理杂志, 2016, 32(11):1958-1965.

[21] Bonnet MH, Arand DL. Clinical effects of sleep fragmentation versus sleep deprivation. Sleep Med Rev, 2003, 7(4): 297-310.

[22] Kimoff RJ. Sleep fragmentation in obstructive sleep apnea. Sleep. 1996;19(9 Suppl):S61-S66.

[23] Hakim F, Wang Y, Zhang SX, et al. Fragmented sleep accelerates tumor growth and progression through recruitment of tumor-associated macrophages and TLR4 signaling. Cancer Res, 2014, 74(5):1329-1337.

[24] Zheng J, Almendros I, Wang Y, et al. Reduced NADPH oxidase type 2 activity mediates sleep fragmentation-induced effects on TC1 tumors in mice. Oncoimmunology, 2015, 4(2):e976057.

[25] Grivennikov SI, Greten FR, Karin M. Immunity, inflammation, and cancer. Cell, 2010, 140(6):883-899.

[26] Almendros I, Gileles-Hillel A, Khalyfa A, et al. Adipose tissue macrophage polarization by intermittent hypoxia in a mouse model of OSA: effect of tumor microenvironment. Cancer Lett, 2015, 361(2):233-239.

[27] Zhang J, Cao J, Ma S, Dong R, et al. Tumor hypoxia enhances Non-Small Cell Lung Cancer metastasis by selectively promoting macrophage M2 polarization through the activation of ERK signaling. Oncotarget, 2014, 5(20):9664-9677.

[28] Cubillos-Zapata C, Martinez-Garcia MA, Campos-Rodriguez F, et al. Soluble PD-L1 is a potential biomarker of cutaneous melanoma aggressiveness and metastasis in obstructive sleep apnea patients. Eur Respir J, 2019, 53(2):1801298.

[29] Cubillos-Zapata C, Avendaño-Ortiz J, Hernandez-Jimenez E, et al. Hypoxia-induced PD-L1/PD-1 crosstalk impairs T-cell function in sleep apnoea. Eur Respir J, 2017, 50(4):1700833.

[30] Cubillos-Zapata C, Balbás-García C, Avendaño-Ortiz J, et al.

Age-dependent hypoxia-induced PD-L1 upregulation in patients with obstructive sleep apnoea. Respirology, 2019, 24 (7):684-692.

[31] 刘远灵,罗少华,欧琼,等.阻塞性睡眠呼吸暂停低通气综合征患者外周血 CD4+T 细胞 PD-1、CTLA-4 表达及 VEGF 的变化研究.中华结核和呼吸杂志,2019,42(4):268-274.

[32] Liu Y, Lao M, Chen J, et al. Short-term prognostic effects of circulating regulatory T-Cell suppressive function and vascular endothelial growth factor level in patients with non-small cell lung cancer and obstructive sleep apnea. Sleep Med, 2020,70:88-96.

[33] Korneev KV, Atretkhany KN, Drutskaya MS, et al. TLR-signaling and proinflammatory cytokines as drivers of tumorigenesis. Cytokine, 2017, 89:127-135.

[34] Carpagnano GE, Spanevello A, Sabato R, et al. Systemic and airway inflammation in sleep apnea and obesity: the role of ICAM-1 and IL-8. Transl Res, 2010, 155(1):35-43.

[35] Schlesinger M, Bendas G. Vascular cell adhesion molecule-1 (VCAM-1)--an increasing insight into its role in tumorigenicity and metastasis. Int J Cancer, 2015, 136 (11): 2504-2514.

[36] Said EA, Al-Abri MA, Al-Saidi I, et al. Altered blood cytokines, CD4 T cells, NK and neutrophils in patients with obstructive sleep apnea. Immunology Lett, 2017, 190:272-278.

[37] Cubillos-Zapata C, Hernández-Jiménez E, Avendaño-Ortiz J, et al. Obstructive Sleep Apnea Monocytes Exhibit High Levels of Vascular Endothelial Growth Factor Secretion, Augmenting Tumor Progression. Mediators Inflamm, 2018.

[38] Hatfield SM, Kjaergaard J, Lukashev D, et al. Immunological mechanisms of the antitumor effects of supplemental oxygenation. Sci Transl Med, 2015, 7(277):277-230.

[39] Steinman L. Conflicting consequences of immunity to cancer versus autoimmunity to neurons: insights from paraneoplastic disease. Eur J Immunol, 2014, 44(11):3201-3205.

[40] Sade K, Fishman G, Kivity S, et al. Expression of Th17 and Treg lymphocyte subsets in hypertrophied adenoids of children and its clinical significance. Immunol Invest, 2011, 40 (6):657-666.

[41] Ye J, Liu H, Zhang G, et al. The treg/th17 imbalance in patients with obstructive sleep apnoea syndrome. Mediators Inflamm, 2012:815308.

[42] Goto H, Kudo E, Kariya R, et al. Targeting VEGF and interleukin-6 for controlling malignant effusion of primary effusion lymphoma. J Cancer Res Clin Oncol, 2015, 141 (3): 465-474.

[43] King HW, Michael MZ, Gleadle JM. Hypoxic enhancement of exosome release by breast cancer cells. BMC Cancer, 2012, 12:421.

[44] Kucharzewska P, Christianson HC, Welch JE, et al. Exosomes reflect the hypoxic status of glioma cells and mediate hypoxia-dependent activation of vascular cells during tumor development. Proc Natl Acad Sci U S A, 2013, 110 (18): 7312-7317.

[45] Ramteke A, Ting H, Agarwal C, et al. Exosomes secreted under hypoxia enhance invasiveness and stemness of prostate cancer cells by targeting adherens junction molecules. Mol Carcinog, 2015, 54(7):554-565.

[46] Umezu T, Tadokoro H, Azuma K, et al. Exosomal miR-135b shed from hypoxic multiple myeloma cells enhances angiogenesis by targeting factor-inhibiting HIF-1. Blood, 2014, 124 (25):3748-3757.

[47] Capello M, Vykoukal JV, Katayama H, et al. Exosomes harbor B cell targets in pancreatic adenocarcinoma and exert decoy function against complement-mediated cytotoxicity. Nat Commun, 2019, 10(1):254.

9 阻塞性睡眠呼吸暂停致靶器官损伤的免疫学机制

李庆云　李诗琪

阻塞性睡眠呼吸暂停（obstructive sleep apnea，OSA）对人群健康的影响越来越受到重视，最新报道显示全球30~69岁的成年人中近10亿人患有OSA，中至重度OSA人数预计接近4.25亿，其中我国人群患病率为8.8%。OSA是心脑血管疾病、2型糖尿病、认知功能障碍及肿瘤发生发展的危险因素。OSA所致靶器官损伤一直为关注重点，是多种慢性疾病的"源头疾病"，2017年世界睡眠日的中国主题"健康睡眠 远离慢病"即源于此。基于OSA特征性病理生理表现慢性间歇性低氧（chronic intermittent hypoxia，CIH）和睡眠片段化（sleep fragmentation，SF）探索靶器官损伤的机制至关重要。特别是近年来关于OSA对免疫系统的影响及相关靶器官损伤的免疫机制的研究逐渐深入，为相关治疗或药物研发提供了新的思路。

一、动脉粥样硬化和内皮细胞功能受损

OSA是心血管疾病的独立危险因素，多种免疫细胞参与CIH所致动脉粥样硬化和内皮细胞功能受损。巨噬细胞具有高度异质性和可塑性，其在不同组织微环境或病理条件下可极化为经典活化的M1型和替代性活化M2型，M1型参与Th1介导的免疫应答，起促炎和杀伤细胞内感染的病原体作用；M2型主要促进Th2相关免疫应答，参与免疫调节，抑制炎症及肿瘤发展等。巨噬细胞极化参与OSA动脉粥样硬化形成的机制包括，CIH促进巨噬细胞前体单核细胞向血管壁募集，诱导单核细胞晚期糖基化终产物受体表达增加，并激活NF-κB信号通路，细胞趋化及黏附能力增强。进一步，CIH下募集的巨噬细胞极化为M1型，吞噬低密度脂蛋白转变成泡沫细胞，促进粥样斑块形成。同时，SF使下丘脑食欲素分泌减少，使中性粒细胞前体细胞中巨噬细胞集落刺激因子表达增加，导致髓系造血异常并表现为Ly-6C^{high}单核细胞、中性粒细胞、巨噬细胞增多，促进动脉粥样硬化发生发展。此外，巨噬细胞胆固醇外流为胆固醇逆向转运的起始环节，OSA患者外周血单核细胞的三磷酸腺苷结合转运体A1表达下降，细胞胆固醇外流受损，加速粥样硬化进程。

T淋巴细胞根据表面标志物不同分为αβT细胞和γδT细胞，αβT细胞又可进一步分为CD4$^+$T细胞及CD8$^+$T细胞。OSA患者T淋巴细胞数目和表型发生显著改变。多数研究表明OSA患者CD4$^+$T细胞数目增加，可能与IL-1β高表达诱导CD4$^+$T细胞分化成熟及增殖相关。亦有研究发现成人和儿童OSA患者CD4$^+$T细胞数量、CD4$^+$/CD8$^+$比值下降，提示免疫功能受损。不过，OSA患者CD8$^+$T细胞数目改变尚无一致结论，可能与不同研究所纳入OSA患者的严重度、实验设计的低氧暴露时间及存在组织特异性有关。OSA患者CD4$^+$T和CD8$^+$T细胞表型和功能改变可直接或通过产生细胞因子导致血管内皮损伤，促进动脉粥样硬化进程。OSA患者共刺激受体OX40和4-1BB高表达的CD4$^+$CD28^{null}亚群增加2.9倍，产生高水平γ干扰素（interferon-γ，IFN-γ）、肿瘤坏死因子（tumor necrosis factor-α，TNF-α）及细胞毒颗粒穿孔素和颗粒酶，促进炎症反应，发挥细胞毒性T淋巴细胞样作用，在动脉粥样硬化斑块形成及发展中起重要作用，同时，T细胞分泌的IL-4及IL-8等亦参与其中。关于内皮细胞损伤的研究显示，OSA患者CD8$^+$T细胞共刺激分子受体CD40L表达增加4.2倍，穿孔素和CD56 NK受体表达显著增加，对内皮细胞具有细胞毒作用，且这一作用呈现OSA严重度依赖性。CPAP治疗则可降低TNF-α和CD40L表达，减轻T细胞杀伤作用，缓解内皮损伤。进一步动物实验研究证实，CIH导致外周血CD4$^+$T和CD8$^+$T细胞凋亡延迟，加重T细胞所致血管内皮损伤。此外，初始CD4$^+$T细胞受抗原及细胞因子调控，进一步分化为Th1、Th2、Th17及调节性T细胞（regulatory T-cells，Tregs），OSA患者存在Th1/Th2相关细胞因子失衡，导致全身炎症反应而参与OSA靶器官的损伤。γδT细胞的作用也受到关注，研究发现，γδT细胞是参与动脉粥样硬化早期病变的最主要T细胞；同时通过高表达L-选择素和TNF-α使γδT细胞对内皮细胞亲和力增高，细胞毒性增加2.5倍。

二、胰岛素抵抗与代谢紊乱

OSA与肥胖、胰岛素抵抗、2型糖尿病及非酒精性脂肪肝炎（NAFLD）等代谢紊乱相关，多种免疫细胞参与其中。研究证实脂肪组织慢性炎症是引起胰岛素抵抗的重要因素，脂肪组织病理变化特征为巨噬细胞浸润和其他免疫细胞，包括T淋巴细胞和肥大细胞，排列成坏死脂肪细胞周围的冠状结构。CIH可诱导巨噬细胞向脂肪组织聚集，并向M1型极化。进一步，M1型巨噬细胞分泌IL-6、TNF-α等炎症因子和NOS2表达，导致脂肪组织炎症并释放游离脂肪酸，胰岛素下游信号通路改变，导致胰岛素抵

抗和代谢紊乱。值得注意的是，CIH 模型恢复常氧后胰岛素抵抗和代谢紊乱不完全可逆，可能与巨噬细胞发生 DNA 甲基化（如 PPARγ）及组蛋白修饰（H3K9ac、H3K27me3）等表观遗传学改变相关。此外，非编码 RNA 参与 CIH 对巨噬细胞的调控，导致 miR-365 的表达水平显著降低，调节 IL-6 的表达，促进非酒精性脂肪肝炎发生发展。

三、恶性肿瘤发生发展

越来越多证据表明 OSA 同肿瘤发生发展密切相关。多项研究报道了 OSA 与特定肿瘤发生风险的关系，包括乳腺癌（$HR\ 2.09, 95\%CI\ 1.06\sim4.02$），中枢神经系统肿瘤（$HR\ 1.71, P=0.027$），鼻咽癌（$HR\ 5.96, 95\%CI\ 2.96\sim11.99$），以及前列腺癌（$HR\ 3.69, 95\%CI\ 1.98\sim6.89$）等。Wisconsin 睡眠队列研究发现轻、中、重度 OSA 患者癌症死亡率分别为未罹患 OSA 组的 1.1、2.0、4.8 倍。因此，探讨 OSA 促进肿瘤发生发展的机制成为近年来研究热点之一，免疫学机制研究也取得了进展。

多个研究关注了肿瘤相关巨噬细胞（tumor-associated macrophages，TAMs）。TAMs 的 M2 型极化促进肿瘤的发生发展，与诸多调节因子相关，如 NF-κB、STAT3、STAT6、Notch、PPAR-γ，以及 c-Myc 等。针对 OSA 致肿瘤发生发展的研究发现，CIH 可致 TAMs 的极性变化，诱导 TAMs 向 M2 型极化。同时 SF 亦可通过 TLR4 信号通路诱导 TAMs 向 M2 型极化，使肿瘤生长加速及侵袭力增加。

OSA 患者 T 细胞改变亦影响肿瘤发生发展，CIH 和 SF 均可诱导细胞毒性 T 细胞数量显著下降，且颗粒酶 B、穿孔素和 IFN-γ 在 CD8$^+$ 肿瘤浸润淋巴细胞中的表达下调，CD8$^+$ T 细胞抗肿瘤的细胞毒效应减弱，而表达 Oct4$^+$ 和 CD44$^+$CD133$^+$ 的肿瘤干细胞增加，进而促进肿瘤生长和侵袭转移。Tregs 细胞通过抑制效应性 T 细胞及抗原呈递细胞等发挥免疫抑制作用，是肿瘤免疫逃逸关键机制之一。研究证实低氧可诱导 Foxp3 高表达，促进 CD4$^+$ T 细胞向 Foxp3$^+$ Tregs 分化。非小细胞肺癌合并 OSA 患者 Foxp3$^+$ Tregs 比率显著高于不合并 OSA 的非小细胞肺癌患者，且 VEGF 及 TGFβ1 高表达，提示 OSA 促进 Tregs 成熟而产生免疫抑制，参与肿瘤发生发展。此外，OSA 患者穿孔素阳性 CD3$^+$ γδT 细胞及恒定型自然杀伤 T 细胞（natural killer T-cells，NKT）减少导致抗肿瘤活性下降，导致肿瘤生长及侵袭性增加。PD-1 是 T 细胞介导免疫反应中重要的抑制性免疫检查点。OSA 患者 CD8$^+$ T 细胞表面 PD-1 表达上调，同 PD-L1 结合诱导淋巴细胞的凋亡，抵抗淋巴细胞的杀伤作用，最终造成肿瘤免疫逃逸。进一步研究提示 OSA 相关的 PD-1 和 PD-L1 表达上调由 CIH 介导而非 SF 介导。

自然杀伤细胞（natural killer cells，NK）是固有免疫的主要组分，NK 细胞无须主要组织相容性复合体的抗原呈递，直接杀伤病毒感染的靶细胞和肿瘤细胞，在肿瘤免疫亦起重要作用。OSA 患者外周血 NK 细胞数量显著下降，因此抗肿瘤免疫功能下降。此外，OSA 影响免疫细胞表型，使单核细胞向免疫抑制表型极化。研究显示，与健康对照和 CPAP 治疗组比较，OSA 患者的单核细胞表面高表达糖蛋白 A 主导的重复序列，分泌 TGF-β 调控 NK 细胞向不成熟表型转变，对肿瘤细胞的细胞毒性减弱，导致肿瘤免疫逃逸。

参 考 文 献

[1] Benjafield AV, Ayas NT, Eastwood PR, et al. Estimation of the global prevalence and burden of obstructive sleep apnea: A literature-based analysis. Lancet Respir Med, 2019, 7(8): 687-698.

[2] Veasey SC, Rosen IM. Obstructive sleep apnea in adults. N Engl J Med, 2019, 380(15): 1442-1449.

[3] Zhou J, Bai W, Liu Q, et al. Intermittent hypoxia enhances THP-1 monocyte adhesion and chemotaxis and promotes M1 macrophage polarization via RAGE. Biomed Res Int, 2018, 2018: 1650456.

[4] Gileles-Hillel A, Almendros I, Khalyfa A, et al. Early intermittent hypoxia induces proatherogenic changes in aortic wall macrophages in a murine model of obstructive sleep apnea. Am J Respir Crit Care Med, 2014, 190(8): 958-961.

[5] Cortese R, Gileles-Hillel A, Khalyfa A, et al. Aorta macrophage inflammatory and epigenetic changes in a murine model of obstructive sleep apnea: Potential role of CD36. Sci Rep, 2017, 7: 43648.

[6] Trzepizur W, Cortese R, Gozal D. Murine models of sleep apnea: functional implications of altered macrophage polarity and epigenetic modifications in adipose and vascular tissues. Metabolism, 2018, 84: 44-55.

[7] McAlpine CS, Kiss MG, Rattik S, et al. Sleep modulates haematopoiesis and protects against atherosclerosis. Nature, 2019, 566(7744): 383-387.

[8] Xu RY, Huang R, Xiao Y, et al. Attenuated macrophage cholesterol efflux function in patients with obstructive sleep apnea-hypopnea syndrome. Sleep Breath, 2015, 19(1): 369-375.

[9] Xie H, Yin J, Bai Y, et al. Differential expression of immune markers in the patients with obstructive sleep apnea/hypopnea syndrome. Eur Arch Otorhinolaryngol, 2019, 276(3): 735-744.

[10] Said EA, Al-Abri MA, Al-Saidi I, et al. Altered blood cytokines, CD4 T cells, NK and neutrophils in patients with obstructive sleep apnea. Immunol Lett, 2017, 190: 272-278.

[11] Su MS, Xu L, Xu K, et al. Association of T lymphocyte immune imbalance and IL-10 gene polymorphism with the risk of obstructive sleep apnea in children with obesity. Sleep Breath, 2017, 21(4): 929-937.

[12] Zhang Z, Wang C. Immune status of children with obstructive sleep apnea/hypopnea syndrome. Pak J Med Sci, 2017, 33(1): 195-199.

[13] Joanna DK, Osińska I, Aleksandra P, et al. T, B, and NKT Cells in systemic inflammation in obstructive sleep apnoea. Mediators Inflamm, 2015, 2015: 161579.

[14] Liu J, Li T, Wu H, et al. Lactobacillus rhamnosus GG strain mitigated the development of obstructive sleep apnea-induced hypertension in a high salt diet via regulating TMAO level and CD4(+) T cell induced-type I inflammation. Biomed Pharmacother, 2019, 112: 108580.

[15] Dyugovskaya L, Lavie P, Lavie L. Lymphocyte activation as a possible measure of atherosclerotic risk in patients with sleep apnea. Ann N Y Acad Sci, 2005, 1051: 340-350.

[16] Dumitriu IE. The life(and death)of CD4+CD28(null)T cells in inflammatory diseases. Immunology, 2015, 146(2): 185-193.

[17] Dyugovskaya L, Lavie P, Hirsh M, et al. Activated CD8+ T-lymphocytes in obstructive sleep apnoea. Eur Respir J, 2005, 25(5): 820-828.

[18] 吕恒娟, 李津娜, 陈宝元, 等. 阻塞性睡眠呼吸暂停低通气综合征模式间歇低氧对大鼠淋巴细胞亚群凋亡的研究. 中华肺部疾病杂志(电子版), 2014, 7(6): 7-9.

[19] Vu DM, Tai A, Tatro JB, et al. γδT cells are prevalent in the proximal aorta and drive nascent atherosclerotic lesion progression and neutrophilia in hypercholesterolemic mice. PLoS One, 2014, 9(10): e109416.

[20] Dyugovskaya L, Lavie P, Lavie L. Phenotypic and functional characterization of blood γδT cells in sleep apnea. Am J Respir Crit Care Med, 2003, 168(2): 242-249.

[21] Khalyfa A, Qiao Z, Gileles-Hillel A, et al. Activation of the integrated stress response and metabolic dysfunction in a murine model of sleep apnea. Am J Respir Cell Mol Biol, 2017, 57(4): 477-486.

[22] Murphy AM, Thomas A, Crinion SJ, et al. Intermittent hypoxia in obstructive sleep apnoea mediates insulin resistance through adipose tissue inflammation. Eur Respir J, 2017, 49(4): 1601731.

[23] Wang Y, Lee MYK, Mak JCW, et al. Low-frequency intermittent hypoxia suppresses subcutaneous adipogenesis and induces macrophage polarization in lean mice. Diabetes Metab J, 2019, 43(5): 659-674.

[24] Ryan S. Adipose tissue inflammation by intermittent hypoxia: mechanistic link between obstructive sleep apnoea and metabolic dysfunction. J Physiol, 2017, 595(8): 2423-2430.

[25] Schaeffer E, Wu W, Mark C, et al. Intermittent hypoxia is a proinflammatory stimulus resulting in IL-6 expression and M1 macrophage polarization. Hepatol Commun, 2017, 1(4): 326-337.

[26] Campos-Rodriguez F, Martinez-Garcia MA, Martinez M, et al. Association between obstructive sleep apnea and cancer incidence in a large multicenter Spanish cohort. Am J Respir Crit Care Med, 2013; 187(1): 99-105.

[27] Chang WP, Liu ME, Chang WC, et al. Sleep apnea and the subsequent risk of breast cancer in women: a nationwide population-based cohort study. Sleep Med, 2014, 15(9): 1016-1020.

[28] Chen JC, Hwang JH. Sleep apnea increased incidence of primary central nervous system cancers: a nationwide cohort study. Sleep Med, 2014, 15(7): 749-754.

[29] Fang HF, Miao NF, Chen CD, et al. Risk of cancer in patients with insomnia, parasomnia, and obstructive sleep apnea: A Nationwide Nested Case-Control Study. J Cancer, 2015; 6(11): 1140-1147.

[30] Nieto FJ, Peppard PE, Young T, et al. Sleep-disordered breathing and cancer mortality: results from the Wisconsin Sleep Cohort Study. Am J Respir Crit Care Med, 2012, 186(2): 190-194.

[31] Khalyfa A, Kheirandish-Gozal, Gozal D. Exosome and macrophage crosstalk in sleep-disordered breathing-induced metabolic dysfunction. Int J Mol Sci, 2018, 19(11): 3383.

[32] Torres M, Martinez-Garcia MA, Campos-Rodriguez F, et al. Lung cancer aggressiveness in an intermittent hypoxia murine model of postmenopausal sleep apnea. Menopause. 2020.

[33] Campillo N, Torres M, Vilaseca A, et al. Role of Cyclooxygenase-2 on intermittent hypoxia-induced lung tumor malignancy in a mouse model of sleep apnea. Sci Rep, 2017, 7: 44693.

[34] Almendros I, Wang Y, Becker L, et al. Intermittent hypoxia-induced changes in tumor-associated macrophages and tumor malignancy in a mouse model of sleep apnea. Am J Respir Crit Care Med, 2014, 189(5): 593-601.

[35] Almendros I, Gileles-Hillel A, Khalyfa A, et al. Adipose tissue macrophage polarization by intermittent hypoxia in a mouse model of OSA: effect of tumor microenvironment. Cancer Lett, 2015, 361(2): 233-239.

[36] Guo C, Buranych A, Sarkar D, et al. The role of tumor-associated macrophages in tumor vascularization. Vasc Cell, 2013, 5(1): 20.

[37] Tang X, Mo C, Wang Y, et al. Anti-tumour strategies aiming to target tumour-associated macrophages. Immunology, 2013, 138(2): 93-104.

[38] Hakim F, Wang Y, Zhang SX, et al. Fragmented sleep accelerates tumor growth and progression through recruitment of tumor-associated macrophages and TLR4 signaling. Cancer Res, 2014, 74(5): 1329-1337.

[39] Akbarpour M, Khalyfa A, Qiao Z, et al. Altered CD8+ T-Cell lymphocyte function and TC1 cell stemness contribute to enhanced malignant tumor properties in murine models of sleep apnea. Sleep, 2017, 40(2).

[40] Wu J, Cui H, Zhu Z, et al. Effect of HIF-1a on Foxp3 expression in $CD4^+ CD25^-$ T lymphocytes. Microbiol Immunol, 2014, 58(7): 409-415.

[41] Liu Y, Lao M, Chen J, et al. Short-term prognostic effects of circulating regulatory T-Cell suppressive function and vascular endothelial growth factor level in patients with non-small cell lung cancer and obstructive sleep apnea. Sleep Med, 2020, 70: 88-96.

[42] Staats R, Rodrigues R, Barros A, et al. Decrease of perforin positive CD3(+) gamma delta-T cells in patients with obstructive sleep disordered breathing. Sleep Breath, 2018, 22(1): 211-221.

[43] Gaoatswe G, Kent BD, Corrigan A, et al. Invariant natural killer T cell deficiency and functional impairment in sleep apnea: links to cancer comorbidity. Sleep, 2015, 38(10):

1629-1634.
[44] Cubillos-Zapata C, Avendaño-Ortiz J, Hernandez-Jimenez E, et al. Hypoxia-induced PD-L1/PD-1 crosstalk impairs T-cell function in sleep apnoea. Eur Respir J,2017,50(4):1700833.
[45] Cubillos-Zapata C, Almendros I, Díaz-García E, et al. Differential effect of intermittent hypoxia and sleep fragmentation on PD-1/PD-L1 upregulation. Sleep,2019:zsz285.
[46] Hernández Jiménez E, Cubillos Zapata C, Toledano V, et al. Monocytes inhibit NK activity via TGF-β in patients with obstructive sleep apnoea. Eur Respir J,2017,49(6):1602456.

10 评估量表在 OSA 患者中的应用

李善群

阻塞性睡眠呼吸暂停低通气综合征（obstructive sleep apnea hypopnea syndrome, OSAHS）以间歇性上气道部分或全部塌陷为特征，导致夜间低氧血症，睡眠觉醒。嗜睡是 OSAHS 患者最主要的日间症状，也是患者生活质量下降的重要因素。OSAHS 在人群中的患病率为 9%～38%。睡眠多导图（PSG）是诊断 OSA 的金标准，但是这种筛查既昂贵又耗时，不适合作为常规筛查手段。与之相比，问卷调查就成了一个不错的筛查手段。同时，鉴于患者也往往需要关注白天嗜睡、困倦、乏力等 PSG 无法反应的主观症状，生活质量和睡眠质量相关的量表也可以发挥 PSG 所不能和发挥的优势。

普适性量表可以用于发现 OSAHS 引起的一般生活质量损害，涉及生理、心理和社会等各个方面，涵盖范围广泛，但也正因如此，其针对性不如睡眠特异性量表。随着生活质量评估量表的发展，又出现了针对 OSAHS 的特异性评价量表，其特点是可以更全面细微地反映 OSAHS 患者的临床症状，以及持续正压通气（CPAP）治疗前后的症状改善。

OSAHS 相关的生活质量评估量表能够很好地评估 OSAHS 患者的疾病史、睡眠状况及生活质量（QOI），并可以在一定程度上反映 OSAHS 所引起的器官功能损害的存在及其严重程度。下面就评估量表在 OSAHS 患者的研究进展进行介绍。

一、OSA 的筛查问卷

柏林问卷（BQ）1999 年制定，用于确定睡眠呼吸暂停的危险因素。该问卷包含 10 个问题，涉及以下 3 个类别：打鼾行为，日间嗜睡或疲劳，肥胖或高血压。以上 3 种类型中至少有 2 种症状持续且频繁（每周 3～4 次）的患者被划分为发展为睡眠呼吸暂停的高危人群。一项包含了 29 个研究结果，9444 名受试者的荟萃分析证实，当 AHI⩾30 时，检测 OSA 的 BQ 最高灵敏度为 97.3%，阴性预测值 NPV 为 95.4%，BQ 对中度 OSA 的检测特异性最高，为 91.7%，当 AHI⩾5 时阳性预测值 PPV 从 11.5% 升高到 91%。MBQ 是 BQ 的改良版本，将 BQ 中的肥胖界值 30kg/m² 更改为了 25kg/m²，在亚洲患者中的评估效果要优于 BQ。

STOP 问卷（SQ）和 STOP-BANG 问卷（SBQ）都是在 2008 年开发的，用于评估 OSA 的风险，作为外科患者术前评估的一部分。SQ 是一种简洁易用、灵敏度高的 OSA 筛查工具，评估指标包括：大声打鼾，疲劳，观察到的呼吸暂停和高血压。如果患者对 2 个或 2 个以上问题的回答是肯定的，SQ 可以将他们划分为患有阻塞性睡眠呼吸暂停的高风险人群。SQ 在 9 项研究（8196 名受试者）中进行评估，结果证实对于中度 OSA 患者，SQ 具有最高的预测敏感性（100%）、特异性（92.3%）和 NPV（100%），而对于轻度 OSA 患者，PPV 的范围为 12.8%～92.5%。

SBQ 包括 4 个主观项目（STOP：打鼾，疲劳，观察到的呼吸暂停和高血压）和 4 个人口统计项目（BANG：BMI，年龄，颈围，性别）。得分为 5～8 的人被归类为 OSA 的高危人群。一项包含了 13 项研究，9584 名 OSA 患者的荟萃分析证实，在 AHI⩾30 时有敏感性和阴性预测值 NPV 最高。在 AHI⩾5 时，阳性预测值 PPV 在 12.2%～93.7%。SBQ 检测中度阻塞性睡眠呼吸暂停的特异性最高（74.7%）。一项 2017 年的荟萃分析指出，与 BQ、STOP 问卷相比，SBQ 是检测轻度、中度和重度 OSA 更准确的工具。

我们课题组的一项研究显示，在合并慢性阻塞性肺病（COPD）的情况下，BQ、MBQ 和 SBQ 的筛查能力会受到肺功能的影响，肺功能越差的患者获得准确诊断的可能性更高。该论文已经于 2020 年发表于"International journal of COPD"(IF=2.8)。

NoSAS 是 2016 年提出，内容较新，问卷计分方式包括：颈围超 40 cm 计 4 分，BMI 在 25～29 计 3 分，BMI⩾30 计 5 分，习惯性打鼾者 2 分，年龄超过 55 岁计 4 分，男性计 2 分，当得分⩾8 分被认为是阳性结果。与现有的筛查评分相比，NoSAS 评分可以帮助临床医生以比目前更高的准确性决定哪些个体应该被进一步的检测，从而减少睡眠障碍性呼吸诊断的漏诊数量和不必要的夜间记录。

No-Apnea 是一种新开发并经过验证的筛查工具，它只包括 2 个客观参数：颈围（NC）和年龄，总分从 0 到 9（分值⩾3 划分为 OSA 高危人群）。在队列研究中证实 No-Apnea 在 OSA 的筛查中，STOP-BANG 或 NoSAS 的表现相似。但针对 No-Apnea 有几点值得强调：①缺乏主观变量，会限制适用范围，特别是在 OSA 患病率较低的地区。②年龄为 55 岁，已经足以将 OSA 诊断为高危人群，可能限制了其在老年人群中的使用。③由于每个参数的评分不同，可能难以采用和实施，特别是在一般临床实践中。

在临床应用中，可以将上述问卷联合其他项目使用，例如 2013 年发表在 Chest 上的一篇研究证实，血清 HCO_3^-

水平增加 STOP-BANG 筛选特异性预测中度/重度 OSA，建议在临床采用两步法初筛 OSA 患者，第一步 STOP-BANG 分数筛选患者，第二步 STOP-BANG 分数≥3 的患者中，检验血清 HCO_3^- 水平是否≥28mmol/L，联合使用，来提高特异性。2017 年发表在 J Clin Anesth 的一篇研究证实，当 STOP-BANG 问卷联合患者的体型时（梨形身材、苹果形身材），STOP-BANG 问卷不仅可以提高对 OSA 患者的筛查。上述问卷表也可用于其他疾病中 OSA 患者的筛查，本课题组前期研究发现，在 AHI 的阈值设为 15 时，和 BQ 相比，SBQ 检测合并哮喘的中重度 OSA 的诊断敏感性较高（84.4% vs.60%），特异性较低（79.5% vs.91%），阳性预测值（PPV）较低（70.4% vs.79.4%），阴性预测值（NPV）较高（90% vs.80%）。在检测哮喘患者中度和重度阻塞性睡眠呼吸暂停方面，SBQ 是一种比 BQ 更好的睡眠问卷。

二、普适性健康量表

（一）36 项简明健康问卷调查（SF-36）

SF-36 量表是美国医学结局研究组（Medical Outcomes Study, MOS）开发的一个评估生命质量的普适性测定量表，它通过 36 个多选问题评估患者目前在 8 个不同领域的健康状况，包括生理功能、躯体疼痛、总体健康、活力、社会功能、情感职能和精神健康，评分和健康状况呈正相关。

2018 年，一项研究表明 OSAHS 对患者生活质量造成的影响与性别有关。研究结果显示，与男性患者相比，同等严重程度的 OSAHS 对女性患者 SF-36 评分的负面影响更严重。该课题还表明女性患者因 OSAHS 共病心血管疾病和脂代谢异常的程度更高，且临床症状更严重，这可能是 SF-36 评分在两性间存在差异的原因之一。

目前已有不少研究将 SF-36 广泛应用于 OSAHS 患者中，目的是评估患者生活质量受损的严重程度和治疗效果（CPAP、口腔矫正器等）。多项研究表明其中活力版块与 OSA 患病的关联是最为紧密的，不过也有例外。2020 年，在一项纳入了 104 例患者的随机对照试验中，对非重度阻塞性睡眠呼吸暂停（OSA）患者采用连续气道正压（CPAP）或双块提下颌夹板（MAS）治疗，并比较其健康相关生活质量（HRQoL）和自我报告睡眠质量的影响。SF-36 问卷被用于评估 HRQoL 和匹兹堡睡眠质量指数（PSQI）评估睡眠质量。研究结果显示，CPAP 治疗组的物理成分得分均有所改善，而 MAS 组的 SF-36 心理成分得分有所改善。两组患者在最终随访时的 SF-36 总评分均无差异。另外，近年，SF-36 也被用于验证一系列 OSA 治疗相关的颌面部手术[例如：矢状支截骨术（SSRO）和下颌骨牵引成骨术（MDO）]对患者生活质量的改善效果，或用于对比各个术式之间效果的区别。

遗憾的是，时至今日各类的课题研究结果均表明 SF-36 与 OSAHS 患者的低通气指数（AHI）指数和病情严重程度无关。因此目前没有证据证明 SF-36 在 OSAHS 的筛查中能有价值。SF-36 的主要应用范围局限于对患者整体生活质量的评估。

（二）诺丁汉健康问卷（NHP）

NHP 是由 Hunt 等研究人员在 1985 年设计的调查问卷，旨在评价健康相关的生活质量；其中包括 38 项条目，评分越高，健康状况越差；其子条目包括精力、疼痛、情感反应、睡眠质量、社交和体能。

研究中发现除了情感反应之外，OSAHS 患者和健康人群的所有子条目都存在显著差异。Meta 分析通过 16 项对照研究发现，CPAP 治疗能够明显改善 OSAHS 患者的 NHP 评分。然而，研究显示在 NHP 不能在 CPAP 治疗时间长短不同的 OSAHS 患者中做出差异。

另外，有研究显示 NHP 的情感反应评分能反映 OSAHS 患者对 CPAP 治疗的依从性。

与 SF-36 相比，HNP 在 OSA 中的应用极其受限。最近的有关 HNP 和 OSA 的论文发表于 2013 年。该研究显示中重度 OSA 患者的 NHP 中的"睡眠""精力"和"情绪反应"得分最高，同时提示患者可通过 NHP 问卷的"活动能力"版块正确评估其活动障碍。

（三）小结

SF-3、NHP 等普适性量表已经广泛应用多种疾病的相关生活质量评估。这些问卷的优点是可以用来比较 OSAHS 和其他呼吸道疾病，如哮喘和 COPD 等给患者造成的影响，以及应用 CPAP 等手段治疗 OSAHS 前后生活质量的改善。

然而，其缺陷也显而易见，即这些问卷通常不包括 OSAHS 患者常见的症状。而且大多数的问卷是为横向比较同一天生活质量的优劣而设计的，因而不能反映疾病治疗过后 QOL 的变化，因此需要有能反映患者的睡眠状态及 QOL 的特异性问卷

三、睡眠特异性问卷

（一）Epworth 睡眠问卷（ESS）量表

ESS 量表由位于澳大利亚墨尔本的 Epworth 医院的睡眠疾病中心于 1990 年设计并投入使用。包含 8 种常见的日常生活状态下嗜睡情况的评估，可反映患者的一般嗜睡状态，一般认为评分＞8 分则说明患者存在白日过度嗜睡问题。许多研究都证实 OSAHS 患者的 ESS 评分显著高于正常人群。

ESS 量表因其简单实用而广泛应用于临床，尤其是 OSAHS 患者。研究表明 ESS 评分与患者的 AHI 及 BMI 高度相关，因此也可以应用于 OSAHS 患者的初筛，临床 SACS 上习惯于以 8 为标志点筛选 OSAHS 患者。2019 年一项研究对比了 ESS 与 SBQ、BQ 和 SACS 筛选 OSAHS 患者的能力，结果显示无论是以 AHI＞5、15、还是 30 为界值，ESS 量表对 OSA 患者的筛查能力都是 4 个量表中最差的，且其 AUC 均＜0.7（AHI＞5：0.609；AHI＞15：0.611；AHI＞30：0.676）。该研究显示 ESS 的敏感性优于特异性，这意味着应用其筛选很可能将许多其他疾病导致的嗜睡问题误诊为 OSA。鉴于 2019 年的一项 Meta 分析显示老年 OSAHS 患者的 ESS 评分显著低于中老年患者，可认为年龄影响了患者对嗜睡的自我评估，因而也会对问卷调查的准确性造成影响。另一篇文献显示 ESS 与 STOP 问

卷的联合应用也没能改善 STOP 问卷对 OSA 的筛查能力。另一项研究显示与非快动眼睡眠依赖型 OSA 患者相比，尽管快动眼睡眠依赖型的 OSA 患者的 AHI 低 2 倍，两组患者的 ESS 评分也并没有区别。

这一系列研究都证实 ESS 在 OSA 患者的筛查中发挥的作用非常有限，但是另一方面 ESS 能够较好地评估颌面部手术或 CPAP 等各种治疗手段对 OSAHS 患者的治疗效果。多项研究表明 CPAP 治疗后多数 OSAHS 患者的 ESS 评分会有不同程度下降，表明其日间嗜睡症状的改善，然而问题是 ESS 评分下降多少才能被认为是有临床意义的改善。目前，有研究者提出 OSAHS 人群中只有 ESS 评分下降超过 6 才能认为患者嗜睡症状得到改善。

Multiple Sleep Latency Test（MSLT）是衡量嗜睡的金标准。有研究证实，和 ESS 是不可相互替代的。一方面，ESS 受心理因素的影响，MSLT 不受心理因素的影响。另一方面，ESS 是主观问卷，不能用于证明或排除困倦，而 MSLT 测量的是客观数据，因此可以用于证实实际的睡眠情况。2017 年的一项研究证实与主观睡眠质量相关问卷 ESS、SSS 相比，MSLT 能更准确地评估 OSA 患者的睡眠障碍与 IL-6 之间的相关关系。

（二）斯坦福嗜睡 SSS 量表

SSS 是一种主观性嗜睡评估量表，把嗜睡程度从轻到重分为 7 个等级，调查对象根据问卷的语言描述选择一个最符合自己嗜睡状态的等级，等级越高，嗜睡状况越严重。1999 年的一项研究提出 SSS 评分和 AHI 存在相关性，且是 OSA 的危险因素之一。后来，研究人员又发现示 SSS 评分不佳也是 OSA 患者死亡的独立危险因素之一。

CPAP，光照疗法和悬雍垂-腭-咽成形术（UPPP）的治疗效果都可以在本量表中得到反映。UPPP 术后患者由 SSS 评价的主观嗜睡症状得到显著改善。而 CPAP 相关的临床研究则证明，尽管 CPAP 治疗能有效地改善 SSS 的评分，但是一旦间断使用 CPAP，即使是停用一天也有可能导致症状的复发。而光照疗法没能通过改善 SSS 评分证实自身改善睡眠的能力。

（三）功能评估性睡眠问卷（functional outcomes of sleep questionnaire，FOSQ）

FOSQ 是为评价白天嗜睡症状对患者日常生活的影响而制定的量表，包含总体劳动能力、社会创造价值、活动水平、警觉性、社会关系及性活动 5 个方面评价患。SSS 评分和 AHI 存在相关性，且是 OSA 的危险因素之一。但是在 2020 年，一项在共患 2 型糖尿病的 OSA 患者中的研究证实比起 ESS，FOSQ 和 PSQI 对高 AHI 的预测能力明显较弱。另一项在共患冠心病的 OSA 患者的研究中发现 FOSQ 与冠心病组患者的 AHI 亦无相关性。这表明 FOSQ 对 OSA 的评估易受共患病的影响。

与 ESS 量表和 SSS 量表相比，包括了患者日常生活因睡眠问题而受到的限制，因此 FOSQ 能更好地反映 OSAHS 患者除夜间睡眠和日间嗜睡问题之外的症状特点。

目前，FOSQ 已被应用于包括 CPAP、口腔矫正、手术在内的多种临床研究里，以评估这些 OSA 治疗方案的效果。值得一提的是，假 CPAP 治疗的研究发现假治疗后 OSAHS 患者的 FOSQ 警觉性和总体舒适度评分都有显著改善。也有研究者在轻度 OSAHS 患者中发现模拟的 CPAP 治疗也可以改善 FOSQ 的评分。这提示 FOSQ 的主观性较强，在用来评估疗效时应该设立对照组。

研究发现，在 OSAHS 患者中 FOSQ 的结果和普适性量表（SIP、SF-36 等）评分相关性较弱，提示二者反映的 OSAHS 患者的特点存在不重合的范围。

（四）匹兹堡睡眠质量指数（pittsburgh sleep quality index，PSQI）

PSQI 是美国匹兹堡大学精神科医生 Buysse 博士等于 1989 年编制的。该量表适用于睡眠障碍患者、精神障碍患者评价睡眠质量，同时也适用于一般人睡眠质量的评估。量表由 9 道题组成，前 4 题为填空题，后 5 题为选择题，其中第 5 题包含 10 道小题。问卷的条目包含了客观评估内容和主观评估内容。

多项研究证实，OSA 患者的 PSQI 评分情况比正常人群糟糕，因此 PSQI 有可能成为 OSA 的潜在筛查工具。2014 年一项 Meta 分析显示，尽管 PSQI 能在 OSA 患者的筛查中发挥一定的作用，但是其诊断的准确性并不是很好，因此不建议单独用于 OSA 的筛查之中。

目前与不少研究都认为 PSQI 可以应用于 CPAP、肌肉锻炼等 OSA 治疗康复手段临床疗效的评估，但是其中不少研究反映其评估效果不如 ESS。

（五）小结

总的来说，与普适性健康量表相比，睡眠特异性量表的劣势在于评分内容往往局限于睡眠质量，不能兼顾其他系统的情况。但也正因如此，它们往往能更准确的区别 OSA 患者和正常人群，是可用于 OSAHS 筛查的潜在工具。遗憾的是其筛查能力往往不如 BQ、SBQ 等专为 OSA 筛查定制的问卷。

目前有部分研究表明，普适性健康量表和睡眠特异性问卷评分之间可能存在相关性。比如 2018－2020 年的几项研究中，研究人员发现 SF-36 心理成分和活动能力部分的得分与 PSQI 和 ESS 整体得分之间存在微弱到中度的相关性。但也有许多研究报告他们没能在普适性健康量表和睡眠特异性问卷中发现相关性。这可能是由于普适性健康量表包含了大量与 OSAHS 和睡眠无关的条目，因而二者的关注点并不一致所致。

四、OSAHS 的特异性评价量表

（一）Calgary 睡眠呼吸暂停生活质量指数（sleep apnea quality of life index，SAQLI）

Calgary SAQLI 是针对睡眠呼吸暂停患者的专用生活质量量表，包括日常活动、社会交往、情感及症状 4 个方面，共 35 个条目。患者在专门医师指导下进行。对每个问题分 7 个等级进行评价，各部分总分除以各自条目总数，即得每部分的分数。量表的总分为 4 部分的平均分，分数越高，相关生活质量越高，范围为 17 分。另外，Calgary 还包括第五个方面，即治疗相关症状，主要用于评估临床治疗 OSAHS 可能出现的不良影响。

这是首个根据 OSAHS 症状特点制定的生活质量相关量表,与既往的 QOL 量表相比,它能较为全面地反映 OSA 患者 QOL 的相关症状,并且能够对治疗前后的症状改变及不同治疗方法的差异作出评估。研究表明 SAQLI 和 SF-36 评分高度相关,并且敏感度高于 FOSQ。

2020 年一项研究表明 SAQLI 的日常功能、社交互动、情绪功能和症状模块的内容效度指数(CVI)值分别为:93、93、96 和 1.00,而问卷的效度分析应用了 exploratory factor。其结果为显示该问卷的信度和效度均较好,可适用于 OSA 患者的筛查和评估。

目前,SAQLI 已经被用于多种 OSA 治疗手段的临床效果的评估,包括上气道手术、颏舌肌及舌下神经电刺激、CPAP 等。Lain 等发现在不考虑治疗相关症状的情况下,CPAP 治疗能够改善 SAQLI 评分。同时,也有研究表明 SAQLI 可用来评价宣传教育在 OSAHS 治疗中的作用。在一项针对 CPAP 治疗的 OSA 患者的对照研究中,医师通过录像和宣传教育给予实验组患者更多的 OSAHS 和 CPAP 治疗的相关信息,发现两组患者在治疗的依从性和 ESS 评分没有明显差异,然而实验组的 SAQLI 评分得到了显著改善。

SAQLI 问卷的完成需要临床医师的指导,其优点在于提高了问卷的可信度;缺点是复杂而且耗时,不同医师的指导方式会影响结果,不利于大规模临床研究。同时,也有研究证实该量表内容冗余,因此需要研制简便自测的 SAQLI,从而满足不同的研究需要。

(二)魁北克睡眠问卷(QSQ)

QSQ 是 OSAHS 特异性问卷,包括 32 个条目,反映 OSAHS 患者白天嗜睡、日间症状、夜间症状、情感、社会交往等方面的状况,每一方面包括 4~7 个条目,每个条目又可以分 7 个等级做答。

目前,QSQ 在临床研究中的应用较少,主要被用于 CPAP 等 OSA 治疗手段等的临床效果的评估。研究表明,从标准应答均数看 QSQ 比 FOSQ 更能反映 CPAP 治疗后的症状改变,因此未来可以在临床试验和工作中推广。

(三)呼吸暂停知识测验(apnea knowledge test,AKT)与呼吸暂停信念问卷(apnea beliefs scale,ABS)

众所周知,患者对自身疾病的认识和信念会影响一系列健康相关因素,包括治疗依从性。因此,量化这些变量以评估其对依从性的影响是十分重要的,特别是对于例如 OSA 这类依赖于自主治疗的慢性疾病。AKT 和 ABS 是两种针对 OSA 患者的特殊问卷,能够评估 OSA 患者对疾病的认识和信念。

有研究证实,在存在自我感觉到呼吸暂停症状的 OSA 患者中其 AKT 和 ABS 的评分更好,同时,这类患者对 CPAP 治疗的依从性也更好。一项研究显示,AKT 和 ABS 评分是患者对 CPAP 治疗依从性的独立影响因素。

五、ICF

世界卫生组织(WHO)从 1996 年开始制定了新的残疾与健康分类——《国际功能、残疾和健康分类》(International Classification of Functioning,Disability and Health,简称 ICF)。ICF 主要从身体结构、身体功能、活动和参与,以及环境这 4 个方面进行全面评估,并对患者的康复治疗效果评价及指导提供重要依据,最终目的是要建立一种统一的、标准化的术语系统,来提供理解和描述功能和残疾的共同框架,便于对功能和残疾进行描述和评估。ICF 所依据的是身体、个体和社会三个水平的健康状态所发生的功能变化及出现的异常,目前主要用于康复患者的评估。

在 2001—2009 年,关于 ICF 的文献多集中于 ICF 概念的研究及传播 ICF 方面,近年来随着 ICF 越来越被人们所熟知,这类文献的数量开始减少。2010 年后,关于 ICF 的临床应用文献的数量呈上升趋势,对于特定人群的信效度检验方面,康复领域的研究成为热点,此外,也可以应用至不同的领域,如临床法医学、康复教育和护理学等。大量研究证实 ICF 对多种疾病的评估具有有效性,可用于各种严重程度的患者,同时作为身体和心理康复的评估标准。随着 ICF 相关系统的陆续开发,ICF 已经被广泛的应用于临床、教育、康复领域,并作为一个框架指导临床实践。

ICF 共包含 1400 多个类别,结合临床 WHO 制定了针对 COPD、肥胖、睡眠障碍和糖尿病的 ICF 核心集,但目前没有针对 OSA 的特定 ICF 核心集。由于 OSA 是一种以肥胖和睡眠障碍为特征的疾病,我们课题组选取针对睡眠障碍和肥胖的 ICF 核心集来评估 OSA 患者的功能和健康状况。通过对 592 名 OSA 患者进行睡眠和肥胖的 ICF 评估,证实睡眠和肥胖两个 ICF 核心集的身体功能这一部分与患者的 BMI、颈围和 AHI 成正相关,在不同严重程度的患者中,这一部分的分数也存在显著性差异,通过对睡眠和肥胖 ICF 核心集进行比较,发现睡眠-ICF 核心集更适用于 OSA 患者,这部分研究成果目前已发表于"Respiratory Research"(IF=3.9)。同时我们课题组用 COPD-ICF 量表对 COPD 患者进行评估,结果证实 COPD 核心集的"活动和参与"这一部分用来评估 COPD 患者的日常活动水平,具有较高的可靠性和有效性,该成果目前发表于"International journal of COPD"(IF=2.8)。

六、结 语

问卷是筛查 OSAHS 患者非常有效的道具,且对 OSAHS 患者进行 QOL 评估是必要的。因为 PSG 诊断较为不便,应用问卷对潜在的 OSA 患者进行筛查是一种有效诊断的方式。同时,随着经济的发展和医学模式的转换,OSAHS 患者会更加关注自身 QOL 的提高,目前临床评估疗效也只是将目标集中在 AHI 变化和最低血氧饱和度等 PSG 指标的客观改变上,因此设计科学的 QOL 量表对患者 QOL 进行全面的个体化的评估,从而更好地指导临床对 OSAHS 进行严重程度分类,对不同的治疗方式进行评估并及时进行调整是十分有必要的。

11 阻塞性睡眠呼吸暂停与肠道菌群

王拢拢 欧琼

阻塞性睡眠呼吸暂停（obstructive sleep apnea, OSA）是最常见的睡眠呼吸疾病，以睡眠期间上气道反复完全或不完全塌陷造成呼吸暂停或低通气、导致夜间间歇性低氧和睡眠片段为主要病理生理。目前普遍认为 OSA 是一种全身性疾病，是高血压的独立危险因素，且与包括冠心病、房颤等其他心脑血管疾病、代谢综合征、认知功能障碍等多系统疾病的发生发展有关。到目前为止，该病发病机制不是十分清楚，遗传因素（上气道解剖结构、形态）、环境因素（增龄、肥胖、烟酒等）的交互作用与 OSA 患者的表型变异密切相关，然而，即使将遗传和环境因素包含在模型中，它们在 OSA 疾病表型的变异中也只占据非常小的比例。因此，探讨 OSA 发病机制中的未知因素，为精准防治提供依据显得尤为重要。

近年研究发现，肠道菌群作为人体内一种微生物与许多疾病的发生发展有关。肠道菌群与 OSA 的关系也备受关注。作为人体最大的微生物群，肠道菌群包含至少 1000 种微生物，数量级达 10^{14}，主要由"5 个门"组成，分别是拟杆菌门、厚壁菌门、放线菌门、变形菌门和 Cerrucomicrobia，其中革兰阴性拟杆菌门和革兰阳性厚壁菌门占据 90% 以上。肠道菌群的结构和功能失调与人体许多疾病发生有关，如胃肠道、神经系统、呼吸系统、心脑血管系统及代谢性疾病。本文简要总结近年 OSA 与肠道菌群关系的研究进展。

一、OSA 动物模型的肠道菌群

许多外部因素或疾病状态可影响肠道菌群，包括饮食、运动、吸烟、喝酒、抗生素和胃肠道疾病等。但是 OSA 对肠道菌群的影响还不清楚，有学者根据 OSA 的睡眠片段化和间歇性低氧特征构建了小鼠模型以明确其对肠道菌群的影响。Poroyko 等先将小鼠暴露于 4 周的慢性睡眠片段化（sleep segment, SF），之后 2 周时间恢复，粪便菌群多样性分析表明，在小鼠 4 周的慢性睡眠片段化之后，厚壁菌门的丰度增加了 20%，拟杆菌门和放线菌门的丰度分别减少了 20% 和 50%；在科的水平上，主要表现为毛螺菌科和瘤胃菌科增加，而乳酸杆菌及双歧杆菌显著减少。当 2 周的睡眠恢复后，毛螺菌科和瘤胃球菌科的丰度返回到睡眠片段化之前的水平，表明肠道菌群改变与睡眠片段化存在相关性。除此之外，慢性睡眠片段化的小鼠食物摄入量增加，胰岛素敏感性下降，内脏脂肪含量及炎症水平增加，肠道屏障功能受损，并将 SF 小鼠的粪便移植到无菌小鼠，得到相似的结果，因此推测慢性睡眠片段可能通过影响肠道菌群进而介导代谢紊乱及机体慢性炎症。与 Poroyko 等的研究结果相似，Bowers 等先将小鼠暴露于 5 d 的睡眠中断中，随后是 4 d 的随意恢复睡眠，在多个时间点测定小鼠粪便微生物组和粪便代谢组，结果表明，睡眠中断的小鼠厚壁菌门/拟杆菌门比例（Firmicutes/Bacteroidetes, F/B）增加，乳酸杆菌属、放线菌门和双歧杆菌属减少，并且代谢组也发生了改变，如胆汁酸代谢，且这些影响的某些方面持续到恢复随意睡眠后的第 4 天。由此认为睡眠片段化或睡眠中断后，肠道菌群失调可能导致机体某些病理变化，并且这些变化甚至可能在睡眠恢复正常后仍然存在。

Moreno-Indias 等评估了模拟 OSA 特征之一的间歇性低氧小鼠模型是否会有粪便微生物群的改变。他们将 10 只小鼠置于慢性间歇性缺氧的环境作为实验组（含有 5% 氧气的空气 20s，室温空气下 40s，6h/d，连续 6 周），10 只正常饲养的小鼠作为对照组，并获得两组的粪便标本进行分析。结果显示，实验组小鼠整体微生物群落结构存在显著改变，与对照组相比，肠道菌群的 α 多样性增加，并且诱发了肠道菌群的改变，表现为厚壁菌门、普氏菌属、帕拉普菌属、脱硫弧菌属及毛螺菌科增加；拟杆菌门、Odoribacter、Turicibacter、消化球菌科及丹毒丝菌科减少。并且发现间歇性缺氧小鼠肠腔内存在明显的缺氧/再灌注循环。这些发现表明，间歇性缺氧暴露后，肠道内总氧含量减少，使专性厌氧菌的生长更具有生态优势，表现为间歇性低氧小鼠组专性厌氧菌相对富集，可能导致肠道某些代谢物质发生改变，进而导致疾病发生发展。这与 Albenberg 等的研究结果是一致的，并且他们用高压氧改善组织氧合后，肠道微生物群组成也发生了改变。既然间歇性缺氧能显著改变小鼠的肠道菌群，那么在恢复正常氧合后，肠道菌群的改变是否可逆呢？Moreno-Indias 等再次重复了上述实验，并且之后两组均给予了 6 周的正常氧合，结果表明，间歇缺氧小鼠的肠道菌群数量和种类与治疗前相似，在正常氧合后，与对照组相比，间歇性缺氧小鼠组拟杆菌丰度显著降低，而厚壁菌门和除铁菌门的丰度显著增加，这些结果表明，模拟 OSA 间歇性缺氧小鼠诱导的肠道菌群的改变或许需要更长时间的正常氧合才能逆转，但这需要进一步研究。

另一项模拟 OSA 间歇性缺氧及高碳酸血症（intermittent hypoxia and hypercapnia,IHH)的小鼠模型结果显示，与对照组相比，IHH小鼠肠道艰难杆菌科、颤螺旋菌属、毛螺菌科、梭菌科增加。

上述动物实验研究表明，模拟睡眠片段化或间歇性缺氧的小鼠均可导致肠道菌群改变。

二、OSA 患者中的肠道菌群

有关肠道菌群与OSA患者中的临床研究不多。新近的一项研究作者Ko等比较了93例不同严重程度的OSA患者其中轻度40例（5＜AHI≤15）、中度23例（15＜AHI≤30）、重度30例（AHI≥30）和正常对照组20例（AHI≤5）的肠道菌群分布，并检测了血中同型半胱氨酸、IL-6(interleukin-6)和TNF-α(tumor necrosis factor alpha)的水平，结果显示不同程度的OSA及对照组肠道菌群在属的水平上，丰度存在显著性差异，并据此用以将OSA患者和正常对照组鉴别开来（ROC－AUC＝0.789）。功能分析发现OSA患者肠道产短链脂肪酸（short-chain fatty acid,SCFA）的细菌减少，有害病原体及IL-6水平增加，肠道乳杆菌属与同型半胱氨酸的水平正相关，然而TNF-α水平在OSA组与正常对照组无明显差异。

另一项研究探索了OSA的特征之一打鼾对肠道菌群的影响，该研究纳入的是2岁打鼾儿童，结果表明，与不打鼾者相比，打鼾者中变形菌门、肠杆菌科、韦荣球菌科丰度更高，F/B比例更高，但由于年龄对肠道菌群存在影响，该研究结果是否可推广到成年打鼾者仍然未知。

另外的临床研究不完全是OSA与肠道菌群，但都是与睡眠相关肠道菌群的研究，其中一项纳入了9名正常体重男性的研究，利用标准化的实验室方案（固定的进餐时间和锻炼时间表），在2个晚上的部分睡眠剥夺（睡眠时间02:45~07:00），并在2个晚上正常睡眠后（睡眠时间22:30~07:00），收集粪便标本，进行微生物组分析。结果表明，厚壁菌门/拟杆菌门比例增加，红蜱菌科和韦荣球菌科丰度增加，软壁菌门丰度下降，然而没有发现对β-多样性的影响，表明短期的睡眠不足可能会对肠道微生物群产生轻微的影响。Liu等探索了急性睡眠-觉醒周期的转变对肠道微生物的影响，该研究纳入了22名20~35岁的志愿者，受试者被要求在实验前至少7d保持正常的作息，然后将常规睡眠时间推迟2~4h，并在第2天早上自然醒来，以模拟睡眠-觉醒周期的转变。粪便样本在3个时间点采集：实验前1天（T0），睡眠时间转换后的第2天早上（T1），以及恢复正常睡眠时间后的第2天（T2）。结果表明，与基线（T0）相比，观察到T1厚壁菌门/拟杆菌门比例有所增加，但是3个时间点的微生物群落没有显著的差异。另一项在人群中限制睡眠的研究也表明睡眠限制后，肠道微生物组成没有发生显著的改变。这些研究结果均提示，在睡眠干预期间，肠道微生物的丰度和多样性只有轻微的改变，甚至没有变化，这可能与对睡眠干预的时间较短及样本量较小有关。

失眠是另一种睡眠障碍类型，国内实施的一项关于失眠对肠道菌群影响的研究显示，失眠导致肠道菌群的α和β多样性均发生显著改变，F/B比例下降，这与睡眠片段化/间歇性缺氧等动物模型上及OSA临床研究得到的结果均不同，可能是由于睡眠障碍的形式不同所造成的病理生理机制不同所致。

除了肠道菌群方面，有学者对OSA与人体其他部位微生物群的关系也做了探索。Lu等通过支气管肺泡灌洗液标本研究了OSA患者下呼吸道微生物群的变化（OSA患者11例/正常对照组8例），结果表明，两组患者微生物组存在明显差异，OSA患者变形杆菌和梭杆菌门丰度高于对照组，而厚壁菌门低于对照组。Wu等使用鼻腔冲洗液标本研究了OSA患者是否存在鼻微生物群的改变，结果显示，与非OSA相比，OSA患者鼻部微生物群富含链球菌、普雷沃菌和韦荣球菌，在CPAP治疗3个月后，鼻微生物群的组成也并未发生明显改变。

目前有限的临床研究结果显示，OSA患者的人体微生物群的组成发生了改变，包括肠道菌群、下呼吸道菌群、鼻咽部菌群，但仍不能明确二者的因果关系。

三、肠道菌群失调介导的OSA 相关性疾病

（一）肠道菌群与OSA诱导的高血压

OSA是高血压独立的危险因素，虽然这种关系已被确立，但OSA导致高血压的具体机制尚不清楚。模拟OSA的小鼠模型存在肠道菌群紊乱，而研究也发现高血压的动物模型及患者中也存在着肠道菌群紊乱，那么肠道菌群是否介导OSA诱导的高血压呢？Durgan等建立的OSA大鼠模型研究结果表明，在高脂饮食情况下，肠道菌群紊乱参与了OSA诱导的高血压的发生，在OSA 7d和14d后，血压分别升高24mmHg和29mmHg（$P<0.05$），并对其粪便菌群进行分析，可见到产生SCFA-丁酸盐的细菌减少。SCFA是膳食纤维的微生物发酵的产物，主要包括丁酸盐、丙酸盐和乙酸盐。在啮齿动物模型中，SCFA是直接的血管扩张剂，具有降低血压的作用。另有一些研究也表明，SCFA的减少可能在高血压的发病中起重要作用。间歇性缺氧/睡眠片段化小鼠构建的OSA动物模型均发现，厚壁菌门丰度增加，拟杆菌门丰度减少，F/B比例增加，已有研究显示F/B增加与产SCFA细菌减少有关。此外，临床研究也显示OSA患者肠道产SCFA的细菌减少。因此可推测OSA所致的肠道菌群紊乱可能通过减少SCFA从而诱导高血压的发生。Ganesh等对此进行了验证：在高脂饮食的背景下，与对照组相比，OSA大鼠1周和2周的收缩压分别显著增加24mmHg和44mmHg（$P<0.05$），当使用益生菌丁酸梭菌或益生元Hylon后，OSA组与对照组血压无显著差异，即未见OSA诱导的高血压。研究还发现OSA后，盲肠中的乙酸盐浓度降低了48%，但是当使用丁酸梭菌或Hylon后，这种变化也消失了。为了进一步验证乙酸盐在OSA诱发的高血压中的作用，研究者在2周时间内将乙酸盐注入OSA大鼠和对照组的盲肠内，结果表明恢复盲肠内乙酸盐的浓度可以预防OSA诱导的肠道炎症和高血压。该实验证明了乙酸盐是OSA诱导高血压的

关键所在。上述研究均表明肠道 SCFA 减少是 OSA 诱导的高血压的因素,因此,我们或许可通过补充益生菌或益生元来提高肠道内 SCFA,进而预防或治疗 OSA 诱导的难治性高血压,但这需要在临床研究中进一步证实。

(二)肠道菌群与 OSA 诱导的动脉粥样硬化

OSA 是心血管疾病的独立危险因素,心肌梗死、脑卒中及外周动脉疾病是与 OSA 相关的心血管病,其主要病理生理基础是动脉粥样硬化。事实上,在慢性间歇性缺氧或者睡眠片段化动物模型中已经发现主动脉内膜中层增厚、弹性纤维网紊乱及促炎免疫细胞的浸润,这种血管重塑及慢性间歇性缺氧/睡眠片段化导致的代谢改变是 OSA 诱导动脉粥样硬化的最重要的危险因素。最近的研究也发现,肠道菌群的产物氧化三甲胺(trimethylamine N-oxide,TMAO)水平增加与不良心血管事件风险及冠状动脉动脉粥样硬化负荷增加有关。Xue 等在高脂饮食的背景下,将 ApoE$^{-/-}$ 或 Ldlr$^{-/-}$ 小鼠分别置于 IHC(intermittent hypoxia and hypercapnia)环境和正常空气中,8 周后,与对照组(正常空气组)相比,IHC 组小鼠检测到更多更大的粥样硬化斑块,通过喂养 TMA(trimethylamine)的抑制剂 DMB(3,3-dimethyl-1-butanol)以减少 TMAO 的生成,发现动脉粥样硬化的程度显著减轻,而 TMAO 主要由普氏菌属(间歇性缺氧小鼠模型中发现普氏菌属丰度增加)产生,因此可推测 OSA 诱导的肠道菌群紊乱可能通过增加 TMAO 水平诱导动脉粥样硬化并加速其进展,这为进一步阐明 OSA 导致动脉粥样硬化找到了新的理论依据,从而可能成为 OSA 诱导的心脑血管疾病治疗的新靶点。

(三)肠道菌群与 OSA 诱导的代谢综合征

肠道菌群紊乱最近被认为是导致代谢性疾病的一个关键因素,由外部因素引起的肠道微生物组成变化会导致肠道细菌和宿主之间的共生关系发生改变,从而促进代谢性疾病的发展,尤其是,肠道微生物群已被认为是通过刺激机体产生低度炎症而导致代谢性疾病。Ko 等的研究发现与对照组相比,OSA 患者循环中 IL-6 的水平显著更高,产 SCFA 的细菌丰度减少,SCFA 具有维持肠屏障完整性的作用,SCFA 水平下降可导致肠道屏障功能受损。Poroyko 等研究显示 SF 小鼠肠道屏障功能受损,内脏脂肪及全身炎症水平增加,伴有胰岛素抵抗。间歇性缺氧小鼠模型即使经长时间的常氧恢复后(6 周),循环脂多糖(lipopolysaccharide,LPS)浓度仍然较高,LPS 是革兰阴性细菌细胞壁的一种成分,是内毒素产生毒性效应的主要生物活性物质,可导致肥胖和胰岛素抵抗。上述实验对象均存在肠道菌群紊乱,我们可推测间歇性缺氧/睡眠片段化或者肠道菌群紊乱致代谢物质的改变(如 SCFA 水平下降)致肠道屏障受损、通透性增加,肠道菌群代谢物通过受损的肠屏障进入循环或者菌群移位,激活炎症级联反应而致机体低度炎症状态,从而导致代谢性疾病。事实上,OSA 肠道菌群紊乱参与代谢综合征的可能机制众多,通过调节肠道菌群紊乱这一始动因素,可能预防 OSA 诱导的代谢综合征。

综上所述,目前在模拟 OSA 间歇性低氧/睡眠片段化的动物模型上发现了肠道菌群与 OSA 存在关联,有限的临床研究结果显示在 OASHS 患者中存在肠道菌群的紊乱,同时,研究显示它们可能通过各种途径导致 OSA 出现高血压、心脑血管疾病及代谢性疾病等并发症。由于肠道菌群在多种疾病的发生发展中起作用,且菌群的变化受很多因素影响,因此,有关 OSA 与肠道菌群的关系仍有待进一步的研究,特别是临床研究。

参 考 文 献

[1] Riha RL, Gislasson T, Diefenbach K. The phenotype and genotype of adult obstructive sleep apnoea/hypopnoea syndrome. Eur Respir J, 2009, 33(3): 646-655.

[2] Farré N, Farré R, Gozal D. Sleep apnea morbidity: A consequence of microbial-immune cross-talk?. Chest, 2018, 154(4): 754-759.

[3] Mashaqi S, Gozal D. Obstructive sleep apnea and systemic hypertension: Gut dysbiosis as the mediator?. J Clin Sleep Med, 2019, 15(10): 1517-1527.

[4] Lynch SV, Pedersen O. The human intestinal microbiome in health and disease. N Engl J Med, 2016, 375(24): 2369-2379.

[5] Poroyko VA, Carreras A, Khalyfa A, et al. Chronic sleep disruption alters gut microbiota, induces systemic and adipose tissue inflammation and insulin resistance in mice. Sci Rep, 2016, 6: 35405.

[6] Bowers SJ, Vargas F, González A, et al. Repeated sleep disruption in mice leads to persistent shifts in the fecal microbiome and metabolome. PLoS One, 2020, 15(2): e0229001.

[7] Moreno-Indias I, Torres M, Montserrat JM, et al. Intermittent hypoxia alters gut microbiota diversity in a mouse model of sleep apnoea. Eur Respir J, 2015, 45(4): 1055-1065.

[8] Albenberg L, Esipova TV, Judge CP, et al. Correlation between intraluminal oxygen gradient and radial partitioning of intestinal microbiota. Gastroenterology, 2014, 147(5): 1055-1063. e8.

[9] Moreno-Indias I, Torres M, Sanchez-Alcoholado L, et al. Normoxic recovery mimicking treatment of sleep apnea does not reverse intermittent hypoxia-induced bacterial dysbiosis and low-grade endotoxemia in mice. Sleep, 2016, 39(10): 1891-1897.

[10] Tripathi A, Melnik AV, Xue J, et al. Intermittent hypoxia and hypercapnia, a hallmark of obstructive sleep apnea, alters the gut microbiome and metabolome. mSystems, 2018, 3(3): e00020-18.

[11] Ko CY, Liu QQ, Su HZ, et al. Gut microbiota in obstructive sleep apnea-hypopnea syndrome: Disease-related dysbiosis and metabolic comorbidities. Clin Sci(Lond), 2019, 133(7): 905-917.

[12] Collado MC, Katila MK, Vuorela NM, et al. Dysbiosis in snoring children: An interlink to comorbidities?. J Pediatr Gastroenterol Nutr, 2019, 68(2): 272-277.

[13] Benedict C, Vogel H, Jonas W, et al. Gut microbiota and glu-

cometabolic alterations in response to recurrent partial sleep deprivation in normal-weight young individuals. Mol Metab, 2016,5(12):1175-1186.
[14] Liu Z, Wei ZY, Chen J, et al. Acute sleep-wake cycle shift results in community alteration of human gut microbiome. mSphere,2020,5(1):e00914-19.
[15] Zhang SL, Bai L, Goel N, et al. Human and rat gut microbiome composition is maintained following sleep restriction. Proc Natl Acad Sci USA,2017,114(8):E1564-E1571.
[16] Liu B, Lin W, Chen S, et al. Gut microbiota as an objective measurement for auxiliary diagnosis of insomnia disorder. Front Microbiol,2019,10:1770.
[17] Lu D, Yao X, Abulimiti A, et al. Profiling of lung microbiota in the patients with obstructive sleep apnea. Medicine(Baltimore),2018,97(26):e11175.
[18] Wu BG, Sulaiman I, Wang J, et al. Severe obstructive sleep apnea is associated with alterations in the nasal microbiome and an increase in inflammation. Am J Respir Crit Care Med, 2019,199(1):99-109.
[19] Durgan DJ, Ganesh BP, Cope JL, et al. Role of the gut microbiome in obstructive sleep apnea-induced hypertension. Hypertension,2016,67(2):469-474.
[20] Nutting CW, Islam S, Daugirdas JT. Vasorelaxant effects of short chain fatty acid salts in rat caudal artery. Am J Physiol, 1991,261(2 Pt 2):561-567.
[21] Yang T, Santisteban MM, Rodriguez V, et al. Gut dysbiosis is linked to hypertension. Hypertension, 2015, 65 (6): 1331-1340.
[22] Durgan DJ. Obstructive sleep apnea-induced hypertension: Role of the gut microbiota. Curr Hypertens Rep, 2017, 19 (4):35.
[23] Pluznick J. A novel scfa receptor, the microbiota, and blood pressure regulation. Gut Microbes,2014,5(2):202-207.
[24] Natarajan N, Hori D, Flavahan S, et al. Microbial short chain fatty acid metabolites lower blood pressure via endothelial g protein-coupled receptor 41. Physiol Genomics, 2016, 48 (11):826-834.
[25] Ganesh BP, Nelson JW, Eskew JR, et al. Prebiotics, probiotics, and acetate supplementation prevent hypertension in a model of obstructive sleep apnea. Hypertension,2018,72(5): 1141-1150.
[26] Carreras A, Zhang SX, Peris E, et al. Chronic sleep fragmentation induces endothelial dysfunction and structural vascular changes in mice. Sleep,2014,37(11):1817-1824.
[27] Cortese R, Gileles-Hillel A, Khalyfa A, et al. Aorta macrophage inflammatory and epigenetic changes in a murine model of obstructive sleep apnea: Potential role of cd36. Sci Rep, 2017,7:43648.
[28] Castro-Grattoni AL, Alvarez-Buvé R, Torres M, et al. Intermittent hypoxia-induced cardiovascular remodeling is reversed by normoxia in a mouse model of sleep apnea. Chest, 2016,149(6):1400-1408.
[29] Tang WH, Wang Z, Levison BS, et al. Intestinal microbial metabolism of phosphatidylcholine and cardiovascular risk. N Engl J Med,2013,368(17):1575-1584.
[30] Senthong V, Li XS, Hudec T, et al. Plasma trimethylamine n-oxide, a gut microbe-generated phosphatidylcholine metabolite, is associated with atherosclerotic burden. J Am Coll Cardiol,2016,67(22):2620-2628.
[31] Xue J, Zhou D, Poulsen O, et al. Intermittent hypoxia and hypercapnia accelerate atherosclerosis, partially via trimethylamine-oxide. Am J Respir Cell Mol Biol, 2017, 57 (5): 581-588.
[32] Koeth RA, Wang Z, Levison BS, et al. Intestinal microbiota metabolism of l-carnitine, a nutrient in red meat, promotes atherosclerosis. Nat Med,2013,19(5):576-585.
[33] Marchesi JR, Adams DH, Fava F, et al. The gut microbiota and host health: A new clinical frontier. Gut, 2016, 65 (2): 330-339.
[34] Cani PD, Amar J, Iglesias MA, et al. Metabolic endotoxemia initiates obesity and insulin resistance. Diabetes, 2007, 56 (7):1761-1772.
[35] Boulangé CL, Neves AL, Chilloux J, et al. Impact of the gut microbiota on inflammation, obesity, and metabolic disease. Genome Med,2016,8(1):42.

12 阻塞性睡眠呼吸暂停患者的炎症损伤与认知功能障碍

欧阳若芸 陈 燕

以往的研究表明,阻塞性睡眠呼吸暂停综合征(obstructive sleep apnea syndrome,OSAS)患者间歇性缺氧(intermittent hypoxia,IH)可引起神经元损伤(尤其是海马和皮质区),导致认知功能障碍。OSAS患者反复出现气道塌陷和阻塞,导致睡眠呼吸暂停和觉醒,从而出现IH和日间嗜睡(excessive daytime sleepiness,EDS),进而导致炎症的发展。而IH介导的炎症可能进一步引发各种类型的认知功能障碍。许多动物实验研究发现,抗炎药物可能对减轻IH引起的认知功能障碍有效。本文阐明了炎症损伤在IH介导的认知障碍发生发展中的作用机制,并对OSAS患者中两者关系的研究进展进行了批判性回顾。

一、OSAS中的炎症

OSAS的主要机制是缺氧和氧化应激(oxidative stress,OS),然而,一些研究表明炎症在其发生发展中也起着至关重要的作用。OSAS患者因慢性间歇性低氧血症(chronic intermittent hypoxia,CIH)、持续缺氧、OS、睡眠碎片化和剥夺而表现为全身和局部炎症。

(一)OSAS的炎症生物标志物水平

许多研究表明,OSAS可导致患者全身和局部炎症。一项荟萃分析指出,OSAS患者的C反应蛋白(C-reactive protein,CRP)、肿瘤坏死因子α(tumor necrosis factor-α,TNF-α)、白介素-6(interleukin-6,IL-6)、白介素-8(interleukin-8,IL-8)、细胞间黏附分子(intercellular adhesion molecules,ICAM)、血管细胞黏附分子(vascular cell adhesion molecule,VCAM)和选择素水平明显升高,表达最突出的炎症因子为IL-1、IL-6和CRP。此外,细胞因子水平的变化与患者的年龄、体重指数(body mass index,BMI)和呼吸暂停低通气指数(apnea hypopnea index,AHI)密切相关。

TNF-α参与睡眠调节,促进非快速眼动睡眠,其在人体内的浓度呈现出昼夜节律性。在经历睡眠碎片化和剥夺后,TNF-α水平增加。Bozic等筛选了50名新诊断的OSAS患者和25名健康对照者,结果显示重度OSAS组的TNF-α、IL-6、高敏C反应蛋白(high-sensitivity C-reactive protein,hsCRP)水平明显高于中度组和健康对照组。

IL-6因可引起血管炎症、促进心血管疾病、糖尿病和认知功能恶化而备受关注;而tau蛋白是一种微管相关蛋白,对正常神经元活动至关重要,且与β淀粉样蛋白(amyloid beta,Aβ)一起参与了神经退行性变和神经元死亡。

CIH可通过上调OSAS患者的tau蛋白磷酸化水平来增加总tau蛋白含量。Motamedi团队研究发现与对照组和轻度OSAS组相比,重度OSAS组tau蛋白和IL-6浓度显著升高。

此外,Svatikova等对OSAS患者的主要急性期血清淀粉样蛋白A(serum amyloid A,SAA)的研究提示中重度OSAS患者的SAA水平比健康人和轻度OSAS患者高出2.5倍,并发现OSAS组正五聚体蛋白-3(pentraxin-3,PTX-3)、IL-33及其可溶性受体ST2(soluble receptor ST2,sST2)的水平均高于对照组,而其他细胞因子如降钙素原(procalcitonin,ProCT)和CRP在各组中呈现了相似水平。

(二)CPAP治疗后的炎症水平

持续气道正压(continuous positive airway pressure,CPAP)通常被认为是OSAS患者的一线疗法。

一些研究表明,经CPAP治疗后OSAS患者的炎症水平显著下降。最近的一项荟萃分析提示,CPAP治疗能显著降低OSAS患者CRP、IL-6、IL-8和TNF-α的水平。更长的治疗时间(>3个月)和足够的依从性(≥4小时/夜)也能更有效地减轻全身性炎症。Schiza等对患者12个月随访期内的CRP水平进行了测定,结果显示CRP浓度在第3个月时逐渐下降,第6个月时急剧下降,此后趋于平稳。Steiropoulos等予以OSAS患者CPAP治疗6个月后,将其分为高依从性组(平均CPAP使用量≥4小时/夜)和低依从性组(平均CPAP使用量<4小时/夜),发现仅前者的血清TNF-α、尿酸(uric acid,UA)水平及CD4$^+$细胞计数有所下降。这些数据表明,只有充足时间的CPAP治疗才能使得机体的炎症水平得到改善。Jin团队的研究发现,OSAS组IL-8、TNF-α、CRP、ICAM-1、VCAM-1和选择素水平升高,而在3个月的CPAP治疗后,炎症因子明显降低。此外,Lu等发现OSAS患者升高的核因子-κB(nuclear factor kappa B,NF-κB)和缺氧诱导因子-1α(hypoxia-inducible factor-1α,HIF-1α)水平在CPAP治疗后下降。然而,许多研究未能证实CPAP治疗对炎症标志物水平有任何显著影响。因此,我们需要更多治疗时间长、依从性好的随机对照实验以阐明CPAP对OSAS患者炎症反应的影响。

(三)OSAS的炎症机制

近几年越来越多的证据表明,OSAS应被视为低级别的慢性炎症性疾病。缺氧和炎症之间存在密切联系。HIF-1α是缺氧诱导的关键转录因子,可激活诱导型一氧化氮合酶(inducible nitric oxide synthase,iNOS)基因表达,促进一氧化氮(nitric oxide,NO)合成。而 NO 在炎症过程的启动和调节中起着关键作用。一些研究表明,OSAS 患者缺氧可能导致脂肪组织炎症,从而产生胰岛素抵抗。瘦素是肥胖的典型生物标志物,主要在白色脂肪组织中产生,在 OSAS 患者中也有所增加。IH 是瘦素的强刺激因子,瘦素水平的失调会促进 OS 和 IL-6 和 TNF-α 的生成,这是 OSAS 独立诱导的。CRP 和 TNF-α 可上调 NF-κB 的转录活性,导致内皮细胞中 VCAM-1 和单核细胞趋化蛋白-1(monocyte chemoattractant protein-1,MCP-1)的表达增加,使得单核细胞-内皮细胞黏附,加剧内皮细胞的炎症反应。

二、OSAS 的认知损害

认知功能是人脑接受外界信息,对其进行加工,然后将其转化为一种内在的心理活动,从而获得知识并加以运用的过程。它包括记忆、注意、推理、语言、计算、执行和视觉空间功能等心理过程,是人类高级神经功能的重要组成部分。OSAS 已被证实可促进认知功能障碍的的产生和发展。无论是成人还是儿童,OSAS 患者的神经认知功能损害都会对其生活质量、学习和工作效率及医疗保健产生不利影响。

(一)OSAS 患者的脑组织损伤与认知功能障碍

OSAS 在广泛认知功能障碍的发生和发展中起着关键作用:如注意力和警惕性、言语和视觉延迟的长期记忆、视觉空间或构造能力及执行功能等。

越来越多的研究表明 OSAS 患者的认知功能障碍与大脑各区域广泛的结构改变相关,如灰质和白质、海马体、丘脑、大脑皮质、脑干、基底节、额叶、颞叶、枕叶和边缘叶、额叶上回、扣带回和小脑。研究发现,灰质和白质完整性的受损与信息处理速度减慢、情绪功能异常甚至是与记忆、注意力和执行功能等认知功能受损相关。此外,OSAS 患者睡眠时 IH 可使得海马结构凋亡和萎缩,从而导致学习、记忆、注意和执行功能的缺陷。Macey 等发现在新诊断、未经治疗的 OSAS 患者中,表现出性别特异性的海马区域体积发生了改变。Cross 等使用磁共振成像(magnetic resonance imaging,MRI)评估了有或无 OSAS 的老年人大脑皮质的厚度和皮质下体积。结果表明,氧饱和度降低与颞叶皮质厚度减少明显关联,从而导致了语言编码的减少。睡眠障碍与右侧中央后回、距状旁回和岛盖部厚度增加及海马体和杏仁核体积增加有关。根据上述两项研究,人们提出一个假说,即皮质厚度的增加和皮质下体积的增大可理解为是一种反应性或适应不良造成的增生或肥大,如脑水肿、炎症、胶质细胞活化甚至是 Aβ 沉积。病变过程中可能因神经细胞的凋亡和神经组织的萎缩,从而导致厚度和体积减少。这种差异提示 OSAS 对大脑完整性的损害可能存在一个明显的时间进程。Canessa 等证实了治疗后认知缺陷的可逆性和相应的脑形态学变化,他们发现左侧海马(内嗅皮质)、左侧后顶叶皮质及右侧额叶上回的灰质体积减少。治疗后,以上区域体积的增加与言语和视觉空间短期记忆、注意力及执行功能的改善有关。因此,坚持 CPAP 和手术等治疗方法不仅可以改善临床症状,还能促进大脑结构的恢复。

(二)OSAS 患者认知功能损伤机制

对 OSAS 和认知缺陷的前瞻性研究及来自观察和实验性研究的结果表明,睡眠片段化和低氧血症是认知功能下降的两个最可能的危险因素。

反复发作的的夜间呼吸暂停导致睡眠中反复觉醒,随后出现 EDS,这是 OSAS 患者的特征之一。最近的一篇综述提示,睡眠片段化和 EDS 主要影响注意力、警惕性、学习和记忆功能,并且缺氧被证明是额叶损伤和执行功能缺陷的重要预测因子。许多研究表明,OSAS 间歇慢性缺氧可能会导致大脑多个区域的神经元损伤,尤其是海马和额叶皮质,从而导致注意力减退、处理速度减慢和执行功能受损。在一项动物研究中,暴露于 CIH 的小鼠脑源性神经营养因子(brain-derived neurotrophic factor,BDNF)的表达显著降低,而 BDNF 水平的下降是导致海马长期可塑性和记忆功能受损的关键因素。

三、炎症在 OSAS 认知功能障碍发展中的作用

与身体其他部位相比,大脑需要消耗更多的能量和氧气,对缺氧更敏感。缺氧导致 OSAS 患者炎症的激活,炎症使得脑内的内皮细胞功能障碍和动脉粥样硬化,从而减少脑血流量,降低神经元的代谢功能和耗氧量。这些变化又可引发神经细胞凋亡和坏死,继而产生各种认知功能障碍。

(一)OSAS 患者炎症与认知功能障碍的关系

Huang 等对 47 名非肥胖 OSAS 儿童和 32 名健康对照儿童的促炎细胞因子和认知状态进行了研究,实验提示 CRP、TNF-α、IL-17 和 IL-23 等细胞因子升高与注意力不集中和警觉能力受损有关。此外,TNF-α、IL-6 和 IL-23 水平升高与执行功能下降有关。Sun 等发现 OSAS 患者的视觉空间、注意力、执行功能和延迟记忆功能都有明显的损伤,重度 OSAS 组 hsCRP、瘦素和 TNF-α 水平升高。在校正 BMI、年龄和教育年限等混杂因素后,蒙特利尔认知评估量表(Montreal cognitive assessment,MoCA)评分与 AHI、氧减饱和度指数(oxygen desaturation index,ODI)及 TNF-α 呈负相关,与最低血氧饱和度正相关。值得注意的是,经 CPAP 治疗后 OSAS 患者的炎症和认知功能障碍均得到了改善。在另一项由 Haensel 等进行的研究中纳入了 39 名未经治疗的 OSAS 患者,他们发现可溶性肿瘤坏死因子受体 1(soluble tumor necrosis factor receptor 1,sTNF-R1)与认知功能受损有关,提示 sTNF-R1 是认知状态的一个重要预测因子。综上所述,以上研究结果表明炎症水平的升高至少部分地促成了 CIH 介导的神经元损伤和认知功能障碍。

(二)CIH 动物中炎症与认知功能障碍的关系

迄今为止,CIH 小鼠已被广泛应用于揭示 OSAS 认知障碍的潜在机制。Dong 等发现七氟烷通过下调海马过氧化物酶体增殖物激活受体 γ(peroxisome proliferators-activated receptor γ,PPAR-γ),扩大了 CIH 大鼠小胶质细胞介导的神经炎症,并且加重了认知功能障碍。在 IH 暴露

和应用七氟烷后,采用 Morris 水迷宫实验检测大鼠的空间学习记忆能力,以及测定海马区 TNF-α、IL-1-α 等促炎因子水平和小胶质细胞活性。结果表明,CIH 大鼠海马内小胶质细胞活性、TNF-α、IL-1-α 水平均升高,而 CIH+七氟烷大鼠海马内升高更明显。值得注意的是,与 CIH 组相比,CIH+七氟烷组大鼠表现出更长的逃避潜伏期来定位隐藏的平台,在目标象限的时间也更少。因此,被七氟烷加重的由小胶质细胞介导的神经炎症在 CIH 诱导的认知功能缺陷的发病机制中起重要作用。Shi 等发现 IH 暴露后,小胶质细胞活性、NF-κB-p65,TNF-α 和 IL-1β 水平及海马神经元凋亡显著增加,另外,他们还发现在体外激活的小胶质细胞中高迁移率蛋白 1(high mobility group box 1,HMGB1)的分泌显著增多。

Darnall 等发现,暴露于 IH 的幼鼠血浆 Gro/CXCL1 水平升高,以及小脑干扰素-γ(interferon-γ,IFN-γ)和 IL-1β 水平升高。此外,与对照组相比,IH 组大鼠髓质中(由神经元死亡和脑外伤后释放)神经元特异性烯醇化酶(neuron-specific enolase,NSE)水平较高。这些发现提示,缺氧介导的炎症和脑损伤可能表现为迟发的执行力缺陷。同样,Block 等解剖了 IH 大鼠的皮质、髓质和脊髓组织,以测定在炎症调节中起重要作用的炎性细胞因子 Toll 样受体 4(toll-like receptor 4,TLR4)的 mRNA 水平。结果表明,IH 干预增强了不同脑区炎症基因的表达,包括 iNOS、环氧合酶 2(cyclooxygenase-2,COX-2)、TNF-α、IL-1β 和 IL-6。此外,因 IH 显著上调的 TLR4 的 mRNA 水平和 TLR4 表达的增加与炎症基因表达高峰的时间一致,提示 TLR4 是 IH 诱导炎症的重要因素。

(三)炎症导致认知功能障碍的深入机制探寻

如前所述,OSAS 中炎症与认知功能障碍密切相关。而过度炎症反应可导致认知功能受损已在许多其他疾病的研究中得到了证实,如脓毒症、阿尔茨海默病、术后认知功能障碍(post-operative cognitive dysfunction,POCD)、脑外伤和脊髓损伤。由此,我们可推断出 OSAS 中炎症是导致认知功能障碍的潜在机制。

血脑屏障(blood-brain barrier,BBB)是一种将中枢神经系统(central nervous system,CNS)与外周环境隔离的物理和生化屏障,它对维持大脑的稳态起着重要作用。由于 BBB 的保护作用,以前人们认为 CNS 不受外周炎症的影响。而现在越来越多的证据表明,外周炎症是通过损伤内皮细胞、破坏 BBB 的完整性和通透性而导致神经炎症的主要因素。许多研究提示,TNF-α 和下游 NF-κB 的释放可以破坏 BBB,促进巨噬细胞向海马体的迁移,激活胶质细胞,最终导致外周手术后的认知障碍。BBB 可选择性地通过大脑内皮细胞中的特异性受体和转运体转运一些炎症细胞因子,如 IL-1β、IL-6 和 TNF-α。炎性细胞因子也可以通过 BBB 不连续的室周区域进入大脑。

胶质细胞是 CNS 中除神经元外的另一大类细胞。小胶质细胞作为 CNS 的免疫细胞,在调节大脑炎症反应中起着重要作用。神经炎症具体表现为胶质细胞的激活。许多研究表明,CIH 和外周炎性因子的侵袭激活了小胶质细胞和星形胶质细胞,导致它们分泌细胞因子(如 IL-1β、IL-6、TNF-α 和 HMGB1)、氧化物、黏附分子和其他信号传导介质。小胶质细胞和星形胶质细胞产生的高水平细胞因子又可加重神经元轴突和突触损伤,增加脱髓鞘,并损害多个 CNS 区域白质的完整性。同时胶质细胞释放的细胞因子可以进一步破坏 BBB 并激活胶质细胞,导致恶性循环。有证据表明,手术动物模型中的炎症反应导致 BDNF 水平降低,这对神经可塑性至关重要。海马与学习和记忆功能有关,由于该区域存在大量炎症介质的受体(如 IL-1β 受体、TNF-α 受体和 HMGB1 受体),似乎对过度神经炎症反应特别敏感。这些研究使我们对炎症状态与特定认知功能之间的潜在关系有了更清晰的认识。然而,炎症导致认知功能减退的深入机制在 OSAS 中却鲜有提及,主要集中在其他疾病上,如阿尔茨海默病、POCD 和脓毒症。因此,需要进一步的临床和动物实验来阐明 OSAS 炎症介导的脑结构损伤和认知改变的确切机制和特异性信号通路。

(四)炎症介导的认知功能障碍的治疗新思路

一些动物体内实验表明,部分抗炎药物能有效地抑制炎症过程并改善认知功能障碍。在幼鼠侧脑室注射抗 HMGB1 抗体可抑制癫痫持续状态后海马区炎性细胞因子合成、小胶质细胞活化和神经元损伤。Terrando 等在手术介导的认知功能下降的动物模型中,发现阻断 TNF-α 可降低下游 IL-1 水平,从而减轻神经炎症和改善认知功能。Toll 样受体是一种重要的免疫受体,可与病原体相关分子模型(pathogen-associated molecular patterns,PAMPs)特异结合,介导炎症反应,几乎与所有炎症相关疾病有关。在阿尔茨海默病小鼠模型中,TLR4 拮抗剂的使用也起到改善神经炎症和认知的作用。非甾体消炎药(nonsteroidal anti-inflammatory drugs,NSAIDs)通过抑制环氧合酶(COX-1 和 COX-2)来阻断前列腺素的合成,从而抑制炎症活动。许多研究已经发现,在动物模型中使用非甾体消炎药,如布洛芬、扑热息痛和帕瑞昔布,可以改善高水平的细胞因子表达(IL-1β、IL-6 和 TNF-α)、胶质细胞活化、海马小胶质细胞增生和认知缺陷。

除上述抗炎药外,α₂ 肾上腺素受体激动剂右美托咪定可降低海马区 IL-1β、IL-6、TNF-α 和 TLR-4 水平,降低胶质细胞活性,逆转神经退行性变和神经元凋亡,从而改善认知功能。Deng 等发现调节 TLR4 表达的阿托伐他汀可减轻神经元损伤,并降低 TLR4 和海马内 TNF-α 和 IL-1β 等下游炎性细胞因子水平。从绿茶中提取的茶多酚(green tea catechins polyphenols,GTPs)可减轻 IH 诱导的空间学习缺陷。此外,GTPs 还降低了 IH 暴露动物的高水平炎症和 OS。Lam 等提出枸杞多糖(lycium barbarum polysaccharides,LBPs)对 IH 诱导的认知障碍大鼠具有神经保护作用,减轻了空间记忆缺陷。亮蓝 G 是一种选择性的 P2X7 受体拮抗剂,通过抑制 CIH 小鼠模型海马的炎症和 OS,可以防止 IH 诱导的神经细胞凋亡和空间学习障碍。替米沙坦是血管紧张素 II 1 型受体阻滞剂,对 CIH 所致海马损伤具有保护作用。Yuan 等发现替米沙坦治疗抑制了 CIH 大鼠模型外周血和海马体炎症和 OS 水平的升高,这一结果表明替米沙坦的神经保护作用可能主要是源于对炎症和 OS 水平的抑制。综上所述,以上研究开启了抗炎药物治疗 OSAS 炎症介导的认知损害的新思路,未来还需要更多的临床研究来验证。

四、结 论

OSAS 患者反复发生的气道塌陷和阻塞引起睡眠中的反复呼吸暂停和周期性觉醒,从而导致 IH 和 EDS,促进了神经炎症的发生发展和继发性认知损害。参与 OSAS 患者认知功能障碍发展的炎性细胞因子包括 IL-1β、IL-6、TNF-α、NF-κB、HMGB1 和 COX-2 等。抗炎治疗可减轻 IH 引起的神经炎症,改善神经认知功能。这些研究结果提示 OSAS 中炎症与认知功能损害之间存在密切关联,为 OSAS 认知功能障碍的治疗提供了新的思路。

参 考 文 献

[1] Nadeem R,Molnar J,Madbouly EM,et al. Serum inflammatory markers in obstructive sleep apnea: a meta-analysis. J Clin Sleep Med,2013,9:1003-1012.

[2] Bozic J,Borovac JA,Galic T,et al. Adropin and Inflammation Biomarker Levels in Male Patients With Obstructive Sleep Apnea:A Link With Glucose Metabolism and Sleep Parameters. J Clin Sleep Med,2018,14:1109-1118.

[3] Motamedi V,Kanefsky R,Matsangas P,et al. Elevated tau and interleukin-6 concentrations in adults with obstructive sleep apnea. Sleep Medicine,2018,43:71-76.

[4] Svatikova A,Wolk R,Shamsuzzaman AS,et al. Serum amyloid a in obstructive sleep apnea. Circulation,2003,108:1451-1454.

[5] Xie X,Pan L,Ren D,et al. Effects of continuous positive airway pressure therapy on systemic inflammation in obstructive sleep apnea: a meta-analysis. Sleep Med, 2013, 14: 1139-1150.

[6] Schiza SE,Mermigkis C,Panagiotis P,et al. C-reactive protein evolution in obstructive sleep apnoea patients under CPAP therapy. Eur J Clin Invest,2010,40:968-975.

[7] Steiropoulos P,Kotsianidis I,Nena E,et al. Long-term effect of continuous positive airway pressure therapy on inflammation markers of patients with obstructive sleep apnea syndrome. Sleep,2009,32:537-543.

[8] Jin F,Liu J,Zhang X,et al. Effect of continuous positive airway pressure therapy on inflammatory cytokines and atherosclerosis in patients with obstructive sleep apnea syndrome. Molecular medicine reports,2017,16:6334-6339.

[9] Lu D,Li N,Yao X,et al. Potential inflammatory markers in obstructive sleep apnea-hypopnea syndrome. Bosnian journal of basic medical sciences,2017,17:47-53.

[10] Murphy AM,Thomas A,Crinion SJ,et al. Intermittent hypoxia in obstructive sleep apnoea mediates insulin resistance through adipose tissue inflammation. European Respiratory Journal,2017,49.

[11] Berger S,Polotsky VY. Leptin and Leptin Resistance in the Pathogenesis of Obstructive Sleep Apnea:A Possible Link to Oxidative Stress and Cardiovascular Complications. Oxidative medicine and cellular longevity,2018,5137947.

[12] Devaraj S,Davis B,Simon SI,et al. CRP promotes monocyte-endothelial cell adhesion via Fcgamma receptors in human aortic endothelial cells under static and shear flow conditions. American journal of physiology Heart and circulatory physiology,2006,291:H1170-H1176.

[13] Feng YM,Thijs L,Zhang ZY,et al. Glomerular function in relation to circulating adhesion molecules and inflammation markers in a general population. Nephrol Dial Transplant,2018,33:426-435.

[14] Macey PM,Prasad JP,Ogren JA,et al. Sex-specific hippocampus volume changes in obstructive sleep apnea. Neuroimage Clin,2018,20:305-317.

[15] Cross NE,Memarian N,Duffy SL,et al. Structural brain correlates of obstructive sleep apnoea in older adults at risk for dementia. Eur Respir J,2018,52.

[16] Canessa N,Castronovo V,Cappa SF,et al. Obstructive sleep apnea: brain structural changes and neurocognitive function before and after treatment. Am J Respir Crit Care Med,2011,183:1419-1426.

[17] Zhou J,Camacho M,Tang X,et al. A review of neurocognitive function and obstructive sleep apnea with or without daytime sleepiness. Sleep Med 2016,23:99-108.

[18] Gagnon K,Baril AA,Gagnon JF,et al. Cognitive impairment in obstructive sleep apnea. Pathol Biol,2014,62:233-240.

[19] Xie H,Yung WH. Chronic intermittent hypoxia-induced deficits in synaptic plasticity and neurocognitive functions:a role for brain-derived neurotrophic factor. Acta Pharmacol Sin,2012,33:5-10.

[20] Huang Y-S,Guilleminault C,Hwang F-M,et al. Inflammatory cytokines in pediatric obstructive sleep apnea. Medicine,2016,95.

[21] Sun L,Chen R,Wang J,et al. Association between inflammation and cognitive function and effects of continuous positive airway pressure treatment in obstructive sleep apnea hypopnea syndrome. Zhonghua yi xue za zhi,2014,94:3483-3487.

[22] Haensel A,Bardwell WA,Mills PJ,et al. Relationship between inflammation and cognitive function in obstructive sleep apnea. Sleep and Breathing,2009,13:35-41.

[23] Dong P,Zhao J,Li N,et al. Sevoflurane exaggerates cognitive decline in a rat model of chronic intermittent hypoxia by aggravating microglia-mediated neuroinflammation via downregulation of PPAR-γ in the hippocampus. Behavioural brain research,2018,347:325-331.

[24] Shi Y,Guo X,Zhang J,et al. DNA binding protein HMGB1 secreted by activated microglia promotes the apoptosis of hippocampal neurons in diabetes complicated with OSA. Brain,behavior,and immunity,2018,73:482-492.

[25] Darnall RA,Chen X,Nemani KV,et al. Early postnatal exposure to intermittent hypoxia in rodents is proinflammatory,

impairs white matter integrity, and alters brain metabolism. Pediatr Res, 2017, 82:164-172.

[26] Block ML, Smith SMC, Friedle SA, et al. Chronic Intermittent Hypoxia Exerts CNS Region-Specific Effects on Rat Microglial Inflammatory and TLR4 Gene Expression. PLoS ONE, 2013, 8.

[27] Terrando N, Eriksson LI, Ryu JK, et al. Resolving postoperative neuroinflammation and cognitive decline. Annals of neurology, 2011, 70:986-995.

[28] Cheon SY, Kim JM, Kam EH, et al. Cell-penetrating interactomic inhibition of nuclear factor-kappa B in a mouse model of postoperative cognitive dysfunction. Scientific reports, 2017, 7:13482.

[29] Kiernan EA, Smith SMC, Mitchell GS, et al. Mechanisms of microglial activation in models of inflammation and hypoxia: Implications for chronic intermittent hypoxia. The Journal of physiology, 2016, 594:1563-1577.

[30] Hong S, Beja-Glasser VF, Nfonoyim BM, et al. Complement and microglia mediate early synapse loss in Alzheimer mouse models. Science(New York, NY), 2016, 352:712-716.

[31] Terrando N, Monaco C, Ma D, et al. Tumor necrosis factor-alpha triggers a cytokine cascade yielding postoperative cognitive decline. Proceedings of theNational Academy of Sciences of the United States of America, 2010, 107:20518-20522.

[32] Balducci C, Frasca A, Zotti M, et al. Toll-like receptor 4-dependent glial cell activation mediates the impairment in memory establishment induced by β-amyloid oligomers in an acute mouse model of Alzheimer's disease. Brain, Behavior, and Immunity, 2017, 60:188-197.

[33] Peng M, Wang Y-L, Wang F-F, et al. The cyclooxygenase-2 inhibitor parecoxib inhibits surgery-induced proinflammatory cytokine expression in the hippocampus in aged rats. The Journal of Surgical Research, 2012, 178:e1-e8.

[34] Zhao W-X, Zhang J-H, Cao J-B, et al. Acetaminophen attenuates lipopolysaccharide-induced cognitive impairment through antioxidant activity. Journal of Neuroinflammation, 2017, 14:17.

[35] Ning Q, Liu Z, Wang X, et al. Neurodegenerative changes and neuroapoptosis induced by systemic lipopolysaccharide administration are reversed by dexmedetomidine treatment in mice. Neurological research, 2017, 39:357-366.

[36] Deng Y, Yuan X, Guo X-l, et al. Efficacy of atorvastatin on hippocampal neuronal damage caused by chronic intermittent hypoxia: Involving TLR4 and its downstream signaling pathway. Respiratory physiology & neurobiology, 2015, 218:57-63.

[37] Burckhardt IC, Gozal D, Dayyat E, et al. Green tea catechin polyphenols attenuate behavioral and oxidative responses to intermittent hypoxia. Am J Respir Crit Care Med, 2008, 177:1135-1141.

[38] Lam CS, Tipoe GL, So KF, et al. Neuroprotective mechanism of Lycium barbarum polysaccharides against hippocampal-dependent spatial memory deficits in a rat model of obstructive sleep apnea. PLoS One, 2015, 10:e0117990.

[39] Deng Y, Guo X-L, Yuan X, et al. P2X7 Receptor Antagonism Attenuates the Intermittent Hypoxia-induced Spatial Deficits in a Murine Model of Sleep Apnea Via Inhibiting Neuroinflammation and Oxidative Stress. Chinese Medical Journal, 2015, 128:2168-2175.

[40] Yuan X, Guo X, Deng Y, et al. Chronic intermittent hypoxia-induced neuronal apoptosis in the hippocampus is attenuated by telmisartan through suppression of iNOS/NO and inhibition of lipid peroxidation and inflammatory responses. Brain Research, 2015, 1596:48-57.

13　ICU获得性衰弱与睡眠障碍的相关性研究

崔越亭　王蓓

ICU获得性衰弱（intensive care unit acquired weakness，ICU-AW）又称ICU获得性肌无力，是ICU患者（特别是ICU老年患者）常见的并发症之一，严重影响患者预后和生活质量。目前，ICU-AW的发病机制尚不明确，国内外现有研究表明ICU-AW是多种因素相互作用的结果。ICU患者由于患有危及生命的疾病、ICU环境、药物镇静或心理压力常导致睡眠障碍，睡眠障碍会产生两个互补的内分泌反应，包括合成代谢激素降低（胰岛素样生长因子1、睾酮和生长激素）和分解代谢激素升高（胰岛素抵抗、糖皮质激素和肌生成抑制素），从而导致蛋白质合成障碍及细胞分裂受阻。因此推测睡眠障碍可导致或加重ICU-AW。笔者就近年来关于ICU-AW与睡眠障碍的相关研究予以综述，以期为将来治疗和预防提供新思路。

一、ICU-AW

（一）ICU-AW概念、流行病学及临床表现

美国胸科学会将ICU-AW定义为"一种在患者危重时发生发展，危重病本身所导致全身性四肢无力的综合征"。包括危重病性肌病（critically illness myopathy，CIM）、危重病性多发性神经病（critical illness polyneuropathy，CIP），以及两者并存的危重病性多神经肌病（critical illness polyneuromyopathy，CIPNM）三个类型。研究发现，约有40%的重症患者发生ICU-AW，其中机械通气患者中约有25%发生ICU-AW，应用糖皮质激素患者中ICU-AW发生率为30%，神经阻滞剂应用患者中ICU-AW发生率约46%，全身炎症反应综合征（systemic inflammatory response syndrome，SIRS）患者ICU-AW的发病率更高达50%~100%，气管插管超过7 d的患者至少有25%会发生ICU-AW。ICU-AW临床表现为四肢对称性无力，脱机困难，腱反射减弱或消失，以四肢近端神经肌肉区域肌无力最明显，呼吸肌也常受累，而眼部及面部肌肉很少受累。因此，经常会观察到ICU患者很少或几乎不产生肢体回缩动作。

（二）ICU-AW相关危险因素

ICU-AW相关的危险因素包括：①制动：肌肉处于制动或无负荷状态时，肌肉纤维开始发生萎缩，长时间制动是导致ICU-AW的常见病因。②相关并发症：脓毒败血症，全身炎症反应综合征，多器官功能衰竭，高血糖和低蛋白血症等均会促进ICU-AW发生发展。③药物：糖皮质激素及神经肌肉阻滞剂的使用，药物的作用主要是影响肌细胞的兴奋性，以及激活肌肉蛋白质水解系统，导致肌肉蛋白质降解增加和肌肉无力。

（三）ICU-AW发病机制

1. 离子通道功能障碍　离子跨膜转运平衡形成静息电位，在静息电位基础上，通过离子通道开放和离子跨细胞膜转运，形成动作电位，激活肌细胞膜兴奋-收缩耦联过程。因此细胞膜离子通道失活及结构异常都将会影响肌细胞膜兴奋-收缩耦联。研究证实，电压依赖性钠通道和钙通道异常所导致肌纤维膜兴奋性下降及兴奋-收缩耦联障碍是ICU-AW的主要因素。另有研究发现，高钾血症和低氧血症可引起周围神经除极，也可导致ICU-AW的发生。

2. 微循环改变　CIP发生的主要机制可能是微循环障碍所导致的神经细胞损伤和轴突变性。研究发现，E-选择素在CIP患者外周神经血管内皮细胞中表达较正常人部分增多，E-选择素可增加微血管通透性，使有害物质从微血管中渗出，从而导致神经内膜水肿，影响周围神经微循环，同时渗出的有害物质也可导致线粒体功能障碍，进一步促进ICU-AW发生。

3. 肌肉失用性萎缩　在ICU中，肌肉失用性萎缩是指由于卧床休息、关节固定、肢体悬吊和机械通气而产生的外周骨骼肌和呼吸肌活动的减少。研究发现，在肌肉失用性萎缩的动物模型中，可以观察到肌肉质量降低和肌纤维横截面积减小。肌肉质量减少的程度可能与肌肉类型相关。研究发现，后肢制动动物的比目鱼肌和腓肠肌相比其他肌肉肌肉质量减少的程度更加明显。研究表明，I型肌纤维是人类日常生活中最常用的肌肉类型，而在肌肉质量减少的过程中，I型肌纤维最先丢失，这一发现可能与ICU-AW的发生相关。肌肉失用性萎缩的病理生理学基础为肌肉蛋白质合成与蛋白质降解之间失衡，导致肌肉蛋白质丢失增多，进一步引发ICU-AW发生。

二、ICU患者睡眠障碍

睡眠主要由两个系统调控：一个是调节24 h周期的生理系统，另一个是确保获得充足睡眠时间的稳态系统。在危重患者中，由于ICU环境、改变睡眠药物的使用、急性疾病（如脓毒症）和先前存在的睡眠障碍等，可能会影响这2个系统正常调节作用。因此，ICU患者经常伴有睡眠周期倒置、睡眠节律紊乱和睡眠效率低下等睡眠障碍表现。

(一)光照水平

在ICU内,日间光照水平范围为30~165勒克斯(lx),夜间光照水平为2.4~145勒克斯(lx),ICU内日间和夜间较高的光照度可改变ICU患者昼夜节律。研究表明,褪黑素是松果体在夜间分泌的一种激素,ICU夜间光照可减少褪黑素分泌,可能导致患者睡眠中断及昼夜节律紊乱。另有研究发现,ICU内严重脓毒症患者尿液中褪黑素代谢产物6-羟基硫酸褪黑素(6-SMT)的排泄无昼夜变化,提示ICU患者可能伴有昼夜节律紊乱及睡眠障碍。Gile J等对持续接受光暴露的动物模型发现,持续光照造成的昼夜节律紊乱可导致动物视交叉上核(SCN)中PER-2基因表达减少及发生精神错乱等。由此可得,ICU内较高的光照水平会导致危重患者睡眠障碍及改变患者精神状态。

(二)噪声

噪声是导致ICU患者睡眠障碍的重要因素之一。噪声最常见来源为医护人员对话、医疗设备警报和护理操作等。世界卫生组织规定医疗环境声级不应超过30 A加权分贝(dBA)。ICU中噪声大约为53~59dBA,峰值噪声大约为67~86dBA,并且ICU内白天和夜间噪声水平相近。研究发现,ICU噪声可降低患者睡眠质量并导致患者缺乏快速眼动(rapid eye movement,REM)睡眠,进一步可导致患者发生认知功能障碍。

(三)镇静

镇静药物的应用会使ICU患者产生非典型脑电图模式,在正常睡眠中很少产生这种脑电图模式。苯二氮䓬类药物和异丙酚是两种γ-氨基丁酸(GABA)受体激动剂,经常用于危重患者镇静。苯二氮䓬类药物可缩短睡眠潜伏期,但会影响睡眠结构,减少睡眠的慢波睡眠(slow wave sleep,SWS)阶段和REM阶段。危重患者通常使用镇静剂联合阿片类药物,阿片类药物同样会抑制SWS阶段和REM阶段,且呈剂量依赖性。Gehlbach等对静脉镇静和镇痛的ICU机械通气患者研究发现,患者有明显颞叶功能紊乱和正常睡眠脑电图严重缺失。右旋美托咪定是一种高选择性的α_2肾上腺素能激动剂,具有剂量依赖性的镇静、镇痛和抗焦虑作用。右美托咪定与其他GABA激动剂相比更能促进正常睡眠。研究显示,右美托咪定能够改善睡眠效率及改变睡眠模式,并能够增加夜间睡眠时间。但是,目前对于ICU患者睡眠障碍、昼夜节律紊乱和镇静剂之间相互关系的研究,仍然存在许多尚未解决的问题。

(四)免疫功能紊乱

褪黑素除了具有调节生物节律作用外,还在免疫反应中发挥着重要作用。研究表明,褪黑素与1型辅助性T细胞(Th-1)的特异性受体结合可促进促炎细胞因子产生与释放,并增强细胞吞噬功能和抗原呈递作用。ICU中光照模式的改变可干扰褪黑素生理分泌,导致ICU患者发生免疫功能紊乱。最近研究发现,在全身炎症反应综合征(systemic inflammatory response syndrome,SIRS)早期,炎症因子的暴露会激活线粒体PGC-1α和SOD2通路,从而抵消线粒体酶学的减少,补偿线粒体功能障碍,增强线粒体生物通路并减少氧化损伤;但SIRS后期且表现为ICU-AW的患者,股外侧肌氧化磷酸化水平降低50%伴有单核细胞和淋巴细胞数量的减少及细胞功能的减弱。该研究提示在SIRS早期和后期对骨骼肌肌肉代谢的影响是不同的,而免疫功能可能是造成这种现象的关键因素。由此推测,免疫功能低下可能会导致ICU-AW发生发展并且不容易被逆转。

(五)其他

1. 制动 ICU患者由于卧床休息、关节固定和肢体悬吊导致肢体活动减少,这会影响患者与环境之间正常的感觉互动。Huber R等对健康志愿者研究发现,短期上肢固定可以减少大脑皮质感觉运动区的局部突触活动,并且能够明显降低同一大脑皮质区域的慢波活动(SWA)。由此可得,制动可通过影响大脑皮质局部突触活动而使其睡眠调节功能发生障碍。

2. 机械通气 睡眠与机械通气之间的相互作用非常复杂。睡眠期间,机体通气需求和吸气做功减少,压力支持通气(PSV)过多会导致睡眠中断。最近的研究表明,在第一次自主呼吸试验(SBT)失败后,与正常睡眠模式患者相比,睡眠模式不典型且REM睡眠缺乏患者所需要的脱机时间更长。研究显示,与未通过SBT或通过SBT后但未拔管的患者相比,通过SBT并成功拔管的患者更容易产生正常的睡眠模式,并且通过SBT并成功拔管的患者通常在夜间接受较低剂量的镇静药物。由此推测,在夜间接受较高剂量镇静药物的患者更可能达不到脱机标准及不能通过SBT,或在临床评估后通过SBT但仍未拔管。由此可见,睡眠障碍可能会影响ICU患者脱机能力,但这种影响的作用机制及过程尚不明确。

3. 精神状态改变 神志不清的危重患者常伴有睡眠障碍。虽然睡眠剥夺被认为是导致神志不清的一个潜在危险因素,但神志不清本身也有可能导致睡眠障碍。SWS睡眠和REM睡眠减少被认为是导致神志不清的原因之一。睡眠障碍和精神错乱之间联系尚不明确,但它们之间可能有共同病理生理机制。

三、ICU-AW与睡眠障碍

肌肉蛋白质合成和降解失衡和细胞因子异常释放等都可造成肌肉萎缩、肌肉无力及神经传导障碍,导致ICU-AW发生发展。研究发现,在睡眠期间机体发生更多的细胞分裂、且所需要的时间更少,蛋白质合成具有明显的昼夜节律变化,并且在睡眠期间出现合成峰值,故目前公认良好的睡眠是愈合恢复的基础。睡眠障碍会导致合成代谢激素分泌减少和分解代谢激素分泌增多,从而导致蛋白质合成及细胞分裂受阻,进一步引发ICU-AW发生发展。

(一)胰岛素样生长因子-1

胰岛素样生长因子-1(insulin-like growth factor 1,IGF-1)是一种多功能细胞增殖调控因子,广泛分布于人体各个组织,在细胞的增殖分化和个体的生长发育中发挥重要的作用。REM期睡眠剥夺及夜间低氧血症可导致血清IGF-1降低。研究发现,IGF-1介导的信号传导可促进肌肉蛋白质合成。在肌细胞中,IGF-1与其受体结合后通过调节雷帕霉素靶蛋白(mTOR)来刺激磷脂酰肌醇3激酶

(PI3K)和蛋白激酶B(Akt)的激活,PI3K/Akt/mTOR信号通路的表达在肌肉肥大时上调,在肌肉萎缩时下调,表明mTOR途径可以促进肌肉蛋白质的合成。同时最近研究证实,mTOR对核糖体蛋白S6激酶1(S6K1)的磷酸化和活化起重要作用。由此推测,mTOR/S6K1信号通路可能控制细胞的转录、翻译、细胞的生长及蛋白质的合成。

(二)肌肉生长抑制素

肌肉生长抑制素(myostatin,Mstn),也被称为生长分化因子-8。Myostatin是一种主要表达于骨骼肌组织的分泌蛋白,可以抑制肌肉细胞的生长和分化,减少肌肉蛋白质的合成。睡眠剥夺可能会上调DNA损伤反应调节基因1(regulated in development and DNA damage response 1,REDD1)的表达并激活泛素-蛋白酶体系统,进而促进Mstn生成。Shaoting Weng等研究 *Myostatin* 基因敲除的小鼠发现,与对照组相比,*Myostatin* 基因敲除小鼠股四头肌和内收肌重量增加,*Myostatin* 基因敲除小鼠的肌纤维数量和体积明显增加,*Myostatin* 基因敲除小鼠组的体重增加明显大于对照组。由此推测,小鼠总体重的增加不仅是局部肌肉质量的增加,而且由于Mstn的减少,肌肉组织萎缩减缓,骨质量增加和某些激素分泌增加引起的。随后的研究还发现Mstn可以抑制细胞增殖相关蛋白的表达,并且能够上调细胞周期依赖性磷酸转移酶抑制因子,进而抑制成肌细胞从G1期向S期转化。敲除 *Myostatin* 基因可将细胞从G2期激活为M期,进而促进肌细胞生长和肌肉质量增加。

(三)生长激素

研究发现,慢波睡眠与生长激素分泌之间呈正向关系,并且随着年龄增长,老年人的生长激素分泌明显降低。生长激素通过促进氨基酸的利用来促进肌肉蛋白质合成,生长激素可进一步通过刺激IGF-1的产生来介导肌肉蛋白质合成。

(四)胰岛素抵抗

研究表明,在睡眠不足的健康成年人对葡萄糖的急性胰岛素反应明显降低,这表明睡眠减少、糖耐量受损和胰岛素抵抗增加之间存在联系。睡眠呼吸障碍,如阻塞性睡眠呼吸暂停,也与胰岛素抵抗增加相关。胰岛素抵抗可能通过抑制PI3K和Akt信号而导致肌肉蛋白质丢失。抑制PI3K/Akt导致肌肉蛋白质水解系统激活,如泛素-蛋白酶体途径和caspase-3,导致肌肉蛋白质降解。

(五)糖皮质激素

在骨骼肌中,糖皮质激素会降低蛋白质的合成速率并增加蛋白质的分解速率,从而导致肌肉萎缩。糖皮质激素对肌肉蛋白质分解代谢作用主要是由肌肉蛋白质水解系统(泛素-蛋白酶体系统,自噬-溶酶体系统和钙蛋白酶系统)的激活引起。糖皮质激素分解代谢作用的严重性和作用机制可能随着年龄的增长而变化,在老年人中尤为显著。部分睡眠不足会引起应激反应,从而增加血液中糖皮质激素水平,进而导致肌肉蛋白质降解增加。

四、小 结

ICU-AW会严重降低危重患者的生存质量,影响危重患者预后。ICU-AW的发生发展与多种危险因素有关,并且涉及多种病理生理机制。彻底了解与睡眠障碍相关的蛋白质合成减少和蛋白质降解增加所涉及的病理生理机制将有助于降低危重患者ICU-AW的发生率及改善危重患者的预后。未来的研究应该以监测危重患者的睡眠质量为主,并早期诊断ICU-AW,以及探讨ICU-AW和睡眠障碍之间是如何相互联系的。以期寻找更佳的干预和治疗位点,为ICU-AW的发病机制、预防或治疗提供新思路。

参 考 文 献

[1] Latronico N, Herridge M, Hopkins R O, et al. The ICM research agenda on intensive care unit-acquired weaknes. Intensive Care Med, 2017, 43(9): 1270-1281.

[2] Elias, Maya N, Munro C L, et al. Sleep and Intensive Care Unit-Acquired Weakness in Critically Ill Older Adults. Dimensions of Critical Care Nursing, 2019, 38: 20-28.

[3] Fan E, Cheek F, Chlan L, et al. An Official American Thoracic Society Clinical Practice Guideline: The Diagnosis of Intensive Care Unit-acquired Weakness in Adults. American Journal of Respiratory & Critical Care Medicine, 2014, 190(12): 1437-1446.

[4] Latronico N, Bolton CF. Critical illness polyneuropathy and myopathy: a major cause of muscle weakness and paralysis. Lancet Neurol, 2011, 10(10): 931-941.

[5] Hermans G, Clerckx B, Van Den Berghe G, et al. Interobserver agreement of medical research council sum-score and handgrip strength in the intensive care unit. Muscle & Nerve, 2012, 45(1): 18-25.

[6] De Jonghe B, Lacherade J C, Sharshar T, et al. Intensive care unit-acquired weakness: risk factors and prevention. Critical Care Medicine, 2009, 37(10 Suppl): 9-15.

[7] Zorowitz R. ICU-acquired weakness: a rehabilitation perspective of diagnosis, treatment, and functional management. Chest, 2016, 150(4): 966-971.

[8] Nardelli P, Vincent JA, Powers R, et al. Reduced motor neuron excitability is an important contributor to weakness in a rat model of sepsis. Exp Neurol, 2016(282): 1-8.

[9] Llano-Diez M, Cheng AJ, Jonsson W, et al. Impaired Ca^{2+} release contributes to muscle weakness in a rat model of critical illness myopathy. Crit Care, 2016, 20(1): 254-261.

[10] Kara Atila, Akin Sakir, Ince Can. Monitoring microcirculation in critical illness. Curr Opin Crit Care, 2016, 22: 444-452.

[11] Bolton CF. Neuromuscular manifestations of critical illness. Muscle Nerve, 2005, 32(2): 140-163.

[12] Reid M B, Judge A R, Bodine S C. CrossTalk opposing view: The dominant mechanism causing disuse muscle atrophy is proteolysis. Journal of Physiology, 2014, 592(24): 5345-5347.

[13] Baehr Leslie M, West Daniel WD, Marshall Andrea G, et al. Muscle-specific and age-related changes in protein synthesis and protein degradation in response to hindlimb unloading in

rats. Journal of Applied Physiology,2017,122:1336-1350.

[14] Suzuki Hideki, Yoshikawa Yuki, Tsujimoto Hisaya, et al. Clenbuterol accelerates recovery after immobilization-induced atrophy of rat hindlimb muscle. Acta Histochem,2020,122:151453-151460.

[15] Fitts RH, Trappe SW, Costill DL, et al. Prolonged space flight-induced alterations in the structure and function of human skeletal muscle fibres. The Journal of Physiology,2010,588(18):3567-3592.

[16] Collop NA, Salas RE, Delayo M, et al. Normal sleep and circadian processes. Crit Care Clin,2008,24:449-460.

[17] Verceles AC, Silhan L, Terrin M, et al. Circadian rhythm disruption in severe sepsis: the effect of ambient light on urinary 6-sulfatoxymelatonin secretion. Intensive Care Med, 2012, 38:804-810.

[18] Gile J, Scott B, Eckle T. The period 2 enhancer nobiletin as novel therapy in murine models of circadian disruption resembling delirium. Crit Care Med,2018,46:600-608.

[19] Simons Koen S, Verweij Eva, Lemmens Paul M C, et al. Noise in the intensive care unit and its influence on sleep quality: a multicenter observational study in Dutch intensive care units. Crit Care,2018,22:250-257.

[20] Gehlbach BK, Chapotot F, Leproult R, et al. Temporal disorganization of circadian rhythmicity and sleep-wake regulation in mechanically ventilated patients receiving continuous intravenous sedation. Sleep,2012,35:1105-1114.

[21] Lu W, Fu Q, Luo X, et al. Effects of dexmedetomidine on sleep quality of patients after surgery without mechanical ventilation in ICU. Medicine(Baltimore),2017,96:23-28.

[22] Papaioannou V, Mebazaa A, Plaud B, et al. Chronomics' in ICU: circadian aspects of immune response and therapeutic perspectives in the critically ill. Intensive Care Med Exp, 2014,2:18-26.

[23] Maestraggi Quentin, Lebas Benjamin, Clere-Jehl Raphaël, et al. Skeletal M-uscle and L-ymphocyte Mitochondrial Dysfunctions in Septic Shock Trigger ICU-Acquired Weak-nessand Sepsis-Induced Immunoparalysis. BiomedResearch International,2017,2017:1-12.

[24] Huber R, Ghilardi MF, Massimini M, et al. Arm immobilization causes co-rtical plastic changes and locally decreases sleep slow wave activity. Nat Neurosci,2006,9:69-76.

[25] Thille AW, Reynaud F, Marie D, et al. Impact of sleep alterations on wea-ning duration in mechanically ventilated patients: a prospective study. E-urRespir,2018,51:24-65.

[26] Younes M, Ostrowski M, Soiferman M, et al. Odds ratio product of sleep EEG as a continuous measure of sleep state. Sleep,2015,38:641-654.

[27] Pinzon Daniel, Galetke Wolfgang. Sleep in the intensive care unit. Som-nologie(Berl),2020,24:16-20.

[28] 徐雁,李舜伟,黄席珍,等. 阻塞性睡眠呼吸暂停综合征患者的认知障碍与胰岛素样生长因子-I间的关系. 中华医学杂志,2002,82(20):1388-1390.

[29] Dattilo, Antunes, H. K. M, et al. Sleep and muscle recovery: Endocrinologic-al and molecular basis for a new and promising hypothesis. medical hypotheses,2011,77(2):220-222.

[30] Ahmed Abdullah R, Owens Raymond J, Stubbs Christopher D, et al. Direct imaging of the recruitment and phosphorylation of S6K1 in the mTORC1pathway in living cells. Sci Rep, 2019,9:3408-3422.

[31] Weng Shaoting, Gao Feng, Wang Juan, et al. Improvement of muscular at-rphy by AAV-SaCas9-mediated myostatin gene editing in aged mice. Ca-ncer Gene Ther,2020:1-16.

[32] Hackett Ruth A, Dal Zeynep, Steptoe Andrew, The relationship between sl-eep problems and co-rtisol in people with type 2 diabetes. Psychoneuroendocrinology,2020,117:46-88.

[33] Reutrakul S, Van Cauter E. Sleep influences on obesity, insulin resistance, and risk of type 2 diabetes. Metabolism,2018:56-66.

[34] Wang X, Hu Z, Hu J, Mitch WE. Insulin resistance acceleratesmuscle prot-ein degradation: activation of the ubiquitin-proteasome pathway by defects in muscle cell signaling. Endocrinology,2006,147(9):4160-4168.

[35] Leproult R, Copinschi G, Buxton O, et al. Sleep loss results in an elevati-on of cortisol levels the next evening. Sleep,1997,20(10):865-870.

14 阻塞性睡眠呼吸暂停相关的恶性心律失常

王 彦

越来越多的研究表明阻塞性睡眠呼吸暂停(obstructive sleep apnea,OSA)是多种心血管疾病发病和死亡的独立危险因素,同时也可严重影响心脏的电活动,发生心律失常,其中恶性心律失常可在短时间内引起血流动力障碍,导致患者晕厥甚至猝死,从而造成严重后果。

一、恶性心律失常定义

恶性心律失常一般指短时间内引起血流动力障碍,导致患者晕厥甚至猝死的心律失常。根据心律失常的程度及性质分类的一类严重心律失常,也是一类需要紧急处理的心律失常。OSA患者中较多见的恶性心律失常主要包括室速(VT)、室扑、室颤(VF)、高度或三度房室传导阻滞(AVB)等。恶性心律失常可在短期内导致严重后果,是心源性猝死(SCD)的首位原因,临床应加强重视,早期识别和积极治疗。

二、OSA基于证据的恶性心律失常

1970年,MacGregor等首先报道Pickwickian综合征患者SCD的相对风险增加23%。1983年,Guilleminault等首次对大型OSA人群(400例)进行24h动态心电图同步多导睡眠监测(PSG),结果发现48%的患者夜间发生心律失常,其中8例持续性室性心动过速,43例窦性停搏(2.5~13s),31例二度AVB。75例频发室性早搏(PVC)(>2次/分)。50例因严重心律失常进行了气管切开术。1997年,黄席珍团队首先报道OSA发作时出现室性异搏占57%~74%,窦性停搏占9%~11%,二度AVB占4%~8%,并指出窦性停搏>3s应引起临床高度重视,当动脉血氧饱和度(SaO_2)<60%时可出现频繁的室性期前收缩或异位性心动过速。在频发OSA周期中,交感神经-副交感神经兴奋性不断变化,恢复呼吸一瞬间,副交感神经兴奋为主转为交感神经兴奋为主的过程中,可使心肌异位兴奋点阈值降低,这种心律失常是引起OSA患者猝死的主要原因。2000年丁殿勋等报道1例OSA患者在急性心肌梗死过程中引起高度窦房、房室阻滞和心脏停搏。另1例在急性心肌梗死基础上每有OSA发作便激发出VT和(或)VF,抗心律失常药和电复律效果欠佳。因此OSA可能不仅是冠心病重要危险因素,也是诱发心肌梗死和激发恶性心律失常较为直接的因素。

(一)快速性恶性心律失常

非持续性室性心动过速(NSVT)定义为连续3个或3个以上PVC,持续时间少于30s。Mehra等发现OSA患者NSVT发生概率为无OSA者的3倍,复杂性室性异搏(complex ventricular ectopic pulses,CVEP)的2倍,即使调整了潜在的混杂因素后,重度OSA患者夜间发生复杂性心律失常的风险为无OSA者的2~4倍。Wang等发现肥厚型梗阻性心肌病患者NSVT患病率随OSA的严重程度而增加(无、轻、中、重度OSA分别为12%、16%、33%和54%)。肥厚型梗阻性心肌病患者OSA的存在及其严重程度与NSVT独立相关,NSVT是该人群SCD和心血管死亡的危险因素。Selim等发现中重度睡眠呼吸障碍(SDB)患者CVEP(包括NSVT、二联律、三联律或四联律)和快速性心律失常(包括VT和室上速)的发生概率是无SDB者的2倍。Mehra等在2911例老年人群中发现SDB严重程度增加与CVEP的风险升高有关。SDB亚型分析发现CVEP与OSA和低氧密切相关。Monahan等调查了2816例SDB患者,其中2%的患者出现心律失常(其中76%为NSVT),且NSVT与先前的呼吸事件存在直接的时间关联。尽管心律失常绝对发生率较低(1次心律失常/4万次呼吸事件),但呼吸事件后90s危险期内NSVT的相对风险显著增加,是正常呼吸后的17.4倍。Koehler等的研究发现有SDB的慢性心力衰竭(CHF)患者NSVT发生率明显高于无SDB者(50%;19%),夜间NSVT的发生率约为白天的2倍,且呼吸暂停低通气指数(AHI)与NSVT相关,因此CHF和SDB的结合易诱发夜间恶性室性心律失常。但Abe等的研究结果发现OSA患者发生NSVT(无、轻、中、重度OSA分别为0、1.0%、1.5%、1.3%)、三度AVB(无、轻、中、重度OSA分别为0、0、0、0.1%)的概率不高($P>0.05$),可能与恶性心律失常发生次数太少有关。Javaheri发现持续性VT与OSA无相关性(对照组和OSA组中持续性VT患者的百分比相似)。Salama等回顾分析了美国3年住院患者18 013 878例,结果发现OSA组VT患病率(2.24%)显著高于无OSA组(1.16%),OSA是VT的独立预测因子($OR=1.22$)。OSA组VF患病率(0.3%)显著高于无OSA组(0.2%),但多变量回归分析后OSA组VF并未显著升高。

动物实验也支持OSA模式间歇低氧(IH)与恶性心律失常的关系。Morand等调查了IH对心肌缺血相关性室性心律失常的发展和严重程度的影响。在体内，暴露于 IH 的大鼠缺血诱导的致死性心律失常的发生率是常氧大鼠的 2 倍。IH 大鼠 VF 总体发生率 66.7% 明显高于常氧大鼠（33.3%）。在体外，IH 大鼠离体心脏在心肌缺血期间 VF 发生率 34.5% 明显高于常氧大鼠（4.2%）。IH 延长校正后的 QT 间期（QTc）和 T 波顶点到 T 波终末点之间的时间（TpTe 间期），增加心室单相动作电位持续时间（APD）梯度并上调心内膜 L 型钙（LTCC）、瞬时受体电位通道（TRPC）1 和 TRPC6 的表达。因此慢性 IH 通过交感神经激活和心室复极改变，透壁 APD 梯度和心内膜钙通道表达改变，促进心肌缺血相关的致死性室性心律失常。

（二）缓慢性恶性心律失常

有关 OSA 导致缓慢性恶性心律失常的研究很少。Maeno 等报道了一例 54 岁男性 OSA 患者，PSG 同时进行的 24h 动态心电图监测显示高度 AVB，心搏停止长达 6.4s。2015 年欧洲心脏协会指南中建议，心动过缓鉴别诊断时应考虑 OSA。睡眠呼吸暂停和 SaO_2 降低可能是 SDB 患者发生 SCD 的危险因素。

（三）置入式心律转复除颤器治疗

置入式心律转复除颤器（ICD）已经广泛应用于临床针对恶性心律失常的治疗，能有效防止院外 SCD 的发生。Bitter 等发现合并 OSA 的 CHF 患者午夜 0 时至凌晨 6 时发生 ICD 除颤电击事件增多，与恶性心动过速事件风险增加相关。Tomaello 等的研究纳入 22 例行 ICD 治疗的 CHF 患者，其中 17 例有 SDB。控制左心室射血分数（LVEF）和心功能分级（NYHA）后，ICD 放电次数与 AHI 正相关（$r=0.718$），与夜间最低 SaO_2 负相关（$r=-0.619$）。AHI 和睡眠中低氧严重程度是恶性心律失常风险的预测指标。Kwon 等对 9 项前瞻性队列研究进行系统回顾和 Meta 分析，评估 SDB 对 CHF 患者 ICD 治疗的影响，结果发现 SDB 与 ICD 治疗风险增加有关（$RR=1.55$）。他们的结论是 SDB 与 CHF 患者的心血管死亡率增加有关，其中恶性室性心律失常可能起重要作用。Bitter 等随访 255 例置入心脏再同步装置后 6 个月的 CHF 患者 4 年，发现中重度 SDB 患者首次监测到室性心律失常和首次心脏复律除颤治疗的时间明显缩短，发生恶性室性心律失常及需要适当心脏复律除纤颤治疗的风险增加，而且等待首次心脏复律除颤治疗的无事件生存期缩短。Raghuram 等的系统回顾纳入 20 项研究，包括 10 项观察性研究，8 项病例对照研究，1 个病例报告和 1 项 CPAP 干预性研究，OSA 导致室性心律失常的心电图预测因子（例如 PVC，QTc 延长，QTcd，T 波改变和心率变异）和 SCD 的风险明显增加。OSA 与 SCD 和适当 ICD 治疗的持续性 VT 独立相关。

（四）心源性猝死

一般人群中 SCD 风险从晨 6 时至中午达到高峰，从午夜至晨 6 时达到低谷。而 OSA 由于神经激素和电生理异常，可能增加 SCD 的风险，尤其在睡眠期间。提示 OSA 和 SCD 之间存在关联的第一项研究是由 Gami 等在 2005 年进行的。他们发现从午夜至凌晨 6 时，46% 的 OSA 患者发生 SCD，明显高于无 OSA 者（21%）和总人群（16%），且 OSA 越严重，夜间 SCD 相对风险越高。Young 等对 1522 例 Wisconsin 睡眠队列进行 18 年的死亡率随访，发现随着 SDB 严重程度增加，心血管死亡率呈明显增加的趋势。未经治疗的重度 SDB 患者死亡风险最高（$HR=5.2$），且不受年龄、性别和体重指数（BMI）的影响。Lee 等发现韩国人 OSA 严重程度与心血管死亡率增加有关。重度 OSA 组心血管死亡率高于非 OSA 组（$HR=4.66$），调整是否接受治疗后仍高于非 OSA 组（$HR=4.19$）。Gami 等在接受 PSG 检查的 10 701 名成年人长达 15 年随访中发现，OSA 的存在可预测 SCD 发作，且 SCD 风险程度可通过 OSA 严重性的多个参数预测，包括 $AHI>20$（$HR=1.60$），夜间平均 $SaO_2<93\%$（$HR=2.93$）、最低 $SaO_2<78\%$（$HR=2.60$）。这些发现提示 OSA 是 SCD 新的危险因素。Shamsuzzaman 等发现先天性长 QT 综合征（LQTS）患者的 OSA 的存在和严重程度与经心率校正的 QT 延长的程度有关，这是 SCD 的重要生物标志。治疗 LQTS 患者的 OSA 可降低 QT 延长，从而降低长 QT 触发 SCD 的风险。Kerns 等前瞻性调查了 558 名血液透析患者中 OSA 与心血管死亡率和 SCD 的相关性，结果发现 OSA 的血液透析患者心血管死亡率和 SCD 的风险增加。在调整了人口统计学和 BMI 后，OSA 与心血管死亡率的高风险相关。调整人口统计学和多种心血管危险因素后，OSA 与 SCD 高风险相关。因此未来的研究应筛查 OSA 并评估以 OSA 为目标的干预措施对终末期肾病死亡率的影响。Koo 等发现冠状动脉旁路移植术患者睡眠呼吸暂停与主要心脑血管不良事件（包括心血管死亡率、SCD 或心脏骤停复苏等）增加独立相关。

三、OSA 诱导恶性心律失常的机制

OSA 通过多种机制导致复杂性心肌损伤。关键因素包括 OSA 相关的自主神经系统波动，其典型特征是呼吸事件时副交感神经活动增强，以及呼吸事件后交感神经活动突然增加，这导致心律失常倾向增加。OSA 诱导心律失常的更直接的病理生理影响包括 IH 和高碳酸血症、睡眠片段和胸内压力波动导致心肌舒张。OSA 可能引发心律失常的中间途径包括全身炎症反应、氧化应激、促血栓形成通路上调和血管内皮功能障碍。这些机制导致心室肥大和功能障碍，在组织和细胞水平上表现为多灶性梗死、心肌细胞肥大、细胞凋亡和炎性浸润。长期 OSA 可引起心脏结构和电重构，导致高血压、心室肥大、纤维化和冠状动脉疾病也易导致室性心律失常。

（一）自主神经功能失衡

OSA 患者连续的自主神经改变可导致恶性心律失常易感性增强。呼吸暂停事件中迷走神经活动增强导致心动过缓，副交感神经系统的激活还可导致 QTc 延长和心室复极异质性增加，表现为 QTc 离散度增加，增加室性心律失常和心脏猝死的风险。随后呼吸暂停结束上气道张力恢复后，继于呼吸中枢交感神经耦合、低氧血症、高碳酸血症和正常肺反射启动交感抑制作用缺乏，引发强烈的交感神经系统反应，导致心动过速和左心室后负荷激增。重

度OSA患者不仅夜间交感神经活动增加，而且白天的交感神经活动也增加。交感神经张力增加导致心率和血压升高，常发生室性异位搏动，副交感神经兴奋转为交感神经兴奋时，迷走神经抑制恶性心律失常的保护作用减弱，室颤阈值降低，易发生恶性心律失常，导致猝死。此外，局部心脏舒张反射和压力反射也可能起作用。

(二) 间歇低氧

低氧血症直接刺激颈动脉体的化学感受器，促进通气和交感神经放电。此外，低氧会导致周围血管收缩，从而增加前负荷和后负荷，改变心室复极化并增加左心室心内膜钙通道的表达，促进心肌缺血时SCD的发生和发展。此外，上气道阻塞终止后再氧合可能导致活性氧簇（ROS）形成。由于钙通道活性改变和微血管缺血，ROS的产生与心律失常有关。

(三) 胸内压力变化

正常人吸气时胸内压通常为$-8cmH_2O$，而OSA患者上气道阻塞产生的胸内负压$<-30cmH_2O$。OSA由于反复的上呼吸道阻塞，导致胸内压力剧烈波动，增加右心室的静脉回流和左室后负荷，降低左心室顺应性并增加心脏跨壁压力，这足以引起心室重构。在动物实验中，OSA期间胸腔内压力波动会导致心室复极变化，而中枢性睡眠呼吸暂停（CSA）则未观察到这种变化，并且主要是由交感神经激活引起的。

(四) 心脏结构和电变化

胸腔内负压增大、IH和长期OSA引起的全身性炎症反应和氧化应激上调可导致心脏结构和电重构。心室重构可能导致左右心室肥大，进而导致收缩和舒张功能障碍。反复缺血性损伤可能会促进心室纤维化。Jiang等的研究表明，OSA可以通过改变钾离子通道的正常功能，导致心肌细胞电位不稳定，从而改变心肌细胞复极，增加QT间期延长和心律失常事件，直至发生恶性心室事件。Sökmen等报道在呼吸暂停阶段TpTe间期、QT间期、TpTe/QT、TpTe/QTc呈增加趋势，在过度通气阶段呈下降趋势，提示心室复极参数的延长可能导致致死性室性心律失常，其研究结果揭示OSA患者睡眠期间可能存在心室复极参数的改变从而增加SCD的风险。

(五) 心肌缺血

低氧血症、心率和血压升高以及左室后负荷增加（由于交感神经活性增强和胸内压力增加）的结合，导致心肌耗氧量增加和供氧量减少之间不平衡。此外，OSA还可引起酸中毒、血管内皮功能障碍、全身炎症反应和氧化应激，这些都可能导致心肌缺血，从而增加室性心律失常和SCD的风险。

四、OSA相关恶性心律失常的心电图预测

可用于评估心室复极的参数是QT间期、QTc、QT离散度（QTd）和复极的透壁离散度，可使用体表心电图TpTe间期来评估。TpTe/QT和TpTe/QTc是代表心律失常的其他心电图指标。OSA患者不仅复极受损，碎片状QRS波（fQRS）是除极异常的标志物。研究已经证实这些参数与室性心律失常和SCD有关。

QT间期代表心室除极和复极的关系，包括折返性心动过速的易感期，它被认为是心室电不稳定的标志，是发生恶性心律失常和SCD的危险因素。QTd是心电图上最大QT间期和最小QT间期之间的差，反映了心室复极化和心肌电不稳定的不均匀性。校正后的QT离散度（QTcd）增加≥60ms是心脏死亡的一个独立的重要危险因素。TpTe间期测量心脏复极跨壁离散度，可通过从心内膜（最长）到心外膜细胞（最短）动作电位持续时间的梯度来解释。TpTe间期延长导致早期后除极的易感性增加，并与VT和SCD风险增加有关。未经校正的TpTe间期>100ms的患者发生SCD的风险增加。fQRS是结构性心脏病患者心血管死亡的预测指标，通过不均匀的底物和（或）局部心肌内/室内传导阻滞反映心室的电活动异常。异常的冲动传导通过折返机制为室性心律失常创造了环境。导致fQRS的机制之一是心脏结构中的细胞凋亡和间质纤维化，这可能是继发于慢性缺氧、代谢异常和氧化应激的结果。

Voigt等发现与健康人群相比，患OSA且无结构性心脏病的患者有更高的QTd或QTcd，这可能是SCD风险增加的标志。Panıkkath等发现SCD患者平均TpTe间期明显高于冠心病对照组。QTc正常者TpTe与SCD仍明显相关。因此得出结论：TpTe间期延长与SCD独立相关，是SCD的重要预测因子。Kilicaslan等也发现中重度OSA患者TpTe间期、TpTe/QT和TpTe/QTc延长。AHI与TpTe间期、TpTe/QT和TpTe/QTc正相关。Sökmen等的研究结果发现在呼吸暂停期间TpTe间期、QT间期、TpTe/QT和TpTe/QTc显著增加，而在呼吸暂停后过度通气期间显著下降。QTc间期在呼吸暂停期间增加，在呼吸暂停后过度通气期间仍持续增加。OSA患者这些心室复极参数的变化可能有助于解释SCD的潜在机制。Schmidleitner等回顾性评估100例准备接受冠状动脉旁路移植术（CABG）的患者，发现其中有SDB的患者TpTe、QTc间期、TpTe/QT延长。独立于已知的心律失常危险因素，SDB与CABG术前的心脏复极异常相关，提示SDB可能导致CABG术后发生恶性室性心律失常的风险增加。Morand等在麻醉大鼠中记录Ⅱ导心电图，结果发现IH诱导大鼠QTc、TpTe间期明显延长，心内膜APD50明显增加。Adar等的研究发现OSA患者（独立于肥胖）中的fQRS，提示心肌电重构。fQRS是OSA患者亚临床左心室功能障碍的独立预测因子，这表明它可以识别出可能存在明显心功能障碍风险的OSA患者。有fQRS的OSA患者中较高的C反应蛋白水平，提示炎症可能在QRS形态改变中起作用。

五、持续气道正压通气治疗

持续气道正压通气（CPAP）治疗缓解与呼吸暂停相关的低氧血症和睡眠结构紊乱，并消除胸内压力波动过大。CPAP在室性心律失常中可能的作用机制包括改善心肌氧

输送,降低交感活动、左心室透壁压和后负荷。通过减少需氧量和增加供氧量,CPAP 可预防缺血性心脏病患者的局部缺血或改善心室复极,并减少心脏交感神经通路。在 CPAP 治疗组中发现夜尿中去甲肾上腺素水平降低支持了这一点。另一种机制可能涉及心室负荷,消除其短暂的机械性扩张,从而减轻电机械分离。已经证明 CPAP 治疗能改善 OSA 患者的心脏参数,如心率、QTd、动脉压及每搏量。此外通过 CPAP 治疗,不良心室重塑和异位减少以及心电图标志物得以改善。

Simantirakis 等招募了 23 例中重度 OSA 患者,所有患者植入能监测心律的可插入式循环记录器持续 16 个月。CPAP 治疗前 47% 的患者夜间频繁发作心脏停搏>3s 和严重心动过缓<40bpm。CPAP 治疗 8 周后发作次数明显减少,此后随访 6 个月中未记录到发作,提示 CPAP 可显著降低严重缓慢性心律失常发作。Bilal 等发现重度 OSA 患者的 QTcd 明显高于对照组,且 QTcd 与 AHI、氧减指数正相关。CPAP 治疗 3 个月后 QTcd 显著降低(从平均 62.48ms 降至 41.42ms)。CPAP 治疗可缩短重度 OSA 患者的 QTcd,因此可降低心律失常和心血管疾病的风险。Dursunoglu 等发现 CPAP 治疗可显著降低无高血压的中重度 OSA 患者 QTcd,改善复极的不均匀性,从而降低心血管发病率。而停止 CPAP 治疗 2 周时 QTc、TpTec 间期长度明显增加,且停止 CPAP 治疗与 QTc、TpTec 间期延长有关,这可能为 OSA 和心律失常乃至 SCD 提供可能的机制联系。Yajima 等发现 CPAP 治疗后 R-R 间期接近正态分布,表明自主神经系统保持平衡。Javaheri 随访 29 例稳定期心力衰竭患者发现 CPAP 治疗无效者各种室性心律失常(VT、PVC、成对)每小时发生次数无显著变化。CPAP 治疗有效者各种室性心律失常减少,VT 从每小时 1.1 降到 0.05,PVC 从每小时 66 降到 18,但无统计学差异。Abe 等发现 CPAP 治疗可显著减少房颤、PVC、窦性心动过缓和窦性停搏的发生,但 CPAP 治疗前后 NSVT 和二度/三度 AVB 无统计学差异,可能与例数太少有关。Craig 等未发现 4 周 CPAP 治疗恶性心律失常的发生率显著降低。Raghuram 等的系统回顾提示没有足够的证据表明 CPAP 治疗显著降低 VT 或 VF。但间接证据表明 CPAP 治疗可预防 SDB 患者(特别是 AHI≥20)的室性心律失常。总体而言,CPAP 治疗的持续时间、治疗依从性、OSA 的严重程度和心脏病理学是影响 CPAP 治疗效果的重要混杂因素。

六、小　结

OSA 与恶性心律失常密切相关,OSA 的长期心血管损害及存在器质性心脏病是其发生的基础。OSA 相关的恶性心律失常诱发机制复杂,且引起特殊的心电图变化,一旦突然发作抢救成功率低,严重威胁生命安全和健康,必须加强重视、早期识别、早期干预。重度 OSA 患者在积极治疗原发病基础上早期应用 CPAP 治疗,避免发展为恶性心律失常甚至 SCD 的风险。

参 考 文 献

[1] MacGregor MI, Block AJ, Ball WC Jr. Topics in clinical medicine: serious complications and sudden death in the Pickwickian syndrome. Johns Hopkins Med J, 1970, 126(5): 279-295.

[2] Guilleminault C, Connolly SJ, Winkle RA. Cardiac arrhythmia and conduction disturbances during sleep in 400 patients with sleep apnea syndrome. Am J Cardiol, 1983, 52(5): 490-494.

[3] 牛楠,戴玉华,黄席珍. 阻塞性睡眠呼吸暂停综合征与心律失常. 中华心血管病杂志, 1997, 25(5): 330-333.

[4] 黄席珍,韩芳,慈书平,等. 睡眠呼吸障碍. 中国实用内科杂志, 1998, 18: 195.

[5] 丁殿勋,杨晔,康建利,等. 阻塞性睡眠呼吸暂停综合征引起冠心病急性发作并激发恶性心律失常三例报道. 天津医药, 2000(03): 140-142.

[6] Mehra R, Benjamin EJ, Shahar E, et al. Association of nocturnal arrhythmias with sleep-disordered breathing: The Sleep Heart Health Study. Am J Respir Crit Care Med, 2006, 173(8): 910-916.

[7] Wang S, Cui H, Song C, et al. Obstructive sleep apnea is associated with nonsustained ventricular tachycardia in patients with hypertrophic obstructive cardiomyopathy. Heart Rhythm, 2019, 16(5): 694-701.

[8] Selim BJ, Koo BB, Qin L, et al. The Association between Nocturnal Cardiac Arrhythmias and Sleep-Disordered Breathing: The DREAM Study. J Clin Sleep Med, 2016, 12(6): 829-837.

[9] Mehra R, Stone KL, Varosy PD, et al. Nocturnal Arrhythmias across a spectrum of obstructive and central sleep-disordered breathing in older men: outcomes of sleep disorders in older men(MrOS sleep) study. Arch Intern Med, 2009, 169(12): 1147-1155.

[10] Monahan K, Storfer-Isser A, Mehra R, et al. Triggering of nocturnal arrhythmias by sleep-disordered breathing events. J Am Coll Cardiol, 2009, 54(19): 1797-1804.

[11] Koehler U, Apelt S, Cassel W, et al. Sleep disordered breathing and nonsustained ventricular tachycardia in patients with chronic heart failure. Wien Klin Wochenschr, 2012, 124(3-4): 63-68.

[12] Abe H, Takahashi M, Yaegashi H, et al. Efficacy of continuous positive airway pressure on arrhythmias in obstructive sleep apnea patients. Heart Vessels, 2010, 25(1): 63-69.

[13] Javaheri S. Effects of continuous positive airway pressure on sleep apnea and ventricular irritability in patients with heart failure. Circulation, 2000, 101(4): 392-397.

[14] Salama A, Abdullah A, Wahab A, et al. Is obstructive sleep apnea associated with ventricular tachycardia? A retrospective study from the National Inpatient Sample and a literature review on the pathogenesis of Obstructive Sleep Apnea.

Clin Cardiol,2018,41(12):1543-1547.

[15] Morand J,Arnaud C,Pepin JL,et al. Chronic intermittent hypoxia promotes myocardial ischemia-related ventricular arrhythmias and sudden cardiac death. Sci Rep, 2018, 8(1):2997.

[16] Maeno K,Kasai A,Setsuda M,et al. Advanced atrioventricular block induced by obstructive sleep apnea before oxygen desaturation. Heart Vessels,2009,24(3):236-240.

[17] Priori SG,Blomström-Lundqvist C,Mazzanti A,et al. 2015 ESC Guidelines for the management of patients with ventricular arrhythmias and the prevention of sudden cardiac death: The Task Force for the Management of Patients with Ventricular Arrhythmias and the Prevention of Sudden Cardiac Death of the European Society of Cardiology(ESC). Endorsed by: Association for European Paediatric and Congenital Cardiology(AEPC). Eur Heart J,2015,36(41):2793-2867.

[18] Bitter T,Fox H,Dimitriadis Z,et al. Circadian variation of defibrillator shocks in patients with chronic heart failure: the impact of Cheyne-Stokes respiration and obstructive sleep apnea. Int J Cardiol,2014,176(3):1033-1035.

[19] Tomaello L,Zanolla L,Vassanelli C,et al. Sleep disordered breathing is associated with appropriate implantable cardioverter defibrillator therapy in congestive heart failure patients. Clin Cardiol,2010,33(2):E27-30.

[20] Kwon Y,Koene RJ,Kwon O,et al. Effect of Sleep-Disordered Breathing on Appropriate Implantable Cardioverter-Defibrillator Therapy in Patients With Heart Failure: A Systematic Review and Meta-Analysis. Circ Arrhythm Electrophysiol,2017,10(2):e004609.

[21] Bitter T,Westerheide N,Prinz C,et al. Cheyne-Stokes respiration and obstructive sleep apnoea are independent risk factors for malignant ventricular arrhythmias requiring appropriate cardioverter-defibrillator therapies in patients with congestive heart failure. Eur Heart J,2011,32(1):61-74.

[22] Raghuram A,Clay R,Kumbam A,et al. A systematic review of the association between obstructive sleep apnea and ventricular arrhythmias. J Clin Sleep Med, 2014, 10 (10): 1155-1160.

[23] Gami AS,Howard DE,Olson EJ,et al. Day-night pattern of sudden death in obstructive sleep apnea. N Engl J Med,2005, 352(12):1206-1214.

[24] Young T,Finn L,Peppard PE,et al. Sleep disordered breathing and mortality:eighteen-year follow-up of the Wisconsin sleep cohort. Sleep,2008,31(8):1071-1078.

[25] Lee JE,Lee CH,Lee SJ,et al. Mortality of patients with obstructive sleep apnea in Korea. J Clin Sleep Med, 2013, 9 (10):997-1002.

[26] Gami AS,Olson EJ,Shen WK,et al. Obstructive sleep apnea and the risk of sudden cardiac death: a longitudinal study of 10,701 adults. J Am Coll Cardiol,2013,62(7):610-616.

[27] Shamsuzzaman AS,Somers VK,Knilans TK,et al. Obstructive Sleep Apnea in Patients with Congenital Long QT Syndrome: Implications for Increased Risk of Sudden Cardiac Death. Sleep,2015,38(7):1113-1119.

[28] Kerns ES,Kim ED,Meoni LA,et al. Obstructive Sleep Apnea Increases Sudden Cardiac Death in Incident Hemodialysis Patients. Am J Nephrol,2018,48(2):147-156.

[29] Koo CY,Aung AT,Chen Z,et al. Sleep apnoea and cadiovascular outcomes after coronary artery bypass grafting. Heart, 2020 May 18:heartjnl-2019-316118.

[30] Marinheiro R,Parreira L,Amador P,et al. Ventricular Arrhythmias in Patients with Obstructive Sleep Apnea. Current Cardiology Reviews,2019,15(1):64-74.

[31] May AM,VanWagoner DR,Mehra R. Obstructive sleep apnea and cardiac arrhythmogenesis: Mechanistic Insights. Chest,2017,151(1):225-241.

[32] Farré R,Montserrat JM,Navajas D. Morbidity due to obstructive sleep apnea: Insights from animal models. Curr Opin Pulm Med,2008,14(6):530-536.

[33] Linz D,Denner A,Illing S,et al. Impact of obstructive and central apneas on ventricular repolarisation: lessons learned from studies in man and pigs. Clin Res Cardiol, 2016, 105 (8):639-647.

[34] Jiang N,Zhou A,Prasad B,et al. Obstructive Sleep Apnea and Circulating Potassium Channel Levels. J Am Heart Assoc,2016,5(8):e003666.

[35] Sökmen E,Özbek SC,Çelik M,et al. Changes in the parameters of ventricular repolarization during preapnea,apnea,and postapnea periods in patients with obstructive sleep apnea Pacing Clin Electrophysiol,2018,41(7):762-766.

[36] Hayashi T,Fukamizu S,Hojo R,et al. Fragmented QRS predicts cardiovascular death of patients with structural heart disease and inducible ventricular tachyarrhythmia. Circ J, 2013,77(12):2889-2897.

[37] Voigt L,Haq SA,Mitre CA,et al. Effect of obstructive sleep apnea on QT dispersion: a potential mechanism of sudden cardiac death. Cardiology,2011,118(1):68-73.

[38] Panikkath R,Reinier K,Evanado AU, et al. Prolonged Tpeak-to-tend interval on the resting ECG is associated with increased risk of sudden cardiac death. Circ Arrhythm Electrophysiol,2011,4(4):441-447.

[39] Kilicaslan F,Tokatli A,Ozdag F,et al. Tp-e interval, Tp-e/QT ratio, and Tp-e/QTc ratio are prolonged in patients with moderate and severe obstructive sleep apnea. Pacing Clin Electrophysiol,2012,35(8):966-972.

[40] Schmidleitner C,Arzt M,Tafelmeier M,et al. Sleep-disordered breathing is associated with disturbed cardiac repolarization in patients with a coronary artery bypass graft surgery. Sleep Med,2018,42:13-20.

[41] Adar A,Kırış A,Bülbül Y,Bektaş H,Acat M,Casim H et al. Association of Fragmented QRS with Subclinical Left Ventricular Dysfunction in Patients with Obstructive Sleep Apnea. Med Princ Pract,2015,24(4):376-381.

[42] Simantirakis EN,Schiza SI,Marketou ME,et al. Severe bradyarrhythmias in patients with sleep apnoea: the effect of continuous positive airway pressure treatment: a long-term evaluation using an insertable loop recorder. Eur Heart J, 2004,25(12):1070-1076.

[43] Bilal N,Dikmen N,Bozkus F,et al. Obstructive sleep apnea is associated with increased QT corrected interval dispersion:

the effects of continuous positive airway pressure. Braz J Otorhinolaryngol,2018,84(3):298-304.

[44] Dursunoglu D,Dursunoglu N. Effect of CPAP on QT interval dispersion in obstructive sleep apnea patients without hypertension. Sleep Med,2007,8(5):478-483.

[45] Rossi VA,Stoewhas AC,Camen G,et al. The effects of continuous positive airway pressure therapy withdrawal on cardiac repolarization:data from a randomized controlled trial. Eur Heart J,2012,33(17):2206-2212.

[46] Yajima Y,Koyama T,Kobayashi M,et al. Continuous Positive Airway Pressure Therapy Improves Heterogeneity of R-R intervals in a Patient with Obstructive Sleep Apnea Syndrome. Intern Med,2019,58(9):1279-1282.

[47] Javaheri S. Effects of continuous positive airway pressure on sleep apnea and ventricular irritability in patients with heart failure. Circulation,2000,101(4):392-397.

[48] Craig S,Pepperell JC,Kohler M,et al. Continuous positive airway pressure treatment for obstructive sleep apnoea reduces resting heart rate but does not affect dysrhythmias:a randomised controlled trial. J Sleep Res, 2009, 18(3): 329-336.

15 减重在睡眠呼吸疾病治疗中的价值

张立强

世界范围内肥胖发病率逐年升高,对健康和社会经济造成重大影响。从1980年到2013年,全球肥胖的患病率成人增加了27.5%,儿童增加了47%。全球21亿人超重(BMI>25 kg/m²),5亿人肥胖(BMI>30 kg/m²)。肥胖对呼吸系统影响众所周知,尤其可导致睡眠呼吸疾病,包括阻塞性睡眠呼吸暂停(obstructive sleep apnea,OSA)和肥胖低通气综合征(obesity hypoventilation syndrome,OHS)。肥胖在睡眠呼吸疾病发病起重要作用,肥胖和睡眠呼吸疾病可对机体多系统产生协同效应,增加并发症的发病率和严重程度,如高血压、糖尿病等心血管疾病危险因素。因此,肥胖管理即减重在睡眠呼吸疾病治疗过程中具有重要价值。

一、肥胖在睡眠呼吸疾病发病中的作用

肥胖是睡眠呼吸疾病的重要危险因素,同时也是主要的可调整危险因素。威斯康星州睡眠队列研究报告显示,BMI增加10%可导致呼吸暂停低通气指数(aponea-hypopneaindex,AHI)增加32%,或者患中重度OSA风险增加6倍。AHI变化与体重减轻程度并不一致,体重减轻10%导致AHI降低26%。肥胖影响睡眠状态下呼吸生理机制如下。

1. 脂肪组织沉积在腹部和胸部,导致肺容量减少,胸壁和肺顺应性降低,肺的静态弹性回缩压增加。中心性肥胖限制了膈肌的运动,胸壁扩张,尤其是仰卧位。除了胸壁的顺应性降低,肺本身的顺应性也降低。因为压缩的肺容积导致双肺底肺不张和小气道闭合,肺部僵硬增加。肺容积减少最大的是呼气储备量(ERV)。肺总量(TLC)在肥胖患者中受影响相对较小,在ERV降低的情况下,吸气量增加反映了这一点。在严重肥胖的情况下,小气道关闭,ERV处于最低临界值时,TLC和吸气量都开始下降。肺容量减少伴小气道关闭有效地增加维持通气所需的呼吸功。

2. 颈部肥胖对OSA发生有重要作用,独立于BMI。研究显示颈围这一人体测量变量与OSA相关最密切。颈部脂肪增加导致咽腔内压力增加,造成上呼吸道阻塞和塌陷。

腹部肥胖和肺容积减少也会降低上气道纵向牵引力,引发上呼吸道塌陷。

3. 正常睡眠通气不足伴发轻度、短暂性高碳酸血症,快速眼动睡眠(REM)期由于通气刺激反应降低,呼吸肌张力显著降低,通气降至最小潮气量。在肥胖患者,已经存在肺容量下降,呼吸功增加,呼吸肌力量相对不足,REM睡眠期通气量降低更突出。肥胖二氧化碳分压水平正常的患者可以持续增强呼吸驱动满足通气需求。持续高碳酸血症的肥胖患者中枢呼吸驱动减弱,通气反应降低,通气水平下降,不经治疗发展至慢性日间低通气。

4. 瘦素通常辅助增强呼吸驱动来克服增加的呼吸负荷,肥胖患者出现瘦素抵抗也可能降低中枢呼吸驱动而加重通气不足。

5. 睡眠呼吸疾病使肥胖患者中的炎症水平进一步升高,交感神经活性和间歇低氧引发的氧化应激反应增强,引起炎症因子反应,与肥胖多余脂肪组织产生炎症反应叠加,使IL-6、TNF-α和CRP水平明显升高。这种慢性低度炎症在OSA和OHS中都可促进胰岛素抵抗和血管内皮功能障碍,可能有助于心血管疾病发病率和致死率的升高。睡眠质量下降可通过饥饿素增强饥饿信号,通过瘦素降低饱食信号,导致食欲增加,高热量食物摄入,显示睡眠片段化可加重肥胖。

二、减重在睡眠呼吸疾病治疗中的价值

1. 减重应作为睡眠呼吸疾病的辅助治疗　除夜间治疗之外,减重可以改善呼吸肌功能、气体交换和血流动力学功能。减重可改善OSA病情,心血管与代谢并发症与生活质量。但很少能完全消除睡眠呼吸紊乱。

美国胸科学会(ATS)推荐OSA的减重治疗是参加综合生活方式干预,包括减少热量饮食,增加体力活动,以及行为心理咨询。这种综合生活方式干预能降低体重5%~8%,明显改善内科并发症。ATS和美国睡眠医学会(AASM)建议考虑药物或减重外科治疗肥胖相关的OSA。BMI至少为30 kg/m²或至少为27 kg/m²的患者有肥胖相关的合并症(包括OSA)应给予除生活方式干预以外的药物辅助治疗。已有证据表明药物对肥胖和肥胖相关OSA患者治疗有效,研究发现奥利司他可以小幅度明显降低体重而改善症状和生活质量,芬特明/托吡酯、利拉鲁肽使用数月可体重减轻,同时显著降低AHI。

减重手术是一种新兴的治疗肥胖的方法,表现为单独

干预降低体重效果最大。手术选择包括胃束带、袖状胃切除术、胃旁路术（Roux-en-Y）或胃分流术（RYGB/OAGB）或双胰分流术。胃束带能明显减轻体重，改善打鼾和日间嗜睡症状，但 AHI 与 OSA 病情无改变。新近一项荟萃分析表明减重手术对 86% OSA 患者有效。另一项研究显示胃旁路手术治疗 132 例肥胖患者，术后 12 个月 OSA 患病率从基线水平的 71% 降至 45%，78% OSA 患者病情减轻，45% 治愈。考虑治疗方案时，减重手术应该作为肥胖相关睡眠呼吸疾病的一种选择。

2. 减重与持续气道正压通气（CPAP）治疗相结合降低血压、血脂，改善胰岛素抵抗较单纯减重和 CPAP 更显著

一项研究将 181 例中重度 OSA 的肥胖患者随机分为 3 组，分别给予 CPAP、减重、减重结合 CPAP 三种治疗方式，治疗 24 周。结果显示减重、减重结合 CPAP 两种治疗方式明显降低 CRP 水平、胰岛素抵抗和血脂水平，单纯 CPAP 治疗上述三种指标无改变；三种治疗方式均降低血压；减重结合 CPAP 治疗改善胰岛素抵抗和血脂水平较单纯 CPAP 治疗更显著；治疗依从性符合要求的患者，减重结合 CPAP 治疗降低收缩压和平均动脉压水平较单纯减重或 CPAP 治疗更明显。此研究提示减重与 CPAP 结合改善肥胖相关 OSA 代谢与心血管合并症效果更好，可更好地起到肥胖睡眠呼吸疾病患者心血管疾病防控效应，改善预后。

鉴于 CPAP 既不能帮助减肥也不能令人信服地改善心血管疾病病情，积极控制肥胖对 OSA 患者至关重要。减肥对改善血压、胰岛素抵抗、血脂和血管炎症已得到充分证实。上述随机对照试验表明体重减轻导致心血管危险因素降低比 CPAP 疗法更突出，因此，强调两种疗法结合的重要性。

3. 减重对肥胖 OSA 患者嗜睡的干预效应

(1) 肥胖患者的嗜睡独立于 OSA：日间嗜睡、肥胖和 OSA 在发达国家是很普遍的现象。用 ESS 嗜睡量表测试 6%～12% 人群存在主观嗜睡。许多发达国家 60% 成人超重（BMI>25kg/m²），1/3 成人肥胖（BMI>30kg/m²），重度肥胖（BMI>35kg/m²）的患者约 30% 日间过度嗜睡。肥胖是 OSA 最大的风险因素，OSA 的发病率为 2%～4%，肥胖人群 OSA 发病高达 30%，所以，似乎 OSA 单独即可解释肥胖人群高发嗜睡。

肥胖与 OSA 密切相关，但是，反映 OSA 轻重程度的 AHI 却与反映主观嗜睡程度的 ESS 量表分值呈弱相关（$r^2<0.3$）。而且，许多 OSA 患者有效治疗 OSA 后仍有一定程度嗜睡，这种嗜睡部分原因可能是 OSA 造成觉醒神经元不可逆损伤所致。但是，肥胖可能是这种嗜睡的重要原因不可忽视。

尽管 OSA 是肥胖患者嗜睡的最重要因素，但是，几项研究已证实肥胖独立于 OSA 与嗜睡相关。有研究比较伴发和未伴发 OSA 的肥胖患者的嗜睡发生状况，发现两类患者嗜睡发生率类似。50% 不伴发 OSA、其他睡眠疾病或肥胖睡眠低通气的重度肥胖患者存在明显日间嗜睡。一项研究显示，重度肥胖患者多次睡眠潜伏期试验中潜伏期更短，多次小睡间清醒时间更少，睡眠时间更长，REM 睡眠更多。新近一项研究对医学中心减重手术的肥胖患者行 ESS 评分，显示 26% 轻度 OSA 患者与 32% 中重度 OSA 患者表现为重度嗜睡（ESS 评分分值>11），但 18% 既不伴发 OSA，也无其他睡眠疾病的肥胖患者也存在重度嗜睡。因此，提示肥胖本身即可致日间嗜睡，并非一定经 OSA 参与。

(2) 经治疗 OSA 患者的残余嗜睡：OSA 有效治疗后，大部分患者日间嗜睡会明显改善。日间嗜睡改善与使用 CPAP 的时间长短存在显著的剂量相关性。但是，相当一部分中重度 OSA 患者即使 OSA 得到充分治疗仍有嗜睡。12%～30% 使用 CPAP≥4 h/每夜的肥胖患者中仍有嗜睡。肥胖患者（平均 BMI=35kg/m²）甚至使用 CPAP 更长时间（每夜≥7h），经维持清醒试验测定 30% 仍存在客观嗜睡，20% ESS 量表分值仍异常。肥胖 OSA 患者存在如此高发嗜睡患病率，单纯源于 OSA 的不可逆损伤证据不充分，应探究可逆性过度嗜睡的病因。

(3) 减重手术对嗜睡的改善效应：日间过度嗜睡的 OSA 患者经减重手术治疗主观嗜睡会显著改善。一项研究表明过度肥胖的 OSA 患者（n=56）经减重手术（胃旁路术）治疗后 1 个月，体重按预期降低了 10～12 磅，同时 ESS 分值从术前严重嗜睡（14 分）降至正常（5 分）。另一项类似的研究显示腹腔镜胃束带术后患者（n=25，平均 BMI 53 kg/m²）ESS 分值从 14 降至 4（正常）。25 例患者中 17 例术前 ESS 评分分值异常（>10），而这些患者中 12 例正在使用 CPAP，术后所有患者停用 CPAP，但是患者 ESS 评分分值都在 10 以下。减重手术使 CPAP 治疗后 ESS 评分分值整体变化较小患者嗜睡改善至正常令人惊人，因为 Meta 分析表明 CPAP 治疗只能改善 ESS 评分 2 分，CPAP 改善 ESS 评分不明显，部分原因可能是纳入了嗜睡轻微的患者的缘故。减重手术改善嗜睡效应似乎更持久，一项研究显示 88% 的患者在减重手术术后 7 年仍维持日间警觉，无嗜睡。总之，减重手术可明显改善 OSA 患者日间嗜睡，但是，患者嗜睡的改善是 OSA 部分纠正的结果？还是饮食调整与外科手术致能量负平衡？通过什么分子机制改善了患者的觉醒状态？这些问题有待进一步回答。

(4) 肥胖导致嗜睡的 OSA 以外的机制。①肥胖与交感神经活性增强：肥胖的一个生理反应——交感神经活性增强可能扰乱夜间睡眠。肥胖和代谢综合征与交感神经系统（SNS）基础水平异常升高相关，交感神经系统活性增强有可能使睡眠片段化而导致白天嗜睡。肥胖，尤其是腹部内脏脂肪增加的肥胖患者有更多去甲肾上腺素释放到全身循环。另一项研究发现，肥胖易感大鼠去甲肾上腺素水平显著降低，下丘脑去甲肾上腺素转换减少，同时 α_2-肾上腺素受体结合减少，提示交感神经调节异常可能参与肥胖致嗜睡机制。②饮食诱导肥胖对觉醒的效应：动物实验研究表明高脂饮食可打破 24 h 睡眠/觉醒模式，伴随白天睡眠时间增多，与肥胖患者睡眠觉醒模式类似，尤其是，进食高脂饮食与高糖类饮食，动物身体活动并无差异，因此，高脂饮食导致的日间嗜睡不应归因于身体活动减少。长时间高脂饮食（6 周）动物 24 h 清醒时间较对照组减少 100min。清醒和睡眠状态转换的次数增加，而两种状态每

次持续时间减少。这种睡眠觉醒模式的变化随着调整至正常饮食,或减轻体重而恢复。另一项研究显示高脂饮食可延长小鼠的昼夜节律,这种节律延长只发生在第 1 周内,以后尽管体重有显著的增加,但节律没有进一步的变化,提示饮食结构也影响节律改变。这些研究表明高脂肪饮食和体重增加可能损害清醒和昼夜节律而参与肥胖患者的嗜睡发病。③代谢对觉醒的调节:觉醒主要受体内平衡、昼夜节律和代谢的调节。代谢调节与觉醒的神经生物学相结合进行觉醒的调节。总体而言,最佳觉醒状态需要睡眠活跃神经元群失活与唤醒活动神经元和靶神经元激活同时发生。神经元划分为唤醒活动神经元是基于睡眠/觉醒状态的神经元单元记录和对激活组神经元的反应。唤醒活动神经元定义为觉醒时表现为活动性增多,睡眠明显减少。当大量唤醒活动神经元被激活时,觉醒就增强了。最近研究显示唤醒活动神经元对环境或生理刺激的反应是独特的。唤醒活动神经元包括基底前脑和脑干胆碱能神经元,下丘脑食欲素能和组胺能神经元,以及脑干多巴胺能、5-羟色胺能和去甲肾上腺素能亚群。拮抗任何一种唤醒神经调节介质信号的药物都可降低觉醒状态。例如,抗胆碱能、抗组胺、抗多巴胺和一些 5-羟色胺能拮抗药物可透过血脑屏障有明显的镇静作用。

食欲素能神经元在许多方面都是独特的唤醒活性神经元。食欲素能神经元的显著但不完全丧失可导致白天过度嗜睡,夜间睡眠中断或睡眠片段化。食欲素能神经元更广泛的缺失导致伴猝倒的发作性睡病。如下所述,这些神经元与摄食行为和代谢反应密切相关。肥胖患者的睡眠模式(白天嗜睡和夜间睡眠片段化)与食欲素功能障碍相关。

最近研究证实睡眠限制对进食与限制进食对睡眠都具有显著影响。睡眠不足会影响瘦素和胃饥饿素的水平和食欲,研究表明睡眠剥夺或限制睡眠 4h/d 可使食欲增强,瘦素水平降低,伴随瘦素分泌峰值变平。每日缩短睡眠时间 1.5 h 持续 2 周可明显增强食欲和增加热量摄入。睡眠限制明显影响进食和体重,反之,限制实验动物进食 4~5d 后可明显缩短睡眠时间,延长觉醒时间,限制进食 6~11d,动物没有明显睡眠。这些研究提示限制进食,减轻体重的同时可增强觉醒反应。人类在营养缺乏时也有类似的觉醒反应,例如胰岛素依赖型糖尿病患者出现严重低血糖,即启动这种保护性反应,从睡眠中觉醒。总之,限制进食与减轻体重可产生显著觉醒反应,进食增加可减少觉醒时间,因此,减少热量摄入是否可改善肥胖患者的日间嗜睡有待进一步研究。

大量肠道激素和脂肪因子会分别对食物摄入和体脂产生反应。总之,肠道激素随进食而水平发生急剧变化,同时,脂肪因子随着脂肪沉积的改变和长期能量平衡而急剧或慢性改变。类似的双向关系存在于进食相关的肠道激素、脂肪因子,睡眠与觉醒的生理活动。例如,进食蛋白质或脂肪,肠促胰酶肽、神经降压素、肠抑制素水平升高,睡眠增多。进食糖类,垂体腺苷环化酶激活肽水平升高,觉醒时间增多。进食糖类、脂肪和纤维类,YY 肽水平升高,睡眠增多。肥胖患者 IL-6、TNF-α 水平升高,睡眠增多,血管紧张素 II 水平升高,REM 睡眠减少。

三、小 结

减重作为睡眠呼吸疾病的一种重要治疗方式,可改善呼吸肌功能、气体交换和血流动力学,改善睡眠呼吸紊乱同时降低血压、胰岛素抵抗、血脂和血管炎症,从而降低心血管疾病等内科并发症,改善预后;其次,可减轻睡眠呼吸疾病的重要症状——日间嗜睡。总之,减重是睡眠呼吸疾病不可或缺的治疗方式。

参 考 文 献

[1] Imran Johan Meurling, Donal O'Shea, John F Garvey. Obesity and sleep: a growing concern. Curr Opin Pulm Medi, 2019, 25(6):602-608.

[2] Webber L, Divajeva D, Marsh T, et al. The future burden of obesity-related diseases in the 53 WHO European-Region countries and the impact of effective interventions: a modelling study. BMJ Open, 2014, 4:e004787.

[3] Ng M, Fleming T, Robinson M, et al. Global, regional and national prevalence of overweight and obesity in children and adults 1980-2013: a systematic analysis. Lancet, 2014, 384:766-781.

[4] Crummy F, Piper AJ, Naughton MT. Obesity and the lung: 2. Obesity and sleep-disordered breathing. Thorax, 2008, 63:738-746.

[5] Piper AJ, Grunstein RR. Obesity hypoventilation syndrome: mechanisms and management. Am J Respir Crit Care Med, 2011, 183:292-298.

[6] Dempsey JA, Skatrud JB, Jacques AJ, et al. Anatomic determinants of sleep disordered breathing across the spectrum of clinical and nonclinical male subjects. Chest, 2002, 122:840-851.

[7] Peppard PE. Longitudinal study of moderate weight change and sleep disordered breathing. JAMA 2000, 284:3015.

[8] Jones RL, Nzekwu M-MU. The effects of body mass index on lung volumes. Chest, 2006, 130:827-833.

[9] Mortimore IL, Marshall I, Wraith PK, et al. Neck and total body fat deposition in nonobese and obese patients with sleep apnea compared with that in control subjects. Am J Respir Crit Care Med, 1998, 157:280-283.

[10] Hudgel DW, Patel SR, Ahasic AM, et al. The role of weight management in the treatment of adult obstructive sleep apnea. An official American Thoracic Society Clinical Practice Guideline. Am J Respir Crit Care Med, 2018, 198:e70-e87.

[11] Bray GA, Fruhbeck G, Ryan DH, Wilding JPH. Management of obesity. Lancet, 2016, 387:1947-1956.

[12] Heymsfield SB, Wadden TA. Mechanisms, pathophysiology,

and management of obesity. N Engl J Med, 2017, 376: 254-266.

[13] Winslow DH, Bowden CH, DiDonato KP, et al. A Randomized, double-blind, placebo-controlled study of an oral, extended-release formulation of phentermine/topiramate for the treatment of obstructive sleep apnea in obese adults. Sleep, 2012, 35: 1529-1539.

[14] Blackman A, Foster GD, Zammit G, et al. Effect of liraglutide 3.0mg in individuals with obesity and moderate or severe obstructive sleep apnea: the scale sleep apnea randomized clinical trial. Int J Obes, 2016, 40: 1310-1319.

[15] Feigel-Guiller B, Drui D, Dimet J, et al. Laparoscopic gastric banding in obese patients with sleep apnea: a 3-year controlled study and follow-up after 10 years. Obes Surg, 2015, 25: 1886-1892.

[16] Dixon JB, Schachter LM, O'Brien PE, et al. Surgical vs conventional therapy for weight loss treatment of obstructive sleep apnea. JAMA, 2012, 308: 1142.

[17] Buchwald H, Avidor Y, Braunwald E, et al. Bariatric surgery: a systematic review and meta-analysis. JAMA, 2004, 292: 1724-1737.

[18] Ashrafian H, Toma T, Rowland SP, et al. Bariatric surgery or non-surgical weight loss for obstructive sleep apnoea? A systematic review and comparison of meta-analyses. Obes Surg, 2015, 25: 1239-1250.

[19] Peromaa-Haavisto P, Tuomilehto H, Kössi J, et al. Obstructive sleep apnea: the effect of bariatric surgery after 12 months. A prospective multicenter trial. Sleep Med, 2017, 35: 85-90.

[20] Aird LNF, Hong D, Gmora S, et al. The impact of a standardized program on short and long-term outcomes in bariatric surgery. Surg Endosc, 2017, 31: 801-808.

[21] Julio A Chirinos, Indira Gurubhagavatula, Karen Teff, et al. CPAP, weight loss, or both for obstructive sleep apnea. N Engl J Med, 2014, 370(24): 2265-2275.

[22] Imran H Iftikhar, Meredith A Donley, Mohammed Al-Jaghbeer, et al. Continuous positive airway pressure plus weight loss for obstructive sleep apnea(OSA), association of cancer with OSA, and hypoglossal nerve stimulation for OSA treatment. Am J Respir Crit Care Med, 2015, 191(7): 845-847.

[23] Lori A Panossian, Sigrid C Veasey. Daytime sleepiness in obesity: mechanisms beyond obstructive sleep apnea-a review. Sleep, 2012, 35(5): 605-615.

[24] Straznicky NE, Lambert EA, Lambert GW, Masuo K, Esler MD, Nestel PJ. Effects of dietary weight loss on sympathetic activity and cardiac risk factors associated with the metabolic syndrome. J Clin Endocrinol Metab, 2005, 90: 5998-6005.

[25] Fuller PM, Gooley JJ, Saper CB. Neurobiology of the sleep-wake cycle: sleep architecture, circadian regulation, and regulatory feedback. J Biol Rhythms, 2006, 21: 482-493.

16 基于标准 PSG 数据的 OSA 临床表型分析

袁海波

持续气道正压通气（continuous positive airway pressure，CPAP）是阻塞性睡眠呼吸暂停（obstructive sleep apnea，OSA）的一线治疗方法，这种方法无创且有效。然而，CPAP 在很多时候会给患者造成不适，导致依从性下降，最终影响治疗效果。在一些国家，由于 CPAP 治疗费用未纳入医疗保险范围，部分患者因难以承担治疗费用，而失去治疗机会。寻求治疗 OSA 患者的其他可替代 CPAP 的治疗方法，长期以来一直是困扰睡眠医生的一个课题。

目前有多种替代 CPAP 的方法，包括口腔矫治器、外科手术、减重、刺激舌下神经、补充氧气疗法和应用新型药物等。这些替代方法对不同病理生理学特征的 OSA 表型治疗效果不同。比如，气道易塌陷的患者对非机械性干预，如氧气和催眠药的联合治疗的反应较差；对于更严重的塌陷和高环路增益的患者，口腔矫治器效果较差；对于代偿性肌肉反应差的患者，药理学上应用地昔帕明刺激咽肌张力最有效。因此，评估 OSA 患者的临床病理生理学表型，可以帮助临床医生选择最合适的治疗方法，并最大限度保证患者的治疗效果。而迄今为止，OSA 患者表型特征的测量方法很多是侵入性的，这些方法仅限于在某些特定的睡眠生理实验室进行研究，不能广泛应用于临床。

为了促进 OSA 患者的个体化精准治疗，一些睡眠专家一直在寻找非侵入性的临床适用技术，并试图从多导睡眠监测这种常规的睡眠监测技术中寻找答案。应用常规睡眠监测研究中所收集的通气信号可以用来量化 OSA 患者的病理生理学特征。一些研究已经证实，在自然呼吸过程中，监测呼吸驱动的能力，可以评估 OSA 患者环路增益（loop gain）和觉醒阈值（arousal threshold），从而间接评估咽部塌陷和咽部神经肌肉代偿能力。咽部塌陷性可以定义为，在正常通气驱动下可以达到的通气量（Vpassive，相当于临界塌陷压力的通气量）；神经肌肉代偿能力是伴随着呼吸驱动力的增加而出现的通气增加的能力（从正常压力水平升高到触发觉醒的水平）。

从标准 PSG 数据中得到 OSA 临床表型的分析，要首先从 OSA 发生的病理生理学原理谈起。

一、OSA 病理生理模型的建立

CPAP 压力滴定量化的金标准方法

受试者佩戴口鼻面罩，置于 CPAP 的治疗水平下，从这一水平 CPAP 骤然降低，用以评估正常呼吸驱动下的通气情况。每次下降后呼吸 2～4 次，当 CPAP 降至一定范围，即可获得通气与 CPAP 压力的曲线图（图 7-16-1）。随后，CPAP 逐渐降低，直到呼吸驱动力提高到接近觉醒阈值的水平，这时咽部舒张肌的活性增加，从这一水平骤然下降到 0 cmH$_2$O，以测量在高位驱动时发生的通气反应。将这种情况下的通气值与被动呼吸的通气值作比较，并将这种差异量化作为咽部代偿的指标。

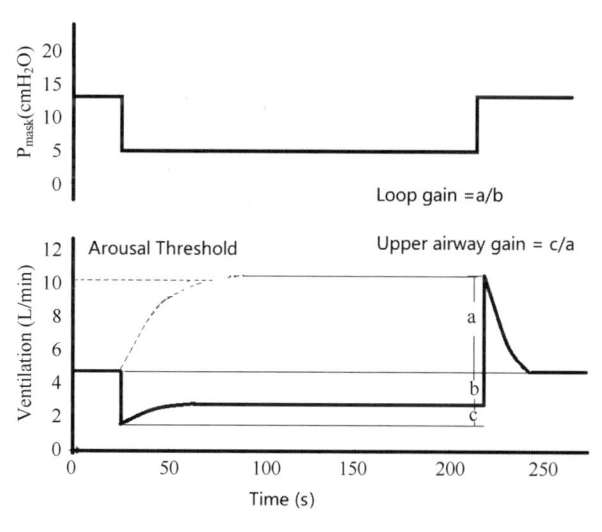

图 7-16-1 CPAP 滴定下通气与呼吸驱动

根据 OSA 发病机制，应用电生理学及工程学分析技术，分别计算出受试者在佩戴口鼻面罩时，面罩压力为零时的通气量 Passive V$_0$，也就是图 7-16-2 中的 B，环路增益（loop gain）采取 1/loop gain 来表示以完成 OSA 模型。计算受试者在呼吸机压力下的通气量图 7-16-2 中的 A，以及觉醒阈值（arousal threshold，TA）。上气道增益即 upper airway gain。如图 7-16-2 所示，环路增益与上气道增益的交点是睡眠中上气道最稳定的交点，如果觉醒阈值落在此交点左侧，受试者将发生 OSA，如果觉醒阈值落在此交点右侧,则受试者发生 OSA 可能较小。如果环路增益与上气道增益没有交点,则觉醒阈值必然落在两条直线上而没有交点,受试者将是一个重度 OSA。

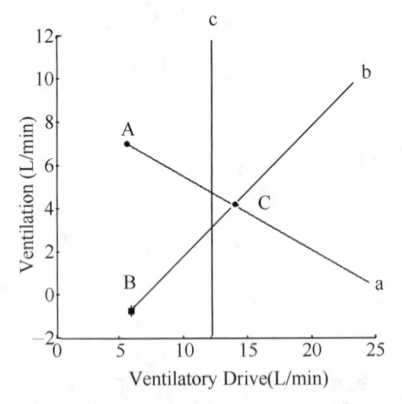

A:ventialtion on CPAP　　　　a:1/loop gain
B:ventilation off CPAP(anatomy)　b:slope of upper airway gain
C:the new, steady of ventilation　c:arousal threshold

图 7-16-2　OSA 模型图

二、标准 PSG 数据的处理

Sand S 等研究者在研究了上气道生理学机制的同时,应用标准 PSG 原始数据,与反映上气道驱动能力的金标准膈肌肌电进行了对比,发现应用标准 PSG 原始数据分析,亦可获得 OSA 临床表型的评估数据。研究者扩展了评估环路增益和觉醒阈值的方法,同时量化咽部塌陷性和神经肌肉代偿能力。并且将从鼻压力获得的通气参数特征与使用密封面罩和呼吸气体流速计评估通气量获得的值进行了比较。发现标准 PSG 的数据可以评估 OSA 患者不同的临床表型。

(一)多导睡眠监测仪的设置

除了常规的多导睡眠图测量(脑电图、眼电图、心电图、胸腹运动、血氧饱和度测定)外,还通过呼吸气流流速计和密封的口鼻面罩来评估通气量。测量食管内膈肌肌电图以评估呼吸驱动力。对原始肌电进行均方根和低通处理,得到分析整合的膈肌肌电信号。根据标准对睡眠、觉醒和呼吸事件进行评分。

(二)量化病理生理学特征的方法

根据上气道病理生理机制进行量化。咽部塌陷性可以用平静呼吸下呼吸驱动时的通气量来评估,通气量较低会造成气道更易塌陷。咽肌代偿是指随着呼吸驱动力的增加而引起通气的改变。具体地说,通气补偿是主动呼吸和被动呼吸之间的差异,其中主动呼吸是最大呼吸驱动下(即觉醒阈值下的呼吸驱动)的通气水平,而被动呼吸是指正常通气驱动下可达到的通气量。根据脑电图觉醒之前的呼吸驱动的中位数来评估觉醒阈值。根据这些原理构建睡眠期间通气与呼吸驱动之间的逐次呼吸的表型图。

通过评估呼吸驱动来量化 OSA 表型特征。如果咽部气道没有阻塞,在睡眠期间可以观察到通气的预期值。当气道畅通时,即在阻塞性呼吸事件之间,可以看到呼吸驱动。使用化学反射反馈控制模型的通气信号来计算呼吸驱动,该模型输出呼吸驱动信号;当气道开放时,调整参数以使驱动信号与呼吸期间的通气信号匹配为最佳。例如,呼吸暂停或低通气期间通气量的减少会导致随后的呼吸驱动的增加,这与呼吸暂停后过度通气的时间进程相一致。在非快速眼动睡眠期(NREM)的每 7 min 为一个窗口进行分析。除了化学反射模型外,还通过数据拟合的附加参数来评估对觉醒的通气反应。

(三)软件对数据的处理与分析

使用 MATLAB 进行数据处理,经过通道选择、EDF 数据读取、xls 文件设定读取与写入,MAT 文件生成、采样频率统一等步骤,接下来进行数据特征提取、曲线生成、数据曲线保存为 .fig 格式,获取 Vpassive, Vactive 及表型分类,患者数据的存取等一系列步骤,完成对多导睡眠图的分析。将睡眠期间的通气和呼吸驱动的数值进行列表及汇总。将呼吸驱动数据整理成十分位数,并取得通气和呼吸驱动中位数。获得平静呼吸及呼吸驱动的通气量中位数和觉醒阈值的通气量中位数。因而在临床上实现非侵入性的 OSA 表型分析,这将有助于 OSA 患者的精确治疗干预。

应用临床案例,能更清楚说明应用 PSG 数据可以实现对 OSA 表型的分析,如图 7-16-3 所示:A、B、C 分别为 3 名重度 OSA 患者。呼吸暂停低通气指数(apnea-hypopnea index,AHI)分别为:68N/h,45N/h 和 42N/h。然而,从临床表型分析,经过软件运算,得出 3 名患者的表型分析数据,并与金标准比较分析,结果呈现一致性。仔细分析这 3 名患者,患者 A 的上气道解剖学结构塌陷性数值低,但是上气道神经肌肉代偿能力很好,觉醒阈值较高;患者 B 的上气道解剖学塌陷性数值比较低,并且上气道神经肌肉代偿能力不好,觉醒阈值较低;患者 C 上气道解剖学塌陷性数值较高,然而神经肌肉代偿能力太差,表现为负值,觉醒阈值较低。由此可见,临床上仅凭 AHI 判断 OSA 病情严重程度并进行治疗是不够的,分析 OSA 的不同表型,才能因病施治。

利用标准 PSG 数据对 OSA 患者进行表型分析的方法,无须侵入性检查,无须 CPAP 操作,可以应用自动化程序处理数据。其分析结果可使临床医生指导患者选取最优化的替代治疗方案。这将使对 OSA 患者的管理从一刀切似的依赖于 CPAP 的治疗,转变为更为精准化的治疗。进一步的临床研究我们需要确定哪种治疗方法对哪种 OSA 患者的表型最为敏感,以期得到更精准的治疗方案。大规模多中心的 OSA 患者数据库的建立,必将为 OSA 临床表型的分类及治疗方案的选择提供更可靠的资料,并为临床 OSA 精准治疗提供理论依据。

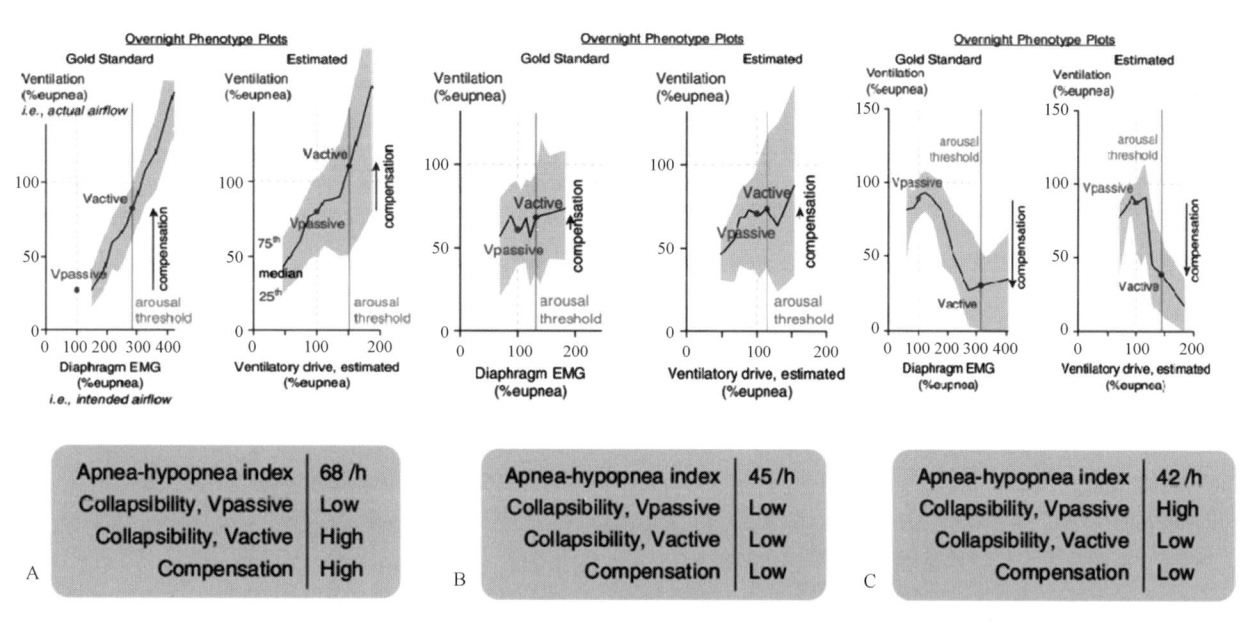

图 7-16-3 三名重度 OSA 患者的不同亚型特征（PSG 与金标准对比）

引自：Sands SA, et al. Phenotyping Pharyngeal Pathophysiology using Polysomnography in Patients with Obstructive Sleep Apnea. Am J Respir Crit Care Med, 2018 May 1, 197(9): 1187-1197.

参 考 文 献

[1] Patil SP, Ayappa IA, Caples SM, et al. Treatment of Adult Obstructive Sleep Apnea with Positive Airway Pressure: An American Academy of Sleep Medicine Clinical Practice Guideline. J Clin Sleep Med, 2019, 15; 15(2): 335-343.

[2] Wellman A, Malhotra A, Jordan AS, et al. Effect of oxygen in obstructive sleep apnea: role of loop gain. Respir Physiol Neurobiol, 2008, 162: 144-151.

[3] Edwards BA, Andara C, Landry S, et al. Upper-airway collapsibility and loop gain predict the response to oral appliance therapy in patients with obstructive sleep apnea. Am J Respir Crit Care Med, 2016, 194: 1413-1422.

[4] Taranto-Montemurro L, Sands SA, Edwards BA, et al. Desipramine improves upper airway collapsibility and reduces obstructive sleep apnoea severity in patients with minimal muscle compensation. Eur Respir J, 2016, 48: 1340-1350.

[5] Joosten SA, Leong P, Landry SA, et al. Loop gain predicts the response to upper airway surgery in patients with obstructive sleep apnea. Sleep, 2017, 40(7).

[6] O'Driscoll DM, Landry SA, Pham J, et al. The physiological phenotype of obstructive sleep apnea differs between Caucasian and Chinese patients. Sleep, 2019, 42(11).

[7] Sutherland K, Kairaitis K, Yee BJ, et al. From CPAP to tailored therapy for obstructive sleep Apnoea. Multidiscip Respir Med, 2018, 13: 44.

[8] Wellman A, Eckert DJ, Jordan AS, et al. A method for measuring and modeling the physiological traits causing obstructive sleep apnea. J Appl Physiol, 2011, 110: 1627-1637.

[9] Wellman A, Edwards BA, Sands SA, et al. A simplified method for determining phenotypic traits in patients with obstructive sleep apnea. J Appl Physiol, 2013, 114: 911-922.

[10] Terrill PI, Edwards BA, Nemati S, et al. Quantifying the ventilatory control contribution to sleep apnoea using polysomnography. Eur Respir J, 2015, 45: 408-418.

[11] Sands SA, Terrill PI, Edwards BA, et al. Quantifying the arousal threshold using polysomnography in obstructive sleep apnea. Sleep, 2018, 41: 1-9.

[12] Sands SA, Edwards BA, Terrill PI, et al. Phenotyping sleep apnea using polysomnography: upper airway collapsibility and responsiveness. Am J Respir Crit Care Med, 2016, 193: A6378.

[13] Sands SA, Edwards BA, Terrill PI, et al. Phenotyping Pharyngeal Pathophysiology using Polysomnography in Patients with Obstructive Sleep Apnea. Am J Respir Crit Care Med, 2018, 197(9): 1187-1197.

第八部分

危重症医学

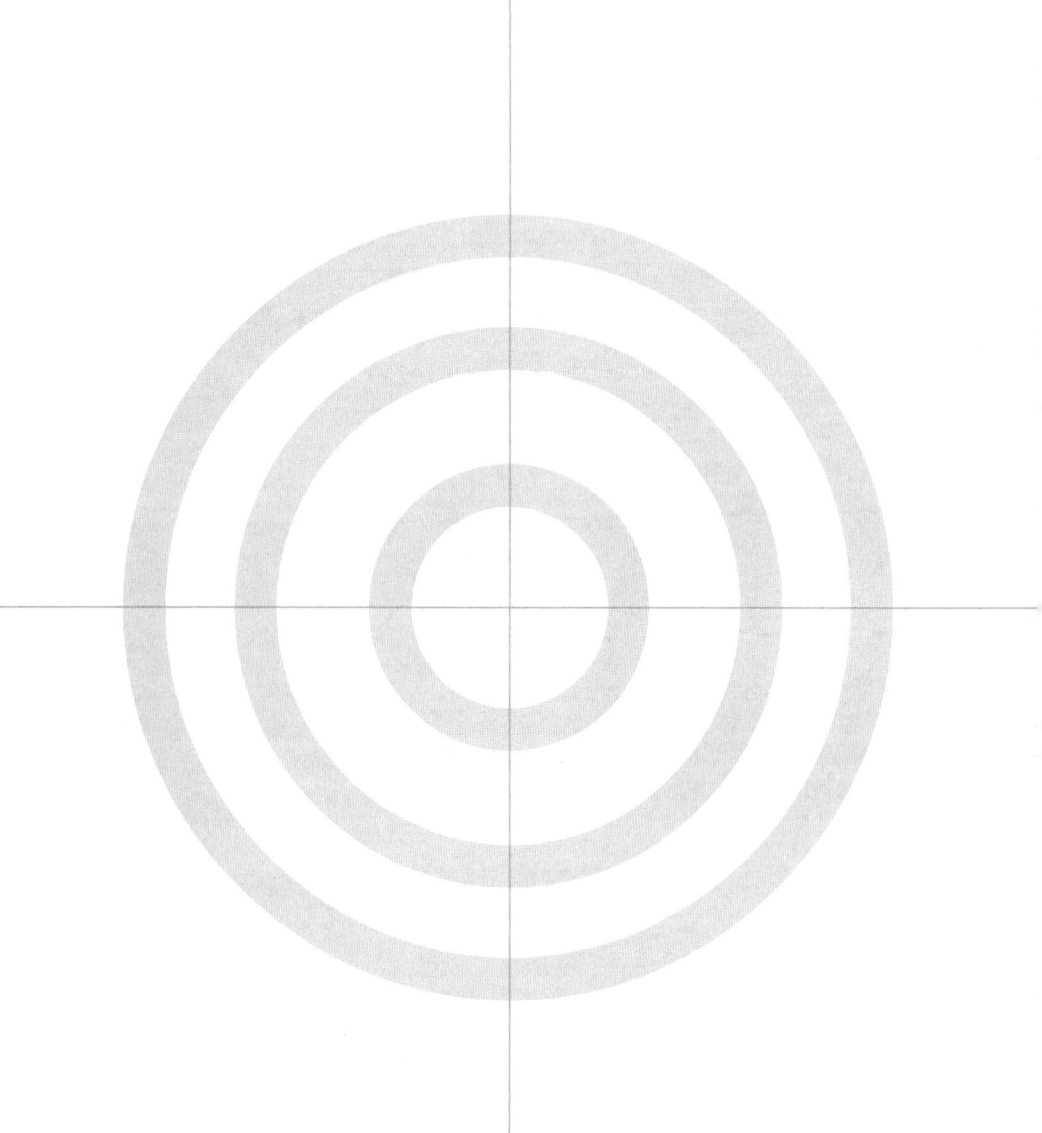

1 新型冠状病毒肺炎呼吸支持介入时机

解立新

2019年度突如其来的新型冠状病毒（2019 novel coronavirus，COVID-2019）感染肆虐中华大地，表现为肺炎的部分患者病情发展隐匿、短期内进展迅速而出现急性呼吸衰竭危及生命。我们在临床救治过程中发现，这个疾病突如其来，与2003年SARS和重症甲流患者比较尤其不同之处，需要我们尽快认识和掌握，尤其是不同呼吸支持手段介入时机和个体化评估，以及呼吸支持手段如何准确应用，将有助于帮助临床医师及时选择有效的呼吸支持手段提高COVID-2019肺炎的临床救治率，降低重症患者的病死率。

呼吸支持的方式

1. 普通氧疗 普通氧疗包括鼻导管、简单开放面罩、文丘里面罩、储氧面罩吸氧等方式，应用于轻度呼吸衰竭（$300>PaO_2/FiO_2 \geqslant 200$）患者的治疗，在治疗过程中要注意观察患者的脉搏氧饱和度（pulse oxygenation saturation，SpO_2）、呼吸频率等指标的变化，目标是使患者SpO_2维持在93%～95%。但是要注意的是，我们在一线工作和救治2019-nCoV感染患者会诊中，经常发现SpO_2为100%的许多轻症患者也在持续进行普通氧疗。众所周知，高氧血症因其产生过氧化会进一步加重对呼吸系统的损伤，甚至会增加病死率，因此氧疗的适应证在临床要受到重视。

2. 经鼻高流量湿化氧疗（high-flow nasal cannula oxygen therapy，HFNC） 随着近些年大家对HFNC的临床价值认识不断深入，在各地救治2019-nCoV感染肺炎合并轻度呼吸衰竭中，HFNC起到了至关重要的作用，与无创正压通气比较，HFNC舒适性更好，患者依从性更高，结合近些年国内外的研究和2019年出版的专家共识，我们建议对轻到中度低氧性呼吸衰竭（$300>PaO_2/FiO_2 \geqslant 150$）的患者可以考虑应用。由于HFNC是完全开放氧疗，虽然通过高流量能够形成一定水平的正压，但很难维持稳定和高水平的呼气末正压，而重症2019-nCoV肺炎患者因弥漫性肺渗出和实变需要一定水平甚至高水平的呼气末正压维持肺泡开放，HFNC难以达到。对$PaO_2/FiO_2<150$的患者要慎重应用，尤其是既往没有心肺基础疾病的患者，如果持续HFNC治疗24 h难以明显改善氧合，建议及时应用无创正压通气甚至气管插管有创正压通气。

3. 无创正压通气（non-invasive positive pressure ventilation，NIPPV） 无创正压通气在因重症肺炎导致低氧性呼吸衰竭临床应用一直有较大的争议，虽然2003年SARS期间NIPPV广泛应用推动了大家对NIPPV的认识，当时应用还有一个重要原因是顾虑气管插管导致院内感染发生。16年过去了，人们对NIPPV的临床价值体会更深，2019年孙兵等在 Crit Care 发表的重症肺炎应用NIPPV与常规氧疗平行对照研究表明，对于氧合指数PaO_2/FiO_2在100～150的中重度低氧性呼吸衰竭患者，NIPPV在改善氧合方面具有明显的优势，但并不能降低气管插管率及ICU和住院病死率，作者认为NIPPV治疗18 h呼吸频率增快（>11L/min）是NIPPV治疗失败的危险因素。另外NPPV治疗成功与失败对没有心肺功能疾病的急性低氧性呼吸衰竭患者差异巨大，若疗效不佳，则持续24 h死亡风险增加6.78倍。另外，针对病毒性肺炎应用NIPPV治疗还要注意双水平正压通气和肺反复萎陷复张可能带来纵隔气肿、气胸的风险。因此，我们建议对$PaO_2/FiO_2 \geqslant 150$的患者可以考虑NIPPV作为普通氧疗和HFNC治疗疗效不佳的替代治疗手段，也可以和HFNC交替应用。对于$150>PaO_2/FiO_2 \geqslant 100$者要慎重应用，并做好随时气管插管准备。$PaO_2/FiO_2<100$者不建议常规应用。

4. 有创正压通气（invasive positive pressure ventilation，IPPV） 有创正压通气是救治重症呼吸衰竭的有效治疗手段，以小潮气通气+一定水平呼气末正压（positive endexpiratory pressure，PEEP）通气为标志的肺保护性通气是治疗重症肺炎继发急性呼吸窘迫综合征（acute respiratory distress syndrome，ARDS）的常规治疗手段，关键的是如何进行PEEP滴定和是否需要常规进行有效肺复张应予以重视和关注。鉴于2019-nCoV重症肺炎肺部表现的不均一性、多形性改变的特点，通过食管压监测跨肺压进行PEEP滴定和维持呼气末跨肺压$\geqslant 0cmH_2O$和吸气末跨肺压$\leqslant 20cmH_2O$的前提下维持有效氧合（$SpO_2>93\%$）。不建议常规进行肺复张，若需要肺复张，建议跨肺压滴定动态监测或通过呼气末二氧化碳分压动态监测更为安全。如果没有食管压监测条件，可在动态评估平台压Pplat$\leqslant 30cmH_2O$和驱动压（Pplat-PEEP）$<15cmH_2O$去设置呼吸机参数，兼顾氧合和呼吸机相关肺损伤之间的平衡。俯卧位通气是能够有效改善患者氧合甚至预后的呼

吸支持手段,其可改善 ARDS 患者通气-血流比例,增加呼气末肺容积,通过肺复张和改变胸壁弹性使通气分布更均匀,在改善氧合的同时降低 VILI 的发生概率。建议对于氧合指数<100、PEEP>10cmH$_2$O 的重症 ARDS 患者进行俯卧位通气,建议每天俯卧位通气时间>12h。如果结合电阻抗(electrical impedance tomography,EIT)技术,通过动态评估肺的实时通气情况,个体化呼吸支持会更为合理和有效。

5. 体外膜肺氧合(extracorporeal membrane oxygenation,ECMO) ECMO 是体外生命支持(extracorporeal life support,ECLS)技术的一种,用于完全替代患者肺和部分替代心脏功能,使其得以充分休息,从而为原发病的诊治争取时间。自 2018 年重症流感以来,近 2 年国内 ECMO 临床应用水平突飞猛进,最新发表的武汉重症 COVID-19 救治有 5% 患者应用了 ECMO 的辅助支持,并有患者成功康复。结合既往治疗 ARDS 患者 ECMO 应用的专家共识,针对本次新型冠状病毒感染的危重型肺炎患者推荐的 ECMO 上机时机是:①早期有创通气<7 d。②仰卧位通气下:PaO$_2$/FiO$_2$≤80mmHg,或尝试俯卧位通气后:PaO$_2$/FiO$_2$≤100mmHg(FiO$_2$>80%,PEEP>10cmH$_2$O)。③吸气项跨肺压>25cmH$_2$O/驱动压>15cmH$_2$O,治疗 24 h 氧合指数无明显改善。④出现严重气压伤(纵隔气肿、气胸等)。需要指出的是,ECMO 的应用没有绝对的禁忌证,要有丰富经验的团队进行操作和维护。

二、呼吸支持治疗的相关建议

1. 疾病严重程度评估 我们在临床救治 COVID-19 患者中发现,一些患者虽然 PaO$_2$/FiO$_2$<200,肺部病变还在进展,但患者主观感觉并没有明显改变,这很容易给医务人员产生错觉,因此对患者病情及时有效进行评估,结合氧合指标、肺部病变动态变化、呼吸频率、活动后心率和氧合指标等进行综合评估,病情变化时及时采取有效呼吸支持等治疗干预手段,避免患者病情突然恶化。

2. 呼吸支持治疗场所 若有条件,所有 PaO$_2$/FiO$_2$<300 的患者建议在 ICU 进行观察治疗。如果条件有限,PaO$_2$/FiO$_2$≥200,接受普通氧疗和 HFNC 治疗的患者可考虑在严密监测下在感染普通病房进行。如果应用 NIPPV 治疗,因 NIPPV 需要很好的人机同步,一定要加强患者生命体征监测和观察人机配合程度。

3. 呼吸支持治疗设备 需要特别指出的是,对于进展的 COVID-19 患者应用 NIPPV 治疗,建议常规选择能够进行空氧混合、提供精确氧供、FiO$_2$>80%、应用 ICU 湿化装置的 ICU 专用无创呼吸机,呼吸支持设备选择在一定程度上能够决定患者的预后。

4. 呼吸支持治疗团队 专业、敬业、有丰富治疗经验的呼吸支持治疗团队直接决定救治成败,建立以呼吸危重症专业医疗-呼吸治疗师-ICU 专科护士为基石,临床药师、康复和心理等专科医师合作的专业团队至关重要。

2 从COVID-19重症病例救治谈俯卧位在ARDS患者中的应用

王导新 马青 邓旺

2019年12月，新型冠状病毒肺炎（novel coronavirus pneumonia，NCP）暴发，并迅速蔓延至世界各个国家，引起大流行，该疾病在2020年2月被世界卫生组织命名为COVID-19。目前突破1500万病例，病死率超60万，COVID-19患者中，重症患者多在发病1周后出现呼吸困难和（或）低氧血症，严重者快速进展为急性呼吸窘迫综合征（acute respiratory distress syndrome，ARDS），严重影响预后。在重症COVID-19患者中，ARDS为最常见的并发症，占重症患者的20%～41%，一旦出现，部分医疗机构的病死率可达74.3%。可见，有效改善COVID-19患者病死率的重点在于提高重症患者的治疗效果，尤其是合并ARDS的患者。

针对ARDS患者，除了寻找引起ARDS的病因，针对病因治疗以外，呼吸支持技术及脏器功能保护是主要治疗手段，其中俯卧位治疗在近年ARDS的临床中得到认可，俯卧位通气由于其体位改变的作用，减轻心脏对左下肺的压力以促进塌陷肺泡的复张，使得背侧肺重新开放，改善肺不张、通气血流比例，增加肺的顺应性，另可促进气道分泌物的引流，从而达到改善ARDS患者的通气氧合的目的。2017年美国胸科学会（ATS）对成年ARDS患者的机械通气指南中推荐，对于严重ARDS患者至少应俯卧12 h/d。并且强调早期使用俯卧位通气（ARDS发病48 h内）。在此，我们通过重症COVID-19患者应用俯卧位辅助，浅谈其在ARDS中的应用。

由Aoyama等发表在 JAMA 的一篇Meta分析选择从数据库建立到2019年5月29日截止，搜索所有采用肺保护性通气的中度至重度ARDS患者的RCT研究，最后纳入25项RCT，包含7743名中重度ARDS患者，对不同的治疗策略进行比较和排序，以确定能降低成年中重度ARDS患者死亡率相关的最佳干预措施。主要结果为28 d病死率，次要结果为发生气压伤的比率。结果显示在评估9项干预措施的7743名患者中有2686名在28 d内死亡，病死率为34.6%；与单独肺保护性通气相比，俯卧位和ECMO可显著降低28 d病死率，俯卧位的RR为0.69（95%CI，0.48～0.99），ECMO的RR为0.60（95%CI，0.38～0.93）；其中18项临床试验报道了气压伤的情况，6258例患者中有448例合并气压伤，气压伤发生率为7.2%。得出结论，与单独肺保护性通气相比，俯卧位显著降低了28 d病死率，表明俯卧位通气可用于中度至重度急性呼吸窘迫综合征患者。

Guérin等的APRONET研究是一项针对ARDS俯卧位通气的前瞻性的流行病学研究，对来自20个国家141个重症监护室的6723名患者中的735名ARDS患者进行分析，分别于2016年4月、7月、10月和2017年1月进行了4次调研。在每个研究日，每个ICU的调查员必须对每个患者进行筛查，记录ARDS患者在俯卧位之前和结束时的氧合指数、呼吸机参数等，并记录并发症和不使用俯卧位治疗的原因。发现101例ARDS患者（13.7%）至少进行了1次俯卧位治疗；轻度、中度和重度ARDS患者俯卧位使用率分别为5.9%（11/187）、10.3%（41/399）和32.9%（49/149）（$P=0.0001$）；首次俯卧位持续时间的中位数为18 h；相较于俯卧位之前，俯卧位结束时患者的PaO_2/FiO_2从101mmHg增加至171mmHg（$P=0.0001$）；而不使用俯卧位治疗的最常见的原因（64.3%）是认为患者低氧血症的程度不够严重；其中12例（11.9%）患者发生并发症。在这次前瞻性国际流行病学研究中发现，32.9%的严重ARDS患者使用了俯卧位治疗，且并发症发生率低，氧合明显增加。在这项研究中，因为各中心提前得到了研究日期的通知，他们可能会有意识地调整自己的做法，医务工作者在病人的选择上可能存在选择偏倚。

显然，众多相关研究的存在证实了ARDS患者能够获益于俯卧位治疗，可以改善其氧合，降低死亡率。已经有足够的循证医学证据证明俯卧位通气治疗在ARDS气管插管、呼吸机辅助通气患者中的正向作用。最近的一项研究描述了COVID-19合并ARDS患者机械通气的呼吸生理，发现新冠肺炎患者仰卧位时同样具有较低的肺顺应性，反之俯卧位可增加肺顺应性和改善氧合，为俯卧位治疗在COVID-19合并ARDS这类患者中的应用提供了理论基础。俯卧位治疗在COVID-19合并ARDS患者中的应用已经得到相关指南的推荐支持。但是如何有效降低新冠肺炎患者的病死率，如何降低重症患者的比率及减轻世界各地ICU的压力，众多学者将视线聚焦于轻、中度ARDS，尚不需要入住ICU行气管插管的清醒患者，早期为这类患者行俯卧位治疗，希望通过提高氧合情况避免病情重症化，降低插管率和病死率。

一项来自意大利的Anna Coppo等发表在 Lancet Respir Med 杂志上的前瞻性的队列研究，对意大利蒙扎圣赫拉尔多医院18～75岁确诊为COVID-19合并ARDS的清醒患者，在接受氧疗或无创通气治疗的同时进行最少持续3 h的俯卧位治疗，收集俯卧位前、恢复仰卧位后10 min和

1 h 后的临床资料,主要研究结果是氧合指数的变化。共入组 56 例患者,俯卧位在 46 例患者(83.9%)中至少维持 3 h 是可行的;俯卧位之后的氧合指数(285.5mmHg)较俯卧位之前(180.5mmHg)明显改善($P<0.0001$);23 例(50%)患者在恢复仰卧位后维持了良好的氧合,然而,这一改善与俯卧位前相比差异不显著(恢复 1 h 后的氧合指数为 192.9 mmHg($P=0.29$)。证明了俯卧位对需要补充氧的清醒 COVID-19 合并 ARDS 患者快速改善氧合指数是可行且有效的,约 50% 患者在恢复仰卧位后维持了良好的氧合。

Chiara Sartini 等的横断面研究选择氧饱和度低于 94% 的 15 例 COVID-19 合并轻、中度 ARDS 患者进行无创通气,如果无创通气效果不佳,在基础上行俯卧位通气,在 2020 年 4 月 2 日进行横断面调查,分别在俯卧位前、俯卧位中(开始后 60 min)和俯卧位结束后 60 min 测量呼吸参数及氧合指数,并随访 14 d 后患者的预后情况。发现与俯卧位前相比,所有患者在俯卧位期间和俯卧位结束后呼吸频率均有所降低($P<0.001$),所有患者俯卧位期间 SpO_2 和 PaO_2/FiO_2 均有改善($P<0.001$),80% 患者俯卧位结束后 1 h 的 SpO_2 和 PaO_2/FiO_2 有所改善($P<0.001$);并且随访 14 d,在 15 例患者中,9 例患者出院,1 例俯卧位后病情好转并停止,3 例继续进行俯卧位通气,1 例插管入 ICU,1 例死亡。

Xavier 等的研究对 24 名无须插管的严重新冠肺炎合并 ARDS 的患者进行俯卧位治疗,于俯卧位之前、俯卧期间、俯卧结束后 6~12 h 测定动脉血气分析,观察动脉血氧分压(PaO_2)在俯卧位治疗前后增加 20% 的患者的比例,及治疗前后 PaO_2 和 $PaCO_2$ 的变化值,可行性(持续俯卧位治疗 1 h、3 h 的患者比例),和持久反应者的比例(相较俯卧位前,治疗后的 PaO_2 增加 20% 以上患者的比例)。发现其中 4 人(17%)对俯卧位的耐受性不超过 1 h,5 人(21%)的耐受性为 1~3 h,15 人(63%)超过 3 h;相比俯卧位治疗前,有 6 例患者(25%)的 PaO_2 在俯卧位期间增加 20%;有 3 例患者(12.5%)在俯卧位治疗结束 6 h 后的 PaO_2 仍增加 20% 以上;在持续治疗 3 h 或以上的患者中,PaO_2 从俯卧位前的平均 73.6mmHg 增加到俯卧位期间的 94.9mmHg($P=0.006$),但在俯卧位结束 6 h 后的 PaO_2 增加并不显著;参与试验的患者无重大并发症发生;在 10 d 随访期结束时,5 例患者需要有创机械通气,其中 4 例患者耐受性不足 1 h。得出结论,在清醒的非插管 COVID-19 合并 ARDS 的患者中应用俯卧位治疗可能有效改善其氧合,避免病情加重及转入 ICU 进一步治疗。

这些研究结果均表明在处于清醒状态下的非插管的 COVID-19 合并 ARDS 的患者中使用俯卧位治疗是可行且有效的,可有效改善患者氧合情况,为俯卧位通气的适应症的扩展提供了一定的临床依据。但是这些研究样本量小,选则的是传染性强的病毒性肺炎为对象,也缺乏对照组的比较,并且研究中的俯卧位时间均比较短,这可能是因为相比气管插管患者,清醒患者能够很好的耐受俯卧位治疗的时间更短。再者,这类患者在俯卧位过程中确实可以改善氧合,但是其作用维持时间通常较短。现有的荟萃分析表明,急性呼吸窘迫综合征患者在发病初期、严重氧合受损和较长时间的俯卧位可以降低死亡率。那么在清醒患者中的短疗程俯卧位到底能否降低插管率及死亡率需要进一步研究。

除治疗方法的有效性外,还应考虑护理方面及体位对 ARDS 患者产生的潜在不良事件和并发症。患者在机械通气的同时接受俯卧位治疗会面临相应的风险,如气管导管意外脱出、气压伤、有限的静脉输液通道、导尿管等导管的弯曲和拉扯、身体压疮、嘴角擦伤、眼周和面部水肿、胃食管反流、过多的痰液和涎流等。在俯卧位时,将柔软的枕头放置在有气管导管及呼吸机通气患者的肩下可以防止气道阻塞,同时接受适当的镇静和神经肌肉阻滞剂,可以使用眼垫让患者闭上眼睛来预防角膜溃疡。患者胃内压力大,胃注食物后发生反流的可能性很大,因此必须密切监测他们的胃内容物的吸入情况,避免因为误吸而加重肺部感染。为了更好的实施俯卧位治疗,真正做到降低并发症的发生率,还需更多合理的护理措施及技术改良去实现。

总之,对 ARDS 患者俯卧位治疗效果的研究明确指出,正确选择开始俯卧位的时机、俯卧位持续的时间长短及并发症的预防都会影响其治疗效果。最优化的俯卧位策略和技术需要进一步大样本、高质量的临床研究去证实。

参 考 文 献

[1] Phelan AL, Katz R, Gostin LO. The novel coronavirus originating in Wuhan, China: challenges for global health governance. JAMA, 2020, 323: 709-710.

[2] Wang D, Hu B, Hu C, et al. Clinical Characteristics of 138 Hospitalized Patients with 2019 Novel Coronavirus-Infected Pneumonia in Wuhan, China. JAMA-J Am Med Assoc Published Online First, 2020.

[3] Shawn Kaku, Christopher DN, Natalie NH, et al. Acute Respiratory Distress Syndrome: Etiology, Pathogenesis, and Summary on Management. Journal of Intensive Care Medicine, 2020, 35(8): 723-737.

[4] An Official American Thoracic Society/European Society of Intensive Care Medicine/Society of Critical Care Medicine Clinical Practice Guideline: Mechanical Ventilation in Adult Patients with Acute Respiratory Distress Syndrome. Am J Respir Crit Care Med, 2017, 195(9): 1253-1263.

[5] Aoyama H, Uchida K, Aoyama K, et al. Assessment of therapeutic interventions and lung protective ventilation in patients with moderate to severe acute respiratory distress syndrome: a systematic review and network meta-analysis. JAMA, 2019, 2(7): e198116.

[6] Guérin C, Beuret P, Constantin J. A Prospective International Observational Prevalence Study on Prone Positioning of ARDS Patients: The APRONET (ARDS Prone Position Net-

work)Study. Intensive Care Med,2018,44(1):22-37.
[7] Pan C, Chen L, Lu C, et al. Lung Recruitability in SARS-CoV-2 Associated Acute Respiratory Distress Syndrome: A Single-center, Observational Study. Am J Respir Crit Care Med,2020.
[8] Bouadma L, Lescure FX, Lucet JC, Yazdanpanah Y, Timsit JF. Severe SARS-CoV-2 infections: practical considerations and management strategy for intensivists. Intensive Care Med,2020,46:579-582.
[9] Anna Coppo, Giacomo Bellani, DarioWinterton, et al. Feasibility and Physiological Effects of Prone Positioning in Non-Intubated Patients With Acute Respiratory Failure Due to COVID-19(PRON-COVID): A Prospective Cohort Study. Lancet Respir Med,2020.
[10] Chiara Sartini, Moreno Tresoldi, Paolo Scarpellini. Respiratory Parameters in Patients With COVID-19 After Using Non-invasive Ventilation in the Prone Position Outside the Intensive Care Unit. JAMA,2020,323(22):2338-2340.
[11] Xavier Elharrar, Youssef Trigui, Anne-Marie Dols, et al. Use of prone positioning in nonintubated patients with COVID-19 and hypoxemic acute respiratory failure. JAMA,2020,323(22):2336-2338.
[12] Mora-Arteaga J, Bernal-Ramǎnrez O, Rodrǎnguez S. The effects of prone position ventilation in patients with acute respiratory distress syndrome. A systematic review and meta analysis. Medicina Intensiva(English Edition),2015,39(6):359-372.
[13] Parisa Ghelichkhani, Maryam Esmaeili. Prone Position in Management of COVID-19 Patients; a Commentary. Archives of Academic Emergency Medicine,2020,8(1):e48.

3 ECCO₂R 促进 ARDS 超保护性通气是否可行？

李鋆璐　邢丽华

正压机械通气是急性呼吸窘迫综合征（acute respiratory distress syndrome，ARDS）患者重要的生命支持措施，但每次正压呼吸肺泡过度膨胀和（或）低通气肺泡开放和塌陷可潜在性进一步加重肺损伤，即呼吸机诱导肺损伤（ventilator-induced lung injury，VILI）。低潮气量（tidal volume，VT）6 ml/kg 标准体重（PBW）及限制平台压（platform pressure，Pplat）<30 cmH₂O 的肺保护性通气策略仍不能避免 VILI 的发生，且可能导致高碳酸血症和呼吸性酸中毒。体外二氧化碳去除（extracorporeal CO₂ removal，ECCO₂R）通过体外气体交换器从血液中去除一定量 CO₂，实现 VT<6 ml/kg，降低 Pplat 和驱动压（⊿P），为控制 VILI 提供生理前提；同时又能保持足够的气体交换，减轻高碳酸血症。1986 年 ECCO₂R 结合低频正压通气首次应用于重度 ARDS，显示出其有效性和安全性。近年来基础和临床医学研究显示，ECCO₂R 微创、安全、高效，ECCO₂R 在 ARDS 救治中的作用越来越多地引起关注。

一、ARDS 超保护性通气

（一）VILI 发生机制

VILI 是机械通气（mechanical ventilation，MV）的一种严重并发症，在病理上不仅表现为肺泡外气体，还包括肺泡上皮和血管内皮的广泛破坏、肺水肿和肺不张等弥漫性肺损伤。VILI 机制包括以下几方面。

1. 容量伤（压力伤）　局部肺过度扩张是导致 VILI 的关键因素。高容量通气可导致肺泡破裂、漏气和严重气压伤（如气胸、纵隔气肿和皮下气肿），还可导致更细微的损伤，表现为肺水肿。接受大潮气量通气的 ARDS 患者致死率和器官衰竭发生率明显高于小潮气量患者。正压通气高气道压导致肺泡和血管间隙之间的压力梯度增大，跨肺压是决定其压力梯度的关键因素。跨肺压等于 Pplat 与胸内压之差，胸内压稳定时，Pplat 是引起气压伤的决定因素。

2. 剪切伤（不张伤）　重复打开和关闭气道和萎陷的肺组织造成损伤，并影响肺表面活性物质及区域组织缺氧情况，导致肺上皮细胞脱落、透明膜形成，诱发肺水肿。一定的呼吸末正压（positive end expiratory pressure，PEEP）通气维持肺容积可以减少剪切伤。

3. 生物伤　上述物理性因素可以直接（通过损伤各种细胞）或间接（通过将这些力转导成上皮细胞，内皮细胞或炎性细胞中细胞信号传导途径的激活）引起各种细胞内炎症因子释放，不仅直接损失肺组织，还可以炎症介质为趋化因子，将细胞（如中性粒细胞）募集到肺释放更多炎症介质，导致全身炎症反应，甚至多器官功能障碍和死亡。

4. 机械功率伤　除了 MV 时的"静态"特征，如 Pplat、VT、PEEP 和 ⊿P 等外，呼吸频率（RR）和流速等 MV 的"动态"特征也会引起肺损伤。机械功=VT×P=VT×（气道阻力×流速+VT/(2×顺应性)+PEEPtot）。研究表明，这是一加速度过程，一旦启动，肺损伤可能会以指数方式增加。降低 MV 强度，从而限制 VILI，需要减少传输到肺部的总机械功率。

对 VILI 的认识深入带来了通气管理目标的根本性改变，从以往的"维持气体交换，同时尽量减少呼吸功"，至现在在"提供维持生命的气体交换，同时尽量减少 VILI"。多种策略用以降低 MV 参数如 VT、Pplat、⊿P、RR 等，现在理念更注重使用更小的潮气量来保护肺部，体外支持技术膜肺氧合（ECMO）、ECCO₂R 为实现肺超保护提供了基础。

（二）肺保护性通气策略及超保护性通气策略（ultra-protective lung ventilation strategy，UPLVS）

ARDS 指南提出保护性通气策略，即 VT 限制为 6 ml/kg PBW，而 Pplat 限制为 30 cmH₂O 以内。ARDS 协作网（ARDSnet）进行的大样本、多中心临床试验及研究显示，这一具有里程碑式的 MV 策略使 ARDS 患者的死亡率降低了 9%，ARDSnet 研究发现，Pplat 越低，患者生存机会越大，提示低 Pplat 更有助于患者预后。然而，有研究表明，尽管 Pplat 值≤30 cmH₂O，仍可能会出现肺泡过度膨胀，导致炎症介质和肺部炎症反应加剧，ARDS 患者仍可能有 VILI 风险。在保护性通气策略下，仍有 30% 的 ARDS 患者 CT 扫描显示有肺泡过度膨胀，同时伴随肺泡灌洗液中炎性细胞因子增加。降低 VT 和 Pplat 也会降低 ⊿P，后者最近被确定为 ARDS 患者死亡的主要危险因素。动物实验研究显示，VT 从 12 ml/kg 到 6 ml/kg 直至 3 ml/kg 有助于减少肺泡上皮细胞和内皮细胞的损伤，一项观察性研究也发现，初始 VT 每增 1 ml/kg 患者死亡率增加 23%，表明 ARDS 初期 VT 的微小变化可能会影响预后。因此，极低潮气量、降低 Pplat 有望进一步降低 VILI，即实施 UPLVS。

UPLVS 主要内容为：超小潮气量（≤4 ml/kg，一般在 2~4 ml/kg）通气及平台压≤20~25 cmH₂O，（高）PEEP 维持肺复张等。

(三)UPLVS 不可避免的高碳酸血症

UPLVS 在控制 VILI 的同时,由于通气量的下降,将不可避免加重高碳酸血症及呼吸性酸中毒,并由此带来潜在的严重不良反应,包括颅内压升高、肺动脉高压、心肌收缩力降低、肾血流降低,以及肺不张和高吸氧浓度等。有证据显示,过低的 VT 结合中等水平的 PEEP 容易导致肺结构的不稳定性和肺泡塌陷等。在 UPLVS 开始 MV 后的最初 48 h 内,二氧化碳(CO_2)分压($PaCO_2$)≥50mmHg 的允许性高碳酸血症会增加 ARDS 患者重症监护病房(ICU)死亡率的风险。因此,UPLVS 时需采取降低 CO_2 水平的措施,近年来采用 MV 与部分体外支持(如 $ECCO_2R$)相结合的方法,将维持生命所需的通气强度降低,CO_2 通过体外循环排出以减轻高碳酸血症。

二、$ECCO_2R$ 在 ARDS 超保护性通气中的应用

(一)$ECCO_2R$ 原理

$ECCO_2R$ 是一种通过体外气体交换器从血液中去除 CO_2 的人工呼吸支持技术。1977 年,德国 Gattinoni L 和 Kolobow T 团队首次将 $ECCO_2R$ 描述为减弱低顺应性呼吸系统中高压/高容量机械通气的工具。$ECCO_2R$ 设备包括放置在中央静脉(V-V 系统)或动脉(A-V 系统)中的引流套管、人工肺和血液回路系统,分为有泵和无泵两种类型。无泵设备只能在 A-V 配置中使用,但是为了确保回路中有足够的血流,需要至少 70 mmHg 的平均动脉压或动静脉压力梯度≥60mmHg,并且必须保持高于 3 L/min/m² 的心指数,重症患者经常出现血流动力学不稳定和(或)心力衰竭,可能会限制此类型设备的使用,因此 $ECCO_2R$ 通常是通过静脉(VV)配置实现的,其中颈内或股静脉为插管首选部位。

目前常用的 $ECCO_2R$ 设备包括 Hemolung 呼吸辅助系统(ALung Technologies,Pittsburgh,USA)、iLA Activve (Xenios,Heilbronn,Germany) 或 Cardiohelp® HLS 5.0 (GETINGE Cardiopulmonary Care,Rastatt,Germany)。设备间的区别主要:①用于膜肺(membrane lung,ML)表面的聚合物。②ML 气体交换表面积(0.5~2 m²)和形状(菱形、圆柱形)。③流量工作范围(0.2~1.8 L/min)。④所用泵的类型(蠕动或离心)。⑤插管的直径和血管通路的构型(动静脉或静脉静脉)。Hemolung 呼吸辅助系统(较低的二氧化碳去除装置)采用横截面积为 0.59 m² 的膜肺,血流量 300~500 ml/min。其他 2 个装置(更高二氧化碳去除装置)采用 1.30 m² 的膜肺,血流量 800~1000 ml/min。

$ECCO_2R$ 功能取决于以下几个因素:ML 的表面积及其特征,进入 ML 的静脉血 PCO_2,以及血液和气体的体外流速。在恒定的动脉 PCO_2 下,ML 的 CO_2 去除量($V_{CO_2}ML$)加上自然肺的 CO_2 去除量($V_{CO_2}NL$)等于产生的 CO_2 通过新陈代谢($V_{CO_2}tot = V_{CO_2}ML + V_{CO_2}NL$)。1L 血液中约含有 500ml 或更多的 CO_2,每分钟产生的 CO_2 量为 200~250ml,因此 500ml/min 的血流量足以清除人体产生的所有 CO_2。因此,$ECCO_2R$ 系统现在可以在相对较低的血流量(300~1000 ml/min)下提供具有临床意义的 CO_2 去除水平。对于 CO_2 去除,除了血流量外对 ML 的膜面积要求也较低,动物实验发现,完全纠正呼吸性酸中毒,仅需要 0.8 m² 以上的膜表面和 750 ml/min 以上的血流量,而更小面积的人工膜仍可通过较低的血流量消除部分 CO_2。因此 $ECCO_2R$ 这种较小流量(0.2~1.8 L/min)及膜面积(0.5~2 m²),所需体外支持系统体积更小,成本更低,所需导管可使用常规双腔导管(15~18Fr),仅需更小侵入性血管通路。另外,由于所需的血液流量低,对全身血流动力学不会产生负面影响。

(二)$ECCO_2R$ 的临床应用

目前 $ECCO_2R$ 适应证及禁忌证并无统一标准,根据现有研究数据,其适应证包括轻度或中度 ARDS、慢性阻塞性肺疾病急性加重期高碳酸血症或其他原因引起的顽固性高碳酸血症。禁忌证包括:急性脑损伤,严重肝功能不全(Child-Pugh 评分＞7)或暴发性肝衰竭,肝素诱导的血小板减少,全身抗凝禁忌证,不能使用股静脉或颈静脉导管,气胸,血小板计数＜50 G/L,以及未征得患者或家属知情同意者。

$ECCO_2R$ 回路通常需要全身性抗凝以防止回路血栓形成,但目前尚不清楚抗凝最佳方法以安全有效地降低出血性并发症。大多以普通肝素抗凝,且国际标准化比值达到 1.5~2.0 倍为标准,且需要对患者进行 $ECCO_2R$ 评估时应考虑是否适合全身性抗凝治疗。对于被认为不适合抗凝治疗(如出血风险,肝素诱发的血小板减少症)的患者,应寻求替代治疗选择,并且应研究局部抗凝治疗(例如枸橼酸抗凝治疗)的安全性和有效性。

(三)$ECCO_2R$ 的并发症

低氧血症恶化的风险被认为是 $ECCO_2R$ 的一个可能缺陷。由于潮气量从 6 ml/kg 降至 4 ml/kg 和 3 ml/kg PBW,应用 $ECCO_2R$ 后需要更高的 FiO_2 补偿平均气道压降低、低通气-灌注比(两者都会促进肺不张)而致的肺泡氧分压较低,和继发于呼吸商降低所致的低肺泡氧分压。此外,还需要更高水平 PEEP 来维持肺复张和功能残余容量,必要时可能需要 $ECCO_2R$ 联合俯卧位通气,或转向高流量 V-V ECMO。

由于 $ECCO_2R$ 设备采用的低血流量,增加了导管和膜血栓形成的风险,即使持续应用抗凝治疗(目标 INR 1.5~2),仍可能在回路中形成血凝块,导致 $PaCO_2$ 迅速增加,甚至出现危及生命的情况,此时需要迅速更换回路,改变呼吸机的设置及通气方式。

$ECCO_2R$ 常见并发包括出血和溶血,小出血事件不影响血流动力学。研究发现,在低于 1 L/min 的血液流速下运行,液压效率将急剧下降至 5%~10%,在这些流速范围内,泵的内部流动再循环率将增加 6~12 倍,由于多次暴露在高剪切应力下,溶血和血小板破坏急剧增加。因此,当泵速低于 2 L/min 时,应谨慎使用,因为循环量大,循环力大,剪切应力大,溶血作用大。

其他 $ECCO_2R$ 相关或潜在相关的并发症包括有气胸、插管部位出血、感染、菌血症、血管闭塞、动脉瘤形成、假性

动脉瘤形成,以及泵、氧合器等出现机械故障。

三、$ECCO_2R$ 在 ARDS 中的应用

(一)$ECCO_2R$ 应用现状

2016年法国一项观察性研究通过电话访问法国附属医院239个ICU在2010—2015年5年间应用$ECCO_2R$情况,结果显示,有35个(15%)ICU至少使用过1次$ECCO_2R$。2019年,法国一项为期2年的多中心前瞻性观察研究对大都市应用$ECCO_2R$的使用情况调查显示,使用率约为单中心每月0.19例,目前$ECCO_2R$使用率仍偏低。

(二)$ECCO_2R$ 对 ARDS 患者机械通气及炎症反应的影响

$ECCO_2R$治疗24h后动脉PCO_2及RR明显下降,动脉pH明显升高。一项动物实验发现,血流量为300 ml/min的静脉$ECCO_2R$能将血液中的CO_2含量降低17%~22%。ECCO2R支持下ARDS通气参数VT可由6 ml/kg降至3 ml/kg。在一项为期2年的多中心前瞻性观察研究对大都市应用$ECCO_2R$的使用情况调查发现,ARDS患者中位VT从5.9 ml/kg降至4.1 ml/kg。2016年3月至2017年6月,法国在5个ICU进行了一项试点研究,结果显示超保护性通气策略下(VT 4 ml/kg,Pplat≤25 cmH_2O) ARDS患者机械通气中PEEP从基线时的(13.4±3.6)cmH_2O显著增加到(15.0±3.4)cmH_2O,驱动压力从(13.0±4.8)cmH_2O降至(7.9±3.2)cmH_2O。平均$PaCO_2$从(43±8)mmHg上升到(53±9)mmHg。平均pH从基线的7.39±0.1下降到7.32±0.10。而PaO_2/FiO_2、呼吸系统顺应及呼吸频率没有改变。在2019年法国一项多中心前瞻性研究,纳入11个ICU中35名中重度ARDS患者实施$ECCO_2R$联合超保护通气治疗,发现约2/3的中低度至重度ARDS患者中可达到超保护通气,驱动压力中位数降低4 cmH_2O,进一步证实了$ECCO_2R$下的超保护通气可行性,但其中1/3患者出现高碳酸血症。同期,在欧洲一项多中心Ⅱ期临床研究证明,$ECCO_2R$有助于超保护通气策略(VT 4 ml/kg,平台压≤25 cmH_2O)的实施,8 h、24 h达成超保护通气的比例分别为78%和82%。提示$ECCO_2R$可能促进中度ARDS患者的低通气的超保护通气策略的实施。

低流量$ECCO_2R$装置强大的病理生理学的合理性促进了ARDS患者实施UPLVS的同时,也可降低机体炎症反应。研究发现$ECCO_2R$治疗下血浆白细胞介素-6(IL-6)、IL-8和肿瘤坏死因子-α(TNF-α)浓度显著降低,支气管肺泡灌洗液(BALF)中IL-6和TNF-α浓度降低,且不影响呼吸力学、气体交换和血流动力学。

(三)$ECCO_2R$ 支持下 ARDS 患者并发症发生情况

法国一项观察性研究通过电话访问法国附属医院239个ICU在2010—2015年5年间应用$ECCO_2R$情况,结果显示,并发症发生率为63%,其中最常见的是出血(45%)和膜功能障碍(18%)。欧洲一项多中心Ⅱ期临床医学研究证明,$ECCO_2R$在实施ARDS超保护通气时,$ECCO_2R$相关不良反应发生率约39%。由此提示$ECCO_2R$并发症发生率较高。

(四)$ECCO_2R$ 支持下 ARDS 患者预后

在2007—2010年在德国8个ICU和澳大利亚2个ICU多中心的前瞻性研究发现,$ECCO_2R$支持下ARDS患者随达到保护性通气(VT降至3ml/kg),但28 d内及60 d内无机械通气天数及死亡率未有改善,仅在严重ARDS患者($PaO_2/FiO_2 \leq 150$ mm Hg)亚组析因分析,发现可改善其60 d内无机械通气时长,死亡率较无$ECCO_2R$支持的ARDS降低,但无统计学意义。欧洲一项多中心Ⅱ期临床医学研究结果显示,$ECCO_2R$联合超保护通气治疗ARDS患者,28 d及出院存活率分别为73%和62%。

总之,$ECCO_2R$微创、有效,改善高碳酸血症优势明显,对于无危及生命低氧血症的ARDS患者可实现超保护性通气。但现有研究多为单中心、队列研究,大多数可用临床数据及当前设备的技术特征和性能均存在差异,迄今为止未有证据显示$ECCO_2R$对ARDS生存的有益影响。因此,在$ECCO_2R$广泛应用之前,还需更多的数据来评估$ECCO_2R$的临床获益与潜在并发症的风险,$ECCO_2R$在ARDS中应用有待随机临床试验进一步论证。

参 考 文 献

[1] Schmidt M, Jaber S, Zogheib E, et al. Feasibility and safety of low-flow extracorporeal CO_2 removal managed with a renal replacement platform to enhance lung-protective ventilation of patients with mild-to-moderate ARDS. Crit Care, 2018, 22(1):122.

[2] Gattinoni L, Pesenti A, Mascheroni D, et al. Low-frequency positive-pressure ventilation with extracorporeal CO_2 removal in severe acute respiratory failure. JAMA, 1986, 256(7): 881-886.

[3] Brower R G, Lanken P N, Macintyre N, et al. Higher versus lower positive end-expiratory pressures in patients with the acute respiratory distress syndrome. N Engl J Med, 2004, 351(4):327-336.

[4] 杨依依,姚尚龙,尚游. 呼吸机相关性肺损伤发病机制研究新进展. 中华危重病急救医学,2016,28(9):861-864.

[5] Bilek A M, Dee K C, Gaver D R. Mechanisms of surface-tension-induced epithelial cell damage in a model of pulmonary airway reopening. J Appl Physiol (1985), 2003, 94(2): 770-783.

[6] Slutsky A S, Tremblay L N. Multiple system organ failure. Is mechanical ventilation a contributing factor?. Am J Respir Crit Care Med, 1998, 157(6 Pt 1):1721-1725.

[7] 孙秀梅,王玉妹,杨燕琳,等. 机械功率在呼吸机相关性肺损伤的研究现状. 中华危重病急救医学,2019,31(12):1549-1551.

[8] Marini J J. Evolving concepts for safer ventilation. Crit Care, 2019,23(Suppl 1):114.

[9] Dreyfuss D, Saumon G. Ventilator-induced lung injury: les-

sons from experimental studies. Am J Respir Crit Care Med, 1998,157(1):294-323.
[10] Frank J A, Gutierrez J A, Jones K D, et al. Low tidal volume reduces epithelial and endothelial injury in acid-injured rat lungs. Am J Respir Crit Care Med, 2002,165(2):242-249.
[11] Terragni P P, Rosboch G, Tealdi A, et al. Tidal hyperinflation during low tidal volume ventilation in acute respiratory distress syndrome. Am J Respir Crit Care Med, 2007,175(2):160-166.
[12] Richard J C, Marque S, Gros A, et al. Feasibility and safety of ultra-low tidal volume ventilation without extracorporeal circulation in moderately severe and severe ARDS patients. Intensive Care Med, 2019,45(11):1590-1598.
[13] Amato M B, Meade M O, Slutsky A S, et al. Driving pressure and survival in the acute respiratory distress syndrome. N Engl J Med, 2015,372(8):747-755.
[14] Villar J, Martin-Rodriguez C, Dominguez-Berrot A M, et al. A Quantile Analysis of Plateau and Driving Pressures: Effects on Mortality in Patients With Acute Respiratory Distress Syndrome Receiving Lung-Protective Ventilation. Crit Care Med, 2017,45(5):843-850.
[15] Needham D M, Yang T, Dinglas V D, et al. Timing of low tidal volume ventilation and intensive care unit mortality in acute respiratory distress syndrome. A prospective cohort study. Am J Respir Crit Care Med, 2015,191(2):177-185.
[16] 朱峰."超"保护性肺通气策略的实践:体外膜氧合与高频振荡通气联合通气模式. 中华结核和呼吸杂志, 2014,37(11):845-848.
[17] Morelli A, Del S L, Pesenti A, et al. Extracorporeal carbon dioxide removal(ECCO$_2$R) in patients with acute respiratory failure. Intensive Care Med, 2017,43(4):519-530.
[18] Moerer O, Harnisch L O, Barwing J, et al. Minimal-flow ECCO$_2$R in patients needing CRRT does not facilitate lung-protective ventilation. J Artif Organs, 2019,22(1):68-76.
[19] Ismaiel N M, Henzler D. Effects of hypercapnia and hypercapnic acidosis on attenuation of ventilator-associated lung injury. Minerva Anestesiol, 2011,77(7):723-733.
[20] Nichol A D, O'Cronin D F, Howell K, et al. Infection-induced lung injury is worsened after renal buffering of hypercapnic acidosis. Crit Care Med, 2009,37(11):2953-2961.
[21] Leypoldt J K, Goldstein J, Pouchoulin D, et al. Extracorporeal carbon dioxide removal requirements for ultraprotective mechanical ventilation: Mathematical model predictions. Artif Organs, 2020,44(5):488-496.
[22] Nin N, Muriel A, Penuelas O, et al. Severe hypercapnia and outcome of mechanically ventilated patients with moderate or severe acute respiratory distress syndrome. Intensive Care Med, 2017,43(2):200-208.
[23] Duscio E, Cipulli F, Vasques F, et al. Extracorporeal CO$_2$ Removal: The Minimally Invasive Approach, Theory, and Practice. Crit Care Med, 2019,47(1):33-40.
[24] Kolobow T, Gattinoni L, Tomlinson T A, et al. Control of breathing using an extracorporeal membrane lung. Anesthesiology, 1977,46(2):138-141.
[25] Del S L, Cypel M, Fan E. Extracorporeal life support for adults with severe acute respiratory failure. Lancet Respir Med, 2014,2(2):154-164.
[26] Goligher E C, Combes A, Brodie D, et al. Determinants of the effect of extracorporeal carbon dioxide removal in the SUPERNOVA trial: implications for trial design. Intensive Care Med, 2019,45(9):1219-1230.
[27] Grasselli G, Castagna L, Bottino N, et al. Practical Clinical Application of an Extracorporeal Carbon Dioxide Removal System in Acute Respiratory Distress Syndrome and Acute on Chronic Respiratory Failure. ASAIO J, 2020, 66(6):691-697.
[28] Camporota L, Barrett N. Current Applications for the Use of Extracorporeal Carbon Dioxide Removal in Critically Ill Patients. Biomed Res Int, 2016,2016:9781695.
[29] Nentwich J, John S. Current techniques for extracorporeal decarboxylation. Med Klin Intensivmed Notfmed, 2019, 114(8):733-740.
[30] Fan E. Extracorporeal CO$_2$ Removal-A Solution in Search of a Problem?. Crit Care Med, 2019,47(1):124-126.
[31] Winiszewski H, Aptel F, Belon F, et al. Daily use of extracorporeal CO$_2$ removal in a critical care unit: indications and results. J Intensive Care, 2018,6:36.
[32] Fanelli V, Ranieri M V, Mancebo J, et al. Feasibility and safety of low-flow extracorporeal carbon dioxide removal to facilitate ultra-protective ventilation in patients with moderate acute respiratory distress sindrome. Crit Care, 2016,20:36.
[33] Boyle AJ, Sklar MC, Mcnamee JJ, et al. Extracorporeal carbon dioxide removal for lowering the risk of mechanical ventilation: research questions and clinical potential for the future. Lancet Respir Med, 2018,6(11):874-884.
[34] Del S L, Fan E, Nava S, et al. ECCO$_2$R in COPD exacerbation only for the right patients and with the right strategy. Intensive Care Med, 2016,42(11):1830-1831.
[35] Gross-Hardt S, Hesselmann F, Arens J, et al. Low-flow assessment of current ECMO/ECCO$_2$R rotary blood pumps and the potential effect on hemocompatibility. Crit Care, 2019,23(1):348.
[36] Deniau B, Ricard JD, Messika J, et al. Use of extracorporeal carbon dioxide removal(ECCO$_2$R) in 239 intensive care units: results from a French national survey. Intensive Care Med, 2016,42(4):624-625.
[37] Augy J L, Aissaoui N, Richard C, et al. A 2-year multicenter, observational, prospective, cohort study on extracorporeal CO$_2$ removal in a large metropolis area. J Intensive Care, 2019,7:45.
[38] Terragni P P, Del S L, Mascia L, et al. Tidal volume lower than 6 ml/kg enhances lung protection: role of extracorporeal carbon dioxide removal. Anesthesiology, 2009, 111(4):826-835.
[39] Livigni S, Maio M, Ferretti E, et al. Efficacy and safety of a low-flow veno-venous carbon dioxide removal device: results of an experimental study in adult sheep. Crit Care, 2006,10(5):R151.
[40] Bein T, Weber-Carstens S, Goldmann A, et al. Lower tidal volume strategy(approximately 3 ml/kg) combined with ex-

tracorporeal CO₂ removal versus'conventional' protective ventilation(6 ml/kg)in severe ARDS: the prospective randomized Xtravent-study. Intensive Care Med,2013,39(5):847-856.

[41] Combes A,Fanelli V,Pham T,et al. Feasibility and safety of extracorporeal CO₂ removal to enhance protective ventilation in acute respiratory distress syndrome: the SUPERNOVA study. Intensive Care Med,2019,45(5):592-600.

[42] Grasso S,Stripoli T,Mazzone P,et al. Low respiratory rate plus minimally invasive extracorporeal CO₂ removal decreases systemic and pulmonary inflammatory mediators in experimental Acute Respiratory Distress Syndrome. Crit Care Med,2014,42(6):e451-e460.

4 脓毒症与免疫失衡：个体化诊疗的希望

赵洪文

脓毒症(sepsis)是一种以感染后器官衰竭为特征的威胁生命的综合征，是住院患者最常见的死亡原因。脓毒症患者的死亡风险随着器官功能障碍程度的加重而增加。有报道，在ICU内脓毒症的发病率高达38%，并且死亡率明显高于非脓毒症患者。如果脓毒症不能及时被发现和正确治疗，可因明显的循环和细胞代谢异常而导致低血压和高乳酸血症，从而发生脓毒症休克(septic shock)，此时患者的住院病死率将进一步增加，可高达40%以上。因此，由于脓毒症和脓毒症休克的高发病率和高病死率，脓毒症已是一个危害人类健康的公共卫生问题，早期发现脓毒症并进行及时恰当治疗是防止其进展到脓毒症休克的关键，也是改善预后的决定因素。

一、脓毒症和脓毒症休克新定义

2016年SCCM和ESICM专家组发布了脓毒症新定义(Sepsis-3.0)和诊断标准。新定义指出，Sepsis是指宿主对感染的反应失控，并引起危及生命的器官功能障碍，其诊断标准为：感染引起危及生命的器官功能障碍(序贯器官衰竭估计评分，SOFA≥2)；脓毒症休克是指感染导致的循环衰竭和细胞代谢异常，是Sepsis的一个亚型，其诊断标准为：Sepsis患者经积极液体复苏后仍需要升压药物维持平均动脉压≥65 mmHg，并且血乳酸>2mmol/L。因此，根据脓毒症定义，感染是脓毒症的触发因素，宿主对感染的反应失调(即炎症/免疫反应失衡)是脓毒症病理生理学的核心。如何根据脓毒症患者的免疫失衡状态进行个体化诊疗来改善预后是临床所面临的问题。

二、免疫系统的功能和构成

免疫系统是人体健康最重要的一道屏障，具有免疫防御(消灭各种入侵的病原体)、免疫监视(识别并清除病变/癌变细胞)、免疫稳定(清理衰老细胞，稳定正常代谢)的功能。人体的免疫系统由先天免疫(或称固有免疫)和适应性免疫(或称获得性免疫)构成，其中，先天免疫是非特异性免疫，构成人体防卫功能的第一道防线，包括：组织屏障、先天免疫细胞(巨噬细胞、树突状细胞、NK细胞、中性粒细胞等)和先天免疫分子(诸如补体、溶菌酶及细胞因子等)；适应性免疫是特异性免疫反应，包括：①T淋巴细胞介导的细胞免疫：经Toll样受体(TLRs)信号途径诱导初始T细胞分化、辅助B细胞生成抗体、增强$CD8^+$细胞毒性T淋巴细胞活性、调节免疫反应和诱导炎症反应。②B淋巴细胞介导的体液免疫：通过补体激活而发生溶菌效应，通过抗体介导的调理作用而促进吞噬细胞吞噬抗原，抗体依赖性细胞介导的细胞毒作用(ADCC)，增强NK、巨噬细胞、中性粒细胞对靶细胞的杀伤作用。一般来说，在脓毒症的发生发展过程中，急性炎症反应主要与先天免疫有关，适应性免疫与免疫抑制和继发感染有关。

三、脓毒症患者免疫状态特点

当机体发生感染时，先天免疫细胞通过其表达的模式识别受体(PRRs)识别致病原相关分子模式(PAMPs)和组织损伤释放的相关分子模式(DAMPs)，引发了一系列炎症反应，包括黏附分子、细胞因子和活性氧(ROS)产物等的上调。当这些抗炎反应上调成功清除病原体时，机体最终恢复组织内环境稳态。然而，如果先天性和适应性反应不能在局部抑制正在进行的感染，感染就会在全身扩散，导致细胞功能障碍和组织损伤，并进一步出现引起危及生命的器官功能障碍，即脓毒症发生。

研究证实，免疫功能失衡是脓毒症发生发展过程中的重要特点。1996年美国学者Bone指出：脓毒症患者的免疫功能状态呈现出促炎反应/抗炎反应失控的动态性变化——Bone假说，即：在病程早期，感染引起机体出现一种难以控制的全身瀑布式炎症反应，机体呈现过度的全身炎症反应(SIRS)，促炎症反应占优势，即免疫亢进；随后，体内代偿性释放抗炎介质过量而引起的免疫功能降低及感染易感性增高，即出现内源性代偿性抗炎反应综合征(CARS)；若SIRS与CARS同时并存又相互加强，则会导致炎症反应和免疫功能更为严重的紊乱，从而对机体产生更强烈的损伤，称为失代偿性炎症反应综合征，也称为混合性拮抗反应综合征(MARS)；在病程后期则转化为抗炎症机制占优势而导致免疫抑制，甚至免疫麻痹，出现不同程度的慢性炎症、获得性的免疫抑制、对院内感染高风险和严重的蛋白分解代谢状态，即持续性炎症免疫抑制及高分解代谢综合征(PICS)。但也有研究发现脓毒症患者免疫反应变化没有明显的时效性，即使严重脓毒症早期机体也不一定表现为SIRS，部分患者表现为

MARS 状态。

人体对感染的免疫反应受很多因素的影响,取决于宿主因素和病原体因素。其中,宿主因素包括:基因型和表型、年龄、性别、合并疾病(诸如糖尿病、肝硬化、肾衰竭、心脏病、慢性阻塞性肺疾病等)、严重免疫抑制(诸如长期激素治疗、肿瘤化疗、HIV 感染、肝移植等);病原体因素包括:病原体种类(病毒、细菌或真菌)、感染部位(肺炎、腹膜炎、泌尿系感染或脑膜炎)和感染的程度和时间等。因此,作为感染(原因)和器官功能障碍(结果)之间桥梁的宿主炎症免疫反应失衡是复杂而异质性的。有作者将脓毒症分为经典脓毒症(高炎症反应型)和非经典脓毒症(低炎症反应型)。高炎症反应被视为经典脓毒症患者器官功能障碍的主要原因,而凝血、免疫、神经内分泌、代谢等因素起次要作用。相反,非经典脓毒症患者器官功能障碍可能是由高龄、免疫抑制、合并慢性基础疾病等其他宿主或由机械通气、镇静、或其他非感染性原因造成的,而炎症反应不明显。

因此,脓毒症患者治疗面临的最大挑战之一是失调宿主炎症免疫反应的异质性,这种异质性是以前脓毒症宿主靶向治疗临床试验失败的原因之一。因此,脓毒症患者必须个体化精确治疗。

四、脓毒症对免疫系统的影响

脓毒症对免疫系统的影响是复杂的,在疾病的发生发展过程中是动态变化的,但许多机制尚不清楚。

(一)脓毒症早期对免疫系统的影响

脓毒症早期先天免疫系统被过度激活而导致过度炎症和随之而来的心血管衰竭。过度炎症是多种先天免疫细胞类型通过其表达的模式识别受体(PRRs)识别病原体相关分子模式(PAMPs)和组织损伤释放的相关分子模式(DAMPs)后释放促炎介质、细胞因子和活性氧(ROS)产物等介导的。与此同时,补体系统、血管内皮和凝血系统的激活导致微循环疾病。这些过程被中性粒细胞胞外诱捕网(NETosis)的释放和炎症细胞焦亡而进一步加剧。中性粒细胞是循环中除单核细胞外主要的先天免疫细胞,由于产生高 ROS,它具有强大的吞噬和细胞内杀伤活性,是早期控制入侵病原体的必需细胞。脓毒症时产生的促炎刺激物(病原体和其他促炎因子)激活系统循环中的中性粒细胞后,上调其促炎基因(如 TNF-α,IL-1α,IL-1β)和抗凋亡基因(如 Bcl-xL,Mcl-1,A1,Bak),从而通过增加吞噬作用和 ROS 产生杀死病原体来增强其抗菌作用。然而,如果中性粒细胞激活后无法控制,通过血管内皮向各种靶器官的迁移、浸润就会增加,从而导致周围组织损伤而发展为多器官功能障碍综合征(MODS)。中性粒细胞的移出增加是由于中性粒细胞的黏附分子(即 β 整合蛋白和 L-选择蛋白)及其同源的内皮细胞的黏附分子(ICAM-1,VCAM-1等)的过度表达所致。

(二)持续的脓毒症对先天免疫系统的影响

脓毒症对先天免疫系统的所有细胞成分都有多种重要的影响。例如,脓毒症迅速引起滤泡树突状细胞、树突状细胞、未成熟巨噬细胞、自然杀伤细胞(NK)细胞和骨髓来源的抑制细胞(MDSCs)大量凋亡。相反,中性粒细胞抵抗脓毒症诱导细胞凋亡的能力较强,这一结果被认为是继发于中性粒细胞活化机制的结果。在最初的中性粒细胞动员和激活后,随后从骨髓释放的中性粒细胞其杀菌功能和细胞因子产生能力均较弱。有研究显示,中性粒细胞亚群释放大量的免疫抑制细胞因子 IL-10。研究表明,包括单核细胞、巨噬细胞和树突状细胞在内的抗原呈递细胞的人类白细胞 DR 抗原(HLA-DR)表达减少是脓毒症的一个标志,这可能会影响将其微生物抗原最佳的递呈给 T 淋巴细胞。此外,中性粒细胞上的程序性细胞死亡 1 配体(PDL-1)表达增加,导致表达程序性细胞死亡 1(PD-1)的 $CD4^+$ 和 $CD8^+$ T 细胞的凋亡增加,这与其他免疫抑制机制一起共同导致脓毒症诱导的免疫抑制的发展。脓毒症休克时,由于中性粒细胞凋亡增加,循环中成熟中性粒细胞数量减少,而未成熟的中性粒细胞数量增加,导致杀灭和清除病原体能力下降。研究表明,血液循环中未成熟中性粒细胞数量的增加与脓毒症不良预后有关。然而,循环中成熟中性粒细胞的减少和未成熟中性粒细胞数量的增加都是造成 MODS 和死亡率增加的原因。

骨髓来源的抑制细胞(MDSCs)是一组髓系含有粒细胞和单核细胞祖细胞的未成熟先天免疫细胞的异质性细胞群。在遇到病原体和炎症因子时,MDSCs 从未成熟的髓细胞中迅速生成和增加,导致 MDSCs 在循环、骨髓、脾脏和淋巴结中增加。MDSCs 通过分泌各种免疫抑制分子(包括 IL-10 和 TGF-β)而对 $CD4^+$、$CD8^+$ T 淋巴细胞发挥免疫抑制作用,并使其向 Th2 免疫反应发展。在脓毒症诱导的免疫抑制中,MDSCs 对 T 细胞免疫反应的抑制进一步增加了脓毒症患者后续感染的易感性。

(三)持续的脓毒症对适应性免疫系统的影响

脓毒症导致 $CD4^+$ 和 $CD8^+$ T 淋巴细胞及 B 淋巴细胞明显减少。由于调节性 T 细胞(TReg)抵抗 Sepsis 诱导细胞凋亡的能力较强,因此,与其他淋巴细胞亚群相比,脓毒症患者血液中 TReg 细胞的比例增加,这有助于形成一个免疫抑制更强的表型。存活的 $CD4^+$ 和 $CD8^+$ T 淋巴细胞要么从促炎 T 辅助性细胞(TH1)表型转变为抗炎 TH2 细胞表型,要么发展为"耗竭"表型,其特征是 PD-1 表达增加和细胞因子分泌减少。$CD4^+$ T 淋巴细胞的 CD28 表达和 T 细胞受体(TCR)多样性的减少,可能导致对入侵病原体的抗菌反应减弱。

五、免疫调理辅助治疗在脓毒症治疗中的地位

目前,脓毒症的治疗通常是支持性治疗,包括液体复苏、血管活性物质、吸氧和抗生素应用等。然而,这些治疗的临床效果并不理想,因此需要探讨新的治疗方法。由于脓毒症患者病原体感染可引起机体免疫反应异常,从过度炎症到免疫抑制,这使得免疫调节辅助治疗成为可能。然而,脓毒症患者的免疫状态在疾病过程中是复杂的、动态变化的。在混合促炎和抗炎反应并随着时间而迅速改变

的复杂情况下,恰当的免疫调理辅助治疗策略依赖于对患者免疫状态的评估能力。如果没有监测和评估患者的免疫状态而进行免疫抑制或免疫增强治疗,就很难改善患者的免疫功能紊乱。

(一)免疫功能状态的评估

脓毒症患者的宿主免疫反应非常复杂,是一个高度个体化的过程,其特征是包括对感染的过度炎症免疫反应和深度免疫抑制。有作者提出,用于脓毒症免疫治疗的有潜力的生物标志物如下。①先天免疫:单核细胞 HLA-DR 的表达,脂多糖刺激的全血细胞产生 TNF,单核细胞 PDL-1 的表达。②适应性免疫:持续严重的淋巴细胞减少,巨细胞病毒或单纯疱疹病毒感染的复活,$CD4^+$ 或 $CD8^+$ 细胞 PD-1 的表达,循环调节性 T 细胞数目,T 细胞产生 γ-干扰素,T 细胞增殖。③先天免疫和适应性免疫:低毒或条件致病菌(如肠球菌、不动杆菌或念珠菌)引起的感染,IL-10/TNF 比率,迟发型高敏反应。其中,脓毒症过程中与过度炎症反应相关的指标包括:促炎介质(TNF-α、IL-1、γ-IFN、IL-6、IL-8 等)、细胞因子和 DAMPs 的释放;免疫细胞的活化,如抗原呈递细胞(APCs);细胞损伤,中性粒细胞胞外诱捕网的释放(NETosis)和细胞焦亡;凝血和补体的激活;血管内皮的活化;丧失屏障功能;微血管血栓。

脓毒症过程中的免疫抑制涉及适应性和先天性免疫系统,其相关指标包括:抗炎介质(IL-4、IL-10、IL-11、可溶性 TNF-α 受体、TGF-β、NO 等)的释放;T 细胞、B 细胞和树突状细胞的凋亡;T 细胞枯竭;PD1/PD-L1 轴的上调;中性粒细胞杀菌功能丧失;APCs 的重编程;HLA-DR 表达降低;Treg 细胞和 MDSCs 的增加。到目前为止,绝对淋巴细胞计数(包括 $CD4^+$ 和 Treg 淋巴细胞)和单核细胞 HLA-DR 表达下降是在多中心研究中应用最多的指标,因为这两种指标的测量方法都是标准化的,而且它们的变化与器官功能障碍和不良后果(院内感染发生或死亡率)有关。此外,监测 MDSCs 和(或)未成熟的中性粒细胞(作为骨髓活动度和慢性低度炎症的标志物)、T 淋巴细胞 PD-1 和单核细胞 PD-L1 的表达(作为抗 PD-1/抗 PD-L1 治疗的潜在分层标志物)是在更大的患者群中进一步验证的良好候选指标。在将来评估脓毒症免疫辅助治疗临床试验的设计中,使用的生物标志物使患者分层是必需的步骤。

(二)脓毒症的免疫抑制治疗

除了感染性病原体的全身播散所带来的威胁,脓毒症早期先天免疫系统的过度激活可导致过度炎症和随之而来的心血管衰竭。因此,阻断先天免疫系统的激活作为脓毒症早期治疗的一个组成部分是很合理的,目前针对脓毒症的过度炎症的临床研究见表 8-4-1。

表 8-4-1 目前针对脓毒症的过度炎症的临床研究(免疫抑制治疗)

治疗	目标分子和主要作用	临床实验编号	主要结局	注释
Anakinra	重组人 IL-1 受体拮抗剂	NCT03332225	28 d 死亡率	另一个研究组在免疫抑制状态下接受 IFNγ 治疗
Adrecizumab	肾上腺髓质素结合抗体	NCT03085758	90 d 以上安全性	只招募血清肾上腺髓质素>70 pg/ml 的患者(2019)
维生素 C(抗坏血酸)	抑制 NF-κB 的激活	NCT02106975	在 96h SOFA 评分的变化	已终止:SOFA 评分无差别(2019)
	抑制 HMGB1 的释放	NCT03680274	28 d 死亡率和器官衰竭	无
	增强趋化性和吞噬作用	NCT03835286	血管加压药的消耗量	无
氢化可的松,抗坏血酸和硫胺素	多效性的免疫调节作用	NCT03509350	无血管加压药和无呼吸机的天数	研究方案已发表(2019)
	抑制 NF-κB 和 AP-1 的激活	NCT03333278	在第 7 天无须血管加压药	研究方案已发表(2019)
		NCT03380507	60 d 死亡率	无
	抑制内皮细胞和中性粒细胞的激活	NCT03540628	2 年死亡率	无
		NCT03828929	30 d 死亡率	无
		NCT03258684	14 d 死亡率	无
克拉霉素	抑制 NF-κB 和干扰素调节因子-3 的激活	NCT03345992	28 d 死亡率	无
多黏菌素 B 血液灌流	通过结合脂质 A 中和脂多糖	NCT01046669	28 d 死亡率	已终止:死亡率无差别(2018)
		NCT01222663	28 d 死亡率	已终止:死亡率无差别(2015)
CytoSorb	清除 PAMPs、DAMPS 和细胞因子	NCT29084247	IL-6 血清水平	已终止:IL-6 水平无差别(2017)
治疗性血浆置换	消除促炎和替换保护分子	NCT03065751	28 d 死亡率	初步研究显示改善血流动力学(2018)

(三)脓毒症的免疫刺激治疗

尽管脓毒症的免疫反应是复杂的、动态变化的,但研究表明,脓毒症患者或多或少、或长或短都存在免疫抑制,这增加了后期感染易感性和死亡风险。有一种可能性就是应用免疫刺激剂治疗可能有助于宿主达到免疫稳态。因此,免疫刺激疗法已成为一种合理的治疗选择。为此,许多分子作为脓毒症的免疫佐剂正被研究(表8-4-2)。

表8-4-2 目前针对脓毒症的免疫抑制的临床研究(免疫刺激治疗)

治疗	目标分子和主要作用	临床实验编号	主要结局	用于初始治疗的免疫生物标志物	注释
GM-CSF	增加中性粒细胞、巨噬细胞和单核细胞的生成和活性	NCT02361528	第28天或ICU出院时ICU获得性感染	单核细胞HLA-DR水平降低(每个细胞<8000单克隆抗体)	
IFNγ	增加白细胞的活性	NCT01649921	LPS刺激的白细胞分泌TNF	无	
		NCT03332225	28 d死亡率	CD-14单核细胞HLA-DR表达<30%	另一个研究组在高炎症状态下接受anakinra治疗
IL-7	促进淋巴细胞增殖和存活	NCT02640807	安全性和免疫重建	≤900淋巴细胞/μl	已终止:耐受良好,淋巴细胞计数增加3倍以上(2018年)
IgG,IgA,IgM	提高对病原体的识别和抗凋亡作用	NCT03334006	第7天MOF评分的提高	IL-6水平>1000 pg/ml	
间充质干细胞	增强细菌清除	NCT02421484	安全性和细胞因子反应	无	已终止:安全,且升高的细胞因子水平无加重(2019)
	限制细胞凋亡	NCT03369275	减少使用机械通气、肾脏替代治疗或血管加压药的天数	无	
	增强损伤修复	NCT02883803	第7天SOFA评分	无	
anti-PD-L1	减少细胞凋亡,促进T细胞反应	NCT02576457	安全性和90 d死亡率	≤1100淋巴细胞/μl	已终止:安全,且无药物诱导的细胞因子释放综合征(2019)

总之,机体免疫反应失调是脓毒症发生发展的重要病理生理机制,脓毒症患者机体对病原体引起的免疫反应异常,从过度炎症到免疫抑制,在疾病过程中是复杂的、动态变化的。因此,免疫调理辅助治疗已成为脓毒症一种合理的辅助治疗选择。但由于脓毒症期间发生的免疫反应的异质性和快速进展,宿主、入侵病原体和感染持续时间等多种特异性因素决定了脓毒症患者是处于主要的高炎症还是低炎症状态,免疫状态评估是脓毒症患者选择免疫治疗的干预类型和免疫治疗成功的前提。只有根据脓毒症患者免疫状态实施个体化精准免疫治疗才能改善患者的预后。然而,目前仍无统一生物学指标能判断免疫辅助治疗介入时机。在抗生素等基础治疗前提下,联合免疫调理辅助治疗将是未来脓毒症治疗的发展方向。

参 考 文 献

[1] Vincent JL, Sakr Y, Sprung CL, et al. Sepsis in European Intensive Care Units: Results of the SOAP study. Crit Care Med, 2006, 34(2): 344-353.

[2] Singer M, Deutschman CS, Seymour CW, et al. The Third International Consensus Definitions for Sepsis and Septic Shock (Sepsis-3). JAMA, 2016, 315(8): 801-810.

[3] Bhan C, Dipankar P, Chakraborty P, et al. Role of cellular events in the pathophysiology of sepsis. Inflammation Research, 2016, 65(11): 853-868.

[4] Bone, RC. Sir Isaac Newton, sepsis, SIRS, and CARS. Crit Care Med, 1996, 24(7): 1125-1128.

[5] Gentile LF, Cuenca AG, Efron PA, et al. Persistent inflammation and immunosuppression: a common syndrome and new horizon for surgical intensive care. J Trauma Acute Care Surg, 2012, 72(6): 1491-501.

[6] Cortes-Puch I. and Hartog CS. Change is not necessarily progress: Revision of the sepsis definition should be based on new scientific insights. Am J Respir Crit Care Med, 2016, 194

(1):16-18.
[7] Deutschman CS. Imprecise medicine: The limitations of sepsis-3. Crit Care Med,2016,44(5):857-858.
[8] Ding R,Meng Y,Ma X. The Central Role of the Inflammatory Response in Understanding the Heterogeneity of Sepsis-3. Biomed Res Int,2018,2018:5086516.
[9] Cohen J,Vincent JL,Adhikari NK,et al. Sepsis: A roadmap for future research. Lancet Infect Dis,2015,15:581-614.
[10] Perner A,Gordon AC,Angus DC,et al. The intensive care medicine research agenda on septic shock. Intensive Care Med,2017,43:1294-1305.
[11] Steinhagen F,Schmidt SV,Schewe JC,et al. Immunotherapy in sepsis-brake or accelerate? Pharmacol Ther,2020, 208:107476.
[12] Del Fresno C,Hidalgo A. Neutrophils acROSs the enemy lines. Immunity,2017,46:335-337.
[13] Nicolás-Ávila JÁ,Adrover JM,Hidalgo A. Neutrophils in homeostasis,immunity,and cancer. Immunity,2017,46:15-28.
[14] Tamayo E,Gómez E,Bustamante J,et al. Evolution of neutrophil apoptosis in septic shock survivors and nonsurvivors. Crit Care,2012,27,415. e1-11.
[15] Shen XF,Cao K,Jiang JP,et al. Neutrophil dysregulation during sepsis:an overview and update. J Cell Mol Med,2017, 21(9):1687 1697.
[16] Sônego F,Castanheira FV,Ferreira RG,et al. Paradoxical roles of the neutrophil in sepsis:protective and deleterious. Front Immunol,2016,7:155.
[17] Kasten KR,Muenzer JT,Caldwell CC. Neutrophils are significant producers of IL-10 during sepsis. Biochem. Biophys. Res. Commun,2010,393:28-31.
[18] Hotchkiss RS,Monneret G,Payen D. Sepsis-induced immunosuppression: from cellular dysfunctions to immunotherapy. Nat Rev Immunol,2013,13(12):862-874.
[19] Wang JF,Li JB,Zhao YJ,et al. Up-regulation of programmed cell death 1 ligand 1 on neutrophils may be involved in sepsis-induced immunosuppression:an animal study and a prospective case-control study. Anesthesiology,2015,122:852-863.
[20] Alves-Filho JC,Spiller F,Cunha FQ. Neutrophil paralysis in sepsis. Shock,2010,34(Suppl 1):15-21.
[21] Bermejo-Martin JF,Tamayo E,Ruiz G. Circulating neutrophil counts and mortality in septic shock. Crit Care,2014,18 (1):407.
[22] Kumar, V. Immunometabolism: Another Road to Sepsis and Its Therapeutic Targeting. Inflammation, 2019, 42 (3): 765-788.
[23] Monneret G,Gossez M,Aghaeepour N,et al. How Clinical Flow Cytometry Rebooted Sepsis Immunology. Cytometry A,2019,95(4):431-441.
[24] Venet F,Lukaszewicz AC,Payen D,et al. Monitoring the immune response in sepsis: A rational approach to administration of immunoadjuvant therapies. Curr Opin Immunol, 2013,25:477-483.
[25] Monneret G,Venet F. Sepsis-induced immune alterations monitoring by flow cytometry as a promising tool for individualized therapy. Cytometry B Clin Cytom, 2016, 90 (4): 376-386.
[26] Hotchkiss RS,Monneret G,Payen D. Immunosuppression in sepsis: A novel understanding of the disorder and a new therapeutic approach. Lancet Infect Dis,2013,13:260-268.
[27] Leentjens J,Kox M,van der Hoeven JG,Netea MG,et al. Immunotherapy for the adjunctive treatment of sepsis:From immunosuppression to immunostimulation. Time for a paradigm change? Am J Respir Crit Care Med, 2013, 187: 1287-1293.

5 重症患者血液净化和抗生素剂量调整——慎思笃行

李国强 蔡湘龙

恰当抗生素治疗可以降低ICU重症感染患者的病死率,适当剂量是恰当治疗的重要方面,联合肾脏替代治疗(renal replacement therapy,RRT)部分患者,由于缺乏抗生素剂量调整的循证医学研究,临床多根据健康成年人药代动力学/药效学(pharmacokinetics/pharmacodynamics,PK/PD)的研究数据进行剂量调整。然而重症患者病理生理改变、RRT治疗导致PK改变,从而改变了到达靶器官抗生素浓度;为达到最佳疗效,重症患者的PD目标也需提高,故既往推荐剂量大多不适合重症患者。因此,为发挥抗感染药物最大抗/杀菌作用,改善患者预后,需对患者病情、抗生素PK/PD,以及RRT对于不同抗生素清除率等方面加以综合考虑与分析,以制订更优的抗生素给药方案。

一、重症患者抗生素剂量个体化调整

(一)抗生素PK/PD和分类

抗生素游离部分能否到达感染部位和维持有效浓度与疗效密切相关,感染部位抗生素浓度是药物进入机体后吸收、分布、代谢和排出过程的综合结果。除血流感染外,临床常见的感染部位多位于血管外,抗生素到达感染部位的能力决定于组织相关因素(如组织血管床面积、紧密连接的存在或有孔毛细血管等)和药物相关因素(如分子量,molecular weight,MW)和血浆蛋白结合率(plasma protein binding,PPB)等。临床疗效是感染部位药物浓度、细菌负荷、细菌生长阶段及最低抑菌浓度(minimum inhibitory concentration,MIC)、最低杀菌浓度(minimum bactericidal concentration,MBC)、抗生素后效应(postantibiotic effect,PAE)等多种因素共同作用的结果,这些因素的任一变化可能会改变抗生素对病原体的作用能力,从而改变临床结果。PK/PD将这些因素整合,目前主要PK/PD指标为:T>MIC、C_{max}/MIC、AUC/MIC及PAE。时间依赖性抗生素与杀菌效果最匹配的PK/PD参数为T>MIC,这类抗生素杀菌作用相对慢,没有或短PAE,典型代表抗生素为β内酰胺类抗生素;浓度依赖性抗生素最佳PK/PD参数为C_{max}/MIC,随抗生素浓度增加,其杀菌作用增加,这类抗生素具有PAE,许多抗生素包括一些氨基糖苷类和喹诺酮类、达托霉素和甲硝唑具有此特征;部分浓度依赖性抗生素还具有时间依赖性杀菌特点,其最佳参数为AUC/MIC,这类抗生素以抑菌剂为主并且具有中长PAE,包括四环素、替加环素、一些氨基糖苷类、喹诺酮类、棘白菌素和三唑类等。

脂/水分配系数(lipid-water partition coefficient)也是一个重要的因素,常用log P表示,是药物在机体内非水相浓度和水相浓度之比的log值(log $P_{O/w}$),根据log P值可以分为水溶性和脂溶性,低log P值为水溶性抗生素,高log P值为脂溶性抗生素。水溶性抗生素(如青霉素类、头孢类、碳青霉烯类、氨基糖苷类、糖肽类、利奈唑胺、多黏菌素和达托霉素)主要分布于血浆和细胞外液,具有表观分布容积(volume of distribution,V_d)低,不能通过脂膜(对细胞内病原体无效)等特点,并多以原形自肾脏清除,肾功能受损会影响水溶性抗生素及其代谢物的排出,为避免药物毒性常需调整剂量,且可以被RRT快速清除,故在治疗时和治疗结束时需要认真评估RRT清除的药物总量,以增加给药剂量。脂溶性抗生素(如喹诺酮类、大环内酯类、替加环素、林可霉素、四环素类、氯霉素和克林霉素)具有V_d大,可以通过脂膜进入细胞(对细胞内菌有效),在细胞内聚集,主要经过肝脏代谢,RRT治疗时只有药物总量的很小一部分会被清除,因而在RRT治疗时或治疗结束后大多没有必要补充剂量。但临床也存在例外,如头孢曲松和苯唑西林为水溶性抗生素,从胆汁排泄;左氧氟沙星和环丙沙星为脂溶性抗生素,而经肾脏排泄。

(二)重症患者抗生素剂量调整

重症疾病的恶化进展不具有线性特点,明显的酸碱平衡失调、重要器官功能改变、基础疾病各异、多种合并用药,加之RRT、体外膜肺等体外治疗措施,以上均会影响所使用抗生素的PK/PD,而影响治疗效果,此外多重耐药菌要求更高的抗生素浓度等,这都给临床医生提出了抗生素剂量个体化的要求。

1. 负荷剂量 抗生素剂量包括负荷剂量和维持剂量,临床给予负荷剂量的目的在于迅速达到治疗浓度目标(therapeutic concentration target,TCT),负荷剂量为V_d和血浆药物浓度的乘积,抗生素负荷剂量与药物分布相关(和药物清除无关),因而,负荷剂量无须考虑患者的肝肾功能。

$$D = C \times V_d \times IBW$$

D剂量,C目标血浆药物浓度,IBW理想体重。

重症患者出现血管内、外容量的改变、血浆蛋白水平下降及器官清除能力的下降,会改变抗生素的V_d和PPB,

休克患者需积极液体复苏治疗,多合并不同程度毛细血管渗漏,液体和蛋白漏出到血管外间隙,V_d 增加,水溶性抗生素主要分布于细胞外间隙,随 V_d 增加,抗生素浓度降低,而脂溶性抗生素主要在细胞内聚集,可以代偿细胞外间隙的被动稀释。V_d 增加重症患者,常规负荷剂量导致 TCT 不能达标,故 V_d 增加时,水溶性抗生素需相应的增加其负荷剂量,以达到 TCT,例如氨基糖苷类抗生素的 V_d 为细胞外液,如出现水肿、渗出液,按照标准千克体重计算的常规剂量会导致剂量不足,增加的细胞外液需要被估算并增加额外剂量。相反,细胞外容积下降导致 V_d 下降,标准剂量估算则会导致过量,如对于肥胖患者,细胞外液与总体重的占比下降,按照常规剂量给予导致肾毒性增加。重症患者实际 V_d 与药物说明书可能不同,不同患者或不同病情也存在差异,故当使用 V_d 估计药物剂量时可能存在谬误,如氨基糖苷类抗生素在重症患者会增加 25% 左右,而万古霉素、甲硝唑和大部分 β 内酰胺类抗生素和正常值接近。对于脂溶性抗生素,重症并不增加 V_d,也不需要增加负荷剂量。

2. 维持剂量　正确的负荷剂量使机体短时间内达到有效血浆药物浓度,而维持剂量可以维持机体在抗生素给药间隔期间保持合适的抗生素浓度,与负荷剂量不同,维持剂量主要与药物清除有关,抗生素的总清除率是包括肝脏、肾脏和其他代谢部位清除率的总和,若重症患者的清除发生改变,如维持剂量仍按常规剂量给予,会导致 TCT 不达标或出现毒性反应。抗生素经肾脏清除占总清除的量是经肾脏排出抗生素维持剂量调整的主要参考指标,经肾脏清除占总清除 25%～30% 以下时,肾功能损伤对药物总清除影响不大,无需调整维持剂量。急性肾损伤损伤程度的准确评价是水溶性抗生素维持剂量调整的关键。研究发现 50% 急性肾损伤患者在 48h 后自行缓解,故如需剂量调整,可以适当延迟至 48h 后,而以 Cockcroft-Gault 和 MDRD 公式计算的血肌酐清除率、肾小球滤过率不准确,重症患者需每日至少计算一次尿肌酐清除率以评估肾小球滤过率。时间依赖性抗生素的 PD 目标为 T/MIC,降低每次给药剂量而非延长给药间隔为恰当方案;而浓度依赖性抗生素,保证负荷剂量达到峰浓度的情况下,应延长给药间隔。肾功能减退时,水溶性抗生素维持剂量需要根据肾功能下降的程度进行相应调整:

$$D = D_N \times CL_{ANUR}/CL_N$$

D_N 为常规剂量,CL_{ANUR} 为无尿时药物清除率,CL_N 为正常药物清除率。

另外,重症患者高动力状态时,肾脏血流增加,肾小球滤过率相应增加,肾脏清除增加(augmented renal clearance,ARC),一般用尿肌酐清除率 $\geq 130\text{ml}/(\min \cdot 1.73\text{m}^2)$ 代表 ARC,临床研究发现经肾脏清除抗生素 ARC 和抗生素浓度不达标有关。重症患者 ARC 为 15%～65.1%,年轻、病情程度轻及心指数增加(孕妇、贫血及脓毒性休克的高动力阶段)、中枢神经系统感染和广泛外伤的重症患者易合并 ARC,ARC 经常被临床医师和药师忽略。

二、RRT 治疗时药物清除:治疗模式相关技术因素

抗生素经 RRT/CRRT 清除与经肾脏清除类似,V_d、PPB、fu 等因素影响清除。临床使用的抗生素 MW 多在 1000Da 以下,仅有很少抗生素 MW 超过 1500Da(替考拉宁为 1880Da),而现在生物合成透析膜孔径较大(5000～20 000Da),CRRT 使用的滤过膜孔径更大(20 000～30 000Da),对于 MW 对药物清除的影响,可以不考虑。仅抗生素的非蛋白结合部分能被滤过,因而高 PPB 的药物被 CRRT 清除的少,再者,V_d 大代表药物只有一少部分分布于血管内,通过肾脏或体外清除技术清除的也少,V_d 越大,被 RRT 清除的药物越少,一般认为,$V_d \leq 1\text{L/kg}$ 可以被体外清除技术清除,而 $V_d \geq 2\text{L/kg}$ 则不能被清除。

(一) 弥散 (diffusion)

在透析(hemodialysis,HD)过程中溶质清除的功效决定于溶质的浓度梯度、透析膜的面积和极性,与对流清除相比,弥散清除随分子量增加而降低,不同滤过膜的弥散清除能力不同,聚丙烯腈(PAN,AN-69)要优于聚酰胺。透析液的饱和度(dialysate saturation,Sd)是指一种药物通过透析膜并溶解于透析液中能力,等于透析液中药物浓度(Cd)除以血浆药物浓度(Cp)。

$$Sd = Cd/Cp$$

药物弥散清除(diffusive drug clearance,CL_{HD})等于 Sd 乘以 Q_D(透析液流速)。

$$CL_{HD} = Sd \times Q_D$$

高分子量药物降低弥散速度,高透析液流速降低弥散时间,上述任一因素增加,Sd 会下降,Sd 理论上只受药物与膜相互作用及膜对蛋白质吸附的影响,当计算体外清除技术药物清除时,Sd 大致相当于非结合部分在总药量的比例,但是需要注意的是,Sd 不是恒定的,Q_D 不同,Sd 也会变化。

(二) 对流 (convection)

目前滤过治疗选择滤器膜材为高通透膜,范围在 20 000～50 000Da,远高于大多数抗生素的分子量,故对流清除不受抗生素分子量影响。药物通过滤器膜的能力为筛选系数(sieving coefficient,SC),为超滤液药物浓度(Cuf)和血浆药物浓度(Cp)的比值,对于大部分抗生素,SC 为抗生素的非蛋白结合部分(SC≈fu,相当于 1-PPB)。

$$SC = Cuf/Cp$$

根据置换液给予位置可分为两种治疗模式:前稀释和后稀释,不同模式会影响溶质清除效率,对于后稀释治疗模式,对流对抗生素的清除($CL_{post-HF}$)即为 Q_{UF} 和 SC 的乘积。

$$CL_{post-HF} = Q_{UF} \times SC$$

对于前稀释治疗模式,由于血浆抗生素浓度在进入滤器之前被置换液稀释,药物清除降低,修正分数(correction factor,CF)影响其降低程度,而 CF 决定于血流速度和前稀释置换液流速。

$$CL_{pre-HF} = Q_{UF} \times SC \times CF$$

$$CF = Q_B / (Q_B + Q_{pre})$$

只有置换液高流速时，不同稀释模式才会对药物清除产生明显影响，这可以部分解释体外实验没有证实前后稀释对清除率有影响，但体内研究发现前稀释 CVVH 清除率低于后稀释，上述公式还提示清除与超滤率成正比，因而药物剂量应根据超滤率进行调整，而在具体临床实践中，超滤率的变化范围要明显超过 SC 的变化，因而，超滤率也是一个更需要重视的方面。

间断血液透析（intermittent hemodialysis, IHD）和 CRRT 是显著不同的，行高通量 IHD 治疗时，具有较大 V_d 的药物可以迅速自血浆清除，但一次血液透析清除的药物总量仅占体内药物总量的一小部分，而在 IHD 治疗之后，血浆药物浓度逐渐恢复，CRRT 的清除作用缓慢但持续，虽短时间内对血浆药物浓度影响不如 IHD 明显，但在治疗过程中始终存在药物在血管内和组织之间的再分布，CRRT 的对流虽然抗生素清除功效低，但治疗强度大，抗生素清除量不一定低于高功效的 IHD。

（三）弥散联合对流

透析滤过（hemodiafiltration, HDF）治疗模式时溶质通过弥散和对流方式清除，此种模式下的计算抗生素清除较困难，特别是在不同的 Q_{UF} 和 Q_D 设置下。CVVHDF 后稀释，药物清除可以通过以下公式估算。

$$CL_{HDF} = Q_{UF} \times SC + Q_D \times Sd$$

如果此时用非蛋白结合部分来代替 Sd，会高估清除。CVVHDF 治疗模式，如果 Q_{UF} 为 400ml/h，Q_D 为 1～2L/h，依据健康志愿者非结合部分数据推算出的清除率和实际测的清除率相比，低 Q_D 基本相符。

溶质通过弥散和对流清除的过程中，弥散和对流存在交互作用，总清除要低于分别行弥散或对流清除之和。CVVHDF 治疗时对流驱动溶质到达透析液，降低了弥散的浓度差，而浓度差是弥散驱动力，Sd 进一步降低，从而降低抗生素清除，此外，弥散清除还受 MW、Q_B、Q_D、和 Q_{UF} 及膜材影响，很难预测，为了避免高估 CL_{HDF}，Choi 建议如下。

$$CL_{HDF} = (Q_{UF} + Q_D) \times Sd$$

（四）高容量（high Volume, HV）血滤

HV-CRRT 在脓毒症患者中使用较多，相比于肾脏剂量 CRRT，HV-CRRT 在药物清除方面有所不同。大部分抗生素的 PK 属于 2 室或 3 室模型，中央室常指血浆室，机体内不同组织为外周室，在标准的低容量 CRRT，药物清除的限速因素为 Q_D 或 Q_{UF}，由于 Q_B 明显超过 Q_D 或 Q_{UF}，药物经过 CRRT 清除的速度和药物自外周室向中央室转移速度基本相似，因而，停止 CRRT 治疗后，药物浓度不会发生反跳；而 HV-RRT 治疗开始后，中央室中非蛋白结合部分药物迅速清除，药物自外周室向中央室快速转移，以万古霉素为例，如果 Q_{UF} 由 14ml/min 提高到 28ml/min，SC 将下降约 30%，Q_D 由 8.3ml/min 提高到 33.3ml/min，Sd 下降 30%，提示将 Q_{UF} 或 Q_D 提高 1 倍，溶质清除能力并非也增加 1 倍，增加的同时，Sd 是下降的，下降幅度与使用的滤器相关，故在 HV-RRT 时药物清除的计算复杂，SC 和 Sd 的变化均需考虑。在 IVOIRE 研究中，140 例重症患者分为 2 组，HV 血滤组[70ml/(kg·h)]和标准容量血滤组[35ml/(kg·h)]在治疗的 96hrs 中，均给予标准剂量（如哌拉西林 16g/d，头孢曲松 2g/d），所有抗生素的平均清除半衰期在高容量血滤组短于标准剂量组。

（五）滤器膜及吸附

药物清除与透析或滤过膜的面积成正比，临床使用的膜面积为 0.5～2.5 m²，聚砜、聚丙烯腈、聚酰胺等生物合成膜孔径大小不影响抗生素清除，滤器膜对抗生素的吸附可能清除药物，不同的滤器膜吸附能力不同，但目前临床缺乏不同滤器对不同抗生素吸附能力的研究，各个指南中也未涉及，从整体来说，吸附对抗生素剂量调整地位不明确，临床也不推荐使用对抗生素有吸附作用的膜材进行 CRRT 治疗。临床因脓毒症休克或急性肝衰竭而行灌流或吸附治疗，在连续性血浆滤过吸附（continuous plasma filtration adsorption, CPFA）治疗模式时，树脂罐可以吸附万古霉素和哌拉西林，但整体上对血中抗生素浓度无影响，固定多黏菌素 B 的灌流器 2h 治疗清除美罗培南接近于 0，也无须因灌流而调整剂量。

三、CRRT 治疗时抗生素剂量调整原则

以肾脏清除为主要途径的抗生素，因 RRT/CRRT 清除部分药物，剂量需要进行相应调整，如经肾脏的清除部分低于 20%，CRRT 对总清除影响不大，则治疗时无须剂量调整，但如合并肝衰，CRRT 占总清除的比率将增加，而需进行剂量调整。抗生素的总清除是机体不同部位清除的总和，其中包括 CRRT 清除的部分，经体外清除技术清除占比（fractional extracorporeal clearance, FrEC）为体外清除技术清除与总清除的比值，如果超过 25%～30%，认为有临床意义，需要调整剂量。

$$Fr_{EC} = CL_{EC} / (CL_{EC} + CL_{nr} + CL_r)$$

其中 CL_{EC} 为体外清除技术的药物清除，CL_{nr} 为非肾途径药物清除，CL_r 为经肾脏药物清除。

从上述公式也可以发现，对于主要经非肾途径清除的药物体外清除技术占比有限，临床意义较小。虽然急性肾衰竭患者的残余肾功能（residual renal function, RRF）临床评估困难，但是在计算总清除时这部分必须考虑，如果 RRF 较好，会明显降低 FrEC，甚至可以忽略体外清除技术的临床意义，而且体外清除技术替代的仅是肾小球滤过功能，而经肾脏清除包括肾小球滤过、肾小管分泌和重吸收，对于主要经肾小管分泌排出的药物，仅根据残余肾功能推算的简单方法是不推荐的。再者，不同的血液净化技术药物清除效率不同，总体上 CVVHDF＞CVVH＞IHD，而且每种抗生素理化特点和 PK 不同，经 CRRT 清除率也不同。

合并急性肾损伤者行 CRRT 治疗时，具体剂量调整根据抗生素类型（时间或浓度依赖性抗生素）、CRRT 清除率等确定。对于时间依赖性抗生素，疗效决定于药物浓度超过 MIC 的时间（T＞MIC），而且对于重症患者，C_{min} 要超过 MIC 的 4～5 倍，因而，最佳剂量调整为缩短用药间隔，保持每次剂量不变。给药间隔可按下面公式估算。

$$Iv_{EC} = Iv_{anu} \times [CL_{NR}/(CL_{EC}+CL_{NR})]$$

Iv_{EC} 是 CRRT 治疗时给药间隔，Iv_{anu} 是无尿时给药间隔。

相反，对于浓度依赖性抗生素，疗效决定于 C_{max} 与 MIC 的比值，最佳疗效为 C_{max}/MIC 达到 8～10 及 AUC/MIC 超过 100，因而，最佳剂量调整应为增大每次用药剂量，保持用药间隔不变。如氨基糖苷类抗生素在无尿非透析患者低剂量使用，随 C_{max} 下降杀菌作用和药物毒性均是降低的，CRRT 治疗时增加剂量，可以获得更好的疗效，CRRT 治疗降低了最低药物浓度（或谷浓度），还相应降低了药物毒性。

$$D_{required} = (C_{max} - C_{actual}) \times V_d \times 体重$$

在 CRRT 清除率方面，如 CRRT 清除药物占总清除较高，应该根据清除的药物量，给予补充剂量，RENAL 研究提示 ICU 中 RRT 治疗患者的 25% 存在抗生素剂量不足。综合 CRRT 药物清除特点、不同抗生素 PK 等，抗生素剂量与用药间隔可通过下述数学公式进行估算。血药稳态浓度（Cp_{ss}）乘以 CL_{EC} 为 CRRT 时每小时经超滤清除的药物量，经 CRRT 清除的药物总量（D_{EC}）如下。

$$D_{EC} = Cp_{ss} \times CL_{EC} \times T_{dur}$$，其中 T_{dur} 为 CRRT 治疗时长。

CRRT 下总的药物剂量包括肾功能减退时推荐剂量和经 CRRT 清除剂量之和：

$$D = D_{anur} + D_{EC} = D_{anur} + Cp_{ss} \times CL_{EC} \times T_{dur}$$

目前，重症患者早期 CRRT 治疗逐渐增加，RRT 治疗对药物清除是有影响的，剂量可按以下公式计算：

$$D_{EC} = Dn \times [P_X + (1-P_X) \times CL_{CRtot}/CL_{CRn}]$$

Dn 是常规剂量，$P_X = CL_{NR}/CL_N$（CL_{NR} 为非肾清除，CL_N 为正常药物清除），CL_{CRtot} 为肾脏肌酐清除率和体外清除肌酐清除率的和，CL_{CRn} 是正常肌酐清除率。这个公式根据实际肌酐清除率的变化动态估算药物清除和调整药物剂量。

上述公式均是建立在复杂数学模型基础上的，多数数学模型在特定情况对某些药物可能适用，而适合所有药物、不同病情和不同治疗状态的数学模型尚不存在。

急性肾衰竭重症患者在 CRRT 时，包括患者因素、疾病、药物类型和治疗模式等多种因素影响药物清除，这些因素因患者而异，即使同一患者，也因病程而异。包括不同抗生素，考虑到各种变量及同时适合所有患者，涵盖 CRRT 不同剂量、不同设备、不同滤器等因素的抗生素剂量调整方案是非常困难的，甚至是不可能的。CRRT 技术的不断发展、脓毒症休克或器官衰竭体外治疗技术的出现及新抗生素的上市，剂量调整方案也需持续更新，目前虽有发布的抗生素剂量调整推荐，但还很有限。所以，重症患者需进行治疗药物浓度检测（therapeutic drug monitoring，TDM），以确保正确负荷剂量和维持剂量。最近的临床研究也证实其在重症患者中具有重要意义，目前 TDM 临床多用于指导氨基糖苷类和糖肽类抗生素的剂量调整，以获得最佳治疗浓度并降低肾毒性，但在其他种类抗生素较少使用，如果不具备 TDM 能力，抗生素的 PK/PD 模型则对于经验性剂量调整至关重要。

四、CRRT 治疗时美罗培南剂量调整循证研究

美罗培南是 β 内酰胺类抗生素，高度水溶性，Vd 为 0.3 L/kg，PPB 为 2%，87% 自肾脏排出，重症感染经验和目标治疗的重要选择。肾脏对美罗培南的排出或肾小球滤过率是影响 PK/PD 的最重要因素，在非 RRT 患者，调整剂量需要根据肌酐清除率和病原体的 MIC 确定，持续泵入给药对 PD 的影响要超过总剂量的影响，总剂量如果确定，持续静脉泵入要优于延长输注和普通输注。病原体不明确的经验性治疗时，如果 CrCL ≥ 90 ml/min，需要 6000mg 持续泵入才能达到 100% 达标概率（probability of target attainment，PTA），而对于铜绿假单胞菌等多重耐药病原体，单药不能达到 PD 目标，需要联合用药。联合 CRRT 治疗时，临床研究没有发现不同治疗模式（CVVHDF、CVVH）、治疗强度影响美罗培南清除，而残余肾功能是影响清除率的主要因素，CL(L/h) = 3.68 + 0.22（残存尿量/100ml），重症感染患者要达到 100%fT > 5 × MIC，需要 1000mg 美罗培南延长 3h 泵入或更高剂量泵入，间隔 8h 一次。慢性肝衰合并脓毒症的患者，肝肾功能同时恶化，进行 CVVHD 治疗时，以铜绿假单胞菌为代表（MIC 为 2 mg/L），常规剂量和给药方式，PTA 不能达标，这时肝衰竭导致 Vd 增加，需要增加负荷剂量和维持剂量或持续给药，PTA 才能达标。

高吸附性聚乙烯亚胺膜百希瑞（oXiris）是近年上市的高吸附膜材，在 CVVHDF 治疗模式（血流速度 200～250ml/min，后稀释，透析液和超滤液流速均为 1.5L/h）时，美罗培南经血液净化清除的速度（7.78L/h）高于 AN69 膜材（6.63 L/h），对于重症感染患者要达到 100%fT > 4 × MIC（MIC：2mg/L），需要 3000mg 美罗培南持续泵入或 2000mg 延长 2h 泵入，间隔 8h 一次。在日本和欧洲一些国家，以聚苯乙烯和聚丙烯的共聚物作为基底纤维的多黏菌素 B 灌流器（DHP-PMX）批准在脓毒症患者中使用，CVVH（血流速度 150～200ml/min，前联合后稀释，超滤液流速均为 1.5～1.8L/h）联合灌流（血流速度 120ml/min，治疗 2h）治疗模式时，美罗培南经灌流清除的速度为 0.04 L/h，2h 清除量仅占总清除量的 1%，因而单纯内毒素吸附治疗时对抗生素的清除可以忽略，也不需要调整剂量。CVVHD（血流速度 160ml/min，透析液流速为 2.8L/h）和 CVVH[血流速度 160ml/min，前联合后稀释 1:2，置换液流速为 35 ml/(kg·h)]时，美罗培南经血液净化清除的速度为 15.1L/h，非血液净化清除为 21.1L/h，对于重症感染患者 100%fT > 4 mg/l，需要 2000mg 间隔 8h 一次的剂量。从美罗培南的循证医学研究可以发现，PK/PD 理论和 TDM 结果不完全一致，但重症患者进行 CRRT 治疗时，无论肾功能损伤程度，对于药敏处于中介的病原体，常规剂量将不能达到 100%fT > 4 × MIC，需要增加剂量和延长输注时间、甚至持续泵入；而肾功能正常或 ARC 患者，因脓毒症 CRRT 治疗时，增加剂量、持续泵入和联合用药是避免治疗失败的选择。

总之,重症患者感染的治疗是一个巨大挑战,临床常用剂量来源于健康成年人,没有考虑到重症患者的明显不同;重症患者存在明显的血流动力学紊乱、器官功能改变、多种基础疾病,这些特点均改变了抗生素的PK,而使得对比健康人的常规剂量产生不同的PD,影响治疗效果;重症患者肾功能改变分为药物肾清除减少和肾脏清除增加;CRRT影响抗生素的清除;根据抗生素CRRT清除的基本原则,可以通过数学公式个体化抗生素的剂量和用药间隔;TDM是剂量调整的重要工具,PK/PD模型和在线软件也是剂量调整的参考工具,重症患者抗生素剂量调整需临床医师慎思笃行。

参 考 文 献

[1] Crass RL, Rodvold KA, Mueller BA, et al. Renal Dosing of Antibiotics: Are We Jumping the Gun? Clin Infect Dis, 2019, 68(9): 1596-1602.

[2] Tsai D, Lipman J, Roberts JA. Pharmacokinetic/pharmacodynamic considerations for the optimization of antimicrobial delivery in the critically ill. Curr Opin Crit Care, 2015, 21(5): 412-420.

[3] Guilhaumou R, Benaboud S, Bennis Y, et al. Optimization of the treatment with beta-lactam antibiotics in critically ill patients-guidelines from the French Society of Pharmacology and Therapeutics (Societe Francaise de Pharmacologie et Therapeutique-SFPT) and the French Society of Anaesthesia and Intensive Care Medicine (Societe Francaise d'Anesthesie et Reanimation-SFAR). Crit Care, 2019, 23(1): 104.

[4] 中国医药教育协会感染疾病专业委员会. 抗菌药物药代动力学/药效学理论临床应用专家共识. 中华结核和呼吸杂志, 2018, 41(6): 409-446.

[5] Jamal JA, Mueller BA, Choi GY, et al. How can we ensure effective antibiotic dosing in critically ill patients receiving different types of renal replacement therapy? Diagn Microbiol Infect Dis, 2015, 82(1): 92-103.

[6] Shaw AR, Chaijamorn W, Mueller BA. We Underdose Antibiotics in Patients on CRRT. Semin Dial, 2016, 29(4): 278-280.

[7] Roberts JA, Abdul-Aziz MH, Lipman J, et al. Individualised antibiotic dosing for patients who are critically ill: challenges and potential solutions. Lancet Infect Dis, 2014, 14(6): 498-509.

[8] Williams P, Cotta MO, Roberts JA. Pharmacokinetics/Pharmacodynamics of beta-Lactams and Therapeutic Drug Monitoring: From Theory to Practical Issues in the Intensive Care Unit. Semin Respir Crit Care Med, 2019, 40(4): 476-487.

[9] Li L, Li X, Xia Y, et al. Recommendation of Antimicrobial Dosing Optimization During Continuous Renal Replacement Therapy. Front Pharmacol, 2020, 11: 786.

[10] Pea F. From bench to bedside: Perspectives on the utility of pharmacokinetics/pharmacodynamics in predicting the efficacy of antifungals in invasive candidiasis. Mycoses, 2020.

[11] Sinnollareddy MG, Roberts MS, Lipman J, et al. Beta-lactam pharmacokinetics and pharmacodynamics in critically ill patients and strategies for dose optimization: a structured review. Clin Exp Pharmacol Physiol, 2012, 39(6): 489-496.

[12] Almulhim AS, Al-Dahneen BA, Alsowaida YS. Pharmacists Knowledge About the Impact of Augmented Renal Clearance on Antimicrobial Dosing in Critically Ill Patients: A Cross-Sectional Study. Infect Dis Ther 2020.

[13] Pea F, Viale P, Pavan F, et al. Pharmacokinetic considerations for antimicrobial therapy in patients receiving renal replacement therapy. Clin Pharmacokinet, 2007, 46(12): 997-1038.

[14] Joukhadar C, Frossard M, Mayer BX, et al. Impaired target site penetration of beta-lactams may account for therapeutic failure in patients with septic shock. Crit Care Med, 2001, 29(2): 385-391.

[15] Ulldemolins M, Roberts JA, Lipman J, et al. Antibiotic dosing in multiple organ dysfunction syndrome. Chest, 2011, 139(5): 1210-1220.

[16] Roberts JA, Joynt GM, Choi GY, et al. How to optimise antimicrobial prescriptions in the Intensive Care Unit: principles of individualised dosing using pharmacokinetics and pharmacodynamics. Int J Antimicrob Agents, 2012, 39(3): 187-192.

[17] Pea F. Plasma pharmacokinetics of antimicrobial agents in critically ill patients. Curr Clin Pharmacol, 2013, 8(1): 5-12.

[18] Blot SI, Pea F, Lipman J. The effect of pathophysiology on pharmacokinetics in the critically ill patient-concepts appraised by the example of antimicrobial agents. Adv Drug Deliv Rev, 2014, 77: 3-11.

[19] Wong G, Sime FB, Lipman J, et al. How do we use therapeutic drug monitoring to improve outcomes from severe infections in critically ill patients? BMC Infect, Dis, 2014, 14: 288.

[20] Logre E, Enser M, Tanaka S, et al. Amikacin pharmacokinetic/pharmacodynamic in intensive care unit: a prospective database. Ann Intensive Care, 2020, 10(1): 75.

[21] Perez-Blanco JS, Saez Fernandez EM, Calvo MV, et al. Amikacin initial dosage in patients with hypoalbuminaemia: an interactive tool based on a population pharmacokinetic approach. J Antimicrob Chemother, 2020, 75(8): 2222-2231.

[22] Gao C, Tong J, Yu K, et al. Pharmacokinetics of cefoperazone/sulbactam in critically ill patients receiving continuous venovenous hemofiltration. Eur J Clin Pharmacol, 2016, 72(7): 823-830.

[23] Udy AA, Baptista JP, Lim NL, et al. Augmented renal clearance in the ICU: results of a multicenter observational study of renal function in critically ill patients with normal plasma creatinine concentrations*. Crit Care Med, 2014, 42(3): 520-527.

[24] Tsai D, Udy AA, Stewart PC, et al. Prevalence of augmented renal clearance and performance of glomerular filtration estimates in Indigenous Australian patients requiring intensive care admission. Anaesth Intensive Care, 2018, 46(1): 42-50.

[25] Morabito S, Pierucci A, Marinelli R, et al. Efficiency of different hollow-fiber hemofilters in continuous arteriovenous he-

modiafiltration. Am J Nephrol,2000,20(2):116-121.
[26] Clark WR,Hamburger RJ,Lysaght MJ. Effect of membrane composition and structure on solute removal and biocompatibility in hemodialysis. Kidney Int,1999,56(6):2005-2015.
[27] Choi G,Gomersall CD,Tian Q,et al. Principles of antibacterial dosing in continuous renal replacement therapy. Crit Care Med,2009,37(7):2268-2282.
[28] Breilh D,Honore PM,De Bels D,et al. Pharmacokinetics and Pharmacodynamics of Anti-infective Agents During Continuous Veno-venous Hemofiltration in Critically Ill Patients: Lessons Learned from an Ancillary Study of the IVOIRE Trial. J Transl Int Med,2019,7(4):155-169.
[29] Pistolesi V,Morabito S,Di Mario F,et al. A Guide to Understanding Antimicrobial Drug Dosing in Critically Ill Patients on Renal Replacement Therapy. Antimicrob Agents Chemother,2019,63(8):e00583-00519.
[30] Mueller BA,Pasko DA,Sowinski KM. Higher renal replacement therapy dose delivery influences on drug therapy. Artif Organs,2003,27(9):808-814.
[31] Page M,Cohen S,Ber CE,et al. In vivo antibiotic removal during coupled plasma filtration adsorption:a retrospective study. ASAIO J,2014,60(1):70-75.
[32] Singhan W,Vadcharavivad S,Areepium N,et al. The effect of direct hemoperfusion with polymyxin B immobilized cartridge on meropenem in critically ill patients requiring renal support. J Crit Care,2019,51:71-76.
[33] Hoff BM,Maker JH,Dager WE,et al. Antibiotic Dosing for Critically Ill Adult Patients Receiving Intermittent Hemodialysis,Prolonged Intermittent Renal Replacement Therapy,and Continuous Renal Replacement Therapy:An Update. Ann Pharmacother,2019.
[34] Roberts DM,Liu X,Roberts JA,et al. A multicenter study on the effect of continuous hemodiafiltration intensity on antibiotic pharmacokinetics. Crit Care,2015,19:84.
[35] Ehmann L,Zoller M,Minichmayr IK,et al. Development of a dosing algorithm for meropenem in critically ill patients based on a population pharmacokinetic/pharmacodynamic analysis. Int J Antimicrob Agents,2019,54(3):309-317.
[36] Isla A,Rodriguez-Gascon A,Troconiz IF,et al. Population pharmacokinetics of meropenem in critically ill patients undergoing continuous renal replacement therapy. Clin Pharmacokinet,2008,47(3):173-180.
[37] Ulldemolins M,Soy D,Llaurado-Serra M,et al. Meropenem population pharmacokinetics in critically ill patients with septic shock and continuous renal replacement therapy:influence of residual diuresis on dose requirements. Antimicrob Agents Chemother,2015,59(9):5520-5528.
[38] Grensemann J,Busse D,Konig C,et al. Acute-on-chronic liver failure alters meropenem pharmacokinetics in critically ill patients with continuous hemodialysis:an observational study. Ann Intensive Care,2020,10(1):48.
[39] Padulles Zamora A,Juvany Roig R,Leiva Badosa E,et al. Optimized meropenem dosage regimens using a pharmacokinetic/pharmacodynamic population approach in patients undergoing continuous venovenous haemodiafiltration with high-adsorbent membrane. J Antimicrob Chemother,2019,74(10):2979-2983.
[40] Onichimowski D,Bedzkowska A,Ziolkowski H,et al. Population pharmacokinetics of standard-dose meropenem in critically ill patients on continuous renal replacement therapy:a prospective observational trial. Pharmacol Rep,2020,72(3):719-729.

6 跨肺压指导的机械通气策略在 ECMO 支持的 ARDS 患者中的应用

孙 兵 王 睿

急性呼吸窘迫综合征(acute respiratory distress syndrome,ARDS)是呼吸衰竭常见的病因,病死率高达 35%~46%。体外膜肺氧合(extracorporeal membrane oxygenation,ECMO)通常作为危重 ARDS 患者的挽救性治疗手段。2018 年发表的 EOLIA(ECMO to rescue lung injury in severe ARDS)随机对照试验显示,与常规机械通气比较,ECMO 未能改善重度 ARDS 患者的预后。然而 EOLIA 研究数据的贝叶斯分析显示,ECMO 治疗后生存获益的可能性很高。Laveena Munshi 等近期发表的荟萃分析也显示,静脉静脉-ECMO(venovenous ECMO,VV-ECMO)可以降低重度 ARDS 患者 60 d 的病死率。因此,近年来 VV-ECMO 救治重度 ARDS 被逐渐推广普及,但在患者的管理方面还存在一些亟待解决的问题,其中机械通气策略的选择就是重要的一项。

VV-ECMO 能够显著改善患者的通气和氧合,在建立 ECMO 之后应尽快下调潮气量、平台压和呼吸频率,个体化的进行呼吸机参数的设置,最大程度地避免或减少呼吸机相关肺损伤(ventilator associated lung injury,VALI)是 ECMO 之后机械通气策略的主旨。床旁跨肺压监测是研究 ARDS 肺部病变特点的有效手段,同时也有助于 ECMO 患者机械通气策略的选择。

一、跨肺压的监测

跨肺压(transpulmonary pressure,Ptp)是直接扩张肺组织的压力,即静态条件下作用于胸膜腔表面对抗肺组织回缩的力量,数值上等于肺泡压与胸腔内压之差。肺泡压可以通过测定气道的平台压代替,由于测定胸腔内压是侵入性的,所以,目前用食管压(esophageal pressure,Pes)来替代胸腔内压。那么,跨肺压可以表达为平台压与食管压的差值。

食管测压管为专门设计的导管,成人测压管在距离导管远端 5~7cm 处有多个小孔,在导管的末端有一个 10cm 长的气囊,可以充气 0.5~2.5ml 膨胀,以防小孔被食管壁和分泌物所堵塞。应用时,经鼻腔将导管置入,使气囊到达胃腔,并向气囊注入气体。临床常用 Baydur 阻断试验辅助验证气囊的合适位置。对于保留自主呼吸的患者,呼气末阻断气道以保证肺容积无变化,当患者出现吸气努力时,气道压和食管压同时降低,此时如两者下降幅度的比值在 0.8~1.2,则说明气囊已置于合适位置。阻断试验的原理是气道阻断时,虽然患者出现吸气努力,但不会发生肺容积和跨肺压的变化,因此理论上气道压和胸腔压的改变应该是一致的。对于没有自主呼吸的患者,可以在呼气末进行气道阻断,同时轻轻挤压患者肋骨,使气道压和食管压同时升高,再计算气道压与食管压变化值的比值。

此外,置入食管压监测导管时,应严密观察患者是否存在咳嗽,或者气道压突然升高的情况,避免导管误入气道。对于咳嗽反射较弱或无自主呼吸的患者,更需要格外注意食管压的监测波形。如果心电伪影很小,同时进行呼气末和吸气末气道阻断时,食管压与气道压的数值十分接近,需要警惕气囊位于气道内。

二、跨肺压指导 ARDS 患者机械通气参数的设置

跨肺压是维持呼气末肺泡开放的关键,呼气末正压(positive end expiratory pressure,PEEP)的设置水平直接影响跨肺压的数值。监测跨肺压可以用于判断 ARDS 患者对 PEEP 的需求,指导机械通气 PEEP 的设置,选择使呼气末跨肺压保持在 0~5 cmH$_2$O 的最小 PEEP 值,避免呼气末肺泡萎陷的同时,最大程度减少剪切伤和气压伤,改善氧合和通气,实现 PEEP 的个体化设置。

Talmor 等在 EPVent(esophageal pressure guided ventilation)-1 研究中比较了两组 ARDS 患者,试验组根据保持呼气末跨肺压 0~10cmH$_2$O 来设定 PEEP 水平,限制吸气末跨肺压＜25cmH$_2$O,避免肺泡过度膨胀,对照组以 ARDSnet 方案的低 PEEP-FiO$_2$(fraction of inspired oxygen)表来设定 PEEP 水平。结果显示,试验组的 PEEP 水平较高,有较好的氧合,呼吸系统顺应性也得到了明显改善,28d 病死率有降低趋势。提示根据患者跨肺压指导机械通气参数的设置更加合理。

此后 Beitler 等继续开展相关研究,于 2019 年发表了 EPVent-2 研究,北美 14 家中心参与了此项随机对照研究,共纳入了 200 例中、重度 ARDS 患者,比较了两种 PEEP

滴定方法,即跨肺压指导和经验性(ARDS network 高PEEP 表)的 PEEP 滴定策略,结果发现跨肺压组并没有改善预后指标,即包括 28d 病死数和无呼吸机天数的综合评分。与 EPVent-1 研究不同,EPVent-2 研究未能证实跨肺压指导的 PEEP 设定能够改善 ARDS 患者临床转归。

EPVent-1 对照组采用了低 PEEP-FiO$_2$ 表,结果与跨肺压组相比,PEEP 水平较低。相反,在 EPVent-2 研究中,对照组采用的是高 PEEP-FiO$_2$ 表,组间 PEEP 差异很小,所以没有阳性的结果,以上结果更加说明了个体化的 PEEP 设置,保持肺泡开放的重要性。

2016 年 Baedorf Kassis 等实现了跨肺驱动压(吸气末跨肺压-呼气末跨肺压)的监测,在对 ARDS 患者实施肺复张后,试验组采用呼气末跨肺压为正值滴定 PEEP,对照组采用 ARDSnet 推荐的 PEEP 设置方法,结果显示存活组患者驱动压和跨肺驱动压明显低于病死组,同时试验组的跨肺驱动压明显低于对照组。这些研究对跨肺压在 ARDS 患者中的临床应用提供了新的思路。

三、跨肺压指导的机械通气策略在 ECMO 患者中的应用

VV-ECMO 支持的 ARDS 患者和单纯机械通气支持的 ARDS 患者存在诸多方面的不同。首先,ECMO 支持的 ARDS 患者氧合和肺脏的顺应性更差,对于机械通气参数设置要求精度更高;其次,ECMO 的支持使得"肺休息"成为可能,但是如何合理地"休息肺"而不导致肺泡塌陷尤为重要。

目前,体外生命支持组织(extracorporeal life Support organization,ELSO)推荐的"休息肺"策略被广泛应用于各个 ECMO 中心,其主要特点为低压力:气道峰压 20~25cmH$_2$O,PEEP 10~15cmH$_2$O;低频率:呼吸频率 10/min;低吸氧浓度:FiO$_2$ 0.3。上述"休息肺"策略 PEEP 水平设置偏低,可能会导致大量肺泡的塌陷,甚至很难再复张,不利于肺的康复。

我们中心也进行了相关的研究,一方面保留"休息肺"策略限制气道峰压和潮气量,另一方面应用跨肺压指导 PEEP 的设置,避免"肺休息"策略低 PEEP 所致的肺萎陷,实现 ECMO 支持的 ARDS 患者个体化的通气参数设置。本研究共纳入了 104 例重度 ARDS 患者,随机分为跨肺压指导的机械通气策略组和肺休息策略组。跨肺压指导的机械通气策略组(跨肺压组)采用 P-A/C 模式,气道峰压<25cmH$_2$O,调节 PEEP 使得呼气跨肺压介于 0~5 cmH$_2$O,呼气频率为 10 次/min,吸入氧浓度<0.5;肺休息策略组(肺休息组)采用 P-A/C 模式,气道峰压 20~25cmH$_2$O,PEEP 10~15 cmH$_2$O,呼吸频率为 10 次/min,吸入氧浓度<0.5。结果显示,跨肺压组 VV-ECMO 成功撤机率明显高于肺休息组(71.2% vs 48.0%;$P=0.017$)。VV-ECMO 支持过程中,跨肺压组驱动压、潮气量和机械能显著低于肺休息组,PEEP 显著高于肺休息组。随着时间推移,跨肺压组白细胞介素-1β、白介素-6 和白介素-8 显著低于肺休息组,白介素-10 显著高于肺休息组。因此,我们认为 VV-ECMO 支持过程中跨肺压指导的通气策略实现了对呼吸机参数的个体化设定,有助于维持肺泡形态,降低了炎症反应,一定程度上能够改善了患者的预后。

四、跨肺压监测存在的问题

1. 体位对于食管压的影响 Washko 等发现,食管压能准确反映直立位健康人群的胸腔内压,但 ARDS 患者均为平卧位,食管会受心脏和纵隔等器官压迫,使得平卧位测量的食管压高于直立位食管压,故应对平卧位测量的食管压进行矫正,但因存在个体差异性,很难统一而论。

2. ARDS 肺组织不均一性对食管压的影响 ARDS 患者肺组织呈现明显的不均一性,导致了胸腔压力自非重力依赖区至重力依赖区呈现一定的压力梯度。然而食管压仅能反映中部肺组织对应的胸腔内压,会高估非重力依赖区的胸腔压力,低估重力依赖区的胸腔内压。那么,用食管压和跨肺压的变化值来代替绝对值,能够消除上述误差。

3. 其他因素对跨肺压监测的影响 跨肺压测定时患者需要充分镇静和镇痛,甚至肌松,避免人机不同步导致的监测误差。当患者存在气胸时,给予胸腔闭式引流胸膜腔的完整性被破坏,测定的跨肺压也存在误差。

综述所述,对于 VV-ECMO 支持的重度 ARDS 患者,如何在减少肺泡塌陷和防止过度膨胀之间寻找平衡依然充满挑战。新的机械通气策略仍在不断探索中,通过监测跨肺压,个体化设置呼吸机参数以适应不同患者呼吸力学特征上的差异,减少进一步的 VALI。虽然跨肺压指导的机械通气策略在单中心的临床试验中已被证明安全有效,依然需要更大规模、多中心、随机对照研究来进一步证实其在 VV-ECMO 支持的重度 ARDS 患者的价值。

参 考 文 献

[1] Bellani G, Laffey JG, Pham T, et al. Epidemiology, Patterns of Care, and Mortality for Patients With Acute Respiratory Distress Syndrome in Intensive Care Units in 50 Countries. JAMA, 2016, 315(8):788-800.

[2] Combes A, Hajage D, Capellier G, et al. Extracorporeal Membrane Oxygenation for Severe Acute Respiratory Distress Syndrome. N Engl J Med, 2018, 378(21):1965-1975.

[3] Goligher EC, Tomlinson G, Hajage D, et al. Extracorporeal Membrane Oxygenation for Severe Acute Respiratory Distress Syndrome and Posterior Probability of Mortality Benefit in a Post Hoc Bayesian Analysis of a Randomized Clinical Trial. JAMA, 2018, 320(21):2251-2259.

[4] Munshi L, Walkey A, Goligher E, et al. Venovenous extracorporeal membrane oxygenation for acute respiratory distress

syndrome:a systematic review and meta-analysis. Lancet Respir Med,2019,7(2):163-172.

[5] Schmidt M,Pham T,Arcadipane A,et al. Mechanical Ventilation Management during Extracorporeal Membrane Oxygenation for Acute Respiratory Distress Syndrome. An International Multicenter Prospective Cohort. Am J Respir Crit Care Med,2019,200(8):1002-1012.

[6] Mauri T,Yoshida T,Bellani G,et al. Esophageal and transpulmonary pressure in the clinical setting:meaning, usefulness and perspectives. Intensive Care Med, 2016, 42 (9): 1360-1373.

[7] Milic-Emili J,Mead J,Turner JM,et al. Improved Technique for Estimating Pleural Pressure from Esophageal Balloons. J Appl Physiol,1964,19:207-211.

[8] Baydur A,Behrakis PK,Zin WA,et al. A simple method for assessing the validity of the esophageal balloon technique. Am Rev Respir Dis,1982,126(5):788-791.

[9] Chiumello D,Consonni D,Coppola S,et al. The occlusion tests and end-expiratory esophageal pressure:measurements and comparison in controlled and assisted ventilation. Ann Intensive Care,2016,6(1):13.

[10] Talmor D,Sarge T,Malhotra A,et al. Mechanical ventilation guided by esophageal pressure in acute lung injury. N Engl J Med,2008,359(20):2095-2104.

[11] Beitler JR,Sarge T,Banner-Goodspeed VM,et al. Effect of Titrating Positive End-Expiratory Pressure(PEEP)With an Esophageal Pressure-Guided Strategy vs an Empirical High PEEP-Fio2 Strategy on Death and Days Free From Mechanical Ventilation Among Patients With Acute Respiratory Distress Syndrome:A Randomized Clinical Trial. JAMA,2019, 321(9):846-857.

[12] Baedorf Kassis E,Loring SH,Talmor D. Mortality and pulmonary mechanics in relation to respiratory system and transpulmonary driving pressures in ARDS. Intensive Care Med,2016,42(8):1206-1213.

[13] Wang R,Sun B,Li X,et al. Mechanical Ventilation Strategy Guided by Transpulmonary Pressure in Severe Acute Respiratory Distress Syndrome Treated With Venovenous Extracorporeal Membrane Oxygenation. Crit Care Med,2020.

[14] Washko GR,O'Donnell CR,Loring SH. Volume-related and volume-independent effects of posture on esophageal and transpulmonary pressures in healthy subjects. J Appl Physiol,(1985)2006,100(3):753-758.

[15] Yoshida T,Amato MBP,Grieco DL,et al. Esophageal Manometry and Regional Transpulmonary Pressure in Lung Injury. Am J Respir Crit Care Med,2018,197(8):1018-1026.

7 肥胖 ARDS 患者的机械通气

曾 勉　何婉媚

社会的稳定与经济的发展给人们带来的不仅是丰富的物质供应,同样给人们带来新的烦恼,就是肥胖。世界卫生组织(WHO)建议体质指数(body mass index,BMI)超过 25 kg/m² 称为超重,超过 30 kg/m² 则定义为肥胖。肥胖不仅只是重量或形体方面的变化,而且是一种病理状态,表现为内脏脂肪堆积、严重代谢紊乱,并可引起全身多脏器异常及疾病。存在急性呼吸窘迫综合征(acute respiratory distress syndrome,ARDS)发生风险的 ICU 患者中,进展为 ARDS 者的 BMI 比没有进展为 ARDS 的患者 BMI 要高,2009 年 H1N1 流感流行的数据显示,严重(BMI>35 kg/m²)和病态肥胖者(BMI>40 kg/m²)ARDS 发病率是正常体重者的 5~15 倍,推测其原因可能与肥胖本身存在呼吸功能异常相关。机械通气是基于人体呼吸力学的产物,也是目前公认的 ARDS 的主要治疗措施。认识肥胖者的呼吸功能有助于指导机械通气在此类患者中的应用。

一、肥胖者的呼吸功能特点

根据脂肪分布类型,肥胖分为中心性和周围性。中心性肥胖者的脂肪主要分布在胸腔、腹腔和内脏器官。胸腹腔脂肪堆积可致胸腹腔压力升高,进而引起横膈上移,胸壁向外扩展范围受限,影响整个呼吸系统的顺应性。Behazin 等对 BMI 超过 38 kg/m² 的严重肥胖者进行镇静肌松、气管插管机械通气(容控)后监测他们的呼吸系统顺应性,发现肥胖者的呼吸系统及肺顺应性均较 BMI<30 kg/m² 的对照组人群显著下降。呼气流速限制亦常见于肥胖患者中。在非插管、自主呼吸的病态肥胖患者中,呼气流速限制在坐位时占 20%~25%,平卧时呈 3 倍增加。呼气流速限制的存在可引起肺动态过度充气,不仅使内源性呼气末正压(iPEEP)增加,呼吸功显著增加,而且会损伤膈肌,进一步影响膈肌的收缩功能。将插管肥胖患者的体位从仰卧位改为坐位可减少呼气流速限制。

即使是无呼气气流受限证据或无肺部基础疾病的肥胖者(BMI≥30 kg/m²),肺功能检查显示无论是采取坐位还是平卧位的体位,肥胖者的肺总容量(total lung capacity,TLC)、肺活量(vital capacity,VC)、功能残气量(functional residual capacity,FRC)均较 BMI 正常组降低,而且功能残气量的下降程度与肥胖程度呈相关性,第 1 秒用力呼气容积(forced expiratory volume in one second,FEV_1)与用力呼气容积(forced vital capacity,FVC)仅轻度下降。受肥胖影响,患者肺基底部往往通气不足,而由于重力缘故,肺基底部的血流较其他部位丰富,造成肥胖患者普遍存在通气/血流匹配失调,血气分析显示氧分压轻度下降及肺泡-动脉氧分压差增加。此外,Behazin 等的研究还发现,气道压和食管压存在显著相关性,严重肥胖者(BMI>38 kg/m²)的患者食管压较 BMI<30 kg/m² 的对照组患者升高,提示严重肥胖者存在气道压升高的情况。

二、肥胖 ARDS 的病理生理特点

肺容积减少、肺顺应性降低和严重通气/血流失调是 ARDS 的主要病理生理改变,这与上述肥胖者的呼吸功能改变极为相似。胸部 CT 显示 ARDS 患者肺重力依赖区(仰卧位时靠近背部的肺区)以肺水肿和肺不张为主,该区域的静水压(叠加压)升高。与此相似的是,由于受胸腹壁、腹部脂肪增加、膈肌上抬、腹腔压力升高等因素影响,肥胖者胸内压明显增高。目前常通过监测食管内压反映胸内压的变化。Chiumello 等的研究证实,肥胖 ARDS 患者呼气末食管内压比非肥胖 ARDS 者高。肺泡内压与胸腔内压的差值为跨肺压,随着胸内压升高,跨肺压下降。跨肺压是肺扩张的压力,跨肺压的降低可引起肺泡萎陷。另一方面,胸腔内压的增高,可引起小气道陷闭,导致肺不张。研究数据显示,肥胖 ARDS 者静水压均值为 15.2 cmH_2O,与 BMI 正常 ARDS 者(均值为 12.9 cmH_2O)具有统计学差异,这意味着肥胖 ARDS 患者比单纯 ARDS 患者存在更为显著的肺水肿、肺不张的情况,通气/血流比例失调更为显著,可能导致愈加明显的低氧。

三、肥胖 ARDS 患者的机械通气策略

在肥胖 ARDS 患者中施行有创机械通气,应该个体化调整呼吸机参数,使 PaO_2 维持在 50~80mmHg,SaO_2 维持在 88%~95%,血气 pH>7.25,对于 ARDS 患者来说是安全的。目前尚无明确依据表明容量控制模式还是压力控制模式更适合,因此,两者模式均可作为临床选择。对于个体化进行呼吸机参数的调整,则可参考以下通气策略。

(一)小潮气量通气

目前多数 ARDS 诊疗指南推荐采用小潮气量通气 4~6 ml/kg 的机械通气保护策略,该策略同样适用于肥胖者。然后,与 BMI 正常者不同的是,若给予肥胖者的潮气量过

低（<6 ml/kg），可能会使肺不张情况加重。Pepin等认为，对于肥胖人群，最适潮气量应该是6～8 ml/kg，并且建议施加外源性PEEP，以减少肺不张；如潮气量设定低于6ml/kg，则需要肺复张＋PEEP的方式以使肺泡重新开放及防止肺泡再次萎陷。值得注意的是，计算潮气量时，应该按照患者的理想体重而不是按实际体重计算，最简单的理想体重计算公式是，男：理想体重（kg）＝身高（cm）－100，女：理想体重（kg）＝身高（cm）－110。这是因为体重与肺容量并不成正比关系，而且上述已提到，大部分肥胖患者已存在TLC及VC下降。2016年Lancet的一篇综述中，通过CT的方法测定比较BMI分别为52 kg/m^{2}及21 kg/m^{2}的2个女性个体的肺容量，发现前者的肺容量为3138 ml，而后者为3196 ml。BMI差距甚大的2个个体，肺容量却差别不大。

当然，在应用小潮气量通气期间，常出现$PaCO_2$升高，此时可以通过调整呼吸机呼吸频率，使通气量适当增加，以维持pH>7.25。

（二）应用外源性PEEP

外源性PEEP，具有抵消内源性PEEP的作用，以及防止气道塌陷，减少肺不张，增加呼气末肺容量，改善呼气流速限制的作用。在外源性PEEP不足的情况下，若肥胖患者存在呼气流速限制，则可能意味着外周气道的周期性塌陷和重新开放，这可能引起气道的损伤。2017年一项研究显示，在BMI>30 kg/m^{2}的ARDS患者中，机械通气过程中施加高PEEP组（10～15 cmH$_2$O）的死亡率比低PEEP组（8～10 cmH$_2$O）低（18％ vs. 32％，P＝0.04），而在BMI<30kg/m^{2}的非肥胖ARDS患者中，则未观察到显著统计学差异（P＝0.13）。可是过高的PEEP可引起肺泡过度膨胀、通气血流比例失调、血流动力学不稳定。一项PROVHILO的欧洲研究将接受潮气量为8ml/kg的腹部术后机械通气患者随机分为2组：低PEEP组（≤2 cmH$_2$O且未进行肺复张）及高PEEP组（12 cmH$_2$O且进行肺复张），研究结果显示，两组在术后5 d内的肺部并发症发生率无显著差异，但是高PEEP组出现更多血流动力学不稳定的情况。另一方面，肥胖患者由于代谢性等因素影响，常合并心脏、高血压等心血管疾病，更容易发生血流动力学紊乱、严重心律失常等并发症，由此限制了PEEP的应用。因此，如何设定最佳PEEP？

目前常采用以下方式设定PEEP：①采用ARDSnet建议的PEEP与FiO$_2$联合调整方案表；该方案有两种：高PEEP/FiO$_2$组合及低PEEP/FiO$_2$组合搭配。②PV曲线法。③肺复张后根据氧合、CT表现、呼吸系统顺应性、肺牵张指数作为判断标准滴定PEEP。④测定呼气末跨肺压滴定PEEP。Jacopo等在对肥胖ARDS肺复张的临床研究中，分别采用上述的三种方式，即低PEEP/FiO$_2$组合（ARDSnet）、肺复张后递减PEEP、递增PEEP并监测呼气末跨肺压来设置最佳PEEP。研究结果显示采用后两种方式滴定PEEP的患者，重力依赖区通气的肺组织比第一种方式增加，此外，采用肺复张后递减PEEP方法组的患者氧合改善最显著。前面已提到，高PEEP与低PEEP对肥胖ARDS生存率影响存在显著差异，Jacopo等的研究是采用低PEEP/FiO$_2$组合，同年发表在JAMA的一篇文章则采用高PEEP/FiO$_2$组合，发现该组合与监测跨肺压滴定PEEP组相比，在60 d生存率方面，两者无明显差异。

上述提到的肺复张滴定PEEP方法，在应用前建议先评估可复张肺容积，因为可复张肺容积越少，肺复张效果不佳，并可能导致肺泡过度扩张充气，肺内分流增加，氧合进一步下降。我国邱海波教授认为，如果随着PEEP增高而肺复张容积不再明显增加，则没有必要选择更高的PEEP。

（三）监测跨肺压及平台压

既往研究认为，高驱动压（平台压与PEEP的差值）与ARDS高死亡率相关，可是该结论并不适用于肥胖ARDS患者。多因素分析结果显示，驱动压并不是肥胖ARDS患者死亡的独立风险因素。即使如此，考虑到驱动压与呼吸机相关性肺损伤的密切相关性，肥胖ARDS患者机械通气过程中，驱动压不宜超过17 cmH$_2$O。相比驱动压，监测跨肺压（肺泡内压与胸腔内压的差值）对肥胖ARDS患者更为重要，这是因为跨肺压是维持呼气末肺泡持续开放的关键。ARDS肥胖患者，由于呼吸系统顺应性降低、胸腔内压升高缘故，即使给予较高的驱动压或高PEEP，肺泡内压明显增高，跨肺压依然不高。在一项纳入16例的急性呼吸衰竭肥胖患者（BMI>35 kg/m^2）机械通气的研究中，通过放置食管气囊监测食管压的方法，测定跨肺压，采用肺复张后递减PEEP方法滴定PEEP，发现这些患者氧合最佳时，呼气末跨肺压>0 cmH$_2$O。Williams等认为，对于严重肥胖、腹腔高压或平台压>30 cmH$_2$O的患者，应该考虑监测跨肺压，并通过滴定最佳PEEP、肺复张、减少潮气量等方法适当降低驱动压。研究表明，当测定跨肺压为负值时，可以预测肺是处于陷闭状态的；当保持跨肺压为正值时，肺驱动压降低。2016年发表在Intensive Care Med的一篇综述，对跨肺压值进行了归纳总结，认为在维持吸气末跨肺压<25 cmH$_2$O、呼气末跨肺压>0 cmH$_2$O的前提下，允许气道峰压>30cmH$_2$O，可有效减少肺泡塌陷、避免剪切伤及气压伤。

也有国外学者依旧将监测平台压作为调整呼吸机参数的目标之一。他们认为对于肥胖ARDS患者，目标平台压应始终<27 cmH$_2$O，或基于腹腔内压调整目标平台压，即校正目标平台压（cmH$_2$O）。

（四）俯卧位通气

通过改变体位的方式使原本处于肺泡陷闭的重力依赖区变为非重力依赖区，使萎陷肺组织相对减少，由此改善通气/血流比值失调及改善氧合。俯卧位通气已经成为ARDS机械通气最常用的辅助手段。Audrey等在Chest发表的单中心、非盲、非随机、观察性临床研究显示：非肥胖组ARDS患者俯卧位后并发症发生的例数与肥胖组无差异，后者在俯卧位后氧合改善更明显。可是，由于肥胖患者常存在胃内压及腹腔内压升高，与俯卧位相关的不良并发症，如胃食管内容物反流误吸、腹腔内压进一步升高及肝、肾功能损伤仍是人们所关心的问题。为避免这些并发症，对肥胖患者俯卧位后在胸部及盆骨处放置承托物（如枕头）支撑，采取反Trendelenburg体位（即头高足低位),可有助于减轻腹部受压,降低腹内压。可是,至今尚缺乏相关研究明确上述操作方法对肥胖者俯卧位腹压的影响,因此,肥胖 ARDS 患者俯卧位通气的安全性仍有待确定。

肥胖患者由于自身的病理生理结构及代谢因素,正常静息状态下会存在肺不张、肺通气/血流失调、呼吸功能减低等情况,使该部分患者在疾病状态下较体重正常者更容易发生 ARDS。鉴于此,更有必要对肥胖 ARDS 机械通气患者采取肺保护性通气策略,如小潮气量通气、最佳外源性 PEEP,以改善肺不张、减轻肺进一步损伤。由于肥胖患者胸内压明显升高,因此监测驱动压的实际作用不如跨肺压。考虑到俯卧位有助于改善通气比例失调,因此在充分考虑俯卧位过程中的细节问题后,仍可在肥胖 ARDS 患者中尝试进行俯卧位通气,并加强观察及注意体位调整。

四、结论与展望

肥胖患者胸腹腔脂肪堆积致胸腹腔压力升高,横膈上移、胸壁向外扩展受限,影响整个呼吸系统的顺应性,因此,肥胖患者呼吸系统病理生理特点同样存在肺容积减少,呼吸系统及肺顺应性降低和通气/血流失调,胸内压增高,肺通气功能减低,呼气流速受限。肥胖 ARDS 患者施行有创机械通气,应该个体化调整呼吸机参数,同样可遵循小潮气量通气的肺保护性通气策略,滴定最佳 PEEP,肥胖不是俯卧位通气的禁忌证。肥胖 ARDS 目前机械通气治疗的临床证据相对较少,需要进一步大数据精准研究评估其机械通气策略有效性和可行性,为肥胖 ARDS 患者提供有效治疗途径。

参 考 文 献

[1] Gong MN, Bajwa EK, Thompson BT, et al. Body mass index is associated with the development of acute respiratory distress syndrome. Thorax, 2010, 65(1):44-50.

[2] 张书娟,韩丽丽,万献尧. 肥胖急性呼吸窘迫综合征患者的临床特点. 中国呼吸与危重监护杂志, 2017, 16(4):421-424.

[3] Behazin N, Jones SB, Cohen RI, et al. Respiratory restriction and elevated pleural and esophageal pressures in morbid obesity. J Appl Physiol(1985), 2010, 108(1):212-218.

[4] Umbrello M, Fumagalli J, Pesenti A, et al. Pathophysiology and Management of Acute Respiratory Distress Syndrome in Obese Patients. Semin Respir Crit Care Med, 2019, 40(1):40-56.

[5] Junhasavasdikul D, Telias I, Grieco DL, et al. Expiratory Flow Limitation During Mechanical Ventilation. Chest, 2018, 154(4):948-962.

[6] Lemyze M, Mallat J, Duhamel A, et al. Effects of sitting position and applied positive end-expiratory pressure on respiratory mechanics of critically ill obese patients receiving mechanical ventilation. Crit Care, Med, 2013, 41(11):2592-2599.

[7] Watson RA, Pride NB. Postural changes in lung volumes and respiratory resistance in subjects with obesity. J Appl Physiol (1985), 2005, 98(2):512-517.

[8] Jones RL, Nzekwu MM. The effects of body mass index on lung volumes. Chest, 2006, 130(3):827-833.

[9] Dixon AE, Peters U. The effect of obesity on lung function. Expert Rev Respir Med, 2018, 12(9):755-767.

[10] Rivas E, Arismendi E, Agusti A, et al. Ventilation/Perfusion distribution abnormalities in morbidly obese subjects before and after bariatric surgery. Chest, 2015, 147(4):1127-1134.

[11] Chiumello D, Colombo A, Algieri I, et al. Effect of body mass index in acute respiratory distress syndrome. Br J Anaesth, 2016, 116(1):113-121.

[12] Pépin JL, Timsit JF, Tamisier R, et al. Prevention and care of respiratory failure in obese patients. Lancet Respir Med, 2016, 4(5):407-418.

[13] Pelosi P, Rocco P, Gama de Abreu M. Close down the lungs and keep them resting to minimize ventilator-induced lung injury. Crit Care, 2018, 22(1):72.

[14] Bime C, Fiero M, Lu Z, et al. High Positive End-Expiratory Pressure Is Associated with Improved Survival in Obese Patients with Acute Respiratory Distress Syndrome. Am J Med, 2017, 130(2):207-213.

[15] Fumagalli J, Santiago R, Teggia Droghi M, et al. Lung Recruitment in Obese Patients with Acute Respiratory Distress Syndrome. Anesthesiology, 2019, 130(5):791-803.

[16] Beitler JR, Sarge T, Banner-Goodspeed VM, et al. Effect of Titrating Positive End-Expiratory Pressure (PEEP) With an Esophageal Pressure-Guided Strategy vs an Empirical High PEEP-Fio2 Strategy on Death and Days Free From Mechanical Ventilation Among Patients With Acute Respiratory Distress Syndrome: A Randomized Clinical Trial. JAMA, 2019, 321(9):846-857.

[17] Gattinoni L, Caironi P, Cressoni M, et al. Lung recruitment in patients with the acute respiratory distress syndrome. N Engl J Med, 2006, 354(17):1775-1786.

[18] 邱海波,许红阳,杨毅,等. 呼气末正压对急性呼吸窘迫综合征肺复张容积及氧合影响的临床研究. 中国危重病急救医学, 2004, (07):399-402.

[19] De Jong A, Verzilli D, Jaber S. ARDS in Obese Patients: Specificities and Management. Crit Care, 2019, 23(1):74.

[20] De Jong A, Cossic J, Verzilli D, et al. Impact of the driving pressure on mortality in obese and non-obese ARDS patients: a retrospective study of 362 cases. Intensive Care Med, 2018, 44(7):1106-1114.

[21] Ball L, Pelosi P. How I ventilate an obese patient. Crit Care, 2019, 23(1):176.

[22] Williams EC, Motta-Ribeiro GC, Vidal Melo MF. Driving Pressure and Transpulmonary Pressure: How Do We Guide Safe Mechanical Ventilation. Anesthesiology, 2019, 131(1):155-163.

[23] Fumagalli J, Berra L, Zhang C, et al. Transpulmonary Pressure Describes Lung Morphology During Decremental Positive End-Expiratory Pressure Trials in Obesity. Crit Care

Med, 2017, 45(8): 1374-1381.
[24] Baedorf Kassis E, Loring SH, Talmor D. Mortality and pulmonary mechanics in relation to respiratory system and transpulmonary driving pressures in ARDS. Intensive Care Med, 2016, 42(8): 1206-1213.
[25] Mauri T, Yoshida T, Bellani G, et al. Esophageal and transpulmonary pressure in the clinical setting: meaning, usefulness and perspectives. Intensive Care Med, 2016, 42(9): 1360-1373.
[26] De Jong A, Molinari N, Sebbane M, et al. Feasibility and effectiveness of prone position in morbidly obese patients with ARDS: a case-control clinical study. Chest, 2013, 143(6): 1554-1561.
[27] Weig T, Janitza S, Zoller M, et al. Influence of abdominal obesity on multiorgan dysfunction and mortality in acute respiratory distress syndrome patients treated with prone positioning. J Crit Care, 2014, 29(4): 557-561.

8 大环内酯类药物的免疫调节作用：在重症患者中的治疗潜力

曾勉 林山

免疫功能失调在重症患者中极其常见，其特征是同时出现过度炎症反应和免疫抑制。过度炎症反应会导致组织损伤和器官衰竭，而免疫抑制则与继发感染和潜伏病毒的再激活密切相关。大环内酯类药物是一类可用于重症监护病房控制感染或缓解胃肠动力障碍的抑菌类抗生素。然而，大环内酯类药物也具有广泛而强大的免疫调节特性，可能具有在不影响关键的抗菌防御屏障能力的情况下纠正危重患者免疫失调的潜力。本文结合目前相关研究进展，阐述大环内酯类药物免疫调节作用在重症疾病中的治疗潜力，并讨论其可能的潜在机制，确定可能从治疗中获益的患者亚群，为临床决策提供一定启示。

一、大环内酯类药物与重症患者免疫失调

危重症患者普遍存在免疫失调。脓毒症就是这种免疫失调的典型例证，其中微生物表达的病原相关分子模式（PAMPs）和损伤相关分子模式（DAMPs）从受损组织中释放，通过结合模式识别受体，包括 Toll 样受体（TLRs）和 Nod 样受体（NLRs），产生强烈的炎症反应，进而可导致器官衰竭。伴随着过度炎症反应发生的同时，免疫抑制和免疫耗竭使个体易发生继发感染和潜伏病毒的重新激活。其他严重疾病（如急性呼吸窘迫综合征，多发伤和急性胰腺炎）的组织损伤也会引起类似的免疫反应。然而在近30年来，尽管进行了大量的基础和临床实验来探索控制这种免疫失调的治疗方法，但至今尚未成功应用于临床实践中。

大环内酯类是一类抑菌类抗生素，通过与细菌核糖体结合来抑制蛋白质合成，对较多的革兰阳性细菌和一些革兰阴性细菌具有广泛的抗菌活性。其中红霉素是一种较常见的大环内酯类药物，同时也是胃动素受体激动剂，在重症监护病房（ICU）常给予较低的剂量以缓解胃肠动力障碍。值得注意的是，大环内酯类药物还具有强大的免疫调节的潜力，可以改变宿主免疫反应。大环内酯类药物可以加快免疫稳态的恢复速度，并维持甚至增强关键的抗微生物防御屏障功能，而不仅仅局限于简单的抑制或刺激免疫反应。或许大环内酯类药物的免疫调节潜能最突出的例子是在弥漫性泛细支气管炎上的应用，这是一种特发性、渐进性的细支气管疾病，而每日小剂量服用红霉素可以逆转这种致命的疾病。目前除了对慢性气道疾病（包括慢性阻塞性肺疾病、囊性纤维化和支气管扩张）有公认的益处外，越来越多的证据表明大环内酯类药物在纠正重症患者免疫失调中同样具有较大的治疗潜力。

二、大环内酯类药物在重症疾病临床前研究中的治疗价值

目前已有研究探讨了大环内酯类药物在肺炎、脓毒症和肺损伤等重症疾病中的免疫调节能力，结果表明：单独或与一种有效抗生素联合使用大环内酯类药物可以调节免疫反应，减轻炎症引起的组织损伤并提高生存率，且与细菌负荷无关。Patel 等研究提示在盲肠结扎和穿孔的脓毒症模型中，尽管两组动物血液中的细菌负荷相似，与单独使用头孢曲松相比，在低于保护剂量的头孢曲松中加入阿奇霉素，使小鼠的存活率翻了1倍；而阿奇霉素的潜在保护作用的机制可能与血浆和肺组织中白细胞介素（IL）-1β、IL-6和肿瘤坏死因子（TNF-α）等促炎细胞因子的浓度降低有关。同样，Yamada 等在多重耐药的鲍曼不动杆菌引起的呼吸机相关性肺炎小鼠模型中发现，所有经阿奇霉素治疗的小鼠均存活，而未经阿奇霉素治疗组中只有不到50%的小鼠得以存活；进一步分析显示这种保护作用同样与阿奇霉素导致的小鼠肺部炎性细胞浸润明显减少有关。在高压通气性肺损伤的小鼠模型中，Amado-Rodríguez 等研究同样发现，克拉霉素减轻了炎症导致的肺损伤及小鼠肺部中性粒细胞等炎性细胞的浸润。而 Weis 等最近的一项研究却显示阿奇霉素在蓝藻肽诱导的急性胰腺炎模型中的益处不大，这可能与疾病严重程度不足有关，但是这并不能否认大环内酯类药物的潜在治疗价值，在其他急性全身性炎性疾病中的使用获益仍需进一步研究。

三、大环内酯类药物在重症疾病临床研究中的治疗价值

（一）重症肺炎

在细菌性肺炎中，局部炎症反应在清除侵袭性病原体方面至关重要，但炎症反应失控又会导致肺损伤、ARDS 以及脓毒症，从而产生不良结局。在 Ceccato 等和 Pons 等的研究中，大环内酯类药物治疗可以显著降低死亡率和炎症反应。Lorenzo 等的研究同样提示在治疗72h后无反应的社区获得性肺炎患者中，18 例接受大环内酯类药物治疗的

患者支气管肺泡灌洗液中细胞因子(IL-6 和 TNF-α)浓度低于接受其他抗生素治疗方案的患者,并且达到临床稳定的时间也比接受其他抗生素方案的患者更短;在临床结局方面,与接受其他抗生素治疗的患者相比,接受大环内酯类药物治疗的患者死亡率显著降低。

肺炎链球菌肺炎是社区获得性肺炎最常见的病因,目前研究显示无论该病原菌株是否对大环内酯类药物耐药,大环内酯类药物治疗获益在肺炎链球菌肺炎中最为明显,可能的机制与抑制肺炎链球菌溶血素的分泌及大环内酯类药物刺激脾脏巨噬细胞细菌库的清除有关。大环内酯类药物还可以抑制群体感应,该机制为细菌用来增加其毒力以应对细菌种群密度变化。由 van Delden 等进行的一项随机对照试验(RCT)研究了阿奇霉素是否可以通过抑制固有的大环内酯类抗药性铜绿假单胞菌定植患者的群体感应来预防呼吸机相关性肺炎,结果显示与对照组相比,阿奇霉素治疗组的呼吸机相关肺炎的发生率下降,但这一发现没有统计学意义。Laserna 等对铜绿假单胞菌导致的社区获得性肺炎的研究,结果未观察到大环内酯类药物治疗组显著获益,且在进入 ICU 后的亚组分析中,同样未观察到大环内酯类药物治疗组死亡率下降,但该研究样本量较小且未对相关混杂因素进行调整,仍需开展大样本的前瞻性研究。

(二)脓毒症

在脓毒症发生发展中,全身性感染会导致严重的免疫失调,即使最初的感染被彻底控制后,免疫紊乱仍然会持续存在。Restrepo 等研究发现肺炎所致的脓毒症中,大环内酯类药物治疗可显著提高 30 d 及 90 d 的生存率,该获益在病原体对大环内酯类抗生素耐药的情况下仍然存在。由 Giamarellos-Bourboulis 等进行的两项 RCT 研究评估了克拉霉素静脉注射对脓毒症的免疫调节作用,该研究为了排除其他抗生素可能带来的潜在生存益处,仅纳入了感染病原体最有可能对大环内酯类药物耐药的感染患者,其中第一项 RCT 纳入了 200 例呼吸机相关性肺炎患者,第二项 RCT 纳入了 600 例疑似或经微生物学证实为革兰阴性脓毒症患者。两项 RCT 研究的主要结局为 28 d 病死率,结果均为阴性,但接受克拉霉素治疗组的临床症状持续时间缩短了 4～5.5 d。而在呼吸机相关肺炎的亚组分析中,24 名接受克拉霉素治疗的感染性休克和多器官衰竭患者在第 4 天血清 IL-10/TNF-α 比值较低,IL-6 水平较高,TNF-α 水平较低,细胞凋亡增加,共刺激分子 CD86 的表达增加。这些研究结果可能表明克拉霉素逆转了免疫抑制和增加了对内毒素的耐受性,并加速恢复免疫系统的稳态。从进一步的分析发现,接受克拉霉素治疗组 90 d 病死率显著降低。综合来看,大环内酯类药物可能有助于机体免疫系统稳态的恢复,并维持针对再入侵病原体的先天性免疫细胞功能。

(三)ARDS

肺炎、脓毒症或其他局部或全身疾病随着疾病的进展可能发展为 ARDS,其病理为肺泡内皮细胞弥漫性损伤,肺泡内皮细胞屏障被破坏,毛细血管通透性增高,富含蛋白质的液体渗出至肺泡腔及肺间质,进而导致非心源性肺水肿及透明膜形成,临床上表现为进行性呼吸困难和顽固性低氧血症,死亡率高。Walkey 等对 235 名 ARDS 患者的研究,结果提示使用大环内酯类药物可降低 180 d 死亡率,并缩短机械通气时间。随后 Kawamura 等研究同样发现了类似的结果,提示静脉注射阿奇霉素辅助治疗对中、重度 ARDS 患者有效,提高 90 d 生存率,并缩短机械通气的时间。Simonis 等对 873 名 ARDS 患者(其中 158 名接受大环内酯类辅助治疗)的研究发现,低剂量大环内酯类药物使 ARDS 患者的院内死亡率降低,但是该获益仅在非肺源性 ARDS 及非炎症表型 ARDS 患者中具有统计学意义。在 Giamarellos-Bourboulis 等对革兰阴性菌导致的脓毒症合并 ARDS 的 RCT 研究中,接受克拉霉素治疗与未接受克拉霉素治疗组的死亡率分别为 28.5% 和 55.9%。相比之下,最近由 Pons 等开展的一项对 7182 名行机械通气的急性呼吸衰竭(包括 ARDS)患者的研究分析发现,其中 1295 人主要以抗生素为目的接受大环内酯类药物治疗,在接受大环内酯类药物的患者与未接受大环内酯类药物的患者之间,死亡率、机械通气持续时间或二次感染发生率方面无显著差异。

四、大环内酯类药物与重症疾病相关的作用机制

大多数大环内酯类药物免疫调节活性的体内研究显示均与肺部炎症有关,但大环内酯类药物与细胞之间相互作用表明它们还可能影响肺外炎症性疾病。由于直接修饰靶细胞,而其他作用最有可能是由于复杂的系统相互作用所引起的,例如,在使用单一的大环内酯类药物治疗后,小鼠的肠道菌群可以在较长的时间内发生改变,这反过来也可以调节免疫反应。此外,大环内酯类化合物还诱导非免疫性效应,增强气道对病原体的抵抗力,改变痰的黏稠度和减少过度分泌,使病原体清除,增强气道上皮完整性,并降低花生酸类的代谢。

(一)对炎症反应启动的影响

在炎症反应的启动过程中,DAMPs 和 PAMPs 通过与 TLR 等模式识别受体相互作用而诱导强烈的免疫反应。已经证实大环内酯可减少树突状细胞和巨噬细胞的 TLR 的表达,其中信号通路包括 NF-κB、p38、ERK 和 JNK 通路,研究表明大环内酯类可以增强 NEMO 抑制剂 IKKζ 的表达,导致 p50 的诱导减少和 NF-κB 核转位的减少,并且大环内酯类还可以抑制核转位所需的 JNK 和 ERK 的磷酸化,降低 NALP3 蛋白的稳定性,从而减少和抑制 NLRP3 炎症小体的激活。这些机制可能是其免疫调节作用的重要的组成部分。

(二)对抗炎因子和促炎因子的影响

与 TLR 结合可激活免疫细胞清楚入侵的病原体。然而,重症患者可能会出现过度的炎症反应,其特征在于促炎细胞因子的大量释放。大环内酯类药物通过减少促炎细胞因子释放和限制免疫细胞迁移来抑制这种反应。大环内酯类药物会减少气道上皮细胞,单核细胞,巨噬细胞,树突状细胞和 T 细胞中 IL-6 和 TNF-α 的分泌。同样,大

环内酯类药物会抑制 NOD 样受体蛋白 3(NLRP3)和 NLRC4 炎性小体的激活，从而减少单核细胞和巨噬细胞对脂多糖刺激或整个细菌的应答，进而抑制 IL-1β 的产生。在革兰阴性和革兰阳性细菌感染模型中，大环内酯类药物可降低血清和支气管肺泡灌洗液中 IL-1β、IL-6 和 TNF-α 的含量，抑制树突状细胞产生 IL-12。

目前大环内酯类药物对抗炎细胞因子的作用比较模糊。有研究发现大环内酯类药物可上调单核细胞和巨噬细胞产生 IL-10，但似乎却抑制 T 细胞和树突状细胞中 IL-10 的表达。在小鼠感染模型中，大环内酯类药物治疗可增加或不改变血清或支气管肺泡灌洗液中 IL-10 的浓度，而这些研究中观察到的 IL-10 增加可能部分来自大环内酯类诱导的髓系衍生抑制细胞(MDSCs)。最近的一项研究表明，IL-10 对于克拉霉素诱导的 MDSC 在致死性休克(由脂多糖注射引起)和流感后肺炎球菌性肺炎模型中的保护作用至关重要。重症患者的过度炎症反应与白细胞的大量募集有关，该过程导致血管渗漏和组织损伤，从而导致器官衰竭。在急性感染和高压通气性肺损伤的小鼠模型中，大环内酯类药物减少了中性粒细胞到肺的募集，从而防止了肺实质的破坏，可能的机制为大环内酯类药物降低生长因子和趋化因子的浓度。总体而言，大环内酯类药物可减少粒细胞和粒细胞和粒-巨噬细胞集落刺激因子的产生，并下调募集中性粒细胞、单核细胞和其他白细胞的趋化因子，如 IL-8(CXCL8)、巨噬细胞炎性蛋白 2(CXCL2)等。此外，大环内酯类药物在体外可减少 CD4$^+$ T 细胞产生 IL-17，这可能进一步降低了中性粒细胞的激活和动员。

(三)对免疫细胞增殖、分化和凋亡的影响

免疫细胞除了被募集到感染部位外，也会增殖以控制感染。然而，危重病患者的免疫反应常受到过度炎症反应和免疫耗竭的影响。大环内酯类药物可以抑制 CD4 T 细胞的增殖，从而抑制炎症反应，其原因可能是多方面的。首先，大量研究表明大环内酯类药物可以下调抗原提呈细胞上共刺激分子的表达，Iwamoto 等研究进一步证实了阿奇霉素可降低体外培养树突状细胞上主要组织相容性复合体 II 类的表达，这种下调与促炎细胞因子的产生减少相结合，可能会减少对 T 细胞增殖的刺激。其次，Iwamoto 等研究还发现 T 细胞暴露于经阿奇霉素处理的树突状细胞产生 γ 干扰素减少，IL-10 分泌增加，这会抑制自分泌的激活和随后的细胞增殖；IL-10 的增加促使 T 细胞向辅助 T 细胞 2 型分化，这提示大环内酯类可以通过使细胞分化向更多的耐受性表型倾斜而进一步抑制危重病人的过度炎症反应。Matsui 等研究证实了这一点，即大环内酯类药物可以促进巨噬细胞和单核细胞向耐受性或 M2 样表型转化。最后，细胞活力的降低也可以解释增殖减弱的原因，有研究发现大环内酯类在较高浓度时可诱导 T 细胞凋亡。

由于危重患者普遍存在 T 细胞、B 细胞、树突状细胞和巨噬细胞凋亡增加，这可能导致进一步的感染，并与多器官衰竭和死亡率增加相关，但研究发现中性粒细胞凋亡的减少或不受影响，而这恰恰延长了过度炎症反应。大环内酯类药物可以通过直接刺激凋亡和抑制粒细胞集落刺激因子的释放来减少中性粒细胞的存活。这种促凋亡作用并不一定削弱对病原体的防御，有研究表明，当中性粒细胞与肺炎链球菌共存时，阿奇霉素并不诱导凋亡；高浓度的阿奇霉素在体外才能诱导树突状细胞、自然杀伤细胞和 CD4 T 细胞的凋亡。然而，这些细胞的凋亡还没有在临床实践中观察到，因此似乎不太可能加剧重症患者的免疫抑制。

(四)对细胞功能的影响

免疫相关细胞通过吞噬作用使细菌内化可以防止传播，促进细菌的杀灭，并且是启动适应性免疫中抗原提呈所必需的过程。Pinder 和 Danikas 等的研究表明，重症患者的细胞吞噬能力显著降低，且与院内二次感染和死亡率增加密切相关。已有研究表明大环内酯类可增强树突状细胞和肺泡巨噬细胞的吞噬能力，Hodge 等发现阿奇霉素可以帮助因疾病而受损的免疫细胞，给予阿奇霉素可以恢复 COPD 患者肺泡和单核细胞来源的巨噬细胞的吞噬力。Persson 等研究进一步发现阿奇霉素在体内外可以保护巨噬细胞因氧化应激诱导的死亡，并改善吞噬小体的稳定性，防止细菌从吞噬小体中逃逸，从而有助于细菌的清除。自噬同样也可以用来杀死病原体，调节免疫反应，防止凋亡。Lai 等同样证实了大环内酯类药物可以增强对病原体的吞噬内杀伤力，如金黄色葡萄球菌，放线菌。经大环内酯类药物处理的中性粒细胞释放更多的抗菌肽，为了杀灭入侵的病原体，中性粒细胞还可以分泌各种储存在体内的抗菌肽。阿奇霉素和克拉霉素还被报道具有降低弹性蛋白酶的活性和增强髓过氧化物酶活性的能力，其进一步提高了自然杀伤细胞的活性，从而发挥杀菌作用。

(五)对细菌的影响

大环内酯类药物除了具有抑制细菌蛋白质合成的直接抑菌作用外，还具有多种机制降低细菌的毒力，即使该菌株对大环内酯类耐药。大环内酯类药物可以抑制肺炎链球菌释放一种帮助细菌免疫逃逸的酶 LytA，进而下调肺炎球菌溶血素，这将导致补体沉积增强，从而促进细菌的杀灭。大环内酯类还可以抑制其他细菌(包括大肠埃希菌，铜绿假单胞菌和真菌)产生毒力因子。在有利的生长条件下，细菌会形成生物膜，从而将其敏感性降到最低程度，并减少对抗生素和免疫细胞的接触。生物膜的形成是留置导管和医疗设备在 ICU 中定植的关键机制，是医院获得性感染的重要毒力因素。大环内酯类药物可抑制包括铜绿假单胞菌，流感嗜血杆菌和表皮葡萄球菌在内的细菌产生生物膜，其中部分机制是通过减少群体感应来实现的。最后，大环内酯类药物还可以抑制细菌对气道上皮的黏附。

大环内酯类还可与其他分子，如类固醇，抗菌肽或小的信号分子偶联，以增强其功能。利用大环内酯类药物在体内相对稳定，并可以在吞噬细胞中聚集，将大环内酯类药物作为向吞噬小体或炎症部位传递药物或信号的优秀载体分子。例如，DP7 是一种有效的抗菌肽，由于其副作用而不能系统给药，而 Li 等研究将抗菌肽与阿奇霉素设计成脂质体，在对耐甲氧西林金黄色葡萄球菌(MRSA)感染期间给予这些脂质体，不仅具有持续的药物释放特性和免疫调节作用，在体内研究小鼠中未观察到明显的副作用及毒性，并且对 MRSA 感染小鼠模型具有良好的抗菌活性；还可以通过上调抗炎因子和趋化因子的表达减少炎症反应，以及协同激活细菌先天免疫反应。

五、新型非抗生素类大环内酯衍生物

抗生素的广泛使用可能会加剧抗菌素耐药性的形成，对大环内酯类药物进行修饰以消除它们的抗菌作用，同时保持或增强它们的免疫调节能力具有良好的未来应用前景。EM703 就是一种非抗生素类红霉素衍生物，可改善铜绿假单胞菌引起的气道感染后小鼠的存活率，可能是通过减少促炎细胞因子的释放。另一种红霉素衍生物 EM900，有研究表明其可以抑制感染诱导的促炎细胞因子的产生、NF-κB 通路的激活及上皮细胞分泌黏液。Balloy 等对阿奇霉素衍生物 CSY0073 研究结果同样显示 CSY0073 可以降低脂多糖诱导的促炎性细胞因子和趋化因子在小鼠肺组织中的浓度。

六、结论与展望

大环内酯类药物强大的免疫调节作用，有望纠正重症患者失控的免疫平衡。但是大环内酯类的免疫调节作用是复杂的，与时间、剂量和疾病的严重程度等密切相关。大环内酯类化合物的抗炎和促修复特性以减轻过度炎症和组织损伤，这可能转化为症状持续时间的缩短和死亡率的降低。然而，尽管利用大环内酯类有益的免疫调节作用是一个诱人的前景，但目前临床证据较少，需要进一步的研究来确定大环内酯类的免疫调节是否可以成为危重患者的有效治疗途径，并确定最有可能受益于大环内酯类免疫调节治疗的临床或免疫学表型。同时，应进一步优化新的非抗生素大环内酯类化合物，在增强其免疫调节潜力的同时，最大限度地减少抗菌素耐药性的产生。

参 考 文 献

[1] Matthay MA, Zemans RL, Zimmerman GA, et al. Acute respiratory distress syndrome. Nat Rev Dis Primers, 2019, 5:18.

[2] Leliefeld P H C, Wessels C M, Leenen L P H, et al. The role of neutrophils in immune dysfunction during severe inflammation. Crit Care, 2016, 20(1):1-9.

[3] Delano M J, Ward P A. Sepsis-induced immune dysfunction: can immune therapies reduce mortality?. J Clin Invest, 2016, 126(1):23-31.

[4] Hotchkiss R S, Monneret G, Payen D. Sepsis-induced immunosuppression: from cellular dysfunctions to immunotherapy. Nat Rev Immunol, 2013, 13(12):862-874.

[5] Kanoh S, Rubin B K. Mechanisms of action and clinical application of macrolides as immunomodulatory medications. Clin Microbiol Rev, 2010, 23(3):590-615.

[6] Kudoh S, Azuma A, Yamamoto M, et al. Improvement of survival in patients with diffuse panbronchiolitis treated with low-dose erythromycin. Am J Respir Crit Care Med, 1998, 157:1829-1832.

[7] Patel A, Joseph J, Periasamy H, et al. Azithromycin in combination with ceftriaxone reduces systemic inflammation and provides survival benefit in murine model of polymicrobial sepsis. Antimicrob Agents Chemother, 2018, 62:e00752-718.

[8] Upadhyay K, Hiregoudar B, Meals E, et al. Combination therapy with ampicillin and azithromycin improved outcomes in a mouse model of group B streptococcal sepsis. PLoS One, 2017, 12:e0182023.

[9] Yoshioka D, Kajiwara C, Ishii Y, et al. Efficacy of β-lactamplusmacrolide combination therapy in a mouse model of lethal pneumococcal pneumonia. Antimicrob Agents Chemother, 2016, 60:6146-6154.

[10] Yamada K, Yanagihara K, Kaku N, et al. Azithromycin attenuates lung inflammation in a mouse model of ventilator-associated pneumonia by multidrug-resistant Acinetobacter baumannii. Antimicrob Agents Chemother, 2013, 57:3883-3888.

[11] Yamashita Y, Nagaoka K, Kimura H, et al. Efficacy of azithromycin in a mouse pneumonia model against hospital-acquired methicillinresistant Staphylococcus aureus. Antimicrob Agents Chemother, 2019, 63: e00149-19.

[12] Amado-Rodríguez L, González-López A, López-Alonso I, et al. Anti-inflammatory effects of clarithromycin in ventilator-induced lung injury. Respir Res, 2013, 14:52.

[13] Weis S, Heindl M, Carvalho T, et al. Azithromycin does not improve disease severity in acute experimental pancreatitis. PLoS One, 2019, 14:e0216614.

[14] Ceccato A, Cilloniz C, Martin-Loeches I, et al. Effect of combined β-lactam/macrolide therapy on mortality according to the microbial etiology and inflammatory status of patients with communityacquired pneumonia. Chest, 2019, 155:795-804.

[15] Pons S, Timsit J-F, Ruckly S, et al. Impact of macrolide therapy in critically ill patients with acute respiratory failure: a desirability of outcome ranking analysis to investigate the outcomerea database. Intensive Care Med, 2019, 45: 1043-1045.

[16] Lorenzo M J, Moret I, Sarria B, et al. Lung inflammatory pattern and antibiotic treatment in pneumonia. Respir Res, 2015, 16(1):15.

[17] Cilloniz C, Albert RK, Liapikou A, et al. The effect of macrolide resistance on the presentation and outcome of patients hospitalized for Streptococcus pneumoniae pneumonia. Am J Respir Crit Care Med, 2015, 191:1265-1272.

[18] Ercoli G, Fernandes VE, Chung WY, et al. Intracellular replication of Streptococcus pneumoniae inside splenic macrophages serves as a reservoir for septicaemia. Nat Microbiol, 2018, 3:600-610.

[19] van Delden C, Köhler T, Brunner-Ferber F, et al. Azithromycin to prevent Pseudomonas aeruginosa ventilator-associated

pneumonia by inhibition of quorum sensing: a randomized controlled trial. Intensive Care Med,2012,38:1118-1125.
[20] Laserna E, Sibila O, Fernandez JF, et al. Impact of macrolide therapy in patients hospitalized with Pseudomonas aeruginosa community-acquired pneumonia. Chest,2014,145:1114-1120.
[21] Restrepo MI, Mortensen EM, Waterer GW, et al. Impact of macrolide therapy on mortality for patients with severe sepsis due to pneumonia. Eur Respir J,2009,33:153-159.
[22] Giamarellos-Bourboulis EJ, Pechère J-C, Routsi C, et al. Effect of clarithromycin in patients with sepsis and ventilator-associated pneumonia. Clin Infect Dis,2008,46:1157-1164.
[23] Giamarellos-Bourboulis EJ, Mylona V, Antonopoulou A, et al. Effect of clarithromycin in patients with suspected Gram-negative sepsis: results of a randomized controlled trial. J Antimicrob Chemother,2014,69:1111-1118.
[24] Walkey AJ, Wiener RS. Macrolide antibiotics and survival in patients with acute lung injury. Chest, 2012, 141(5): 1153-1159.
[25] Kawamura K, Ichikado K, Takaki M, et al. Adjunctive therapy with azithromycin for moderate and severe acute respiratory distress syndrome: a retrospective, propensity score-matching analysis of prospectively collected data at a single center. Int J Antimicrob Agents,2018,51:918-924.
[26] Simonis FD, de Iudicibus G, Cremer OL, et al. Macrolide therapy is associated with reduced mortality in acute respiratory distress syndrome (ARDS) patients. Ann Transl Med, 2018,6:24.
[27] Ruiz V E, Battaglia T, Kurtz Z D, et al. A single early-in-life macrolide course has lasting effects on murine microbial network topology and immunity. Nat Commun, 2017, 8(1): 1-14.
[28] Iwamoto S, Kumamoto T, Azuma E, et al. The effect of azithromycin on the maturation and function of murine bone marrow-derived dendritic cells. Clin Exp Immunol,2011,166.
[29] Matsui K, Tamai S, Ikeda R. Effects of macrolide antibiotics on Th1 cell and Th2 cell development mediated by Langerhans cells. J Pharm Pharm Sci,2016,19:357-366.

[30] Lin SJ, Kuo ML, Hsiao HS, et al. Azithromycin modulates immune response of human monocyte-derived dendritic cells and $CD4^+$ T cells. Int Immunopharmacol,2016,40:318-326.
[31] Namkoong H, Ishii M, Fujii H, et al. Clarithromycin expands $CD11b^+$ $Gr-1^+$ cells via the STAT3/Bv8 axis to ameliorate lethal endotoxic shock and post-influenza bacterial pneumonia. PLoS Pathog,2018,14(4):e1006955.
[32] Feng Y, Liu B, Zheng X, et al. The protective role of autophagy in sepsis. Microb Pathog,2019,131:106-111.
[33] Pinder EM, Rostron AJ, Hellyer TP, et al. Randomised controlled trial of GM-CSF in critically ill patients with impaired neutrophil phagocytosis. Thorax,2018,73:918-925.
[34] Danikas DD, Karakantza M, Theodorou GL, et al. Prognostic value of phagocytic activity of neutrophils and monocytes in sepsis. Correlation to CD64 and CD14 antigen expression. Clin Exp Immunol,2008,154:87-97.
[35] Hodge S, Hodge G, Brozyna S, et al. Azithromycin increases phagocytosis of apoptotic bronchial epithelial cells by alveolar macrophages. Eur Respir J,2006,28:486-495.
[36] Lai P-C, Schibler MR, Walters JD. Azithromycin enhances phagocytic killing of Aggregatibacter actinomycetemcomitans Y4 by human neutrophils. J Periodontol,2015,86:155-161.
[37] Li Z, Wang X, Chen Y, et al. Novel antimicrobial peptide-modified azithromycin-loaded liposomes against methicillin-resistant Staphylococcus aureus. Int J Nanomedicine, 2016, 11:6781-6794.
[38] Kasetty G, Bhongir RKV, Papareddy P, et al. The nonantibiotic macrolide EM703 improves survival in a model of quinolone-treated Pseudomonas aeruginosa airway infection. Antimicrob Agents Chemother,2017,61:1-11.
[39] Kalonji NL, Nomura K, Kawase T, et al. The non-antibiotic macrolide EM900 inhibits rhinovirus infection and cytokine production in human airway epithelial cells. Physiol Rep, 2015,3:e12557.
[40] Balloy V, Deveaux A, Lebeaux D, et al. Azithromycin analogue CSY0073 attenuates lung inflammation induced by LPS challenge. Br J Pharmacol,2014,171:1783-1794.

9 感染性疾病与炎症风暴

李 丹

炎症风暴又名细胞因子风暴（cytokine storm），1993年首次提出用来描述移植物抗宿主（GVHD）的效应；2003年开始用于描述流感病毒感染中的大量炎性因子分泌，随后逐渐被发现存在于各种感染，因此在脓毒症领域被广泛研究。在自身免疫疾病领域，炎症风暴经常与"噬血细胞性淋巴组织细胞增生症"（HLH）和"巨噬细胞活化综合征"（MAS）这两个名词紧密联系使用。实际上，目前，炎症风暴并没有统一的、确切的定义，通常认为是指疾病导致细胞因子产生自放大的级联反应，而极端数量的炎症介质可导致脏器的损伤和功能衰竭。COVID-19的流行，使炎症风暴这个名词再次出现在讨论的中心。不同疾病引起的炎症风暴均有其炎症因子集合的不同特点，而本文仅讨论感染性疾病中的炎症风暴。

病原体致病的免疫机制经过数十年的研究、积累，已经取得了非常大的进步。尽管具体的机制仍不完全清楚，但已经明确，感染造成的损害不仅是由致病微生物导致的直接损伤，机体在抵抗致病因素时的过度反应也是造成损伤的重要原因，极端状况下，可能是导致机体死亡的主要因素。要深入了解感染过程中由什么细胞释放了什么炎症因子，就有必要先来了解一下感染过程中机体免疫活化的过程。

一、机体抗感染免疫的分子机制

病原体入侵机体后，首先激活的是天然免疫系统。天然免疫系统主要由组织屏障、固有免疫细胞和固有免疫分子组成。固有免疫细胞的主要成分是血细胞，包括单核细胞、巨噬细胞、中性粒细胞、嗜酸性粒细胞和嗜碱性粒细胞，还有自然杀伤（NK）细胞。固有免疫细胞通过表面的模式识别受体（PRRs）识别病原微生物的病原相关分子模式（PAMPs），通过固定的信号传导，导致一系列蛋白的激活/磷酸化，放大炎症信号，激活相关的免疫细胞，清除病原菌。PRRs所识别的致病分子模式除了PAMPs，还包括内源性坏死细胞释放的损伤相关分子模式（DAMPs）（图8-9-1）。目前为止，脊椎动物确认了4种PRRs，包括

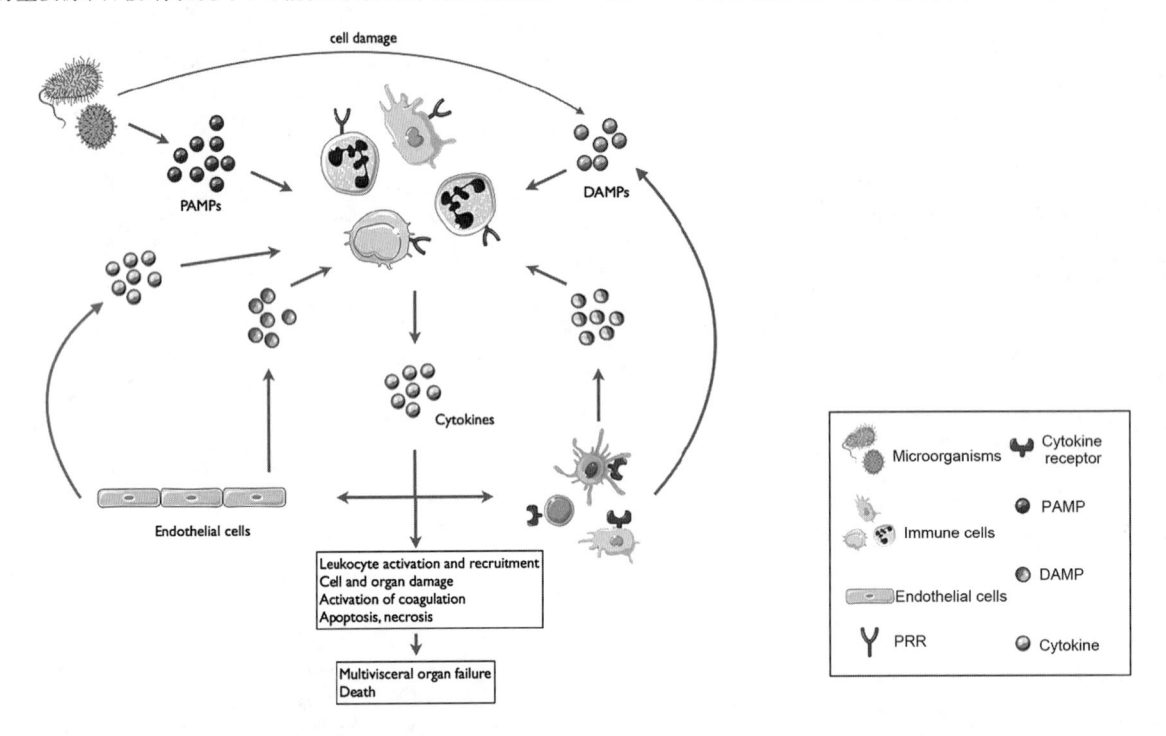

图 8-9-1 脓毒症时细胞因子的级联反应（引自 CHOUSTERMAN B G, SWIRSKI F K, WEBER G F. Cytokine storm and sepsis disease pathogenesi）

TLRs、NLRs、RLRs 和 CLRs。目前研究较确切的是 TLRs 和 NLRs 的信号传导。TLR 主要有 10 种亚型,其中 TLR1、2、4、5 和 6 主要表达在细胞膜上,识别来自胞外病原体 PAMPs;而 TLR3、7、8 和 9 位于胞质内,主要识别来自病毒和细菌的核酸等 PAMPs。PAMPs 或 DAMPs 与 TLR 结合后,可通过 MyD88 依赖途径和 TRIF 信号通路途径激活下游级联活化信号通路,如 MAPK、NF-κB、IRF3、IRF7 等,进而产生多种细胞因子如:IL-1β、IL-6、IL-8(趋化因子)、IL-18、TNF-α 等(图 8-9-2)。NOD 样受体(NOD like receptor,NLR)是一类含核苷酸结合寡聚域的蛋白质家族,广泛存在于人细胞胞质内,是重要的模式识别受体之一。NLR 的信号传导主要有受体相互作用蛋白 2(NLR-RIP2,receptor interacting protein 2)介导的信号途径和炎症小体介导的信号途径。①NLR-RIP2 信号通路是 NOD1 和 NOD2 相关的信号通路,配体激活 NLR 后,募集 RIP2 进一步激活 MAPK 和 NF-κB 信号通路。②炎症小体信号通路中研究最清楚的是 NLRP3 炎症小体。多种 PAMPs、DAMPs(如 LPS、细菌 RNA、尿酸盐、热休克蛋白等)被 NLRP3 识别并结合,导致 NLRP3 寡聚化,进一步结合 pro-Caspase-1,形成炎症小体,使 pro-Caspase-1 转变为成熟的 Caspase-1,进一步剪切 pro-IL-1β、pro-IL-18,形成活化的 IL-1β、IL-18(图 8-9-3)。

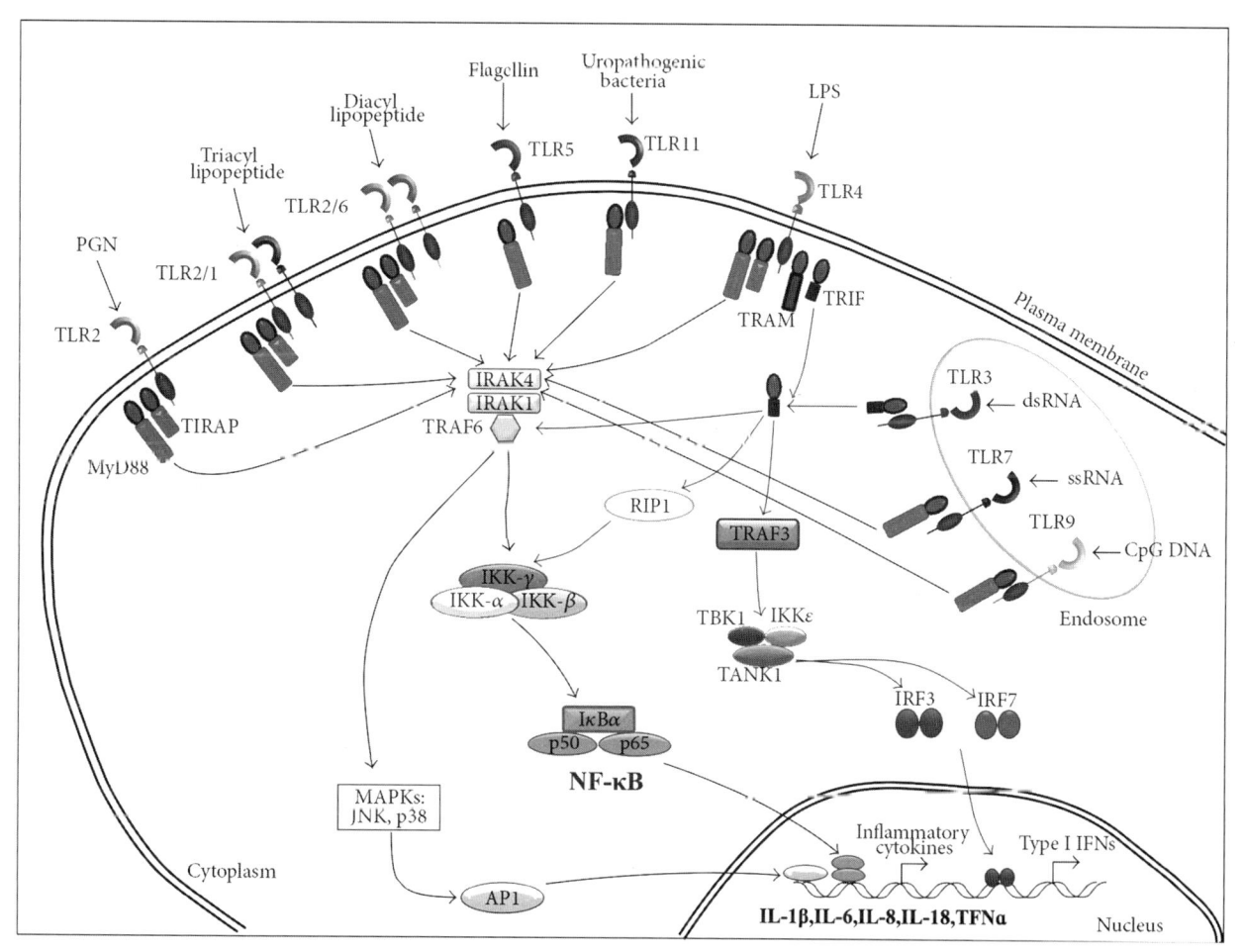

图 8-9-2 TLR 信号传导通路。TLR 信号以依赖于 MyD88(黑色箭头)和依赖于 TRIF(蓝色箭头)的方式激活下游信号。MyD88 信号通路导致 MAPKs、NF-κB 激活,而 TRIF 信号通路导致 IRF3、IRF7 和 NF-κB 激活(根据 OVIEDO-BOYSO J, BRAVO-PATINO A, BAIZABAL-AGUIRRE V M. Collaborative action of Toll-like and NOD-like receptors as modulators of the inflammatory response to pathogenic bacteria 修改)

二、炎症风暴相关的细胞因子

天然免疫对病原体的清除是无特异性的,适量的细胞因子的释放有助于病原体清除及诱导后续的适应性免疫反应,即淋巴细胞的抗原特异性克隆扩增。而不恰当的过量的细胞因子水平并不利于诱导适应性免疫应答,并且会对机体造成损伤。目前认为炎症风暴主要与天然免疫反应失控关系比较密切。所涉及的细胞因子主要有以下几类:白细胞介素、肿瘤坏死因子、干扰素、趋化因子和生长因子。

(一)白细胞介素

白细胞介素(interleukin,IL)是感染过程中释放的最重要的一组细胞因子。主要由白细胞和内皮细胞分泌。白介素主要负责细胞信号传递,依据白介素活化后的生物学效应,可以分为促炎因子和抗炎因子。促炎白细胞介素

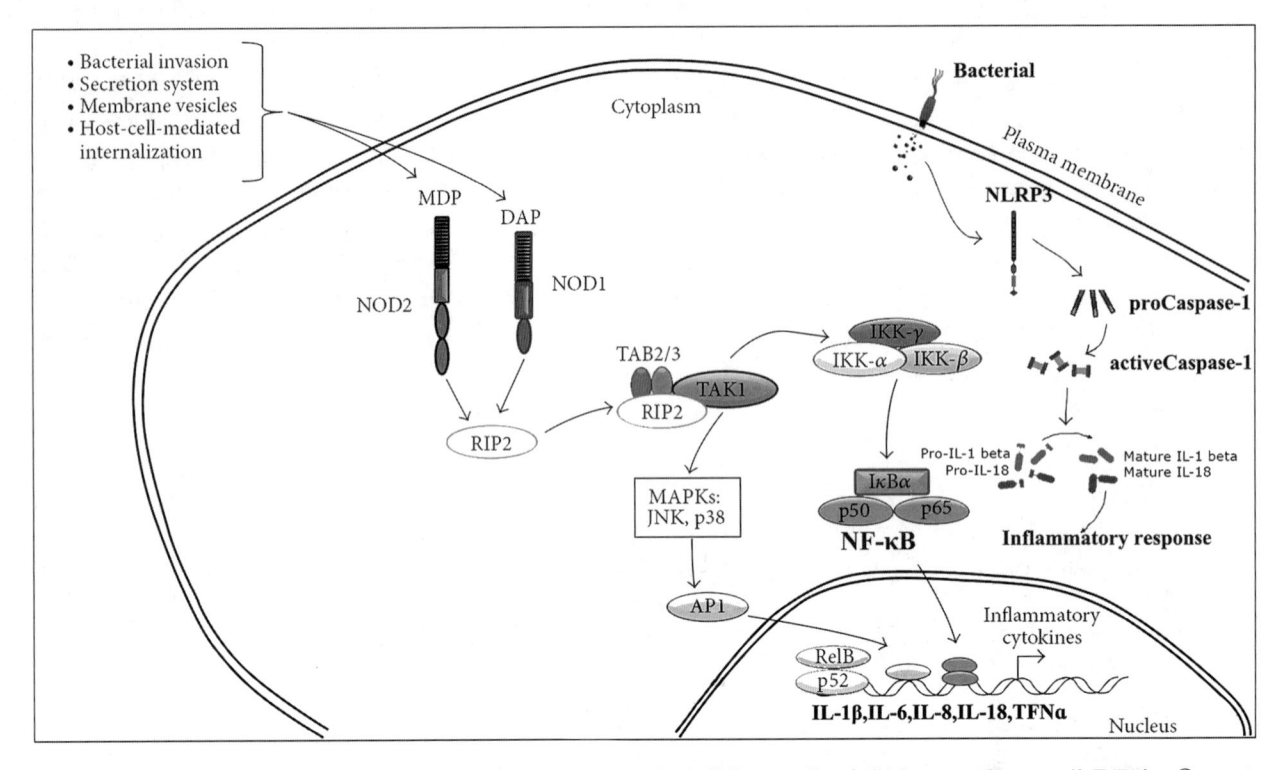

图 8-9-3 NLR 信号传导通路。①NLR-RIP2 信号通路：NOD1 和 NOD2 激活，募集 RIP2 进一步激活 MAPKs 和 NF-κB 信号通路。②NLRP3 炎症小体信号通路：配体被 NLRP3 识别并结合，导致 NLRP3 寡聚化，进一步结合 pro-Caspase-1，形成炎症小体，使 pro-Caspase-1 转变为成熟的 Caspase-1，进一步剪切 pro-IL-1β、pro-IL-18，形成活化的 IL-1β、IL-18（根据 OVIEDO-BOYSO J，BRAVO-PATINO A，BAIZABAL-AGUIRRE V M. Collaborative action of Toll-like and NOD-like receptors as modulators of the inflammatory response to pathogenic bacteria 修改）

主要导致细胞活化、增殖、趋化免疫细胞或组织损伤，而抗炎白细胞介素主要是抑制炎症过度活化，促进损伤组织的修复，维持机体稳态。目前研究较多且相对明确的促炎细胞因子包括 IL-6、IL-1β、IL-8（详见趋化因子）、IL-12 和 IL-17。抗炎因子主要有白介素 1 受体拮抗剂（IL-1RA）和 IL-10。

1. IL-6　IL-6 是目前在炎症风暴中作用确切的促炎因子，针对 IL-6 的单克隆抗体在治疗自身免疫性疾病方面已取得了明确的疗效。当 PAMPs 或 DAMP 或其他刺激因子（如 IL-1、TNF-α、异常增多的凝血因子Ⅶa、凝血酶）作用于巨噬细胞、血管内皮细胞、间充质细胞、成纤维细胞等，可迅速产生 IL-6，进一步诱导急性期免疫反应。正常情况下，IL-6 的表达受转录和转录后机制严格调控。IL-6 受体主要分为可溶性细胞因子受体（soluble IL-6R，sIL-6R）和膜结合型细胞因子受体（membrane IL-6R，mIL-6R），后者主要表达于一些免疫细胞、气道上皮细胞、肝细胞等。IL-6 与 mIL-6R 结合后，诱导下游 gp130 蛋白同源二聚化，进一步活化下游的 JAK/STAT 和 Ras/MAPK 信号通路，促使转录因子如 STAT3 核内转位，调控 IL-6 效应基因的表达。对于细胞表面不表达 IL-6R 的细胞，IL-6 可以通过与 sIL-6R 结合，首先形成 IL-6/sIL-6R 复合物，该复合物可以结合到细胞表面上的 gp130，并诱导 gp130 蛋白同源二聚化，后续的信号通路与 mIL-6R 的信号传导基本一致。IL-6 通过 sIL-6R 进行信号传导的方式称为跨细胞信号传导（trans-signaling）。由于 sIL-6R 可以随着体液循环到身体各处，而 gp130 分布广泛，几乎所有细胞都表达，因此"trans-signaling"有助于 IL-6 将局部的应激信号传导至全身各处。

以脓毒症为例，已经有研究表明，脓毒症患者体内高浓度 IL-6 与预后不佳密切相关（图 8-9-4）。IL-6 能迅速诱导肝脏产生 CRP、血清淀粉样蛋白 A、抗胰蛋白酶、肝杀菌肽、纤维蛋白原、血小板生成素和补体 C3 等多种蛋白质，有助于机体限制和清除病原体。但是，IL-6 可直接或通过诱导血管内皮生长因子（VEGF）诱导内皮细胞上血管内皮细胞钙黏附素的分解，导致血管通透性增加，大量炎性因子渗出，损伤组织。IL-6 上调内皮细胞上的补体 C5a 受体，增加内皮细胞对 C5a 的反应性，进一步增强血管通透性。IL-6 还诱导单核细胞表面组织因子（tissue factor，TF）表达增加，触发凝血级联反应，激活凝血酶，形成纤维蛋白凝块，导致微血栓形成。凝血酶诱导血管内皮细胞表达 IL-6，而 IL-6 增加 MCP-1 和 IL-8 的合成，从而触发单核细胞和中性粒细胞向病变部位募集。IL-6 还会抑制穿孔素和颗粒酶 B 来抑制 NK 细胞的细胞毒活性。此外，IL-6 可以减弱心肌收缩，导致心肌功能障碍。因此，IL-6 的多重作用与脓毒症时组织缺血、缺氧、弥散性血管内凝血（DIC）、多器官功能障碍密切相关。

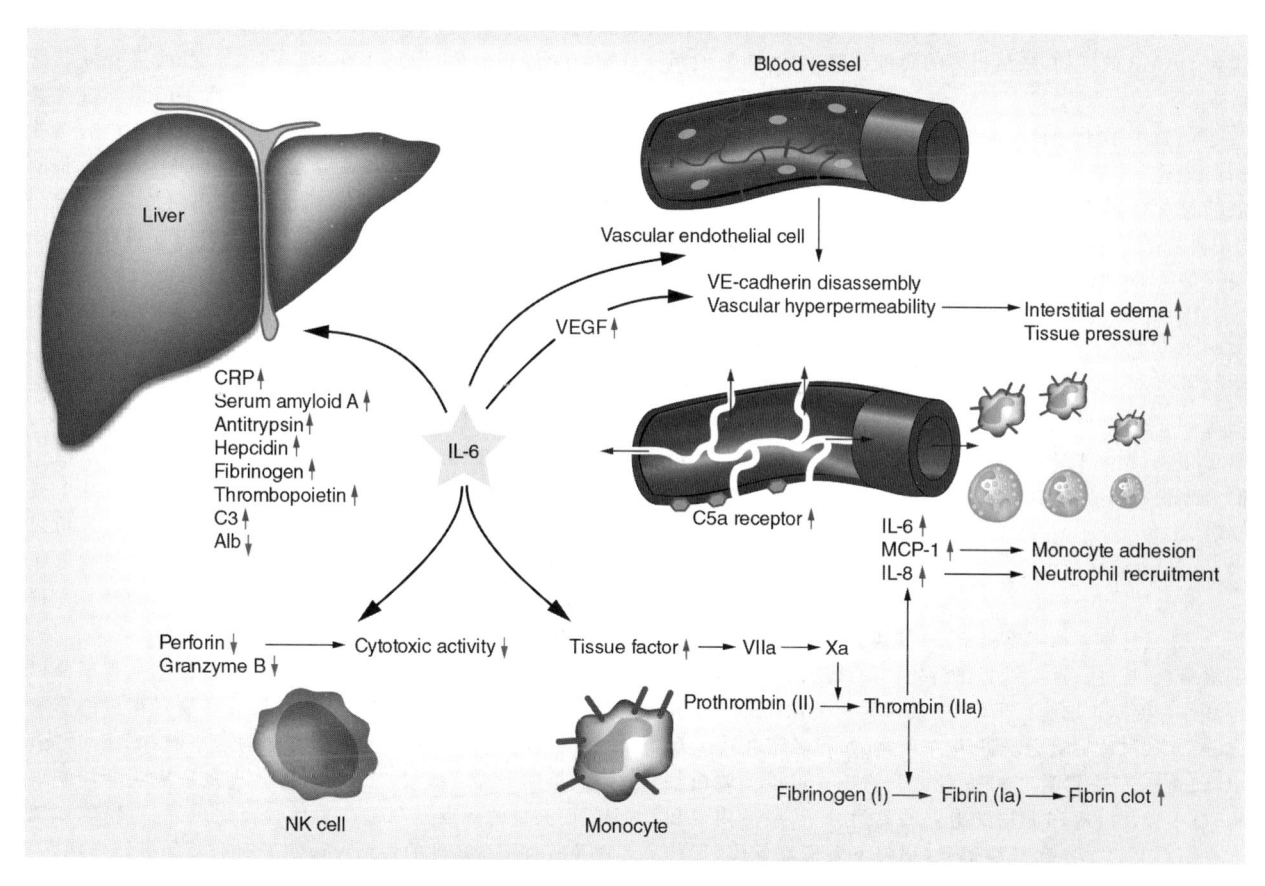

图 8-9-4 IL-6 在脓毒症中的作用机制。①IL-6 迅速诱导肝脏产生 CRP、血清淀粉样蛋白 A、抗胰蛋白酶、肝杀菌肽、纤维蛋白原、血小板生成素和补体 C3 等多种蛋白质。②IL-6 直接或通过诱导血管内皮生长因子(VEGF)诱导内皮细胞上血管内皮细胞钙黏附素的分解,导致血管通透性增高,损伤组织。③IL-6 上调内皮细胞上的 C5a 受体,增加内皮细胞对 C5a 的反应性,从而进一步增强血管通透性。④IL-6 还诱导单核细胞表面组织因子表达,触发凝血级联反应,激活凝血酶,形成纤维蛋白凝块。⑤凝血酶诱导血管内皮细胞表达 IL-6,而 IL-6 增加 MCP-1 和 IL-8 的合成,从而触发单核细胞和中性粒细胞向病变部位募集。⑥IL-6 还通过减少穿孔素和颗粒酶 B 来抑制 NK 细胞的细胞毒活性。CRP:C 反应蛋白;MCP-1:单核细胞趋化蛋白-1;NK:自然杀伤细胞(引自 LIU Q, ZHOU Y H, YANG Z Q. The cytokine storm of severe influenza and development of immunomodulatory therapy)

高水平 IL-6 与病毒感染(流感、SARS、MERS 和 COVID19)的不良预后同样有密切相关性。但有动物实验表明 IL-6 同时可以提高流感病毒清除和感染组动物的存活率,白细胞介素 6 缺陷小鼠的中性粒细胞不足,病毒的清除延缓,并伴随严重的肺损伤。

2. IL-1 家族成员 是先天免疫和炎症的中枢介质,具有多种局部和全身效应,在多种炎症性疾病中起关键作用。大多数 IL-1 家族成员是促炎因子(IL-1α,IL-1β,IL-18,IL-33,IL-36),而部分有抗炎作用(IL-1ra,IL-36ra,IL-37 和 IL-38)。IL-1β 与 IL-18 前体无活性,须经 caspase-1 剪切后,裂解成 IL-1β 和 IL-18(图 8-9-3)释放到胞外才具有活性。多数是由炎症小体(特别是 NLRP3)被病原体激活后产生的。IL-1β 与相关受体结合后,通过 JNK 和 p38-MAPK 通路,增加 NF-κB 的活性。IL-1β 促进扩增级联反应,诱导多种炎症因子的表达,如 IL-6、IL-8、MCP-1、COX-2、IκBα、IL-1α、IL-1β 和 MKP-1。

在脓毒症期间,死亡患者的 IL-1β 水平显著高于存活者,提示高水平的 IL-1β 与脓毒症预后负相关。在流感病毒感染早期,IL-1β 的高表达可以促进康复,可能的机制为:IL-1R 激动后启动流感特异性细胞毒性 CD8+T 细胞应答和产生 IgA 应答,提高病毒的清除率。但在感染后期 IL-1β 持续高表达,可导致致死性的炎症反应。IL-18 在病毒感染后,可以促进病毒特异性 CD8+T 细胞产生特定细胞因子和增强自然杀伤细胞的细胞毒作用清除病毒,改善病毒感染者的预后。同时,还有研究表明,IL-18R 信号通路也能负向调节 IFN-α 的产生,因此,其在细胞因子风暴的发展中似乎扮演着复杂的角色。

有研究表明,IL-1 在 COVID-19 患者呼吸功能恶化之前已经出现显著的表达升高。其余促炎细胞因子均是在出现呼吸功能障碍症状后才诱导产生。这个结果提示 IL-1 可能在 COVID-19 相关肺损伤免疫病理的早期进展中起作用。另外,IL-1 和 TNF-α 可以促进 Th17 细胞分化、发育,因此,COVID-19 患者体内 Th17 相关细胞因子含量明显增加,而 Th17 相关因子是典型的致免疫病理损伤和血管通透性增加的因子。

IL-33 组成性表达于上皮细胞。静止细胞中,IL-33 主要位于细胞核,可直接结合 NF-κB,阻碍其激活的基因转录。病毒感染呼吸道上皮后,诱导上皮细胞产生 IL-33,并致上皮细胞损伤,将细胞核内 IL-33 分泌到细胞外。IL-33 作为 DAMP 的一种,激活更多的免疫细胞,引起明显的组织损伤。

3. 抗炎因子　目前研究较多的抗炎细胞因子主要包括白介素1受体拮抗剂(IL-1RA)和IL-10。IL-1RA由免疫细胞或上皮细胞分泌,并与IL-1R结合,有阻断IL-1α或IL-1β炎症信号的作用。IL-1RA治疗改善了由多菌腹膜炎或革兰阴性杆菌肺炎引起的脓毒症的临床表现。

IL-10是经典的抗炎细胞因子,在细菌和病毒感染过程中对先天免疫和获得性免疫起负性调节作用。具有阻断髓系免疫细胞分化,减弱 NK 细胞和 T 细胞产生炎性细胞因子的能力。IL-10 作为抗炎标志物,与IL-6 水平呈正相关,提示抗炎与促炎关系密切。高IL-10水平可能与感染状态下机体为恢复自身稳态而启动的代偿性机制有关。

(二)肿瘤坏死因子α

肿瘤坏死因子α(TNF-α)是一种典型的促炎细胞因子,也是最早发现的细胞因子,通过其受体TNFR1诱导T细胞凋亡,是可以直接引起细胞死亡的细胞因子,因此,它也被称为促凋亡细胞因子,一度被认为是炎症风暴的主要成分。体、内外实验均表明,细菌产物(如脂多糖(LPS)、肽聚糖)可以有效刺激 TNF-α 释放。TNF-α 可以上调白细胞、血小板及内皮和上皮细胞上的黏附分子,激活内皮和上皮细胞上的血栓和纤溶信号,增强下游炎症反应,促使血管扩张剂如一氧化氮的生成和释放增多。这种作用会导致局部损伤,但是对抵抗局部和侵袭性细菌感染也是至关重要的。

临床发现,脓毒症患者的TNF-α水平会升高,且升高水平与脓毒症严重程度密切相关。在动物模型中,单独使用TNF可以产生类似脓毒症症状的心脏、血管、肺、肾和肝脏功能障碍。部分COVID19患者的研究报道表明TNF-α与T细胞计数呈负相关。推测TNF-α可能是T细胞存活或增殖的负调节因子。然而,也有研究报告COVID19患者重型和危重型患者的TNF-α水平没有显著差异。

通过小鼠脓毒症模型发现,早期选择性使用TNF拮抗剂(如抗TNF血清、抗TNF抗体)可以增加存活率,减少器官损伤。高致病性H5N1感染的动物模型进一步提示了机体对TNF-α的反应可能主要影响了病毒导致机体致病的概率,而不影响清除病毒的效率。

(三)干扰素

干扰素是天然免疫的重要角色,同时参与适应性免疫。主要功能是抑制病毒复制。因此,针对干扰素的研究更多集中在病毒感染性疾病领域。依据其分子结构特征、受体特异性及生物学活性分为三大类。Ⅰ型干扰素主要发挥干扰病毒复制的作用,包括IFN-α、IFN-β。IFN-α主要由单核-巨噬细胞产生;IFN-β主要由成纤维细胞产生。Ⅲ型干扰素即IFN-λ(包括IL-28、IL-29),与Ⅰ型干扰素有相似的功能,也可由多种细胞产生。病毒感染呼吸道上皮细胞后,同时被巨噬细胞、树突状细胞和单核细胞上的PRRs(如TLR3、7、8)识别,通过一系列信号传导,促进干扰素的合成分泌。Ⅰ型干扰素(IFN-α/β)/Ⅲ型干扰素(IFN-λ)与相应受体结合后,通过JAK-STAT途径启动信号级联反应,导致干扰素刺激基因(ISGs)转录,产生的相关蛋白具有强大的抗病毒活性,直接抑制受感染上皮细胞内病毒的复制。其中IFN-λ的受体主要在上皮细胞表达,因此,Ⅲ型干扰素虽然有重要的抗病毒活性,但作用比较局限。而Ⅰ型干扰素除了对上皮细胞的影响外,还可以促进颗粒酶B的产生,促进病毒清除。另一方面,病毒也可以通过不同的机制减少Ⅰ型干扰素的释放,以此减弱天然免疫的效果,并进而影响适应性免疫细胞的扩增。

IFN-γ是唯一的Ⅱ型干扰素,主要由活化的Th1细胞和几乎所有的CD8⁺T细胞和NK细胞产生。因此,IFN-γ更多见于适应性免疫阶段。IFN-γ信号通路主要依赖于JAK1、JAK2、p38MAPK和STAT1,并诱导IRF1或Smad7等因子表达。其功能除了直接抗病毒之外,还可以促进树突状细胞的活化,增强其他免疫细胞的细胞毒作用,诱导B细胞产生抗体等。是T细胞发挥抗原特异性抗病毒作用的重要免疫分子。

从对流感病毒的研究开始,到后来的冠状病毒感染以及如今的COVID19患者,干扰素延迟释放对预后的影响一直被津津乐道,并从机制上研究的越来越深入。首先,疾病早期干扰素释放缺乏或延迟会直接造成病毒控制不利,而大量的病毒复制是产生后续炎症风暴、淋巴细胞凋亡及所有不良事件的根源。而除了对病毒的直接作用,干扰素本身还通过直接作用及间接作用对T细胞免疫起到双向调节的作用。一方面,Ⅰ型干扰素可以通过调节抗原呈递细胞功能有助于适应性淋巴细胞的克隆增殖;另一方面,还可以通过多种机制抑制T细胞的克隆增殖,比如,可通过活化NK细胞介导的细胞毒活性直接杀死效应T细胞;慢性的Ⅰ型干扰素暴露可以产生大量免疫调节型细胞因子,诱导凋亡受体表达,限制T细胞活化。进一步研究发现,TCR活化与INF信号启动的时间的先后顺序是导致T细胞后续克隆增殖或凋亡的关键,如果TCR活化在先,则INF对T细胞的作用表现为促增殖,抗凋亡;而如果INF信号活化在先,则INF对T细胞的作用表现为促凋亡,抗增殖。这种机制提示了当干扰素作用于活化的T细胞时,会进一步促进细胞增殖,而当T细胞不能有效活化,INF持续存在的情况下,则会促进细胞凋亡。

(四)趋化因子

趋化因子(chemokines,CKs)是一类由免疫细胞分泌的小分子细胞因子,具有诱导附近反应细胞定向趋化的能力,多数为可溶的小分子(8～12 kDa)蛋白。除了募集免疫细胞外,还能激活免疫细胞。与细胞因子能广泛作用于多种细胞不同,趋化因子与细胞的作用都是特异性的。根据其氨基酸序列和两个半胱氨酸残基之间的间距,趋化因子分为四类:CC、CXC、CX3C和XCCKS。在感染性疾病中研究最多的趋化因子是MCP-1/CCL2、CXCL8/IL-8。CKs诱导白细胞聚集到感染部位,清除细菌和死亡细胞并诱发炎症反应。缺乏CKs或其受体会导致免疫抑制,并使机体更容易受到致死性感染。在炎症风暴形成的过程中,趋化因子通过对其他细胞和细胞因子的激活间接参与组织损伤。

(五)生长因子

参与细胞因子风暴产生的最多的生长因子是造血靶向集落刺激因子(CSFs):粒细胞巨噬细胞集落刺激因子(GM-CSF)、巨噬细胞集落刺激因子(MCSF)和粒细胞集落刺激因子(G-CSF)。此外,在 IL-3 等其他因素的共同作用下,CSFs 还会诱导髓系细胞增殖、分化。大量扩增、激活的细胞有助于合成更多的细胞因子,从而促进细胞因子风暴形成。此外,除了直接作用外,CSF 还可以通过增强免疫细胞对 IL-1β 或 TNF-α 等早期分子的应答而发挥功能作用。以上机制的发现主要来源于脓毒症研究领域。

三、COVID-19 重症病例与炎症风暴

目前席卷全球的 COVID-19 是继 2003 年 SARS 和 2009 年 MERS 之后的又一次更为严重的冠状病毒引起的传染病疫情,现定性为全球大流行病。已明确病原体为 SARS-CoV-2。近半年之内,全球科学家对 SARS-CoV-2 感染的发病机制及治疗措施贡献了井喷式的研究成果。其中对炎症风暴的研究是人们普遍关注的焦点之一,现总结如下。

在此次疫情的早期,我国的曹彬教授就在总结了 41 例 COVID-19 重症病例的临床和实验室特点时,提出了炎症风暴与疾病严重程度有关,之后世界各国的研究进一步证实了 COVID-19 重症病例中炎症风暴的存在。目前研究表明,炎症风暴与 COVID-19 患者的急性呼吸窘迫综合征(ARDS)、多器官功能衰竭(MODS)有密切关系。SARS-CoV-2 侵入呼吸道上皮后,在细胞内迅速复制、扩散,进一步感染更多免疫细胞。在感染的早期,临床上测得的炎症指标急剧升高,COVID-19 患者的循环中可检测到高水平的 TNF-α、IL-1β、IL-1Ra、sIL-2Rα、IL-6、IL-10、IL-17、IL-18、IFN-γ、MCP-3、M-CSF、MIP-1a、G-CSF、IP-10 and MCP-1,意味着天然免疫的迅速激活。这些细胞因子的水平结合临床表现可以将患者区分成轻、中、重型,重型患者循环中的细胞因子以 IL-1β、IL-1Ra、IL-6、IL-7、IL-10、IP-10 和 TNF-α 为主。当细胞因子含量升高到一定程度,机体出现了 ARDS、DIC 或 MODS 时,我们则称为"炎症风暴"。

天然免疫活化的另外一个组成部分是固有免疫细胞释放大量的趋化因子。在 COVID19 患者的 BALF 中检测到了上调的趋化因子的转录水平,包括中性粒细胞趋化因子(CXCL8、CXCL1、CXCL2、CXCL10、CCL2、CCL7),以及单核巨噬细胞趋化因子(CXCL6、CXCL11、CCL2、CCL3、CCL4、CCL7、CCL8、CCL20)。这样的结果与病理发现相一致,即患者肺组织内主要为中性粒细胞和单核巨噬细胞浸润,而淋巴细胞数目很少。快速复制的病毒会造成干扰素释放延迟,阻碍适应性免疫的激活,进一步延缓了病毒的清除。病毒通过持续激活固有免疫细胞而招募更多的中性粒细胞和单核巨噬细胞浸润到肺组织引起组织损伤,并释放大量炎症因子,引发第二轮细胞因子风暴的出现。(图 8-9 5)这通常出现在 COVID19 疾病的后期阶段(7~10 d),表现为病情(如发热、气短)出乎意料的突然加重,伴随着红细胞沉降率、C 反应蛋白、铁蛋白等急性期炎症反应标志物的升高,凝血障碍和细胞裂解。这些表现非常类似于肿瘤患者应用 CART 细胞治疗时出现的细胞因子释放综合征(cytokine release syndrome,CRS),或者反应性噬血细胞性淋巴组织细胞增生症(reactive hemophagocytic lymphohistiocytosis,reHLH)。reHLH 在临床上多继发于病毒感染,而仅见于 3%~4% 的脓毒症患者。有人把重症 COVID19 患者的免疫失调分成两种类型:一种是由 IL-1β 介导的巨噬细胞活化综合征(MAS),MAS 通常被认为是一种继发的 HLH;另一种是由 IL-6 驱动的免疫细胞功能失调,主要表现为 CD14 单核细胞表面 HLA-DR 缺失,造成抗原呈递缺陷,包括 NK 细胞在内的广泛的淋巴细胞减少。

四、抗炎症风暴的相关治疗

最早开始研究对抗炎症风暴治疗的感染性疾病是脓毒症,1904 年,William Osler 在"现代医药进展"一书中提到,对脓毒症更有效的治疗可能在于免疫调节。第一个被尝试的免疫抑制治疗无疑是糖皮质激素,但到现在为止,仍然没有大规模证据质量高的临床研究能证明糖皮质激素在脓毒症治疗中的作用。如果说糖皮质激素的失败在于它作用的广泛性,那么后来靶向性治疗的失败则让人们进一步看到了感染引起的炎症风暴的复杂性。在确认了 TNF-α 和 IL-1β 是主要的炎症因子之后,20 世纪后期进行了多项阻断细胞因子来治疗脓毒症的临床研究,但是随后陆续得到的阴性结果挫败了研究者的热情,使抗炎症风暴的免疫治疗研究沉寂了一段时间。总结这些临床研究失败的原因,除了与患者难以在足够早的时机入组之外,还与宿主与病原体交互作用的复杂性有关。我们很难把炎症风暴看作一个独立的疾病,它可能是许多不同种类疾病在后期的一个共同类似的表现,因此同一种治疗不可能适用于所有的情况。由此人们意识到细胞因子风暴的治疗想要开启新的时代,必然需要更加个体化的精准治疗。

从 2019 年末开始,人们结合以往的经验,针对 COVID-19 的炎症风暴开展了多种多样的临床实践,临床研究和基础研究,包括应用干扰素、糖皮质激素、丙种球蛋白、IL-6 单克隆抗体、氯喹、羟氯喹、乌司他丁、干细胞、血液净化治疗等。这些治疗均在部分患者或者动物模型中取得了一些效果,都有望在适当的时机成为改善 COVID-19 病死率的手段。值得进一步尝试的治疗还包括 IL-1 家族受体拮抗剂、IFN-λ 拮抗剂、TNF 阻断剂、IFN-α/β 抑制剂,抑制单核巨噬细胞招募其他免疫细胞等。同时我们也知道,相比于单一一种治疗,阻断炎症风暴更加依赖于综合治疗,包括有效的病毒清除,精准的应用时机,支持治疗获取的时间等。

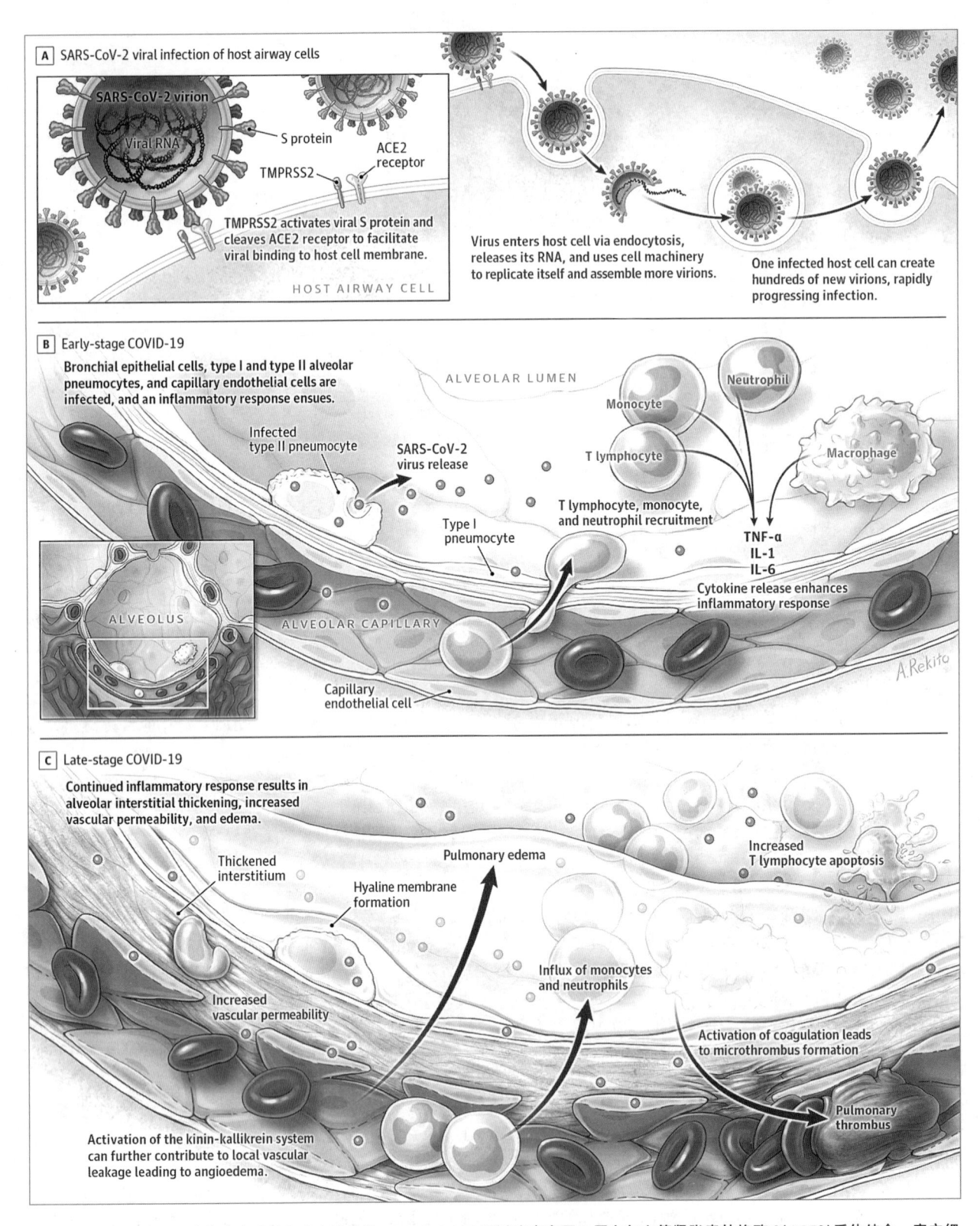

图 8-9-5　SARS-CoV-2 感染宿主后的免疫病理机制。SARS-CoV-2 通过病毒表面 S 蛋白与血管紧张素转换酶 2(ACE2)受体结合。宿主细胞中的 TMPRSS2 通过裂解 ACE2 和激活 SARS-CoV-2 的 S 蛋白进一步促进病毒的内化。在感染早期,病毒复制活跃,感染快速播散。感染部位炎症因子招募的单核细胞和中性粒细胞及感染细胞和肺泡巨噬细胞释放大量促炎因子,诱导和趋化中性粒细胞和单核细胞对病变部位浸润,加重局部损伤。晚期由于促炎细胞因子的激增,导致肺泡细胞屏障功能受损、内皮细胞受损,导致微血管内多发血栓形成、肺水肿、透明膜形成。最终导致肺通气功能障碍和急性呼吸窘迫综合征[引自 WIERSINGA W J, RHODES A, CHENG A C, et al. Pathophysiology, Transmission, Diagnosis, and Treatment of Coronavirus Disease 2019(COVID-19): A Review]

参考文献

[1] Cavaillon J M. Exotoxins and endotoxins: Inducers of inflammatory cytokines. Toxicon,2018,149:45-53.

[2] Chousterman B G,Swirski F K,Weber G F. Cytokine storm and sepsis disease pathogenesis. Semin Immunopathol,2017, 39(5): 517-28.

[3] 龚非力. 医学免疫学. 北京:科学出版社,2014.

[4] Oviedo-Boyso J,Bravo-Patino A,Baizabal-Aguirre V M. Collaborative action of Toll-like and NOD-like receptors as modulators of the inflammatory response to pathogenic bacteria. Mediators Inflamm,2014.

[5] Magrone T,Jirillo E. Sepsis: From Historical Aspects to Novel Vistas. Pathogenic and Therapeutic Considerations. Endocrine,metabolic & immune disorders drug targets,2019,19 (4): 490-502.

[6] Van Der Poll T,Van De Veerdonk F L,Scicluna BP,et al. The immunopathology of sepsis and potential therapeutic targets. Nat Rev Immunol,2017,17(7): 407-420.

[7] Tanaka T,Narazaki M,Kishimoto T. Immunotherapeutic implications of IL-6 blockade for cytokine storm. Immunotherapy,2016,8(8): 959-970.

[8] Jones S A,Scheller J,Rose-John S. Therapeutic strategies for the clinical blockade of IL-6/gp130 signaling. J Clin Invest, 2011,121(9): 3375-3383.

[9] Weber A,Wasiliew P,Kracht M. Interleukin-1(IL-1) pathway. Science signaling,2010,3(105): cm1.

[10] Guo X J,Thomas P G. New fronts emerge in the influenza cytokine storm. Semin Immunopathol, 2017, 39(5): 541-550.

[11] Ong E Z,Chan Y F Z,Leong W Y,et al. A Dynamic Immune Response Shapes COVID-19 Progression. Cell Host Microbe, 2020,27(6): 879-882. e2.

[12] Wu D,Yang X O. TH17 responses in cytokine storm of COVID-19: An emerging target of JAK2 inhibitor Fedratinib. J Microbiol Immunol Infect,2020,53(3): 368-370.

[13] Carriere V,Roussel L,Ortega N,et al. IL-33,the IL-1-like cytokine ligand for ST2 receptor, is a chromatin-associated nuclear factor in vivo. Proceedings of the National Academy of Sciences of the United States of America,2007,104(1): 282-287.

[14] Couper K N,Blount D G,Riley E M. IL-10: the master regulator of immunity to infection. J Immunol, 2008, 180(9): 5771-5777.

[15] Hotchkiss R S,Monneret G,Payen D. Sepsis-induced immunosuppression: from cellular dysfunctions to immunotherapy. Nat Rev Immunol,2013,13(12): 862-874.

[16] Gupta S,Bi R,Kim C,et al. Role of NF-kappaB signaling pathway in increased tumor necrosis factor-alpha-induced apoptosis of lymphocytes in aged humans. Cell Death Differ, 2005,12(2): 177-183.

[17] Huang C,Wang Y,Li X,et al. Clinical features of patients infected with 2019 novel coronavirus in Wuhan,China. Lancet, 2020,395(10223): 497-506.

[18] Chen G,Wu D,Guo W,et al. Clinical and immunological features of severe and moderate coronavirus disease 2019. J Clin Invest,2020,130(5): 2620-2629.

[19] Li Y,Hu Y,Yu J,et al. Retrospective analysis of laboratory testing in 54 patients with severe-or critical-type 2019 novel coronavirus pneumonia. Lab Invest,2020,100(6): 794-800.

[20] Szretter K J,Gangappa S,Lu X,et al. Role of host cytokine responses in the pathogenesis of avian H5N1 influenza viruses in mice. J Virol,2007,81(6): 2736-2744.

[21] Romero C R,Herzig D S,Etogo A,et al. The role of interferon-γ in the pathogenesis of acute intra-abdominal sepsis. J Leukoc Biol,2010,88(4): 725-735.

[22] Crouse J,Kalinke U,Oxenius A. Regulation of antiviral T cell responses by type I interferons. Nat Rev Immunol,2015, 15(4): 231-242.

[23] Chousterman B G,Boissonnas A,Poupel L,et al. Ly6Chigh Monocytes Protect against Kidney Damage during Sepsis via a CX3CR1-Dependent Adhesion Mechanism. Journal of the American Society of Nephrology: JASN, 2016, 27(3): 792-803.

[24] Robben P M,Laregina M,Kuziel W A,et al. Recruitment of Gr-1+ monocytes is essential for control of acute toxoplasmosis. J Exp Med,2005,201(11): 1761-1769.

[25] Yang Y S C,Li J,Yuan J,et al. Exuberant Elevation of IP-10,MCP-3 and il-1ra during sars-cov-2 infection is associated with disease severity and fatal outcome. Medrxiv,2020,2020 (3).

[26] Huang C W Y,Li X,Ren L,Zhao J,et al. Clinical features of patients infected with 2019 novel coronavirus in wuhan,china. Lancet Lond Engl,2020,395:497-506.

[27] Zhou ZRL,Zhang L,et al. Overly exuberant innate immune response to sars-cov-2 infection. Available at ssrn: Https://ssrn.com/abstract=3551623.

[28] Yao XH,Li TY,He ZC,et al. [A pathological report of three COVID-19 cases by minimal invasive autopsies]. Zhonghua bing li xue za zhi = Chinese journal of pathology,2020,49 (5): 411-417.

[29] Wiersinga W J,Rhodes A,Cheng A C,et al. Pathophysiology,Transmission, Diagnosis, and Treatment of Coronavirus Disease 2019(COVID-19): A Review. Jama,2020.

[30] Karakike E,Giamarellos-Bourboulis E J. Macrophage Activation-Like Syndrome: A Distinct Entity Leading to Early Death in Sepsis. Front Immunol,2019,10(55).

[31] Giamarellos-Bourboulis EJ,Netea MG,Rovina N,et al. Complex Immune Dysregulation in COVID-19 Patients with Severe Respiratory Failure. Cell Host Microbe, 2020, 27(6): 992-1000.

[32] Hahn EO,Houser HB,Rammelkamp CH,et al. Effect of cortisone on acute streptococcal infections and poststreptococcal complications. J Clin Invest,1951,30(3): 274-281.

[33] Sprung C L,Annane D,Keh D,et al. Hydrocortisone therapy for patients with septic shock. The New England journal of

medicine,2008,358(2):111-124.

[34] Abraham E, Wunderink R, Silverman H, et al. Efficacy and safety of monoclonal antibody to human tumor necrosis factor alpha in patients with sepsis syndrome. A randomized, controlled, double-blind, multicenter clinical trial. TNF-alpha MAb Sepsis Study Group. Jama,1995,273(12):934-941.

[35] Clark M A, Plank L D, Connolly A B, et al. Effect of a chimeric antibody to tumor necrosis factor-alpha on cytokine and physiologic responses in patients with severe sepsis--a randomized, clinical trial. Critical care medicine,1998,26(10):1650-1659.

[36] Fisher C J, Jr, Dhainaut J F, Opal S M, et al. Recombinant human interleukin 1 receptor antagonist in the treatment of patients with sepsis syndrome. Results from a randomized, double-blind, placebo-controlled trial. Phase III rhIL-1ra Sepsis Syndrome Study Group. Jama, 1994, 271 (23): 1836-1843.

[37] Behrens E M, Koretzky G A. Review: Cytokine Storm Syndrome: Looking Toward the Precision Medicine Era. Arthritis Rheumatol,2017,69(6):1135-1143.

[38] Arabi Y M, Shalhoub S, Mandourah Y, et al. Ribavirin and Interferon Therapy for Critically Ill Patients With Middle East Respiratory Syndrome: A Multicenter Observational Study. Clin Infect Dis,2020,70(9):1837-1844.

[39] Omrani A S, Saad M M, Baig K, et al. Ribavirin and interferon alfa-2a for severe Middle East respiratory syndrome coronavirus infection: a retrospective cohort study. Lancet Infect Dis,2014,14(11):1090-1095.

[40] Zumla A, Chan J F, Azhar E I, et al. Coronaviruses-drug discovery and therapeutic options. Nat Rev Drug Discov,2016,15(5):327-347.

[41] Chen N, Zhou M, Dong X, et al. Epidemiological and clinical characteristics of 99 cases of 2019 novel coronavirus pneumonia in Wuhan, China: a descriptive study. Lancet,2020,395(10223):507-513.

[42] Xu X, Han M, Li T, et al. Effective treatment of severe COVID-19 patients with tocilizumab. Proceedings of the National Academy of Sciences of the United States of America,2020,117(20):10970-10975.

[43] Gao J, Tian Z, Yang X. Breakthrough: Chloroquine phosphate has shown apparent efficacy in treatment of COVID-19 associated pneumonia in clinical studies. Bioscience trends,2020,14(1):72-73.

[44] 广东省科技厅及广东省卫生健康委磷酸氯喹治疗新冠状病毒肺炎多中心协作组.磷酸氯喹治疗新型冠状病毒肺炎的专家共识.中华结核和呼吸杂志,43(2020-02-20).

[45] Wang H, Liu B, Tang Y, et al. Improvement of Sepsis Prognosis by Ulinastatin: A Systematic Review and Meta-Analysis of Randomized Controlled Trials. Frontiers in pharmacology,2019,10:1370.

[46] Ju M, He H, Chen S, et al. Ulinastatin ameliorates LPS-induced pulmonary inflammation and injury by blocking the MAPK/NF-κB signaling pathways in rats. Molecular medicine reports,2019,20(4):3347-3354.

[47] Uccelli A, De Rosbo N K. The immunomodulatory function of mesenchymal stem cells: mode of action and pathways. Ann NY Acad Sci,2015,1351:114-126.

[48] Ben-Mordechai T, Palevski D, Glucksam-Galnoy Y, et al. Targeting macrophage subsets for infarct repair. Journal of cardiovascular pharmacology and therapeutics,2015,20(1):36-51.

[49] Lee J W, Fang X, Krasnodembskaya A, et al. Concise review: Mesenchymal stem cells for acute lung injury: role of paracrine soluble factors. Stem Cells,2011,29(6):913-919.

[50] 徐凯进,蔡,沈毅弘,等.2019 冠状病毒病(COVID-19)诊疗浙江经验.浙江大学学报(医学版),2020.

[51] Zuccari S, Damiani E, Domizi R, et al. Changes in Cytokines, Haemodynamics and Microcirculation in Patients with Sepsis/Septic Shock Undergoing Continuous Renal Replacement Therapy and Blood Purification with CytoSorb. Blood purification,2020,49(1-2):107-113.

[52] Shimabukuro-Vornhagen A, G Del P, Subklewe M, et al. Cytokine release syndrome. Journal for immunotherapy of cancer,2018,6(1):56.

[53] Shakoory B, Carcillo J A, CHATHAM W W, et al. Interleukin-1 Receptor Blockade Is Associated With Reduced Mortality in Sepsis Patients With Features of Macrophage Activation Syndrome: Reanalysis of a Prior Phase III Trial. Critical care medicine,2016,44(2):275-281.

[54] Lagunas-Rangel F A, Ch Vez-Valencia V. High IL-6/IFN-γ ratio could be associated with severe disease in COVID-19 patients. J Med Virol,2020.

[55] Channappanavar R, Fehr A R, Vijay R, et al. Dysregulated Type I Interferon and Inflammatory Monocyte-Macrophage Responses Cause Lethal Pneumonia in SARS-CoV-Infected Mice. Cell Host Microbe,2016,19(2):181-193.

[56] Mcdermott J E, Mitchell H D, Gralinski L E, et al. The effect of inhibition of PP1 and TNFα signaling on pathogenesis of SARS coronavirus. BMC systems biology,2016,10(1):93.

第九部分

肺功能检查

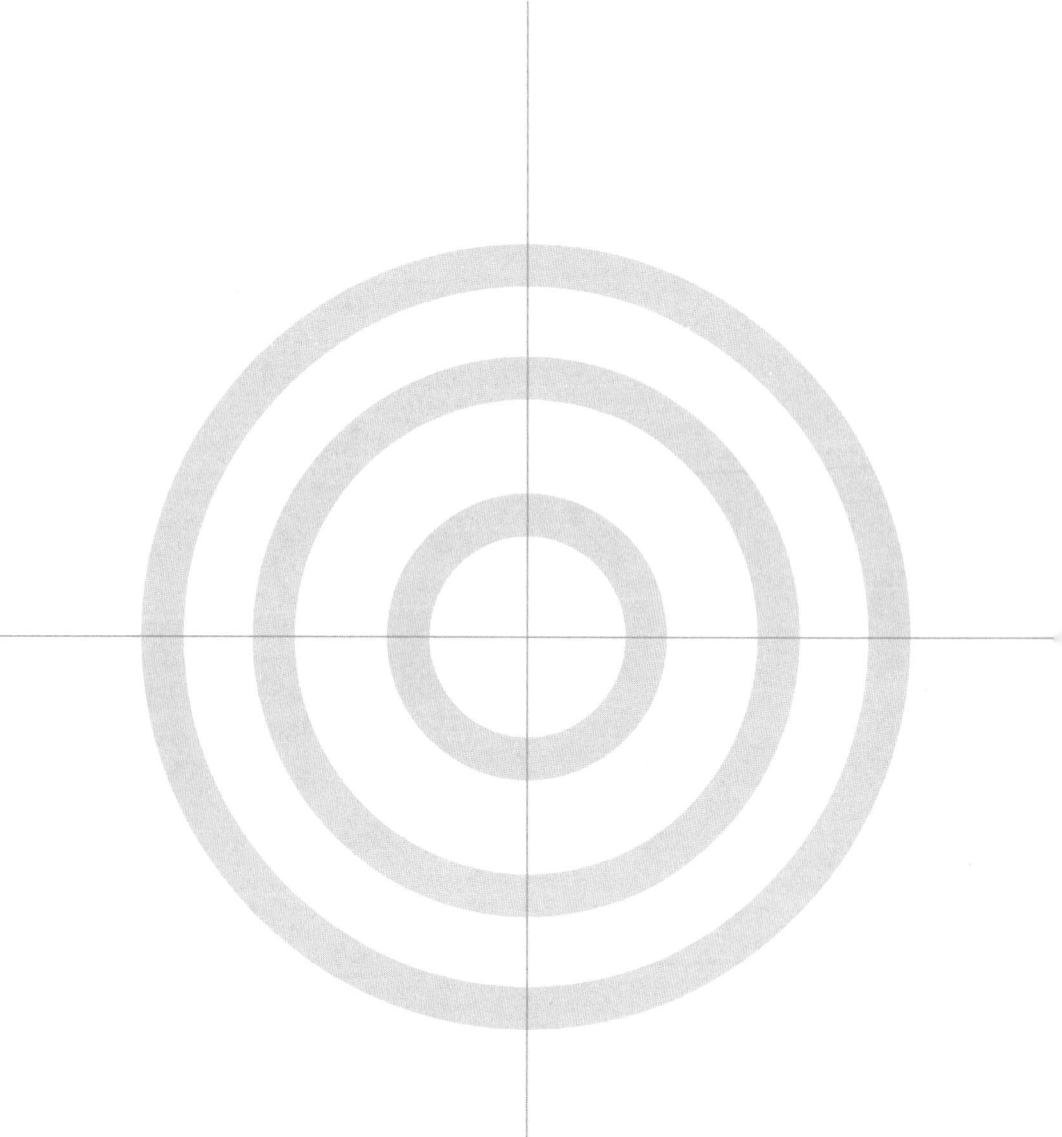

1 膈肌功能评价与训练方法研究进展

刘国梁

膈肌是人最重要的呼吸肌肉，参与生命维持，并作为核心肌参与姿势控制、增加腹内压、促进心肺功能恢复及淋巴回流等。膈肌功能的研究越来越受到临床重视。膈肌功能障碍最常见为膈肌疲劳(diaphragmatic fatigue)，是指膈肌产生力量和(或)速度的能力下降，这种能力的下降可通过休息而恢复。膈肌无力(diaphragmatic weakness)是指休息后膈肌产生力量和(或)速度的能力亦不能恢复。严重者出现膈肌麻痹。

一、膈肌的解剖结构

膈肌的解剖结构呈拱形，由中心腱、肋间部和脚部三部分组成，中心腱包括心包下部；肋条间部附着于肋骨边缘并终止于中心腱；脚部分为起止，其于第2～3腰椎的左、右2个膈脚，其纤维终止于中心腱。膈肌在组织学中属骨骼肌，由不同类型的肌纤维混合组成，通常按肌纤维的收缩时间和代谢特征分为肌纤维分为慢收缩纤维(I类)和快收缩纤维(II类)两种类型。I类慢收缩纤维肌质网数目较少，ATP酶活性较低，线粒全含量丰富，主要靠有氧氧化方式获得能量供应，收缩速度及最大收缩速度较慢，有较高的耐疲劳能力。II类快收缩纤维分为IIA和IIB两个亚型，IIA型为快速氧化糖酵解型纤维，线粒体含量较多，能以有氧氧化和糖酵解两种方式获得能量供应，具有一定的耐疲劳能力；IIB型为快速糖酵解纤维，线粒体含量较少，主要以糖酵解方式获得能量供应，具有快收缩能力，耐疲劳能力很低。

二、膈肌疲劳的发病机制

膈肌疲劳的发生是多因素相互作用的结果，主要包括：①呼吸中枢的驱动不足引起的膈肌疲劳，但亦可能是呼吸中枢为防止呼吸肌的进一步损伤而产生的驱动力调整现象。②神经肌肉疾病，包括衰老、Guillain-Barre综合征及各种肌病导致。③膈肌收缩初长度的改变，如胸腔积液、肺气肿等可导致膈肌低平，初长度增长其机械收缩力下降。④膈肌工作负荷增加，一些气道疾病导致气道阻力增加，膈肌的工作负荷增加导致疲劳。⑤膈肌能量供需紊乱及代谢障碍，如低氧血症、脓毒血症等可影响膈肌能量供应及代谢导致膈肌疲劳。

三、膈肌疲劳的分类及临床表现

依据膈肌活动的驱动，膈肌疲劳可分为：因呼吸中枢的驱动不足所致，比如麻醉、药物过量等导致的中枢性疲劳，以及由神经疾病、神经肌肉传递、兴奋-收缩耦联障碍等引起外周性疲劳。根据膈肌收收缩的力频率曲线关系，膈肌疲劳又可分为高频疲劳和低频疲劳两类。高频疲劳指在＞60 Hz电刺激下肌力特别低，疲劳发生快，肌力下降严重，主要与神经-肌肉接头传递障碍有关；低频疲劳指在＜25 Hz电刺激下肌力特别低，力频率曲线右移，疲劳持续时间长，主要与肌肉本身的兴奋-收缩耦联障碍有关。

膈肌疲劳症状主要表现有气短、乏力、胸闷、吸气不足感、呼吸费力等呼吸困难表现，一些患者表现为咳痰困难、咳嗽无力，可伴有腰背痛、腹胀、胃食管反流，严重者有呼吸浅快、二氧化碳潴留、腹部反常呼吸运动等。在一些高危人群中应注意以上临床表现，及时进行膈功能评价。膈肌功能评价对于进行有效的疾病管理、康复及阻止膈肌功能损伤相关并发症的发生具有重要意义。

四、膈肌功能评估

膈肌功能可依据临床表现及辅助检查进行评价。尽管有大量证据表明呼吸肌功能障碍是很多患者常见的器官衰竭形式，并与不良的近期及远期预后相关，但临床医师经常忽视膈肌疲劳的诊断。对于重症患者，理论上任何需要机械通气的患者都应被认为存在膈肌无力的危险。有几个具体的临床情况能够表明存在膈肌功能异常，虽然仅仅依靠临床表现评估膈肌功能是不全面的，但这应该是对患者进行进一步评估的重要一步，这可以在床边很容易的实施评估并尽早识别危重患者的膈肌无力。

1. 最应引起注意的体征是腹部反常矛盾呼吸运动，表明可能存在膈肌无力。当患者处于仰卧位时，最容易发现腹部矛盾呼吸运动；重症患者在呼吸肌撤机试验间期或在患者接受低水平压力支持通气时亦可观察到腹部矛盾呼吸运动。但也有可能在没有固有的膈肌功能障碍的情况下，显著的呼气肌活动也可诱发膈肌矛盾运动，这种情况下还需要进行其他测试来确认是否存在真正的膈肌功能障碍。重症机械通气患者在脱机困难时,尽管肺部浸润、胸部检查经数天的治疗有所改善,仍应考虑膈肌功能障碍。对于反复出现不明原因呼吸衰竭的患者,也应考虑严重膈肌无力的可能性。值得注意的是那些既往没有肺部疾病病史,但有高碳酸血症呼吸衰竭和 X 线胸片正常的患者,应考虑严重膈肌功能障碍的临床情况。这些患者可能存在未确诊的原发性神经肌病过程,如肌萎缩侧索硬化、吉兰-巴雷综合征、慢性炎症性脱髓鞘性多发性神经病、重症肌无力、原发性肉碱缺乏症、糖原贮积病、多发性肌炎或包涵体肌炎。这些疾病的表现上可能存在较大的异质性,由呼吸肌无力引起的急性呼吸衰竭可能是这些疾病的主要临床表现,如果不能早期诊断,患者则可能失去求治的机会。

2. 膈肌功能辅助检查评估包括结构和功能学两方面。功能学测量包括最大吸气压(MIP)、最大呼气压(MEP)、跨膈压(Pdi)及肺功能检查等;膈肌结构的静态和动态成像方法包括荧光透视、X 线胸片、CT 和磁共振成像(MRI)及膈肌超声检查等。由于目前尚缺乏严格的实验评价和大规模、多中心的临床调查研究数据,对于应用以上评估方法尚无统一的诊断标准,需要根据临床情况参照辅助检查进行评估和诊断。

3. 肺功能测试中常用肺活量、功能残气量、肺总量等作为评价膈肌功能的初筛检测指标。对于机械通气患者,评估其肺部和呼吸系统功能的简单床边指标,即呼吸系统静态顺应性、吸气气道阻力和快速浅呼吸指数(RSBI)也非常有用。当机体单侧膈肌功能紊乱时通常肺活量中度下降,低于 75% 预测值,仰卧位时会再下降 10%～20%,而功能残气量和肺总量保持不变;当双侧膈肌功能紊乱时肺活量通常为 50% 预测值,仰卧位时再降低 30%～50%,并且肺部量下降而功能残气量可能升高。肺功能测试简单、方便,为诊断膈肌功能障碍提供参考依据,但其特异性较低,并且受患者配合程度影响,因此临床常结合其他检测方法评价膈肌功能。

4. 力学指标测试包括最大呼气压(MEP)、最大吸气压(MIP)测试和跨膈压(Pdi)。最大吸气压(MIP)指在功能残气位时受试者用最大力量吸气产生的口腔压。MIP 男性不低于 80 cmH$_2$O,女性不低于 60 cmH$_2$O。当 MIP>80 cmH$_2$O 时可排除膈肌无力,当 MIP 下降至 60% 预计值时,提示单侧膈肌麻痹;MIP 下降至 30% 预计值时提示可能存在累及双侧膈肌情况。

经鼻吸气压(SINP)也能反映吸气肌功能,较 MIP 特异性更高,两者联用可降低 20% 假阳性率。

跨膈压(Pdi)是指腹内压与胸内压差值,通过操作食管胃导管来测定胃内压(代表腹内压)及食管内压(代表胸内压)。膈神经刺激产生的跨膈压是评价膈肌功能的金标准,通常认为当跨膈压<15cmH$_2$O 时存在膈肌功能障碍。Pdi 是直接反映膈肌力量的良好指标,跨膈压可检测平静呼吸时膈肌功能,也可在最大经鼻吸气时或联合膈神经刺激综合评价膈肌收缩功能。

力学指标测试然受患者主观用力程度影响,跨膈压测定是一种有创性操作,由于暴露射线的危险或仪器操作复杂、技术要求高等原因,这些测量方法推广应用均一定的局限性。

5. 影像学检查中,X 线透视可以实时观察膈肌运动状态,对评价膈肌功能紊乱具有一定价值。当发现一侧膈肌出现矛盾呼吸时即可考虑存在该侧膈肌功能存在麻痹或疲劳可能。该方法在诊断膈肌功能紊乱时存在一定假阳性率,约有 6% 的正常人会出现膈肌矛盾运动。当患者一侧膈肌无力时会出现膈肌矛盾运动,而当患者存在双侧膈肌无力时,X 线透视下则不易发现膈肌矛盾运动,这种情况下 X 线透视有可能低估了患者病情。当 X 线胸片发现右侧膈肌高度超过左侧 2cm 以上,或出现左、右两侧膈肌齐高时可考虑存在单侧膈肌麻痹,但胸部 X 线片不能区别如胸腹腔占位性疾病等所致继发性膈肌功能障碍,X 线胸片评价膈肌功能障碍的敏感性约为 90%,特异性只有 44%。对于膈肌器质性占位疾病,胸部计算机断层扫描(CT)可以更清楚发现膈肌占位,更准确显示其位置、大小、形态等,并且可以鉴别诱发膈肌升高的病变原因。对于显示膈肌结构及诊断膈肌周围病变性质,磁共振成像(MRI)检查具有明显优势,并可测定不同体位下吸气相与呼气相膈肌移位、运动速率及左、右肺叶同步性等,在有技术条件的单位可以用于膈肌功能检查。超声检查评估膈肌功能具有以上影像学方法相同的精确性,且具有无创、安全、操作容易等优点。特别是病情严重的患者在紧急情况下无法转运至放射科,超声可快速准确地评估膈肌功能,在膈肌功能评价方面中的应用日益广泛。

B 型超声及 M 型超声都可用于评价膈肌功能,B 型超声主要反映膈肌厚度,M 型超声能评价一段时间内膈肌运动情况。一般选取右侧肋弓下腋前线与锁骨中线之间进行超声检查,通过评价膈肌位置、运动幅度及膈肌厚度等判断是否存在膈肌功能障碍。超声检测的膈肌厚度平均为 0.3 cm(0.12～1.18 cm)。膈肌厚度比为(最大呼吸膈肌厚度－平静呼吸时膈肌厚度)/最大呼吸时膈肌厚度×100%,其正常下限为 20%,为常用的较敏感的膈肌功能检测指标。由于超声检查无创、便捷,常用于评估卧床患者膈肌功能,并能辅助评估机械通气患者呼吸肌功能指导疾病预后及辅助脱机。

6. 膈肌的电生理检测可以通过评估膈肌电信号活动情况来评价膈肌功能,表面肌电图及针极肌电图检测具有相同的检测效度。膈肌肌电图是诊断膈肌疲劳非常敏感的方法,可直接于体表进行测定,在膈肌疲劳早期即有改变。膈肌表面肌电信号分析参数中,临床上常采用时域分析参数均方根值等、能量频域分析参数中位频率等来检测膈肌疲劳程度。膈肌表面肌电检测也可结合膈神经刺激方法,膈肌复合肌肉动作电位变化能较好地反映患者呼吸功能变化。也可同时监控肋间外肌和腹直肌等相关呼吸肌参与度等方法,检测呼吸肌在自主通气过程中的参与度有助于指导机械通气患者脱机。膈肌肌电频谱范围为 20～350Hz,其中 20～40Hz 为低频范围,150～350Hz 为高频范围。膈肌疲劳时,高低频电活动比率和中位频率均可降低。

五、膈肌功能训练方法

研究近些年来取得了较大的进展,对于一些锻炼方法的认识也在逐步深入。膈肌的锻炼有非特异性和特异性两种。非特异性方法可以通过游泳、跑步、上楼梯等运动实现对膈肌的锻炼。通过深慢呼吸法、吹气球、缩唇呼吸、腹式呼吸操、体外膈肌起搏、经阻力呼吸器呼吸锻炼等可以对膈肌进行特异性锻炼。通过锻炼可以使膈肌肌纤维数量增加、体积增大、毛细血管床增多、蛋白质合成增多、糖原含量升高,从而增强膈肌的氧化、抗氧化能力,提高膈肌的抗疲劳程度,降低膈肌疲劳的发生率。新近研究发现,吸气肌训练在提高膈肌和辅助呼吸肌力与耐力方面具有明显的优势,在重症患者及慢阻肺患者中取得了较为可靠训练效果。吸气肌训练方法可有效改善机械通气患者的最大吸气压,增强呼吸肌肌力与耐力,缩短机械通气时间和脱机时间,改善其氧合状态,降低病死率,减少ICU住院时间,改善患者医疗结局。针对膈肌疲劳,可以应用充分膈肌休息的方法改善膈功能,但常常收效不不显著。如何科学有效地进行膈肌康复仍是临床研究的重要课题。

参 考 文 献

[1] Bordoni B, Morabito B, Simonelli M. Ageing of the Diaphragm Muscle. Cureus, 2020, 12(1): e6645.

[2] Dres M, Dube BP, Mayaux J, et al. Coexistence and impact of limb muscle and diaphragm weakness at time of liberation from mechanical ventilation in medical intensive care unit patients. Am J Respir Crit Care Med, 2017, 195(3): 57-66.

[3] Demoule A, Molinari N, Jung B, et al. Patterns of diaphragm function in critically ill patients receiving prolonged mechanical ventilation: a prospective longitudinal study. Ann Intensive Care, 2016, 6(1): 75.

[4] Supinski GS, Westgate P, Callahan LA. Correlation of maximal inspiratory pressure to transdiaphragmatic twitch pressure in intensive care unit patients. Crit Care, 2016, 20(1): 77.

[5] Larsson L, Friedrich O. Critical illness myopathy (CIM) and ventilator-induced diaphragm muscle dysfunction (VIDD): acquiredmyopathies affecting contractile proteins. Compr Physiol, 2016, 7(1): 105-112.

[6] Dres, M; Demoule, A. Monitoring diaphragm function in the ICU. Curr Opin Crit Care, 2020, 26: 18-25.

[7] Aguilera, Garcia Y; Palkar, A, et al. Assessment of Diaphragm Function and Pleural Pressures During Thoracentesis. Chest, 2020, 157(1): 205-211.

[8] Bissett B, Leditschke IA, Green M, et al. Inspiratory muscle training for intensive care patients: a muhidisciplinary practical guide for clinicians. Aust Crit Care, 2019, 32(3): 249-255.

[9] Vorona S, Sabatini U, A1 Maqbali S, et al. Inspiratory muscle rehabilitation in critically ill adults: a systematic review and meta. analysis. Ann Am Thorac Soc, 2018, 15(6): 735-744.

2 2019ATS/ERS 肺量计检测标准变迁

杨文兰

一、背景与简介

肺量计是最常用的肺功能检测方法,广泛用于在肺部疾病诊断功能监测。2005 年,ATS 与 ERS 联合发表肺量计的指导标准。随着设备和计算能力的改进,许多新的研究试验实施更严格的质量控制措施,需要对 2005 年的肺量计技术标准进行更新,以更好地应用这项检测技术。由 ATS 与 ERS 联合小组专家依据肺功能测试标准、实验室质控要求、不断发展的国际标准及已发表的相关评述,同时收集患者测试感受的文献,发表了 2019 年肺量计检测标准。

肺量计检测是一项生理学检测,用以测定受试者最大吸气和呼气时的气体容量。在文中,操作者(operator)是指挥试验完成的人员。患者(patient)是指被测试者,需注意的是,不是所有人都是患者,测定(maneuver)是指 VC 吸气和呼气测定过程。必须(must)是指必须符合标准的要求。应该(should)是指不是强制但应是最好的举措。这些标准是指肺量计临床应用中必须达到的最低标准,但不适用于所有情况,比如临床研究或职业监测等。

二、方　法

ATS 和 ERS 工作组成员由科学家和内科医师组成,他们有制定国际指南和标准的经验,有临床肺功能检测的经验和专业知识,发表相关研究论著。所有潜在利益冲突都按照 ATS 和 ERS 的规则和程序进行披露和管理。引用 2004 年至 2018 年期间的相关 190 篇直接相关,382 可能相关的论著。另外,2018 年和 2019 年有 12 份参考文献也纳入其中。

三、患者体验

为收集患者在肺量计测定时所面对的问题和经验,一项由欧洲呼吸基金会(The European Lung Foundation)在 2018 年 8 月和 9 月进行的调查结果显示,80% 被调查者表示对检测难度大多或完全接受,有 31% 被调查者认为,对于"即使感觉到没有任何气体出来,也要继续吹气"是中等或严重的问题。

四、适应证与禁忌证

(一)适应证

肺量计是评估呼吸健康的基本检测。可以评估疾病对肺功能的影响,气道反应性,监测病情,以及治疗干预的效果,评估手术风险,许多肺部疾病的预后。较 2005 年有一定变化。肺量计适应证见表 9-2-1。

表 9-2-1　肺量计适应证

诊断
用于评估症状、体征或不正常的实验室异常的=结果
用于评估疾病造成的生理功能改变
用于筛选有肺病疾病风险的个体
用于评估术前风险
用于评估预后
监测
用于评估对治疗干预的反应
监测疾病进展
监测患者疾病的急性加重及加重后的恢复
监测人们暴露于有害物质的不利影响
监测已知有肺毒性作用的药物的不良反应
伤残评估
康复管理中的一部分,对患者进行评估
保险评估的一部分,对患者进行评估
出于法律原因对个人进行评估
其他
临床研究和试验
流行病学调查
预计值公式的推导
危险职业的就业前肺部健康监测
在开始有风险的体育活动前进行健康状况评估

(二)相对禁忌证

肺量计检测有一定的体力要求。用力呼气动作可增加胸腔内压、腹腔内压和颅内压。肺量计测定时产生的胸腔内最大压力会影响腹部、腔内的器官、静脉回流和体循环的血压、胸壁和肺的扩张。用力动作会增加心肌的需求。肺量计的相对禁忌证见表 9-2-2。有潜在禁忌证的患者在基层医疗机构被禁止检查,但在能够及时得到救诊的机构,在经验丰富的操作者指挥下完成操作。

此外，肺量计检测需要患者积极参与，对指令不能充分理解、不愿配合的患者，往往达不到最好结果。

表9-2-2 肺量计的相对禁忌证

心肌需求增加或血压变化
1周内的急性心肌梗死
低血压或严重高血压
显著的心房/心室心律失常
失代偿的心力衰竭
没有控制的肺动脉高压
急性肺源性心脏病
临床不稳定肺栓塞
与强迫呼气/咳嗽相关的晕厥史
由于颅内压/眼压升高
脑动脉瘤
4周内进行过脑部手术
近期症状持续的脑震荡
1周内眼部外科手术
由于鼻窦和中耳压力的增加
1周内鼻窦手术、中耳手术或感染
由于胸内和腹内压的增加
气胸
4周内行胸部手术
4周内行腹部手术
妊娠晚期
感染控制问题
活动性或疑似传染性呼吸道感染或全身感染，包括肺结核
易引起感染传播的身体状况，如咯血，显著的分泌物增多，口腔损伤或口腔出血

五、实验室细则

必须记录环境温度，大气压和日期时间。

测试应在安静舒适的环境中进行，采用直立坐位，肩膀微微向后，下颌轻微抬起。椅子有扶手（晕厥发生时预防侧面跌倒），没有轮子，可调节高度，确保患者平放在地板。应为儿童或体型小的成人提供小号的椅子或可升起的脚蹬。测试要求使用鼻夹，或者人为捏住鼻孔。如果采用其他体位，应在报告中说明。在成人、肥胖者及儿童的研究中发现，站立位的结果与坐位的结果相似。Fowler's位（抬起头和躯干）比仰卧位或Crook's位（膝盖抬起）产生更高的测定值。多数研究显示，健康受试者，或有呼吸、循环、神经肌肉疾病患者，或者肥胖者，采用直立位，可得到更高的 FEV_1 和 FVC 值。然而，四肢瘫痪的脊髓损伤患者，仰卧位比坐位可得到更高的 FEV_1 和 FVC 值。

六、卫生及感染控制

感染控制的目的是在肺功能检测期间，阻止患者与工作人员之间传染病的传播。有记录的案例非常少，但这种可能性是真实存在的。感染可能通过直接接触过滤器、鼻夹、手持传感器、椅子扶手、阀门或管道的近端表面发生传播。测试期间，患者吹进仪器的气体产生的气溶胶可排入房间中，造成间接感染。

操作者在接触新患者前，必须洗手或用手部消毒剂。即使使用一次性手套仍需洗手和手部消毒，在测试新患者前需更换新手套。患者初次进入检查室，可能会接触各种物品表面，许多肺量计是手持式的，也需要使用手部消毒液或凝胶。

在多数设备中，使用一次性、内置肺量计过滤器已成为标准做法。此外，咬口是过滤器的一部分，可以减少肺量计的污染。一次性物品包括过滤器，咬口，鼻夹，手套在测试结束后需要处置抛弃。

在直接接触咬口、管路、呼吸阀或肺量计表面，须立即洗手。当操作可能被污染的设备和（或）操作者手上有任何开放的伤口或溃疡时，操作者应该戴手套。

制造厂家应详细说明他们仪器的清洗和消毒方法，包括推荐化学试剂的种类和浓度，对操作者采取的安全措施。

对于结核或疑似结核、咯血、口腔病变或其他已知的传染性疾病患者，需要额外的防范措施。如单独为受感染患者测试的仪器；或在工作日结束时对此类患者进行检测，以便有时间进行肺量计的拆卸和消毒；或在患者自己的房间进行检测，并为操作人员提供充分换气和适当的保护措施。消毒卫生措施在ATS肺功能实验室管理和程序手册中有更详细的描述。

七、仪器设备

制造厂商需确保所有肺量仪需符合更新后的ISO26782标准。目前更新为ISO26782:2009，上次更新于2016年，计划2021年再次更新。虽然ISO26782中没有明确规定，但不允许在ISO 26782附件C规则外重新校准肺量计。虽然根据ISO26782第七部分，要求仪器的准确性、线性、重复性在±3%以内，根据ISO 26782附件C中测试文件要求，用3L定标筒定标时，仪器的最大误差在±2.5%以内。如果将来的ISO26782版本明确可容许最大误差为±2.5%，可能会用更低的值。

八、图形显示

所有容量-时间曲线和流量-容积曲线均需显示，操作者需目测检查每一次测量质控。对于流量-容积曲线，呼气流量必须向上绘制，呼气容积必须向右绘制。在流量和容积比例必须保持2:1的纵横比，2 L/s的流量和1 L的容积在各自的轴上必须有相同的距离。应将多次测试的图形依次显示出来。

九、BTPS矫正

肺量计所有的结果必须经BTPS（体温，环境大气压，饱和水蒸气)矫正。环境温度记录的精确度±1℃。环境温度变化过快(30 min内>3℃)时,需要连续的温度矫正。

温度是肺量计或流量传感器变化的一个影响因素。对于容积肺量仪,如果使用环境温度,而不是仪器内部设定温度,FEV1和FVC的误差可以达到6%。因此,使用容积肺量仪,应对每次呼吸测定都测定温度。

十、仪器质量保证

关注仪器质量和定标是测定质控的重要部分。最低要求如下:①定标结果的维护记录,②设备修理和维护记录,③计算机硬件及软件更换升级记录,④设备改变和移动的记录(如职业调查)。如有任何变化,在进行检测之前必须再次进行定标校准和质量控制程序。设备质量控制的关键要素见表9-2-3。

表9-2-3 设备质量控制(用于基于容量和流量的传感器)

肺量计
每日进行低、中、高流量的校准验证;校准验证失败,要进行检查和补救(表11-2-4),并再次校准验证
如果在肺功能测定中使用过滤器,那么在重新校准和验证时也必须使用
在校准验证失败后,制造商推荐的间隔时间内,均须重新校准
如果校准误差的变化≥6%或平均值超过±2SD,则按照制造商的说明,检查和清洗(如有必要)肺量计;检查错误(表9-2-4)并重新校准肺量计
按制造商规定的时间间隔进行例行检查和维护
3L定标筒
每天检查活塞停止的位置,没有黏滞或停顿
根据制造商推荐的间隔周期按时定标,误差在±0.015L以内
每月进行定标筒泄露检查
文件
所有质量控制发现,维修和调整,硬件和软件更新的日志
软件更新后的参考值计算的验证

定标过程可以确定经传感器测定的流量和容量与实际流量和容量的关系。定标验证是确保仪器的定标误差在容许范内(误差在±3%,肺量计±2.5%及定标筒±3%)。当定标误差超过±2SD或变化≥6%,可能提示肺量计需要清洗、维护或修理,制造商需设置明确的警示。定标验证必须每日进行,如制造商有特殊规定,定标频次会更多。肺量计软件应能够生成定标报告,包括每次定标的结果,定标失败的次数,定标要素的变化。定标验证时,变异超过±2SD时,系统需有警示提示。

用于定标和验证的3L筒,全程误差应在±0.015L或±0.5%,制造商必须提供在定标筒误差范围内的定标间隔时间。定标筒必须室温下放置。定标时,操作者为稳定定标筒而握住筒身,会造成温度升高,导致测定出现差错。操作者应注意,定标过程中,定标筒意外调整或变化,会导致定标异常。定标筒每月必须进行泄露试验,出口处用软木塞塞住,用超过定标筒最大容量的气体量进行清空或填充。定标筒掉落或损坏不能进行定标。

定标验证每天至少一次,使用3L定标筒,在0.5~12L/s流量范围下,每个流量要拉推3次,时间0.5~6s。如果测定时使用过滤器,定标和定标验证时也需使用。每个流量下测定的容量在吸入和呼出时误差应在±3%(容量型肺量计只测呼出气)。对于使用一次性传感器的设备,必须每天对每个患者检测的新传感器进行检测。

ATS的肺功能实验室管理和程序手册包括了生物定标:一位健康不吸烟的个体进行多次肺量计测定。生物定标不能用定标筒取代。操作者应了解他们自己的FEV_1和FVC,当怀疑仪器有问题时,可以进行快速粗略的检查。

表9-2-4 校准验证失败的潜在原因

肺量计功能的微小变化,需要随后的重新校准来调整校准系数
肺量计与定标筒的连接上有泄漏
在零流量校订过程中,有气流通过肺量计
未能在一次平滑的动作中完全填充和清空定标筒
定标筒出现故障(如活塞漏气、活塞移位、定标筒掉落损坏)
肺量计传感器内有碎片阻塞或操作者在握持肺量计时手造成的堵塞
传感器、咬口、过滤器和(或)呼吸管装配不当
室温与定标筒温度的差异
环境温度和(或)压力的数据输入错误

十一、操作者细则

正如Ruppel与Enright所观察的"有3个得到高质量肺功能数据的关键要素:精准的设备,一个可接受重复测量的患者/受试者和一个可以让患者有最大表现、有动力的技术人员。在规范化领域,技术人员最不被人关心。"操作者对患者的指导着重要的作用。

观察并与患者互动从而得到最佳结果是操作者的职责,这需要训练与经验。肺量仪定性测试的培训课程可在多个国家找到,它们将引领操作者遵循着ATS/ERS标准,短时培训与跟踪随访非常重要。操作者的培训,认证和继续教育是必要的。

十二、患者细则

记录患者的年龄,身高和体重(穿着室内衣物且不穿鞋)。年龄必须以年为单位,且精确到小数点后1位。身高以厘米(cm)为单位,且精确到小数点后1位,体重读取到最近的0.5 kg;在一些区域,它们以磅和英寸作为测量单位。身高必须以去鞋身高为准,对于无法站直的患者,身高通过尺骨长来估算(通常用在小孩身上)或手臂展开的长度。尺骨长度应用卡尺测量以防止卷尺测量引出的误差。对于一个25岁及以上,且曾在同一设备下测量过可靠身高的患者,在1年随访内无须再次测量身高。

出生性别与种族应在患者信息中作为肺量仪测试的需求。患者性别应告知出生性别,而不是认知性别。不准确的出生性别将导致错误的诊断与治疗。全球肺功能倡议将种族划分为白种人（即，欧洲血统），非洲美国人，东北亚洲人，东南亚洲人，以及其他/混合。如果出生性别（或）种族没有公开，操作者必须告知报告者，并显示出所用的默认预计值。

十三、患者所需准备

患者应在测试前避免表 9-2-5 所示的活动，且在预约时提前告知患者这些需求。当他们到达时，所有事项必须被检查，并且任何偏差必须被报告。

患者在测试前与测试中应尽可能保持放松。患者应被要求穿着合身的衣服。合适的义牙可以不取出。2001 年一项研究表明不取出义齿肺功能结果会更好，但 2018 年的一项更大样本的研究表明当义齿被移除时，FVC 将平均增加 0.080 L。

测试前停用短效或短效支气管扩张剂是由医疗专业人员决定的。如果用来诊断肺部疾病，在测试前停用支气管扩张剂是有用的。当评估已有治疗方案的疗效，支气管扩张药一般不需要停用。

应在预约检查时提前告知患者停用药物的注意事项。操作者须记录将会影响肺功能的药物，检查前最后使用的口服、吸入或注射药物的种类与剂量。操作者应记录观测到的迹象与症状，比如咳嗽，喘息，呼吸困难或发绀。

表 9-2-5　肺功能测定前需避免的行为

测试前 1 h 吸烟、和（或）电子烟、和（或）水烟（避免烟雾吸入导致的支气管痉挛）
在测试前 8 h 内使用麻醉药物（避免配合、理解和机体动作问题）
测试前 1 h 内进行剧烈运动（避免潜在的运动诱发的支气管痉挛）
穿着过于限制胸部和腹部扩张的衣服（避免体外限制对肺功能的影响）

十四、FEV_1 和 FVC 操作

1. 测定过程　肺量计测定吸气和呼气过程，FVC 测定有 4 个明确的阶段：①最大吸气，②爆发式呼气，③持续完全呼气，最大可达 15 s，④最快吸气至最大肺容积位。肺量计测定结果的变异性大多与吸气不足、吸气至 TLC 发生变化、呼气提前结束、用力程度不同有关。

操作者须证明采用了表 9-2-6 中的适宜技术和操作规程。当流量零点矫正结束，患者含住咬口，听从指挥，正常或放松呼吸。操作者确认患者姿势正确，鼻夹在适当的位置，嘴唇包紧咬口。患者不能用嘴呼吸时，可使用面罩。对某些情况如气管切开或鼻部切除者，操作者可使用密闭面罩、管路接口或阻断阀，并进行记录。

2. 最大吸气　吸气动作必须迅速，吸足气后的任何停顿应≤2 s。当吸气动作减慢，或从 TLC 位呼气有 4～6 s 停顿，会导致 PEF 或 FEV_1 减低。

操作者应该站在一个能看到患者和测试设备显示的位置，但应观察患者本人已经充分吸气。应观察患者的头部和面部，指示患者"尽力深吸气"（而不是"进行深呼吸"）。吸气时，操作者用"更多，更多，更多"这样的词汇来指导患者。眉毛抬高，眼睛睁大，有时头部开始抖动，这些均提示患者最大吸气。一个看起来不舒服的患者不太可能处于完全吸气状态。

3. 最大呼气　在完全吸气的情况下，应该毫不犹豫地提示患者"爆发吹气"，而不仅仅是"吹气"，然后鼓励他或她完全呼气。在检查过程中，操作者同时观察患者和电脑显示，以确保患者最大限度地努力。当到达平台期或用力呼气时间（FET）达到 15 s 时，肺量计系统必须向操作者和患者发出提示信号。如果患者有晕厥的迹象应停止测定。避免在测定过程中，患者用力过大（4 s 之后）可使一些呼气量增大，并可能防止声门关闭和避免晕厥。一些限制性肺病患者和高弹性回缩力的年轻患者可以迅速清空他们的肺，不能维持呼气平台持续 1 s。操作者需要识别这种患者的流量-容积图的凸出形态，并将其与提前终止呼气区分开来。

4. 用力呼气后最大吸气　用力呼气完成后，患者应继续含紧吹口，操作者再次指导患者迅速吸气至肺总量位。这是一个测定用力吸气 VC（FIVC）的动作。最大的努力吸气至 TLC 完成流量-容积环。在适当的指导下，认知和神经运动功能正常的 2.5 岁儿童就能够接受的肺活量测定。见表 9-2-6。

表 9-2-6　FVC 操作程序

洗手*（或使用认可的洗手液）
患者准备
给患者分发洗手液
确认患者身份、年龄、出生年月日、性别、种族等
不穿鞋测量体重和身高
询问表 9-2-5 所列的活动、药物使用情况及申请单上标记的任何相关禁忌证；注意呼吸道症状
指导和演示测试
确认咬口和鼻夹的位置
正确的姿势，头稍微抬高
快速吸气至吸足气体
尽全力呼气至完全呼出气体
尽全力吸气至完全吸足
确认患者理解并愿意遵守指示
操作过程
患者的姿势是否正确
连接鼻夹，含住咬口，嘴唇包紧咬口
正常呼吸
快速吸足气至 TLC，停顿时间≤2 s
保持直立姿势，尽最大的努力呼气，直到不再有空气排出为止
最大努力吸气至吸足气体
如有必要，重复指令，努力指导
重复至少 3 次，成人通常不超过 8 次
检查 FEV_1 和 FVC 的重复性，必要时进行更多的操作

(续表)

操作过程(仅有呼气设备)
患者的姿势是否正确
使用鼻夹
快速吸足气至TLC,停顿时间≤2 s
含住咬口,嘴唇包紧咬口
保持直立姿势,尽最大的努力呼气,直到不再有空气排出为止
如有必要,重复指令,大力指导
重复至少3次,成人通常不超过8次
检查FEV₁和FVC的重复性,必要时进行更多的操作

十五、检测内评估

下列标准被作为客观标准,来评测检查中是否达到最大的努力和可接受的 FEV1 和(或)FVC。然而,在某些情况下,不符合所有标准的测定可能是患者在这种情况下所能做的最好的测定,尽管 FEV1 和(或)FVC 测量在技术上是不可接受的,但可应用于临床(如"可使用的")(表9-2-7)。

出于时机的考虑,呼气起始点由外推容积法来确认(图9-2-1)。容量-时间曲线,在 PEF 点上,根据 PEF 斜率,画一条切线,它与横坐标上的交点为时间零点,是所有时间相关测量的起点。外推体积(BEV)是指从最大肺容积到时间零点时呼出的气体,为了确保 FEV1 来自最大的努力,BEV 必须是<5% FVC 或 0.100L,以数值最大的为准。与 2005 年的标准比较,数值由 0.150L 减低至 0.100L。犹豫时间(thehesitation time)是指从最大吸气点到时间零点的时间,应小于 2 s。BEV 超过极限时 FEV1 和 FVC 测量是不可接受的,也不可用的。较大的 BEV 通常会导致错误的增高的 FEV1 值。上呼吸道阻塞或神经肌肉疾病患者往往不能快速增加呼出气流,可导致 BEV 增高。对于此类患者,操作者必须有能力判断 BEV 的可接受性。

容量-时间曲线必须包括用力呼气开始起点(时间零点)前 1 s 或在最大吸气点之前开始,以最先发生的为准。系统应该显示 BEV 值。检查流量-容积曲线,选择有满意起始点的曲线。PEF 出现在呼出气流急剧上升并接近时间零点处,峰流量从 10% 至 90% 的时间应≤150 ms,但对于上气道阻塞的患者,这个时间值增高。

表9-2-7 对FEV1与FVC的可接受性,可用性,与可重复性标准

可接受性与可用性标准	可接受标准 FEV1	可接受标准 FVC	可用性标准 FEV1	可用性标准 FVC
BEV 必须≤5%FVC 或 0.100 L,以较高者为准	是	是	是	是
没有错误的零点流量设置	是	是	是	是
呼出的第1秒内没有咳嗽*	是	否	是	否
声门不得在呼出后第1秒内闭合*	是	是	是	是
声门不得在呼出1秒后闭合*	否	否	否	否
必须达到下列3项EOFE指标下的1个	否	是	否	是
1. 呼出平稳(在呼出最后 s≤0.025L)				
2. 呼出时间≥15 s				
3. 在可重复范围内 FVC 大于最大的先前观测的 FVC†				
咬嘴或肺活量计不得有堵塞迹象	是	是	否	否
不得有泄漏迹象	是	是	否	否
若 EOFE 后最大吸入值大于 FVC,则 FIVC-FVC 必须≤0.100 L 或 5%FVC,以较高者为准‡	是	是	否	否
可重复性标准(用于可接受的 FVC 和 FEV1 值)				
6 岁以上:2 个最大 FVC 值间的差≤0.150 L,且 2 个最大 FEV1 值间的差≤0.150 L				
6 岁及以内:2 个最大 FVC 值间的差≤0.100 L 和 10%最大值,以较高者为准,且 2 个最大 FEV1 值间的差≤0.100 L 和 10%最大值,以较高者为准				

注:BEV. 外推容积;EOFE. 用力呼气结束;FEV0.75. 第 0.75 秒的用力呼出气容积

* 评分系统(表9-2-7)为报告解读者提供信息,当检查结果没有达到可接受标准时,是否符合可用性的标准

† 当患者无法呼出足够长时间以达到平台时(比如,有高弹性回缩或限制性肺疾病的儿童),或当患者在达到平台前吸气或咬嘴脱落。对于操作间的可接受度,判断应用支气管扩张剂前后的测试集合,在可重复范围内 FVC 大于最大的先前观测的 FVC

‡ 尽管最大呼气这项操作被强烈的建议,如缺失,其检查结果仍可进行可接受性判断,除非存在胸外阻塞

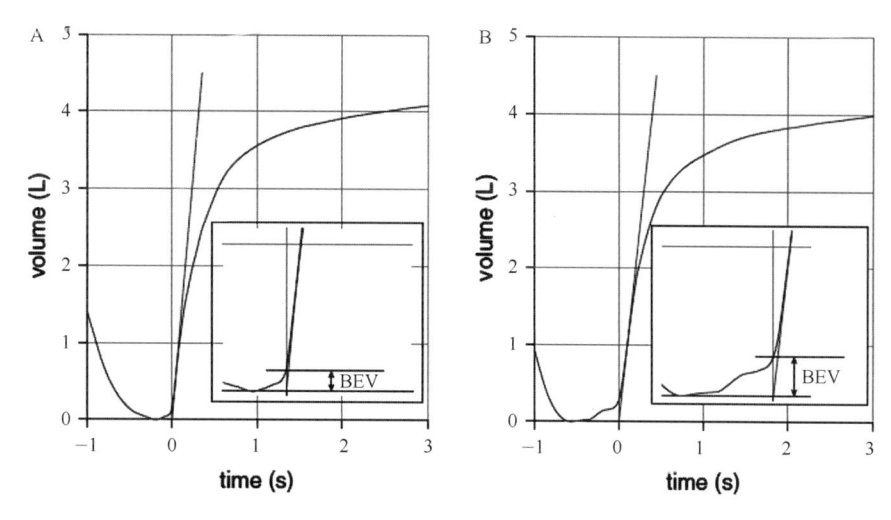

图9-2-1 外推容积(back-extrapolated volume, BEV)。在容量-时间曲线上,通过画一条斜率等于最高流量且通过最高流量点的一条直线,时间零点由这条线与时间轴的交点确定。BEV为时间零点前呼出的气体,A. 是0.136 L(可接受),B. 是0.248 L(不可接受)。对于此患者,BEV极限是5%FVC,即0.225 L

十六、呼气的终止

以前的标准使用测试终止(end of test)缩写"EOT"表示用力呼气(end of forced expiration EOFE)结束。这些标准强调了在用力呼气后进行最大吸气的重要性。因此,用力呼气的终点并不是检查的结束,本标准使用EOFE。

EOFE需满足以下3个推荐指标中的1条(图11-2-2)。

1. 在至少1 s内,容量变化<0.025L(一个"平台")。这是呼气完成最可靠的指标。当呼气达到这一标准,系统需同时有实时显示和音频报警。注意声门关闭可能会提前终止呼气,使其FVC不能被接受,即使显示的呼气时间很长。

2. 患者达到了15 s的FET。当呼气达到这一标准,系统需同时有实时显示和音频报警。对于气道阻塞或老年患者,通常会有更长FETs;但是,超过15 s的FETs很少会改变临床判断。1994年ATS肺活量测定标准使用"用力呼气有合理持续时间"作为EOFE的指标,并建议12~15 s就足够。一项对成年人(平均年龄67岁)的研究发现,超过95%的阻塞患者FET<15 s,95%的正常受试者FET<11 s。不宜多次长时间呼气,可能导致头晕、晕厥、过度疲劳和不适感。

3. 有患者用力呼气不能达到平台期(如有高弹性回缩力的儿童或限制性肺疾病患者)。在这种情况下,患者反复测得相同的FVC,以此判断是否达到EOFE。在可重复性容许的范围内,必须在多个测试中,观察到的最大FVC,来判断测定是否可接受。如果支气管扩张药使用前或使用后,没有呼气平台,且FET<15 s,与后续的测定指标比较,可以判断FVC达到可接受的EOFE标准。如果在可重复性范围内或大于后续的FVC,该检测可接受。因此,在分别判断支气管扩张药前和支气管扩张药后的多个测试时,如果所有FVC没有呼气平台,FET<15 s,在可重复性的容范围内,最大FVC被认为符合EOFE标准。操作者应警惕,患者是否有感到不适的任何迹象,如果患者明显不舒服或接近晕厥,应终止操作。

不符合任何EOFE可接受标准的检测视为不被接受。然而,在1 s后提前终止的测定,其FEV1可被接受。对于6岁或6岁以下的儿童,在0.75 s后提前终止的测定,FEV0.75(最初0.75 s内的用力呼气量)是可接受的。

注意,没有最小FET的要求。研究显示,对于气流阻塞和年老的患者,要达到2005年ATS/ERA要求的呼气平台,是有一定难度的。该标准排除了多数的患者,但对预测值的影响很小。一项针对老年人(平均年龄63岁)的大型职业健康研究发现,尽管由经过训练的操作人员鼓励延长呼气时间,有53%的肺活量测定操作仍未达到稳定水平不能达到呼气平台。然而,在另一项研究中,90%的严重肺功能损害患者能够满足这个标准。其他大型成人研究发现,超过95%的人在呼气时间超过6 s后达到平台。由训练有素、有监督的操作人员参加一项大型临床试验发现,94%的COPD患者能够满足1994年ATS肺功能标准规定的呼气平台标准。

2005年ATS/ERS要求最小FET,导致一些有效的检测不被接受。在一项对1631名10~18岁健康儿童的研究中,仅18%检测达到2005标准中最小FET标准。但是,由于取消了最FET标准,操作人员必须提高警惕,以评估呼气是否完成或提前终止。

如果EOFE之后的最大吸气容量(FIVC)大于FVC时,提示患者没有从TLC开始呼气。

如果FIVC-FVC 0.100L,或5%的FVC(以两者中较大者为准,FEV1和FVC测量是不可接受的。

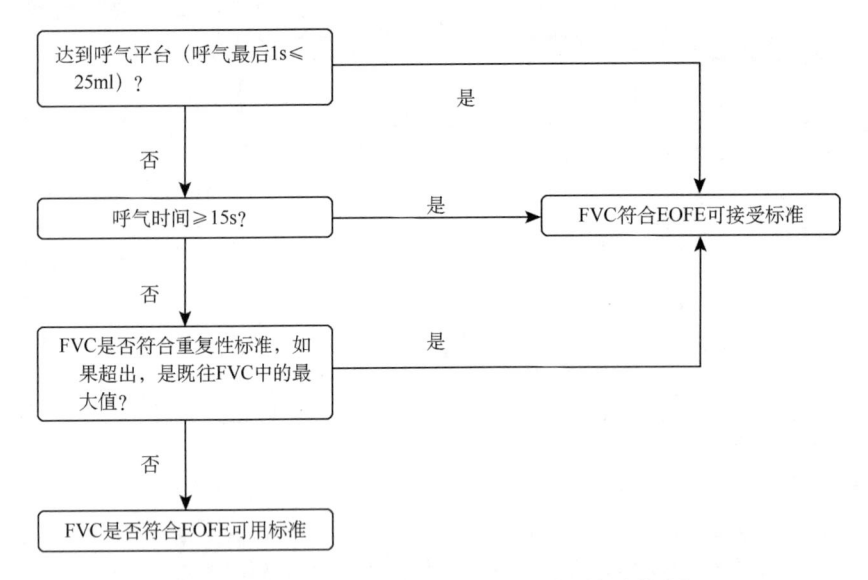

```
                达到呼气平台（呼气最后1s≤
                25ml）？
                          │
                         否│              是
                          ▼              ──────────┐
                    呼气时间≥15s？   ──是──►        │
                          │                        ▼
                         否│              FVC符合EOFE可接受标准
                          ▼                        ▲
                  FVC是否符合重复性标准，如         │
                  果超出，是既往FVC中的最   ──是────┘
                  大值？
                          │
                         否│
                          ▼
                  FVC是否符合EOFE可用标准
```

图 9-2-2 概述 FVC 用力呼气结束（EOFE）接受标准的流程

* 如果在当前支气管扩张药试验之前或之后，无以往的 FVC 值，则此次 FVC 暂时满足 EOFE 可接受标准

测定过程的第 1 秒中，出现咳嗽会影响的 FEV1 测量值，这样 FEV1 既不能接受也不能使用，但是，FVC 可能是可以接受的。

声门关闭或提前终止，如吸气或从咬口移开，则 FVC 不可接受，如果它发生在前 1 s，则 FEV1 不可接受和不可用。与此类似，呼气过程中的前 0.75 s 出现中断，则 FEV 0.75 不可接受和不可用。

嘴部不能有漏气。如果患者不能包紧咬口，可能需要使用凸起形状的咬口，或由操作者协助以保证足够的密封。

咬口阻塞（如舌头咬口的前面，或牙齿放在咬口的前面，或咬变形）可能会影响装置或患者的测定。手持式肺量计因放置不当也会造阻塞。

在错误的流量零流量水平下进行测定，会低估或高估 FEV1 和 FVC。

向操作者反馈。测定系统软件必须在每次检测结束后，向操作员提供明确的反馈，表明 FEV1 和 FVC 的可接受性。操作人员必须有能力否定可接受性提示，注意没有被软件检测到的泄漏，咳嗽，不充分的吸气或呼气，或错误的零流量标定。

必须保留所有可接受或可用的 FEV1 和（或）FVC 的操作记录，因为对某些患者来说，他们的最佳表现可能只产生可用但不符合可接受标准的数据。

十七、测定间的评估

支气管扩张药前和支气管扩张药后的测试目标是目标是达到最少 3 个可接受的 FEV1 和 3 个可接受的 FVC 测量值。注意，可接受的 FEV1 和可接受的 FVC 测量值不一定来自同一测定曲线。操作者必须确保在 2 次动作之间有足够的时间让患者充分恢复，并同意进行另一次最努力的动作。对于 6 岁以上的患者，当最大和次大 FVC 差异≤0.150 L，6 岁或以下且＜0.100 L 或最大 FVC 的 10%（以较大者为准），FVC 有可重复性。对于 6 岁以上的患者，当最大和次大 FEV1 差异≤0.150 L，6 岁或以下且＜0.100 L 或最大 FEV1 的 10%（以较大者为准），FEV1 有可重复性。如果 3 次测试不符合这些标准，必须尝试更多的测试，在成人可达 8 次，儿童可能可以做更多的测试（图 9-2-3）。

达到可重复的结果是患者有最大 FEV1 和 FVC 的最好指标。可重复性的分级，可被量化（见测试质量分级），体现检测结果的可信度。根据重复性标准，确定何时需要更多的操作。大多数情况下，患者能够而且会达到比这些标准更好的重复性。研究发现，大多数成年人的 FVC 和 FEV1 可重复性在 0.150 L 以内，儿童的 FVC 和 FEV1 可重复性在 0.150 L 或 0.100 L 以内。

十八、最大测定次数

8 次是实际操作的上限。在几个用力呼气的动作后，疲劳会开始对患者造成伤害，而额外的测定不会获得更高的测定值。在少见情况下，患者随后的每一次都可能出现 FEV1 或 FVC 的逐渐减少。如果一个可接受的 FEV1 值较起始值减低至 80% 以下，为患者的安全，应终止试验程序。测试儿童时，可能需要超过 8 次尝试，因为每次尝试都可能不是一个完整操作。在尝试完整测试前，儿童可以练习不同阶段的动作。操作人员鼓励儿童热情和努力完成检查，避免使儿童在测试中筋疲力尽或灰心丧气。

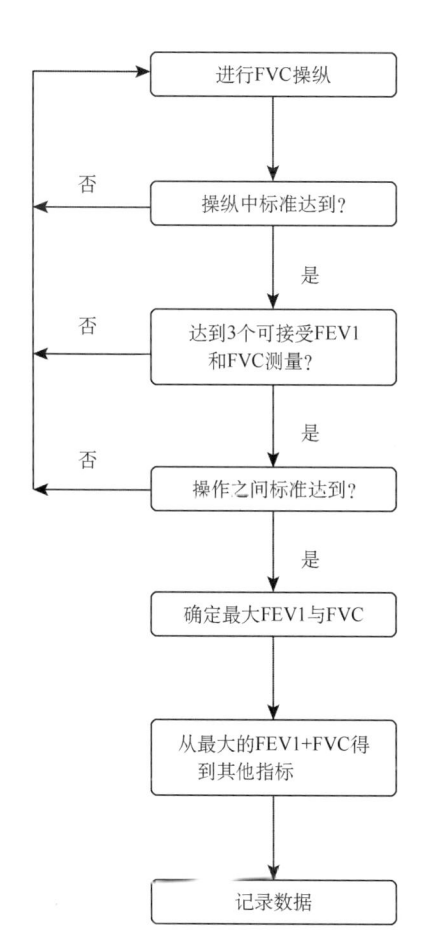

图 9-2-3 概述可接受性和重复性标准的应用流程

量计测定,但在做决定时,需考虑肺功能的基线变异性重要性。通过连续肺量计测定来监测肺功能,特别是对阻塞性肺疾病患者,随访用药后的变化更有意义。

表 9-2-8 支气管扩张药停用时间

气管扩张药	停药时间(h)
SABA(如沙丁胺醇)	4~6
SAMA(如异丙托溴铵)	12
LABA(如福莫特罗或沙美特罗)	24
超LABA(如茚达特罗、维兰特罗或奥洛他特罗)	36
LAMA(如噻托溴铵、梅草碱、阿地铵或格隆铵)	36~48

注:支气管扩张药后试验的停药时间要短于甲胆碱激发试验的停药时间,这些药物的支气管保护作用比支气管扩张效应有的更持久的作用。对于双支气管扩张药,停药时间以长效支气管扩张药的为准。

LABA. 长效 β_2 激动剂;LAMA. 长效毒蕈碱拮抗剂;SABA. 短效 β_2 激动剂;SAMA. 短效毒蕈碱拮抗剂

十九、支气管扩张药反应性试验

早先,使用"可逆性试验","可逆性试验"有时会误产生气道阻塞完全消除的推断,为避免这一误解,本标准使用"支气管扩张药反应性试验"。支气管扩张药反应性试验是指,通过 FEV1 和 FVC 的变化来测定支气管扩张药使用后气流改善的程度。这个试验常作为肺功能测试的一部分进行。支气管扩张药、剂量和使用方式的选择取决于临床医师的试验目的。

如果测试目的是为了解患者的肺功能是否可以通过治疗来改善,那么患者在测试前可以继续使用原有的治疗药物。如果该试验用于诊断或确定肺肺功能在使用支气管扩张药物后是否有任何变化,那么需要临床医师指导患者在基线试验前停止使用支气管扩张药物。表 9-2-8 列出了各种支气管扩张药的停药时间。停药时间是基于对各种的支气管扩张药药效持续效应的研究。吸入皮质类固醇和白三烯调节剂不须要停药。重要的是在检查前通知和提醒患者停止用药,并在检查时确认停止用药。

因为正常的基线肺功能不能排除支气管扩张药的反应,给药前和给药后都应进行肺量计检测。因此,临床医师可能会选择不进行支气管扩张药反应性试验而进行肺

二十、测定程序

按照如前所述的质控标准,患者首先进行用药前肺功能测定,需有 3 个可接受的 FEV1 和 FVC 值。然后,按照仪器内设定方案的指定方法,吸入定量的支气管扩张药。方案指定的等待时间过后,行肺功能测定,需有至少 3 个可接受的 FEV1 和 FVC 值。每个进行支气管扩张剂反应性测试的机构必须有一份书面的测试方案。罕见情况下,支气管扩张药后被错误地编码为支气管扩张药前。肺量计系统必须允许操作者改变用药前后测试的顺序,这样就不会失去那些好的测试,患者也不需要再做一次。当操作者进行用药后的第一次肺功能测定,系统须显示自用药前最后一次测定以来所经过的时间。如果小于支气管扩张药效应的所需时间,则系统必须向操作者提供警示信息。

二十一、报告数值

支气管扩张药使用前和后的测量结果要分别列出(表 9-2-9)。从所有可接受测定中,选择最大 FVC 和 FEV1 值(如果没有可接受值,则从可用值中选择最大的数值)。FEV1/FVC 比值选最大 FVC 和最大的 FEV1,尽管 2 个数值可能来自不同的测定曲线。如果使用支气管扩张药,要报告与用药前数值相比,用药后 FEV1 和 FVC 的百分比变化和绝对值变化。最近的研究表明,使用 FEV1 占预计值百分比的变化量,或 FEV1 的 z-分数的变化量,来评估支气管扩张药反应性,避免了性别和身高的偏差。

FIVC 是用力呼气后的立即吸气的最大吸气量。PEF 是从肺总量位毫无犹豫地最大用力呼气所达到的最高流量,最大值须符合表 9-2-7 中列出的可接受标准 FEV1 标准。

FET 是测量从时间零点到呼气平台结束的秒数,或最大用力呼气后开始吸气的秒数,或患者松开咬口的时间,取最短的时间。FET 不包括呼气末任何流量为零的时期。报告采用最大 FVC 测试曲线的 FET。对于气流梗阻的患者,FVC 与 FET 密切相关。用使支气管扩张药后 FVC 的明显变化可能是由于 FET 的变化引起的。

FEVt 是从时间零点开始到 ts 后,用力呼气所呼出的最大容积。6 岁或 6 岁以下儿童的气道相对于他们的肺容量相对较大,可在 1 s 内完成呼气,因此,使用 FEV0.75 和 FEV0.5。在 6 岁或更小的儿童中,FEV0.75 的数值与 FEV1 相似。关于学龄前儿童肺功能测试,ATS/ERS 声明指出应报告 FEV0.75 和 FEV0.5 的数值。然而,FEV0.75(而不是 0.5)GLI 参考值适用于 3~7 岁儿童的,6 岁或更小的儿童应报告 FEV0.75,如果 FET>1 s,则 FEV1 也应报告。

平均用力呼气流量,即呼气中段流量（$FEF_{25\sim75}$）,从 FEV1 和 FVC 之和最大的测定曲线中测得。值得注意的是,高度依赖于 FVC 测量的有效性和呼气力的程度。在比较支气管扩张剂使用前后的 $FEF_{25\sim75}$ 数值时,可能需要进行容量调整。

表 9-2-9　测量参数（支气管扩张药前后分别出具测试报告）

参数	单位
FVC	升(L)
FEV1	升(L)
FEV1/FVC	小数点后 2 位
PEF	升/秒(L/s)
FET	秒(s)
FIVC	升(L)
≤6 岁的儿童	
FEV0.75	升(L)
FEV0.75/FVC	小数点后 2 位

在 BTPS(体温、环境大气压和饱和水汽)矫正后,容量以升为单位,PEF 以 L/s 为单位,精它们确到小数点后 2 位。肺量计必须测定这些参数,并按照 ATS 标准格式的显示报告。尽管 FEV1、FVC 和 FEV1/FVC 是强制性的,但操作者必须能够配置报告,使其包含其他可选变量,比如 FEV6,FEV1/FEV6,FEV0.5,平均用力呼气流量,呼气中段流量（FVC 在 25%~75%用力呼气流量）

FET. 用力呼气时间；FEV0.75. 第 0.75 s 用力呼气量；FIVC.；用力吸气 VC；PEF. 呼气峰流量

二十二、其他衍生指标

FEV1/FEV6 被证实在成人的气道阻塞诊断中是有用的。记录 FEV6 相对于 FVC 有更好的重复性,对患者体能需求更低,更不容易引发晕厥,可提供更具体的 EOFE。必须选择合适的 FEV6 参考值。在 50%VC 的 FEF 值与吸气到 50%VC 的比值（FEF50/FIF50）有时会被用来作为上呼吸道阻塞的一个指示。所有所需获取与存储数据的表格可以在网上获取。

ATS 标准报告形式应被作为肺量仪系统的默认报告形式。对于所有年龄段的默认参考值应由 GLI 参考公式给出,尽管人们也可以有其他选择。除了总结报告,报告解读者也要有获取查看所有测定的权限。来自每个测试阶段的流量和(或)容积数据必须可以被导出,并给设备管理者提供足够信息以得出结论,并绘制出每次测定的容量-时间及流量-时间曲线。系统应有能力将数据导出,可以 pdf 形式保存,也可以离散数据形式保存,用于 HL7 国际发布 2 标准临床文档体系结构,或快速健康互通性资源记录。不同仪器记录的数据,包括输入受试者姓名、编码和测试结论,可被识别获取并接收。2019ATS 国际协会的一个研究机构开始研发互通线路图,集成不同仪器记录到的肺功能数据。

二十三、测试阶段质量的评价标准

技术标准的设定可帮助每个患者达到可能的最佳值。肺量仪结论非常依赖患者的配合。

ATS 推荐的肺量仪评价系统,是由 Hankinson 及其同事建立发展改良而来。"U"被记作"可用的"值。FEV1 与 FVC 被分别评价（表 9-2-10）。这些评价被用在支气管扩张药系列整体测试上而非单独的操作上,并且在支气管扩张药后被分别确定。

在这个评价系统中,报告解读者根据获得的信息,根据标准判断结果的可接受性,可用性,与可重复性,选择所有测试中的最佳值。一些患者也许不能满足这些可接受和可重复标准以达到 A 级,但是这些结论仍然在临床上十分有用。肺量仪操作可能会引发咳嗽反应,且在一两次尝试后,患者也许不能够进行下一次可接受检查。当评分没有达到 A 且最好测试时,翻译者的临床判断在翻译结论时会变得更重要。尽管一些曲线可接受或可使用,评分等级低于 A,操作者最重要的目的是必须一直让每位患者达到最佳的测试结果。

表 9-2-10　FEV1 和 FVC 评分系统（分别评分）

级别	测定次数	重复性：>6 岁	重复性：≤6 岁
A	≥3 可接受	0.150L 以内	0.100L 以内*
B	2 可接受	0.150L 以内	0.100L 以内*
C	≥2 可接受	0.200L 以内	0.150L 以内*
D	≥2 可接受	0.250L 以内	0.200L 以内*
E	≥2 可接受	>0.250L	>0.200L
	或 1 次可接受	N/A	N/A
U	0 次可接受及≥1 次可用	N/A	N/A
F	0 次可接受及 0 次可用	N/A	N/A

N/A. 不适用；重复性级别分别适用于对支气管扩张药前和支气管扩张药后的系列测定。可重复性标准用于 2 个最大的 FVC 值和 2 个最大的 FEV1 值之间的差异。U 级表示所获得的测量值仅可用,而不可接受。尽管在 A 级之下,一些操作可能是可以接受或可用的

*或最高值的 10%,以较大者为准；只适用于 6 岁或以下儿童

不能根据质量控制的分级错误地判断受试者肺功能的健康状况。操作者应告知患者这些分级仅代表他们吹气的一致性。

二十四、VC 与深吸气量测定

VC 是 TLC 和残余气体之间的容量。慢 VC 可由两种方法获取。呼气 VC(EVC)是从 TLC 到 RV 慢慢呼出的气体体积。吸气 VC(IVC)是从 RV 到 TLC 慢慢吸入的气体体积。这些操作是非用力的,除了即将达到 RV 或 TLC,此时需要额外的气力。

深吸气量(IC)是从平静呼气末(即 FRC)缓慢而没有犹豫地吸气到最大吸气位(即 TLC)的吸入气量。IC 是评价肺过度充气的一个间接指标,评估药物干预与物理训练下的 FRC 变化。

二十五、设 备

为了测量 VC 和 IC,肺活量计必须符合 FVC 测定的上述要求。VC 通过常规肺活量计或用以静态肺容量仪器及其他仪器来测量。测定过程必须显示吸入与呼出过程。除去对吸入和呼出前的操作,必须记录 VC 测定的完整过程,以确定患者达到是否呼气用力的平稳状态。

二十六、测试流程

对于慢 VC,最多测定 8 次。VC 测定应于 FVC 前进行,由于有肌肉疲劳的可能及容积效应,经过最大吸入,一些严重气道阻塞的患者会回到一个虚高的 FRC 或 RV 位。测定 VC 时可以测量 IVC 或 EVC 值(图 9-2-4)。IVC 与 EVC 测定的重要差别可在气道阻塞的患者中观察到。

患者应放松,正坐且鼻夹到位,正常呼吸直到呼气末肺容积变得平稳。操作者应鼓励患者平稳地吸入和呼出最多的气体。对于健康的受检者,应在 5~6 s 充分最大吸入和呼出气体。呼吸道阻塞的患者将花更长时间,但呼出应在 15 s 后结束。呼气不能过慢,会导致 VC 被低估。操作者应仔细观察患者以确保他/她的嘴唇紧封咬口,无异物堵塞,鼻夹到位且无漏出,达标 TLC 与 RV 位。当平稳呼吸末肺容量出现或存在 10 次潮气时,系统应有语音或视觉提示,在 IVC 或 EVC 测定时,当呼气到 RV 位,或呼出时间达到 15 s 时,系统应有第二次语音(指蜂鸣)或视觉提示。

对于测定时的评估,嘴巴或鼻子处不可漏气且喉舌处无堵塞。如果吸入时用力不足、犹豫、声门过早关闭,吸气太慢,IC 都会被低估。

对于测定评估,和用力肺活量一样,最少要有 3 个可接受 VC 测定。最大和次大 VC 间的差距>0.150 L 或 10%VC,以较小的为准,对 6 岁以上的或>0.100 L 或 10%VC,以较小为准,对 6 岁及以下的,应被进行更多测定。满足可重复标准需要进行最多 8 次测定,且在测定间有足够充分的休息时间,操作者与患者同意开始进行下一次测定。变化量太大,常是由不完全呼吸导致的。对于 VC,3 次可接受测定中,应采用最大值。对于没有达到稳定呼气末肺容量的测定,不能得出 IC 值。对于 IC,应采用可接受测定的平均值。

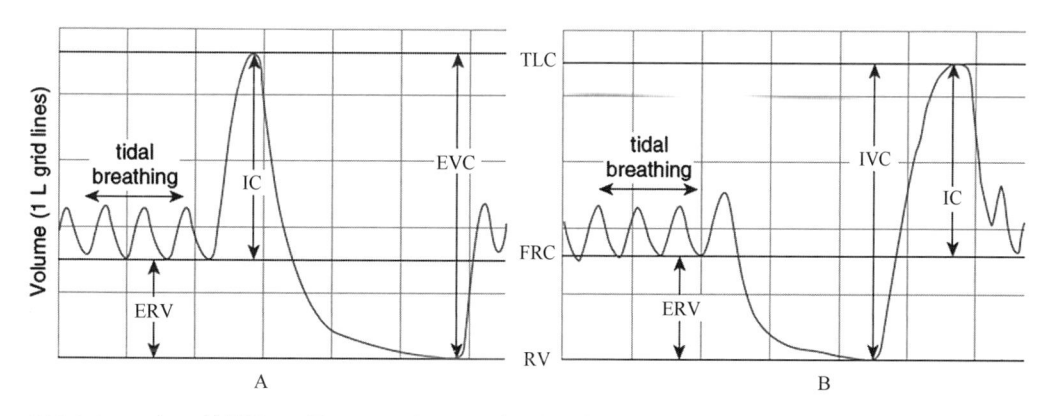

图 9-2-4 VC 与 IC 的测量;VC 用 EVC(A)或 IVC(B)来测量。在这些例子里,体积轴的分隔为 1 L,而时间轴的分隔为 5 s。ERV. 补呼气量;EVC. 呼气 VC;IC. 深吸气容量;IVC. 吸气 VC;RV. 残气

二十七、进一步研究

对于儿童和成人的 BEV 可接受标准,需要进一步分析,制定可接受的循证标准。对于气流阻塞患者的 FETs,应制定更好的可接受标准,用力呼气时间太短会对疾病的诊断造成影响。基于 1979 年的专家意见,EOFE 平台标准是≤0.025 L/s,该标准需要进一步验证。其他未知因素包括测试之间的最佳休息时间,咬口形状(圆形、椭圆形和喇叭形)的影响。家用肺量计和峰值流量监测需要更新标准。慢肺活量 VC 测定的等级评定系统也需要进一步更新和评测。研究也表明,使用远程医疗系统持续监控培训,可以有效地评价和监测在初级健康中心完成的肺量计检查的质量。

二十八、其他潜研究

虽然 FEV1 和 FVC 是肺量计的主要参数,但在流量和容积数据中包含了更多的信息。不断改进分析方法,使用新方法测量容积和流量,可提高潜在风险人群的早期诊断。

利用流量和容积信号分析的曲线形状,测量呼气流量-容积曲线凹度,这对评估儿童哮喘和囊性纤维化是有用一定价值。曲线的斜率在轻度 COPD 也有一定应用价值。关于计算新的时间零点,可使用递归、分段线性回归技术的断点方法进行确定。

更先进的流量和容量数据分析已被提出,以协助肺量计进行自动化质量评估,并自动检测早期终止、咳嗽、额外呼吸和可变流量等错误。使用机器学习系统,辨别可接受曲线,性能接近的水平专家。

有研究显示,孤立的 FEV3/FVC 比值降低提示轻度肺功能损害,检测早期气流限制时,FEV1/FEV6 减低比 FEV1/FVC 具有更高的灵敏度。已获得 FEV1/FEV6、FEV3/FEV6 和 FEV3/FVC 正常值低限。使用呼气过程中前 2~3 s 的数据预估 FVC 可能有助于确定是否达到 EOFE,或在 EOFE 未达到时,为 FVC 提供替代方法。成像技术有可能在不直接接触患者的情况下监测肺容量,对不能或不愿使用咬口的患者进行检测。

3 呼出气一氧化氮检测技术的现状与指南变迁

逯 勇

1980年，Furchgott和Zawadzki在《自然》杂志上提出一氧化氮（NO）的作用，揭开了NO研究的序幕。1991年，Lars E. Gustafsson教授首次报道从人呼出气中检出NO。1993年Kjell Alving教授首次报道哮喘患者呼出气中NO水平比正常人明显升高。随后，1998年，诺贝尔医学及生理学奖授予了R. F. Furchgot t，L. J. lg narro和F. Murad三人，颁奖词中，评审委员对一氧化氮给了极高的评价："这是首度发现一种气体可在人体中成为信号分子"。近40余年，越来越多的研究专注于如何应用呼出气一氧化氮（eNO）这个气道炎症标记物于临床，但气道NO含量非常低（10^{-9}），要准确检出气道不同节段NO水平，并保证其正确反映气道炎症水平，就需要一套完整的技术流程和技术标准。本文试从NO检测技术与临床研究的进展、现状和指南要求的变迁进行说明，以供参考。

一、呼出NO的内涵和外延

（一）FeNO的内涵

分步呼出气一氧化氮（FeNO）指，呼气末吸入NO含量＜5ppb空白气体至肺总量后，以50ml/s对抗5～20cmH_2O阻力经口呼气10s，采集后3s平台期气体样本测得的NO浓度，以10^{-9}（part per billion，ppb）为单位，可描述下气道Th2通路炎症水平。

NO由气道上皮细胞产生，弥散进入气道，随呼气动作排出，是一个呼气流速依赖的指标，同一受试者以不同流速呼气时检测到的结果不同，检测时呼气的流速以毫升每秒（ml/s）表示，以下标形式在FeNO右下角标注。临床指南接受用于描述气道炎症的FeNO为50ml/s下测得的，不经标注或特别说明时，FeNO默认为$FeNO_{50}$。

（二）呼出NO的外延

广义上包括从口、鼻呼出或抽吸出，或经过计算得到的NO相关参数，如图9-3-1所示。

由于NO易向周围组织弥散，尤其在17级以下支气管，为精确计算气道NO水平，1998年Tsoukias教授开发了气道NO双室模型。需要说明除FeNO和FnNO外，其他指标都不能直接测得，而需在不同流速下多次检测，再基于两室模型计算获得。

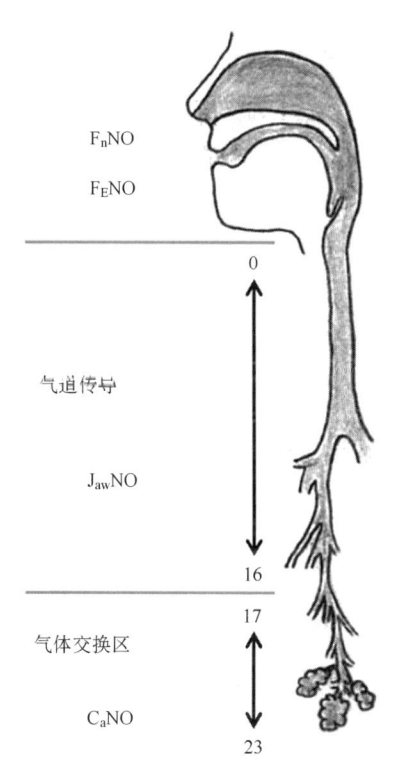

图9-3-1 不同NO指标反映了肺脏不同部位的NO浓度

a）FnNO：通常为经鼻抽吸气体流速为5ml/s状态下，抽出气体中NO的浓度，表示为$FnNO_5$

b）CaNO：肺泡和肺腺泡中NO的浓度，单位为ppb

c）CawNO：气道壁组织中NO的浓度，单位为ppb

d）DawNO：NO从气道壁扩散至气道的能力，单位为ml/s

e）JawNO：除肺泡中NO外，气道中NO总的含量，主要反映主支气管到终末支气管中的NO浓度（JawNO=（CawNO-CANO）×DawNO），如CaNO值为0，JawNO=CawNO×DawNO

二、FeNO检测技术逐渐成熟并确定关键技术细节

1. 1997年，ERS首先发表关于呼出气和鼻NO检测的共识，强调了检测技术流程的标准化，指出吸入NO空白气体是"最标准化的方法"，建议以低速度、对抗阻力呼气，保证软腭上抬以防止鼻腔气体污染。提及鼻NO检测两种可能的方法。第一次比较全面地介绍和分析了关于

呼出气 NO 检测技术和影响因素的诸多问题，提出了统一 NO 检测技术标准的重要性。

2. 1999 年，美国 ATS 发表了成人和儿童呼出 NO 和鼻 NO 的联机和离线检测的标准化程序共识。明确要求成人联机检测使用 NO 含量<5ppb 的空白气体作为吸入气体，不使用鼻夹，吸气到肺总量；对抗 5~20cmH₂O 阻力呼气以关闭软腭；呼气流速 50ml/s±10%，以平衡检测敏感性和受试者舒适程度；呼气相洗脱期需 6 s，其后的平台期至少 3 s；连续检测之间受试者需休息至少 30 s。离线检测提高了检测的便捷性和传感器的利用率，但存在下气道以外的气体污染、样本储存引入的错误和无法及时进行反馈与技术评估等劣势。重申了>12 岁儿童需按照与成人同样的技术要求进行联机检测。儿童离线检测强调排除鼻 NO 干扰，保证平稳呼气。明确表示鼻部气道和血流复杂，影响 NO 的产生和吸收，缺乏评价和比较标准。该共识较 2 年前发表的 ERS 共识就联机 FeNO 检测方面明确了部分推荐；对离线和潮气检测方式及鼻检测，仍未能就诸多关键问题提供确切的推荐。

3. 2005 年 ATS 和 ERS 联合发表了关于联机和离线检测下气道 NO 和鼻 NO 标准检测流程的共识。

（1）成人 FeNO 联机检测，明确了临床对 FeNO 存在需求。列举了影响 FeNO 结果的非疾病相关患者因素，包括年龄/性别、之前进行肺功能检测、气道口径、食物和饮料、昼夜节律、吸烟、感染、检测前运动、药物。推荐吸气相吸入 NO<5ppb 空白气体至肺总量或接近肺总量，不用鼻夹，不要屏气，立即进入呼气相。强调 FeNO 检测可重复性和标准化至关重要：必须保持 5~20cmH₂O 的正压呼气；推荐 50ml/s±10% 为标准呼气流速；确保进入平台期，<12 岁儿童至少呼气 4 s，>12 岁儿童和成人至少呼气 6 s；进入平台后保持 3 s 以采集 150ml 气体检测 NO 水平。

（2）离线 FeNO 检测的共识，联机和离线检测结果即使在流速匹配的情况下也不同，不能互换。离线方法存在三个潜在的问题，包括下气道以外气体的污染、样品存储引入的错误、无法实时反馈和即时技术评估。离线采集气体先经口吸入 NO<20ppb 的气体至肺总量，不要屏气，无须鼻夹，立即对抗一定阻力以 350ml/s 左右（315~385ml/s）气流速呼入特定的储存装置中，如图 9-3-2 所示。样本储存容器必须不与 NO 反应，也不被 NO 渗透，并在 12 h 内进行检测。

（3）儿童联机和离线呼出气 NO 的共识，4~5 岁以上儿童优先选择一口气的联机检测。离线检测应使用 50ml/s 恒定呼气流速，保持至少 5cmH₂O 口腔压强，用不与 NO 反应的气体收集容器。2~5 岁儿童可选联机潮气检测，呼气流速应为 50ml/s。由于存在方法学问题，检测结果不能等同于一口气联机检测，正常参考值尚未建立。

（4）鼻 NO 标准化检测的共识，鼻部腔隙复杂，每一部分都可能产生 NO，无法为其来源提供证据。上气道 NO 检测技术标准化方法的评价与比较尚不成熟。推荐从一侧鼻孔稳定流速抽气，同时在对抗至少 10cmH₂O

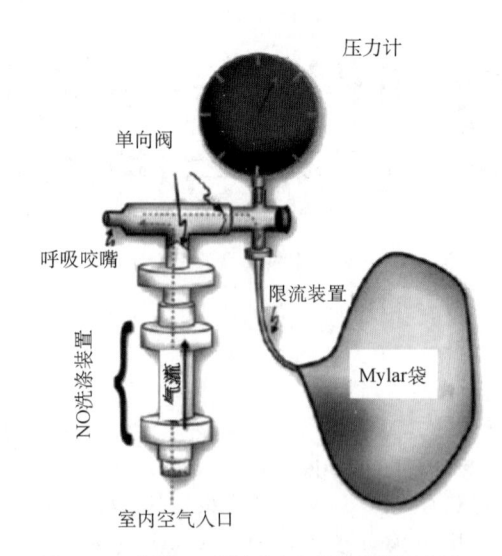

图 9-3-2 离线 NO 检测呼出气采集装置示意图

吸入气体通过 NO 洗涤装置，呼气流速和压力由一个嵌入式压力计和限流装置控制

下缓慢经口呼气的检测方式。鼻 NO 可能的影响因素包括环境气体、体位、年龄、性别、体型/体表面积、体育锻炼、鼻的局部因素、吸烟、药物等。纤毛运动障碍综合征（PCD）患者可出现鼻 NO 下降，鼻 NO 可能成为其筛查项目。

（5）为理解流速对 FeNO 的影响建立了两室模型。

（6）测量 FeNO 设备的共识，大部分使用化学发光法，目前用于成人和儿童临床精确测量 FeNO 和鼻 NO 所需的最低标准如表 9-3-1 所示。潮气检测设备尚无共识。NO 离线检测的设备在灵敏度、准确性和范围的要求与联机检测相同。与样本接触的分析仪和系统组件的材料不能释放 NO，也不能与 NO 反应。

表 9-3-1 NO 分析仪所规定的质量标准

参数	FeNO	鼻 NO
灵敏度	1ppb（噪声<0.5ppb）	10ppb
信噪比	≥3:1	同呼出 NO
准确度	优于 1ppb	优于 10ppb
范围	(1~500)ppb	(10~50)ppm
仪器响应时间*	<500ms	<500ms
系统滞后时间†	需由研究者测量和研究	同 FeNO
漂移	<1%满量程/24h	同 FeNO
重现性	优于 1ppb	优于 10ppb
流通传感器	需由制造商测量并在出版物中报告	同呼出 NO

*为从一个方波信号引入起，直至达到 90% 最大信号之间的延迟，包括电子延迟和由于样本的引入导致的固有仪器物理延迟，但不包括管线长度；†为由于样本在一个特定的应用系统或设置中通过管线和接口的通过时间导致的延迟

2005年ATS/ERS共识是到目前为止对NO检测技术流程和技术细节最完整和详尽的一版,其对联机FeNO检测的技术要求和影响因素进行了相当准确的表述,对离线和潮气采样方式进行了介绍并分析了其存在的主要问题;对于鼻NO的检测中的存在的问题及其复杂性进行了描述,但未提出完整的解决方案;提到了两室模型和小气道(肺泡)NO检测,但未形成共识。

4. 2017年ERS发表肺部疾病呼出生物标记物技术标准。

(1)高度认可了2005年ATS/ERS共识,对相关术语澄清如表9-3-2。

表9-3-2 气道NO相关各生物标记物及其定义

指标	特征
FeNO	通常为经口呼气流速为50ml/s状态下,口呼出气体中NO的浓度,表示为:FeNO$_{50}$,单位为ppb
FnNO	通常为经鼻呼气流速为5ml/s状态下,鼻呼出气中NO的浓度,表示为:FnNO$_s$;如鼻呼气流速为50ml/s状态下,表示为:FnNO$_{50}$
G$_A$NO	肺泡或肺腺泡中NO的浓度,单位为ppb
CawNO	气道壁组织中NO的浓度,单位为ppb
DawNO	NO从气道壁扩散至气道的能力,单位为ml/s
JawNO	除肺泡中NO外,气道中NO总的含量(JawNO=(CawNO-C$_A$NO)×DawNO),如C$_A$NO值为0,JawNO=CawNO×DawNO
V$_{NO}$	NO清除率,单位为pl/s或nl/s
V$_E$	呼气流速,单位为ml/s

(2)认可了FeNO作为哮喘表型和管理的生物标记物,认可了高的FeNO$_{50}$在判断Th2型炎症中的价值,其与哮喘急性发作和吸入激素反应性相关。

(3)FnNO检测也是流速依赖性的,通常采样气体流速应为5ml/s。联机FnNO检测的最佳测量技术尚未确定,FnNO尚无可用的参考值,目前仅被证明可用于PCD。

(4)CaNO用于描述肺泡/小气道NO水平,基于不同流速测得的呼出NO不同气道节段贡献不同,在两室模型的基础上计算得到CaNO。无论采取线性或非线性计算方式都需要在至少3种不同的流速下检测呼出NO,每种呼气流速都要在稳定流速情况下进行2次检测并在平台期采样并计算平均值,全部三种或四种流速下的检测结果代入公式计算。但遗憾的是,未就检测流速种类和具体流速达成共识。健康人CaNO研究结果无法直接应用于患者,且存在矫枉过正,尚无可用的参考值。

(5)检测设备:化学发光设备需要每月进行标准气体校准、每天归零、整机年检,昂贵的价格限制了临床和家庭使用。基于电化学法的手持设备(<1kg)可提供(5~300)ppb的检测范围,精确度为±5ppb或±10%,专门用于FeNO$_{50}$的检测,与化学发光技术获得FeNO$_{50}$结果的差异为±(4~10)pp,适用于常规临床检测。

呼出NO检测技术经历了30年的发展,FeNO联机检测基本成熟,关键技术指标已经达成共识并标准化,电化学检测技术已成为临床常规;但离线和潮气技术、FnNO、CaNO等指标检测方法尚未标准化,部分关键技术问题尚未解决,新的检测手段也仍在开发中。

三、临床指南和共识逐步认可FeNO作为气道炎症生物标记物

1. 2011年ATS发表呼出气一氧化氮(FeNO)检测的临床应用指南,作为首部提出FeNO参考值范围、临床用途、数据解读的指南,明确了:

(1)推荐FeNO用于判断气道嗜酸性粒细胞炎症。

(2)推荐FeNO用于确定可能由气道炎症造成的慢性呼吸道症状的激素反应性。

(3)建议在需要时用FeNO支持哮喘诊断。

(4)建议使用切点值而不是参考值来解释FeNO水平。

(5)推荐12岁以下儿童将年龄作为FeNO的影响因素。

(6)推荐将低FeNO定义为<25ppb(儿童<20ppb),表示受试者存在嗜酸性粒细胞炎症的可能性低,糖皮质激素治疗有效的可能性低。

(7)推荐将高FeNO定义为>25ppb(儿童>20ppb),表示受试者存在嗜酸性粒细胞炎症的可能性高,糖皮质激素治疗有效的可能性高。

(8)推荐FeNO在25~50ppb(儿童20~35ppb)时参照临床情况进行谨慎解读。

(9)推荐将持久性和(或)高过敏原暴露作为高FeNO水平的相关因素。

(10)推荐FeNO用于哮喘患者气道炎症评估。

(11)建议50ppb以上FeNO升高超过20%或50ppb以下FeNO升高超过10bbp判定为明显升高。

(12)建议50ppb以上FeNO下降至少20%或50ppb

以下 FeNO 下降至少 10bbp 判定为明显降低。

FeNO 的优势是无创、便捷、可重复，严重气道阻塞患者相对容易进行，提供了气道炎症信息，为传统临床工具（病史、查体、肺功能）增添了新的维度。该指南就健康人在 50ml/s 流速下联机检测的 FeNO 水平采集了大量样本，涉及 6 项研究共 8441 例，其中 7340 例来自 NIOX 设备，详见表 9-3-3。结合哮喘症状与 FeNO，对相应的临床判断提出了建议，详见表 9-3-4。

表 9-3-3　在健康受试者中开展呼气流速为 50ml/s 时呼气一氧化氮浓度值的研究

作者和参考文献编号	N	给出参考值的组	"正常值"(ppb)	分析仪
Kharitonov 2003(75)	59	成人和儿童的混合人群	平均 16.3ppb，ULN 33	NIOX（Aerocrine AB, Stockholm, Sweden）
Buchvald 2005(76)	405	儿童：年龄 4～17 岁 数据还可根据年龄进行分层	平均 9.7ppb 95%CI 上限：25.2	NIOX（Aerocrine AB, Stockholm, Sweden）
Olivieri 2006(77)	204	男性，非吸烟者，非哮喘患者 女性，非吸烟者，非哮喘患者 （注：未考虑特应性）	4.5～20.6 3.6～18.2 （注：引号内的数值为第 5 和第 95 百分位数）	(CLD88, Ecomedics, Switzerland)
Olin 2007(69)	3376	随机人群 1131 例从未吸烟受试者，未报告任何哮喘症状，干咳或使用吸烟皮质类固醇治疗	见表 9-3-2	NIOX（Aerocrine AB, Stockholm, Sweden）
Travers 2007(78)	3500	男性，非吸烟者，非特应性 男性，非吸烟者，特应性 男性，吸烟者，非特应性 男性，吸咽者，特应性 女性，非吸烟者，非特应性 女性，非吸烟者，特应性 女性，吸烟者，非特应性 女性，吸烟者，特应性	9.5～47.4 11.2～56.5 7.5～38.4 8.8～45.9 7.5～37.4 8.8～44.6 5.9～30.5 6.9～36.4 （注：引号内的数值为 90% 置信区间）	NIOX（Aerocrine AB, Stockholm, Sweden）
Dressel 2008(79)	897	男性，非吸烟者，非特应性，165cm 男性，非吸烟者，特应性，165cm 男性，吸烟者，非特应性，165cm 男性，吸烟者，特应性，165cm 女性，非吸烟者，非特应性，160cm 女性，非吸烟者，特应性，160cm 女性，吸烟者，非特应性，160cm 女性，吸烟者，特应性，160cm	19.5 29.1 12.2 18.3 15.7 23.5 9.9 14.7	(NOA 280, Sievers, Boulder, CO)

表 9-3-4　FeNO 结果解释概况：症状指咳嗽和（或）喘鸣和（或）呼吸急促 *

	$FE_{NO}<25$ppb （儿童中为<20ppb）	$FE_{NO}(25～50)$ppb ［儿童中为(20～35)ppb］	$FE_{NO}>50$ppb （儿童中为>35ppb）
	诊断		
过去 6[+] 周内出现症状	不太可能为嗜酸粒细胞性气道炎症 其他诊断 不太可能自 ICS 治疗获益	应谨慎 评价临床应用环境 监测 FE_{NO} 随时间的变化	出现嗜酸粒细胞性气道炎症可能 自 ICS 治疗获益
	监测（诊断为哮喘的患者中）		
出现症状	可能为其他诊断 不太可能自升高 ICS 治疗剂量中获益	持续性过敏原暴露 依从性或吸入给药技术较差 ICS 治疗剂量不足 恶化风险 类固醇耐药	

	$FE_{NO}<25ppb$ （儿童中为<20ppb）	FE_{NO} 25~50ppb [儿童中为(20~35)ppb]	$FE_{NO}>50ppb$ （儿童中为>35ppb）
未出现症状	ICS治疗剂量适当 依从性较好 逐步降低ICS治疗剂量	ICS治疗剂量适当 依从性较好 监测FE_{NO}的变化	停用ICS治疗或降低剂量可能导致复发 依从性或吸入给药技术较差

ICS. 吸入皮质类固醇；* FeNO检测结果可作为病史、体格检查及肺功能检查的辅助措施

2. 关于FeNO用于哮喘诊断，2015年西班牙哮喘管理指南首次将FeNO纳入哮喘诊断流程，以50ppb作为切点值。随后，2017年底发表的英国NICE NG80指南也将FeNO纳入哮喘诊断流程，并第一次作为成人哮喘诊断的必检项目，将诊断切点设定为≥40ppb（儿童≥35ppb），详见图9-3-3。NICE NG80指南指出，不要在未进行客观检查的情况下仅依靠症状诊断哮喘，不要仅依靠特应性疾病史诊断哮喘；不要使用过敏原皮肤点刺试验、血清总IgE和特异性IgE、外周血嗜酸性粒细胞计数、运动激发试验（对17岁及以上成人）作为哮喘诊断依据；可用于哮喘诊断的实验室检查包括FeNO、肺量计、支气管舒张试验、峰流速变异率，使用组胺或乙酰甲胆碱的直接支气管激发试验是最后的选项，且在儿童和17岁以下青年不进行激发试验。与常见哮喘诊断策略不同，对于疑似哮喘患者，即使肺量计呈阻塞性表现且舒张试验阳性，如没有FeNO支持存在活跃的气道炎症，仍不能诊断哮喘；即使肺功能未发现阻塞性表现也不能除外哮喘，需要联合FeNO和峰流速变异率进行评估，必要时进行激发试验。

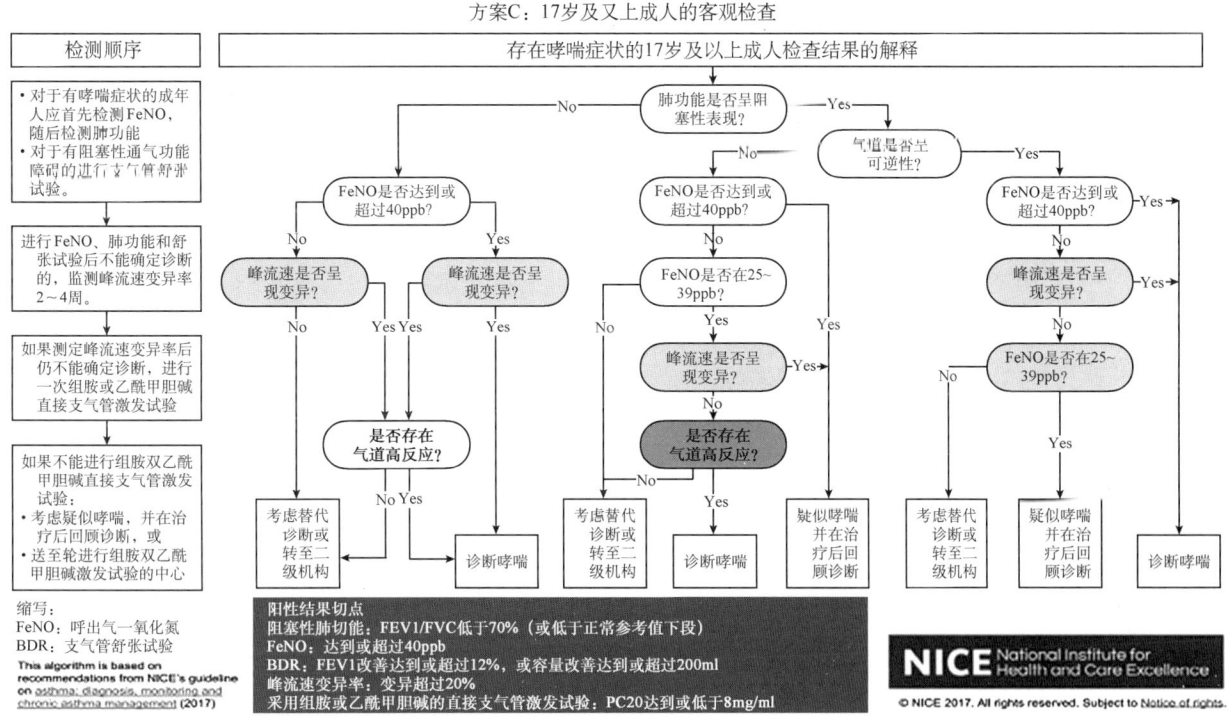

图9-3-3 2017年英国NICE NG80指南将FeNO列入成人哮喘诊断流程并作为必检项目

3. 关于FeNO用于气道炎症评估、抗炎治疗反应性的预判等方面，更多国外指南更早提出了指导性意见。2014年日本成人哮喘指南指出，FeNO升高提示嗜酸性粒细胞气道炎症，反映嗜酸性粒细胞炎症水平，监测气道炎症，高FeNO还提示对激素治疗反应性好。日本指南还指出，在CVA中存在FeNO升高，而在AC中FeNO不升高。2016年的苏格兰-不列颠哮喘管理指南支持用FeNO发现和确定嗜酸性细胞炎症，并指出FeNO可帮助发现依从性不良的患者。详见表9-3-5。2017年发表的德国哮喘诊疗指南也支持FeNO作为Th2通路气道炎症生物标记物用于哮喘管理。2019年ERS和ATS联合发表的重症哮喘管理指南中指出，FeNO≥19.5ppb支持12岁以上的成人和青年重症哮喘患者更可能从抗IgE治疗中获益；FeNO>25ppb提示杜匹鲁单抗可降低激素依赖型重症哮喘患者口服激素的剂量。

表 9-3-5　FeNO 区分哮喘气道炎症类型及预测治疗反应性

FeNO(pb)		判断 EOS 炎症类型	预测 ICS 治疗反应性
成人和>12岁儿童	<12岁儿童		
>50	>35	很可能	可能对 ICS 反应性良好
25~50	20~35	有可能,结合临床综合判断	对 ICS 反应性需结合临床综合判断
<25	<20	不太可能	可能对 ICS 反应性不佳

4. 对于 FeNO 技术及其临床应用,中国指南和共识较早进行了介绍。2013 年《支气管哮喘控制的中国专家共识》提示 FeNO 可作为气道炎指标。2015 年《无创气道炎症评估支气管哮喘的临床应用中国专家共识》对 FeNO 进行了详细介绍,就其方法学、质量控制、结果判读及临床应用等方面提出了指导意见。共识认可 FeNO 是一种诊断和监测炎症性气道疾病的重要标记物,与嗜酸性粒细胞炎症相关;推荐 FeNO 作为哮喘支持性诊断工具;支持 FeNO 用于鉴别哮喘患者炎症分型和预判激素反应性,认可并引用了 2011 年 ATS 指南提出的 FeNO 切点值;支持 FeNO 用于判断吸入糖皮质激素治疗反应性和依从性,并用于评估哮喘控制水平,高 FeNO 或较缓解期 FeNO 水平升高>40% 提示哮喘未控制或嗜酸性气道炎症恶化;参考 2011 年 ATS 指南,列表说明了 FeNO 检测对于激素治疗期间哮喘管理的意义。详见表 9-3-6,表 9-3-7。

表 9-3-6　根据 FeNO 变化情况判断激素治疗疗效

FeNO 水平基线(ppb)	转基线改变	激素反应性
成人和>12岁儿童>50 <12岁儿童>35	较基线下降>20%	反应性好
成人和>12岁儿童<50 <12岁儿童<35	较基线下降>10ppb	反应性好

表 9-3-7　FeNO 检测对于激素治疗期间哮喘管理的意义

FeNO 水平	成人<25ppb (儿童<20ppb) 炎症已控制	成人 25~50ppb (儿童 20~35ppb) 炎症未控制	成人>50ppb (儿童>35ppb) 炎症未控制
有症状	·对增加 ICS 反应性差 ·其他诊断/合并诊断	·依从性差/吸入技术差 ·ICS 剂量不足 ·未经治疗的小气道疾病 ·持续过敏原暴露 ·罕见:激素抵抗	·依从性差/吸入技术差 ·ICS 剂量不足 ·未经治疗的小气道疾病 ·持续过敏原暴露 ·罕见:激素抵抗
无症状	·足够的 ICS 剂量 ·依从性好 ·可以减少 ICS 剂量	·潜在未控制的气道炎症 ·监测 FeNO 和症状水平的变化 ·不要减低激素剂量,除非患者无症状且 FeNO 水平持续稳定 ·已控制的炎症	·依从性差/吸入技术差 ·表明有未经控制的气道炎症,接下来可能导致症状和急性加重的风险 ·不能减少/停止 ICS,否则会引起复发,需评估 FeNO 趋势 ·持续过敏原暴露

在随后发表的《支气管哮喘防治指南(2016 年版)》中再一次认可 FeNO 作为评估气道炎症和哮喘控制水平的指标,也可用于判断吸入激素治疗的反应,介绍了 2011 年 ATS 推荐的参考值,并指出连续测定、动态观察 FeNO 变化的临床价值更大,详见表 9-3-8。2017 年发表的《儿童肺功能及气道非创伤性炎症指标系列指南(七):呼出气体一氧化氮监测》,参考西方重要指南,就 FeNO 在儿科的应用进行了梳理,推荐 FeNO 用于判断儿童哮喘炎症类型和嗜酸粒细胞性炎症水平;判断 ICS 治疗的有效性及依从性;评估哮喘控制水平和预测哮喘急性发作,指导哮喘治疗方案调整;并提出了 FeNO 水平判断气道炎症类型和指导哮喘治疗决策的参考标准(表 9-3-8)。

2019 年中国过敏性哮喘诊治指南(2019 年)是目前最新的中国哮喘相关指南,指明了过敏性哮喘、2 型炎症、嗜酸粒细胞炎症、与 FeNO 升高的关系,并明确 FeNO 在 2 型炎症为主哮喘的诊断和长期管理中价值更大,值得推荐,证据级别为 A 级。FeNO 测定的临床意义为:辅助哮喘诊断与鉴别诊断,预测 ICS 治疗反应性,评估 ICS 治疗依从性,区别气道炎症类型和评估气道炎症水平,评估哮喘控制水平,预测哮喘急性发作风险及指导哮喘治疗方案调整。

5. FeNO 在慢性咳嗽领域进行的研究起步较晚,但相对于国际指南,国内的进展相对更为突出。早在《咳嗽的诊断与治疗指南(2015)》中就将 FeNO 称为"近年来开展的一项无创气道炎症检查技术",并提出"FeNO 增高(>32ppb)提示嗜酸性粒细胞性炎症或激素敏感性咳嗽(如 EB 或 CVA)可能性大"。在该指南提供的慢咳病因诊断流程中,FeNO 以诱导痰细胞学检查的替代手段出现,详见图 9-3-4。

表 9-3-8 FeNO水平判断气道炎症类型和指导哮喘治疗决策的参考标准

类型	成人<25ppb(儿童<20ppb)	成人 25~50ppb(儿童 20~35ppb)	成人>50ppb(儿童>35ppb)
有症状	考虑其他诊断/合并诊断	a 检查过敏原 b 检查依从性或吸入技术 c 升阶梯抗炎治疗	a 检查过敏原 b 检查依从性或吸入技术 c 升阶梯抗炎治疗,特别是当伴有血嗜酸细胞计数增高时,或考虑小颗粒ICS d 若为ICS耐受性哮喘,则需要添加全身性的抗炎治疗
无症状	如果哮喘已被控制至少3~6个月,考虑ICS降阶梯治疗	a 检查过敏原 b 检查依从性或吸入技术 c 如无发作史,维持治疗剂量 d 如果有发作史,升阶梯抗炎治疗	a 检查过敏原 b 检查依从性或吸入技术 c 停用ICS治疗或降低剂量可能导致急性加重 d 升阶梯治疗,特别是伴有血嗜酸细胞计数增高时

注:FeNO:呼出气一氧化氮;成人:>12岁;ppb:十亿分之一(10^{-9});ICS:吸入糖皮质激素 FeNO:fractional exhaled nitric oxide,adult:more than 12 years old;ppb:part per billion;ICS:inhaled corticosteroid

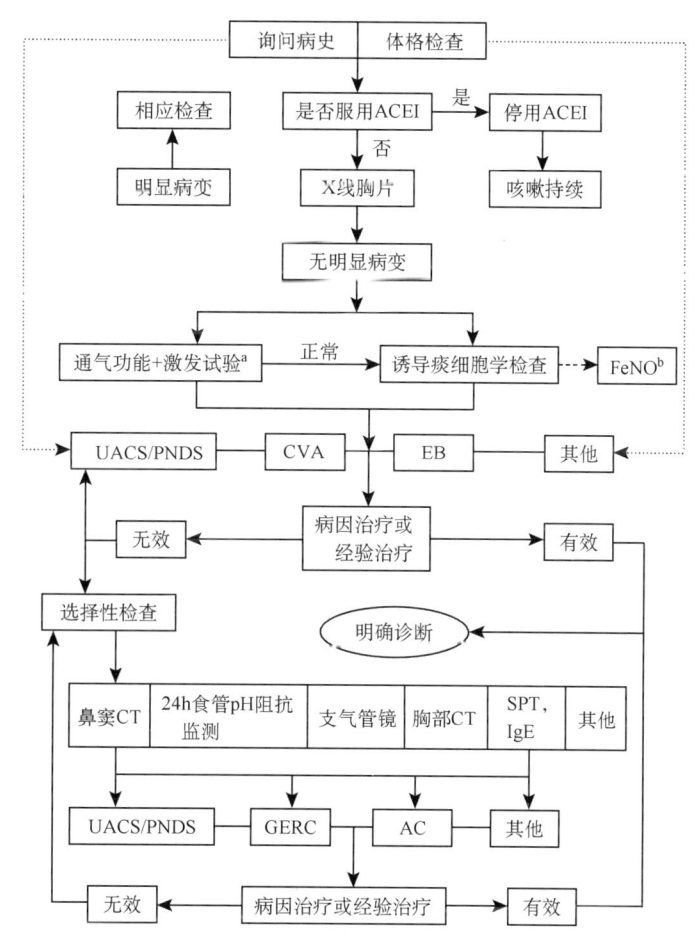

图 9-3-4 慢性咳嗽病因诊断流程

在2019年发表的《咳嗽基层诊疗指南(实践版·2018)》中,重申了FeNO可作为诱导痰细胞学检查的补充,FeNO>32ppb提示嗜酸粒细胞性气道炎症和激素敏感性咳嗽。2020年正式发表的ERS慢性咳嗽诊疗指南中也对FeNO进行了介绍,并尝试使用FeNO解决临床问题,但总体看来,国外指南对FeNO在慢性咳嗽方面应用的态度仍较为保守。

6. GINA虽然不是指南,但其由独立专业组织提供,筛选和报告哮喘领域研究的年度进展,并给出临床建议。2002年GINA报告就对气道NO进行了描述,随着相关研究增多,GINA逐步认可FeNO作为气道炎症评估指标、预估抗炎治疗反应性、用于妊娠哮喘管理可获益、高FeNO是哮喘急性发作独立危险因素等,但同时在某些问题上仍保持谨慎态度。2020年GINA对FeNO的态度变化不大,表示认可 FeNO 在 2 型气道炎症的哮喘患者中升高,但不能仅依靠单次 FeNO 结果确诊或除外哮喘;FeNO 测量方法对大多数 5 岁以下儿童不适用,主要作为研究工具;虽然提出了 1~5 岁儿童 FeNO 正常参考值已发表,但仅引用了一个研究,且该研究使用离线潮气方法(非联机方法)、样本量小(53 例,且来自同一城市)、结果离散且趋势不明显,参考价值有待讨论;认可 FeNO 是区分哮喘和 COPD 的手段之一;认可 FeNO 升高是哮喘急性发作的独立危险因素;认可 FeNO 用于指导治疗可减少儿童、青少年急性发作率;认为 FeNO 检测可以支持起始 ICS 治疗的决策,但不能否定 ICS 治疗策略;支持 FeNO 识别重症哮喘中 2 型炎症表型的患者、评估重症哮喘患者依从性、预测奥马珠单抗反应性、指导抗 IL-4R 治疗和减少 OCS 用量。

随着 FeNO 相关临床数据积累,各国指南对 FeNO 的临床价值逐渐认可,使用范围也从评估气道炎症和支持哮喘诊断,逐渐发展到了气道炎症管理的全过程,但在某些重要问题上仍需进一步研究,如 FeNO 指导抗炎治疗的具体方案等。

四、呼出气 NO 相关指标技术和临床指南/共识现状

气道各 NO 标记物的临床应用现状见表 9-3-9。

表 9-3-9 气道各 NO 标记物的临床应用现状

检测指标	有无标准流程	参考值	参考值来源	总样本量(N)	是否被指南推荐	应用范围
FeNO 联机检测	有	成人:25~50ppb 儿童:20~35ppb	ATS 2011	N=8441	推荐	临床
FeNO 离线检测	有	无	—	—	不推荐	科研
FeNO 潮气检测	无	无	—	—	不推荐	科研
FnNO	无	无	—	—	限制使用	PCD
CaNO	无	无	—	—	不推荐	科研
CawNO	无	无	—	—	不推荐	科研
DawNO	无	无	—	—	不推荐	科研
JawNO	无	无	—	—	不推荐	科研

五、现存问题与研究展望

1. 部分关键技术障碍

(1)FeNO 检测技术成熟,但仍需受试者配合,一方面由于流速依赖性的特点,检测过程需要患者持续保持稳定的呼气流速以获得能够真实反映气道炎症水平的采样;另一方面,需要对抗足够的呼气阻力以关闭软腭,避免鼻 NO 的干扰;且呼吸转换需避免屏气等。这些都需要受试者的配合,存在年龄过小或病情过重无法配合的情况。离线或潮气采样不能解决这些问题。离线检测需遵循联机检测的各项标准,不能降低对受试者配合的要求,且气体样本保存困难。潮气检测也无法解决呼气流速和软腭开放对检测结果的影响,且其检测结果与联机检测无法保持一致,也无法解决受试者配合的问题。需要进一步技术革新以解决部分受试者配合困难的问题。

(2)FnNO 虽然已被部分指南接受作为 PCD 筛查工具,但 PCD 患者的鼻 NO 的产生速度和鼻窦内储存量都普遍低于健康人,即在 PCD 筛查中,主要关心的是 FnNO 是否较低,而即使 FnNO 在正常范围也不能拒绝 PCD 的可能,需要完善其他检查项目。如尝试用 FnNO 描述升高的上气道炎症水平(如鼻炎、鼻窦炎等)则存在受炎症情况下鼻窦开口狭窄影响的问题。鼻窦是相对固定的骨性腔隙,与下气道(具有良好弹性能够主动改变容积的肺)不同,鼻窦腔内部气体流速接近 0,NO 主要通过鼻窦开口弥散到鼻前庭,从鼻前庭开口检测到 NO 的浓度同时受到鼻窦内 NO 含量和鼻窦开口的影响。上气道炎症活跃时,如发生鼻窦开口狭窄或关闭,则 FnNO 的结果可能没有随炎症的活跃而升高,反而呈现出断崖式下降,严重影响临床判断。

(3)CaNO 尝试描述小气道炎症,但其并不是实测值,而是基于不同流速下 $FeNO_x$ 结果依两室模型推算出的。两室模型能否精确反映大、小气道之间的关系仍需进一步确认。计算 CaNO 所需的流速种类和数值未定,计算方法尚未统一,尚未解决校正数据过程中矫枉过正的问题。由于 CaNO 是通过不同流速间 $FeNO_x$ 的差异推算,需要流速差异足够大,受试者能否耐受较高的流速和连续多次检测也需要考虑。

(4)需要对不同检测技术及设备间结果的一致性进行检验。目前广泛应用的是电化学法,一些设备比较研究发现了较大的数据差异,影响比照参考值范围的结果判读和炎症监测过程中前后结果的比较,进而影响临床决策。一些新方法的检测结果一致性仍需要重视和解决。

2. 临床应用中存在的问题和可能的研究方向

(1)正常参考值范围:已有研究显示,FeNO 可能存在年龄差异,儿童期的差异比较明显,2011 年 ATS 指南已就儿童与成人给出了不同参考值。但现有数据大部分基于西方人。近年来一些研究显示中国健康人群 FeNO 水平可能与西方人不同,需要较大规模的研究数据支持产生中

国人FeNO参考值范围,并回答在不同炎症背景、污染程度、季节和环境过敏原水平下FeNO与炎症水平和气道炎症性疾病的关系等问题。

(2)炎症水平判断和疾病诊断的切点:以西班牙哮喘诊疗指南和英国NICE NG80指南为代表的部分国外指南在哮喘诊断过程中引入了FeNO,但FeNO主要反映Th2通路气道炎症,难以准确描述非Th2通路气道炎症,这就要在诊断时就敏感性和特异性进行选择和取舍。对于CVA同样存在这个问题。FeNO在气道炎症性疾病的诊断、炎症分型,以及指导下一步诊疗决策中能起到积极的作用,但具体方案和切点值仍需要在不同人群中进行深入的研究和探讨,还可能涉及与其他指标相配合的具体方法。

(3)参考FeNO进行炎症管理和抗炎药物剂量调整的具体方案:大量指南和共识认可FeNO作为气道炎症标记物,但指导抗炎治疗的具体方案仍需讨论。一些研究显示,FeNO用于哮喘管理在减少急性发作风险上并没有获得统计学意义的结果,但这些研究的设计和统计方法差别较大,特别是部分研究没有将不同炎症类型受试者分别讨论,可能稀释了研究结果。GINA高度认可参考FeNO进行妊娠哮喘患者炎症管理的MAP研究,但其是否为最佳方案,能否够适用于全部哮喘人群,能否应用于其他气道炎症性疾病,仍然需进一步研究。

(4)在亚急性咳嗽和慢性咳嗽中的应用:已有指南推荐FeNO作为慢咳气道炎症标记物筛选嗜酸性粒细胞炎症为主(可能包括EB和一部分CVA患者)的患者,并提出了用于筛选激素敏感性咳嗽的参考值。但国际指南对FeNO的推荐尚未取得完全一致,仍需进一步数据支持。而对于亚急性咳嗽,FeNO在部分病毒感染后可能升高,且不一定随症状消失回到基线水平;感染后咳嗽使用FeNO指导抗炎治疗的可行性、安全性和切点值仍需进一步探讨。

(5)COPD和ACO中FeNO的应用:大部分COPD不是Th2通路气道炎症为主的,且急性加重多与感染有关,对全体COPD患者使用FeNO进行气道炎症管理存在障碍。有研究显示,ACO患者FeNO水平高于COPD,FeNO升高的COPD患者接受抗炎治疗后急性加重风险降低,但如何应用仍需继续探讨。

(6)其他领域:不断有研究者在FeNO应用范围上进行尝试,如在围术期、肺部肿瘤、放射性肺损伤、其他气道炎症性疾病、气道不同节段炎症评估、FeNO与其他呼吸相关指标的联合应用等方面,但研究的质量、数量和相关数据的总结等方面还有待提高。

呼出NO相关指标作为气道炎症标记物已得到基本认可,联机FeNO检测技术基本成熟,具有安全、无创、快捷、量化、重复性好等优势。FeNO应用于哮喘、慢性咳嗽等气道炎症性疾病的诊断、炎症分型、炎症水平评估和管理、支持抗炎治疗决策、评估和改善抗炎治疗依从性、评估和降低炎症活跃风险等方面都获得了初步认可和长足的进步。关于呼出气NO检测技术的一些问题和临床应用仍然需要更广泛和深入持续研究与总结。

4 肺龄指标适用于推广普及肺功能检查及呼吸慢病防控

郑劲平　梁晓林

一、肺龄的概念

肺龄即肺的年龄，指通过年龄来量化肺的生理功能水平。肺龄主要通过肺量计检查指标如FEV1的水平来估算。以第1秒用力呼气容积（FEV1）为例，对应同等FEV1水平的相同性别和身高的健康非吸烟者的年龄即为测量个体的"肺龄"。健康人正常情况下其肺龄应与实际年龄一致，若肺龄大于实际年龄，提示肺功能下降，出现了"早衰"。肺龄与实际年龄的差异大小可提示其肺功能"衰退"的程度。

二、肺龄的优点

由于肺龄通过肺量计检查指标来估算，因此肺龄也可视为肺量计检查结果的一个简化形式。相对于肺功能检查报告中各种复杂的指标，肺龄的优点在于简单、易懂，可以协助医师向患者解释肺功能结果，让患者更清晰地认识到自身的肺功能水平和病情严重程度，从而提高医疗的依从性。肺龄可作为肺功能检查结果解释的一个补充，而且尤其适合用于基层医疗机构。

三、肺龄的计算方法

1985年Morris等首次提出了肺龄的概念，并建立了肺龄的计算公式。该计算公式利用了原有的肺量计指标预计值公式，将受检者实测的FEV1数值和其身高代入FEV1的预计值公式中，反推计算得到的年龄值即为该受检者的肺龄。其后，有学者对肺龄的计算方法进行了改进，利用大量健康非吸烟者的肺量计检查数据，将健康人的实际年龄看作是肺龄，以FEV1等肺量计指标和身高作为自变量，通过多元回归分析建立肺龄的预测模型。该计算方法不仅可提供估算的肺龄均值，还可提供个体的肺龄正常区间，有利于更准确地解读肺龄。目前与肺龄计算公式相关的研究仍较少，仍未有基于大样本数据、适用于中国人群的肺龄计算公式。

四、肺龄在慢性阻塞性肺疾病中的应用

慢性阻塞性肺疾病（简称慢阻肺）目前是世界第4顺位死因。最新的流调数据显示，我国慢阻肺患者人数约1亿，40岁以上成人慢阻肺发病率高达13.7%。慢阻肺的高患病率和高病死率给我国社会带来了对于慢阻肺患者管理的巨大需求，慢阻肺的防治工作已刻不容缓。作为慢阻肺诊疗和评估的重要工具，近年来，早期进行肺功能筛查的重要性也得到强调。目前，肺功能检查已纳入了常规体检项目，在《"健康中国2030"规划纲要》中也倡导40岁及以上或疾病高危人群应每年进行肺功能检查，由此可见，未来肺功能检查的应用将不断增加且向基层医疗机构普及。但肺功能检查的结果涉及众多呼吸专科指标，其结果的解读对于普通大众甚至是基层医务人员而言较为困难，而肺龄则可让大众更容易理解其肺功能检查结果，因此有助于医患沟通及患者教育，提高患者的疾病严重程度的认识和对治疗的依从性，从而促进慢阻肺患者的慢性管理工作。

加强控烟工作，推动戒烟宣传和干预也是慢性呼吸疾病防治的重要工作内容，而大样本的随机对照试验研究表明，告知患者其肺龄相对于告知其FEV1的原始数值，更能激励吸烟者戒烟。因此，使用肺龄可提高吸烟者等高危患病人群的戒烟动力，从而早期预防慢性呼吸疾病的发生。综上，肺龄在慢性呼吸疾病的防治中具有一定的应用前景。由于目前仍缺乏基于中国人群的肺龄估算公式，有必要进行建立中国人群的肺龄估算公式的相关研究，并进一步探索肺龄在慢性呼吸系统疾病管理中的价值。

参 考 文 献

[1] Morris J F, Temple W. Spirometric "lung age" estimation for motivating smoking cessation. Prev Med, 1985, 14 (5): 655-662.

[2] Yamaguchi K, Omori H, Onoue A, et al. Novel regression equations predicting lung age from varied spirometric parameters. Respiratory Physiology & Neurobiology, 2012, 183 (2):

108-114.
[3] Wang C, Xu J, Yang L, et al. Prevalence and risk factors of chronic obstructive pulmonary disease in China (the China Pulmonary Health [CPH] study): a national cross-sectional study. Lancet, 2018, 391(10131): 1706-1717.
[4] Parkes G, Greenhalgh T, Griffin M, et al. Effect on smoking quit rate of telling patients their lung age: the Step2quit randomised controlled trial. BMJ, 2008, 336(7644): 598-600.

5 新冠肺炎患者的呼吸功能评估和康复

郭 健 刘锦铭

一、COVID-19患者肺损伤机制

新型冠状病毒病(COVID-19)简称新冠肺炎,已成为国际关注的突发公共卫生事件。与当年的SARS不同,新型冠状病毒的传播形式更隐蔽、传播速度更快、传染力更强。新冠病毒主要侵及肺部,COVID-19尸体解剖显示新冠病毒主要引起深部气道和肺泡损伤为特征的炎症反应,在电镜下支气管黏膜上皮和Ⅱ型肺泡上皮细胞胞质中可见冠状病毒颗粒,免疫组化染色显示部分肺泡上皮和巨噬细胞呈新型冠状病毒阳性。COVID-19侵及肺部发生的基本病理生理机制主要是新冠病毒与机体细胞膜上的血管紧张素转换酶2(angiotensin converting enzyme 2,ACE2)结合后侵染宿主细胞,ACE2在人体各个组织广泛表达,在Ⅱ型肺泡上皮表达尤为丰富,所以新冠病毒感染人体后可引起以肺脏损伤为主的全身多器官损伤。新冠病毒在进入细胞后进行病毒复制、扩增、释放的同时启动机体的防御反应;病毒在肺内复制,直接破坏肺组织细胞,造成肺内局部的炎症反应,导致肺组织充血水肿,引起局部和全身的炎症反应、氧化应激、组织、细胞缺氧等;部分患者肺内诱导细胞浸润和细胞因子过度表达,产生炎性因子风暴。患者感染新冠病毒后临床表现不一,轻者可无明显临床症状,重者可发展为急性呼吸迫综合征(acute respiratory distress syndrome,ARDS)、脓毒症休克、难以纠正的代谢性酸中毒及多器官衰竭等,严重者导致死亡。

二、COVID-19患者呼吸功能评估

由于新冠病毒主要侵及肺部,引起肺损伤,造成COVID-19患者呼吸功能下降,所以对这部分患者进行呼吸功能评估不仅可以了解患者肺损伤严重情况,还可进一步指导后续康复治疗。因此我们亟需一些评估手段来了解COVID-19患者呼吸功能情况。

(一)呼吸功能评估项目

评估项目应针对患者存在的功能障碍进行评估,项目包括但不限于:①呼吸功能评估,包括呼吸困难指数量表(常用的是Borg呼吸困难量表)、常规肺功能(pulmonary function test,PFT)评估,主要指标:VC(肺活量)、FVC(用力肺活量)、FEV1(第1秒用力肺活量)、FEV1/FVC、RV(残气)、TLC(肺总量)、DLco(肺一氧化碳弥散量)、Rtot(气道阻力)等。②运动功能评估,包括6 min步行试验(6 minutes walking test,6MWT)、心肺运动试验(cardiopulmonary exercise test,CPET)、2 min踏步试验及台阶试验等。③日常生活活动能力评估。④心理功能评估,主要是抑郁自评量表及焦虑自评量表等。其中,PFT及CPET是目前较为重要的用来评估COVID-19患者呼吸功能变化的检测方法。

PFT是检测呼吸系统疾病的重要辅助手段,可以将肺部的功能生理指标进行准确测量,检查诊断的过程相对较短,诊断准确度较高。肺功能主要用于检测呼吸道的通畅程度、肺容量的大小,对于早期检出肺损伤及气道病变,评估患者肺损伤的严重程度,评定药物或其他治疗方法的疗效,鉴别呼吸困难的原因,诊断病变部位、评估后期患者肺康复治疗有重要的临床价值。

CPET是一种客观评价循环、呼吸功能和运动耐力的无创性检测方法,综合应用呼吸气体实时监测分析技术、电子计算机和活动平板或功率踏车技术,实时检测在不同负荷下机体摄氧量(VO_2)和二氧化碳排出量(VCO_2)的动态变化,从而客观、定量、全面地评价循环、呼吸功能和运动耐力。心肺运动试验不同于肺功能,它不但可以动态观察患者呼吸功能储备,还可以研究循环系统的储备功能。是目前世界上应用较为普遍的综合评价机体心肺功能的检查手段。因此国外已将CPET检测技术应用于疾病的早期诊断、临床治疗的疗效、评估呼吸、循环系统和心肺康复方案制订等领域。

然而,PFT和CPET操作具有一定特殊性,过程中均存在一定的感染风险。需要采集患者呼出气体的容积和流量。操作过程中患者可能会出现咳嗽、咳痰、打喷嚏、牙龈出血、口腔开放性损伤,可能会发生血液、体液或分泌物等喷溅。尤其在患者用力呼气过程中,产生较大呼气流量会使污染物雾化到空气中,如果检测者是潜在COVID-19患者,会使病原体通过直接接触或气溶胶传播,发生医-患或者患-患之间的交叉感染。

因此,针对新冠肺炎患者进行呼吸功能评估虽然至关重要,但如何在呼吸功能评估过程中严格做好防控消毒措施,防止疾病的进一步传播扩散是我们必须攻克和解决的关键性问题。迫切需要我们严格做好受试者和检查室的准备、检测人员的防护、仪器的清洗和消毒等措施。

(二)疑似或者确诊COVID-19患者的呼吸功能评估

这部分患者传染性很强,必须在具备负压条件的检查

区域才能进行肺功能测定。我们推荐针对该类人群采用一人专用的简易肺功能仪来进行检测。简易肺功能仪专人使用,配备在COVID-19患者身边,通过视频等方法对其讲解使用方法,患者在负压病房或者其他隔离处即可自行完成检测,同时通过物联网技术和医疗信息技术,由患者把肺功能数据从检查仪器终端上传至肺功能医师工作终端,再由肺功能医师进行线上报告审核与电子签名,然后传输至医院信息化管理系统,实现肺功能报告无纸化电子档案管理,杜绝COVID-19传播风险。

部分简易肺功能仪采用"高灵敏度压差传感检测部件＋呼吸过滤装置"整体抛弃式使用方案,可有效克服医-患、患-患交叉感染的潜在风险。检测通气咬嘴套件是可以全面杜绝交叉感染的,采用双重空气隔离技术,能保证受试者呼出的气体停留在取压孔柱而短时间内不会与传感器部分的空气进行分子交换,达到隔离的作用。虽然简易肺功能仪独特的双重隔离专利技术能最大程度的减少感染风险,疫情期间仍建议一台测试仪一人使用,并且在测试后对仪器整体可采用酒精棉片擦拭消毒,减少和避免仪器手柄等空气暴露部分的潜在细菌病菌污染。

简易肺功能仪的优势就是简易便携,随时随地可以监测肺功能,且监测数据可通过系统云端大数据共享,根据医疗机构需求,统计检查结果及日常数据管理;医院可远端实时了解检查情况,同质化检查报告、相关量表化数据和曲线图形、质控信息等支持多中心联合筛查及分级诊疗模式。简易肺功能仪主要监测的指标包括用力 FVC、FEV1、FEV1/FVC 等,可以用来动态监测 COVID-19 患者肺功能,从而来评估疑似或确诊 COVID-19 患者的呼吸功能,便于出院后的制订康复方案及后续随访观察。

(三)COVID-19 治愈患者的呼吸功能评估

目前,大量 COVID-19 患者已得到及时有效的诊治,治愈后出院,这些患者肺脏损伤严重程度不一,评估这部分人群的呼吸功能、通气有效性及运动耐力有非常重要的临床价值。

这部分患者是根据国家卫健委颁布的新型冠状病毒感染的肺炎诊疗方案第 7 版诊疗方案确诊的 COVID-19 患者,并已经治愈,治愈标准:体温恢复正常 3 d 以上;呼吸道症状明显好转;肺部影像学显示急性渗出性病变明显改善;连续 2 次痰、鼻咽拭子等呼吸道标本核酸检测阴性(采样时间至少间隔 24 h)。并在出院 1 个月后进行复测,连续 2 次痰、鼻咽拭子等呼吸道标本核酸检测阴性(采样时间至少间隔 24 h)。

虽然这些患者已经达到临床治愈,但无法完全排除其复阳的可能。因此在对这类人群进行肺功能检查时仍要严格做好操作人员的防护、仪器的清洗和消毒、检查室的消毒等措施。建议这类患者在肺功能检测前需提供 1 周内 2 次核酸检测阴性的报告。

对治愈患者进行肺功能检查时应注意以下几点要求:

1. 操作人员在接诊过程要求受试者全程佩戴口罩,执行二级防护措施,做好个人防护。正确穿戴和脱摘用来防护的一次性乳胶检查手套、帽子和医用防护口罩,佩戴护目镜和防护服或隔离衣。严格执行手卫生;肺功能人员在诊疗过程中,未发现明显污染物时可以使用速干手消毒剂。任何情况下,接触患者血液、唾液或痰液等体液后,都应该立即严格按照《医务人员手卫生规范》的要求执行手卫生。每完成 1 例受试者均应更换手套并严格执行手卫生消毒。

2. 受试者进行肺功能检测过程中,一人一个房间,测定时使用一次性咬嘴和呼吸过滤器,用后统一销毁。

3. 操作者尽量向受试者详细讲解动作要领,减少受试者的测试次数,提高效率,缩短检查时间;同时检查操作者的座位方向应与受试者相同,切勿与受试者面对面就坐,以免受试者的呼出气直接排向操作者。

4. 每完成一名患者检测后,对常规肺功能仪器的管道、流量传感头、阀门、接口及呼吸面罩等配件需进行拆卸清洗和消毒:应用中性的戊二醛消毒液充分接触和浸泡 10～20 min(流量传感头中的密封圈不能进行浸泡消毒)。对于无法进行浸泡消毒的部分及肺功能仪器主机表面、仪器手柄、操作台面等物体进行表面消毒:每完成 1 例受试者的检查操作,可使用 75% 乙醇擦拭 2 遍,作用 3 min。

5. 检查室的消毒:操作中建议使用移动式空气消毒机进行消毒;每位患者检测完毕后在无人状态下持续使用紫外线照射消毒,每次≥30 min。但由于某些体描仪的箱体材质是树脂玻璃,长期使用紫外线照射可能出现裂纹,因此,针对此类材质的体描仪,建议用布遮挡玻璃再进行紫外线消毒。

三、COVID-19 患者呼吸功能康复

随着我国对 COVID-19 疫情的有效管控,新发病例显著减少,大部分患者治愈出院,但是我们发现部分 COVID-19 出院患者仍存在气促、喘憋等呼吸系统症状,这也是造成他们身体功能受限的主要原因。因此对 COVID-19 出院患者进行肺功能损害评估和呼吸功能康复成为工作重点。国家卫生健康委员会也在《关于做好新型冠状病毒肺炎出院患者跟踪随访工作的通知》中提到要为重症、危重症出院患者提供肺功能损害评估。所以对 COVID-19 患者制订长期的个性化的呼吸康复方案迫在眉睫。

近年来,呼吸康复医学在临床得以广泛应用,是由一系列科学有效的健康促进方法组成,通过规范的 PFT 或者全身功能的康复评估如 CPET 后开展的个体化治疗方案。呼吸康复训练操作简单便捷(居家可以完成)、效果确切,适用人群广泛,其逐渐被医护人员和患者认可。呼吸康复主要内容包括运动训练、呼吸肌训练、教育及心理行为干预、氧疗和无创通气、营养治疗等。其中,呼吸肌和运动训练是肺康复中最重要的组成部分,对治疗效果起到关键性作用。前文提到新冠病毒主要引起肺损伤,导致患者出现呼吸功能、运动耐力等下降。呼吸康复可以提高 COVID-19 患者心肺活动耐力,改善呼吸功能和心理状态,还有利于患者逐步地恢复参与社会活动的能力。研究表明,在疾病急性期的病情稳定阶段,呼吸康复介入越早预后越好。

虽然 COVID-19 是乙类传染病,但是按甲类传染病管理,考虑到确诊患者都是在定点医院进行救治,同时对重

症和危重症的住院患者主要以挽救生命的疾病救治为主,所以呼吸康复主要针对出院患者来实施。

依据《新型冠状病毒肺炎疫情期间康复诊疗工作综合指导意见(第2版)》的要求,根据康复医学的原理,对患者肺炎的相关症状、心肺活动耐力、体能和日常生活活动进行简要的评估,个体化制订了康复诊疗规范,以改善不同病情阶段患者的整体功能,促进生活质量的全面提高。

(一)出院患者的界定

符合《新型冠状病毒感染的肺炎诊疗方案(试行第7版)》的疑似病例/确诊病例的诊断标准,经治愈出院的患者。

(二)出院患者的呼吸康复目标、措施及评估

1. 呼吸康复目标 旨在改善肺功能、减轻患者的呼吸困难、乏力等症状、提高运动耐力及生活质量、改善患者心理障碍及社会适应能力等。

2. 呼吸康复措施

(1)呼吸训练:包括以下三方面。

1)呼吸模式训练:包括体位管理、调整呼吸节奏及呼吸模式、胸廓活动度训练、调动呼吸肌群参与等技术。具体包括①缩唇呼吸:嘱患者用鼻子缓慢吸气,呼气时嘴型像吹蜡烛或者气球一样,缓慢呼气延长时间。5~10次/min,3~5 min为一组,3~5组/d。②体位管理主要是改善呼吸困难的姿势:当出现气促时,身体保持半前倾姿势,同时配合缩唇呼吸调整呼吸频率。③胸廓活动度训练主要通过胸廓扩张训练:不论患者处坐位、半卧位还是站立位均可完成此训练,嘱患者将双手置于胸部,吸气时用胸廓将双手推开,可在相应区域给予轻微的阻力以增强抗阻意识,视自身情况憋气几秒钟,再将气体缓慢呼出。5~10次/min,3~5 min为一组,3~5组/d。

2)吸气肌训练:采用初始负荷为最大吸气压的30%,5次吸气为一组,2次吸气时间间隔大于6s,每日训练做6组,每组中间休息1 min。

3)排痰训练:咳痰困难的患者,可应用主动循环呼吸技术首先,嘱患者平静状态下进行腹式呼吸,鼻吸气,口呼气,此阶段可重复多次,以达到呼吸稳定的状态;其次,嘱患者吸气,屏气3 s,再呼气,再屏气3 s,直到达到最大吸气量;再次,经口呼出,此阶段可做2~3次;最后,嘱患者呵气1~2次进行排痰。在排痰过程中出现不适,应停止,并休息,必要时及时就医。

(2)运动训练如下

1)有氧运动:有氧运动是一项个性化的训练项目,建议包括运动频率(frequency)、运动强度(intensity)、运动时间(time)和运动类型(type)4个要素,即FITT原则。出院患者可在家进行有氧运动,遵循的原则是循序渐进,由低强度到中等强度逐步进阶。运动频率为1周3~5次,运动时间以10~30 min为宜。

CPET是评定有氧运动强度的有效方法,达到最大耗氧量(VO_2 max)20%~40%的运动量为低强度,60%~80%的运动量为高强度。在运动过程中,患者应用Borg呼吸困难评分表进行自评,并监测血氧饱和度,血氧饱和度低于90%时应及时停止训练。在此过程中如遇喘憋、乏力、心悸、站立不稳等不适应,应及时停止训练活动进行休息,必要时及时就医。

2)力量训练:力量训练有助于增强患者的肌肉力量,减轻呼吸困难等症状,提高日常生活活动能力。力量训练推荐使用渐进性的抗阻训练法,初期可采用徒手力量训练的方式,再循序渐进到轻重量。每个目标肌群的训练频率是每周2~3次,每次1~3组。

3)平衡训练:此项训练主要针对合并平衡功能障碍的患者,应予以平衡训练,可在专业康复治疗师指导下的徒手平衡训练、平衡训练仪等。

(3)日常生活活动干预:主要在出院1个月后进行。对于新冠肺炎患者建议出院4周后需要关注社会参与度等较高级别日常活动能力,建议采用工具性日常活动能力(购物、外出活动、食物烹调、家务活动、洗衣服、服用药物等)进行评定,并采取针对性治疗。需综合考虑患者在完成这些活动时的心理及躯体功能能力,可以通过模拟现实场景进行训练,发现患者参与日常生活的障碍点,在专业人员指导下进行针对性的干预。

(4)心理康复:此外心理建设也是新冠肺炎患者康复的重要组成部分,可在心理咨询师参与下进行康复辅助,主要解决的心理问题主要包括情绪问题、认知问题、人际问题及睡眠问题等。

(5)营养支持:对于重症、长期卧床、合并多种基础疾病的患者,应特别注意营养不良风险,一旦发现营养不良问题,及时请营养专家进行营养学评估,并且遵照营养专家的建议调整膳食方案。

目前随着治愈出院人数逐渐增加,新冠肺炎疫情防控工作已经进入一个新阶段。临床上主要以救治为主,而患者出院后逐步转向以功能康复为主,康复治疗将进一步发挥重要作用。因此对患者进行针对性的康复医学评估,制定科学、可行的规范化治疗方案,以更好地促进患者全面恢复身心功能、生活质量和社会参与能力至关重要。

参 考 文 献

[1] 国家卫生健康委办公厅,国家中医药管理局办公室.新型冠状病毒感染的肺炎诊疗方案(试行第7版).国卫办医函[2020]184号,2020年3月3日.

[2] Wan Yushun, Shang Jian, Graham Rachel, et al. Receptor recognition by novel coronavirus from Wuhan: An analysis based on decade-long structural studies of SARS. Journal of Virology,2020,7(94).

[3] Younan P, Iampietro M, Nishida A, et al. Ebola virus binding to Tim-1 on T lymphocytes induces a cytokine storm. mBio, 2017,8(5):e00845-17.

[4] 高钰琪.基于新冠肺炎病理生理机制的治疗策略.中国病理生理杂志,2020:1-5.

[5] Miller M R, Crapo R, Hankinson J, et al. General considerations for lung function testing. The European Respiratory

Journal,2005,26(1):153-161.
[6] Graham Brian L, Steenbruggen Irene, Miller Martin R, et al. Standardization of Spirometry 2019 Update. An Official American Thoracic Society and European Respiratory Society Technical Statement. American Journal of Respiratory and Critical Care Medicine,2019,200(8):e70-e88.
[7] 高怡,郑劲平.肺功能检查的感染预防与控制.中华结核和呼吸杂志,2005(7):486-488.
[8] 宋元林,李丽.肺功能检查交叉感染预防和控制.中国实用内科杂志,2012,32(8):601-604.
[9] 复旦大学附属中山医院新冠肺炎诊治专家组,宋元林.复旦大学附属中山医院新型冠状病毒肺炎疑似病例诊治方案(2020 v.1).中国临床医学:1-3.
[10] 周怡,王巍,易宾,等.预防SARS患者肺功能检查的交叉感染.中华医院感染学杂志,2003(11):8.
[11] 刘洁,张静,白春学.物联网医学在肺功能随访与监测中的应用.中华结核和呼吸杂志,2014,37(4):316-317.
[12] 国家卫生健康委员会.医疗机构内新型冠状病毒感染预防与控制技术指南(第1版)国卫办医函〔2020〕65号[EB/OL].
[13] 国家卫生健康委员会,医务人员手卫生规范(WS/T313-2019)[Z].2019年11月.
[14] 高怡,郑劲平.呼吸过滤器在肺功能实验室中的应用.国际呼吸杂志,2006,26(11):825-829.
[15] 郑劲平,高怡.肺功能检查实用指南.北京:人民卫生出版社,2009
[16] 中华人民共和国卫生部.医疗机构消毒技术规范(WS/T 367—2012)[Z],2012年4月.
[17] 中华人民共和国卫生部.医院空气净化管理规范(WS/T 368—2012)[Z],2012年4月.
[18] 国家卫生健康委办公厅.关于做好新型冠状病毒肺炎出院患者跟踪随访工作的通知.国卫办医函〔2020〕142号,2020年2月.
[19] 中华人民共和国国家卫生健康委员会,国家卫生健康委办公厅.新型冠状病毒肺炎疫情期间康复诊疗工作综合指导意见(第二版)[EB/OL].(2020-02-18)[2020-03-16].http://www.carm.org.cn/Home/Article/detail/id/2597.html.
[20] VatwaniArchana. Pursed Lip Breathing Exercise to Reduce Shortness of Breath. Archives of physical medicine and rehabilitation,2019,100(1):189-190.
[21] Marques A, Pinho C, De Francesco S, et al. A randomized controlled trial of respiratory physiotherapy in lower respiratory tract infections. Respiratory Medicine,2020,162(2):58 65.
[22] Ang M, Yuping Y, Yin X, et al. Chest physiotherapy for pneumonia in adults. Cochrane Database Syst Revi,2010(2):CD006338.
[23] Garber C E, Blissmer B, Deschenes M R, et al. American College of Sports Medicine position stand: quantity and quality of exercise for developing and maintaining cardiorespiratory, musculoskeletal, and neuromotor fitness in apparently healthy adults: guidance for prescribing exercise. Med Sci Sport Exerc,2011,43(7):1334-1359.
[24] Ngai J C, Ko F W, Ng S S, et al. The long-term impact of severe acute respiratory syndrome on pulmonary function, exercise capacity and health status. Respirology,2010,15(3):543-550.
[25] Zalevli S, Karaali H K, Ilgin D, et al. Effect of home based pulmonary rehabilitation in patients with idiopathic pulmonary fibrosis. Multidiscip Respir Med,2010,5(1):31-37.

6 不同肺功能检测在小气道阻塞中优劣敏感性的对比及小气道的靶向药物治疗

苗丽君　黄凤祥

肺是一个分支结构，从气管(第1代)一直分支到肺泡(第23代)。小气道是指内径小于2mm的细小支气管，是由气道分支的第4～13代产生的(平均第8代)，通常位于第8代气道至呼吸性细支气管，占肺总体积的98.8%。小气道可以看作是由膜性细支气管、呼吸性细支气管和肺泡管形成的气流系统。膜性细支气管包括终末细支气管，被覆带有纤毛的柱状上皮细胞，呼吸性细支气管上皮由柱状上皮过渡到立方形上皮，通向被覆扁平上皮的肺泡管和肺泡囊。小气道具有管腔纤细，管壁菲薄，纤毛上皮细胞减少，无软骨支撑等特点，所以管腔在受到损伤时容易狭窄和闭塞。

一、小气道的病理改变与肺功能的关系

(一)慢阻肺(COPD)患者的小气道组织病理改变与肺功能的关系

COPD患者的气道在香烟烟雾、病毒、细菌等因素的刺激下引起免疫反应、成纤维细胞修复和细胞外基质之间相互作用，导致的主要病理改变如下。

1. 气道重塑　当气道管壁及黏膜遭受损伤后，基底细胞充当纤毛和分泌细胞的前体细胞，但是香烟烟雾等有害颗粒使基底细胞发生上皮间质转化(EMT)，COPD患者气道发生异常的上皮重塑，常见变化包括杯状细胞化生，基底细胞增生和鳞状化生。EMT在COPD小气道上皮细胞中持续存在。研究表明：与非吸烟对照组相比，COPD小气道上皮细胞中的肌成纤维细胞标志物α平滑肌肌动蛋白和波形蛋白增加，并且与气流受限负相关，紧密连接蛋白、闭合蛋白、Zona occludens-1和E-钙黏蛋白的水平降低。另外，在COPD小气道中存在纤维化，黏膜及管壁的厚度增加，细胞外基质蛋白(ECM)沉积增加。Eurlings等结果显示，与吸烟对照相比，GOLD Ⅱ期和GOLD Ⅳ期COPD患者的小气道壁总胶原蛋白水平显著增加。ECM的降解受基质金属蛋白酶(MMP)等内源性蛋白酶的调节。因此，MMP和金属蛋白酶组织抑制剂(TIMPs)之间的平衡对于ECM稳态至关重要。慢性阻塞性肺疾病、肺气肿患者肺组织破坏的潜在原因是与炎症相关的MMPs(MMP-2，MMP-9和MMP-12)增加，导致MMPs和TIMPs之间的

失衡，弹性纤维的形成和修复缺陷。COPD中其他重要的ECM变化包括(小的)气道壁中胶原蛋白沉积增加及胶原蛋白原纤维的结构变化，小气道外膜中核心蛋白聚糖沉积缺乏等。

2. 黏液堵塞　在正常肺的较小气道中，纤毛细胞和杯状细胞均较少，Club细胞变为气道表面的常见细胞。香烟烟雾相关的有毒颗粒和气体会损害上皮并破坏黏膜表面的紧密连接，从而降低黏膜纤毛清除率并增加上皮通透性。这些结构变化包括杯状细胞和鳞状细胞化生，纤毛细胞数量减少和黏膜下腺肥大。电子显微镜研究表明，在慢性支气管炎的受试者中，在健康气道中观察到的覆盖在气道表面的不连续的黏液斑块被连续黏液层所替代。香烟烟雾中的化合物(如丙烯醛)会直接或通过激活表皮生长因子受体(EGFR)增加黏液的产生。小气道中杯状细胞的增生、纤毛细胞的消失及残留纤毛功能的降低，有助于黏液渗出物积聚。另外，慢阻肺患者气道黏液的固体含量增加，其生物物理特性改变为不易清除的高黏度的弹性黏液。黏液分泌过多会导致物理气流阻塞或留存病原微生物而引起小气道功能障碍，从而进一步促进组织炎症和破坏。研究表明，COPD患者中小气道的黏液阻塞与疾病严重程度和早期死亡风险相关。

3. 免疫细胞浸润　大量研究表明COPD小气道中巨噬细胞、中性粒细胞、$CD4^+$和$CD8^+$ T细胞的数量增加，小气道中淋巴滤泡数量随COPD严重程度而增加。有研究报告显示，COPD中FEV1下降与巨噬细胞、PMN、$CD4^+$和$CD8^+$ T细胞及B细胞浸润气道有关。此外，一项将肺功能正常的吸烟者的肺组织与COPD患者的肺组织(GOLD 1-4)进行比较的研究表明，在严重(GOLD 3)和非常严重(GOLD 4)COPD中，炎症免疫细胞浸润与第三淋巴器官形成的急剧增加有关。这些均提示了先天性免疫和适应性免疫参与了COPD的发生和发展。

(二)支气管哮喘患者的小气道组织病理改变与与肺功能的关系

哮喘的本质是气道的慢性炎症，这种炎症可累及大、小气道。通过手术标本或经支气管活检等侵入性的技术手段已经证明，哮喘的炎症和重塑也发生在哮喘患者的周围气道。在因哮喘严重恶化而死亡的患者的周围气道中

发现了剧烈的炎症细胞浸润、管腔堵塞和气道结构异常。网状基底膜(RBM)是气道重塑的标志，由沉积的细胞外基质蛋白(ECM)组成，主要包括胶原蛋白、纤连蛋白和蛋白聚糖(PGs)等。一些研究发现，轻度哮喘患者的小气道中也存在气道炎症、气道重塑和增多的基质沉积，这表明小气道是所有严重程度阶段的疾病发生病理改变的累及部位。小气道受累是哮喘发展的先决条件。小气道功能障碍增加了未控制疾病的风险，并预测哮喘恶化的风险增加，还与重要的临床表现有关，如气道高反应性、夜间哮喘、严重哮喘、运动诱发的哮喘、哮喘症状增加等有关。

二、小气道阻力在气道总阻力中的地位的历史变迁

小气道阻力是否在气道总阻力中占主要地位，对这个问题的认识经历了一个发展变化的过程。最早是瑞士的生理学家弗里茨·罗勒(Fritz Rohrer)在1915年提出的小气道是是阻碍正常气流的主要部位、是气道阻力形成的主要因素的假说，受到了广泛关注。1963年魏贝尔(Weibel)出版的关于人体肺形态的经典著作，提供了定量的解剖信息，表明随着气道分支越分越细，气道的总横截面积越大。后来，Macklem和Mead通过将导管放置在直径<2 mm的气道中并测量气道直径的方法直接测量了气道阻力。这项开创性的研究表明，直径<2 mm的气道实际上占喉部以下总阻力的不到10%。此后不久，Hogg、Macklem和Thurlbeck等研究了肺气肿患者死亡后的气道阻力，发现小气道阻力较健康人增加了4～40倍。进一步，他们使用死后的支气管造影图显示黏液堵塞及小气道的狭窄和闭塞是与阻力大幅度增加相关的关键病理特征。这些发现推动了Mead在1970年发表了开创性的社论，认为小气道是正常肺内的一个静默区域，在该区域中疾病可以在多年内积累而不会被发现。而当肺气肿发生以后，这些小气道又成为肺气肿气道阻塞的主要部位。

正常健康人气道的横截面积从气管中的总面积2.5mm^{2}迅速增加到终末细支气管中的大约180mm^2。在肺气肿患者中，基于显微CT成像的技术发现，终末支气管的数目、平均管腔横截面面积、最小的管腔直径都减少或缩小。Koo等报道尽管没有肺气肿，但终末和呼吸性细支气管数量减少了，提示了小气道病变早于肺气肿。在GOLD 1级患者中，终末和呼吸细支气管的减少分别为29%和41%，在GOLD 2级患者中，分别为40%和53%。另有研究发现，在IV期COPD肺中，有90%的末梢细支气管闭塞。根据泊肃叶定律，气道阻力与气道半径的四次方成反比，所以健康受试者中大部分气流阻力位于近端气道中，而小气道阻力只占气道总阻力的10%左右。当小气道狭窄和闭塞时，半径减小50%，电阻会增加16倍。也有研究认为：气道可以看作是并联电路布置，使用以下公式计算每次气道产生的总阻力：1/RT = 1/R1 + 1/R2 + 1/R3 + 1/R4，以此类推，可以得出50%的气道阻塞才能使气道阻力加倍。总之，COPD小气道阻力增加(≥4倍)主要是由于较多的小气道直径的总体减小所致。FEV1随着年龄的增长而逐渐下降的原因是，随着时间的推移，终末细支气管的并行减法可能对总阻力几乎没有影响，直到大量气道被破坏为止。因此小气道被称为"沉默地带"，对小气道敏感而及时的功能检测对发现疾病的早期阶段有重要作用。

三、小气道的功能障碍的肺功能检测及各自优缺点对比

(一)肺量计测定

肺量计检查是肺功能检查中最常用的检查。第1秒用力呼气容积(forced expiratory volume in one second, FEV1)是肺通气功能的最主要指标之一。在健康人，气道阻力发生的主要部位在第4～8级气道。因此，FEV1在主要反映大、中气道的功能，慢阻肺患者肺通气功能损害的严重程度依据FEV1进行判断。FEV1/FVC是判断气流阻塞的主要指标，但不能准确反映阻塞的程度。最大呼气中期流量(maximal mid-expiratory flow, MMEF)又称用力呼气中期流量(FEF 25%～75%)是判断小气道阻塞的主要指标。然而，FEF25%～75%具有内在可变性和对肺容量的依赖性，使其在临床上的应用存在问题。其一：FEF25%～75%敏感性不够，如FEV1/FVC＞75%，即使小气道发生了病理改变，FEF 25%～75%亦呈现正常值。其二：受FVC的影响大，且FEF25%～75%不经肺活量校正，重复性差。实际上，美国胸科学会已建议FEF25%～75%不能用于诊断小气道功能障碍(SAD)。有研究认为，FEV3/FVC比值可作为小气道疾病评估的可选检测指标。James E等对第三次国家健康与营养检查调查(NHANES III)中从不吸烟者和现吸烟者的数据库进行分析，发现对于不吸烟者来说，从20～80岁这60年的年龄跨度上，FEV1/FVC从85.8%下降至74.2%，而1-FEV3/FVC从2.2%增加至12.6%。FEV3/FVC与年龄的相关性高于FEV1/FVC。而对于现吸烟者FEV1/FVC进一步降低，1-FEV3/FVC进一步升高，并且随着年龄的增长，FEV3/FVC的变化大于FEV1/FVC。1-FEV3/FVC用于评估长时间常数肺单位改善比率，当FEV1/FVC下降时，FEV3/FVC下降，1-FEV3/FVC上升。而这些指标比FEF25%～75%更为敏感。Gibbons等建议组胺刺激后FVC的变化比FEV1的下降在探测哮喘患者的小气道功能障碍中更优，FVC下降表明小气道关闭和气体潴留。一项对入选国家研究所的《严重哮喘研究计划》中患者的研究发现，FVC与RV/TLC呈负相关。这表明(至少在小组级别)FVC在评估SAD方面有一定的实用性，特别是FVC易检测，因此可作为连续评估来监测SAD。其他具有被建议用于评估小气道疾病包括FVC与减慢肺活量的比率(SVC)。

肺容量检查是评估气道陷闭和肺过度充气的敏感的检测方法，RV是测定小气道功能障碍的重要指标，可能在哮喘发生异常肺容量之前异常增高，其与哮喘患者小气道阻力相关。相较于TLC，RV/TLC对判断小气道陷闭更为敏感。

(二)体描法

体描法肺容量检查尤其适用于气道阻塞严重、气体分布不均的受试者,是评估肺容量的气体潴留和肺过度充气的敏感方法。肺过度充气可以被认为是呼气末肺容积的异常升高。气道变窄导致呼气时间延长,气道过早闭合导致气体滞留。FRC的高值,RV或RV/TLC表示肺过度充气,提示存在SAD。体描法比用力呼气流量检测小气道阻塞更灵敏。研究发现:在哮喘患者中,在肺量计测定异常之前就可以出现RV升高。而应用孟鲁司特治疗后,哮喘症状改善与RV降低有关,但与肺量计参数无相关性。Sorkness等研究证实,RV/TLC比值在重度哮喘患者高于非重度哮喘患者,与FVC成反比。在慢阻肺中,因气体潴留导致TLC升高,RV/TLC对于气体潴留可能是更有用的标记物。要注意的是:正常值的上限随年龄、性别而变化,因此对气体潴留的评估预测值可能比绝对值会准确。

体描法在进行肺容量检测的同时还可以测定气道阻力,常用指标有:气道阻力(Raw)、气道传导率(Gaw)、比气道阻力(sRaw)、比气道传导率(sGaw)。体描法气道阻力的测定因综合考虑了气流驱动压的影响,因此对气道阻塞的判断更为敏感和精确。但是,它不能区分阻塞的部位、不局限于小气道的检测限制了它在远端气道诊断和监测中的应用。

比气道阻力(sRaw)在气道的阻塞、阻塞的可逆性判断方面更有价值。sRaw分为总比气道阻力(sRtot)和有效比气道阻力(sReff),与sReff相比,sRtot更能敏感地反映外周气道功能失调。如果将流量绘制在垂直轴上,变换容积绘制在水平轴上,就获得了闭合曲线,即比气道阻力环,呼吸环倒数的斜率代表比气道阻力。分析比气道阻力环的形式能提供相关的病理生理信息。陡峭的曲线排除气流阻塞。曲线平坦表示阻塞,可能是吸气或呼气期。环的展开表明通气的不均一性,可能是气体陷闭或肺气肿和支气管炎。如果呼吸部分呈高尔夫球拍状,代表肺弹性阻力下降和气体滞留,在肺气肿、慢性气道阻塞中常见。中央气道狭窄或阻塞,环呈现腊肠形状;膈肌升高、肥胖和或呼气末关闭,环呈"V"形;上气道阻塞时环呈现明显"S"形。

(三)一口气氮冲洗法(SBNW)和重复呼吸氮冲洗法(MBNW)

一口气氮冲洗法(SBNW)始于1960年,使用惰性气体冲洗技术检测外周气道通气的不均一性(III相斜率)和气道闭合(闭合容积),因此能够间接检测气道阻塞患者小气道的功能性病变。氮气法的呼出曲线在X-Y记录仪上是一条上扬型曲线,曲线分为4个相。第I相来自解剖无效腔的呼出气,不含指标气体,氮为零。第II相为肺泡与无效腔的混合气,指示气体浓度急剧上升,曲线斜行向上。第III相为各区域肺泡呼出气,由于各区域气体同步呼出,呼出气中的指示气体浓度大致相同,曲线呈高浓度上的水平线,有肺泡坪之称。第IV相下肺小气道开始闭合,具有最低氮浓度的重力依赖性肺区域中的气道关闭,从上肺呼出含较高浓度的指示气体,曲线徒然上升成上扬型。

第III相与第IV相连接点是下肺小气道开始关闭的标记,该点至呼气终点的肺容量称闭合容积(CV),闭合容积与残气之和称闭合容量(closing capacity, CC)。一般用CV/VC%及CC/TLC%来表示,以实测值占正常预计值加以判断。正常值CV=0.40L,CC=1.90L,CC/TLC=32%。临床上小气道有阻塞性病变时,呼气时小气道容易闭合,使闭合容积增加,可用作早期诊断;III相斜率(SIII)增加,氮浓度差($\triangle N_2/L$)的增高提示气体分布不均,见于肺气肿患者。在一些吸烟者中,闭合体积和III相斜率都是异常的。而且,这些异常与纯传导性(膜性)及呼吸性细支气管的病理异常较FEF25%~75%具有良好的相关性。

SBNW指数已被用于哮喘和COPD的评估和治疗反应。与健康对照组相比,FEV1正常的哮喘患者CV和III期斜率增加。此外,病情加重的频率与SIII相关,提示SIII可能是控制不良患者的一个敏感指标。此外,严重、激素依赖性哮喘患者的SBNW指数比轻、中度哮喘患者有更明显的变化。在吸烟者可见到CV增加,提示SBNW对气道的早期变化很敏感,但是在COPD中使用该指标是有争议的。Buist等证明,在9~11年的随访中,许多肺量计功能正常但小气道指数异常的吸烟者并没有继续发展为阻塞性肺功能。尽管有敏感性,但SBNW对小气道病变并不是特异的。每一代传导气管的变化也会影响III相斜率。因此,虽然可以推断正常的SIII表明不存在小气道疾病,但该测试无法定位病理的解剖位置。

MBNW是在SBNW技术上的一种改进。其中的一常用指标肺清除指数(LCI)常用来测量肺内混合气体的效率。研究发现:气道阻塞和过度通气患者的LCI均值为12.6高于健康对照组的7.0。根据肺的理论模型已提出MBNW可用于区分源自肺泡腔(sacin)及较近端的传导气道(Scond)的通气不均匀性,其中,Scond由逐步冲洗过程中发生的呼吸次数函数的III相斜率的逐渐增加计算得出,而Sacin由Scond校正的初始阶段III相斜率计算得出。计算Sacin和Scond可以表明不均匀性的起源是在外周气道还是在中央气道。尽管Scond和Sacin并未与气道和实质的病理变化直接相关,但各种建模研究表明,这些指标能反映出肺泡和气道的功能变化。Verbanck等研究表明:DLCO和CT显示有肺气肿的COPD患者较没有显示肺气肿的患者Sacin更高,吸入组胺后产生的支气管收缩可增加Scond,但对Sacin无作用。对于有10年以上吸烟史的吸烟者来说可见到Sacin和Scon的异常,而肺功能检查只有在吸了20年.包烟之后才会变得异常。提示Sacin和Scond在反映早期的气道改变方面其敏感性要优于肺量计法。William McNulty等认为从理论上讲,任何第一代传导性气道的异常都可能导致Scond的异常,因此它并不只局限于小气道。另外,理论建模是对正常受试者进行了气道疾病定位的建模,可能与疾病状态不同,因此解剖定位可能并不准确。

(四)脉冲振荡技术(impulse oscillometry system IOS)

IOS是在FOT基础上发展起来的,其是通过外部发生器产生矩形电磁脉冲,通过扩音器转变为各种频率的机械波叠加在被检者静息呼吸上,滤除由自主呼吸产生的低频部分,连续记录在外加振荡频率下的气道压力与流速,测得一系列阻抗参数值。

呼吸阻抗（Impedance，简称Zrs），俗称呼吸阻力，是指呼吸的黏性阻力、弹性阻力和惯性阻力的总和。Rrs代表呼吸阻抗中的黏性阻力部分。R5代表气道总阻力，R20代表中心气道阻力，其值正常应在预计值的150%以内；周边气道阻力很小，用R5-R20代表。在健康人，Rrs与振荡频率无关，当存在气道阻塞时，Rrs成为频率依赖性。电抗（Xrs）代表呼吸阻抗中弹性阻力和惯性阻力之和。X5代表周边弹性阻力，其预计值与实测值之差不大于0.2kPa/(L·s)为正常。Xrs取决于肺的弹性和惯性特性，与频率依赖有关。在低频时，Xrs为负，主要代表肺的弹性阻力。在高频下，Xrs为正，由肺的惯性阻力决定。在某个地方弹性和惯性相等且相反，Xrs为0，这称为共振频率（Fres），它是支气管功能检查中最为敏感的指标，其敏感度为FEV1的2倍。正常人Fres不超过10Hz。电抗面积（AX）包括从最低频率到Fres的电抗曲线下的面积，在任何肺部周围疾病中也会增加。

1. IOS与气道疾病　在气道阻塞性疾病及小气道疾病方面可见到IOS参数异常。在支气管哮喘患者中，可见到R5、Fres和AX升高，而X5值更负。在支气管激发试验中，观察到类似的反应。FEV1降低20%相当于X5降低50%，这已被证明X5是识别支气管高反应性的更敏感参数。一项对2054名COPD（GOLD标准）、233位非吸烟对照和322位吸烟者的研究显示：COPD与R5，R5-R20和电抗增加有关。但是，有5%～10%的具有正常肺活量测定法的吸烟者具有"异常"的IOS。这些受试者的FEV1较低（但正常），是年龄较大、重度吸烟的患者，反映出IOS能检测出肺活量测定法无法诊断的早期小气道疾病。尽管早期COPD的Rrs确实有所增加，电抗可以更好地鉴定疾病的严重程度并且与其他参数包括FEV1和过度通气的关系有更密切的关系。

2. IOS参数与临床症状存在相关关系　Tomoshi-Takeda等使用IOS和肺活量测定仪评估了哮喘患者近端和外周气道功能与健康状况，呼吸困难和疾病控制之间的关系。结果证明，通过IOS评估，除了近端气道功能（R20）外，外周气道功能（R5-R20和X5）与健康状况（生活质量评分AQLQ，圣乔治评分SGRQ），呼吸困难评分（BDI）和疾病控制（哮喘控制问卷ACQ评分）显著相关。相比之下，肺活量指数（FEV1）对健康状况或呼吸困难没有显著影响。这提示IOS指数与肺活量指数相比与临床症状的关系更大。

3. IOS与肺量计在检测敏感性的比较　在一些研究中已经报道，IOS能够识别肺活量方法未检测到的远端气道阻力增加，从而将健康受试者与呼吸系统疾病患者区分开。有研究者对世界贸易中心（WTC）倒闭后，出现新发的呼吸道症状而肺活量测定法显示正常气道功能的174名患者进行了调查研究，发现这些患者通过射线照相可以看到支气管壁增厚和空气滞留，表明这些有症状个体可能具有常规肺活量测定法（包括MEF 25%～75%）无法检测到的远端气道功能异常。通过IOS对他们进行检测，发现尽管肺活量测定结果正常，但在5 Hz，5~20 Hz的平均电阻和电抗面积（AX）均有增加，支气管扩张后电阻和电抗恢复正常。IOS较肺活量测定能更好地反映出小气道的功能。因此，当肺活量测定结果正常时，IOS对远端气道功能的检查对于评估有职业和环境危害的受试者可能具有重要的价值。

钟南山院士研究小组在使用EB-OCT进行客观评估的基础上，比较了肺活量测定法和IOS在重度吸烟者和COPD中小气道疾病的诊断价值。发现Fres和外周气道阻力（R5-R20）的诊断价值高于FEV1%预测值和MMEF，可以区分从未吸烟者与重度吸烟者及Ⅰ型COPD患者的重度吸烟者中的小气道疾病。Piorunek等对COPD患者和对照组进行了肺量计和IOS测定，旨在评估R5-R20，MMEF和FEV3/FVC在评估慢性阻塞性肺部小气道阻塞中的作用。结果显示COPD患者的FEV3/FVC和MMEF显著降低，R5-R20差值增大；这种变化取决于气道阻塞的严重程度。R5-R20反映MMEF的敏感性为84%，特异性为44.2%，PPV为72.4%，NPV为61.3%。因此，R5-R20差值在评估小气道阻塞方面优于肺活量测定法。R5-R20反映MMEF的高灵敏度使IOS方法对检测轻度肺损伤特别有用，而肺活量FEV3/FVC比值的高特异性使其有助于排除小气道阻塞。因此，这两种方法是互补的。

IOS检查方便，少受患者配合影响，重复性好，在识别早期小气道疾病较肺量计更加敏感。与体描相比，其阻力测定有很好的特异性，能区分阻塞发生的部位（中心或周边）、严重程度及呼吸动力学特征等，更有助于疾病的早期诊断。主要的局限性是缺乏参考值以及对不同疾病状况的广泛评估。另一个限制可能是其成本和缺乏便携性。因此，缩小外形尺寸，使其便于携带的技术的发展将使IOS在常规临床实践中成为肺活量测定的可行替代方案。

（五）呼出气一氧化氮（eNO）

呼出气一氧化氮（eNO），是气道炎症生物标志物。一方面，eNO变化早于肺功能的变化与临床症状，可用于早期诊断。另一方面，由于嗜酸性炎症时显著升高，可用于炎症分型。另外其还可以预测激素疗效、管理预后等。eNO表现出流量依赖性，呼气流速不同反映不同部位的气道炎症，低流速（50ml/s 口呼气测定）时，检测FeNO主要反映的是大气道炎症，高流速（50～350ml/s 多口气变流速呼气测定）时，检测CaNO主要反映的是肺泡及周边的小气道炎症，10ml/s流速单鼻孔抽气时检测FnNO反映上气道炎症。

FeNO已广泛应用于哮喘的临床研究和实践。无论是在稳定期还是在病情加重期，中央气道似乎都是NO产生的主要场所。严重哮喘患者的肺泡内NO浓度升高，与肺泡嗜酸性炎症和其他小气道功能障碍相关。刘琳等发现哮喘患者小气道功能异常组FeNO、lgE、EOS、阻抗面积（AX）及Fres水平明显高于小气道功能正常组，提示FeNO水平和IOS指标是诊断哮喘小气道功能异常的敏感特异性指标，二者联合能更好的评估哮喘患者小气道的功能。FeNO在COPD中的作用尚不明确。有研究报道FeNO与FEV1和氧饱和度负相关。国内董燕等对喘息的患者检测发现在排除哮喘影响后，FeNO与吸烟、ICS、FEV1/FVC、MEF25、MEF50、MEF75仍呈负相关，并提示当老年人 FeNO>40.5 ppb 时可判断为老年性小气道功能障碍。

周围呼吸道炎症和功能障碍是 COPD 发病机制中的关键因素。一氧化氮的呼出肺泡部分（CaNO）是肺周围炎症的间接生物标志物。Lehtimaki 等证实，肺泡炎患者的肺泡 NO 水平高于哮喘患者，哮喘患者的支气管 NO 水平高于前者。在肺泡炎患者中，肺泡 NO 与转移因子和肺泡体积相关，而哮喘患者支气管 NO 与哮喘患者的高反应性有关。两组患者使用类固醇治疗后 FeNO 均有改善，表明干预治疗后 FeNO 有反应。Santus 等研究发现：在 COPD 中，CaNO 与气道阻力、RV/TLC 和 FEV1 存在相关关系，在应用 LABA 后，FeNO、CaNO 均比基线显著降低，CaNO 的变化与肺活量的变化和 RV/TLC 相关，而与 FEV1 无关。证明了在 COPD 中，CaNO 水平与周围气道功能障碍程度之间存在直接相关性。CANO 水平减少与反映空气滞留的功能参数的改善有关。

eNO 由于其操作简单、无创、重复性好等广泛应用于临床。然而，要注意 NO 在肺泡和气道腔之间的反向扩散，NO 会从气道向下扩散到肺泡，从而使肺泡 NO 升高，气道测量 NO 减少。在气道狭窄或闭塞的疾病状态下，NO 反向扩散较少，导致 FENO 较高，肺泡浓度较低。还应该注意的是，吸烟、饮食、环境、运动、烟酒都会影响 eNO 的测量值，检测时要注意这些影响因素。

四、小气道功能检测的对比及存在的问题

上述的小气道功能检测方法各有自己的优缺点，而目前小气道的肺功能检测没有一个统一的"金标准"。Usmani 等检索 Pubmed 数据库，对使用不同的方法进行小气道功能研究的相关文献进行梳理，在 837 篇文章中筛选出有价值的 17 篇文献，它们使用不同的 SAD 判定标准，甚至同一测量方法采用的判定标准也不一致。比如肺量计法，有以 FEF25%～75%＜60% 预计值，或 FEF25%～75%＜预计值-1.64 RSD，RV/TLC＞预计值+1.64 RSD 等。不像 FEV1 在经过数十年的发展形成了明确的人口数据，有明确的判定标准，其他小气道功能检测方法很多尚处于婴儿期，还需要大量的人口数据。

在上述的几种 SAD 检测方法中，有研究对比了它们的敏感性。Postma 等招募了 2014 年 6 月 30 日至 2017 年 3 月 3 日期间应用不同的检测方法评估的 773 名哮喘患者和 99 名对照组患者，发现哮喘患者的 SAD 患病率取决于所用的测量方法，MBNW 法检测的肺泡通气异质性（Sacin）相关的 SAD 发生率最低，IOS 法和肺活量测定法对临床 SAD 评分的影响最大。提示 IOS 法和肺活量测定法检测 SAD 的敏感性要强 MBNW。更多的研究则显示联合不同的检测方法能提高 SAD 的敏感性和准确率。除了肺功能检测之外，近年来 HRCT、显微 CT 在判断小气道结构及气体潴留方面取得了很大进步，为 SAD 的检测提供了客观依据，若 HRCT、显微 CT 联合肺功能检测可能对 SAD 的判断更为客观和准确。

五、基于小气道病理和肺功能的关系看小气道的靶向治疗

小气道是阻塞性肺疾病的重要病变位点，在病理上可表现为上皮细胞的损伤、上皮间质转化、杯状细胞增生、黏膜下腺体肥大、细胞外基质沉积、多种炎症细胞浸润、小气道平滑肌细胞增殖等导致小气道重塑、纤维化、黏液的阻塞导致气道阻力的增加，并且有证据表明 SAD 发生于 COPD 病程发展的早期，是肺气肿发展的先兆，也是哮喘发展的先决条件，其炎症程度与疾病的严重程度有关，在任何有效治疗这种疾病的治疗策略中也需要将远端肺作为目标，针对小气道的治疗策略可能会降低疾病发生发展的速度。笔者认为从小气道的病理来看小气道的靶向研发主要集中于下面几个方面。

（一）靶向小气道的吸入疗法

气道树的连续分支降低了气流速度，会增加吸入空气中颗粒物的暴露，固体颗粒的扩散速度比气体慢，因此会增加微粒物质与小气道的接触时间。一方面这是小气道在有害烟雾刺激下容易发生病变的原因，同时也是药物靶向治疗的理论所在。吸入颗粒的大小决定了它们在呼吸道中的沉积，较大的颗粒沉积在口咽、气管和上支气管树中，而较小的颗粒可以到达远端气道，因此优化吸入疗法可以提高向小气道的输送。加压定量吸入器中的氢氟烷推进剂已允许制造溶液制剂，以确保更大比例的颗粒沉积在肺部而不是口咽部。另外，可以增加超细成分以实现向小气道的更大输送。目前，有提供超细 ICS/LABA 或 ICS/LABA/LAMA 的吸入疗法。尽管这些组合吸入器已在临床试验中证明了有效的功效，但仍需要针对与 COPD 相关的其他机制为目标的新型疗法

（二）靶向 EMT

支气管上皮作为化学、物理和免疫刺激的屏障，诱导损伤和随后的修复反应，以维持组织的稳态。呼吸道上皮受伤后，需要用分化的细胞类型重新上皮化才能恢复正常功能。然而，COPD 发生异常的上皮重塑。在上皮再形成过程中，基底细胞充当纤毛和分泌细胞的前体，但是吸烟改变了基底细胞的转录程序，导致异常的修复过程。EMT 在 COPD 小气道上皮细胞中持续存在；TGFβ、Wnt、ILK 和其他通路与 EMT 有关，但在吸烟者和 COPD 的气道中还几乎没有具体的研究工作，关注涉及的 EMT 相关转录因子通路的研究有可能为小气道保护与修复提供新的策略。

（三）靶向气道黏液的产生

COPD、哮喘患者气道中有黏液的过度产生和黏液的堵塞，有证据表明气道黏液过量产生是与 COPD 相关的能力下降的关键，但尚无特异性和有效的药物可直接有效地阻断慢性支气管炎或任何其他形式的呼吸道疾病中黏液过量产生。大环内酯类药物（如阿奇霉素），磷酸二酯酶-4 抑制剂（如罗氟司特），抗氧化剂/还原剂（如 N-乙酰半胱氨酸）和糖皮质激素可能减少 COPD 恶化的次数，大概是基于慢性支气管炎的缓解。但是，这些药物似乎在气道上皮细胞水平上对体内黏液产生没有特异性和直接的作用。

这些药物似乎更有可能通过免疫系统起作用,从而下调可能刺激上皮细胞黏液产生的免疫细胞衍生的细胞因子,甚至这些间接作用也可能相对较弱。同样,新的生物制剂通常基于抗细胞因子/细胞因子受体单克隆抗体(mAb),它们也针对免疫反应,而不是直接作用于产生黏液的气道上皮细胞的。

气道祖上皮细胞(APEC)是基底细胞的一种类型,APEC 功能的增强与 COPD 患者 IL-33-基底细胞数量的增加有关,MAPK13 是 APEC 向黏液细胞过渡的主要调节剂,APEC 依赖的 IL-33 或相关细胞因子的释放可能会引起气道高反应性和黏液生成,同时 IL-13-IL-13R 与 MUC5AC 黏蛋白的基因表达特征也相关,靶向 APEC 来减弱气道黏液产生、应用 MAPK13 抑制剂控制上皮干细胞生长和分化及相关的细胞因子的调节、积极研究改变杯状细胞数量的确切分子途径等可能为治疗带来新的策略。

(四)靶向 ECM

COPD 小气道中存在纤维化,黏膜及管壁的厚度增加,细胞外基质蛋白(ECM)沉积增加。小气道 ECM 的沉积与肺功能有密切关系。ECM 蛋白的主要产生者是成纤维细胞和活化的肌成纤维细胞,其次是气道平滑肌和气道上皮细胞。ECM 的降解受内源性蛋白酶的调节,其中 MMP 是肺中的主要类型。紊乱的 ECM 发展和稳态在 COPD 发展中有重要作用,需要弄清确切的疾病驱动机制,并确定新的潜在的干预目标。

(五)靶向细胞因子和免疫反应

COPD 小气道中存在炎症细胞、免疫细胞的浸润及淋巴滤泡的生成,而且随 COPD 严重程度而增加,哮喘患者小气道也存在炎症细胞的浸润,外周血及肺泡灌洗液中检测到细胞因子的升高。COPD 中靶向中性粒细胞炎症和促炎细胞因子如 IL-8、TNF-α、IL-1 等的疗效似乎不尽人意,而且导致不良事件的增加,而靶向嗜酸性炎症已经证明了其有效性,并且没有增加不良事件。嗜酸性炎症在哮喘中很常见,但在 COPD 中发病率较低,且与特应性增高无关。因此,COPD 嗜酸性炎症的机制尚不清楚,但提供了一个潜在的治疗靶点。寻找探索与适应性免疫或上游调控分子可能提供新的治疗靶标。

总之,小气道的病理改变导致了小气道的阻力增加,与气道疾病发生发展有重要关系,应用无创性的肺功能检测可以帮助我们早期诊断,同时基于小气道病理与肺功能的关系为我们提供的未来研究探索治疗的靶标。

参 考 文 献

[1] Mullen JB, Wright JL, Wiggs BR, et. al. Reassessment of inflammation of airways in chronic bronchitis. Br Med J(Clin Res Ed),1985,291(6504):1235-1239.

[2] Nakano Y, Wong JC, de Jong PA, et. al. The prediction of small airway dimensions using computed tomography. Am J Respir Crit Care Med,2005,171(2):142-146.

[3] Dolhnikoff M, da Silva LFF, de Araujo BB, et al. The outer wall of small airways is a major site of remodeling in fatal asthma. J Allergy Clin Immunol,2009,123:1090-1097.

[4] den Otter I, Silva LFF, Carvalho ALN, et al. High-affinity immunoglobulin E receptor expression is increased in large and small airways in fatal asthma. Clin Exp Allergy,2010,40:1473-1481.

[5] Caramori G, Oates T, Nicholson AG, et al. Activation of NF-kappaB transcription factor in asthma death. Histopathology,2009,54:507-509.

[6] Nihlberg K, Andersson-Sjoland A, Tufvesson E, et al. Altered matrix production in the distal airways of individuals with asthma. Thorax,2010,65:670-676.

[7] Martin RJ. Therapeutic significance of distal airway inflammation in asthma. J Allergy Clin Immunol, 2002, 109:S447-S460.

[8] Ueda T, Niimi A, Matsumoto H, et al. Role of small airways in asthma: investigation using high-resolution computed tomography. J Allergy Clin Immunol,2006,118:1019-1025.

[9] Hogg JC, McDonough JE, Suzuki M. Small airway obstruction in COPD: new insights based on micro-CT imaging and MRI imaging. Chest,2013,143(5):1436-1443.

[10] Gelb AF, Williams AJ, Zamel N. SPirometry FEV1 vs. FEF25%~75%. Chest J,1983,84:4734.

[11] Boggs PB, Bhat KD, Vekovius WA, et al. Volume adjusted maximal mid-expiratory flow (Iso-volume FEF25%-75%): defifinition of "Significant" responsiveness in healthy, normal subjects. Ann Allergy,1982,48:1378.

[12] American Thoracic Society. Lung function testing: selection of reference values and interpretative strategies. Am Rev Respir Dis,1991,144:1202-1218.

[13] Hansen JE, Sun X-G, Wasserman K. Discriminating measures and normal values for expiratory obstruction. Chest J,2006,129:36977.

[14] Gibbons WJ, Sharma A, Lougheed D, et al. Detection of excessive bronchoconstriction in asthma. Am J Respir Crit Care Med,1996,153:5829.

[15] M. Contoli, M. Kraft, Q. Hamid, et al. Do small airway abnormalities characterize asthma phenotypes? In search of proof. Clin Exp Allergy,2012,42:1150-1160.

[16] Perez T, Chanez P, Dusser D, et al. Small airway impairment in moderate to severe asthmatics without significant proximal airway obstruction. Respir Med,2013,107:1667-1674.

[17] Kraft M, Cairns CB, Ellison MC, et al. Improvements in distal lung function correlate with asthma symptoms after treatment with oral montelukast. Chest J,2006,130:1726-1732.

[18] Sorkness RL, Bleecker ER, Busse WW, et al. Lung function in adults with stable but severe asthma: air trapping and incomplete reversal of obstruction with bronchodilation. J Appl Physiol,2008,104:394403.

[19] Buist AS, Ghezzo H, Anthonisen NR, et al. Relationship between the single-breath N test and age, sex, and smoking habit in three North American cities. Am Rev Respir Dis. 1979,120(2):305-318.

[20] Cosio M, Ghezzo H, Hogg JC, et al. The relations between structural changes in small airways and pulmonary-function tests. N Engl J Med,1978:1277-1281.

[21] Bourdin A, Paganin F, Pre'faut C, et al. Nitrogen washout slope in poorly controlled asthma. Allergy,2006,61:85-89.

[22] Battaglia S, den Hertog H, Timmers MC, et al. Small airways function and molecular markers in exhaled air in mild asthma. Thorax,2005,60:63944.

[23] Buist AS, Vollmer WM, Johnson LR, et al. Does the single-breath N2 test identify the smoker who will develop chronic airflflow limitation? Am Rev Respir Dis,1988,137:293-301.

[24] Verbanck S. Physiological measurement of the small airways. Respiration,2012,84:17788.

[25] Fähndrich S, Lepper P, Trudzinski F, et al. Lung clearance index is increased in patients with COPD-LCI measurements in the daily routine. J Pulm Respir Med,2016,6(3):354.

[26] Verbanck S, Schuermans D, Meysman M, et al. Noninvasive assessment of airway alterations in smokers: the small airways revisited. Am J Respir Crit Care Med,2004,170(4):414-419.

[27] Verbanck S, Schuermans D, Van Muylem. et al. AVentilation distribution during histamine provocation, J Appl Physiol (1985),1997,83(6):1907-1916.

[28] William McNulty & Omar S. Usmani Techniques of assessing small airways dysfunction, European Clinical Respiratory Journal,2014,1:1,25898.

[29] Bailly C, Crenesse D. Evaluation of impulse oscillometry during bronchial challenge testing in children. Albertini M Pediatr Pulmonol,2011,46(12):1209-1214.

[30] Shinke H, Yamamoto M, Hazeki N, et al. Visualized changes in respiratory resistance and reactance along a time axis in smokers: a cross-sectional study. Nishimura Y Respir Investig,2013,51(3):166-174.

[31] Takeda T, Oga T, Niimi A, et al. Relationship between small airway function and health status, dyspnea and disease control in asthma. Respiration,2010,80:120-126.

[32] Oppenheimer BW1, Goldring RM, Herberg ME. et al. Distal airway function in symptomatic subjects with normal spirometry following World Trade Center dust exposure. Chest,2007,132(4):1275-1282.

[33] Su ZQ, Guan WJ, Li SY, et al. Significances of spirometry and impulse oscillometry for detecting small airway disorders assessed with endobronchial optical coherence tomography in COPD. Int J Chron Obstruct Pulmon Dis, 2018, 13: 3031-3044.

[34] Piorunek T1, Kostrzewska M2, Stelmach-Mardas M, et al. Small Airway Obstruction in Chronic Obstructive Pulmonary Disease: Potential Parameters for Early Detection. dv Exp Med Biol,2017,980:75-82.

[35] Van Veen IH, Sterk PJ, Schot R, et al. Alveolar nitric oxide versus measures of peripheral airway dysfunction in severe asthma. Eur Respir J,2006,27:951-956.

[36] 刘琳. 应用呼出气一氧化氮联合脉冲振荡肺功能评估哮喘患者小气道功能的研究. 山东大学学报医学版,2017:1-67.

[37] 董燕,王晓玲,倪瑾华,刘后芹. 呼出气一氧化氮诊断老年小气道功能障碍的应用价值. 中国老年学杂志,2020,40(8):1634-1636.

[38] Lehtimaki L, Kankaanranta H, Saarelainen S, et al. Extended exhaled NO measurement differentiates between alveolar and bronchial inflflammation. Am J Respir Crit Care Med,2001,163:1557-1561.

[39] Santus P, Radovanovic D, Mascetti S, et al. Effects of Bronchodilation on Biomarkers of Peripheral Airway Inflammation in COPD. Pharmacol Res,2018,133:160-169.

[40] Usmani OS, Singh D, Spinola M, et al. The prevalence of small airways disease in adult asthma: A systematic literature review. Respir Med,2016,116.

[41] Postma DS, Brightling C, Baldi S, et al. Exploring the relevance and extent of small airways dysfunction in asthma (ATLANTIS): baseline data from a prospective cohort study. Lancet Respir Med,2019,7(5).

7 支气管激发试验可疑阳性患者的长期跟踪随访研究

周明娟

近年来哮喘患病率在全球范围内有逐年增长的趋势。目前，全球哮喘患者至少有3亿人，中国哮喘患者约3000万人。支气管哮喘是一种异质性疾病，由多种细胞包括嗜酸性粒细胞、肥大细胞、T淋巴细胞、中性粒细胞、平滑肌细胞、气道上皮细胞等，以及细胞组分参与的气道慢性炎症性疾病。其临床表现为随时间不断变化的呼吸道症状病史，如反复发作的喘息、气急、胸闷或咳嗽等症状，常在夜间及凌晨发作或加重，多数患者可自行缓解或经治疗后缓解，同时伴有可变的气流受限和气道高反应性，随着病程的延长可导致一系列气道结构的改变，即气道重构。患者符合上述症状同时具备气流受限客观检查中的任一条，并除外其他疾病所引起的喘息、气急、胸闷和咳嗽，可以诊断为哮喘。支气管激发试验阳性是临床确诊缓解期哮喘最常用的检测手段，尤其是对于肺通气功能正常或者轻度阻塞的患者（FEV1＞70％），其临床价值高于支气管舒张试验，但要注意结合治疗反应，即抗哮喘治疗有效，临床上亦要注意假阴性的可能。

临床上亦常见支气管激发可疑阳性的患者，中华医学会呼吸病学分会肺功能专业组2014年在《肺功能检查指南（第三部分）——组织胺和乙酰甲胆碱支气管激发试验》提出，支气管激发试验可疑阳性的诊断标准：即吸入最大剂量或最高浓度的激发剂后，FEV1下降15％～20％，无气促喘息发作。支气管激发可疑阳性的患者气道反应性较高，通常建议治疗后2～3周后复查，必要时2个月后复查。但临床医师对支气管激发可疑阳性患者并未引起足够的重视，复查率低，很多此类患者没有得到有效治疗，导致患者进展到真正哮喘阶段才开始规范治疗，错失早期诊治时机。

通过全面检索中英文数据库，目前国内外尚无支气管激发试验可疑阳性患者的长期随访性研究，更缺乏探讨影响支气管激发试验可疑阳性患者预后转归结局相关因素的文献报道。仅有的几篇关于支气管激发试验可疑阳性患者的随访研究，不是随访时间太短，就是研究样本量较小。如郭云霞对71例乙酰甲胆碱支气管激发试验可疑阳性患者进行了回顾性分析发现按哮喘治疗后，61例（87％）患者症状改善，9例无效，该研究时间较早，既无随访时间，也无支气管激发试验复查结果。又如王辉等对82例组胺支气管激发试验可疑阳性患者按照哮喘正规治疗13d的短期疗程复查，68例（82.9％）支气管激发试验转为阴性，14例仍为可疑阳性，但该研究随访时间太短成为缺陷。

我院对49例支气管激发可疑阳性患者进行了为期6个月的随访研究，发现转阴性者20例（40.8％），转阳性者2例（4.1％），仍然可疑阳性者4例（8.2％），并且不同性别、BMI、病程、有无过敏性鼻炎家族史、有无哮喘家族史及是否服用中药、白三烯受体拮抗剂、口服糖皮质激素、氨茶碱缓释片、抗胆碱能药物、抗生素与支气管激发试验可疑阳性转阴无关；但另外23例患者（接近总例数50％）拒绝复查支气管激发试验，结果未知，导致研究例数较少。

我院肺功能科长期对支气管激发试验可疑阳性的患者进行跟踪随访，研究目的是探讨影响支气管激发试验可疑阳性患者的预后转归因素，以期为此类患者预防发展到哮喘阶段提供临床依据。患者均来自于我院呼吸科门诊患者，西药、中药或者三伏贴等穴位贴贴敷等治疗措施不限。支气管激发试验检查采用德国耶格 MS Diffusion 肺功能仪及 APS 定量雾化激发系统，患者签署肺功能检测知情同意书后，按肺功能指南操作流程。所有患者检测前均按时停用解痉平喘抗炎和抗过敏药物，经德国耶格 APS 定量雾化装置让患者吸入从低到高递增浓度的组胺或乙酰甲胆碱激发剂溶液，吸入后每次间隔60～90s后复测肺通气功能，如果吸入最大剂量或最高浓度的激发剂后，FEV1下降15％～20％停止检测。期间因为组胺和乙酰甲胆碱限购改用定量雾化改良高渗盐水支气管激发试验，该激发试验流程和组胺或乙酰甲胆碱支气管激发试验流程相似，经德国耶格 DeVilbiss 646 大功率 APS 定量雾化杯吸入固定浓度4.5％氯化钠雾化溶液，每次雾化吸入60～90s后检测FEV1，如果FEV1下降范围在10％～15％停止检测。记录所有患者的症状、体征，并给以相应对症处理，登记患者联系方式并预约复查支气管激发试验，患者复查所用的激发剂同初次支气管激发试验检查时所用。

本研究共纳入128例支气管激发试验可疑阳性患者，7例患者用组胺，35例患者用乙酰甲胆碱，86例患者用高渗盐水。患者年龄10～69岁，平均年龄（34.9±13.9）岁，男性47例，女性81例，平均病程（80.1±147.9）周。本研究共有92例患者参加复查，11例患者因登记的联系方式更改或有误，无法取得联系，25例患者诉临床症状已缓解，拒绝回院复查支气管激发试验，无死亡病例。回院复查病例中有8例患者3个月后转阳性，2例患者6个月后转阳性，3例患者1年后转阳性，合计13例患者转阳性，总转阳性为10.16％；8例患者3个月仍然可疑阳性，7例患者6个月后仍然可疑阳性，3例患者1年后仍然可疑阳性，1例患者1年后仍然可疑阳性,合计19例患者仍然可疑阳性,占总人数百分比为14.84%;48例患者3个月后转阴性,5例患者6个月后转阴性,1例患者1年后转阴性,1例患者2年后转阴性,5例患者3年后转阴性,合计60例患者转阴,总转阴率为46.69%,转阴率与我院前期6个月的随访研究相似,转阴率明显高于我院另外一项针对哮喘患者规范治疗2年的随访研究,该研究中哮喘患者的转阴率仅为17.02%,这也提醒我们在发现支气管激发试验可疑阳性而未能确诊哮喘时,最好先按照指南建议,在排除受试者配合欠佳、激发剂及测试仪器问题,排除病毒或者支原体等引起的上呼吸道感染、长期吸烟、接触臭氧等情况引起的一过性气道反应性增高的情况后,要结合患者的临床症状、病史、过敏史和家族史进行综合评估是否需要按哮喘规范治疗或其他治疗,治疗后复查支气管激发试验,复查为阳性者可以按哮喘治疗方案规范用药,定期复查;复查仍为可疑阳性者建议诊断性治疗后定期复查;复查转阴者可以考虑排除哮喘。

我们认为肺功能检查除加强质控,重视筛查,降低哮喘、慢阻肺等疾病的漏诊率外,复查也非常重要,尤其是对缓解期无症状哮喘和隐匿性哮喘患者而言,支气管激发试验不仅是确诊的重要手段,也是了解其治疗后气道反应性是否改善的重要客观指标,为哮喘早期临床诊断和疗效评估提供了有力的支持证据,并建议积极复查和治疗支气管激发试验可疑阳性患者,预防此部分患者进一步进展为哮喘患者。

参 考 文 献

[1] 中华医学会呼吸病学分会哮喘学组.支气管哮喘防治指南(2016年版).中华结核和呼吸杂志,2016,39(9):675-697.

[2] 中华医学会呼吸病学分会肺功能专业组.肺功能检查指南(第三部分)——组织胺和乙酰甲胆碱支气管激发试验.中华结核和呼吸杂志,2014,37(8):566-571.

[3] 郭云霞.支气管激发试验可疑阳性病人71例用药后结果分析.中国社区医师·医学专业,2010,12(23).

[4] 王辉,王玉梅,施恋,等.82例支气管激发试验可疑阳性患者接受正规哮喘治疗后的情况分析.中国伤残医学,2015,23(1):118-120.

[5] 谢涵,陈远彬,周明娟,等.146例支气管激发或舒张试验可疑阳性患者随访6个月肺功能转归调查.中国全科医学,2020,23(10):1-6.

[6] 许银姬,周明娟,梁桂兴,等.咳嗽变异性哮喘患者规范治疗2年的随访研究.广东医学,2016,12:2104-2107.

8 人工智能结合肺量计检查在慢性呼吸疾病中的应用

王译民　简文华　高　怡　郑劲平

据世界卫生组织报道,哮喘和慢性阻塞性肺疾病(chronic obstructive pulmonary disease,COPD)已经成为影响全球的严重卫生问题,目前全球共有约2.35亿哮喘患者,每年约有25万患者死于哮喘,其中超过80%的死亡患者来自低收入及中低收入国家。同时,每年有超过300万患者死于COPD,其中超过90%患者来自低收入及中低收入国家。一项中国7个地区的调查发现,COPD在40岁以上成年人中的患病率为8.2%,但直到疾病发展到晚期,许多COPD仍未被诊断,COPD患者的诊断率仅为31%。肺量计检查是肺功能检查最重要的项目之一,对慢性呼吸疾病早期诊断、疾病进展、远程随访具有重要评估作用,人工智能(artificial intelligence,AI)结合肺量计检查在慢性呼吸疾病中的应用具有重要意义。

本文综述了AI结合肺量计检查在慢性呼吸疾病中的应用进展。本文介绍了AI结合肺量计检查在慢性呼吸疾病诊断中的应用,在慢性呼吸疾病肺功能进展趋势中的预测作用,AI结合肺量计检查在远程医疗中的应用,以及AI结合肺量计检查在呼吸领域应用的未来展望。

一、AI结合肺量计检查诊断慢性呼吸疾病

(一)单独结合肺量计检查

肺量计检查是诊断慢性呼吸疾病最重要的检查之一,可早期诊断慢性呼吸疾病。来自比利时鲁汶大学的Janssens博士团队重点研究了AI算法结合肺量计检查在慢性呼吸疾病诊断中的应用。他们用多元回归分析支气管舒张后的流量-容积曲线(flow-volume curve,F-V curve)以诊断严重吸烟者是否存在肺气肿。运用贝叶斯、k-近邻算法(k nearest neighbors,kNN)、决策树、径向基神经网络、支持向量机(support vector machines,SVMs)结合肺量计检查流量-时间曲线(flow-time curve,F-T curve)诊断COPD并判断严重程度,其中SVM表现最优,其敏感性、特异性、准确率分别为85%、98.1%、88.2%,但此研究的算法验证选用的内部交叉验证,对于算法表现验证效果较差,未来可考虑增加外部数据库验证算法表现。随后他们运用决策树基于ATS/ERS判读策略结合肺量计检查和弥散功能对COPD、哮喘、过度换气综合征、间质性肺病、神经肌肉疾病、肺血管疾病、上气道阻塞进行诊断预测,基于简单规则的ATS/ERS判读策略仅有38%的确诊率,对COPD的诊断准确率稍高,对其他类型的呼吸疾病很难明确诊断,结合决策树算法后确诊率可以提高到68%,对于各类常见呼吸疾病诊断敏感性和特异性也较高。在此基础上,通过扩大样本量和增加肺功能项目,AI算法对慢性呼吸疾病的总体确诊率提升到82%,对比来自欧洲16家医疗机构120名呼吸专家确诊率44.6%,AI明显提高了呼吸疾病的确诊率,可作为一个强大的诊断决策工具。

(二)同时结合其他临床资料

AI结合肺量计检查对疾病的诊断可通过增加临床资料信息、影像学检查和其他客观检查来提高诊断准确率。为诊断哮喘和COPD,一项研究以贝叶斯算法、逻辑回归、神经网络、SVM、kNN、决策树和随机森林以哮喘和COPD患者的临床资料和肺量计检查共22项特征为预测指标,发现肺量计检查中的MEF 25%~75%是对哮喘诊断最重要的因素,而COPD患者最重要的因素为吸烟史。另一项研究将受试者的39类呼吸音与肺量计检查的指标作为特征输入,SVM、kNN、逻辑回归和决策树等算法可用于诊断COPD,仅输入呼吸音时其准确率为83.6%,结合肺量计检查FEV1、FVC后AI诊断准确率可提升至100%。Tomita等比较了深度学习的深度神经网络(deep neural network,DNN)算法与逻辑回归、SVM等经典机器学习算法在诊断成人哮喘上的表现,通过患者症状、肺量计检查和支气管激发试验、气道反应性、呼出气一氧化氮(fractional exhaled nitric oxide,FeNO)等预测指标来诊断哮喘和COPD,DNN对成人哮喘的诊断准确率为0.98,显著高于SVM的0.82和逻辑回归的0.94,DNN可在未来诊断慢性呼吸疾病中发挥更大作用。部分哮喘患者通过医师依据临床症状进行诊断,存在过度诊断的问题。针对这一现象,一项基于566名哮喘和非哮喘患者的研究利用多元逻辑回归结合症状、反复发作史、过敏史和喘鸣音构建评分系统并结合支气管舒张后1秒率小于0.7用于诊断哮喘,通过AI算法可更有效的预测成人哮喘并给出及时就医的指导意见。另一项研究运用聚类分析结合肺量计检查、支气管舒张试验、气道阻力等可将儿童哮喘患者分为不同严重程度亚群。以上研究AI算法在肺量计检查的基础上结合其他临床资料可更好的诊断慢性呼吸疾病。

(三)专家系统

来自波黑的国际伯奇大学研究者通过构建专家诊断系统可在临床中自动识别哮喘和COPD,专家系统学习患

者临床症状问卷和肺量计检查,将哮喘和COPD从健康人中区分出来,对哮喘和COPD诊断的敏感性为96.45%,特异性为98.71%,肺功能检查正常者可达到98.71%的准确率。该专家系统的良好表现建立在实验室前期大量研究的基础上。另一项研究也构建专家系统诊断慢性阻塞性呼吸疾病,包括慢性支气管炎、肺气肿和有气道阻塞的哮喘,通过支气管舒张试验和X线检查结合症状特征,这一专家系统总准确率可达到97.5%。

二、AI结合肺量计检查预测慢性呼吸疾病发展趋势

AI结合肺量计检查除运用于慢性呼吸疾病诊断,还可进行COPD分型并分析肺功能发展趋势。一项多中心的研究以线性混合效应模型对4167名随访肺量计检查超过20年的患者数据进行学习,用于预测FEV_1和1秒率下降趋势,并将算法转化为应用程序,对慢性呼吸疾病患者气流受限的趋势进行预测。来自中国的学者基于小样本也构建了COPD进展趋势的预测模型,仅将肺量计检查中的1秒率<0.8作为预测的一个指标,其余预测指标来自于临床资料和其他客观检查。AI还被用于儿童哮喘控制情况的预测,通过FVC、FEV_1、1秒率、FEF 25%~75%和FeNO等指标,人工神经网络(artificial neural network,ANN)可分别对哮喘未控制和控制的预测达到100%和79.6%的准确率。单独运用强迫振荡检查或结合肺量计检查,机器学习可预测哮喘和COPD,这些研究重点在于开发强迫振荡检查在AI预测慢性呼吸疾病中的应用价值。AI结合肺量计检查还可用于预测囊性纤维化的短期预后情况,研究运用贝叶斯算法对英国约99%的囊性纤维化患者进行分析,对患者是否适合进行肺移植提供依据。

三、AI结合肺量计检查的远程医疗

目前国内外均有简易肺量计仪供基层医院和患者选用,但其判读、质控、仪器校准等变异率大、精确度低,仪器质量参差不齐,且部分医院的肺量计较为老旧,短期内又没有更换的必要,因此开发高质量的AI模型结合肺量计检查在远程医疗中具有重要意义。通过开发AI基于肺量计检查的远程应用,可减少门诊量、减少仪器费用、增加患者舒适度。

(一)肺量计检查指标远程监测

基于智能手机的设计和开发使肺量计检查可通过卷积神经网络实时显示FEV1、FVC、1秒率、PEF、F-V曲线和F-T曲线对结果正常和疾病做出分类,其对正常的分类可达100%,对疾病的诊断可达到80%。基于iphone5s开发的肺量计仪致力于仅用手机来完成肺量计检查,相较于简易肺量计仪,其预测PEF、FEV1、FEV6、FVC、FEV1的错误率差异在1%~10%,患者能更简单更经济的完成健康监测。其他基于手机的家用肺量计仪开发通过直接在手机上内置麦克风完成患者呼气时流量的记录。对着手机屏幕用力呼气,可脱离传统肺量计检查的方式来预测对FVC、FEV1、1秒率,其平均百分比误差与智能手机式肺量计仪、医疗机构用肺量计仪的平均百分比误差分别为4.6%、3.1%和3.5%,该仪器仅能预测相关指标,不能输出F-V曲线和V-T曲线。个人用肺功能监测装置可完成对哮喘患者的监测,通过手持式外接手机装置收集FEV1、FEV6和F-V曲线,并携带检测呼吸产生的一氧化氮(nitric oxide,NO)、一氧化碳(carbon monoxide,CO)和氧气(oxygen,O_2)的化学测量仪。

(二)慢性呼吸疾病远程诊断和管理

部分手持式肺量计仪的设计可输出曲线和指标并给出简单诊断,如非COPD的诊断,诊断过程需通过远程联结医师来完成。应用遥测设备、人工神经网络和模糊分析的专家系统结合手机应用程序可对健康人、哮喘患者和COPD患者进行区分,通过分析患者症状和肺量计检查给出疾病诊断。基于联结医师、患者的慢性病管理平台,通过平台监测患者体重、血压、血糖、心电图、肺功能、氧饱和度等指标,完成对慢性心力衰竭、糖尿病、COPD的远程管理。安卓系统可构建电子健康系统结合肺量计仪、专家诊断系统对哮喘和COPD做出诊断,基于780位患者的评估其诊断准确率达97.32%。分类和回归数算法利用COPD患者在家的电子监控数据包括FEV1、氧饱和度、体重等参数对COPD患者第二天的急性发作风险进行预测,其准确率、特异性和敏感性分别为71.8%、80.4%和61.1%。

四、小结与展望

未来,AI结合肺量计检查可在我国慢性呼吸疾病普查和随访中发挥重要作用。首先可在基层医疗机构进行大范围的慢性呼吸疾病的普查,主要是在成人COPD和儿童哮喘中的应用中发挥作用;其次,AI结合肺量计检查可对患者疾病控制情况进行长期监测,并构建与医师的交互平台,实时给患者提供医疗指导和服务;再次,AI结合肺量计检查可对COPD患者急性加重的次数和频率进行预测,可在应用程序中提醒患者做好应对措施;最后,AI结合肺量计检查除诊断常见慢性呼吸疾病,还可对一些罕见病、诊断困难的肺部疾病进行开发应用。本文讨论了AI结合肺量计检查在慢性呼吸疾病中的应用进展,同时探讨了AI结合肺量计检查应用的未来展望。由于我国庞大的慢性呼吸病患者数量及慢性阻塞性肺疾病的早期诊断率低等现实情况,使得AI结合肺量计检查在慢性呼吸疾病的应用中具有良好前景。AI结合肺量计检查可辅助基础医疗机构完成慢性呼吸疾病的普查,帮助慢性呼吸疾病患者进行疾病的自我管理,以达到减轻慢性呼吸疾病所带来的经济和卫生负担的目的。

参 考 文 献

[1] Chronic respiratory diseases. World Health Organization. https://www.who.int/health-topics/chronic-respiratory-diseases#tab=tab_1.

[2] Zhong N, Wang C, Yao W, et al. Prevalence of chronic obstructive pulmonary disease in China: a large, population-based survey. Am J Respir Crit Care Med, 2007, 176(8): 753-760.

[3] Topalovic M, Das N, Burgel PR, et al. Artificial intelligence outperforms pulmonologists in the interpretation of pulmonary function tests. Eur Respir J, 2019, 53(4).

[4] Das N, Topalovic M, Janssens W. Artificial intelligence in diagnosis of obstructive lung disease: current status and future potential. Curr Opin Pulm Med, 2018, 24(2): 117-123.

[5] Topalovic M, Laval S, Aerts JM, et al. Automated Interpretation of Pulmonary Function Tests in Adults with Respiratory Complaints. Respiration, 2017, 93(3): 170-178.

[6] Topalovic M, Exadaktylos V, Decramer M, et al. Modelling the dynamics of expiratory airflow to describe chronic obstructive pulmonary disease. Med Biol Eng Comput, 2014, 52(12): 997-1006.

[7] Topalovic M, Exadaktylos V, Peeters A, et al. Computer quantification of airway collapse on forced expiration to predict the presence of emphysema. Respir Res, 2013, 14: 131.

[8] Pellegrino R, Viegi G, Brusasco V, et al. Interpretative strategies for lung function tests. Eur Respir J, 2005, 26(5): 948-968.

[9] Spathis D, Vlamos P. Diagnosing asthma and chronic obstructive pulmonary disease with machine learning. Health Inform J, 2019, 25(3): 811-827.

[10] Haider NS, Singh BK, Periyasamy R, et al. Respiratory Sound Based Classification of Chronic Obstructive Pulmonary Disease: a Risk Stratification Approach in Machine Learning Paradigm. J Med Syst, 2019, 43(8): 255.

[11] Tomita K, Nagao R, Touge H, et al. Deep learning facilitates the diagnosis of adult asthma. Allergol Int, 2019, 68(4): 456-461.

[12] Tomita K, Sano H, Chiba Y, et al. A scoring algorithm for predicting the presence of adult asthma: a prospective derivation study. Prim Care Respir J, 2013, 22(1): 51-58.

[13] Fitzpatrick AM, Teague WG, Meyers DA, et al. Heterogeneity of severe asthma in childhood: confirmation by cluster analysis of children in the National Institutes of Health/National Heart, Lung, and Blood Institute Severe Asthma Research Program. J Allergy Clin Immunol, 2011, 127(2): 382-389.

[14] Badnjevic A, Gurbeta L, Custovic E. An Expert Diagnostic System to Automatically Identify Asthma and Chronic Obstructive Pulmonary Disease in Clinical Settings. Sci Rep, 2018, 8(1): 11645.

[15] Badnjevic A, Gurbeta L, Cifrek M, et al. Pre-classification process symptom questionnaire based on fuzzy logic for pulmonary function test cost reduction. Singapore: Springer Singapore, 2017, 608-616.

[16] Badnjevic A, Gurbeta L, Cifrek M, et al. Classification of asthma using artificial neural network. Electronics and Microelectronics (MIPRO), 2016: 387-390.

[17] Badnjevic A, Koruga D, Cifrek M, et al. Interpretation of pulmonary function test results in relation to asthma classification using integrated software suite. Electronics and Microelectronics (MIPRO), 2013: 140-144.

[18] Badnjevic A, Cifrek M. Classification of Asthma Utilizing Integrated Software Suite. Cham: Springer International Publishing, 2015: 415-418.

[19] Badnjevic A, Cifrek M, Koruga D. Classification of Chronic Obstructive Pulmonary Disease (COPD) Using Integrated Software Suite. Cham: Springer International Publishing, 2014: 911-914.

[20] Badnjevic A, Cifrek M, Koruga D, et al. Neuro-fuzzy classification of asthma and chronic obstructive pulmonary disease. BMC Med Inform Decis Mak, 2015, 15(3): S1.

[21] Braido F, Santus P, Corsico AG, et al. Chronic obstructive lung disease "expert system": validation of a predictive tool for assisting diagnosis. Int J Chron Obstruct Pulmon Dis, 2018, 13: 1747-1753.

[22] Castaldi PJ, Boueiz A, Yun J, et al. Machine Learning Characterization of COPD Subtypes: Insights From the COPDGene Study. Chest, 2020, 157(5): 1147-1157.

[23] Chen W, Sin DD, FitzGerald JM, et al. An Individualized Prediction Model for Long-term Lung Function Trajectory and Risk of COPD in the General Population. Chest, 2020, 157(3): 547-557.

[24] Guo YI, Qian Y, Gong YI, et al. A predictive model for the development of chronic obstructive pulmonary disease. Biomed Rep, 2015, 3(6): 853-863.

[25] Pifferi M, Bush A, Pioggia G, et al. Monitoring asthma control in children with allergies by soft computing of lung function and exhaled nitric oxide. Chest, 2011, 139(2): 319-327.

[26] Amaral JLM, Lopes AJ, Veiga J, et al. High-accuracy detection of airway obstruction in asthma using machine learning algorithms and forced oscillation measurements. Comput Methods Programs Biomed, 2017, 144: 113-125.

[27] Amaral JLM, Lopes AJ, Faria ACD, et al. Machine learning algorithms and forced oscillation measurements to categorise the airway obstruction severity in chronic obstructive pulmonary disease. Comput Methods Programs Biomed, 2015, 118(2): 186-197.

[28] Amaral JLM, Lopes AJ, Jansen JM, et al. Machine learning algorithms and forced oscillation measurements applied to the automatic identification of chronic obstructive pulmonary disease. Comput Methods Programs Biomed, 2012, 105(3): 183-193.

[29] Amaral JLM, Faria AC, Lopes AJ, et al. Automatic identification of Chronic Obstructive Pulmonary Disease Based on forced oscillation measurements and artificial neural net-

works. Conf Proc IEEE Eng Med Biol Soc, 2010, 2010: 1394-1397.

[30] Faria ACD, Veiga J, Lopes AJ, et al. Forced oscillation, integer and fractional-order modeling in asthma. Comput Methods Programs Biomed, 2016, 128:12-26.

[31] Badnjevic A, Cifrek M, Koruga D, et al. Neuro-fuzzy classification of asthma and chronic obstructive pulmonary disease. BMC Med Inform Decis Mak, 2015, 15(Suppl 3):S1.

[32] Muskulus M, Slats AM, Sterk PJ, et al. Fluctuations and determinism of respiratory impedance in asthma and chronic obstructive pulmonary disease. J Appl Physiol(1985), 2010, 109(6):1582-1591.

[33] Alaa AM, van der Schaar M. Prognostication and Risk Factors for Cystic Fibrosis via Automated Machine Learning. Sci Rep, 2018, 8(1):11242.

[34] Trivedy S, Goyal M, Mohapatra PR, et al. Design and Development of Smartphone-enabled Spirometer with a Disease Classification System Using Convolutional Neural Network. IEEE Trans Instrum Meas, 2020:1.

[35] Larson EC, Goel M, Boriello G, et al. SpiroSmart: using a microphone to measure lung function on a mobile phone. Pennsylvania: Association for Computing Machinery, 2012: 280-289.

[36] Zubaydi F, Sagahyroon A, Aloul F, et al. MobSpiro: Mobile based spirometry for detecting COPD Conference(CCWC), 2017:1-4.

[37] Carspecken CW, Arteta C, Clifford GD. TeleSpiro: A low-cost mobile spirometer for resource-limited settings. 2013: 144-147.

[38] Kwan AM, Fung AG, Jansen PA, et al. Personal Lung Function Monitoring Devices for Asthma Patients. IEEE Sens J, 2015, 15(4):2238-2247.

[39] Rasyid MUHA, Kemalasari, Sulistiyo M, et al. Design and Development of Portable Spirometer. (ICCE-TW), 2018: 1-2.

[40] Granulo E, Bear L, Gurbeta L, et al. Telemetry System for Diagnosis of Asthma and Chronical Obstructive Pulmonary Disease(COPD), 2016.

[41] Fanucci L, Donati M, Celli A, et al. Advanced multi-sensor platform for chronic disease home monitoring, 2015: 646-651.

[42] Gurbeta L, Badnjevic A, Maksimovic M, et al. A telehealth system for automated diagnosis of asthma and chronical obstructive pulmonary disease. J Am Med Inform Assoc, 2018, 25(9):1213-1217.

[43] Mohktar MS, Redmond SJ, Antoniades NC, et al. Predicting the risk of exacerbation in patients with chronic obstructive pulmonary disease using home telehealth measurement data. Artif Intell Med, 2015, 63(1):51-59.

9 侵入性心肺运动试验在不明原因呼吸困难鉴别诊断中的应用

洪谊 高怡 郑劲平

劳累性呼吸困难是呼吸科、心内科等患者的常见主诉。临床上大多数患者通过查体、影像学、肺功能和实验室检查等常规检查来确定病因。但这些检查通常是在静息状态或者无明显症状的情况下进行的。呼吸困难在普通人群中占1/4，有10%~20%的病例经过多项检查仍不能明确病因，被定义为不明原因呼吸困难。

心肺运动试验(cardiopulmonary exercise test, CPET)通过测量运动时肺内气体交换，同步评估心血管和呼吸系统对运动的应激反应，与其他诊断性试验只评价单一器官系统不同，CPET可同步评价运动相关的各器官系统的功能。CPET中，摄氧量(VO_2)是评估受试者有氧能力的金标准，二氧化碳当量斜率(VE/VCO_2 slope)、摄氧效率斜率(OUES)等指标可反映呼吸效率。然而，CPET不能直接测量心脏充盈压力、肺动脉压(PAP)或心排血量(CO)，无法区分射血分数保留的心力衰竭(HFpEF)、运动诱发性肺动脉高压(ePH)和非心脏原因的呼吸困难。因此，非侵入性运动试验无法为某些不明原因呼吸困难的患者提供明确的诊断。

侵入性心肺运动试验(invasive cardiopulmonary exercise test, iCPET)是一种伴有代谢和血流动力学测定的运动试验，通过肺动脉导管和桡动脉导管，可以得到患者运动过程中血流动力学及血气的改变情况，直接获取心室充盈压、PAP、CO、肺功能及氧的运输和利用情况。iCPET将CPET呼出气体分析技术与有创性运动评估相结合，为评估运动耐量下降的原因提供了最可靠、直接的方法，现已逐渐成为不明原因呼吸困难和运动受限原因的金标准诊断方法。

一、iCPET的适应证

目前iCPET主要用于鉴别常用方法不能诊断的亚临床性疾病包括运动诱发的肺动脉高压、早期的舒张性心力衰竭、前负荷不足、线粒体肌病等导致的运动耐量受损等。黄玮等的回顾性研究，评估了一个多学科呼吸困难评估中心(MDEC)2011—2014年用iCPET来诊断不明原因呼吸困难的潜在病因的诊断效果。结果显示，患者确诊时间大幅减少，检查项目也明显减少，不仅使患者得到早期诊治，有利于预后，且诊治费用也减少。

二、iCPET的操作流程

(一)操作步骤

1. 右侧颈内静脉(9-Fr血管鞘)和右侧桡动脉(如4-Fr监测导管)置管。

2. 通过咬口或面罩收集呼吸气体，测量VO_2，并以此计算Fick CO。整个运动试验都进行呼出气体分析。

3. 准备并冲洗7-Fr楔形球囊(BW)，然后通过侧臂适配器将微压力计(MM,2-Fr)插入球囊尖端导管。

4. 将BW插入右心房。将MM调至充满液体的导管处，获得右心房压(RAP)。

5. 在每一运动阶段测量和记录桡动脉管、右IJ鞘(RAP)和BW的压力。

6. 将BW送入右心室，确认MM无漂移，然后记录压力。

7. 将BW送入肺动脉(PA)。确认MM没有漂移，记录压力。同时从PA、SVC(排除左至右分流)和桡动脉行取血气。标注采血时间，以与呼出气气体分析Fick法测的CO对应。

8. 在冲洗打开的情况下，将BW送到肺小动脉远端(PCWP)。通过波形分析、透视表现、血氧饱和度>94%法确认PCWP位置。传递压力，确认MM没有漂移，并记录压力。

9. 将脚放入踏板中，放松30 s后，在PCWP位置进行记录。

10. 开始运动方案(20W)。如不同时进行影像学监测，该阶段的持续时间为3 min，如进行，需留足够的时间进行图像采集，则持续5 min。运动2~4 min后，与静息水平一样测压力及血气。

11. 进入下一个阶段，老年呼吸困难患者，通常使用20 W/3 min的递增量直到峰值。

12. 在每个递增阶段结束前30 s测量PCWP、PA、RAP、PAP和动脉/PA血样采集。获得各阶段Borg劳累评估量表得分和Borg呼吸困难评分。

13. 当患者达症状限制性最大运动时(即Borg劳累评估量表得分>16，Borg呼吸困难评分>6)，则重复步骤11和12。呼吸交换比>1.05提示患者已尽最大努力。

14. 所有结果都测量后停止运动，停止后1 min测量恢复期压力值。

15. 获取所有数据后,将患者的脚从功率自行车踏步取下,并将 BW 导管从鞘中取下。

(二)记录数据

iCPET 记录的数据主要包括静息状态和峰值运动状态下的心率(bpm)、收缩压(mmHg)、mBP(mmHg)、右房压(mmHg)、mPAWP(mmHg)、PAWP V 波(mmHg)、肺动脉收缩压(mmHg)、mPAP(mmHg)、CO(L/min)、CO 储备(%)、mPAP/CO slope、PAWP/CO slope、SVR、PVR、血红蛋白、动脉血氧饱和度、PaO_2、肺动脉血血氧饱和度、肺动脉血 PaO_2、VO_2、VO_2/Kg、AVO_2 diff、呼吸交换率、乳酸等。

(三)血流动力学的正常范围

静息状态和运动状态时血流动力学指标的正常范围见表 9-9-1。

表 9-9-1　血流动力学指标的正常范围

指标	静息状态(mmHg)	运动状态(mmHg)	注　释
RAP	0~6	<15	运动的正常范围不明确
mPAP	≤20	<30 TPR<3WU	50 岁以上正常人通常>30mmHg,但 TPR 不高
PA/CO slope	—	<3	仰卧位运动试验不适用
PAWP	<15	<25	有文献显示静息正常值≤12 或≤15
PAWP/CO slope	—	<2	仰卧位运动试验不适用
PVR	<2~3	<2~3	一般正常<2,值>3 意味着临床风险增加
CI/CO	2.2~4.0	>4.8×△VO2	VO_2 每增加 1 ml/min,CO 预期增加 6 ml/min**

* TPR:全肺阻力;** 心排血量储备预计值等于 $6×\Delta VO_2$。心排血量储备为测量值减去静息 CO 除以心排血量储备预计值。这个比率被称为运动因子,应该是 0.8 或 80%

(四)注意事项

1. 运动试验需室内正常环境中进行,可根据需要调整设定运动试验方案,结果解读也需综合考虑。

2. 注意安全性问题。患者在进行 iCPET 前需要考虑影响肺动脉或桡动脉导管置入的安全因素,包括血小板减少、抗凝状态、深静脉通路、异常的 Allen 测试同时需要受过培训的专业医师、运动生理师、护士共同协作。

3. 需仔细测量和综合评估所测参数,包括压力大小及其波形改变、血气分析和乳酸值、呼吸气体分析、心排血量及 AVO_2 diff 等。

4. 压力测定需在呼气末进行,因此时胸腔压力接近零,肺处于功能储备状态,气流不易影响心内压力。特殊情况,如使用了 PEEP 的 COPD 患者,同时测呼气末和吸气末平均压。

5. 可选择直立位和仰卧位,首选仰卧位。

三、iCPET 的结果解释与疾病诊断

与 CPET 不同的是,iCPET 运动前置入的肺动脉导管和桡动脉置管,这一区别可提供完整的运动和静息的血流动力学参数,肺动脉和外周动脉的血气分析。结合心血管功能、呼吸功能和代谢功能进行综合评估,不同疾病有各种特征性的表现(表 9-9-2),为此可对原因不明的运动导致的呼吸困难进行鉴别诊断,包括早期诊断舒张性心力衰竭、运动诱发的肺动脉高压、前负荷衰竭、线粒体肌病等多种疾病。

表 9-9-2　iCPET 用于特殊疾病的诊断及解释

诊断	诊断标准	注　释
射血分数保留的心力衰竭(HFpEF)	静息 PAWP≥15mmHg,或运动时 PAWP≥15mmHg 或 △PAWP/△CO slope>2mmHg/(L·min)	CO 储备可能减少[a] AVO_2 diff 可能减少[b]
静息或运动诱发的肺动脉高压(ePH)	静息 mPAP≥20mmHg,或尽力运动时 mPAP≥30mmHg 同时 TPR>3WU 或 △PAWP/△CO slope>3mmHg/(L·min)	定义为毛细血管前、后或混合;PVR≥3WU 为毛细血管前 pH;运动时的 PVR 截断值尚不明确
肺或呼吸受限	静息或运动诱发的低氧血症;呼吸储备<15%pred	在室内监测;不能依赖指脉氧仪,ABG 监测不可少
伴射血分数降低的心力衰竭(HFrEF)	压力测试标准同 HFpEF(同上);CO 储备可能下降;AVO_2 diff 可能减少	验证真实的 CO 储备限值,帮助评估 HfrEF 是否需进行移植术
二尖瓣或三尖瓣返流	RAP 或 PAWP 波形出现大 V 波;RAP、PAWP 随运动增加,意味着恶化	要同时做超声心动图或运动心动图来评估返流的严重程度

(续 表)

诊断	诊断标准	注 释
二尖瓣狭窄	PAWP-LV压力阶差随运动增加;运动性毛细血管后肺动脉高压的发生或恶化	考虑到PAWP高估了真实压力阶差,二尖瓣流入梯度需要同时进行超声心动图检查
心脏前负荷不足	心排血量储备减少[a];同时Peak RAP<8mmHg,PAWP<14mmHg,mPAP<30mmHg	考虑POTS或自主神经或肾上腺功能不全
线粒体疾病	峰值VO_2降低,肺动脉血血氧饱和度高于预计值;AVO_2diff下降,但乳酸增加;心排血量储备高,>150%pred	运动时应保持正常的充盈压和PAP,某些严重功能失调患者也可以出现

Ao.动脉;AVO_2diff.动静脉氧含量差;CO.心排血量;LV.左心室;PA.肺动脉;PAP.肺动脉压力;PAWP.肺动脉楔压;POTS.直立性心动过速综合征;RAP.右心房压;TPR.全肺阻力;VO_2.摄氧量;WU. Woods Units.

运动中[a]ΔCO应当>$\Delta VO_2 \times 4.8$;[b]AVO_2diff应增加到接近血浆血红蛋白的水平

参 考 文 献

[1] Guazzi M. The ultimate diagnosis of unexplained dyspnoea on exertion: Stay tuned on invasive cardiopulmonary exercise testing and beyond. Eur J Prev Cardiol, 2017, 24 (12): 1308-1310.

[2] ATS/ACCP Statement on cardiopulmonary exercise testing. Am J Resp Crit Care, 2003, 167(2): 211-277.

[3] Guazzi M, Adams V, Conraads V, et al. EACPR/AHA Scientific Statement. Clinical recommendations for cardiopulmonary exercise testing data assessment in specific patient populations. Circulation, 2012, 126(18): 2261-2274.

[4] Maron BA, Cockrill BA, Waxman AB, et al. The invasive cardiopulmonary exercise test. Circulation, 2013, 127 (10): 1157-1164.

[5] Tolle JJ, Waxman AB, Van Horn TL, et al. Exercise-induced pulmonary arterial hypertension. Circulation, 2011, 118 (21): 2183.

[6] Huang W, Resch S, Oliveira R K, et al. Invasive cardiopulmonary exercise testing in the evaluation of unexplained dyspnea: Insights from a multidisciplinary dyspnea center. European Journal of Preventive Cardiology, 2017, 24(11): 1190-1199.

[7] Andersen MJ, Olson TP, Melenovsky V, et al. Differential hemodynamic effects of exercise and volume expansion in people with and without heart failure. Circ Heart Fail, 2015, 8 (1): 41-48.

[8] Obokata M, Kane GC, Sorimachi H, et al. Noninvasive evaluation of pulmonary artery pressure during exercise: the importance of right atrial hypertension. Eur Respir J, 2020, 55(2).

[9] Oldham WM, Lewis GD, Opotowsky AR, et al. Unexplained exertional dyspnea caused by low ventricular filling pressures: results from clinical invasive cardiopulmonary exercise testing. Pulm Circ, 2016, 6(1): 55-62.

[10] Melamed KH, Santos M, Oliveira RKF, et al. Unexplained exertional intolerance associated with impaired systemic oxygen extraction. Eur J Appl Physiol, 2019, 119 (10): 2375-2389.

[11] Guazzi M, Arena R, Halle M, et al. 2016 Focused update: clinical recommendations for cardiopulmonary exercise testing data assessment in specific patient populations. Circulation, 2016, 133(24): e694-e711.

10 围术期气道反应测定与手术安全性管理

赵桂华 张 娜

随着生命时间延长及外科技术的迅猛发展,越来越多的气道高反应患者,尤其是支气管哮喘患者会经历手术治疗。围术期指从患者决定接受手术治疗开始,到手术治疗直至基本康复,在术前5~7 d至术后7~12 d。支气管痉挛是围术期最常见的并发症之一,而对于气道高反应患者,更容易在围术期发生气道平滑肌痉挛,主要影响因素为支气管哮喘及气道痉挛史、麻醉、手术方式及气管插管等。所以围术期气道反应测定与手术安全性密切相关,精准的术前评估可以减少术中、术后并发症,提高手术成功率,缩短平均住院日,降低再住院率和手术风险,同时减少患者的医疗花费等。近年来,加强康复外科(enhanced recovery after、surgery,ERAS)理念在全球应用已取得良好的效果。呼吸系统管理是ERAS重要环节而且贯穿围术期的全程。加强围术期气道管理的理念越来越得到外科临床医师的重视,国际的COPD全球防治倡议(the global initiative for chronic obstructive lung disease,GOLD)和哮喘全球防治倡议(GlobalInitiative for Asthma,GINA)强调了COPD和哮喘患者术前充分气道管理的重要性。随着国内《胸外科围手术期气道管理专家共识》,以及《多学科围手术期气道管理专家共识》的相继出台,我国对术前肺功能检查及围术期的气道管理也越来越重视。有研究表明,外科手术患者合并肺部并发症的机会较多,特别是有基础呼吸道疾病的高危患者,更应引起足够的重视。就哮喘患者而言,围术期支气管痉挛的发生率国内外报道不一,国内报道的发生率为10%左右,国外发生率低于1.7%,但均较非哮喘患者发生率高。围术期支气管痉挛一旦出现,可导致严重的缺氧和二氧化碳潴留,继而导致缺氧性脑损伤、心肺功能衰竭甚至呼吸心搏骤停,严重危及患者生命。据美国麻醉医师协会统计呼吸系统索赔案中2%与支气管痉挛有关,其中70%死亡。因此我国2016版的哮喘诊治指南也明确指出围术期哮喘管理目标主要为降低围术期哮喘急性发作风险。但由于围术期哮喘多发生于普通外科、骨科、胸外科等非呼吸专科科室,外科医师呼吸专科知识相对缺乏,对围术期哮喘的认识与警惕性远低于专科医师,所以在围术期进行气道反应测定与筛查在降低支气管痉挛风险发生方面极其重要,同时也是加速肺康复的主要内容。

一、气道反应性测定

气道反应性(airway responsiveness,AR)指气管和支气管受各种物理、化学、药物、变应原等刺激后所引起的气道阻力变化。正常气道对轻微刺激不发生收缩反应或仅有微弱反应,是正常生理反应。气道高反应性(airway hyperresponsiveness,AHR)指气管和支气管受轻微物理、化学、药物、变应原等刺激后,气道阻力明显增大的现象。它是基于气道变态反应性炎症的一种病理生理状态。支气管激发试验是通过化学、物理、生物等人工刺激,诱发气道平滑肌收缩,并借助肺功能指标的改变来判断支气管是否缩窄及其程度的方法,是检测气道高反应性最常用、最准确的临床检查。目前,《全球哮喘防治创议(GINA)》,中国的《支气管哮喘防治指南》和《咳嗽的诊断与治疗指南》等都将支气管激发试验阳性列为不典型支气管哮喘或咳嗽变异性哮喘的重要诊断条件之一,也是哮喘治疗效果评估的重要方法之一。特异性支气管激发试验(specific bronchial provocation test)指吸入已知的、不同浓度的特定变应原溶液,测定气道收缩反应,判断气道反应性的试验。非特异性支气管激发试验(non-specific bronchial provocation test)指吸入不同浓度激发剂,测定气道收缩反应,判断气道反应性的试验。临床上常用激发剂为乙酰甲胆碱和组胺等。

二、气道高反应诱发支气管痉挛的病理生理机制

人类所有正常气道均保持轻度张力性收缩。这种支气管平滑肌张力主要通过迷走传出神经来维持,应用抗胆碱药物可有效地消除这种张力。气道阻塞性疾病患者具有特征性的气道高反应性,其病理特点是气道非特异性慢性炎症,表现为气道平滑肌肥厚与增生。气流阻力与气道半径呈负相关,气道口径的改变能显著影响气道阻力,已狭窄气道口径的进一步小可能导致气道阻力增高,气体流动的速度显著下降,引起不同程度的气道阻塞。研究提示机体气道高反应性的主要因素是气道上皮细胞连接损害,使刺激屏障消失,从而刺激物更易接近内皮下受体,产生平滑肌收缩。气道张力受自主性(胆碱能与肾上腺素能)神经、非肾上腺素能和非胆碱能神经及感觉受体的影响。自主神经和感觉受体主要通过副交感途径来改变支气管平滑肌张力。支气管痉挛性疾病患者这些受体对有害刺激的阈值降低,可引起进行性反射性支气管收缩。以哮喘患者为例,最具特征性的病理生理改变是以不同程度

的嗜酸性粒细胞、肥大细胞和 $CD4^+$ T 淋巴细胞浸润为主的慢性气道炎症和以内皮基膜增厚、气道平滑肌增殖、杯状细胞肥大增生及新生血管生成等为主的气道重塑,慢性气道炎症与气道重塑又是哮喘患者 AHR 的主要原因,表现为当气道受到较轻刺激时即发生明显的支气管痉挛。长期的慢性气道炎症和气道重塑导致患者呼气相和吸气相阻力均增高,肺内气体排出受阻致内源性呼气末正压(PEEPi)升高。若病情控制不佳,肺组织因长期呈过度充气状态,吸气肌收缩能力将不同程度受损,尤以膈肌功能的损害为著。增高的肺容积使患者呼吸时额外增加了弹性阻力和呼吸做功,极易诱发呼吸衰竭。此外,气道炎症、黏液堵塞、增生的平滑肌收缩等加剧了患者通气/血流比值失衡和低氧血症的发生。围术期由于处于应激状态,气道及全身炎症反应进一步加重,使支气管和细支气管内黏液分泌增加,加重气道狭窄及 AHR,因而哮喘患者发生支气管痉挛的风险大大增加。

三、气道高反应诱发支气管痉挛的诱因

1. 高危人群　①近期上呼吸道感染,②吸烟,③哮喘与支气管痉挛史,④慢性支气管炎、肺气肿患者。
2. 促发因素　①高位硬膜外麻醉,牵拉、疼痛、咳嗽等神经反射。②分泌物对呼吸道的刺激,浅麻醉下气管内吸痰/插管、导管过深、套囊过度膨胀等均可造成支气管痉挛,③应用了具有兴奋迷走神经、增加气道分泌物、促使组胺释放的麻醉药、肌松药或其他药物,如硫喷妥钠、琥珀胆碱、低分子右旋糖酐等。
3. 术前气道炎症未控制　主要与多种炎症介质和细胞因子介导的气道重塑、AHR 及气管平滑肌收缩有关。
4. 其他　包括肥胖、肺部感染、手术部位、麻醉深度/平面、应激程度、胃食管反流等。

四、气道反应测定等肺功能检查指标在围术期的临床应用

外科治疗是众多疾病获得根治的主要方法,但术中及术后并发症是影响患者围术期快速康复及术后生存质量的主要因素,甚至威胁患者生命。患者术前肺功能状态直接与术后并发症相关,因此,肺功能检查是手术患者安全性评估常规检查项目,特别是胸腹部术前必备检查之一。准确的术前肺功能评估及肺康复训练是预防术后并发症的主要措施。

(一)肺的通气功能

肺通气功能(ventilation function)测定单位时间内肺脏吸入或呼出的气量,反映呼吸道的通畅性。目前临床工作中术前评估肺功能的重要指标是第 1 秒用力呼气容积(forced expiratory volume in one second, FEV_1)和用力肺活量(forced vital capacity,FVC)。肺通气功能很差的患者往往不能耐受麻醉或手术,因此肺通气功能检查是术前评估必不可少的一部分。肺通气功能正常且无哮喘及其他过敏性疾病个人史及家族史的患者手术风险较低。肺通气功能下降者,第 1 秒用力呼气量占预计值百分比 $FEV_1\%$ 预计值 $<80\%$ 相对手术安全; $FEV_1\%$ 预计值 $<50\%\sim60\%$ 者手术风险高。FEV_1 下降是判断阻塞性肺通气功能障碍程度的非常有价值指标,预测手术风险,哮喘患者 $FEV_1\%$ 预计值 $>80\%$ 相对手术安全; $FEV_1\%$ 预计值 $<40\%$ 为手术禁忌。需要注意的是,尽管部分患者 FEV_1 及呼气峰流速(peak expiratory flow, PEF)正常,但小气道功能低下也预示气道高风险;还有一些患者小气道各项指标均正常,也有术中或术后发生气道痉挛,引起哮喘发作。患者个人过敏史及是否有哮喘或过敏性疾病家族史对预测 AHR 有一定意义。临床上发现此类患者尽管术前肺功能正常,术中及术后也容易有 AHR 发生。英国胸科协会(British Thoracic Society, BTS)指南要求接受肺叶切除术患者术前的 FEV_1 不应低于 1.5 L 和接受全肺切除术患者术前 FEV_1 不应低于 2 L。由于身高、年龄、活动强度、体重等因素会影响 FEV_1 绝对值的测定,因此,FEV_1 绝对值不能绝对地真实评价肺外科手术的风险。而 $FEV_1\%$ 则是比 FEV_1 绝对值更个体化的评价指标,很多科学家和临床工作者关注其对肺癌手术的安全性的预测价值,并进行了一系列研究。其中一项研究表明,若患者接受手术前 $FEV_1\%<30\%$,患者手术后发生肺部相关并发症的概率为 43%,而 $FEV_1\%>60\%$ 者并发症发生率仅为 12%。另一项研究表明:每当 FEV_1 下降 10%,接受手术的患者术后发生肺部相关并发症的概率升高 1.1 倍,而发生心血管并发症的概率升高 1.3 倍。所以 $FEV_1\%$ 是可以独立预测肺切除术后肺部并发症的指标,并且优于 FEV_1 绝对值。从而,学界认同 $FEV_1\%=60\%$ 是术后发生肺部并发症概率的阈值,或者 $FEV_1\% \geq 80\%$,那么可以不必进行其他评价就可以实施肺切除手术。经典的文献还同时将预计术后肺功能(predicted postoperative pulmonary function, PPOP)PPO-$FEV_1\%$pred$<40\%$ 作为评估手术高风险的阈值。(PPO-$FEV_1\%$ 计算公式:对于肺切除患者,PPO-FEV_1=术前检测 $FEV_1\times$(1-所切除侧肺功能所占功能比例)。

(二)一氧化碳弥散量(capacity carbon monoxide diffusing amount, DLCO)

患者术前接受肺弥散功能的测定能有效的反映患者肺部可以使用的肺泡膜总体面积、厚度及肺毛细血管容积的情况。20 世纪 80 年代一位学者进行了一项临床试验揭示,若患者术前 DLCO$<60\%$,那么其术后发生肺部并发症的概率大概为 40%,同时死亡的概率为 20%,并表示 DLCO 可以应用为术前评价肺切除手术风险大小的重要因素。国内一项研究分析了 1014 例肺癌手术患者,对于 FEV_1 绝对值在正常范围内的肺癌患者来说,弥散功能低于正常范围仍然是术后在短期内出现并发症的独立危险指标。在患者有肺癌的患者中,FEV_1 与 DLCO 之间相关性不是很强,即使是手术之前测定 FEV_1 绝对值正常的肺癌患者也可能有弥散功能受损的情况出现。于 2009 年发布的 ERS/ESTS 指南建议 DLCO 检测应当作为接受肺部手术患者术前常规检测的指标。对于拟行肺部手术的患

者目前国际指南均同时使用 FEV₁ 和 DLCO 进行评估,并同时计算 PPO-FEV1 和(预计术后肺功能)PPO-DLCO。ERS/ESTS 指南初筛标准仍然采用术前 FEV₁ 和 DLCO,如均>80%预计值,则无须进一步评估,可行预期手术;而 ACCP 指南则在初筛时,就要求切除范围进行 PPO-FEV₁ 和 PPO-DLCO 的计算和评估,如均>60%的预计值,则无需进一步评估,可行包括全肺在内的手术治疗。(PPO-DLCO 计算公式:对于全肺切除患者,PPO-DLCO=术前检测 DLCO×(1-所切除侧肺功能所占功能比例)。当 PPO-FEV₁ 或 PPO-DLCO 介于 30% 和 60% 之间,则建议行运动试验检查。

(三)气道反应性

哮喘患者第 1 秒末用力呼气容积(FEV₁)<70%预计值、用力肺活量(FVC)<70%预计值、或 FEV₁/FVC<65%预计值,是患者围术期气道梗阻性并发症高发的预测因子。FEV₁<80%预计值可用以评估哮喘患者经标准剂量 sABA 治疗后支气管可逆程度,若患者支气管可逆程度>15%,则多提示哮喘症状控制不佳。这类患者术中或术后气道梗阻性并发症发生率较症状控制良好者增加数倍。Groeben 等研究表明,未经治疗的哮喘患者,即使术前肺功能指标正常,气管内局麻后行纤支镜引导下气管插管,其 FEV₁ 下降可高达 50% 以上,提示未经长程抗感染治疗哮喘患者常伴有 AHR,使其对气管插管、术中恶性刺激所致的神经反射及药物治疗的反应性难以预测。这种现象在年轻哮喘患者,尤其是小儿更为显著。对未诊断哮喘,但存在可疑症状(如持续性咳嗽和严重的过敏性疾病)的患者,在行择期手术前应行支气管激发试验,以评估气道反应性,优化术前治疗,降低围术期支气管痉挛风险。

围术期安全有效的气道管理是保证手术成功的关键环节。拟行择期手术患者应在术前 1 周接受临床症状、肺功能及必要的气道反应性评估,以利于较好控制哮喘症状,降低气道的高敏状态,降低气道痉挛的发生,改善肺功能,提高手术的安全性。术前充分询问病史,请呼吸内科、麻醉科等多学科联合会诊,共同评估气道情况。根据患者肺功能检查结果、个人病史及家族过敏史,预测围术期气道并发症风险,并提前治疗干预控制相关疾病症状,预防术中及术后 AHR 的发生。对于 COPD 及其他咳痰症状明显的患者,可同时术前给予气道管理药物,如糖皮质激素、支气管扩张药、肾上腺素及康复训练指导等。术前对哮喘患者进行围术期风险评估和内科治疗指导,对减少患者术中支气管痉挛和术后并发症的发生、缩短住院时间、改善患者预后极为重要。目前外科患者术前肺功能检查对确定手术方式、明确手术切除范围、制定麻醉措施,在提高围术期生活质量及减少肺部并发症发生率和病死率等方面发挥着不可替代作用。仅仅应用临床的肺功能检查仍不能满足临床需要,以肺通气功能指标占主要方面的肺功能检查不能完全真实地反映肺功能状态,我们必须从单纯的肺通气和换气功能联合到气道反应检测,甚至更进一步做运动心肺功能检测、核素扫描等检测和 X 线检查等,同时密切结合临床,早预测患者对于承受手术的能力,更好地判断心肺功能和气道反应性的状况,从而为患者制订个体化最佳治疗方案,降低支气管痉挛的发生率,减少手术风险,推动围术期快速康复,以取得更好的临床效果,提高患者的生存质量为最终目的。

参 考 文 献

[1] 中华医学会呼吸病学分会哮喘学组. 支气管哮喘防治指南(2016 年版). 中华结核和呼吸杂志,2016,39(9):675-697.

[2] GLOBAL INITIATIVE FOR ASTHMA. Global Initiative for Asthma(GINA)2017 Global Strategy for Asthma Management and Prevention[EB/OL],2018,10-18.

[3] 支修益. 胸外科围手术期气道管理专家共识(2012 年版). 中国胸心血管外科临床杂志,2013,20(3):251-255.

[4] 多学科围手术期气道管理专家共识(2016 年版)专家组. 多学科围手术期气道管理专家共识(2016 年版). 中华胸部外科电子杂志,2016,3(3):129-133.

[5] Warner DO,Warner MA,Barnes RD,et al. Perioperative respiratory complications in patients with asthma. Anesthesiology,1996,85(3):460-467.

[6] Kannan JA,Bernstein JA. Perioperative anaphylaxis:diagnosis, evaluation, and management. Immunol Allergy Clin North Am,2015,35(2):321-334.

[7] 郑劲平. 支气管激发试验检查//肺功能学-基础与临床. 广州:广东科技出版社,2007.

[8] GINA ScienceCommittee. Guidelines:Global strategy for asthma management and prevention,Global Initiative for Asthma(GINA)2014. http://www.ginasthma.org/.

[9] 中华医学会呼吸病学分会哮喘学组. 支气管哮喘防治指南(支气管哮喘的定义、诊断、治疗和管理方案). 中华结核和呼吸杂志,2008,31:177-185.

[10] 中华医学会呼吸病学分会哮喘学组. 咳嗽的诊断与治疗指南(2009 版). 中华结核和呼吸杂志,2009,32:407-413.

[11] SAcHDEV G,NAPOLITANO LM. Postoperative pulmonary compljcations:pneumonia and acute respiratory failure. Surg Clin North Am,2012,92(2):321-344.

[12] MCTIER L,BOTTI M,DuKE M. Patient participation in pulmonary interventions to reduce postoperatiVe puhnonary complications following cardiac surgery. Aust Crit Care,2016,29(1):35-40.

[13] BTS guidelines:guidelines on the selection of patients with lung cancer for surgery. Thorax,2001,56(2):89-108.

[14] Berry MF,Villamizar-Ortiz NR,Tong BC,et al. Pulmonary function tests do not predict pulmonary complications after thoracoscopic lobectomy. Ann Thorac Surg,2010,89(4):1044-1051,1051-1052.

[15] Ferguson MK,Siddique J,Karrison T. Modeling major lung resection outcomes using classification trees and multiple imputation techniques. Eur J Cardiothorac Surg,2008,34(5):1085-1089.

[16] Brunelli A,Kim AW,Berger KI,et al. Physiologic evaluation of the patient with lung cancer being considered for resectional surgery:Diagnosis and management of lung cancer,3rd

ed: American College of Chest Physicians evidence-based clinical practice guidelines. Chest, 2013, 143 (5 Suppl): e166S-e190S.
[17] Brunelli A, Charloux A, Bolliger CT, et al. ERS/ESTS clinical guidelines on fitness for radical therapy in lung cancer patients(surgery and chemo-radiotherapy). Eur Respir J, 2009, 34(1):17-41.
[18] Ferguson MK, Little L, Rizzo L, et al. Diffusing capacity predicts morbidity and mortality after pulmonary resection. J Thorac Cardiovasc Surg, 1988, 96(6):894-900.
[19] Schuurmans MM, Diacon AH, Bolliger CT. Functional evaluation before lung resection. Clin Chest Med, 2002, 23(1): 159-172.
[20] Celli BR. What is the value of preoperative pulmonary function testing. Med Clin North Am, 1993, 77(2):309-325.
[21] Gass GD, Olsen GN. Preoperative pulmonary function testing to predict postoperative morbidity and mortality. Chest, 1986, 89:127-135.
[22] Warner DO, Warner MA, Offord KP, et al. Airway obstruction and perioperative complications in smokers undergoing abdominal surgery. Anerthesiology, 1999, 90:372-379.
[23] Milledge JS, Nunn JF. Critetir of fitness for anaesthesia in patients with chronic obshuctive lung diseases. BMJ, 1975, 3: 670-673.
[24] Gmeben H, Schlicht M, Stieglitz S, et al. Both local anesthetics and albuterol pretreatment affect reflex bronchocon striction in volunteers with asthma undergoing awake fiberoptic intubation. Anesthesiology, 2002, 97:1445-1450.
[25] Bishop MJ, Cheney FW. Anesthesia for patients with asthma. Anesthesiology, 1996, 85:455-456.

11 医院血气分析 POCT 管理

张旭华

血气分析是指对血液中具有生理效应的气体成分和含量,以及酸性和碱性物质等进行测定分析的技术过程。通过监控机体的氧气及氧合状况、二氧化碳水平、酸碱平衡状态、电解质、血糖及血乳酸等,可以衡量肺通气及肺换气功能,长久以来一直是肺功能检查的重要组成部分,同时还可以间接反映出中枢对呼吸及血液循环系统的调节功能,心血管系统的运输能力及血细胞功能,肝、肾等主要脏器代谢功能,评价呼吸衰竭、缺氧类型及程度、体液酸碱平衡、离子平衡状态、有机酸代谢等,常用于疾病的诊断与鉴别诊断、病情严重程度评估、治疗效果评价、通气策略制定、危急重症患者管理、麻醉手术及机械通气患者监护等。可以说,血气分析是对肺、心、脑、肝、肾等机体主要器官、组织、系统功能的一个综合反映,广泛应用于临床各科。血气分析检查是急重症患者抢救和监护过程中的关键性指标,临床认可度越来越高,可谓必不可少、不可或缺,同时因其具有自动化、小型化、快捷化、低保养、高性价比等特点,近年来也已成为床旁检测的重要组成部分。在临床实践中,血气分析测定结果往往直接关乎着患者的诊疗工作,其准确性及整个环节的质量控制就显得尤为重要。

一、POCT 概述

即时检测(point-of-care testing,POCT)是指主实验室之外,靠近检测对象并能及时报告结果的小型移动设备的检测。亦称及时检测(timely testing)、床旁检测(bedside testing)、患者身边检测(near-patient testing)、医师诊所检测(physicians' office testing)、家用检测(home use testing)、实验室外检测(extra-laboratory testing)、分散检测(decentralized testing)等,是医院检测自动化和简单化发展趋势下的产物,涵盖所有在医院内、临床实验室之外进行的临床检测项目。比如血气分析、血糖、心肌梗死三项(肌钙蛋白、肌红蛋白、肌酸激酶同工酶)、脑钠肽(利钠肽)、凝血酶原时间(PT)和国际标准化比值(INR)测定等。POCT 是体外诊断器械(IVD)的一个细分行业,凭借便捷、快速的优势,实现在患者身边快速取得诊断结果。中国的 POCT 市场现在还是一个尚未被满足需求的巨大的蓝海市场,国内企业的进口替代才刚刚开始。目前似乎仅限于检验检测,未来包含的内容一定会更加广泛。比如床旁影像、床旁心电、峰流速仪、便携式肺功能仪、无创呼吸机等医学诊疗技术都可能纳入其中。因为,所有这些床旁检测设备的应用都需要质量控制与规范化管理。

二、血气分析 POCT 管理目的和的意义

快速检测结果可以帮助医生快速诊断,挽救生命,特别是针对危急重症患者,快速准确的血气分析结果能为临床医师争取宝贵的诊治时间。血气分析的每一项重要参数,比如 pH、PaO_2、$PaCO_2$、BE、AB/SB、ISE、Glu、Lac 等都关乎着患者的病情,决定了下一步需要采取的紧急医疗干预措施,特别是当患者存在呼吸衰竭、严重的呼吸性或代谢性酸碱失衡、电解质紊乱、乳酸酸中毒等,甚至达到危急值的情况。这些情况本身即可导致或加重原本复杂的临床现象,甚至危及生命。目前,医院 POCT 约占总检查数量的 25%,而且每年仍以 12% 的速度在增长,发达国家比例很高。比如,德国血气分析有 80% 是通过 POCT 检测的,国内很多高等级医院的血气分析检测也基本都能达到或超过了这个水平。POCT 血气分析仪更是遍布诸多临床科室,比如急诊科、麻醉科、手术室、心胸外科、烧伤科、普外科、神经外科、呼吸与危重症医学科、心血管内科、神经内科、肾脏内科、透析室、儿科、各种重症监护室(ICU、CCU、RICU、EICU、PICU、NICU、UICU、AICU、BICU、TICU、OICU、CPICU、CSICU、NSICU……)等。POCT 血气分析检测为临床诊治工作带来了极大的便利,目前仍处于快速增长的势头。但同时,由于医院血气分析仪数目众多、品牌型号繁杂、测定原理各异、上机操作随意、质控管理混乱、结果时有失控。因为临床科室血气分析操作人员构成复杂,多数操作人员为临床医护人员,缺乏质量控制意识和相关知识,所以,全方位加强临床科室血气分析检查的规范化管理具有非常重要的意义。

三、传统检查与 POCT 的区别

在过去医院的传统检测方法中,大量的时间被耗费在分析的前、后阶段,即治疗周转时间(therapeutic turn around time,TTAT)。检测工作经历了患者准备、材料准备、操作者准备、标本采集、标本储存与转运、标本交接、检测设备准备、上机检测、结果分析、报告传送等,最后临床医师才能获得结果。过程复杂而冗长,各个环节发生差错的概率及标本本身的变化都在逐步增加,都可能会对结果

造成严重影响。常见的影响因素可以归纳为管理问题、人员问题、质量控制问题、仪器问题、物料问题、检测报告问题等几个方面。研究显示,对于血气分析检测而言,分析前标本问题往往是导致结果偏离的主要因素。而POCT的中间环节明显减少,特别是减少了标本储存与转运、标本交接、实验室结果分析与报告传送等环节,极大地降低了差错概率和标本变化的影响,而且临床医师可及时得到检测结果,迅速采取治疗措施。

(一)POCT的优势

1. 检测地点优势 靠近患者,便于提供个性化的医疗服务。

2. 现场分析优势 减少周转环节,避免差错,准确性更好,便于患者的监护和管理。

3. 设备配置优势 小型化、移动化、简单化、经济化、免维护。

4. 检测结果优势 近乎适时提供,更能准确反映患者的实际情况。

5. 人力资源优势 节省人力,优化资源。

(二)POCT的劣势

1. 设备问题劣势 设备众多,原理不同,厂家要求各异。

2. 质量控制劣势 质控体系不完善或欠缺,甚至失控。

3. 技术水平劣势 操作者技术水平参差不齐,特别是对标本的处理。

4. 科室管理劣势 科室管理不到位甚至是管理盲区,操作者责任心不强。

5. 医院管理劣势 难以实现规范化、统一化和同质化。

6. 成本核算劣势 多为试剂包和测试片,成本价值高,且不适宜同一标本的复检等。

四、血气分析POCT管理的相关内容和质量管理体系的建立

通常情况下,医院血气分析POCT质量管理体系建设应该包括以下内容。

(一)组织管理

医院成立POCT管理委员会,含POCT管理小组和质量控制小组,负责管理医院所有POCT的开展、质量控制等相关工作。主管院长领导,医务处、护理部负责行政及人员管理,主实验室与临床业务科室负责具体实施,器械设备科提供后勤保障。

(二)操作人员资质管理

医院临床科室从事POCT的操作人员应该具备必须的资质,包括具备卫生专业技术职称,经专门的POCT培训并考核合格,由医院POCT管理委员会或管理小组认定具有做好相应PODT检测工作的专业能力,并获得医院职能部门授权。建立POCT人员档案,包括从业者医、技、护师执业资质、POCT培训记录、考核结果、医院授权证明等。

(三)POCT仪器和耗材管理

选用的POCT仪器、试剂和耗材应当符合国家食品药品监督管理局的有关规定,建议同一POCT项目最好使用同一个厂家的仪器、试剂和耗材。同一品牌的POCT设备大部分也都有厂家自己研发的POCT质量管理方案,比如美国沃芬的iQM、丹麦雷度的AQURE、德国西门子的RAPIDComm质量管理系统等,有的甚至还具有兼容的功能。建立设备档案,包括仪器说明与相关合格证书、校准报告、维护与保养记录、质量控制记录、耗材管理登记等。

(四)质量控制保障

1. 规章制度的建立 开展血气分析POCT的临床科室,必须建立健全各项血气分析POCT质量管理规章制度、工作职责、应急预案和血气分析POCT操作人员培训考核制度等。

2. 建立健全标准操作程序文件(standard operation procedure,SOP) 主要包括患者准备、标本采集流程、标本存储与转运、血气分析检测方法原理、仪器品牌、试剂耗材保存更换、检测操作规程、结果分析和报告、室内质量控制、室间质量评价、检测比对、仪器校准和维护、干扰因素和注意事项、经过验证的项目性能规格、超出可报告范围的处理程序等。所有文件需要POCT管理小组审核签字后,方可实施。

3. 日常管理 血气分析POCT操作人员必须认真做好日常质量控制,填写相关质量控制记录,接受POCT管理小组检查。包括厂商定期(每月1次)对血气分析POCT仪器进行的巡回质量检查、检测、维护与保养。设备日常定标、校准与模拟质控。电极、气体、试剂等耗材配件的购置、存放与使用等。

4. 室内质量控制 每台血气分析POCT设备必须按照行业规范或医院POCT管理委员会及厂方的规定,定期进行外部质控品的检测,通过质控图进行室内质量控制。做好室内质量控制记录和失控的分析与处理。室内质控结果超出范围不能进行标本测定,应当找出失控原因并及时纠正,重新进行质控测定,直至获得正确结果。

5. 室间质量评价 主实验室负责组织全院POCT血气分析仪的室间质评申报、上报室间质评结果及结果回报分析等,并上报POCT管理委员会。对于室间质评不合格的仪器或项目不能进行临床检测,必须查找不合格原因,待问题解决检测合格后方可进行临床检测。

6. 比对 医院所有血气分析POCT要进行全院统一比对。每个血气分析POCT设备均应使用新鲜患者样本与医院主实验室内室间质评合格的同类项目进行比对,每6个月至少进行1次,比对结果满足相关要求并上报POCT质量管理委员会。比对方案要具有科学性。

7. 记录 血气分析POCT操作人员必须做好各种日常性记录工作。医院所有的POCT血气分析设备均应有项目验证记录、样品检测原始记录、室内质量控制记录(包括原始数据和质控判断)、比对记录、室间质量评价记录、仪器使用维护校准记录、与质量有关的投诉和处理意见记

8. 检查指导　POCT 管理委员会或管理小组应经常组织专家对临床所有血气分析 POCT 工作进行质量控制检查和技术指导,根据实际应用情况做出取舍决定。

(五)血气分析 POCT 结果报告

血气分析 POCT 结果报告应当参考《医疗机构临床实验室管理办法》对检测报告的相关要求和规定,注重方便患者,保护患者隐私,符合病历书写和保存规范原则。POCT 结果报告单上须注明"POCT"字样,检测仪器统一编号、操作人员签名、标本检测日期和时间。

(六)生物安全管理

血气分析 POCT 操作人员在各个环节中,都必须严格执行标准操作规程,严格遵守医院院感部门的各项管理规定,注重个人防护和设备清消工作,正确处理医疗废物,防止院感发生保障安全。

五、血气分析 POCT 管理相关要求

血气分析 POCT 管理的相关要求,各种认证机构目前主要采用的是美国临床实验室改进修正法案 88(Clinical Laboratory Improvement Amendment,CLIA 88)、美国病理学家协会(College of American Pathologists,CAP)和国家临床实验标准委员会(National Committee for Clinical Laboratory,NCCLS)等对血气分析的质量控制要求,明确规定实验室至少没 8h 检测一个水平的质控物,至少每 30m 进行 1 次校准,每 24h 检测 1 次 2~3 个水平的质控物,每日对质量控制进行评估,建立质量控制(QC)和质量改进(QI)文件。国际医疗卫生机构认证联合委员会(the Joint Commission International,JCI)对血气分析 POCT 质量管理还提出了同质化的要求。主实验室 POCT 靶机应该参加并通过国家临检中心每个年度组织的针对第三方质控品的室间质量评价。医院也可以根据自身的实际情况和发展需求等,结合当地卫生行政管理部门制定的规章制度,建立自己的血气分析 POCT 质量管理体系。

六、血气分析 POCT 相关人员资质、培训和考核

医院血气分析 POCT 操作人员,基本都是临床医护人员,不具备系统的医学检测技术相关知识,未接受过专业训练,质量控制意识淡薄,必须接受全面系统的上岗前培训与考核,取得相应的技术操作和结果报告资质。由医院职能部门组织实施,包括厂商培训、实验室培训、考核和资质授权等。

(一)厂商培训

由工程师负责执行,内容主要是设备安装、使用操作规程、试剂存放与更换、仪器常规保养与维护、常见故障分析与处理、质量控制操作流程、注意事项等。

(二)实验室培训

由血气分析检测专业人员负责执行,内容主要是 POCT 管理的目的与意义、血气分析的临床应用、标本要求、标本采集、存放和处理规程、血气分析影响因素、误差分析与处理、结果解读与报告签发、生物安全与个人防护、室间质评与比对、POCT 标准程序性文件的编写、执行与保存等。

(三)考核与资质授权

考核工作同样由医院职能部门组织实施,包括理论考核和技能操作考核,只有考核合格后方能由医院相关部门授权准许从事 POCT 检测工作。医院所有的血气分析 POCT 临床科室,应当委派专人负责本科室的血气分析 POCT 相关工作,具备从事血气分析 POCT 工作资质和授权,服从医院 POCT 管理委员会的领导,执行各项规章制度,建立并完善各种 POCT 工作的程序性文件,认真做好本科室的血气分析 POCT 相关工作,自觉接受监督和检查。

总之,血气分析 POCT 是医院临床各科常用的检测设备,为了保障其正常运行、规范化应用、充分发挥作用,应当严格各个环节的质量控制管理。通过多轮次的 PDCA(即计划、执行、检查、处理 4 个阶段)循环,不断提高血气分析 POCT 标准化、规范化和同质化管理水平。

参 考 文 献

[1] Larkin BG,Zimmanck RJ. Interpreting arterial blood gases successfully. Aron,2015,102(4):343-357.

[2] 徐建新,顾敏晔,胡晓波,等.浅谈国内外 POCT 智能技术的发展.中华检验医学杂志,2017,40(12):983-984.

[3] Anthony L,Gonzalez D,Lori S,et al. Blood gas analyzers. Topics in Companion Animal Medicine,2016,31(1):27-34.

[4] 全球 POCT 产业发展现状及 2014 年中国 POCT 产业发展前景展望.产业信息网,2014-09-01.

[5] Rambaldi M,Baranzoni MT,Coppolecchia P,et al. Blood gas and patient safety:Considerations based on experience development in accordance with the risk management perspective. Clin Chem Lab Med,2007,45(6):774-780.

[6] Laboratory Quality Control Based on Risk Management:approved guideline Document EP23-A,Clinical and Laboratory Standards Institute,Wayne,PA,USA,2011.

[7] Application of Risk Management to Medical Devices,document 14971,International Organization for Standardization,Geneva,Switzerland,2007.

[8] 杨红玲,龙燕,张小玲.利用全面质量管理工具实现床旁血糖仪和血气分析仪的标准化管理.中华检验医学杂志,2013,10(36):876-879.

[9] Risk Management Techniques to Identify and Control Laboratory Error Sources,approved guideline document EP18-A2,Clinical and Laboratory Standards Institute,Wayne,PA,USA,2010.

[10] 中华医学会检验分会,卫生部临床检验中心,中华检验医学杂志编辑委员会.POCT 临床应用建议》.中华检验医学杂志,2012,35:10-16.

[11]《医疗机构临床实验室管理办法》.卫医发[2006]73号.

[12] US Department of Health and Human Services Medicare, Medicaid and CLIA Programs: regulations implementing the Clinical Laboratory Improvement Amendment of 1988. Final rule. Fed Register,1992,57(40):7002-7186.

[13] NCCLS. Statistical quality control for quantitative measurement: principles and definitions. Second edition. Approved guideline C24-A2. Wayne,PA:NCCLS,1998.

[14] Joint Commission International. Joint Commission International accreditation standards for hospital. New York: Joint Commission Resources,2014:1-296.

[15] 项盈,付启华,蒋黎敏.血气分析即时检验质量管理实践.检验医学,2017,32(10):911-916.

12 肺功能检查临床应用研究进展(2019—2020年)

邓 琳 郑劲平

肺功能检查是呼吸系统疾病诊断、疗效判断、预后评估、监测随访及早期干预等的重要临床检查。本文回顾了2019—2020年与肺功能检查相关的文献,总结了研究现状、新冠疫情防控、全国推广工作、指南标准更新、技术及临床应用等方面的进展。

一、肺功能检查文献研究现状

肺功能检查是呼吸疾病研究和临床评估的一个重要诊断工具,与其相关的国内外文献在逐年增加,对此我们检索了从2019年1月1日到2020年6月1日收录在国内外数据库PubMed和中国生物医学文献服务系统(SinoMed)的文献。通过跨库检索肺功能检查、肺功能等关键词,同时进行标题/摘要检索,在PubMed上得到6540条文献,浏览后发现有1110条文献与肺功能研究密切相关,其中主要与慢性阻塞性肺疾病(简称慢阻肺,COPD)、哮喘等相关的文献有254条;在SinoMed上得到6632条文献,与肺功能密切相关的文献有1678条,其中与慢阻肺、哮喘等相关的文献有913条。对比国内外研究的检索结果发现,尽管国内数据库收录的文献较国外多,但部分文献中的肺功能检查与我国中医中药疗效评估相关,且多数文献并未被PubMed收录。

二、新型冠状病毒肺炎疫情期间肺功能研究

2019年12月,新型冠状病毒肺炎(COVID-19)在我国湖北省武汉市全面暴发,并在全国及全球范围内迅速蔓延,疫情十分严峻,于2020年3月11日,世界卫生组织(WHO)宣布新型冠状病毒大流行。新型冠状病毒主要经呼吸道飞沫及密切接触传播,人群普遍易感且传染性强,进行肺功能检查可能增加医务人员和受检者之间的传播风险,这就导致肺功能检查的开展工作难以进行。但肺功能检查是临床诊断、评估及监测呼吸系统疾病的主要检查方式之一,因此临床上开展肺功能检查仍是必要的。为了指导医务人员疫情期间的肺功能检查防控工作,2020年4月,中国医师协会呼吸医师分会肺功能与临床呼吸生理工作委员会和中华医学会呼吸病学分会呼吸治疗学组肺功能专业组发表了《新型冠状病毒肺炎疫情防控期间开展肺功能检查的专家共识》,强调做好预防与控制措施,降低感染风险,为医务人员开展肺功能检查工作提供参考,国外专家认为尽管目前尚不清楚新型冠状病毒(SARS-CoV-2)感染与肺功能间的关系,提出了临床和研究对肺功能检查的需求。

为进一步研究COVID-19患者的肺功能变化,Mo和Jian等通过分析110例新冠肺炎康复期患者出院时的肺功能结果,发现在新冠肺炎患者中,弥散功能受损是最常见的肺功能异常,其次为限制性通气功能损害,且均与疾病的严重程度相关,首次总结了新冠肺炎出院患者的肺功能特点,并指出在新冠肺炎出院患者的随访中应纳入肺功能检查,尤其是病情较重的出院患者。

三、全国肺功能检查推广工作进展

2019年4月,钟南山院士、郑劲平教授等多位呼吸领域专家共同打造了《走进肺功能——肺功能检查》在线医学课程,这一课程基于人卫慕课平台,共设40个知识点,并及时调整和更新课程内容,实现在线视频学习、资源共享、习题解答、考试及互动讨论等,且针对新冠疫情,还新增了疫情防控专题,如《新冠肺炎疫情防控期间开展肺功能检查指引》等,得到医学界专家学者的广泛认可,不仅获得了《第二届人卫慕课在线课程与教学资源比赛微视频》本科组的一等奖,同时还被评选为《广东省本科高校在线开放课程》疫情阶段在线教学的优秀案例,并获得课程类一等奖。这一线上课程的开展,不仅推动肺功能检查技术的教育培训,还更进一步地促进了我国肺功能检查的推广和普及。

四、肺功能检查指南的更新

肺量计检查(也称肺通气功能检查)是最常用的肺功能检查,临床上多用于评估、诊断和监测肺功能,其检查质量的好坏往往会影响临床医生对患者病情的判断。为规范肺量计检查技术,提高肺功能检查质量,2019年美国胸科协会(ATS)及欧洲呼吸协会(ERS)更新了肺量计检查的技术规范指南,对2005年指南进行修订。在测试标准方面,新指南用"强迫呼气终止(end of forced expiration,EOFE)"替换"测试终止(end of test)",同时将原标

准中的"呼气时间≥3s（10岁以下儿童）或≥6s（10岁以上受试者）"改为"呼气时间>15 s"。在质量控制方面，新指南不仅对测试的可接受性标准及可重复性标准进行调整，还新增了测试的可用性标准，即尽管第1秒用力呼气容积（FEV1）和（或）用力肺活量（FVC）测试在技术上是不可接受的，但在临床上仍有提示作用，并在这一基础上，新增"U"质控等级（为至少有一次可用但没有可接受的测试）。在图形规范方面，对流量-容积和容积-时间图的图表格式进行调整，如在容积-时间图中，时间轴须从零点前1s开始。此外，尤其需要关注的是，指南对流量-容积曲线（F-V曲线）的吸气相提出了新要求：受试者在呼气起始应快速完成最大吸气量（FIVC），且吸气时间（包括停顿时间）应<2 s，在EOFE时再次快速完成FIVC，还指出当FIVC与FVC的差值>0.1L或5%FVC时，则认为该次测试不可接受。但部分学者认为这一指南仍存在部分问题。Arce提出操作人员须确保在使用支气管扩张药前和后的呼气时间保持一致，否则会影响患者FVC的变化，同时还指出仪器软件应具备接受或拒绝来自不可接受的操作的单个FVC和FEV1值的能力，才能完成U等级的判断。同年，我国新增发表了"肺功能检查报告规范——肺量计检查、支气管舒张试验、支气管激发试验"指南。指南主要内容为肺功能报告内容和格式的推荐、结果解读、检查质量评估分级系统及报告规范用语等，同时还给出了标准版、简易版及窄幅版3种报告示范格式，对我国的肺功能检查报告进行统一，且标准化的报告可加强检查的质量控制，进而促进我国肺功能检查的规范化进程。

强迫振荡技术（forced oscillation technique，FOT）是一种简单的测量和研究呼吸系统力学特征的方法，可通过平静的潮气呼吸来获得相应的参数。近年来，FOT的使用越发广泛，ATS及ERS在2020年发布了相关的技术规范指南，相较2003年的技术规范，此次指南新增了FOT的质控程序，并对审查了支持支气管舒张试验和激发试验的阈值。此外，还更新了成人和儿童的阻抗预计值，为临床检查提供一个更适合的标准。

五、肺功能检查技术及人工智能解读的发展

近年来，物联网医学发展迅速，不断推动着慢性呼吸系统疾病的远程管理、监测、个体化治疗等水平的提高。肺功能检查与物联网医学的结合，将更好地促进肺功能检查技术的发展和推广。哮喘是呼吸系统最常见的慢性疾病之一，许多患者经过药物治疗后仍有症状，可能原因是部分患者没有坚持哮喘的持续治疗，或治疗方案并不适于此部分患者，故实时监控病情变化并及时调整治疗方案是必需的。Ljungberg等运用AsthmaTuner（基于云端的数字化自我管理系统的应用程序），使用蓝牙肺量计仪对失控哮喘患者的症状和肺功能进行自我监测，并同时对患者病情变化自动进行药物调整，指出相比门诊随访这一常规治疗，AsthmaTuner能提高哮喘患者的症状控制，且依从性能得到相应的改善。除哮喘外，特发性肺纤维化（IPF）也能通过物联网对患者进行随访、监测。Moor等纳入90例IPF患者，将其分为家庭监测组和标准护理组，通过一个基于云端的平板电脑和手持式肺量计仪，对FVC的变化进行实时监测，同时调整治疗方案，认为家庭肺量计检查是可行的，能为临床医生提供可靠的结果，且基于云端的电子健康工具是具有潜力的，能为IPF患者提供更多的个性化治疗。

随着大数据时代的来临和计算机技术的快速发展，人工智能（artificial intelligence，AI）和机器学习技术（machine learning techniques）在医学上的应用更加广泛。在呼吸医学领域中，主要是应用于对胸部成像、肺病理切片和肺功能测试等生理数据的解释。已有研究表明，结合肺功能检查结果和临床变量的机器学习框架能提高呼吸系统疾病诊断的总体准确性，Delclaux也认为人工智能辅助临床诊断是有必要的，相较呼吸内科医师，AI在报告判读和疾病诊断上更具优势，但同时也需更多的研究去验证。Das等针对2019年肺量计检查技术规范新指南中的测试可接受性和可用性标准，运用CNN（卷积神经网络）的机器深度学习方法，对ATS/ERS肺量计标准实行自动化质量控制，同时还结合技术人员的视觉经验，发现AI的使用可促进指南中测试可接受性和可用性标准的应用标准化。但Gonem等指出将AI应用于肺功能检查是有前提的，需基于一个大型的医学训练数据集进行开发，而这正是目前已有研究所欠缺的部分。因此，将AI和机器学习技术运用到临床之前，仍需大量的临床数据和研究佐证，并进一步挖掘其未来发展的潜力。

六、肺功能正常值的研究

基于大样本健康人群获得的肺功能正常预计值及方程，有助于准确判断肺功能结果，并可对疾病做进一步诊断。2012年，全球肺功能专责工作组（GLI）发表了多种族肺功能预计值方程GLI2012，为验证方程的适用性，各国针对其各自的人群进行研究。Agarwal等通过对1258名印度西部健康成人的肺功能数据进行了分析，发现当使用GLI2012方程时，部分受试者会被归为正常值下限，指出使用这一方程可能导致呼吸疾病的过度诊断。而相反，Blake等收集了930份3~25岁健康受试者的肺功能数据，样本来自澳大利亚的原住民和托雷斯海峡岛民，发现GLI2012其中的混合方程适于澳大利亚的原住儿童和年轻人，指出GLI方程在原始族群之外仍具有普遍性。在我国台湾，则以757名5~18岁的健康儿童为研究对象，发现东南亚人的预计值方程与此人群的肺功能检查数据并不完全相符，指出GLI方程未来仍需增加和更新非白种人群的数据。上述研究，都对GLI2012方程进行了验证，但在样本的人群选择或年龄的覆盖范围上存在着不足，为进一步研究GLI方程的普遍性和适用性，仍需在种族更广泛、年龄跨度更大的人群中去验证。

七、临床应用新进展

(一)正常值下限 vs 固定阈值 0.70

慢阻肺是一种常见的、可防可治的呼吸系统疾病,其特征是气道和(或)肺泡异常引起的持续呼吸道症状和气流受限。在临床上诊断气流受限的标准是:在肺量计检查中使用支气管舒张药后 1s 率(FEV1/FVC)比值仍<0.70。但这一固定阈值的使用仍存在争议。在最新的慢性阻塞性肺疾病全球创议(GOLD)2020 指南中,仍推荐延用固定阈值 0.70 作为评判气流受限的标准。0.70 这一固定阈值是基于专家意见确定的,并无研究数据佐证,为验证这一阈值,Bhatt 等基于 4 个美国普通人群 15 年随访的队列证据,共纳入 24012 份成人的肺功能数据,结果显示吸烟亚组的最佳比率阈值为 0.70,不吸烟亚组最佳比率阈值为 0.74,指出在预测与慢阻肺相关的住院和死亡率上,0.70 仍然比正常值下限(LLN)更准确。针对这一研究,Miller 等认为,0.70 固定阈值不应被鼓励使用,因它不能对与年龄相关的正常肺功能下降和异常肺功能损害进行区分,相反,LLN 更能说明年龄与肺功能的相关性。Vestbo 等则认为应继续延用固定阈值 0.70,虽然目前对于固定阈值和 LLN 的使用仍无明确定论,但 Bhatt 的研究使得固定阈值 0.70 更具信服力。但这一研究仍存在部分不足,其中需关注的一点是研究中的肺功能数据是源于支气管舒张前的,这与 GOLD2020 指南中基于舒张后 FEV1/FVC 比值判断是否气流受限相悖,故还需要获得进一步去补充验证。

(二)肺功能正常人群应予以关注

临床上,存在一部分有慢性呼吸道症状但肺功能正常(FEV1/FVC>0.70)的患者,既往 GOLD2001 指南曾将肺功能正常但存在咳嗽或咳痰的个体定义为 GOLD 0 期,把这部分患者划入慢阻肺早期,但因无完整证据表明处于 0 期的患者必然会往 1 期发展,故在 GOLD2006 指南中 0 期不再被包含在分期内。但实际上,存在慢性呼吸道症状但肺功能正常的人群所占的比例还是比较大的。Puhan 等基于丹麦人群随机选择了 108 246 名 20~100 岁个体,记录 2003—2018 年其因急性发作加重、肺炎、呼吸系统疾病及全因死亡导致的住院,通过评估这些因素的风险,发现在队列中多达 32%(30890)的人群存在慢性呼吸道症状但肺功能正常,指出在没有已知气道疾病但肺功能正常的人群中,其慢性呼吸道症状与呼吸系统疾病住院和死亡有关,且有症状的不吸烟人群,即使肺功能正常,也可能患有早期慢阻肺或存在其他潜在的呼吸系统疾病。值得注意的是,目前临床上对这部分人群仍无明确的管理和治疗方案,尽管如此,临床医师仍需留意这一人群,关注他们疾病的变化和进展,及时给予相应的干预措施,避免严重不良事件的发生。

(三)小气道功能障碍

除上述肺功能检查正常但存在症状的人群外,临床医生也同样关注经肺功能检查诊断为小气道功能障碍(SAD)的人群。在我国肺功能检查指南中,将最大呼气中期流量(MMEF)、用力呼出 50% 肺活量时的瞬间呼气流量(FEF 50%)及用力呼出 75% 肺活量时的瞬间呼气流量(FEF 75%)3 项指标中有 2 项低于 LLN 时诊断为 SAD。近年来,随着强迫振荡、重复呼吸氮冲洗及 CT 扫描成像技术等的不断发展和使用,关于 SAD 的研究越来越多,并发现 SAD 与慢阻肺和哮喘密切相关,但目前仍无一种明确的检查方法,可对小气道功能障碍进行诊断、衡量、监测。中国成人肺部健康(CPH)研究通过多阶段分层抽样纳入我国 2012 年 6 月至 2015 年 5 月 10 个省市 50479 名成年人的肺量计结果,把 SAD 定义为 MMEF、FEF 50% 和 FEF 75% 中至少有 2 项指标低于预测值的 65%,并将 SAD 分为舒张前 SAD(吸入支气管舒张剂前 FEV1 和 FEV1/FVC 比值正常,即 FEV1 大于预计值的 80% 和 FEV1/FVC 比值大于预计值的 70%)和舒张后 SAD(吸入支气管舒张剂后 FEV1 和 FEV1/FVC 比值正常),结果显示 SAD 的患病率为 43.5%,舒张前 SAD 患病率为 25.5%,舒张后 SAD 的患病率为 11.3%;且经多因素回归分析可发现在 SAD 人群中,吸烟、暴露于高浓度的直径<2.5μm(PM2.5)的颗粒物和体质指数(BMI)增加 5kg/m^2 是主要的可预防的危险因素,提示肺量计定义的 SAD 在我国成年人群中非常普遍,应引起重视。但研究中使用 65% 作为诊断 SAD 的截断值,仍需更多的研究证据支持。而 Postma 等进行了一项为期一年的多国前瞻性队列研究,在 2014—2017 年期纳入 697 例严重哮喘患者和 99 例无气道阻塞患者,通过综合肺功能检查(包括肺量计检查、强迫振荡检查、肺容积检查等)的各项指标,定义了 SAD 评分,并发现这一评分与哮喘的控制、急性发作病史和疾病的严重程度显著相关,指出在所有严重哮喘患者中均存在 SAD,且在 GINA5 分期的患者中发病率最高。通过这两项研究,启示临床医师:基于 SAD 较高的患病率,早期识别和诊断 SAD 是必要且急切的,而当单一检查方法或单一指标无法诊断 SAD,可综合多项检查多项指标进行分析,且 SAD 的准确识别和诊断更为早期干预治疗的增加了可能。

(四)体重影响肺功能水平变化

肺功能水平往往与个体的性别、年龄、身高及种族等有关,临床上使用的正常肺功能预计值则是根据个体的性别、身高、年龄推导得到,但鉴于目前全球范围内肥胖及超重人群(包括儿童)逐渐增加,体重与肺功能的关系再次引起重视。在 ALSPAC 研究中,纳入 6964 名 7~15 岁儿童的体重和身体成分轨迹,结合相应的肺功能结果,首次发现儿童和青春期的瘦体重(LBM)与青春期男孩、女孩较高的肺功能水平有关,脂肪含量只与男孩较低的肺功能相关,认为儿童和青少年的身体成分可影响肺功能的发展。但体重仅仅与儿童和青少年有关吗?ECRHS 研究发现体重变化与成年后的肺功能下降也有关。这项研究基于欧洲和澳大利亚 12 个国家 26 个中心的人群数据,对 3673 名 20~44 岁受试者进行为期 20 年 3 个周期(1991—1993,1999—2003,2010—2014)的随访,并纳入对应的体重和肺功能结果,通过分析不同体重变化下的肺功能轨迹,发现中、高体重增加会加速 FVC 和 FEV1 的下降,而体重减轻则可减缓 FEV1 的下降,表明超重和肥胖对肺功能存在负面影响,但可通过减肥来降低肺功能下降的速度。因此,当患者(包括患儿)的肺功能发生变化时,临床医师除了要判断患者是否存在器质性病变,也要关注其本身体重的变化,同时鼓励并协助他们建立健康的生活方式。

(五)环境暴露引起肺功能下降

肺功能的改变,不仅取决于个体本身因素,还与环境因素息息相关。在GOLD2020指南中指出,慢阻肺持续的呼吸症状和气流受限,通常是由有毒颗粒和气体的显著暴露引起的,其中香烟烟雾暴露是最常见的,研究发现吸烟的慢阻肺患者其肺功能随年龄的增长而加速衰退。随着公共健康卫生知识的普及,吸烟人群的数量逐渐下降,但戒烟后的人群其肺功能是否能恢复到正常人水平,抑或是继续下降?基于这一假设,NHLBI研究整合了以普通社区人群为基础的9个队列,共25352名17~93岁的成年人参与7年的随访研究,通过分析随访得到的肺量计检查数据,指出与从不吸烟者相比,已戒烟者和低强度吸烟者的肺功能下降速度更快,且经观察发现,在戒烟后,其肺功能的加速退仍持续数十年,表明接触香烟烟雾并无一个安全水平,戒烟是减少健康危害的最有效手段。这一研究,再次强调戒烟的重要性,提示临床医师在对慢阻肺患者进行全面评估和诊治时,还应劝导和鼓励患者戒烟,加强健康教育的宣传。除了香烟暴露,还有研究发现当汽车尾气中的柴油废气与过敏原共同暴露后,会降低FEV1,导致肺功能下降,且在粒子耗竭后,这些不利影响仍然存在。而在日常工作中,长期接触并暴露于气体、烟雾、粉尘、芳香族溶剂等危险因素中,也可能导致肺功能下降。Alif等通过2002—2008年随访期间完成的肺功能检查和终身工作历史日程,纳入767名45~50岁的受试者,并对每个受试者的工作接触暴露量进行汇总,分析数据后发现接触芳香族溶剂后,FEV1的下降幅度较大,尽管女性比男性接触较少,但其下降会更明显,指出暴露于芳香族溶剂与肺功能下降有较大的相关性,且女性具有更大的敏感性,认为未来有增加发生阻塞性气道疾病的风险可能。同样的,英国的一项大型前瞻性研究更是指出了6种特定职业与慢阻肺发生风险增加有关。这警示我们:无论是环境暴露还是职业暴露,我们需对这些危险因素采取相应的措施,政府和国家部门需出台相应的防控策略,尽量减少相关因素的接触暴露。

八、小 结

综上所述,新冠肺炎疫情期间肺功能检查工作可在防控措施下继续开展。肺功能检查工作进一步得到推广和普及。肺功能检查技术和报告规范指南得到更新与完善,GLI2012适用性和普遍性还在继续验证。固定阈值0.7仍是慢阻肺诊断的标准,应关注存在慢性呼吸道症状但肺功能正常的人群,小气道功能障碍可通过综合多指标来诊断。肺功能变化不仅与体重有相关性,还受到环境暴露的影响。肺功能检查在与物联网、AI联合应用的探索道路上又向前迈进了一大步。

参 考 文 献

[1] 新型冠状病毒肺炎疫情防控期间开展肺功能检查的专家共识. 中华结核和呼吸杂志,2020,43(4):302-307.

[2] Hull James H,Lloyd Julie K,Cooper Brendan G,Lung function testing in the COVID-19 endemic. Lancet Respir Med,2020.

[3] Mo Xiaoneng, Jian Wenhua, Su Zhuquan, et al. Abnormal pulmonary function in COVID-19 patients at time of hospital discharge. Eur. Respir. J,2020.

[4] Graham Brian L,Steenbruggen Irene,Miller Martin R,et al. Standardization of Spirometry 2019 Update. An Official American Thoracic Society and European Respiratory Society Technical Statement. Am. J. Respir. Crit. Care Med,2019,200:e70-e88.

[5] Arce Santiago C,On the 2019 Spirometry Statement. Am. J. Respir. Crit. Care Med,2020,201:626-627.

[6] 中国呼吸医师协会肺功能与临床呼吸生理工作委员会,中华医学会呼吸病学分会呼吸治疗学组.肺功能检查报告规范——肺量计检查、支气管舒张试验、支气管激发试验. 中华医学杂志,2019,99(22):1681-1691.

[7] King Gregory G,Bates Jason,Berger Kenneth I,et al. Technical standards for respiratory oscillometry. Eur Respir J,2020,55.

[8] Ljungberg Henrik,Carleborg Anna,Gerber Hilmar,et al. Clinical effect on uncontrolled asthma using a novel digital automated self-management solution: a physician-blinded randomised controlled crossover trial. Eur. Respir. J,2019,54.

[9] Moor Catharina C,Mostard Rémy L M,Grutters Jan C,et al. Home Monitoring in Patients with Idiopathic Pulmonary Fibrosis: A Randomized Controlled Trial. Am. J. Respir. Crit. Care Med,2020.

[10] Gonem Sherif,Janssens Wim,Das Nilakash,et al. Applications of artificial intelligence and machine learning in respiratory medicine. Thorax,2020.

[11] Topalovic Marko,Laval Stefan,Aerts Jean-Marie,et al. Automated Interpretation of Pulmonary Function Tests in Adults with Respiratory Complaints. Respiration,2017,93:170-178.

[12] Delclaux Christophe,No need for pulmonologists to interpret pulmonary function tests. Eur. Respir. J,2019,54.

[13] Das Nilakash,Verstraete Kenneth,Stanojevic Sanja,et al. Deep learning algorithm helps to standardise ATS/ERS spirometric acceptability and usability criteria. Eur RespirJ,2020.

[14] Agarwal Dhiraj,Parker Richard,Pinnock Hilary,et al. Normal spirometry predictive values for the Western Indian adult population. Eur. Respir. J,2020.

[15] Blake Tamara L,Chang Anne B,Chatfield Mark D,et al. Global Lung Function Initiative-2012 'other/mixed' spirometry reference equation provides the best overall fit for Australian Aboriginal and/or Torres Strait Islander children and

young adults Respirology,2020,25:281-288.
[16] Chang Sheng-Mao,Tsai Hui-Ju,Tzeng Jung-Ying,et al. Reference equations for spirometry in healthy Asian children aged 5 to 18 years in Taiwan. World Allergy Organ J,2019,12:100074.
[17] Global Initiative for Chronic Obstructive Lung Disease. Global strategy for diagnosis, management, and prevention of COPD [Internet] [updated 2020]. Available from: goldcopd.org/gold-reports/.
[18] Bhatt Surya P,Balte Pallavi P,Schwartz Joseph E,et al. Discriminative Accuracy of FEV1:FVC Thresholds for COPD-Related Hospitalization and Mortality. JAMA, 2019, 321:2438-2447.
[19] Miller Martin R, Stanojevic Sanja. FEV1:FVC Thresholds for Defining Chronic Obstructive Pulmonary Disease. JAMA,2019,322:1609-1610.
[20] Vestbo Jørgen, Lange Peter. Accuracy of Airflow Obstruction Thresholds for Predicting COPD-Related Hospitalization and Mortality:Can Simple Diagnostic Thresholds Be Used for a Complex Disease? JAMA,2019,321:2412-2413.
[21] Çolak Yunus, Nordestgaard Børge G, Vestbo Jørgen, et al. Prognostic significance of chronic respiratory symptoms in individuals with normal spirometry. Eur. Respir. J,2019,54.
[22] Puhan Milo A. Chronic respiratory symptoms but normal lung function:substantial disease burden but little evidence to inform practice. Eur Respir J,2019,54.
[23] 中华医学会呼吸病学分会肺功能专业组. 肺功能检查指南（第二部分）——肺量计检查. 中华结核和呼吸杂志,2014,37(7):481-486.
[24] van den Berge Maarten, Ten Hacken Nick H T, Cohen Judith, et al. Small airway disease in asthma and COPD:clinical implications. Chest,2011,139:412-423.
[25] Xiao Dan,Chen Zhengming,Wu Sinan,et al. Prevalence and risk factors of small airway dysfunction,and association with smoking, in China: findings from a national cross-sectional study. Lancet Respir Med,2020.
[26] Postma Dirkje S,Brightling Chris,Baldi Simonetta,et al. Exploring the relevance and extent of small airways dysfunction in asthma(ATLANTIS): baseline data from a prospective cohort study. Lancet Respir Med,2019,7:402-416.
[27] Peralta Gabriela P, Fuertes Elaine, Granell Raquel, et al. Childhood Body Composition Trajectories and Adolescent Lung Function. Findings from the ALSPAC study. Am J Respir Crit Care Med,2019,200:75-83.
[28] Peralta Gabriela P, Marcon Alessandro, Carsin Anne-Elie, et al. Body mass index and weight change are associated with adult lung function trajectories:the prospective ECRHS study. Thorax,2020,75:313-320.
[29] Fletcher C,Peto R. The natural history of chronic airflow obstruction. Br Med J,1977,1:1645-1648.
[30] Oelsner Elizabeth C, Balte Pallavi P, Bhatt Surya P, et al. Lung function decline in former smokers and low-intensity current smokers: a secondary data analysis of the NHLBI Pooled Cohorts Study. Lancet Respir Med,2020,8:34-44.
[31] Wooding Denise J,Ryu Min Hyung, Hüls Anke, et al. Particle Depletion Does Not Remediate Acute Effects of Traffic-related Air Pollution and Allergen. A Randomized, Double-Blind Crossover Study. Am J Respir Crit Care Med, 2019, 200:565-574.
[32] Alif Sheikh M,Dharmage Shyamali,Benke Geza,et al. Occupational exposure to solvents and lung function decline: A population based study. Thorax,2019,74:650-658.
[33] De Matteis Sara,Jarvis Deborah,Darnton Andrew,et al. The occupations at increased risk of COPD: analysis of lifetime job-histories in the population-based UK Biobank Cohort. Eur Respir J,2019:54.

第十部分

纵隔与胸膜疾病：诊断技术

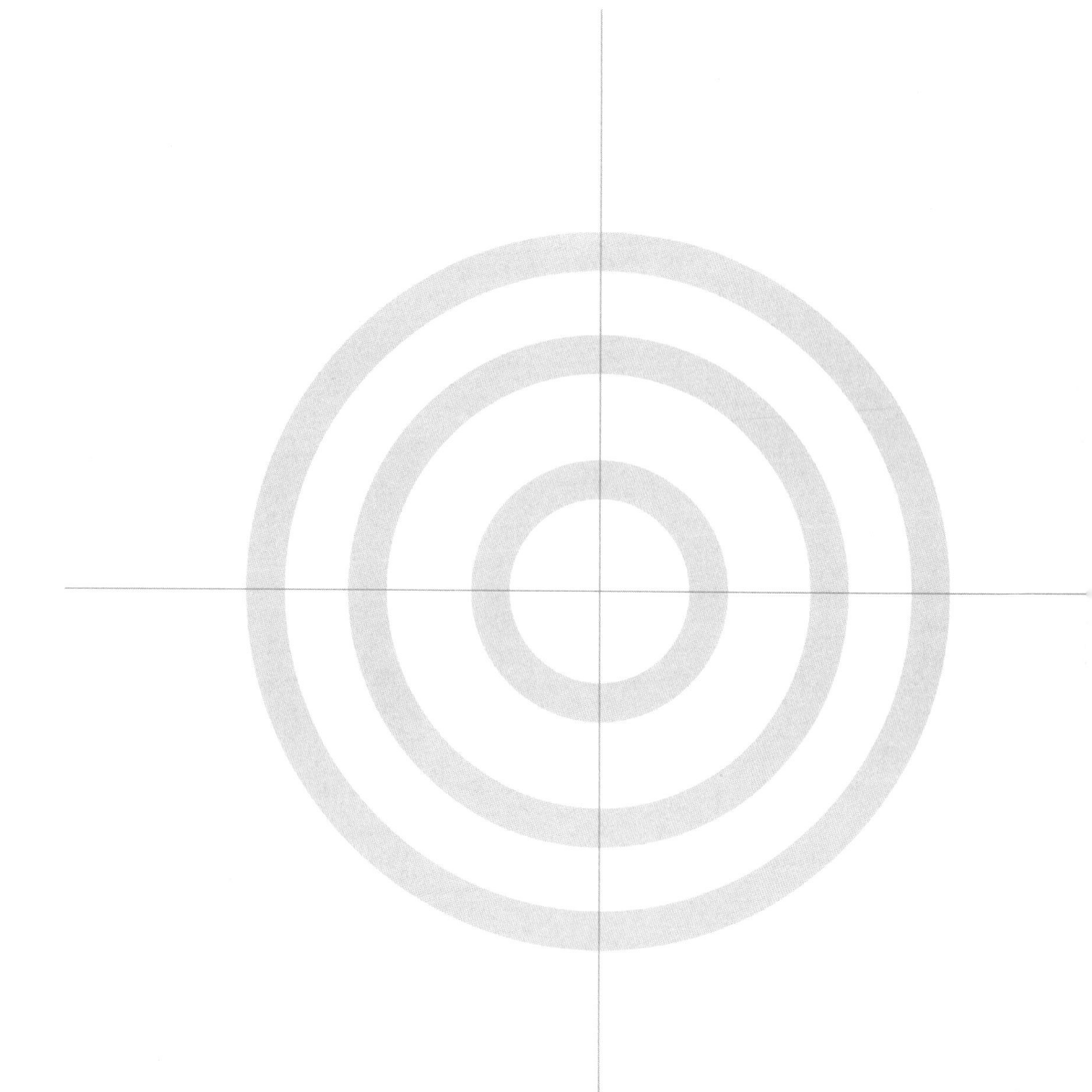

1 生物学标志物在渗出性胸腔积液诊断的研究进展

曾惠清　陈小蓉

胸腔积液(pleural effusion,PE)是呼吸系统的常见病和多发病,可分为漏出液和渗出液;最常见的渗出性 PE 病因为结核病、恶性肿瘤和肺炎,三种病因占所有病例的55%。进一步区分胸腔积液尤其是渗出性 PE 的病因是临床诊治的焦点和难题,常需要通过其他有创性检查如胸膜活检或胸腔镜检查,但是其阳性率及并发症的发生率依赖于操作者的技术水平,且病情重者难于进行。随着研究的深入,越来越多的生物学标志物展现出对 PE 的诊断及鉴别诊断的潜在价值。本文总结常见的渗出性 PE 病因的生物学标志物的研究进展。

一、结核性胸腔积液

(一)腺苷脱氨酶(adenosine deaminase,ADA)

ADA 是一种广泛分布于机体各组织中的核苷酸氨基水解酶,其活性与淋巴细胞的增殖分化以及激活有关。结核性胸膜炎(tuberculous pleural effusion,TPE)时由于胸膜局部的 T 淋巴细胞受到结核分枝杆菌抗原的刺激,使其增殖和分化,胸腔积液中 ADA 活性明显升高。最新荟萃分析发现,在 16 项研究共计 4147 例患者中,ADA 诊断 TPE 的敏感性为 93%,特异性为 92%,阳性似然比为 12,阴性似然比为 0.08,曲线下面积为 0.968。也就是说,ADA 对 TPE 有较高的诊断价值,而 ADA 水平≥40U/L 是最广泛接受的 TPE 的诊断指标。老年患者的 ADA 水平可能偏低,细菌性胸膜感染(尤其是并发的肺炎旁 PE 和脓胸)和淋巴瘤的 ADA 水平可能升高。ADA 临床诊断的准确阈值和准确性尚不清楚。Aggarwal AN 等回顾了 ADA 在 TPE 中的诊断性能,结果表明,常用的 40U/L 的 ADA 阈值具有较低的阴性似然比,可能更有助于排除 TPE 的诊断;相反地,当 ADA 阈值高于 65U/L 时,其阳性似然比较高,并且 TPE 患病率的阳性预测值较高,这样的阈值可能更助于确认而排除 TP 的诊断效能较差。另外,有研究发现,检测 PE 中的 ADA-2 水平(ADA-2 是 ADA 的主要同工酶)提高了 TPE 时总 ADA 诊断的特异性;然而,由于目前可用的 ADA-2 测定方法没有标准化,而且,它在大多数情况下对总 ADA 水平的影响很小,因此并没有得到广泛应用。

(二)白介素-27(interleukin 27,IL-27)

IL-27 是 IL-12 家族的一员,主要由抗原提呈细胞产生,能促进 T 细胞增殖并向 T 辅助淋巴细胞(Th1)细胞方向分化和分泌 γ 干扰素。Ye 等探讨 IL-27(+)CD4(+)T 细胞进入胸膜间隙的机制时发现,IL-27 可通过激活 STAT 3 信号传导通路,显著的促进了胸膜间皮细胞的增殖,并且完全阻止了由 IFN-γ 诱导的胸膜间皮细胞的凋亡,进而影响 TPE 的发展。截止到目前,有三项荟萃分析报告了 IL-27 对 TPE 的诊断意义,其中最具代表性的一项,共纳入了 1157 例 PE 患者,结果显示:IL-27 诊断 TPE 的诊断阈值为 591.4ng/L,敏感性和特异性分别为 93.8%和 91.7%,故其诊断效能是值得肯定的,可作为诊断 TPE 的生物标志物。但检测 PE 中 IL-27 成本较高,且其缺乏被公认的最佳诊断阈值,因此 IL-27 检测在 TPE 诊断中应用仍较少。

(三)干扰素-γ(interferon-γ,IFN-γ)和 IFN-γ 释放试验(IGRAs)

IFN-γ 是 CD4$^+$ T 淋巴细胞释放的一种细胞因子。IFN-γ 能使巨噬细胞聚集,且增加巨噬细胞对结核杆菌的杀菌能力,进而消灭结核分枝杆菌控制感染播散。因此 IFN-γ 也被认为是诊断 TPE 的生物学标志物之一。在一项纳入 22 项研究总计 2883 位患者的荟萃分析报道了 IFN-γ 诊断 TPE 的敏感性为 89%,特异性为 97%。同样地,因其检测成本较高,缺乏相应的准确的临床诊断阈值,在临床上的应用也受到限制。相反,IGRAs 是一种体外免疫检测结核杆菌感染的新方法,结核感染 T 细胞酶联免疫斑点试验(T-SPOT.TB)是 IGRAs 的一种,通过酶联免疫斑点技术检测体内是否存在结核分枝杆菌致敏的 T 淋巴细胞。目前临床上通常使用外周血 T-SPOT.TB 检测,但是诊断价值意义不大。Li 等纳入了 9 项研究进行 Meta 分析,结果显示 PE 中的 T-SPOT.TB 对 TPE 的诊断的敏感性为 93%,特异性为 90%;认为 PE 中的 T-SPOT.TB 作为一种独立的诊断结核性胸膜炎的方法是足够准确的。另一些学者认为,PE 中检测 T-SPOT.TB 具有相当大的异质性,而且没有发现任何有显著影响的协变量;因此,无论是对全血样本还是 PE 样本,对怀疑患有 TPE 的患者诊断准确性较差。总之,PE 中的 T-SPOT.TB 对 TPE 的诊断价值仍存在很多争议。

二、恶性胸腔积液(malignant pleural effusion,MPE)

(一)癌胚抗原(carcinoembryonic antigen,CEA)

CEA 是在结肠癌和胚胎组织中提取的一种肿瘤相关

抗原,在恶性肿瘤患者体内存在于恶性肿瘤细胞的表面,在胸腔积液、腹水等多种体液中均可检出。在大部分肺腺癌患者中,血清和胸腔积液中 CEA 含量升高;另外,CEA可促进肿瘤的发生和转移,并且 CEA 对转移性腺癌导致的 MPE 的诊断灵敏性为 61%~91%。在初次诊断时,约 15%的肺癌患者就已经出现 PE,50%的肺癌患者在疾病过程中会出现 PE,且 PE 中 CEA 水平与血清 CEA 水平呈正相关,常在 MPE 中检测出的 CEA 含量也相应升高。有学者为证实 CEA 在 PE 中的诊断价值,通过检测 PE 中的 CEA 及胰岛素样生长因子结合蛋白 2(IGFBP-2)的水平,发现当 CEA 临界值为 16.43μg/L 时,敏感性为 63.2%,特异性为 100.0%;Nguyen AH 等回顾了 PE 中积液的多种肿瘤标志物在 MPE 中的诊断效能,当采用特异性最高的诊断阈值时,其敏感性只有 54.9%;这说明 CEA 具有较高的特异性,但其敏感性较低,限制了其诊断价值。因此,临床上建议联合检验血清中不同的肿瘤标志物;而单独使用某一种肿瘤标志物是不够的诊断准确性的临床使用。EnzN 等发现 CEA 水平可提高胸水细胞学阴性 MPE 患者的诊断敏感性,为肺结节楔形切除术的随访提供有价值的信息。目前有关 CEA 诊断 MPE 的胸腔积液标志物的研究仍有如下不足:①研究中设定的诊断阈值较高,但并不具有绝对的诊断特异性,而且,为了让胸水标志物能够起到帮助诊断的作用,则任何良性胸腔积液都不应超过设定的诊断阈值。②部分研究中存在良性胸腔积液,良性胸腔积液与恶性胸腔积液较容易区分开,这使得胸水标志物的诊断价值被高估。

(二)血管内皮生长因子(vascular endothelial growth factor,VEGF)

VEGF 是一种高二聚体糖蛋白,具有广泛的生物学功能,包括刺激细胞分化迁移存活,以及调节血管通透性和血管生成。由于 VEGF 在 MPE 形成过程中发挥重要作用,对 PE 中 VEGF 含量进行检测,有助于明确 PE 的性质。GU 等发现 VEGF 临界值为 297.06ng/L 时,VEGF 诊断 MPE 的敏感性为 80.0%,特异性为 96.7%,MPE 中 VEGF 含量明显高于良性组($P<0.01$),且在恶性中表达程度比良性更高。陈先梦等的荟萃分析发现 VEGF 诊断 MPE 具有较高的灵敏性(72%)和特异性(80%),可作为恶性胸腔积液非侵入性诊断的辅助工具。WU 等尝试新的胸水标志物联合诊断,发现当 VEGF 含量>214pg/ml 且蛋白质含量>3.3g/dl 时,MPE 的诊断敏感性为 92.6%,特异性为 78.6%。以上研究的结果均表明 VEGF 除了对 MPE 有较高诊断敏感性和特异性外,当与其他胸腔积液标志物联合检测可以提高其诊断价值。Mohajeri A 等发现 VEGF 在晚期非小细胞肺癌患者的 MPE 中高表达,并且 MPE 中的 VEGF 浓度越高,晚期非小细胞肺癌患者发生远处转移的风险就越高,说明 MPE 中 VEGF 水平可能是判断晚期非小细胞肺癌患者预后的重要指标之一。

(三)凝集素(intelectin,ITLN)

ITLN 是广泛存在于自然界的一大类非免疫来源、无酶活性的多价糖类结合蛋白,能使细胞发生凝集。人 ITLN-1 则是 2003 年 Yang 等发现的,它是一种腹膜网膜脂肪组织特异性分泌的蛋白因子,可以结合乳铁蛋白,参与铁代谢。既往的研究表明 ITLN-1 在糖尿病、心血管系统疾病、哮喘、骨骼运动系统疾病及恶性肿瘤等疾病中发挥作用。Wali 等研究证实恶性胸膜间皮瘤(malignant pleural mesothelioma,MPM)细胞中 ITLN-1 的表达高于正常细胞 139 倍以上。Tsuji 等则研究发现 MPM 患者 PE 中 ITLN-1 的水平明显升高,ITLN-1 在细胞的胞浆而非胞核中表达;双相型 MPM 患者的上皮样间皮瘤细胞表达 ITLN-1 而肉瘤样间皮瘤细胞则不表达 ITLN-1;绝大部分研究对象的 PE 比血浆中表达更多的 ITLN-1,血清与 PE 中 ITLN-1 的表达水平不相关;上皮样型 MPM 患者比肺癌、肺结核患者在 PE 中表达更高水平的 ITLN-1。该研究为今后以免疫组化技术鉴别诊断上皮样型 MPM 提供了新的可能。目前有关 ITLN 的试验主要都集中在动物模型及细胞水平,其在人体中的作用机制研究尚少,其在 PE 中的诊断价值同样值得进一步的探索。

(四)可溶性程序性死亡配体 1(soluble programmed death-ligand 1,sPD-L1)

程序性死亡受体(programmed death-1,PD-1)又称 CD279,是 I 型跨膜糖蛋白,是重要的免疫抑制受体。而程序性死亡配体(programmed death ligand 1,PD-L1)是其配体之一,两者结合可抑制 T 细胞的增殖和 IL-2、IL-10、γ 干扰素等相关细胞因子的分泌。多种肿瘤中均存在 PD-L1 的表达,通过与肿瘤微环境相互作用,PD-L1 发挥免疫抑制作用。因此,PD-1 和 PD-L1 可作为诊断 MPE 的重要生物学标志物,但对送检标本中恶性肿瘤细胞数的要求较高,临床上更多用来作为恶性肿瘤治疗的靶点及监测疗效。近年来有研究表明,PD-L1 除能以膜性形式存在外,还可以在血液、PE 等体液中被检测到其可溶性成分,即 sPD-L1。Howitt E 等发现,同一患者 PE 中 sPD-L1 的表达高于外周血,且其对 MPE 诊断敏感性、特异性也明显提高。国内,王鹏也报道了 sPD-L1 在非小细胞肺癌患者血清中的表达高于良性肺部疾病患者。后来,冀玉珍等对比了良、恶性 PE 患者中 sPD-L1 的水平,结果显示,MPE 中 sPD-L1 水平明显高于良性 PE,当以 1.33ng/ml 作为临床诊断阈值时,其诊断 MPE 的敏感性和特异性较高。因此,sPD-L1 是良恶性 PE 诊断与鉴别诊断有意义的生物学标志物之一。

三、肺炎旁胸腔积液(parapneumonic pleural effusions,PPE)

(一)C 反应蛋白(C-reactive protein,CRP)

CRP 是一种急性期炎性反应蛋白,主要调控炎症部位的应答反应及对抗创伤、感染部位释放的溶蛋白酶,其在多种感染性疾病的诊断和鉴别诊断有较多的报道。张雪漫等研究结果显示 CRP 可以用来区分肺炎患者是否合并了胸腔感染,以及区分 UPPE 还是 CPPE,后者中 CRP 值可升高。赵俊等发现在感染性 PE 中,CRP 水平在 PPE 中明显高于 TPE,提示 CRP 在感染性 PE 中的鉴别价值。有研究报道 PPE 中 CRP 含量明显高于 MPE,CRP<

20mg/L 在 MPE 中敏感性 50%、特异性 89%, CRP>45mg/L 在良性 PE 中敏感性 44%、特异性 95%。目前许多研究是多种标志物联合 CRP 对于感染性 PE 的诊断价值分析，对于 CRP 增高，同时 PE 中性粒细胞增高的患者，诊断 CPPE 的特异度是比较高的。如果 CRP>100 mg/L，同时 pH<7.20 或血糖<3.33mmol/L，诊断 CPPE 的特异度为 97%。若联合检测 PE 中触珠蛋白对良、恶性 PE 的鉴别有良好价值。

(二)降钙素原(procalcitonin, PCT)

PCT 是一种无激素活性的降钙素前体物质，在细菌性肺炎时呈中到重度升高，而在病毒感染、肿瘤、结缔组织病等非感染性疾病时多不增高。有研究证实血清 PCT 水平对局限性肺部感染和全身感染的病因诊断、鉴别诊断和病原学诊断都有一定辅助价值。国内研究也提示 PPE 和脓胸患者血清 PCT 水平均显著升高，而对 PE 中的 PCT 的研究报道较少，Lin 等观察到胸腔积液中的 PCT 浓度与血浆 PCT 浓度相关，不同疾病患者体液和血浆中的 PCT 浓度变化是一致的，局部炎症也会引起全身性的 PCT 浓度变化。PE 中的 PCT 对 PPE 的诊断价值存在争议，黄宇筠等研究显示，PPE 中 PCT 水平明显高于 TPE 患者，有利于鉴别诊断；而邱跃灵等认为，不能将 PCT 视作二者的鉴别指标，因为其在 TPE 及 PPE 患者中的敏感性和特异性均较低。有荟萃分析结果提示血清 PCT 的结果比 PE 中 PCT 的结果更具有诊断价值。

(三)乳酸脱氢酶(Lactate dehydrogenase LDH)

LDH 是参与糖无氧酵解和糖异生的重要酶，当机体某部位的组织受到损伤时，LDH 就会从细胞内进入血液或组织液中，从而检测值升高，是反映炎症反应的重要指标之一，但对病因诊断的特异性较差。许多临床疾病中均发现血 LDH 升高，如肺梗死、恶性贫血、休克及肿瘤转移所致的胸腔积液及腹水。以往的研究就报道血清 LDH 升高可以用作败血症和癌症患者的诊断和不良预后标志物。PE 中 LDH 是区分 CPPE 与 UPPE 的常用生物标志物，而 PE 的 LDH 水平升高可能具有特定的诊断意义，尤其是对脓胸。PPE 早期为无菌浆液性渗出，PE 的 LDH 水平较低，随病情加重可表现为脓性渗出，LDH 水平进行性升高，典型脓胸的 LDH>1000U/ml。PE 与血清的 LDH 比值可能为鉴别 PE 性质的重要补充手段，有研究发现在脓胸中 LDH 及其与血清比值很高，原因可能是化脓性胸膜炎的病灶直接在胸壁上，LDH 的释放无须经过血液循环而直接进入 PE 中。

四、未来研究中具备潜力的生物学标志物

新兴的生物学标志物涉及基因组学(DNA)、转录组学(所有 RNA 类型)、蛋白质组学和代谢组学(小分子或代谢产物)，其利用高通量方法探索大量潜在的未知生物标志物，这些技术由于种种原因尚未在临床应用。下面是一些示例。

(一)外泌体 miRNA

外泌体(exosomes)是细胞通过内吞-融合-外排等一系列生物学机制产生并通过主动分泌作用排出细胞外的囊性小泡，其本质是脂质双分子层，里面含有 miRNA 及多种蛋白成分，参与调节细胞各项生理功能。Tamiya H 等通过实时定量反转录聚合酶链式反应(RT-PCR)对患者胸腔积液中的外泌体 miRNA 进行检查，结果表明，MPE 组中的 miRNA-182 与 miRNA-210 表达水平明显高于良性胸腔积液组，其敏感性与特异性分别为 92.7%、73.3% 和 58.5%、93.3%。说明这两种 miRNA 是 MPE 潜在的诊断生物标志物。

(二)小分子代谢产物

质子磁共振谱(proton nuclear magnetic resonance spectroscopy, 1H-NMR)可以无创的定量检测 PE 中小分子的代谢情况。通过 1H-NMR 检测不同类型 PE 中小分子代谢产物的变化，可以对疾病诊断和治疗提供一定的帮助。Wang 等采用 1H-NMR 对共计 58 例患者(其中 20 例为 TPE、20 例为 MPE、18 例为漏出性 PE)PE 中的小分子代谢产物的变化进行检测，结果发现，TPE 组中枸橼酸、乳酸、肌酸及醋酸的含量明显低于 MPE，且 TPE 中的脂质含量明显高于漏出性 PE 组，MPE 组也表现出氨基酸含量明显降低的趋势。从另一方面说明了 1H-NMR 在不同类型的 PE 中识别小分子生物化学特征的可行性，具有良好的应用前景。

五、小结和展望

近年来，随着生物医学技术的进步，越来越多的生物学标志物被发现和运用，这将为临床工作提供更多、更好的选择，为基础医学研究带来新的认识，同时，更多无创的、更加便宜、快捷和高效的检查将使患者获益更多。

参 考 文 献

[1] Porcel JM, Esquerda A, Vives M, et al. Etiology of pleural effusions: analysis of more than 3,000 consecutive thoracenteses. Arch Bronconeumol, 2014, 50(5):161-165.

[2] 郑建，欧勤芳，刘袁媛，等. 结核性胸膜炎患者结核特异性 T 淋巴细胞的免疫应答及其迁徙作用. 中华传染病杂志, 2013, (12):715-718.

[3] Palma RM, Bielsa S, Esquerda A, et al. Diagnostic Accuracy of Pleural Fluid Adenosine Deaminase for Diagnosing Tuberculosis. Meta-analysis of Spanish Studies. Arch Bronconeumol, 2019, 55(1):23-30.

[4] Jeon D. Tuberculous pleurisy: an update. Tuberc Respir Dis (Seoul), 2014, 76(4):153-159.

[5] Porcel JM, Esquerda A, Bielsa S. Diagnostic performance of adenosine deaminase activity in pleural fluid: a single-center experience with over 2100 consecutive patients. Eur J Intern Med, 2010, 21(5):419-423.

[6] Aggarwal AN, Agarwal R, Sehgal IS, et al. Adenosine deaminase for diagnosis of tuberculous pleural effusion: A systematic review and meta-analysis. PLoS One, 2019, 14(3): e0213728.

[7] Bielsa S, Palma R, Pardina M, et al. Comparison of polymorphonuclear-and lymphocyte-rich tuberculous pleural effusions. Int J Tuberc Lung Dis, 2013, 17(1): 85-89.

[8] Ye ZJ, Xu LL, Zhou Q, et al. Recruitment of IL-27-Producing CD4(+)T Cells and Effect of IL-27 on Pleural Mesothelial Cells in Tuberculous Pleurisy. Lung, 2015, 193(4): 539-548.

[9] Li M, Zhu W, RSU K, et al. Accuracy of interleukin-27 assay for the diagnosis of tuberculous pleurisy: A PRISMA-compliant meta-analysis. Medicine(Baltimore), 2017, 96(50): e9205.

[10] Liu Q, Yu YX, Wang XJ, et al. Diagnostic Accuracy of Interleukin-27 between Tuberculous Pleural Effusion and Malignant Pleural Effusion: A Meta-Analysis. Respiration, 2018, 95(6): 469-477.

[11] Wang W, Zhou Q, Zhai K, et al. Diagnostic accuracy of interleukin 27 for tuberculous pleural effusion: two prospective studies and one meta-analysis. Thorax, 2018, 73(3): 240-247.

[12] Jiang J, Shi HZ, Liang QL, et al. Diagnostic value of interferon-gamma in tuberculous pleurisy: a metaanalysis. Chest, 2007, 131(4): 1133-1141.

[13] Li ZZ, Qin WZ, Li L, et al. Accuracy of enzyme-linked immunospot assay for diagnosis of pleural tuberculosis: a meta-analysis. Genet Mol Res, 2015, 14(3): 11672-11680.

[14] Aggarwal AN, Agarwal R, Gupta D, et al. Interferon Gamma Release Assays for Diagnosis of Pleural Tuberculosis: a Systematic Review and Meta-Analysis. J Clin Microbiol, 2015, 53(8): 2451-2459.

[15] Enz N, Fragoso F, Gamrekeli A, et al. Carcinoembryonic antigen-positive pleural effusion in early stage non-small cell lung cancer without pleural infiltration. J Thorac Dis, 2018, 10(5): E340-E343.

[16] Woo CG, Son SM, Han HS, et al. Diagnostic benefits of the combined use of liquid-based cytology, cell block, and carcinoembryonic antigen immunocytochemistry in malignant pleural effusion. J Thorac Dis, 2018, 10(8): 4931-4939.

[17] Tozzoli R, Basso SM, D'Aurizio F, et al. Evaluation of predictive value of pleural CEA in patients with pleural effusions and histological findings: A prospective study and literature review. Clin Biochem, 2016, 49(16-17): 1227-1231.

[18] 周晓明,康大海,侯闻,等. 胰岛素样生长因子结合蛋白2和癌胚抗原对恶性胸腔积液与结核性胸腔积液的鉴别诊断价值分析. 实用心脑肺血管病杂志, 2017, 25(01): 95-98.

[19] Nguyen AH, Miller EJ, Wichman CS, et al. Diagnostic value of tumor antigens in malignant pleural effusion: a meta-analysis. Transl Res, 2015, 166(5): 432-439.

[20] Chen Y, Mathy NW, Lu H. The role of VEGF in the diagnosis and treatment of malignant pleural effusion in patients with non-small cell lung cancer (Review). Mol Med Rep, 2018, 17(6): 8019-8030.

[21] Gu Y, Zhang M, Li GH, et al. Diagnostic values of vascular endothelial growth factor and epidermal growth factor receptor for benign and malignant hydrothorax. Chin Med J (Engl), 2015, 128(3): 305-309.

[22] 陈先梦,孙耕耘. 血管内皮生长因子对恶性胸腔积液诊断价值的Meta分析. 中华肺部疾病杂志(电子版), 2017, 10(1): 29-34.

[23] Wu DW, Chang WA, Liu KT, et al. Vascular endothelial growth factor and protein level in pleural effusion for differentiating malignant from benign pleural effusion. Oncol Lett, 2017, 14(3): 3657-3662.

[24] Mohajeri A, Sanaei S, Kiafar F, et al. The Challenges of Recombinant Endostatin in Clinical Application: Focus on the Different Expression Systems and Molecular Bioengineering. Adv Pharm Bull, 2017, 7(1): 21-34.

[25] Yang RZ, Lee MJ, Hu H, et al. Identification of omentin as a novel depot-specific adipokine in human adipose tissue: possible role in modulating insulin action. Am J Physiol Endocrinol Metab, 2006, 290(6): E1253-1261.

[26] Wali A, Morin PJ, Hough CD, et al. Identification of intelectin overexpression in malignant pleural mesothelioma by serial analysis of gene expression(SAGE). Lung Cancer, 2005, 48(1): 19-29.

[27] Tsuji S, Tsuura Y, Morohoshi T, et al. Secretion of intelectin-1 from malignant pleural mesothelioma into pleural effusion. Br J Cancer, 2010, 103(4): 517-523.

[28] Böger C, Behrens HM, Mathiak M, et al. PD-L1 is an independent prognostic predictor in gastric cancer of Western patients. Oncotarget, 2016, 7(17): 24269-24283.

[29] Muro K, Chung HC, Shankaran V, et al. Pembrolizumab for patients with PD-L1-positive advanced gastric cancer (KEYNOTE-012): a multicentre, open-label, phase 1b trial. Lancet Oncol, 2016, 17(6): 717-726.

[30] Wang L, Wang H, Chen H, et al. Serum levels of soluble programmed death ligand 1 predict treatment response and progression free survival in multiple myeloma. Oncotarget, 2015, 6(38): 41228-41236.

[31] Howitt BE, Shukla SA, Sholl LM, et al. Association of Polymerase e-Mutated and Microsatellite-Instable Endometrial Cancers With Neoantigen Load, Number of Tumor-Infiltrating Lymphocytes, and Expression of PD-1 and PD-L1. JAMA Oncol, 2015, 1(9): 1319-1323.

[32] 王鹏. 血清可溶性分子B7-H4检测在非小细胞肺癌中的应用. 检验医学, 2013, 28(12): 1140-1141.

[33] 冀玉珍,刘晓良,侯淼. 可溶性程序性死亡分子配体1在肺癌胸腔积液中的水平及临床意义. 检验医学, 2017, 32(2): 99-103.

[34] 张雪漫,王廷杰. 46例脓胸的临床分析和诊治体会. 临床肺科杂志, 2005, (2): 234.

[35] 赵俊,陈毅斐. 血清CRP、ADA、SAA联合检测在鉴别感染性胸腔积液中的价值. 医学新知杂志, 2017, (5): 453-455.

[36] Garcia-Pachon E, Soler MJ, Padilla-Navas I, et al. C-reactive protein in lymphocytic pleural effusions: a diagnostic aid in tuberculous pleuritis. Respiration, 2005, 72(5): 486-489.

[37] Porcel JM, Bielsa S, Esquerda A, et al. Pleural fluid C-reactive protein contributes to the diagnosis and assessment of severity of parapneumonic effusions. Eur J Intern Med, 2012, 23(5): 447-450.

[38] 黄建达,蔡挺. C反应蛋白、触珠蛋白在胸腔积液鉴别诊断中

的价值.临床内科杂志,2001,(3):192-193.
[39] Porcel JM. Pleural fluid tests to identify complicated parapneumonic effusions. Curr Opin Pulm Med,2010,16(4):357-361.
[40] 陈孝谦,汪铮,李秀.血清降钙素原对渗出性胸腔积液病因的鉴别价值.临床肺科杂志,2013,(8):1146-1448.
[41] Lin MC,Chen YC,Wu JT,et al. Diagnostic and prognostic values of pleural fluid procalcitonin in parapneumonic pleural effusions. Chest,2009,136(1):205-211.
[42] 黄宇筠,黄鑫炎,罗益锋,等. HS-CRP、PCT 在鉴别类肺炎性与结核性胸腔积液的研究.实用医学杂志,2013,(22):3666-3667.
[43] 邱跃灵,麦转英.降钙素原与 CA125 联合检测对结核性胸腔积液的诊断价值.临床肺科杂志,2012,(9):1640-1641.
[44] He C,Wang B,Li D,et al. Performance of procalcitonin in diagnosing parapneumonic pleural effusions:A clinical study and meta-analysis. Medicine(Baltimore),2017,96(33):e7829.
[45] Fantin VR,St-Pierre J,Leder P. Attenuation of LDH-A expression uncovers a link between glycolysis, mitochondrial physiology,and tumor maintenance. Cancer Cell,2006,9(6):425-434.

[46] Lee J,Lee SY,Lim JK,et al. Radiologic and laboratory differences in patients with tuberculous and parapneumonic pleural effusions showing non-lymphocytic predominance and high adenosine deaminase levels. Infection,2015,43(1):65-71.
[47] 鄢斌,刘军.联合检测血清及胸水 LDH、ADA、CEA、CA153 对胸水性质的鉴别价值.现代医药卫生,2009,(10):1505-1507.
[48] Tamiya H,Mitani A,Saito A,et al. Exosomal MicroRNA Expression Profiling in Patients with Lung Adenocarcinoma-associated Malignant Pleural Effusion. Anticancer Res,2018,38(12):6707-6714.
[49] Zennaro L,Vanzani P,Nicolè L,et al. Metabonomics by proton nuclear magnetic resonance in human pleural effusions:A route to discriminate between benign and malignant pleural effusions and to target small molecules as potential cancer biomarkers. Cancer Cytopathol,2017,125(5):341-348.
[50] Wang C,Peng J,Kuang Y,et al. Metabolomic analysis based on 1H-nuclear magnetic resonance spectroscopy metabolic profiles in tuberculous, malignant and transudative pleural effusion. Mol Med Rep,2017,16(2):1147-1156.

2 结节病的诊治进展

吴琳颖　王悦虹

结节病(sarcoidosis)是一种原因不明的以非干酪样坏死性上皮细胞肉芽肿为病理特征的多系统的肉芽肿性疾病,以肺部受累最为常见,也可累及皮肤、眼、心脏、神经、周围淋巴结等。结节病的发病呈世界性分布,其临床表现缺乏特异性,诊断需结合临床表现、影像学检查和病理学表现。结节病目前尚无根治性的治疗方法,糖皮质激素仍然是首选治疗。本文主要对结节病的流行病学特点、病因、临床表现、诊断及治疗的进展做一综述。

一、流行病学特点

结节病的发病率和流行率及其临床表现在不同地理区域、不同性别、不同种族和年龄组之间有很大差异。结节病的发病率在北欧国家及非裔美国人中最高,分别为(11～24)/10万和(18～71)/10万,而在亚洲国家中最低,约为1/10万。在同一国家,结节病的分布因地理区域而异,人口密度低的地区结节病的患病率较高。国外数据表明结节病平均发病年龄为40～55岁,男性(30～50岁)比女性(50～60岁)的发病年龄更小,男女患病比例为1.20:1.75。我国的结节病发病率较低,平均发病年龄为47.96岁,男女比例为1:1.6。

二、病因

结节病的病因目前尚不清楚。许多研究表明,遗传易感性、环境因素及生活方式与结节病的发展相关。

(一)遗传因素

遗传易感性是疾病风险的重要组成部分。有结节病家族史的患者发生结节病的风险增加3.7倍,且随着患病亲属数量的增加,患病风险也增加。据估计,结节病的遗传率为39%。人类白细胞抗原(Human leukocyte antigen,HLA)编码的2型主要组织相容性复合体(type 2 major histocompatibility complex,MHC II)是导致不同种族患者疾病易感性和表型的主要因素。

(二)环境因素

美国的一项回顾性研究发现了与结节病相关的多种环境暴露,包括发霉环境、杀虫剂职业暴露和从事农业工作。另外,铸铁工人(接触二氧化硅粉尘)和消防员等职业也被认为是危险因素。病原体也可能诱发结节病,有研究观察到结节病患者组织中微生物DNA和蛋白质抗原增加。并且,分枝杆菌的一些病原体相关的分子模式如分枝杆菌过氧化氢-过氧化物酶、超氧化物歧化酶A、索状因子等能够诱导小鼠肺肉芽肿。总之,许多研究表明吸入性的环境因素,如微生物性气溶胶和一些无机物,都可能诱发结节病。

(三)生活方式

吸烟者发生结节病的风险较低,可能原因是吸烟与T淋巴细胞功能和巨噬细胞吞噬活性的抑制有关,吸烟可能通过干扰巨噬细胞淋巴细胞的活化过程,从而影响肉芽肿的形成。然而,值得注意的是,吸烟与结节病之间的负相关性在亚洲人群中尚未观察到,可能在不同地区或人群中,结节病的病因不同。

肥胖人群发生结节病的风险较高,其具体机制尚未明确。肥胖患者脂肪细胞过度分泌瘦素是可能的原因之一。瘦素是一种具有免疫调节作用的促炎脂肪因子,能够维持自身反应性细胞增殖,从而增加自身免疫和结节病的风险。

三、临床表现

结节病是一种多系统疾病,几乎可以波及体内所有器官,30%～60%的结节病患者在发现本病时并无明显的症状和体征。结节病有急性、亚急性和慢性型表现,较为急性发病时,20%～50%可表现为Löfgren综合征,即结节红斑、双侧肺门淋巴结肿大和多发性关节疼痛。

(一)肺结节病

90%以上的结节病患者有肺内或者胸腔内淋巴结的受累,呼吸道症状较轻,常见症状包括干咳、呼吸困难、喘息等,多伴有全身症状,如发热、乏力和体重减轻。肺功能主要表现为限制性通气功能障碍并伴有弥散功能下降和小气道功能受限。

肺结节病典型的影响学表现为双侧肺门、纵隔淋巴结肿大伴或不伴肺内浸润。肺内改变早期为肺泡炎表现,继而发展为肺间质浸润,晚期发展为肺间质纤维化。根据胸部X线表现,结节病可分为5期(Scandding分期):0期为X线无异常表现,常表现为肺外结节病;Ⅰ期为仅有肺门和(或)纵隔淋巴结肿大,而肺部无异常;Ⅱ期表现为肺部弥漫性病变伴有肺门淋巴结肿大;Ⅲ期为肺部弥漫性病变而不伴有肺门淋巴结肿大;Ⅳ期表现为肺纤维化伴有蜂窝肺形成、肺囊肿和肺气肿等改变。

(二)皮肤结节病

16%~32%的结节病患者有皮肤受累,分为特异性和非特异性两种。结节性红斑最常见,为非特异性皮肤表现,多为结节病的早期表现,多发生于女性。典型的结节性红斑表现为无痛、红斑隆起的皮肤损害,多见于前臂和下肢。特异性皮肤表现包括斑片或结节性病变、冻疮样狼疮、斑丘疹、皮肤斑点、鱼鳞癣、溃疡、瘢痕组织等。狼疮样皮损常见于慢性进展性结节病,并可累及多器官。有趣的是,文身部位易形成肉芽肿。

(三)心脏结节病

至少有2%~7%的结节病患者有明显的心脏受累,而隐匿性心肌受累可能>20%。并且,心脏结节病可在无肺部或全身受累及的情况下发生。心脏结节病是结节病患者突然死亡的重要原因,因此早期诊断和治疗至关重要。其临床表现并无特异性,包括束支传导阻滞和完全性房室传导阻滞充血性心律失常、心肌病所致的心力衰竭等。由于大量的肉芽肿浸润及心肌纤维化,心脏结节病患者死亡的主要原因是室性心律失常、高度的房室传导阻滞或进行性的心力衰竭。

(四)神经系统结节病

4%~10%的结节病患者有神经系统受累。结节病可侵犯神经系统的任一部分,最常见的受累部位是脑神经、脑膜、脑实质、脊髓、下丘脑和垂体。累及下丘脑垂体时可能导致各种内分泌失调,包括高催乳素血症、睾酮水平下降、促卵泡激素或促黄体生成素下降,以及尿失禁,而脑垂体的磁共振成像并不一定显示异常。

(五)眼结节病

葡萄膜炎是结节病最常见的眼部表现,在黑种人和亚洲结节病患者中的发生率为10%~30%。多达1/3的结节病葡萄膜炎患者没有症状,也有的患者出现视力受损和眼部疼痛。

(六)其他器官受累

肝脏受累表现为不明原因发热、腹痛,少数患者可有血清转氨酶、碱性磷酸酶或胆红素升高。脾脏受累会导致脾大,多无症状。肾脏结节病的发生率为5%,常见1,25-双羟维生素D过度产生,导致血钙和尿钙水平增高。结节病性关节炎通常以侵犯大关节为主,表现为单发或多发的关节炎。

四、结节病的诊断

(一)血清生物标志物

血清血管紧张素转换酶(serum angiotensin converting enzyme,SACE)是典型的结节病生物标志物。ACE是由结节病肉芽肿中的上皮样细胞产生,SACE水平被认为是反映肉芽肿疾病负担的生物标志物。然而,ACE对于诊断和评估结节病的预后作用还有待商议。SACE用于结节病的诊断在不同人群中的敏感性为41%~100%,特异性为83%~99%。并且,SACE的水平受检验试剂、受检人群、ACE抑制剂的应用及个体ACE基因的变异等的影响。虽然SACE水平升高意味着诊断结节病的可能性增高,但将SACE作为单独的结节病诊断检测,其特异性不足。尽管如此,SACE可能在疾病活动的评估中发挥作用。当SACE超过正常上限2倍时,其诊断结节病的特异性高。

其他血清生物标志物包括反映$CD4^+$T辅助细胞的激活,如血清白细胞介素2受体(Serum interleukin 2 receptor,sIL 2R),趋化因子CXCL9、CXCL10和CXCL11;反映巨噬细胞的活化,包括壳三糖酶、溶菌酶和血清淀粉样蛋白A(serum amyloid A,SAA)。基于现有的数据,壳三糖酶和sIL 2R最有望作为结节病疾病活动的生物标志物。SAA在诊断中具有潜在的生物标志物作用,在结节病或非结节病的肉芽肿性疾病中,肉芽肿活检标本染色及血清检测SAA具有很高的特异性。

(二)基因标志物和新兴的生物标志物

前期的研究已经发现结节病与特定基因相关,包括HLA-I、HLA-II、白细胞介素1α等的基因多态性。全基因组关联研究(genome wide association studies,GWAS)及免疫芯片检测证实了一些与结节病相关的单核苷酸多态性(single nucleotide polymorphism,SNP),包括与annexin A11、RAB23、NOTCH4、BTNL2、HLA-B、HLA-DB1及白细胞介素23-R相关的SNPs。但是,一些SNPs的具体生物学意义仍不清楚,这也是GWAS的局限性。全基因组分析有助于更深入地了解结节病和其他疾病,超越特定的生物标志物并以系统生物学方法发现结节病的发病机制和治疗靶点,是一种有前景的方法。

在一项比较正常肺组织和结节病患者的肺组织基因表达的研究中发现,不仅Th1免疫反应相关基因上调,调节巨噬细胞来源的金属基质蛋白酶12和ADAM样decysin-12基因也都有所上调。由于组织样本的基因表达检测需要进行活检,因此近年有学者研究外周血的基因表达分析是否能够作为检测结节病组织肉芽肿性炎的替代物,用于诊断结节病和监测疾病的活动。

(三)影像学检查

HRCT是评估结节病肺部受累的主要成像方法。对于有Löfgren综合征的患者,仅通过X线胸片和观察疾病的病程即可诊断,然而在大多数其他疑似结节病的患者中,HRCT可显示支持诊断的特征,如支气管血管串珠征。此外,HRCT能够显示肺实质受累的程度,并发现继发性的并发症,如纤维化、曲霉感染、肺动脉高压等。HRCT显示的纤维化程度结合肺功能参数,能够提供重要的预后信息。

PET/CT显示结节病受累部位代谢活性增强,相比于其他影像学检查更为敏感,能够帮助判断是否累及全身其它部位,并用于指导诊断性活检。但当存在恶性肿瘤、肺结核、恶性肉瘤样变、感染等时,PET/CT也显示代谢活性增强,因此其特异性较低。一项回顾性研究发现,PET/CT扫描的SUVmax值(maximum standardized uptake value)与英夫利昔单抗用于复发性肺结节病的治疗前后用力肺活量的改变明显相关,说明PET/CT对于预测这类患者英夫利昔单抗的治疗效果有一定的价值。

基于生长抑素受体的PET/CT也可用于结节病的检查,2型生长抑素受体(somatostatin receptor,SSTR)在结节病患者中由巨噬细胞和上皮样细胞表达。在心脏结节病患者中,基于 SSTR 的 PET/CT 与心脏磁共振(cardiac nuclear magnetic resonance,CMR)有 96% 的一致性。

(四)支气管镜检查

支气管镜检查是肺结节病的一个重要诊断方法,可以显示典型的支气管内肉芽肿性改变,如鹅卵石样变。支气管镜活检是一种简单、安全的方法,可用于组织学的确诊。研究表明,即使没有肉眼可见的支气管异常,活检也有 20% 的概率发现非坏死性肉芽肿。支气管肺泡灌洗液(bronchoalveolar lavage fluid,BALF)同样能为诊断提供支持性证据,并有助于排除其他原因。BALF 中淋巴细胞增多,$CD4^+$ T 细胞/$CD8^+$ T 细胞比值升高(>3.5)或 $CD4^+$ $CD103^+$ T 细胞/$CD4^+$ T 细胞比值降低(<0.2),同时结合患者的临床特征也支持结节病的诊断。

超声支气管镜引导下经支气管针吸活检(endobronchial ultrasonography-guided transbronchial needle aspiration,EBUS-TBNA)和常规的 TBNA 有助于鉴别恶性肿瘤(特别是淋巴瘤)或感染等引起的纵隔和(或)肺门淋巴结病变。EBUS-TBNA 检测肉芽肿的诊断率比支气管镜经支气管肺活检高 27%。

(五)肺功能检查

肺功能虽然不是结节病诊断性的检查,但对于评估肺部病变的严重程度,监测疾病的进展以及对治疗的反应极为重要。肺结节病通常有三种类型的肺功能异常,包括阻塞性、限制性和混合性通气功能障碍,伴或不伴弥散功能损害。因此,肺活量测定,尤其是用力肺活量(FVC)和第 1 秒用力呼气容积(FEV1)、肺总量(TLC)等的测量是临床最常用的方法。

五、结节病的治疗

结节病在开始治疗前首先要考虑是否能够先观察而不予治疗,大多数的结节病患者无须治疗,病情可自然缓解,而且治疗本身也会带来许多不良反应。一般在以下情况时考虑给予治疗,并首选口服糖皮质激素:严重的眼、神经或心脏结节病,顽固性高血钙症,有症状的Ⅱ期结节病,肺功能进行性下降的Ⅱ期结节病,Ⅲ期结节病,合并脾功能亢进。

(一)糖皮质激素

糖皮质激素已用于肺结节病的一线治疗超过 60 年,目前仍然是最常用的治疗方案。对于累及肺外器官的严重结节病,通常需要应用糖皮质激素治疗。糖皮质激素的初始剂量通常泼尼松 20~40mg/d,对于肺结节病的起始剂量通常比传统建议的小。在最初的 3 个月内宜使用>15mg/d 的剂量,对糖皮质激素有反应的患者通常在 2~4 周即可观察到病情改善。当糖皮质激素剂量<15mg/d 时,结节病可能复发。研究表明对于肺结节病,相对短暂的治疗初期后,并迅速将每日泼尼松剂量减少到 15mg 以下,可以改善治疗效果与药物毒性之间的平衡。流行病学数据显示,在结节病人群中,肥胖、高血压、糖尿病、高胆固醇血症和骨质疏松等的发病率明显增高,但目前不能确定这些是由于结节病本身还是由皮质类固醇的使用或混杂因素引起的。

(二)二线治疗药物

甲氨蝶呤(methotrexate,MTX)、硫唑嘌呤(azathioprine,AZA)、来氟米特(leflunomide)和霉酚酸酯常被视为结节病的二线治疗方法。MTX 是二线药物中研究最广泛和最常用的药物,多用于难治性结节病和不能耐受糖皮质激素副作用的患者。MTX 也是唯一一种经过随机双盲对照试验评估的具有减少糖皮质激素用量的效果的药物。该研究发现,MTX 对于减少类固醇剂量(corticosteroid-sparing effect)和改善急性肺结节病症状有效。AZA 对慢性结节病的疗效与皮质激素相当,但不良反应明显减少。一项病例对照研究比较了 MTX 和 AZA 治疗肺结节病的效果,两种药物在肺功能和皮质类固醇用量减少方面均有改善,但 AZA 的副作用发生率更高。一项回顾性研究表明,来氟米特有助于减少类固醇的使用量,在疾病进展的情况下,可作为单药疗法或附加疗法。MTX 的主要不良反应为肝肾毒性,由于 MTX 能够在血管外液中积聚,在发生胸腔积液或腹水的时应谨慎使用。外周神经病变是来氟米特一个不可忽视的副作用,并且在糖尿病的患者中更常见。

(三)肿瘤坏死因子拮抗剂

英夫利昔单抗(infliximab,类克)是一种肿瘤坏死因子(tumor necrosis factor,TNF)抗体,由于其是人源化的小鼠 IgG 抗体,它比其他 TNF 拮抗剂具有更强的免疫原性,发生过敏性反应的发生率更高,并可能导致抗嵌合抗体的产生,从而导致疗效丧失、免疫复合物型血清病、白细胞破坏性脉管炎。因此,建议联合使用 MTX、来氟米特或其他免疫抑制剂,以减少产生抗嵌合抗体的概率。在一项随机双盲安慰剂对照研究中,英夫利昔单抗耐受性好,对肺结节病的治疗有效,且用力肺活量较低、呼吸困难较重和患慢性疾病较多的患者受益更加明显。

阿达木单抗(adalimumab)是全人源化的抗体,过敏反应较英夫利昔单抗少。阿达木单抗对于因英夫利昔单抗治疗过程中因抗抗体形成或不耐受而导致继发治疗失败的个体也有效果。

(四)抗疟药物

一般来说,抗疟药物在肺结节病治疗中较少应用,通常更广泛用于治疗维生素 D 代谢紊乱、轻度至中度皮肤结节病,偶尔也用于上呼吸道结节病的治疗。羟氯喹由于毒性较低,最常被使用,但氯喹是抗疟药物中唯一进行过随机试验并对肺结节病有作用的药物。研究显示,氯喹可以降低肺结节病的复发风险并降低肺功能下降的速度。尽管如此,抗疟药物对肺结节病的作用通常仅用于辅助治疗,以增加保留糖皮质激素的方案。

(五)利妥昔单抗

利妥昔单抗(rituximab)是一种靶向 B 淋巴细胞 CD20 的单克隆抗体,能够使 B 淋巴细胞耗竭,并能调控调节性 T 淋巴细胞活性。在一项小型的前瞻性病例分析中,利妥昔单抗能够改善一些难治性肺结节病患者的肺功能,但利妥昔单抗用于治疗肺结节病仍然需要进一步的研究。

结节病的病因目前尚不明确,遗传易感性、环境和生活方式可能与结节病的发展相关。结节病的临床表现多种多样,随着新技术和新疗法的采用,结节病的诊断、评估和治疗已得到很大提高。虽然关于结节病的发病机制近年来有一些新的见解,但目前还没有专门针对结节病开发的新疗法,糖皮质激素仍然是结节病治疗的一线药物。随着越来越多的人认识到皮质激素对治疗结节病的毒副作用,降低糖皮质激素用量的药物的使用可能会增加,个性化的治疗策略有益于提高患者生活质量和并降低治疗的毒副作用。

参 考 文 献

[1] Milman N, Selroos O. Pulmonary sarcoidosis in the Nordic countries 1950-1982. Epidemiology and clinical picture. Sarcoidosis, 1990, 7(1): 50-57.

[2] Baughman R P, Field S, Costabel U, et al. Sarcoidosis in America. Analysis Based on Health Care Use. Ann Am Thorac Soc, 2016, 13(8): 1244-1252.

[3] Morimoto T, Azuma A, Abe S, et al. Epidemiology of sarcoidosis in Japan. Eur Respir J, 2008, 31(2): 372-379.

[4] Yoon HY, Kim HM, Kim YJ, et al. Prevalence and incidence of sarcoidosis in Korea: a nationwide population-based study. Respir Res, 2018, 19(1): 158.

[5] Deubelbeiss U, Gemperli A, Schindler C, et al. Prevalence of sarcoidosis in Switzerland is associated with environmental factors. Eur Respir J, 2010, 35(5): 1088-1097.

[6] Arkema EV, Cozier YC. Epidemiology of sarcoidosis: current findings and future directions. Ther Adv Chronic Dis, 2018, 9(11): 227-240.

[7] 汪小鹏,赵妍妍,黎春艳,等. 1303例肺结节病临床荟萃分析. 现代中西医结合杂志, 2013, 22(18): 2009-2011.

[8] 王宇,曹悦鞍,彭朝胜等. 结节病患者155例临床分析. 临床肺科杂志, 2012, 17(09): 1577-1578.

[9] Rossides M, Grunewald J, Eklund A, et al. Familial aggregation and heritability of sarcoidosis: a Swedish nested case-control study. Eur Respir J, 2018, 52(2).

[10] Newman LS, Rose CS, Bresnitz EA, et al. A case control etiologic study of sarcoidosis: environmental and occupational risk factors. Am J Respir Crit Care Med, 2004, 170(12): 1324-1330.

[11] Chen ES, Moller DR. Etiology of sarcoidosis. Clin Chest Med, 2008, 29(3): 365-377.

[12] Swaisgood CM, Oswald-Richter K, Moeller SD, et al. Development of a sarcoidosis murine lung granuloma model using Mycobacterium superoxide dismutase A peptide. Am J Respir Cell Mol Biol, 2011, 44(2): 166-174.

[13] Ungprasert P, Crowson CS, Matteson EL. Smoking, obesity and risk of sarcoidosis: A population-based nested case-control study. Respir Med, 2016, 120: 87-90.

[14] Scadding JG. Sarcoidosis, with Special Reference to Lung Changes. Br Med J, 1950, 1(4656): 745-753.

[15] Judson MA. The Clinical Features of Sarcoidosis: A Comprehensive Review. Clin Rev Allergy Immunol, 2015, 49(1): 63-78.

[16] Saygin D, Karunamurthy A, English J, et al. Tattoo reaction as a presenting manifestation of systemic sarcoidosis. Rheumatology(Oxford), 2019, 58(5): 927.

[17] Sayah DM, Bradfield JS, Moriarty JM, et al. Cardiac Involvement in Sarcoidosis: Evolving Concepts in Diagnosis and Treatment. Semin Respir Crit Care Med, 2017, 38(4): 477-498.

[18] Culver DA, Ribeiro Neto ML, Moss BP, et al. Neurosarcoidosis. Semin Respir Crit Care Med, 2017, 38(4): 499-513.

[19] Valeyre D, Prasse A, Nunes H, et al. Sarcoidosis. Lancet, 2014, 383(9923): 1155-1167.

[20] Chopra A, Kalkanis A, Judson MA. Biomarkers in sarcoidosis. Expert Rev Clin Immunol, 2016, 12(11): 1191-1208.

[21] Katchar K, Eklund A, Grunewald J. Expression of Th1 markers by lung accumulated T cells in pulmonary sarcoidosis. J Intern Med, 2003, 254(6): 564-571.

[22] Chen ES, Song Z, Willett MH, et al. Serum amyloid A regulates granulomatous inflammation in sarcoidosis through Toll-like receptor-2. Am J Respir Crit Care Med, 2010, 181(4): 360-373.

[23] Bargagli E, Bennett D, Maggiorelli C, et al. Human chitotriosidase: a sensitive biomarker of sarcoidosis. J Clin Immunol, 2013, 33(1): 264-270.

[24] Tomita H, Sato S, Matsuda R, et al. Serum lysozyme levels and clinical features of sarcoidosis. Lung, 1999, 177(3): 161-167.

[25] Adrianto I, Lin CP, Hale JJ, et al. Genome-wide association study of African and European Americans implicates multiple shared and ethnic specific loci in sarcoidosis susceptibility. PLoS One, 2012, 7(8): e43907.

[26] Fischer A, Ellinghaus D, Nutsua M, et al. Identification of Immune-Relevant Factors Conferring Sarcoidosis Genetic Risk. Am J Respir Crit Care Med, 2015, 192(6): 727-736.

[27] Judson MA, Marchell RM, Mascelli M, et al. Molecular profiling and gene expression analysis in cutaneous sarcoidosis: the role of interleukin-12, interleukin-23, and the T-helper 17 pathway. J Am Acad Dermatol, 2012, 66(6): 901-910.

[28] Koth LL, Solberg OD, Peng JC, et al. Sarcoidosis blood transcriptome reflects lung inflammation and overlaps with tuberculosis. Am J Respir Crit Care Med, 2011, 184(10): 1153-1163.

[29] Walsh SL, Wells AU, Sverzellati N, et al. An integrated clinicoradiological staging system for pulmonary sarcoidosis: a case-cohort study. Lancet Respir Med, 2014, 2(2): 123-130.

[30] Vorselaars AD, Crommelin HA, Deneer VH, et al. Effectiveness of infliximab in refractory FDG PET-positive sarcoidosis. Eur Respir J, 2015, 46(1): 175-185.

[31] Göktalay T, Çelik P, Alpaydın A, et al. The Role of Endobronchial Biopsy in the Diagnosis of Pulmonary Sarcoidosis. Turk Thorac J, 2016, 17(1): 22-27.

[32] Heron M, Slieker WA, Zanen P, et al. Evaluation of CD103 as a cellular marker for the diagnosis of pulmonary sarcoidosis.

Clin Immunol,2008,126(3):338-344.

[33] Von Bartheld MB,Dekkers OM,Szlubowski A,et al. Endosonography vs conventional bronchoscopy for the diagnosis of sarcoidosis:the GRANULOMA randomized clinical trial. Jama,2013,309(23):2457-2464.

[34] Coker RK. Guidelines for the use of corticosteroids in the treatment of pulmonary sarcoidosis. Drugs,2007,67(8):1139-1147.

[35] Dumas O,Boggs KM,Cozier YC,et al. Prospective study of body mass index and risk of sarcoidosis in US women. Eur Respir J,2017,50(4).

[36] Baughman RP,Winget DB,Lower EE. Methotrexate is steroid sparing in acute sarcoidosis:results of a double blind,randomized trial. Sarcoidosis Vasc Diffuse Lung Dis,2000,17(1):60-66.

[37] Vorselaars ADM,Wuyts WA,Vorselaars VMM,et al. Methotrexate vs azathioprine in second-line therapy of sarcoidosis. Chest,2013,144(3):805-812.

[38] Sahoo DH,Bandyopadhyay D,Xu M,et al. Effectiveness and safety of leflunomide for pulmonary and extrapulmonary sarcoidosis. Eur Respir J,2011,38(5):1145-1150.

[39] Kremer JM,Lee RG,Tolman KG. Liver histology in rheumatoid arthritis patients receiving long-term methotrexate therapy. A prospective study with baseline and sequential biopsy samples. Arthritis Rheum,1989,32(2):121-127.

[40] Martin K,Bentaberry F,Dumoulin C,et al. Peripheral neuropathy associated with leflunomide:is there a risk patient profile?. Pharmacoepidemiol Drug Saf,2007,16(1):74-78.

[41] Drent M,Cremers JP,Jansen TL,et al. Practical eminence and experience-based recommendations for use of TNF-α inhibitors in sarcoidosis. Sarcoidosis Vasc Diffuse Lung Dis,2014,31(2):91-107.

[42] Baughman RP,Drent M,Kavuru M,et al. Infliximab therapy in patients with chronic sarcoidosis and pulmonary involvement. Am J Respir Crit Care Med,2006,174(7):795-802.

[43] Crommelin HA,Van Der Burg LM,Vorselaars AD,et al. Efficacy of adalimumab in sarcoidosis patients who developed intolerance to infliximab. Respir Med,2016,115:72-77.

[44] Baltzan M,Mehta S,Kirkham TH,et al. Randomized trial of prolonged chloroquine therapy in advanced pulmonary sarcoidosis. Am J Respir Crit Care Med,1999,160(1):192-197.

[45] Sweiss NJ,Lower EE,Mirsaeidi M,et al. Rituximab in the treatment of refractory pulmonary sarcoidosis. Eur Respir J,2014,43(5):1525-1528.

3 恶性胸膜病变光动力治疗现状与探索

冯起校 陈昉 麦仲伦 任玺 冯缤

恶性胸膜病变包括胸膜原发性恶性肿瘤及胸膜转移瘤。原发性胸膜恶性肿瘤以恶性胸膜间皮瘤(MPM)为代表,通常预后极差,标准一线治疗方案的总体生存时间中位数约为13个月。继发性胸膜恶性肿瘤则来源于包括肺或远处肿瘤的胸膜转移。恶性胸膜肿瘤侵犯胸膜可导致恶性胸腔积液(MPE)的产生,20%~40%的肺癌及乳腺癌会发展成MPE,间皮瘤MPE的发生率最高,MPE的出现意味着患者进入肿瘤晚期,生存时间短、生活质量低、临床预后差,平均生存时间仅为4~7个月。目前胸膜恶性病变患者的临床预后仍不乐观,主要采用姑息治疗,其中以积极的局部治疗获益最为显著,旨在改善患者生活质量,缓解呼吸困难和(或)胸痛,尽可能延长患者生存时间。目前局部治疗恶性胸膜病变的方法主要有胸腔置管引流并注药、胸膜剥除术、胸膜固定术、胸膜腹膜分流、胸腔热灌注等,但均难以在疗效、副作用、可行性及费用中达到理想的平衡状态,寻找新方法是当前研究的重点,而胸膜热消融技术、胸膜光动力疗法等在恶性胸膜病变的治疗中逐渐展现出了优势。

光动力疗法(photodynamic therapy,PDT)通过肿瘤组织对光敏剂的选择性吸收和潴留,然后用合适波长和剂量的光来激发光敏剂产生细胞毒性物质来杀伤肿瘤细胞,从而达到治疗目的。随着各种新型光敏剂、激光器的研究成功,光动力学疗法的技术也愈发成熟,光动力的临床应用范围也逐步拓展。光动力疗法于1993年在加拿大获准治疗膀胱癌,也是获得的全球第一个批证,此后又在美欧和亚洲多国获得多个肿瘤适应证批证,2006年获得中国CFDA批准。目前我国PDT治疗的临床研究和应用涉及皮肤肿瘤和癌前病变、头颈部肿瘤、脑部肿瘤、胸部肿瘤、消化系统肿瘤、泌尿生殖系统肿瘤、四肢骨与软组织恶性肿瘤。其中关于胸部肿瘤的研究起源于20世纪80年代初,北京结核病医院率先开展关于PDT治疗支气管肺癌的研究。虽然针对恶性胸膜病变的光动力治疗研究仍缺乏前瞻性、多中心、大样本的研究成果,但已有临床观察发现光动力治疗在恶行胸膜疾病中具有值得肯定的疗效。

一、光动力疗法的机制

PDT疗法有三大因素:光敏剂、可见光、组织氧,其中光敏剂为核心因素。几乎所有用于PDT的药物都是血红素(卟啉)的衍生物,因为卟啉是共轭的(包含多个双键),它们可以非常有效地吸收可见光波长,并将能量转换为化学反应。目前光敏剂的发展已经经历三代。第一代光敏剂主要是血卟啉类,第二代光敏剂为二氢卟吩类,目前应用较多的第二代光敏剂是是5-氨基乙酰丙酸(5-aminolevulinicacid,5-ALA),它是光敏剂内源性卟啉Ⅸ(protoporphyrinⅨ,PPIX)的前体,可进入靶细胞的线粒体内,在机体血红素合成的过程中代谢成为PPIX从而发挥光敏剂的作用,因为ALA绕过在血红素合成途径中第一(抑制)反馈的步骤,从而允许PPIX累积到非常高的水平。第三代光敏剂则是第二代的光敏剂偶联上不同的靶向分子,如单克隆抗体,以提高其靶向性,降低PDT治疗过程中的不良反应。此外,科研人员也开始了对新型光敏剂的开发研究,Sophia和Richard Lunt夫妇合作,首次证实了阴离子能够独立的控制光敏剂的细胞毒性和光毒性,发现了一组适用于PDT的理想配对,不但具有高光毒性,细胞毒性几乎可以忽略不计。PPIX在目标癌症或癌前细胞中积累后,用规定量的光照射以激活PPIX。在氧气存在下,PPIX的光活化会在线粒体和周围膜内诱导Ⅱ型光氧化细胞内反应,其中分子氧转化为单线态活性氧(ROS),过量的胞内ROS的存在最终导致靶细胞死亡。为了实现良好的光激活,所选的光源必须在与PPIX吸收光谱中的主要峰相对应的波长处发射足够的能量,通常选择630 nm和635nm(红色)波长。

PDT的早期研究集中于PDT杀死癌细胞的物理和生化机制,并假设高细胞内PPIX水平和高光强度对于良好的杀灭肿瘤是必需的,但研究和临床经验表明,较低的PPIX和光强度也能很好地发挥作用,这表明先前无法识别的机制及免疫系统可能参与PDT的治疗反应。首先,PDT主要通过凋亡、坏死和(或)自噬直接杀死原发部位的恶性细胞。其次,PDT破坏了与肿瘤相关的血管系统的内皮细胞,局部血流量显着减少从而导致肿瘤死亡。这两种机制负责最初的肿瘤消除,这种早期局部炎症反应可以激活免疫系统,进一步触发了第三种抗肿瘤机制,通过诱导免疫原性细胞凋亡,可能也包括诱导非免疫原性细胞凋亡,从而促进清除治疗部位中剩余的肿瘤细胞。在后续的阶段中,也可能发展出适应性免疫记忆,且研究表明,低光量PDT与常规光量PDT相比可以诱导更强的抗肿瘤免疫效应并建立有效的免疫记忆,从长远来看,能够预防肿瘤复发和肿瘤转移。

二、恶性胸膜病变光动力疗法与其他治疗的协同作用探索

关于胸部肿瘤的病例报告描述了成功将PDT用作辅助治疗,PDT协同手术治疗可缩小手术范围,甚至使初始不可手术患者重获手术适应证,对于非小细胞肺癌伴胸膜转移,美国宾夕法尼亚大学2004年的一项Ⅱ期试验表明,手术后接受光动力治疗者比未接受光动力治疗者的中位生存时间显著延长。PDT联合放/化疗可增加放/化疗敏感性。尽管尚无高质量的研究将PDT与其他呼吸内镜下的消融疗法进行比较,但如果适当使用,它们似乎都能相似程度改善临床症状,且PDT可作为非热疗法使用而不会增加气道着火或穿孔的风险,同时PDT和近距离放射疗法比其他方式持续时间更长。有小范围观察发现多种方式组合的呼吸内镜介入治疗生存率较单一治疗有显著提高。尽管支持上述观点的多为气道内光动力的案例,基于同样的原理,仍有罕见病例报告描述了使用PDT治疗非小细胞肺癌,胸腺瘤和间皮瘤的胸膜播散。在欧洲和加拿大的光动力指南建议PDT治疗前轻柔去除病变上的坏死物,冯起校教授团队在临床应用中也发现在PDT治疗前清除病灶表面坏死物能增大PDT治疗效能,这可能是因为清除病灶表面坏死物可使病灶更好暴露于氧气,大量分子氧通过光化学反应转化为单态氧活性氧后可发挥更好的疗效。同理,高压氧治疗也对提高PDT治疗效能有积极作用。

通常PDT疗法的肿瘤组织破坏深度为5~10mm,因此PDT可杀灭表面细胞,同时保护下层组织,使其适合治疗表面扩散的恶性肿瘤,比如弥漫性胸膜转移。但是胸膜转移瘤除了表现为胸膜表浅浸润外,还多同时伴有大小不等结节,甚至融合成片,又正是由于辐射光对组织的穿透深度仅几毫米,难以使光动力反应深入肿瘤组织核心,故不能达到有效的肿瘤杀伤深度。我们假设,在内科胸腔镜下用热消融技术消除肉眼所能辨认的肿瘤病灶后,再进行光动力治疗可进一步杀灭微小及残留肿瘤病灶,从而提高胸膜转移瘤的控制率和患者的生存率。此外,使用激光及温和的局部热疗(将皮肤/黏膜温度升高至40~42℃)被证实可增加PPIX的合成、增加光敏剂的渗透率并增强PDT的治疗反应,因此我们有理由相信胸膜热消融技术可能直接增强胸膜光动力治疗的反应。热消融技术包括氩等离子体凝固术(argon plasma coagulation, APC,又称氩气刀)、激光和高频电等,可以对肿瘤进行电切、电凝。冯起校教授团队从2014年5月至2018年12月期间观察了125例确诊胸膜转移瘤伴恶性胸腔积液患者,其中胸腔穿刺置管引流并腔内注药者50例,内科胸腔镜下非消融组28例,热消融组治疗胸膜转移瘤者47例(其中激光治疗22例,APC治疗25例),发现热消融组的胸水控制有效率、患者中位生存时间均高于非消融组及置管引流组,并且未见严重不良反应。在热消融组内对比,APC组又优于激光治疗组。因此内科胸腔镜下利用APC治疗胸膜转移可能是一种有效、安全的治疗手段。在2019年中国内镜大会上,冯起校及其团队发表的关于光动力方法治疗肺癌胸膜转移瘤的论文中报道了使用氩气刀配合光动力方法治疗胸膜转移瘤的方法。中国台湾的Ke-Cheng Chen等回顾性研究18例手术联合光动力治疗胸膜转移的肺癌和胸腺瘤患者,3年生存率和5年生存率分别为68.9%和57.4%,比较手术加PDT治疗肺癌胸膜转移患者与手术加化疗或靶向治疗患者($n=51$)发现,PDT组存活率与非PDT组患者中位生存时间分别为39.0个月和17.6个月($P<0.047$)。我国王洪武教授在2017年出版的著作《支气管镜介入治疗》当中提到1例内科胸腔镜下氩气刀结合光动力治疗恶性胸膜间皮瘤的病例,患者73岁男性,左胸膜多发结节,肺功能差,不能耐受外科手术,在内科胸腔镜下先将胸膜上肿物用APC烧灼,后再进行PDT治疗,患者术后恢复良好,症状明显改善,存活8个月。王洪武教授在2008年还报道过利用APC联合PDT治疗晚期梗阻性非小细胞肺癌18例,结果CR 4例(22.22%),SR 13例(72.22%),MR 1例(5.56%),有效率明显高于单纯APC组和单纯PDT组。基于上述观察结果,内科胸腔镜下氩气刀联合光动力治疗可能是一种治疗恶性胸膜病变的有效方法。

胸膜面积广泛,为PDT治疗造成困扰,外科手术后辅助PDT治疗恶性胸膜病变通常选择胸顶、后纵隔、后胸壁、前纵隔、前胸壁、侧胸壁及膈面7个固定照射位点以均匀覆盖整个胸腔,而内科胸腔镜下的胸膜光动力治疗则更依赖自荧光支气管镜的"可视化"指导。自荧光摄像头可以将无法用白光区分的病变可视化。与正常组织或良性病变发出的绿色自发荧光相反,肿瘤部位显示为清晰可见的粉红色团块,转移性肿瘤或弥散性病变也同样可见。利用荧光支气管镜诊断性照射寻找残留病灶,为PDT治疗提供指引,明确病灶部位后针对性行光照治疗,既可减少对正常组织的过度杀伤作用,同时不易遗漏肿瘤病灶。临床观察发现,在第1次光照治疗24h后复查并清理坏死物后再次行自荧光支气管镜检查,可见病灶范围缩小、颜色变浅,根据残留病灶情况可选择进一步复照以达到根治的疗效。

有关使用这些联合治疗方案的建议仍需等待更大的临床试验结果的支持。

三、恶性胸膜病变光动力疗法的方法要点探索

定义PDT治疗剂量可能很复杂,因为它涉及局部光通量,局部光敏剂浓度和局部组织氧合作用高度相互依赖且动态变化。治疗剂量不足可能会导致治疗不彻底,而过量则可能会严重损害周围的健康组织。目前,大多数PDT治疗都是根据光敏剂的说明书剂量(通常为3~5mg/kg)进行的。但当PDT治疗以固定的入射光剂量进行时,由于光敏剂的药物学和组织光学特性,患者之间和患者内部不同部位差异很大,组织中的实际PDT剂量可能会有显着变化。因此,在充氧条件下,组织PDT剂量是PDT治疗结果的良好预测指标,因为它说明了局部光敏剂浓度和光通量的变化。结合正在进行的卟啉类光敏剂介导的PDT用于胸膜间皮瘤的Ⅱ期临床试验,Yi Hong Ong等开发了一种能够在PDT期间同时测量光通量率和光敏剂浓度的仪器。

利用实时监测手段,使用相同剂量的2mg/kg的光敏剂,同一名患者的局部光敏剂浓度可以相差2.9倍,而患者之间的局部敏化剂浓度可以相差8.3倍。其中测得的局部光敏剂浓度范围为1.13~9.38mg/kg;最低的是胸膜腔的尖部位,最高的是胸壁前壁部位,从所有部位测得的局部光敏剂浓度的平均值和中位数分别为(3.94±2.01)mg/kg和(3.37±2.01)mg/kg。基于上述研究成果,使用实时PDT剂量监测法来指导治疗似乎更符合精准治疗的需求。

根据光敏剂药品说明书,应在注射后40~50 h镜下引入光源。在实践中,大多数介入专家通常在注射后24~72 h(多为48 h)安排光照。这样可使敏化剂集中在肿瘤细胞中,并洗净正常的黏膜,从而将对相邻非恶性组织的损害降至最低。肿瘤中的浓度在5~7 d仍能达到足够的治疗量,因此在注射光敏剂一周内补充照射仍能起到光动力治疗的效果。

超越常规,新的光敏剂应用方法也在逐渐被开发。2020年6月天津医科大学总医院冯靖教授报道了首例浸入式(免避光)即刻光动力治疗恶性胸腔积液案例,内科胸腔镜术前经皮试及抗过敏及镇痛预处理后在患者患侧卧位状态下直接经胸腔置管注入预计喜泊芬,内科胸腔镜下取壁层胸膜活检,经ROSE确认性质后即刻行胸膜光动力治疗。即刻光动力治疗的出现也为临床恶性胸膜疾病光动力治疗推开了新的探索之路。

光照剂量的选择与肿瘤范围相关,柱状光导纤维更适合胸膜光动力的病灶覆盖,选择纤维长度应超过肿瘤边缘1cm,选取630mm或635nm红色激光,在目前组织能量密度监测尚未普及的前提下,大多数专家在实践中及研究中选择能量密度为200J/cm²。术后通常需要留置28~32F胸腔引流管以充分引流胸腔内坏死物。

四、恶性胸膜病变光动力治疗的展望

近年来,随着光敏剂及光源技术的不断发展,光动力疗法的基础研究和临床应用也逐步深入和拓展,在肿瘤应用方面已取得丰富经验。恶性胸膜病变光动力治疗起源于外科手术后的辅助治疗,正逐渐向内科发展,治疗方法也不断更新,临床上发现恰当的光动力治疗可使者获益,光动力疗法也从外科辅助治疗逐渐成为局部治疗的主要手段之一。但在恶性胸膜病变光动力与其他治疗的联合方案,及光动力的技术规范方面仍迫切需要更多的数据支持。

参 考 文 献

[1] Cantini L, et al. Emerging Treatments for Malignant Pleural Mesothelioma: Where Are We Heading? Front Oncol, 2020, 10:343.

[2] Davies H, E Y, C Lee. Management of malignant pleural effusions: questions that need answers. Curr Opin Pulm Med, 2013, 19(4):374-379.

[3] 李黎波,罗荣城. 具有靶向作用的微创治疗-肿瘤光动力治疗在中国的临床应用. 第九届中国肿瘤微创治疗学术大会, 2013, 中国河南郑州. 11.

[4] Hasan T, O. B. M. A. ed. Photodynamic therapy of cancer. In Cancer Medicine, 9th ed. 2017:537.

[5] Kennedy J C, R H Pottier. Endogenous protoporphyrin IX, a clinically useful photosensitizer for photodynamic therapy. J Photochem Photobiol B, 1992, 14(4):275-292.

[6] Broadwater D, et al. Modulating cellular cytotoxicity and phototoxicity of fluorescent organic salts through counterion pairing. Sci Rep, 2019, 9(1):15288.

[7] Beltran, HI, et al. Preclinical and Clinical Evidence of Immune Responses Triggered in Oncologic Photodynamic Therapy: Clinical Recommendations. J Clin Med, 2020. 9(2).

[8] 刘浩林,等. 低光参量肿瘤靶向光动力疗法的免疫效应及其机制. 中国激光医学杂志, 2019, 28(6):351-357.

[9] Akopov A, et al. Preoperative endobronchial photodynamic therapy improves resectability in initially irresectable(inoperable) locally advanced non small cell lung cancer. Photodiagnosis Photodyn Ther, 2014, 11(3):259-264.

[10] Lee J E, et al. A case of small cell lung cancer treated with chemoradiotherapy followed by photodynamic therapy. Thorax, 2009, 64(7):637-639.

[11] Santos RS, et al. Bronchoscopic palliation of primary lung cancer: single or multimodality therapy? Surg Endosc, 2004, 18(6):931-936.

[12] Dang J, et al. Manipulating tumor hypoxia toward enhanced photodynamic therapy (PDT). Biomater Sci, 2017. 5(8):1500-1511.

[13] Haak CS, et al. Ablative fractional laser enhances MAL-induced PpIX accumulation: Impact of laser channel density, incubation time and drug concentration. J Photochem Photobiol B, 2016, 159:42-48.

[14] Ishida, N., et al. Heating increases protoporphyrin IX production in normal skin after delivery of 5-aminolevulinic acid by iontophoresis. Photodermatol Photoimmunol Photomed, 2009, 25(6):333-334.

[15] Chen KC, et al. Pleural Photodynamic Therapy and Surgery in Lung Cancer and Thymoma Patients with Pleural Spread. PLoS One, 2015, 10(7):e0133230.

[16] 周云芝,等. 氩气刀联合光动力学疗法治疗恶性气道狭窄18例. 中国肿瘤, 2008(11):973-975.

[17] Kitada M, et al. Photodynamic diagnosis of pleural malignant lesions with a combination of 5-aminolevulinic acid and intrinsic fluorescence observation systems. BMC Cancer, 2015, 15:174.

[18] Ong YH, et al. PDT dose dosimetry for Photofrin-mediated pleural photodynamic therapy(pPDT). Phys Med Biol, 2017, 63(1):015031.

4 恶性胸腔积液的免疫微环境与免疫治疗新思路

曾运祥 汪金林

恶性胸腔积液（MPE）常继发于多种恶性肿瘤，如肺癌、淋巴瘤、乳腺瘤和恶性间皮瘤等，以继发于肺癌的 MPE 最为常见。MPE 预后较未发生 MPE 者更差，患者预期寿命仅为 3～12 个月。对于近年新兴的抗肿瘤治疗药物，如 EGFR-TKIs、PD-1/PD-L1 抑制剂，MPE 患者的治疗反应也更差。MPE 的临床特点与其特殊的肿瘤微环境（TIME）相关，目前已有部分研究指出调控 TIME 的免疫微环境对 MPE 的治疗具有一定的作用。本文将对恶性胸腔积液的免疫微环境和免疫治疗方面进行归纳和整理。

一、MPE 的发病情况及治疗现状

临床上，MPE 是由恶性肿瘤侵犯胸膜引起，常见于肺癌、乳腺癌、淋巴瘤和恶性间皮瘤等恶性肿瘤，多为恶性肿瘤的晚期并发症，以肺腺癌（lung adenocarcinoma，LA）患者最常见。MPE 患者的预后取决于多种因素，例如年龄、体能状态、肿瘤类型、肿瘤分期、共存疾病、胸腔积液成分，以及原发肿瘤对抗肿瘤治疗的反应情况。总体来说，MPE 患者的预后较非 MPE 的转移性癌症患者差。有研究表明，对于存在远处转移的晚期 NSCLC 患者，出现 MPE 是 1 年和 2 年总生存率降低的独立预测因素；另有 1 篇纳入了 417 例患者的系统评价显示，在发现 MPE 后患者的中位生存期仅为 4 个月；目前指南指出，继发于 LA 的 MPE（MPE）患者预期寿命仅为 3～12 个月。

目前，MPE 的治疗方法包括化疗等抗肿瘤治疗及最佳支持治疗。由于化疗等疗效较差，副作用较大，因此有相当一部分 MPE 患者往往只采取最佳支持、局部治疗等姑息疗法，如胸腔置管引流术、胸膜固定术、胸膜切除术、分流术、胸膜内纤溶药物治疗。抗肿瘤治疗方面，由于 MPE 对传统的全身性化疗的反应不尽如人意，近些年在抗肿瘤方法也有一些新的尝试。基于有研究表明，血管内皮因子（vascular endothelial growth factor，VEGF）是形成 MPE 的关键细胞因子，贝伐珠单抗是一种重组抗 VEGF 单克隆抗体，非鳞状 NSCLC 引起的 MPE 可能对贝伐珠单抗有反应。一项涵盖 21 个的小样本回顾性队列研究发现，联用传统化疗的非鳞状 NSCLC 合并 MPE 的患者对静脉应用贝伐珠单抗的反应率为 71.4%，在 23.8% 的患者观察到了肿瘤的缩小。另一项随机对照的队列研究表明，在 72 位 NSCLC 合并 MPE 的受试者中，胸腔内联合注射贝伐珠单抗与顺铂的治疗有效率较单用顺铂高（83% vs. 50%）。

然而，VEGF 单克隆抗体并不能改善患者的长期生存率。同样，EGFR 突变型 NSCLC 并发 MPE 的患者可能对 EGFR-TKIs 治疗有反应，一项队列研究表明，具有 EGFR T970M 突变的患者对奥希替尼的反应率约 61%，而无此突变的患者反应率仅为 20%；另一项研究也发现，接受吉非替尼的 EGFR 突变型 MPE 患者，虽然 12 个月的无进展生存率较标准对照组显著要长（24.9% vs. 6.7%），但大部分患者在 1 年后对 EGFR-TKIs 治疗耐药，并快速恶化。因此，MPE 患者治疗难度大，预后不良，生存期短，现有治疗方法改善有限，其发病机制研究对于这类疾病的治疗具有重要的意义。

二、MPE 肿瘤免疫微环境与免疫调节疗法

如前所述，MPE 患者的不良预后可能与其独特的病理生理学特性相关，一方面，MPE 包含悬浮的肿瘤细胞，这些细胞缺乏肿瘤脉管系统的支持，具有天然的"血肿瘤屏障（blood-tumor barrier）"，一般的抗肿瘤药物难以通过静脉给药到达，因此降低了抗肿瘤药物的递送效率。另一方面，MPE 具有特殊的肿瘤免疫微环境（tumor immune microenvironment，TIME），TIME 中的免疫细胞在特定情况下也为肿瘤的"免疫逃逸（immune escape）"提供了便利。免疫逃逸的悬浮肿瘤细胞可以附着在胸膜上，依赖 TIME 中的营养物质及促血管生存因子的支持进一步在胸膜上成长，甚至远处转移，影响预后。研究表明，TIME 中的调节性 B 淋巴细胞（Bregs），可以分泌促肿瘤细胞因子，Breg 浸润可促进肿瘤的进展；而 TIME 中的调节性 T 淋巴细胞（Tregs）或也通过减少细胞免疫而与肿瘤恶化相关；TIME 中的 CD8$^+$ T 细胞，其穿孔素表达较少，杀伤肿瘤能力弱，且在分化成熟前更易凋亡，导致具有抗肿瘤效应的成熟细胞不足；TIME 中抗原呈递细胞（antigen-presenting cells，APCs）对肿瘤细胞的抗原识别和呈递能力均有减弱。因此，TIME 中的固有免疫及获得性免疫的减弱，是肿瘤逃逸的重要机制之一。

通过调控 MPE-TIME，增强其免疫细胞对肿瘤细胞的识别及杀伤能力，成了一个潜在的研究热点。例如，Yang 等证明 TIME 中 M2 肿瘤相关巨噬细胞（M2-TAMs）可以被辐射的肿瘤细胞释放的微粒极化为 M1-TAMs，并显示出增加的 PD-L1 表达，增强了后续联合抗 PD-1 治疗的作

用,对耐顺铂的 MPE 小鼠模型起到肿瘤消融的作用。同样在临床试验中,胸膜腔内输注具有抗癌活性的肿瘤浸润淋巴细胞(TILs)对 MPE 的临床疗效优于顺铂。也有研究提到,IL-2 可通过促进体内淋巴细胞亚群的活化和增殖来抑制 MPE 中的肿瘤细胞。但是,目前的免疫佐剂在安全性上仍存在问题,其针对免疫系统的调节具有非特异性,或有可能造成过度的系统性炎症反应,例如过量的 IL-2 会导致患者发热,寒战和其他症状。因此,尽管免疫调节剂具有潜在的改善 MPE 的治疗效果,仍有必要提高其有效性及安全性。

三、纳米硒对 MPE 肿瘤免疫微环境的免疫调节作用

纳米药物由于具有激活固有免疫及获得性免疫应答作用而发挥抗肿瘤的作用,目前已用于抗癌治疗。硒元素对于真核生物的生长发育必不可少,传统的含硒佐剂也广泛使用于免疫调节。相比于前者,纳米硒(SeNPs)具有良好的生物相容性及低毒性的优点,是多种药物的优良载体,同时也可充当免疫调节佐剂。具体而言,SeNPs 良好的生物相容性,甚至可帮助其穿透血脑屏障,利用此特性,螯合了放疗增强剂或抗肿瘤药物的 SeNPs,便可增强对中枢神经系统肿瘤的杀伤能力。

除了作为药物载体增强抗肿瘤药物或放疗的功效,SeNPs 也通过调节免疫系统发挥抗肿瘤作用。例如,通过调控肿瘤相关巨噬细胞功能,SeNPs 可抑制淋巴瘤增殖;通过升高促炎细胞因子 IFN-γ、TNF-α 和 IL-2 的水平及增加 NK 细胞的活性来诱导有效的免疫反应,SeNPs 在动物水平上展示了对乳腺癌的杀伤及减少转移的作用;广州呼吸健康研究院及其合作课题组前期研究也发现,SeNPs 预处理的 γδT 细胞显著上调了 NKG2D、CD16 和 IFN-γ 等细胞毒性相关分子的表达,同时下调了 PD-1 表达,在细胞及动物水平上均具有更强的杀灭癌症和抑制肿瘤生长的功效。进一步的,我们发现对免疫治疗反应较差的 MPE 患者,其血清硒含量较低,收集 MPE 患者的胸腔积液并在体外用 SeNPs@LNT 处理,发现 SeNPs 可促进 NK、Th1、Tc、γδT 和 B 细胞的增殖,并抑制 Th2、Treg 和抑制性 NK 细胞的表达,提示 SeNPs 具有在体外激活 MPE-TIME 中免疫系统的功能,或具有潜在的治疗 MPE 的作用。因此,SeNPs 具有通过调节免疫系统发挥治疗 MPE 的潜在作用。

四、结 论

恶性胸腔积液预后不良,常规治疗效果差,肿瘤微环境特殊,免疫调节治疗或对其治疗有所帮助。纳米材料,尤其以纳米硒为代表,具有潜在的免疫调节作用,或有通过调节免疫系统发挥治疗 MPE 的潜在作用。

参 考 文 献

[1] Moro-Sibilot D, Smit E, de Castro Carpeño J, et al. Outcomes and resource use of non-small cell lung cancer (NSCLC) patients treated with first-line platinum-based chemotherapy across Europe: FRAME prospective observational study. Lung Cancer, 2015, 88(2): 215-222.

[2] Bray F, Ferlay J, Soerjomataram I, et al. Global cancer statistics 2018: GLOBOCAN estimates of incidence and mortality worldwide for 36 cancers in 185 countries. CA: a Cancer Journal for Clinicians, 2018, 68(6): 394-424.

[3] Ferreiro L, Suárez-Antelo J, Valdés L. Pleural procedures in the management of malignant effusions. Annals of Thoracic Medicine, 2017. 12(1): 3.

[4] Morgenstern D, Waqar S, Subramanian J, et al. Prognostic impact of malignant pleural effusion at presentation in patients with metastatic non-small-cell lung cancer. Journal of Thoracic Oncology, 2012, 7(10): 1485-1489.

[5] Feller-Kopman DJ, Reddy CB, DeCamp MM, et al. Management of malignant pleural effusions. An official ATS/STS/STR clinical practice guideline. American Journal of Respiratory and Critical care Medicine, 2018, 198(7): 839-849.

[6] Masago K, Fujimoto D, Fujita S, et al. Response to bevacizumab combination chemotherapy of malignant pleural effusions associated with non-squamous non-small-cell lung cancer. Molecular and Clinical Oncology, 2015, 3(2): 415-419.

[7] Du N, Li X, Li F, et al. Intrapleural combination therapy with bevacizumab and cisplatin for non-small cell lung cancer-mediated malignant pleural effusion. Oncology Reports, 2013, 29(6): 2332-2340.

[8] Verma A, Chopra A, W Lee Y, et al. Can EGFR-Tyrosine Kinase Inhibitors (TKI) alone without talc pleurodesis prevent recurrence of malignant pleural effusion (MPE) in lung adenocarcinoma. Current Drug Discovery Technologies, 2016, 13(2): 68-76.

[9] Mok TS, Wu Y-L, Thongprasert S, et al. Gefitinib or carboplatin-paclitaxel in pulmonary adenocarcinoma. New England Journal of Medicine, 2009. 361(10): 947-957.

[10] Psallidas I, Kalomenidis I, Porcel JM, et al. Malignant pleural effusion: from bench to bedside. European Respiratory Review, 2016. 25(140): 189-198.

[11] Light R, Hamm H. Malignant pleural effusion: would the real cause please stand up? European Respiratory Journal, 1997, 10(8): 1701-1702.

[12] Guo M, Wu F, Hu G, et al. Autologous tumor cell-derived microparticle-based targeted chemotherapy in lung cancer patients with malignant pleural effusion. Science Translational Medicine, 2019. 11(474): eaat5690.

[13] Liu D, Lu Y, Hu Z, et al. Malignant pleural effusion supernatants are substitutes for metastatic pleural tumor tissues in EGFR mutation test in patients with advanced lung adenocarcinoma. PloS one, 2014, 9(2).

[14] Patel AJ, Richter A, Drayson MT, et al. The role of B lym-

phocytes in the immuno-biology of non-small-cell cancer. Cancer Immunology, Immunotherapy, 2020:1-18.

[15] Budna J, Kaczmarek M, Frydrychowicz M, et al. Regulatory T cells in malignant pleural effusions subsequent to lung carcinoma and their impact on the course of the disease. Immunobiology, 2017, 222(3):499-505.

[16] Prado-Garcia H, Aguilar-Cazares D, Flores-Vergara H, et al. Effector, memory and naive CD8$^+$ T cells in peripheral blood and pleural effusion from lung adenocarcinoma patients. Lung Cancer, 2005, 47(3):361-371.

[17] Bremnes RM, Busund L-T, Kilvær TL, et al. The role of tumor-infiltrating lymphocytes in development, progression, and prognosis of non-small cell lung cancer. Journal of Thoracic Oncology, 2016, 11(6):789-800.

[18] Wan C, Sun Y, Tian Y, et al. Irradiated tumor cell-derived microparticles mediate tumor eradication via cell killing and immune reprogramming. Science Advances, 2020, 6(13): eaay9789.

[19] Chu H, Du F, Gong Z, et al. Better clinical efficiency of TILs for malignant pleural effusion and ascites than cisplatin through Intrapleural and intraperitoneal infusion. Anticancer Research, 2017, 37(8):4587-4591.

[20] Murthy P, Ekeke CN, Russell KL, et al. Making cold malignant pleural effusions hot: driving novel immunotherapies. OncoImmunology, 2019, 8(4):e1554969.

[21] Wang C, Ye Y, Hu Q, et al. Tailoring biomaterials for cancer immunotherapy: Emerging trends and future outlook. Advanced Materials, 2017, 29(29):1606036.

[22] Avery JC, Hoffmann PR. Selenium, selenoproteins, and immunity. Nutrients, 2018, 10(9):1203.

[23] Chang Y, He L, Li Z, et al. Designing core-shell gold and selenium nanocomposites for cancer radiochemotherapy. ACS Nano, 2017, 11(5):4848-4858.

[24] Song Z, Liu T, Chen T. Overcoming blood-brain barrier by HER2-targeted nanosystem to suppress glioblastoma cell migration, invasion and tumor growth. Journal of Materials Chemistry B, 2018, 6(4):568-579.

[25] Gautam PK, Kumar S, Tomar M, et al. Selenium nanoparticles induce suppressed function of tumor associated macrophages and inhibit Dalton's lymphoma proliferation. Biochemistry and Biophysics Reports, 2017, 12:172-184.

[26] Yazdi M, Mahdavi M, Kheradmand E, et al. The preventive oral supplementation of a selenium nanoparticle-enriched probiotic increases the immune response and lifespan of 4T1 breast cancer bearing mice. Arzneimittelforschung, 2012, 62(11):525-531.

[27] Hossein Yazdi M, Mahdavi M, Setayesh N, et al. Selenium nanoparticle-enriched Lactobacillus brevis causes more efficient immune responses in vivo and reduces the liver metastasis in metastatic form of mouse breast cancer. DARU, 2013, 21(4).

[28] Hu Y, Liu T, Li J, et al. Selenium nanoparticles as new strategy to potentiate γδ T cell anti-tumor cytotoxicity through upregulation of tubulin-α acetylation. Biomaterials, 2019, 222:119397.

第十一部分

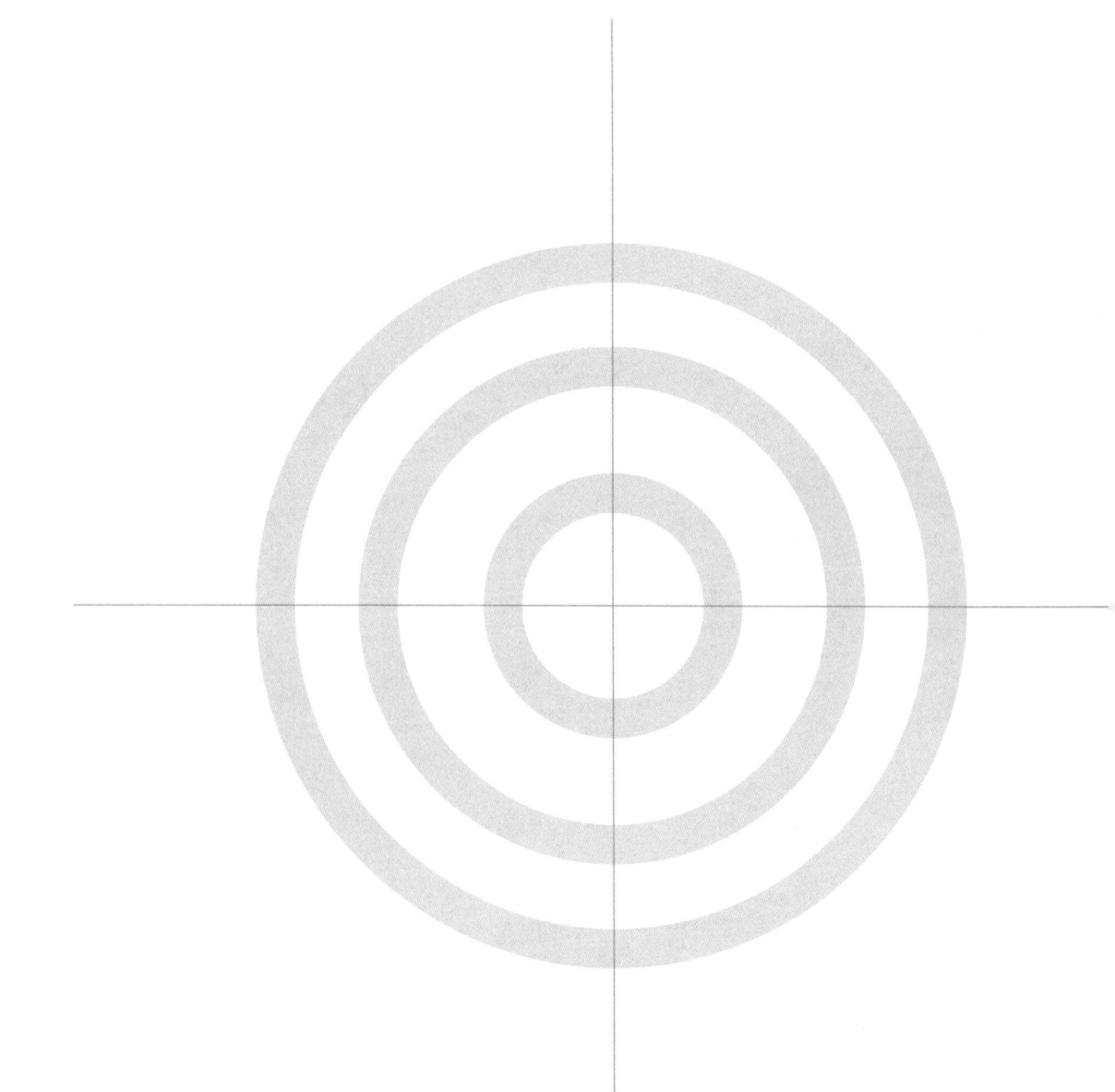

介入呼吸病学

1 关于介入呼吸病学与转化医学的几点思考

钟志成 李 静 崔景华

介入呼吸病学是现代呼吸病学的一门重要亚学科,以可弯曲支气管镜为代表,包括CT、超声、硬质支气管等器械,通过气管或微小创口对特定病变进行诊断与治疗。介入呼吸病学采用微创技术,在传统呼吸内科学和外科学之间开辟新的领域,为呼吸系统疾病的诊断和治疗发挥巨大的、不可替代的作用。转化医学是连接基础和临床的学科,从基础研究结果向临床科学转化,从临床问题形成科学问题进行基础研究,基础、临床双向转化的科学,核心将医学生物学基础研究成果有效地转化可在临床实际应用的理论、技术、方法和药物。

一、国外转化医学情况

1996年Geraghty J提出转化医学后,总结国内外转化医学形式,主要分成3种主要模式:①以美国国立转化医学促进中心为例的国家级平台模式;②以欧洲先进转化医学研究基础设施为例的项目实施模式;③以美国和中国的转化中心为例的单体转化中心模式。

美国国立卫生研究院(National Institutes of Health, NIH)通过设立临床与转化科学基金项目(clinical and translational science award,CTSA)建立国家级平台模式及单体转化医学中心模式。2006年临床和转化科学基金项目 Clinical and Translational Science Awards,CTSA)首批成立12家临床和转化医学中心,2012年全美成立了60余家临床和转化医学中心,这些中心通常紧密依托大学和医学中心。NIH对临床研究管理特点包括:①资助基金计划性强,资助方向重点明确;②针对性强,重视社会影响大、影响范围广的常见病与多发病;③与时俱进,资助急需解决的问题,对疾病预防资助力度大。项目实施通过依托研究型医院、建立院内研究室管理制度,采用实验室主管制度,又称独立研究人(principle investigator,PI)负责制,数字化建设制度等方式。拖进了研究成果的转化应用,同时为美国培养医学人才,保证全球生物医药领域的持久领先地位。

欧洲多国政府和科学组织施行项目实施模式,设定战略项目欧洲先进转化医学研究基础设施(The European Adavcanced Translational Research Infrastructure in Medicine,EATRIS)。EATRIS为保持欧洲在生物医学研究和医疗行业的竞争力,提供分子成像和跟踪、疫苗、生化标记、小分子研究、创新药物研发等转化服务。EATRIS通过促进多国政府合作伙伴、科研合作伙伴,整合资源,根据新的医疗需求,动态调整自身转化研究培训与教育,提高基础研究的转化速度。多国合作,统筹共同部署研究基础设施,节约成本提高效率,同步加快转化速度。

二、我国转化医学发展的现况

转化医学在我国起步晚,建立形成初级单体转化医学中心模型,通过合作或挂靠等形式,以综合性医院或相关科研机构为主题,成立各具特色的转化医学中心。根据《"十三五"国家科技创新规划》,科技部、国家卫生计生委等机构共同开展国家临床医学研究中心,目的为了加强各中心建设,从而实现我国医学创新能力、加快我国卫生与健康科技成果转化能力,为实现健康中国战略目标提供有力支撑。而我国内临床与转化中心以医院本身所开展的临床科研活动为主,整合本身中心诊疗优势,依靠自身临床资源优势与企业协助完成转化。以我国首个综合性国家级转化医学中心为例,转化医学国家重大科技基础设施(上海)项目由上海交通大学和上海交通大学医学院附属瑞金医院共同承担建设,2017年与上海联影医疗科技共识建立医疗设备创新研究和技术转化基地,与上海市闵行去政府成立医疗机器人研究院,开展医疗机器人创新研究;与上海市黄浦区建立医学健康创新园区,为临床研究机构、创新药物研发提供综合产业服务。

我国转化医学发展面临多方挑战,存在诸多发展障碍:①转化医学的复杂性:转化医学需要在临床和实验室进行性研究,需要配合运行机制、教育体制等诸多因素,需要整合各部门、各学科共同解决转化医学所涉及的知识产权、转化方案、临床前工作、临床实验涉及经费筹备等各项问题。②研究耗资巨大:研究来源经费多源,但每个渠道都有局限性。国内转化医学中心建设资金不足,大多依靠科研项目进行建设,不稳定性。③研究人员缺乏:目前缺乏转化医学科研教学模式,需要培养与转化医学相符的集学术型与专业型能力于一体的复合型医学人才。④转化医学研究机构的组织结构与机制问题:目前缺乏基础科学家与临床研究人员分离,导致一定程度的学术障碍。⑤知识产权保护与利益分配:知识产权与利益的合理分配是保证持续性创新的关键,目前我国的知识产权虽有立法,但在具体专利人的相关保障仍未充分。⑥转化效果不佳:对科研成果转化25%通过外部知识产权服务机构转化,25%

通过产学联盟转化,50%通过转让产权进行转化,以技术转让与他人合作转化为主,转化途径少,形式单一。

我国转化医学模式发展现况,发展有自身特点,包括自身的领域范围、运行模式和评价体系。杨静等通过系统评价总结,分析我国转化医学现况。转化医学研究领域中,涉及领域有科研管理、中医药领域、学科服务模式,儿科领域,病理生理学实验平台等。转化医学模式运行方式多样,包括转化医学科研管理创新模式、全维式交叉协同转化医学科研组织模式、转化医学科研模式、转化医学体系下的学科服务模式。目前尚未形成自身明确的评价体系,崔银河提出应对科研成果开展动态价值评估,并遵循公正、客观原则,做到整个评价指标体系全面、细化和量化,提高科研人员积极性和继发创造力,促进学科之间交融与渗透,推进转化医学跨学科研究,实现科研成果快速普及与转化。目前,我国转化医学模式的构建需要借鉴美国和欧洲的经验,探索适合我国转化医学发展模式,寻找适合标准、统一的转化医学模式和临床转化评价体系,形成科学、规范的方法探索合适的实践模式,促使转化医学发展和实施。

三、介入呼吸病学的发展及转化医学方向

介入呼吸病学近些年各技术发展活跃,逐步形成经气道介入、经皮经胸腔介入、经肺血管介入、经食管介入诊疗技术,形成4D介入呼吸病学(4D IP)技术体系。近些年,随着对各种技术普及及熟悉,我国积极总结自身经验,形成介入呼吸病学各操作技术的专家共识、指南,且配合呼吸与急危重症科专科医师培训,逐步形成呼吸介入单项规范化进修培训基地,已逐步改善了技术不规范、培训不规范等问题。Robert Garland 介入呼吸病中心的设计提出在操作室规划额外设计用于"技术研发"的空间。但我国介入呼吸病学发展,存在缺乏基础研究、缺乏拥有自主产权的产品、研发和转化能力滞后等问题,各种呼吸介入器械、材料多依赖进口,如内镜,国产医用内镜市场占有率低,主要由日本、德国等国家占有市场。

笔者根据介入呼吸病学各种诊疗技术的发展模式,大致分成以下几种方式:①借助新的辅助技术:如窄光谱成像、荧光的特殊光染色提高病灶活检阳性率;径向超声引导肺外周病灶检查,气道内超声引导经支气管针吸活检用于肺癌诊断及分期、纵隔病变诊断;②从其余介入学科如心内科介入、消化内镜等技术引入呼吸介入使用:如光学相关断层扫描术开始用于眼科检查、心脏冠脉血管评估,现可用于中央气道至气道的管腔及气道壁的各层结构(包括内膜、黏膜下层。平滑肌、腺体、软骨等)的观察;共聚焦显微镜最初被用于胃肠道黏膜检查,先用于外周小气道、肺组织观察;光动力治疗开始用于皮肤治疗,先可用于气道内早期治疗、气道内肿物、晚期肺癌姑息治疗;③现有的技术的再改良:用于气道狭窄治疗的气道支架,从20世纪80年代第一代金属支架出现,随着材料学发展,逐步调整改良形成硅酮支架、覆膜支架、Y形支架等各类型支架;④影像学技术及计算机智能运算的发展:通过数字图像和医学交流系统(DICOM)结核,形成支气管镜导航系统,可对气管和支气管树进行无创评价,评价支气管狭窄,引导支气管到达肺外周病变的位置,可联合电磁、X光引导病灶标记、活检及治疗;⑤寻找新的自然孔道或微小创口进行介入诊疗;LungPro全肺诊疗导航系统引导,通过Flex-Needle建立直达全肺病灶的隧道,实现全肺病灶的诊断及后续治疗;近些年建立经气管、经血管相关介入诊疗。

随着更多的新科技及技术发展,包括手术机器人、人工智能、3D打印技术、5G技术、远程医疗等技术,新材料的发明,干细胞的运用,都会成未来呼吸介入病学改变的方向。达芬奇机器人具有高度放大的三维视觉,有自由度精确控制的机械臂,使手术视野的图像更清晰,提高手术的精确度;新冠疫情期间,上海市胸科医院使用Microport MedBot微创支气管手术机器人完成首例用于新冠肺炎诊疗的支气管镜肺泡灌洗,为高传染性呼吸系统疾病的诊疗提供更安全的工具,多国多公司均在逐步开发内镜操作机器人;5G技术传输数据量大,避免了远程通信延迟的风险,联合手术机器人,可提供远程医疗、远程手术等可能,通讯技术改善为远程内镜操作提供一种可能性;3D打印术前可病变气管,能用于复杂的病变,更高水平还原操作场景,可用于复杂手术的风险评估,降低手术并发症;可以针对特定病变,3D打印定制个性化的气道支架、封堵器,更贴合个体化诊疗需求;通过3D打印聚乳酸作为原材料的肺癌放射粒子^{125}I治疗肺癌。聚己内酯已经美国食品药品监督管理局(FDA)批准,被广泛用作3D打印的理想材料来源,与仿生水凝胶联合运用3D打印技术可制作人工气管,有较好的生物相容性,为间充质干细胞提供黏附和增殖空间。

综上所述,介入呼吸病学是呼吸病学重要分支,发展迅速,但仍面临着很多有待解决的问题。为解决临床问题提出科学假设,为基础医学提供科学问题,从基础研究寻找解决临床问题的方法,通过为基础转化和临床研究双向转化,医学科技创新在成果转化的助力下,最终目的提高总体医疗水平、满足患者的健康需要、提高全人类的健康水平。

参 考 文 献

[1] 郭述良,李一诗,江瑾玥.呼吸学科应大力推进4D介入呼吸病学技术体系建设.重庆医学,2019,48(7):1084-1088.

[2] 李静.介入呼吸病学——方兴未艾.循证医学,2016,16(6):329-331.

[3] Geraghty J. Adenomatous polyposis coli and translational medicine. Lancet,1996,348(9025):422.

[4] 陈丹霞,安嘉璐,田玲.转化医学主要模式及其比较研究.医学分子生物学杂志,2014,(4):208-213.

[5] 孙枫原,王俊男,程志远,等.美国先进临床研究管理模式的介绍及启示.转化医学杂志,2019,8(1):29-32.
[6] 李冬凉,赖昱臣,张薇薇,等.我国转化医学国家重大科技基础设施建设初探.上海交通大学学报(医学版),2020,40(6):701-706.
[7] 栗美娜,刘嘉祯,张鹭鹭,等.转化医学的发展困境及模式探讨.中国医院管理,2014(10).
[8] 杨静,黄亮,俞丹,等.我国转化医学模式的循证评价.转化医学杂志,2017,6(5):285-290.
[9] 陈晓冰,吴晓婷,张建军.基于转化医学理念培养医学研究生科研能力的研究.教育教学论坛,2020,(30):310-312.
[10] 高胜利,高淑红.我国转化医学学科建设中存在的问题及对策.医学与社会,2013,26(8):95-96.
[11] 李汝德,赵晓英,刘洋,等.转化医学视角下某省级医院科研投入产出分析.卫生软科学,2019,33(8):23-25,35.
[12] 崔银河,姜海.我国转化医学科研模式运行管理研究.科学管理研究,2016,34(5):25-27,39.
[13] 中华医学会呼吸病学分会介入呼吸病学学组.成人诊断性可弯曲支气管镜检查术应用指南(2019年版).中华结核和呼吸杂志,2019,42(8):573-590.
[14] 北京健康促进会呼吸及肿瘤介入诊疗联盟.恶性中心气道狭窄经支气管镜介入诊疗专家共识.中华肺部疾病杂志(电子版),2017,10(6):647-654.
[15] 中华医学会呼吸病学分会.良性中心气道狭窄经支气管镜介入诊治专家共识.中华结核和呼吸杂志,2017,40(6):408-418.
[16] 林江涛,农英,李时悦,等.支气管热成形术手术操作及围手术期管理规范.中华结核和呼吸杂志,2017,40(3):170-175.
[17] 介入呼吸病学理论与实践.天津:科技翻译出版社,2017.
[18] 蔡天智,陈婧婧.2015年我国内窥镜贸易分析.中国医疗器械信息,2016,22(11):21-25.
[19] Häussinger K, Becker H, Stanzel F, et al. Autofluorescence bronchoscopy with white light bronchoscopy compared with white light bronchoscopy alone for the detection of precancerous lesions: a European randomised controlled multicentre trial. Thorax,2005,60(6):496-503.
[20] 罗为展,钟长镐,陈愉,等.灰阶超声声像特征对肺门纵隔恶性淋巴结的预测价值.中华结核和呼吸杂志,2014,37(12):924-927.
[21] Tsuboi M, Hayashi A, Ikeda N, et al. Optical coherence tomography in the diagnosis of bronchial lesions. Lung Cancer,2005,49(3):387-394.
[22] Thiberville L, Salaün M, Lachkar S, et al. Human in vivo fluorescence microimaging of the alveolar ducts and sacs during bronchoscopy. Eur Respir J,2009,33(5):974-985.
[23] 中国抗癌协会肿瘤光动力治疗专业委员会.呼吸道肿瘤光动力治疗临床应用中国专家共识.中华肺部疾病杂志(电子版),2019,12(4):409-415.
[24] Folch EE, Pritchett MA, Nead MA, et al. Electromagnetic Navigation Bronchoscopy for Peripheral Pulmonary Lesions: One-Year Results of the Prospective, Multicenter NAVIGATE Study. J Thorac Oncol,2019,14(3):445-458.
[25] Weiser TS, Hyman K, Yun J, et al. Electromagnetic navigational bronchoscopy: a surgeon's perspective. Ann Thorac Surg,2008,85(2):S797-801.
[26] Herth FJ, Eberhardt R, Sterman D, et al. Bronchoscopic transparenchymal nodule access (BTPNA): first in human trial of a novel procedure for sampling solitary pulmonary nodules. Thorax,2015,70(4):326-332.
[27] Sterman DH, Keast T, Rai L, et al. High yield of bronchoscopic transparenchymal nodule access real-time image-guided sampling in a novel model of small pulmonary nodules in canines. Chest,2015,147(3):700-707.
[28] 安芳芳,荆朝侠,彭燕,等.达芬奇机器人的"前世、今生、来世".中国医疗设备,2020,35(7):148-151,168.
[29] 杨罗伟,杨同卫.达芬奇手术机器人临床应用的伦理学研究.工程研究-跨学科视野中的工程,2020,12(3):286-292.
[30] Peters BS, Armijo PR, Krause C, et al. Review of emerging surgical robotic technology. Surg Endosc,2018,32(4):1636-1655.
[31] 刘晓军,蓝新颜,蓝孝全,等.3D打印在胸腔镜肺上叶切除术制定术前计划中的应用.中国现代手术学杂志,2019,23(3):196-200.
[32] 梁娅男,张建华.3D打印与组织工程技术在气管替代治疗中的应用与热点.中国组织工程研究,2020,24(5):780-786.
[33] 方曙,周金华,杨涵,等.基于桌面级3D打印机的放射性粒子肺癌植入导板的剂量学验证.介入放射学杂志,2020,29(4):397-402.
[34] Chang JW, Park SA, Park JK, et al. Tissue-engineered tracheal reconstruction using three-dimensionally printed artificial tracheal graft: preliminary report. Artif Organs,2014,38(6):E95-E105.
[35] Edelman ER, FitzGerald GA. A decade of Science Translational Medicine. Sci Transl Med,2019,11(489).

2 支气管镜新技术在肺小结节诊断中的应用策略

白 冲

肺结节为小的局灶性、类圆形、影像学表现密度增高阴影,可单发或多发,不伴肺不张、肺门肿大和胸腔积液。孤立性肺结节无典型症状,常为单个、边界清楚、密度增高、直径≤3 cm且周围被含气肺组织包绕的软组织影。直径<8mm的肺结节可称为亚厘米结节,直径<4mm的肺结节称之为微结节。目前,随着薄层CT检查的广泛应用,肺结节检出率越来越多,虽然周围型肺癌一般表现为肿块或结节,但是,肺结节并不等于肺癌。肺结节探查手术24%~30%术后病理诊断为良性疾病。近年来,伴随着支气管镜设备和技术的不断研究、开发和临床应用,如虚拟导航支气管镜(Virtual Navigation Bronchoscopy,VNB)、电磁导航支气管镜(Electromagnetic Navigation Bronchoscopy,ENB)、支气管腔内超声小探头(RP-EBUS)和超细支气管镜等,显著改善支气管镜在周边肺部结节的诊断率。除此之外,其他的综合导引技术还包括X线透视、带引导鞘管的超声小探头(R-EBUS with guide sheath,EBUS-GS)等。随着诊断率不断提高,经人体自然腔道的内镜微创操作逐渐成为临床研究热点,但如何将上述各种导引技术有机结合,获得更高的诊断率,且操纵风险又可控制在较低水平,是目前探索和研究重点。

一、传统支气管镜

1. 支气管镜肺泡灌洗术(BAL) 是利用支气管镜向相应支气管肺泡内注入生理盐水并随即吸出,收集肺泡表面衬液,检查其细胞成份和可溶性物质的一种方法。可用于周围型肺癌诊断。熊瑛等比较选择性BAL相活检对周围型肺癌的诊断作用,结果85例周围型肺癌患者支气管肺泡灌洗液中癌细胞阳性率78.8%,远高于钳取活检(44.7%)和刷检(40.0%)。

2. 经支气管镜肺活检(TBLB) 是肺周围部位肿块、结节性病灶及肺部弥散性浸润病灶病因诊断的有效方法,可采用电透引导或无电透引导操作。美国胸科医师学会(ACCP)指南表明,可弯曲支气管镜检查对<2mm肺外周结节的敏感性为34%,>2mm的为63%。绝大多数细胞学样本均可用于分子学检测,但依赖于样本中肿瘤细胞的绝对数(>100个)、所占比例、保存程度,以及检测方法的敏感性。要进行分子学检测,建议平均抽吸、活检4次;细胞团块和核心组织样本更适合基因突变分析和ALK检测;如肿瘤负荷不足,可选用细胞学玻片来检测EGFR等基因突变。支气管镜获得的标本也可用于PD-L1检测,Stoy等报道22例患者通过支气管镜检查获得初始(81.8%)和疾病进展(18.2%)诊断,20例患者(90.9%)PD-L1测试成功,72.7%的样本采集是通过EBUS-TBNA,9.1%是周边结节针吸活,在PD-L1测试成功率不同采样方法之间(P=0.99)或针大小(P=1.00)无统计差。快速现场细胞学评估(Rapid on-site examinations,ROSE)有助于评估靶病灶样本中肿瘤细胞负荷,因此如需进行分子检测,推荐使用ROSE。

对于部分病灶,CT引导下行TBLB对中央病灶及淋巴结的诊断敏感性较传统支气管镜检查明显提高(见表11-2-1);影响诊断准确率的主要因素是病灶的直径,当病灶直径>3cm时,其诊断率为88%,而当病灶直径≤3cm时,其诊断率仅为33%。

表11-2-1 CT引导与传统电透下TBLB诊断率比较

		CT引导支气管镜	传统支气管镜	P值
周围病灶	敏感性	71%	76%	1.00
	NPV	44%	43%	
中央病灶或纵膈淋巴结	敏感性	100%	67%	0.26
外周淋巴结	敏感性	100%	64%	0.09

二、虚拟支气管镜导航(VNB)

1. LungPoint—增强现实(AR)导航系统 是一种将真实世界和3D模型信息"无缝"集成的技术。利用患者CT数据,定制化3D建模,并在原有在支气管镜下直视的现实影像与建模信息匹配(包括路径、血管、气道尺寸、病灶位置等信息),实现视觉化指导支气管镜的临床诊疗工作。识别并选定标记病灶,自动计算出3条到达病灶点的路径。在已发表的荟萃分析中,所有导航的平均诊断率为70%,而LungPoint的诊断率达到80%。研究结果显示:图像引导导航,可提高查找正确气道和靶向定位的能力。虚拟支气管镜导航的临床价值在于精确的靶向定位,它可以测距:提供到达靶点和气道壁的距离;也可以测直径:提供气道直径的测量数据。

2. LungPro—全肺诊疗导航系统 可以实现对气道外

病变部位特别是X光下不可见的外周孤立性肺小结节的精准定位，建立直接通往气道外病变部位的通道，以实现全肺的诊断及后续治疗。来自德国海德堡大学Herth等研究表明，使用支气管镜经肺实质进行肺结节活检的方法安全可靠，所有的病例均得到满意病理结果，平均每例取材3.3份，实施的穿刺最远的通道已达90mm。

三、超声支气管镜（EBUS）

是用超声支气管镜或将微型超声探头通过支气管镜进入气管、支气管管腔，通过实时超声扫描，获得气管、支气管管壁各层次及周围相邻脏器的超声图像，从而进一步提高诊断水平。EBUS技术自诞生以来发展十分迅速。随着内镜医师使用EBUS的经验增多，诊断率与活检数量均有所提高。EBUS探头将支气管镜与超声探头结合在一起，用于观察包括结节、血管、淋巴结等结构。EBUS检查较为安全，因EBUS引起的缺氧、呼吸衰竭、纵隔气肿、气胸、出血、心脏并发症等发生率低（0～3%）。

对于判断肺癌患者是否适合手术治疗，准确的分期非常重要，CT和PET可以鉴别纵隔淋巴结病变，但特异性不高；纵隔镜检查是分期的金标准，但以EBUS-TBNA进行纵隔和肺门淋巴结穿刺，则更微创、更安全。关于EBUS-TBNA诊断纵隔分期的准确性，Miami大学Sylvester综合肿瘤中心，入选了完成EBUS-TBNA检查以诊断或分期为目的的NSCLC患者151例患者，其中69例进行淋巴结分期，结果在准确性上EBUS-TBNA对比CT，为94%对77%（$P=0.004$）；EBUS-TBNA对比PET，为96%对73%（$P=0.019$），提示相对于CT和PET，EBUS-TBNA用于纵隔分期准确率更高，62%的患者可以避免进行胸腔镜或纵隔镜检查。对比EBUS-TBNA与纵隔镜方法评估2R、2L、4R、4L组淋巴结相比，EBUS-TBNA敏感性更高（91%，88%），确诊率更高（92%，89%）。因此，欧洲胸外科医师协会已经修订了指南，对于纵隔淋巴结的诊断，推荐EBUS-TBNA作为一线方法。对于气道附近、支气管镜无法直接显示的肺部病变，EBUS诊断准确率高达94%。当然，考虑到EBUS-TBNA的阴性预测率比较低，因此对于阴性或无法诊断的患者还是需要采用更积极的探查方法。EBUS-TBNA已成为病理性诊断纵隔淋巴结肿大的标准。针吸活组织有助于快速进行病理检查，诊断符合手术适应症后立即进行病灶切除。

四、导向鞘引导的超声内镜（EBUS-GS）

该技术是利用EBUS将微型超声探头通过支气管镜进入远端，通过实时超声扫描，获得周围肺病灶及其相邻脏器的超声图像，并在EBUS的引导下，通过鞘管对周围肺组织病灶进行活检，从而进一步提高诊断水平。

2004年Kurimoto等首次报道了EBUS-GS技术能提高对肺周围型病变的诊断价值。EBUS-G采用环扫探头。最常用的Olympus公司生产的超细超声探头有两种型号：UM-S20-20R和UM-S20-17S。引导鞘套装包括引导鞘，配套活检钳及细胞刷。操作过程可以在全身麻醉或局部麻醉下进行，根据之前的影像学先大致定位病变。经鼻或口置入支气管镜，超细探头和导向鞘通过气管镜的工作通道，进入支气管远端，对周围病变目标使用EBUS指导定位。一旦超声确定支气管镜所处位置和引导鞘所处位置合适，则撤出超细超声探头，留置导向鞘于病灶内。使用导鞘可以帮助保持气管镜位置固定，进行反复插入细胞刷或者活检钳进行刷检或者活检，甚至进行病变部位的穿刺活检。

对于周围型肺癌病灶，经支气管镜将微型超声探头进入病灶，获得EBUS图像，其诊断率高达87%；而探头靠近病灶，EBUS图像诊断率为42%，活检阳性率为82%。李明等对75例患者，78处肺周围结节进行EBUS引导下进行活检，结果恶性疾病的诊断率84.4%；而提高诊断率的影响因素包括：病灶直径>20mm、超声下病灶包绕探头、CT影像见支气管征、病灶近中心。Steinfort等对18个研究，1420例患者进行荟萃分析，结果显示EBUS对于肺外周病灶诊断特异1.00（95% CI 0.99～1.00），敏感性0.73（95% CI 0.70～0.76）阳性似然率26.84（12.60～57.20），阴性似然率0.28（0.23～0.36）。EBUS结合经支气管镜穿刺，可以增加周围型病灶的诊断准确诊断从51%提高到91%，没有观察到并发症。

EBUS联合多种方法可提高诊断的准确性。我们对41例患者行EBUS，结果诊断阳性率为68.3%（28/41），其中综合导引技术采用小探头+引导鞘管组60.0%（15/25），小探头+透视组50%（2/4），小探头+引导鞘管+透视组87.5%（7/8），虚拟支气管镜+小探头+引导鞘管+透视组100%（4/4）。

五、电磁导航（ENB）

ENB是周围病灶的靶向导航工具，它以CT作为路标进行导航，以精确的工具进行定位和操纵。通过详细精确的单元信息（包括小型化的传感器、166次/秒捕捉信息）及涵盖的CT图像，精准导航对准靶点。ENB运用iLogic虚拟支气管镜专用软件和设备（Super DimensionTM, Medtronic），该技术将CT图像与实时支气管镜检查相结合，操作者使用胸部CT扫描生成患者的肺支气管图像，并利用三维定向装置到达气道指定位置后，定位装置伸出支气管镜的末端，从而进入更远端的小气道。另外，计算机中可以存储多个通向单个结节的通路图，可以提高活检的诊断率。

Dale等比较CT引导下肺活检与ENB引导下肺活检。CT引导下肺活检敏感性81%～97%，气胸发生率15%，其中40%需置管；而ENB引导下肺活检其敏感性70%，与CT引导下肺活检敏感性无差异，但ENB引导下肺活检气胸发生率仅为1.6%。Eberhardt等联合EBUS与ENB对外周肺结节的诊断，共有118例患者入组，EBUS+ENB为88%，高于EBUS 69%，或ENB 59%（$P=0.02$），而并发症中气胸发生率5%～8%，认为EUBS和ENB联合检查方式使得支气管镜检查的诊断率接近 CT 引导下经皮肺穿刺的结果,且具有安全性较好的优势。ENB 检查技术已经受到越来越多的关注,但是 EBN 最大的缺点是检查费用昂贵。

影响 ENB 诊断准确性的因素包括:胸部 CT 图像,病变部位和大小,全身麻醉及 ROSE 的准确率。ENB 实现诊断的 78 例患者(包括 64 例恶性和 14 例良性),ENB 诊断敏感度和精确度分别为 0.69 和 0.76;唯一影响诊断的因素是支气管能否达到病变部位($P = 0.002$),没有并发症的报道。越大的结节 ENB 的诊断率越高,研究表明,当结节小于或大于 2 厘米时,诊断率分别为 61% 和 83%,然而,即使病变较小(<15 mm),ENB 活检的诊断成功率也有近 70%。研究发现全身麻醉较之于局麻可以稍提高诊断率(57.5%,69.2%);当 ENB 联合 ROSE 诊断时,ENB 对纵隔和肺部周围病变的诊断率为 89.5%。尽管 ENB 的主要适应症之一是对肺部外周病变的评估,同时 ENB 也可用于诊断纵隔淋巴结病。ENB 在诊断纵隔淋巴结病方面优于传统的 TBNA,ENB 诊断纵隔淋巴结病的诊断率为 72.8%,而传统 TBNA 诊断率为 42.2%。

六、其他

(一) DSA-Dyna-CT + 支气管镜

DSA-Dyna-CT 是一种锥形束投照/数字平板 DSA 计算机重组断层影像设备;原理是 X 线发生器以较低的射线量(通常球管电流在 10 mA 左右)围绕投照体做环形数字式投照。然后将围绕投照体多次数字投照、重组后进而获得三维图像。其特点是射线剂量低,迅速重建各种三维图像(包括血管、软组织和肺等)。2015 年 12 月,长海医院在德国 Wolfgang Schmidt 教授协助下,完成亚洲首例 DSA-Dyna-CT 重建下支气管镜实时导航肺外周结节活检术肺外周小结节活检、亚洲首例 DSA-Dyna-CT 重建经支气管及经皮会师实时导航肺外周结节活检术、亚洲首例新型 Twin-Stream 高频通气应用无痛麻醉支气管内镜手术操作。

(二) 支气管镜下建立经肺实质到达结节的通道技术 (bronchoscopic transparenchymal nodule access, BTPNA)

是一种新的针对肺结节的取样技术。2014 年首次在动物试验中验证了可行性,2015 年发表了第一次 BTPNA 人体试验的报道:在 12 患者中有 10 位患者创建了 BTPNA 隧道路径,期间没有不良事件发生。10 例(83%)均获得足够的活检组织,且与手术切除的组织学吻合。

(三) 共聚焦荧光显微镜 (confocal fluorescence microscopy, CFM)

光学活检系统——Cellvizio(共聚焦微探头影像仪)也已开展了前期的研究,并有望在临床广泛应用。CFM 是通过活体组织的显微镜图像来观察气道和肺泡在体内的显微机构,以此鉴别良性和恶性改变。CFM 的优势在于可以与所有支气管内镜匹配的共聚焦显微内镜,能够匹配并完善所有肺导航系统;实时用细胞级影像观察肺部组织,利用肺部自体荧光物质(无须造影剂);可检查整个支气管束直达肺泡。

(四) Auris 机器人内镜系统

2016 年 5 月 FDA 批准了第一个由 Auris Surgical 公司研发的医用远程操控 ARES(Auris 机器人内镜系统)机器人,可用于疾病诊断和治疗。Auris Surgical 公司是由机器人行业领导者 Intuitive Surgical 公司(曾制造了广为人知的达芬奇机器人)的联合创始人 Fred Moll 所创立的一家初创公司。2014 年末,Auris Surgical 公司在哥斯达黎加圣何塞的一家医院进行了有关机器人支气管镜的小型临床试验。首席研究员 José Rafael Rojas Solano 博士指出这次临床试验是首次在人类身上进行测试,该测试中采用的机器人可以采用支气管镜对患者进行诊断,从而判断患者是否出现支气管病变或肺部是否疑似出现癌症。研究表明,Auris 机器人在参与试验的 15 名患者的气管中发挥相应作用,且无副作用。在最终确诊有癌症的 9 位患者中,该机器人获得了其中 8 位的活检组织。这项研究使得这种非常有应用前景的技术在肺癌的诊断和治疗领域迈出了第一步。

七、小结

呼吸内镜在肺结节诊断中手段多,价值大,需根据患者病情及本单位条件选择,随着新技术新方法不断出现,必将出现更多的临床诊断方法。EBUS 和 ENB 提高了周围肺结节活检的诊断准确性。鉴于这一趋势,呼吸内镜以其确诊率高、风险小的特点,在评估支气管肺癌方面具有至关重要的地位,并为组织活检提供了更加安全有效的方法。目前我国对支气管镜技术的研究多为单个单位,将来的研究需要多个中心联合参与,以期获得更好的研究结果。

参考文献

[1] MacMahon H, Naidich DP, Goo JM, et al. Radiology 2017; 284:228-243 Guidelines for Management of Incidental Pulmonary Nodules Detected on CT Images: From the Fleischner Society 2017. Radiology, 2017, 284(1): 228-243.

[2] Krochmal R, Arias S, Yarmus L, et al. Diagnosis and management of pulmonary nodules. Expert Rev Respir Med, 2014, 8 (6): 677-691.

[3] 熊瑛,李国平,王宋平,等. 选择性支气管肺泡灌洗液相活检对周围型肺癌的诊断作用. 中华现代内科学杂志, 2006, 3: 78-79.

[4] Chinese Thoracic Society, Chinese Alliance against Lung Cancer. Chinese expert consensus statement on issues related to small specimen sampling of lung cancer, 2017, 6 (4): 219-230.

[5] Stoy SP, Rosen L, Mueller J, et al. Programmed death-ligand 1 testing of lung cancer cytology specimens obtained with bronchoscopy. Cancer Cytopathol, 2018, 126(2): 122-128.

[6] Ost D, Shah R, Anasco E, et al. A randomized trial of CT fluoroscopic-guided bronchoscopy vs conventional bronchoscopy in patients with suspected lung cancer. Chest, 2008, 134(3): 507-513.

[7] Roetting M, Gompelmann D, Herth FJF. Thermic and chemical procedures for bronchoscopic lung volume reduction. J Thorac Dis, 2018, 10(Suppl 23): S2806-S2810.

[8] Um SW, Kim HK, Jung SH, et al. Endobronchial ultrasound versus mediastinoscopy for mediastinal nodal staging of non-small-cell lung cancer. J Thorac Oncology, 2015, 10: 331-337.

[9] Kurimoto N, Miyazawa T, Okimasa S, et al. Endobronchial ultrasonography using a guide sheath increases the ability to diagnose peripheral pulmonary lesions endoscopically. Chest, 2004, 126: 939-963.

[10] Eberhardt R1, Ernst A, Herth FJ. Ultrasound-guided transbronchial biopsy of solitary pulmonary nodules less than 20 mm. Eur Respir J, 2009, 34: 1284-1287.

[11] 李明, 王昌惠. 支气管超声下经引导鞘肺活检术诊断肺周围性病变的价值. 中华结核和呼吸杂志, 2014, 37: 36-40.

[12] Steinfort DP, Siva S, Leong TL, et al. Systematic Endobronchial Ultrasound-guided Mediastinal Staging Versus Positron Emission Tomography for Comprehensive Mediastinal Staging in NSCLC Before Radical Radiotherapy of Non-small Cell Lung Cancer: A Pilot Study. Medicine (Baltimore), 2016, 95(8): e2488.

[13] Skovgaard Christiansen I, Kuijvenhoven JC, et al. Endoscopic Ultrasound with Bronchoscope-Guided Fine Needle Aspiration for the Diagnosis of Paraesophageally Located Lung Lesions. Respiration, 2018.

[14] Huang HD, Ning YY, Zhang W, et al. Multiple guided technologies based on radial probe endobronchial ultrasound for the diagnosis of solitary peripheral pulmonary lesions: a single-center study, 2017, 8(17): 3514-3521.

[15] Dale CR, Madtes DK, Fan VS, et al. Navigational bronchoscopy with biopsy versus computed tomography-guided biopsy for the diagnosis of a solitary pulmonary nodule: a cost-consequences analysis. J Bronchology Interv Pulmonol, 2012, 19(4): 294-303.

[16] Eberhardt R, Morgan RK, Ernst A, et al. Comparison of suction catheter versus forceps biopsy for sampling of solitary pulmonary nodules guided by electromagnetic navigational bronchoscopy. Respiration, 2010, 79(1): 54-60.

[17] Patrucco F, Gavelli F, Daverio M, et al. Electromagnetic Navigation Bronchoscopy: Where Are We Now? Five Years of a Single-Center Experience. Lung, 2018.

[18] Karnak D, Cileda ğ A, Ceyhan K, et al. Rapid on-site evaluation and low registration error enhance the success of electromagnetic navigation bronchoscopy. Ann Thorac Med, 2013, 8: 28-32.

[19] Pritchett MA, Schampaert S, de Groot JAH, et al. Cone-Beam CT With Augmented Fluoroscopy Combined With Electromagnetic Navigation Bronchoscopy for Biopsy of Pulmonary Nodules. J Bronchology Interv Pulmonol, 2018, 25(4): 274-282.

[20] Silvestri GA, Herth FJF, Keast T, et al. Feasibility and safety of bronchoscopic transparenchymal nodule access in canines: a new real-time image-guided approach to lung lesions. Chest, 2014, 145(4): 833-838.

[21] Herth FJ, Eberhardt R, Sterman D, et al. Bronchoscopic transparenchymal nodule access (BTPNA): first in human trial of a novel procedure for sampling solitary pulmonary nodules. Thorax, 2015, 70(4): 326-332.

3 TTS气道支架的基础与临床研究

蒋军红

中央气道是指气管、隆突、左右主支气管及中间段支气管，结核、气道良性肿瘤、气管支气管软化、气管插管或气管切开等良性疾病，肺癌、食管癌、甲状腺癌等恶性疾病发病初或治疗过程中会出现中央气道狭窄，导致肺不张和呼吸困难、影响患者后续的治疗。快速缓解患者的呼吸困难，提高其生存质量，呼吸介入治疗是其必要手段。目前中央气道狭窄的介入治疗手段主要有：支气管镜下肿瘤消融技术（冷冻、激光、氩等离子体凝固、高频电刀等），后装放疗、气道内支架（硅酮支架和金属支架）置入等可以缓解气道阻塞症状，改善患者的生活质量，为后续的肿瘤治疗提供机会。

恶性肿瘤引起的中央气道狭窄根据其生长的情况可分为：①管腔内生长（管内型）②管壁浸润型（混合型）；③管外压迫性（外压型）。由于气道内支架适合管内型、混合型和管外型，其在介入治疗手段中有极其重要的作用。自膨胀性镍钛合金气道支架具有强度高、耐腐蚀、组织相容性好、无毒性、有形状记忆效应等特性。其对中央气道恶性病变的作用已非常明确，对气道阻塞症状的改善率达到78%~98%。良性气道狭窄的主要原因有肉芽组织增生、瘢痕挛缩、软骨结构破坏塌陷等，气道软骨的塌陷所导致的气道狭窄，目前只有支架才能解决，但是支架置入后的并发症限制了在良性气道狭窄患者的使用。美国食品和药物管理局发表声明警告，只有当患者不适合手术、硬支气管镜或硅酮支架置入术时，才应该考虑置入金属支架。

目前国内使用的镍钛记忆合金支架主要有：Ultraflex支架（美国Bostonscience公司生产）、OTW支架（南微医学科技有限公司）。有文献报道，国产镍钛支架及进口Ultraflex支架释放的一次性成功率仅为76%左右，即便经过及时调整或取出后重新放置，仍有5.9%~15.4%的患者支架置入失败。在目前临床广泛常用的自膨胀性镍钛金属支架的基础上，本报告者进行了结构上的突破性改进，发明了一种新型的经软性支气管镜直接释放的支架置入系统，获得国家发明专利和实用新型专利（专利号ZL201510010262.0和ZL201520013352)，转化成临床产品，并且获得中国FDA的上市许可（注册许可证号20193130362、20183130361）和欧盟销售许可（Tracheal Stent CN19/41071），经支气管镜工作孔道（through the scope,TTS）气道支架解决了气道支架可以在气管镜直视下释放的问题。本文详细的介绍TTS支架的结构和力学特性、TTS气道支架置入方法、有关TTS支架进行的动物和临床试验的研究结果。

一、TTS气道支架的结构和力学特性

经支气管镜工作孔道（through the scope,TTS）释放的自膨胀性镍钛合金支架系统主要由外管、中管、内芯、前后手柄、助推管、固定锁和支架等几部分组成。外管直径2.65 mm，表面有支架实际长度的标志，助推管靠近后手柄部分有一个1 cm的尺度标志提示支架还有1 cm的长度在置入器内。内芯为0.6 mm×1 100 mm镍钛合金导丝，其头端为一金属橄榄头，便于通过狭窄段而不损伤气道黏膜。内芯和中管之间的空间可以容纳镍钛记忆合金支架。

TTS气道支架是由单根直径0.22 mm镍钛丝编织而成，有裸支架和全覆膜支架两种型号。TTS裸支架直径≤18 mm，TTS覆膜支架直径≤16 mm。TTS支架两端的丝材折返点为小尖头，便于将支架装入TTS置入器。TTS支架两端设有回收线，回收线是从支架两端第二个网格穿过支架一周，可在利用回收线调整支架位置的同时不影响支架的正常张开，支架两端呈内收状态，便于必要时移除支架。置入器可以通过支气管工作孔道，在支气管镜直视下释放，避免了置入器和气管镜并行影响通气的问题，尤其解决了在紧急状态下快速气道开发，挽救患者的生命。

自膨式镍钛合金支架（self-expandablemetallicstents,SEMs）不但具有良好的组织相容性，而且还具有独特的形状记忆特性，在低温状态下可明显变形，加温到一定温度后又可恢复原有形状，并在形状恢复过程中产生较大的支撑力。SEMS支架的主要力学性能指标包括：①径向支撑力：支架能够有效扩张狭窄的管腔所需要的支撑力。影响支架径向支撑力的主要因素是径丝的直径、编织的头数、导程及覆膜情况。在头数和导程不变的情况下，径丝直径越细，支架径向支撑力越小；在导程和丝径不变的情况下，头数越多，支架径向支撑力越大；在头数和丝径不变的情况下，导程越小径向支撑力越大；覆膜后支架的支撑力增大，主要是因为支架的丝材的交叉点被固定，导致力臂变短，径向支撑力加大。②长度变化率（短缩率）：当支架从被压缩的置入器中进行释放时，支架会从压缩长度逐步恢复至其原始长度。③纵向柔顺性：适应各种管腔内的弯曲情况，从而与管腔形状相顺应。

体外测试结果表明，TTS支架和OTW支架的径向支撑力相当，但TTS支架的柔顺性相比于OTW支架更好，有利于支架适应不同结构的气道（图11-3-1）。

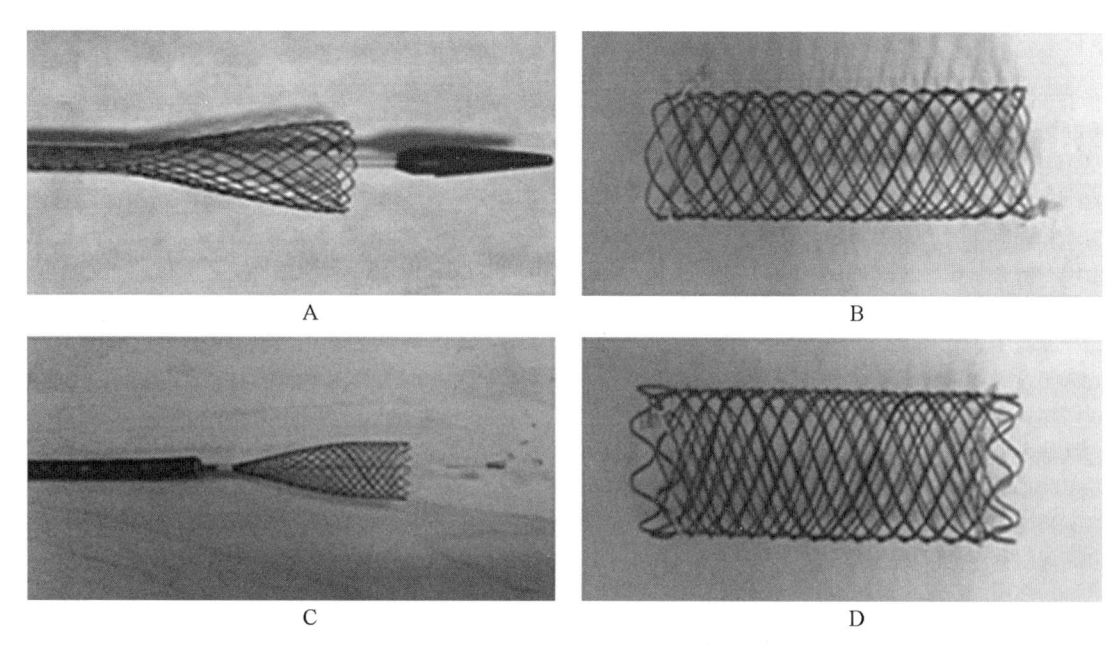

图 11-3-1　OTW 和 TTS 支架结构图

注：A. OTW 支架置入器结构图；B. OTW 圆支架；图 C. TTS 支架置入器结构图；D. TTS 支架

二、TTS 气道支架的置入方法

TTS 支架释放方法根据支气管镜是否能越过狭窄的病变部位分为两种，可称为支气管镜穿越法和置入器穿越法。

1. 支气管镜穿越法　操作者操作支气管镜越过狭窄的病变部位并在支气管镜直视下将置入器沿支气管镜工作孔道插入到狭窄病灶的远端，此时，要求助手松开置入器上的固定锁，左手固定好内芯、右手缓慢后撤外管，先释放出支架的头端，待操作者在支气管镜直视下将支架调整到合适的置入位置后，助手再缓慢后撤置入器外管，与此同时，操作者同步后退支气管镜。当入器的外管前手柄到达标志 B 时，如操作者观察到支架近端业在狭窄病变上端，表示支架位置基本合适，可告知助手继续后撤外管直至支架完全释放。支架完全释放后，为了避免橄榄头回撤时勾住支架造成移位，需在直视下将置入器外管小心地向前推进到内芯橄榄头处，然后再将置入器从支气管镜工作孔道退出，并将支气管镜保留在气道内观察释放后的支架位置和病灶情况。支架释放后的最佳位置为支架两端均能越过狭窄上、下段，两端各超出各 0.5 cm。

2. 置入器穿越法　在支气管镜不能通过狭窄段的情况下，操作者将支气管镜停留在狭窄段的上方，由助手将置入器沿支气管镜工作孔道向狭窄病灶远端推送，直至可在支气管镜下看到标志 A 在狭窄段的上端。此时由助手松开固定锁，固定好内芯，缓慢后撤外管释放支架，当入器外管前手柄到达标志 B 时，如操作者镜下观察到支架近端的位置基本合适，嘱助手继续后撤外管直至支架完全释放。支架完全释放后，为了避免橄榄头回撤时勾住支架造成移位，需在直视下将置入器外管小心地向前推进到内芯橄榄头处，然后再将置入器从支气管镜工作孔道退出并将支气管镜保留在气道内观察释放后的支架位置和病灶情况。支架释放后的最佳位置为支架两端均能越过狭窄上、下段，两端各超出各 0.5 cm。

三、TTS 支架在实验兔良性气道狭窄中的应用研究

近年来，外伤后气管插管、气管切开患者越来越多，结核病的高发等，致使良性气道狭窄的发生率增高，目前针对良性气道狭窄的治疗主要有球囊扩张、冷冻治疗、激光等手段，气道支架由于其支架相关并发症限制了在良性气道狭窄的应用，自膨胀性镍钛合金气道支架可以有效的扩张气道，改善由于气道狭窄引起的呼吸困难。但是由于支架植入后的相关并发症，如肉芽形成、瘢痕挛缩、气管变形、分泌物潴留等限制了在良性气道狭窄中的应用。我们研究团队成功的建立了良性兔气道狭窄模型，在此基础上进行了支架相关的试验研究。

合理选择现有的气管支架能否降低支架相关并发症的发生？我们选择南微医学生产的定制气管支架，在气管狭窄动物模型上留置 A 组（支架直径与气管横径之比≤1）和 B 组（支架直径与气管横径之比≥1.2）两种不同直径气管支架。通过气管镜下、大体标本、病理标本和蛋白组学研究比较观察置入后支架相关并发症随着植入后不同时间点的发生情况。从而为临床选用合适直径的气管支架提供理论依据。我们观察到①良性兔狭窄气道内留置不同直径支架后，置入 2 周时支架内及支架两端可见少量肉芽，不引起管腔狭窄。第 4 周时肉芽进一步增生，B 组开始出现支架两端的瘢痕挛缩，随着时间推移，瘢痕挛缩进一步加重，A 组两端无明显的瘢痕挛缩。②支架留置 12 周

内，B组气管变形发生率100%（24/24）明显高于A组4.8%（1/21），$P<0.05$，具有统计学意义。B组两端瘢痕挛缩发生率45.8%（11/24）明显高于A组9.5%（2/21），$P<0.05$，具有统计学意义。③B组植入后气管组织MMP9呈上升趋势，而A组气管组织呈先升后下降趋势。由我们的研究结果我们认为合理的支架直径的选择会降低气管变形和瘢痕挛缩的发生率。

在小样本的临床研究中我们发现植入TTS支架的痰液驻留和两端肉芽增生有所减少，为了进一步明确TTS两端结构的改变是否能带来并发症的减少？我们选择了同样条件的兔子建立气管狭窄模型，选择狭窄超过50%的兔分别植入同样直径的TTS支架和OTW支架，随访观察实验兔肉芽组织增生导致管腔狭窄30%以上A组6.25%（1/16），B组50%（6/12），$P=0.023(<0.05)$有统计学差异。动物实验进一步证实TTS支架的两端剪切力的降低会导致肉芽增生程度的降低。

四、TTS气道支架在恶性气道狭窄患者的临床研究

由于新型支架置入器的结构的改变，会导致支架在置入器内部的真实长度发生变化，同时，伴随有操作步骤的改变，这些是否会影响支架的正常释放，尚不明确。为了进一步评估新型气道支架植入系统的释放方法的优效性和安全性，我们进行的一项多中心TTS和OTW在治疗恶性气道狭窄的置入方法的优效性临床研究（ChiCTR-IOR-17011431），由苏州大学附属第一医院、江苏省人民医院、厦门市第二医院、温州医科大学附属第一医院、青岛大学附属医院、南通市第一人民医院六家全国呼吸介入做的很好的医院参与，共入组148例恶性气道狭窄的患者，2:1比例分别入组于TTS支架和OTW支架组，研究得出两组入组患者无论是年龄、狭窄程度、支架尺寸的选择等方面都没有差异，TTS和OTW支架在恶性气道狭窄的植入时间分别为$1.79±1.14$和$4.37±1.80$（$P=0.0000$），两组释放成功率是100%，研究认为TTS支架的释放方法简便所导致，其释放方法也便于内镜医师掌握。

有关TTS支架的并发症我们单中心观察了TTS支架置入6个月内的最常见的并发症包括分泌物潴留（25%，9/36）、肉芽组织增生（13.9%，5/36）、肿瘤生长（13.9%，5/36）和咯血（8.3% 3/36），移位（8.3%，3/36）仅发生在覆膜支架内，未发生支架断裂的现象。

总之，TTS支架的释放方法具备以下优点：①避免了原有的操作方式中导丝在支气管镜引导到狭窄段后，在推镜过程中有操作者误把导丝再次带出体外的风险。②避免了原有支架置入器释放方式中需要患者和医师摄入射线的危害。③避免了原有的在喉罩和全麻麻醉方式下释放支架需要短暂脱离呼吸机以给患者带来的相关风险。④避免了原有支架置入器释放时支架置入器和支气管镜并行对患者鼻腔黏膜的损伤。⑤置入器通过工作钳道释放，对呼吸通气的影响较前减少，另外，TTS气道支架相比于OTW支架支架两端结构的改变可以有效的减少肉芽增生的严重程度。这些研究为支架在临床的合理选择提供依据，也为研发新型支架提供理论支撑。这些临床研究数据进一步证实了TTS支架在危急重气道狭窄患者使用具有更大应用价值，为新型支架提供最佳的临床治疗方案，为国产金属支架的合理、规范化使用、操作指南提供临床研究数据，从而进一步推动介入肺脏病诊疗技术的发展。

参 考 文 献

[1] Ernst A, Feller-Kopman D, Becker HD, et al. Central airway obstruction. Am J Respir Crit Care Med, 2004, 169: 1278-1297.

[2] Ost DE, Ernst A, Grosu HB, et, al. Therapeutic Bronchoscopy for Malignant Central Airway Obstruction Success Rates and Impact on Dyspnea and Quality of Life. Chest, 2015, 147 (5): 1282-1298.

[3] 曾伟杰, 支晓兴, 孟猛, 等. 气管支架材料置入后的生物力学特点及其生物相容性. 中国组织工程研究与临床康复, 2009, 13(13): 2573-2576.

[4] Chin CS, Litle V, Yun J, et al. Airways stent. Ann Thorac Surg, 2008, 85(2): S792-796.

[5] Wilson GE, Walshaw MJ, Hind CRK, et al. Treatment of large airway obstruction in lung cancer using expandable metal stents inserted under direct vision via the fibreoptic bronchoscope. Thorax, 1996, 51: 248-252.

[6] Mark-E Lund, Force Seth. Airway Stenting for Patients With Benign Airway Disease and the Food and Drug Administration Advisory. Chest, 2007, 132(4): 1107-1108.

[7] Madden BP, Park JES, Sheth A. Medium term follow up post deployment of Ultraflex expandable metallic stents in the management of endobronchial pathology. Ann Thorac Surg, 2004, 78: 1898-1902.

[8] Xie BX, ZhYM, ChenC, et al. Outcome of TiNi stent treatments in symptomatic central airway stenoses caused by Aspergillus fugmigatus infections after transplation. Transplant Proc, 2013, 45(6): 2366-2370.

[9] 钟维农, 赵子文, 陈裕胜 等, 国产推送释放式与进口拉线释放式镍钛合金支架治疗气道狭窄比较. 中国内镜杂志, 2004, 10(2): 57-60.

[10] 蒋军红. 经支气管镜工作孔道释放的气道支架及置入方法, 中华结核和呼吸杂志, 2020, 43(1), 73-75.

[11] Jiang Jh, Zeng Dx, Wang Chg, et al. A Pilot Study of a Novel through-the-Scope Self-Expandable Metallic Airway Stents Delivery System in Malignant Central Airway Obstruction. Canadian Respiratory Journal, 2019; 7828526.

4 硅酮支架的现场加工技巧与应用

柯明耀

自20世纪80年代首次被用于治疗中央型气道狭窄后,硅酮支架(Dumon支架)已被广泛应用于西方发达国家,并被作为评价其他各种新型支架治疗气道狭窄效果优劣的"金标准"。Dumon硅酮支架于2014年3月引进我国,虽然在国内的应用仅有短短的6年多时间,但国内许多医院已经开展了此项技术,积累了比较丰富的临床应用经验,并尝试通过现场加工技巧做了一些创新性应用,其中有些创意属于国际首创。

一、硅酮支架的特点

(一)硅酮支架的优点

1. 硅酮支架的最主要优点是可以现场加工　与金属支架不同,硅酮支架可进行现场加工,通过现场加工大大增加了适应证,减少了并发症。

2. 硅酮支架另一个吸引人的优点是容易取出　当支架没有治疗价值、出现明显并发症或出现损坏时,均需要给予取出。硅酮支架不管放置气道内多长时间,均可以通过硬镜轻松取出。该类支架的这一优点解除了临床医师对放置支架的主要后顾之忧。

3. 硅酮支架的第三个优点是肉芽生长较轻　与金属支架比较,硅酮支架对气道壁的刺激相对较轻,因此肉芽增生相对轻。

4. 硅酮支架的其他优点　由可长期置入级硅酮制造,长达12年之后仍具备良好的生物相容性及耐受性;光滑表面,分泌物较容易清除;边缘斜边设计对黏膜纤毛清除有帮助;防滑钉设计减少移位;可提供多种直径(5～20mm)及长度(10～110mm);对射线影响小,不影响MRI检查;长期放置一般不会导致管壁破裂;支架腔内不会再狭窄等。

(二)硅酮支架的缺点

1. 需要硬镜放置、置入难度较大;需要备有硬镜镜管、支架置入及抓取设备,需要掌握硬镜技术;相应型号的硬镜镜管必须插到病变部位,支架必须能放置到位。如果没有掌握好适应证及做好充分的支架置入前准备,支架放置的失败率较高,置入时也容易导致管壁破裂或瘘口扩大。

2. 适形性差:可能导致支架与管壁成角,造成支架对管壁的切割、损伤管壁、管腔狭窄;治疗气道瘘时可能因适形性差导致支架壁与管壁贴合不紧密,影响支架的封堵效果。

3. 在国内按客户需求定制费时长,可行性差。

4. 其他缺点:管壁厚,放置后影响管腔内径,分泌物潴留乃较明显,一般需要支气管镜定期清除;直管型支架容易移位等。

二、硅酮支架的现场加工技巧

(一)现场加工的目的与要求

通过现场加工以使支架适应气道结构及病变特点,提高治疗效果,减少并发症,并增加硅酮支架的临床应用适应证。现场加工要求准备好所需的器材,掌握物理学相关知识,掌握缝合技术、裁剪技巧,熟练掌握支架置入技术与技巧。

(二)现场加工内容

1. 基础现场加工　根据病变范围现场剪裁确定支架长度,根据气道特点重塑支架各个边缘的形状,为减少对管壁的刺激对支架边缘进行磨边,为避免阻塞支气管开口采用专用剪孔器或剪刀对支架壁进行开孔,根据是否需要固定支架及治疗目的灵活对防滑钉进行处理,去除部分或全部防滑钉,或减少防滑钉的厚度。

2. 改变支架直径、角度　为与管腔大小形状适型,去除部分管壁并加以缝合,以使直管支架中间形成角度或缩小部分支架的直径;纵向剪除部分管壁可缩小支架直径,横向剪除部分管壁可以使直管支架形成角度。

3. 套接支架(支架环)　包括外套接及内套接、外套接:硅酮支架外套接硅酮支架(支架环)增加支架的外径,包括中间套接、边缘套接(同时增加长度);外套接能够增加支架的外径,使支架与管壁贴合更为紧密,具有增强封堵效果、减少支架外分泌物潴留、防止支架移位、增加支架支撑力等作用。内套接:硅酮支架内套接硅酮支架,使直管型支架变成类似于沙漏状支架的一半,包括上套接、下套接;内套接通过减小支架直径并增加支架总长度,以适应气道管腔结构或减少支架上下缘的肉芽生长。

4. 自制硅酮封堵支架　通过缝合Y支架一个分支远端,使远端管腔闭合,可用于封堵中心支气管管腔,治疗支气管胸膜瘘(主支气管、中间、叶支气管)、顽固性咯血(经内科、血管介入或外科处理无效或不宜采用)、治疗气道壁瘘、内科肺减容、难治性气胸等。自制硅酮封堵支架想法的来源:通过支架封堵气道管腔治疗气道瘘、咯血等,具有较大的临床应用价值;金属封堵支架几乎没有生产许可证,使用有压力;金属封堵支架需要提前定制,定制的规格不一定适合;硅酮封堵支架在国内难以定制;支架材质的特点,使得自制硅酮封堵支架具有可行性。硅酮封堵支架的规格及设计:根据支气管镜检查结果选择合适规格的Y硅酮支架(Novatech),确定Y支架其中的一个支气管分支作为封堵支;Y支架三个分支分别命名为主支、封堵支、侧分支;通过缝合封堵支远端制成硅酮封堵支架。根据检查结果确定各分支的长度、直径及封堵支远端的形状,必要时采用套接技术扩大支架外径以确保支架与管壁贴合紧密;为保证达到完全封堵,应做到封堵支完全紧贴管壁,或者主支及侧分支同时完全紧贴管壁。封堵支的长度根据拟封堵支气管的长度确定,一般短于支气管5mm,以避免放置后贴合不紧或导致瘘口扩大;封堵支直径应比拟封堵支气管内径大10%左右,当支气管内径大于14mm时利用套接技术套入一段5mm长内径14mm的硅酮支架环。主支及侧分支的长度根据拟放气道的长度确定,一般在2~3cm;主支及侧分支的直径尽可能与气道内径一样或稍大,支架直径太小时可通过套接技术扩大其外径。硅酮封堵支架的现场制作及放置:确定支架规格及仔细设计后,采用手术刀片、剪刀及直尺等工具对支架进行准确的现场裁剪;根据需要给予套接支架环,通过套入5mm长内径与支架外径一致的硅酮支架环以扩大外径,可在1~3个分支上套接支架环;采用血管缝合线连续锁边缝合支封堵支的远端使管腔完全闭塞,缝合间距小于2mm;支架缝合后经75%乙醇消毒,装入折叠系统;经硬镜将支架释放到相应位置,直视下采用硬质抓钳或异物钳调整及固定支架。

5. 自制硅酮封堵器　把硅酮支架片缝合到直管硅酮支架一端使管腔闭合,根据拟封堵支气管管腔长度直管硅酮支架长度可选择1~3cm;主要用于封堵中心气道管腔,用于治疗肺部远端出血及支气管胸膜瘘;为防止封堵器移位,一般需要联合使用金属或Y形硅酮支架。

三、硅酮支架的常规应用

(一)正确应用硅酮支架的前提

了解硅酮支架的特性及优缺点,掌握好临床应用适应证;针对不同的病变性质、部位、范围,考虑硅酮支架是否适合放、放什么规格、放置的难度、需要放置体内的时间(短暂、长期);根据患者的头颈及口咽部特点,判断硬镜插入的难度;根据患者身体状况及重要脏器的功能状态,判断全身麻醉下硬镜放置支架围术期的风险大小。

(二)硅酮支架的常规应用

1. 良性气道狭窄　是硅酮支架的主要适应证。瘢痕性狭窄者一般采用硅酮支架长期放置,良性外压性狭窄者可采用硅酮支架暂时或长期放置,管壁软化性狭窄者可采用硅酮支架长期放置,良性增生性狭窄一般不放置支架。

2. 恶性气道狭窄　对于支架放置一段时间后可能需要取出的恶性狭窄,宜优先选择硅酮支架;位于隆突区域的复杂恶性气道狭窄可考虑放置硅酮支架;对于金属支架放置后效果不佳或并发症严重者,可考虑更换硅酮支架。

3. 气道壁瘘　在同样与瘘口周围管壁贴合良好的情况下,硅酮支架疗效更好、治疗时间更长,应优先选择;对食管支架导致的、或合并良性狭窄的气道壁瘘,首选硅酮支架。因适形性差或直径限制等导致支架与瘘口附近管壁贴合不紧,部分气道壁瘘病例不宜采用硅酮支架;在硬镜插入困难、支架放置难以到位、放置中存在使瘘口扩大的危险等情况下也不宜选择硅酮支架。

(三)常规应用的临床评价

1990年Dumon首次报道了带有防滑钉的改良后硅酮支架在治疗外压性气道狭窄中可取得良好的临床效果,随后此类支架被命名为Dumon支架并正式应用于临床。一项多中心临床研究随访了1058名气道狭窄患者,共置入1574枚支架,其中恶性气道狭窄的608枚,支架置入后患者症状得到明显缓解,良、恶性气道阻塞患者的中位随访时间分别是14个月和4个月,结果发现9.5%的患者发生气道移位,8%的患者有肉芽形成,4%患者黏液阻塞气道。而在Cavaliere等研究中,Dumon支架置入的并发症发生率更低,共有393枚支架置入306名恶性气道狭窄的患者,随访发现仅5%患者发生支架移位,1%的患者观察到肉芽形成。此后Dumon支架被广泛的应用于气道病变,尤其是气道狭窄中,越来越多的证据表明其可有效缓解气道狭窄症状,且较为安全。近期Ozgul等报道了Y形硅酮支架在7名慢性阻塞性肺疾病合并呼气性中心气道萎陷(Expiratory central airway collapse,ECAC))中的应用,结果发现,尽管硅酮支架对FEV1的改善并不明显,但改良的英国医学研究委员会呼吸困难量表(modified Medical Research Council,mMRC)评分得到显著改善,其中4名患者观察到一般健康状态评分的改善,这提示硅酮支架可能缓解ECAC症状,改善患者体力状态,为COPD合并ECAC患者提供新的治疗选择。

随着Dumon支架在临床的推广,其适用范围也再扩大。Dumon支架已不局限用于治疗气道狭窄,在气道消化道瘘中也取得了令人满意的疗效。2004年Duta等人回顾性分析了Y形Dumon支架改善恶性气道狭窄或气道瘘的疗效,该研究纳入了86名恶性病变累积气管隆突的患者,其中27名(31.4%)为气道食管瘘,结果提示Dumon支架置入后患者的临床症状得到显著缓解,支架放置中位时间为92.5±77.5 d(3~577 d),且并发症可耐受。Mitsuoka等人对Dumon支架在35名气道病变患者中的临床疗效进行回顾性分析,其中包括6例食管气管瘘患者,结果发现,3名患者的气道瘘口得到完全封堵,另外3名患者症状显著缓解。此外,本中心通过观察发现Dumon支架治疗气道消化道瘘封堵效果良好,并不亚于金属支架,且操作安全,并发症可接受,与金属支架相比,更适用于需长期放置支架的患者。本中心还对比观察了Dumon硅酮支架与金属覆膜支架治疗气道胸腔胃瘘的近期疗效。硅酮支架组21例,共置放Y形支架18枚,直管形2枚,沙漏状1枚;金属支架组17例,共置放镍钛合金Y形支架11枚(3例放置双Y形支架)、直管型5枚,不锈钢Y形支架4枚。术后1个月评价疗效:硅酮支架组完全缓解5例(23.8%),部分缓解12例(57.1%),无效4(19.0%),有效率80.9%;金属支组完全缓解 3 例(17.6%)，部分缓解 10 例(58.8%)，无效 4 例(23.5%)，有效率为 76.5%；两组有效率相差不显著($P>0.05$)。主要并发症均为痰液潴留、肉芽增生等。认为 Dumon 支架治疗气道胸腔胃瘘效果与金属覆膜支架相当，且受咳嗽影响轻；对于支架可与瘘口附近气道管壁贴合良好的病例，建议优先选择 Dumon 支架。

四、自制硅酮封堵支架临床应用评价

Dumon 支架材质的特点，使得现场制作硅酮封堵支架具有可行性。硅酮封堵支架封堵效果可靠、不易损坏、并发症较轻、取出容易、可长期放置，临床上可用于封堵一个肺叶甚至一侧肺，在治疗支气管胸膜瘘、顽固性咯血等具有一定的特色及优势。

支气管胸膜瘘是临床十分棘手的问题，硅酮封堵支架置入后将胸腔与气道分隔，避免气道内分泌物反复进入胸腔造成胸腔持续感染，也阻隔了胸腔内脓液或冲洗液进入气道引起肺部感染，为脓胸的冲洗创造了条件。本中心采用自制硅酮封堵支架治疗支气管胸膜瘘 15 例(封堵左主及右中间支各 4 例、右上叶 3 例、右主 3 例、右下叶 1 例)，其中 11 例瘘口大于 5mm；12 例在硅酮封堵支架置入后得到完全封堵，3 例封堵不完全。脓胸短期内治愈 10 例，明显减轻 5 例。目前采用类似硅酮封堵支架用于治疗支气管胸膜瘘仅有极少的文献个案报道。硅酮支架在肺部出血的应用乃未见报道，本中心在临床诊疗过程中，积累了一些硅酮封堵支架用于治疗顽固性咯血的经验，共治疗顽固性咯血 14 例(封堵左主治疗左肺顽固性出血 5 例，封堵右主治疗右肺出血 4 例、封堵右上叶及左上叶各 2 例、右中间支气管 1 例)，支架放置后均完全封堵管腔，12 例咯血完全停止，仅 2 例乃有少量咯血。此外，本中心还采用硅酮封堵支架行内科肺减容 1 例。患者曾于 1 年前行右上叶活瓣肺减容，术后气急明显减轻，主要肺功能指标上升 1 倍，6min 步行距离增加了 2 倍，但疗效于 6 个月后逐渐降低，治疗 1 年后症状及主要指标均恢复到治疗前状态。此次取出活瓣，采用硅酮封堵支架封堵右上叶，随访 4 个月，其效果与放置活瓣基本一致，右上叶完全不张。30 例自制硅酮封堵支架的主要并发症有痰液潴留、肉芽增生、肺部感染，未见支架封堵支管腔裂。

完全封堵管腔是硅酮封堵支架取得疗效的关键，封堵支远端良好的缝合及支架与管壁的紧密贴合是完全封堵的基本条件。Y 形支架的三个分支都与管壁贴合紧密时封堵效果最理想，封堵支完全紧贴管壁、或者主支及侧分支均完全紧贴管壁也可取得完全的封堵效果。常用的 Y 硅酮支架只有 4 个固定的规格，因此支架直径太小时经常需要采用套接技术扩大支架外径以确保与管壁贴合紧密。预计封堵支可以完全封堵所在支气管管腔时，因封堵效果已经得到保证，其他分支可以不追求与管壁紧密贴合；但对于封堵支短而难以与管壁紧密贴合者，为达到完全封堵效果，可通过套接一段硅酮支架环以扩大主支及侧分支外径从而确保与管壁贴合紧密。总之，硅酮封堵支架自制可行、放置可行、疗效确切，不失为治疗支气管胸膜瘘及顽固性咯血一种安全、有效、微创的方法。鉴于目前国内外尚无关于硅酮封堵支架应用的大宗病例报道，还需临床进一步的应用及观察。

参 考 文 献

[1] Dumon JF. A dedicated tracheobronchial stent. Chest, 1990, 97(2):328-332.

[2] Lee P, Kupeli E, Mehta AC. Airway stents. Clin Chest Med, 2010, 31(1):141-150.

[3] Dumon MC, Dumon JF, Perrin C, et al. Silicone tracheobronchial endoprosthesis. Rev Mal Respir, 1999, 16(4 Pt 2): 641-651.

[4] Cavaliere S, Venuta F, Foccoli P, et al. Endoscopic treatment of malignant airway obstructions in 2,008 patients. Chest, 1996, 110(6):1536-1542.

[5] Karush JM, Seder CW, Raman A, et al. Durability of Silicone Airway Stents in the Management of Benign Central Airway Obstruction. Lung, 2017, 195(5):601-606.

[6] Dumon Silicone. Y-Stenting in Malignant and Nonmalignant Central Airway Obstruction. Chest, 2013, 133, 144(4):801A.

[7] Ozgul MA, Cetinkaya E, Cortuk M, et al. Our Experience on Silicone Y-Stent for Severe COPD Complicated With Expiratory Central Airway Collapse. J Bronchology. Interv Pulmonol, 2017, 24(2):104-109.

[8] Dutau H, Toutblanc B, Lamb C, et al. Use of the Dumon Y-stent in the management of malignant disease involving the carina: a retrospective review of 86 patients. Chest, 2004, 126(3):951-958.

[9] Mitsuoka M, Sakuragi T, Itoh T. Clinical benefits and complications of Dumon stent insertion for the treatment of severe central airway stenosis or airway fistula. Gen Thorac Cardiovasc Surg, 2007, 55(7):275-280.

[10] 吴雪梅，柯明耀，罗炳清，等. Dumon 支架治疗气道消化道瘘 31 例近期疗效观察. 国际呼吸杂志, 2016, 36(4):292-296.

[11] MingYao Ke, Rui Huang, LianCheng Lin, et al. Efficacy of the Dumon™ Stent in the Treatment of Airway Gastric Fistula: A Case Series Involving 16 Patients. Chinese Medical Journal, 2017, 130(17):2119-2120.

[12] Watanabe S, Shimokawa S, Yotsumoto G, et al. The use of a Dumon stent for the treatment of a bronchopleural fistula. Ann Thorac Surg, 2001, 72:276-278.

[13] Junli Zeng, XuemeiWu, MeihuaZhang, et al. Modified silicone stent for difficulttotreat massive hemoptysis: a pilot study of 14 cases. Journal of Thoracic Disease, 2020, 12(3):956-965.

5 呼吸介入转化医学研究

张冀松　陈恩国

1992年美国《Science》杂志首次提出 B to B(bench to bedside,从实验室到病床)概念,1994年再次提出"转化医学"概念,创造性地将基础学科与临床学科结合起来。B to B概念的提出将临床中遇到的实际问题转变为基础科研中的研究方向,从而推动研究成果向临床应用快速转化。在现代呼吸病学的专业领域中,介入呼吸病学是最为活跃也是发展最为迅速的亚专科之一。伴随着人工智能技术、新兴材料技术、医用影像技术等学科的快速发展,各种呼吸介入相关的诊断及治疗技术更新迭代、层出不穷,这为实现呼吸介入转化医学提供了良好的培育土壤。本文将从呼吸介入诊断及呼吸介入治疗两大领域,浅谈笔者关于呼吸介入转化医学的一些理念和看法。

一、介入诊断

(一)超细支气管镜设备在肺外周结节诊断中的作用

随着医疗配套的进步和人民健康意识的增强,胸部CT的普及率日益增加。对普通人群进行定期胸部CT筛查,发现约有25%人群检出肺结节,其中大部分(96.4%)是良性的;对高危人群进行定期的胸部CT筛查,可以早期识别肺癌并降低约20%的死亡率。一旦检出肺结节,患者最迫切的要求就是精准评估肺结节性质,以指导后续治疗。在临床实践中,很难实现单靠影像学表现来明确肺部结节的性质,更多的临床医师需要获取病理确诊。传统获取肺结节病理的方式有三类,包括外科手术、CT引导下经皮肺穿刺活检和经可弯曲气管镜活检。外科手术常常使得取材过程复杂化,极大增加患者的精神及经济负担,并有相对较多的并发症。CT引导下经皮肺穿(Transthoracic percutaneous needle aspiration,TTNA))有着相对较高的阳性率(76%~97.4%),但实践中存在一些问题,双肺无法同时穿刺、存在CT辐射、气胸发生率高(25%~40%)、大咯血发生率在1%~5%,此外对于部分磨玻璃样肺结节、靠近心脏或大血管的结节及过小的结节仍然不适用。在过去,通常只有病变侵犯中央气道后,气管镜才有机会取到组织标本。随着计算机成像技术、人工智能技术、材料技术及微电子技术等多项核心技术的迅速发展,性能优越的超细支气管镜的面世使得对部分外周肺结节的取材得以实现。

现有内镜下辅助肺外周结节诊断的技术非常多,包括虚拟及电磁导航技术、气道内超声引导技术、辅助透视技术等。其诊断效率取决于几个因素,包括病变的大小和位置(上叶和下叶)、透视的使用、放射状探头相对于病变的位置(在病变内或邻近)及使用的导航系统的类型。然而,关于诊断率是否与支气管镜外径有关的数据有限。传统的支气管镜(conventional bronchoscopy,CB)外径为4~6mm,只能插入到段或亚段支气管,即使采用多种辅助技术,也难以保障活检钳顺利到达亚段以外的病灶。目前各临床机构中的主流气管镜先端外径多在3.9~6.0mm范围内,其直径大小决定了目前主流支气管镜最多只能到达6~8级支气管,而4mm以下直径的支气管所在的肺外周区域仍为"诊断盲区"。日本奥林巴斯公司最新研发的一款超细支气管镜BF-MP290F,先端外径细达3mm,保障转向灵活,工作通道直径1.7 mm,可以插入不带鞘的超声探头,并且可以达到更远级别的细支气管。曾有研究报道,超细支气管镜(Ultra-thin bronchoscopy,UTB)和CB在诊断率上没有差异,进一步分析发现在该研究中没有使用透视技术,可能因此影响诊断率差异。在另一项研究中,与CB(外径,4 mm)相比,原型UTB对PPL提供了更高的诊断率(74% vs. 59%)。这项研究结合虚拟导航技术。2020年2月最新报道的一项日本研究,单纯比较了超细支气管镜与传统支气管镜在肺外周诊断率的差异,这也许对本文的探讨更有启发意义。该研究共进行了890次支气管镜检查,其中UTB 142例,CB 112例,分别有76名和39名患者得到明确诊断;其中UTB组的中位检查时间明显长于CB组(24min vs. 20min;$P=0.01$)。UTB组PPL的诊断率显著高于CB组(74.5% vs. 59.1%;$P=0.04$)。对于直径小于10 mm的结节的两组的诊断率均明显降低。比较病变部位,下叶的诊断率高于上叶。特别是,UTB组下叶S6的诊断率明显高于CB组[15/19例(78.9%) vs.4/11例(36.3%),$P=0.04$];两组均显示了良好的安全性。

综上所述,我们认为超细支气管镜设备在肺外周结节的诊断中具有积极意义。但目前仍缺乏各方面性能均优越的设备。例如现有的日本奥林巴斯公司最新研发的超细支气管镜BF-MP290F,先端外径细达3mm,保障转向灵活,但牺牲了成像清晰度,为电子及纤维复合镜。另外一款高端超细支气管镜BF-XP190,尖端3.1mm,但工作孔道直径只有1.2mm,大部分尺寸的活检钳和径向超声探头被限制入内,使得临床便捷性大为下降。BF-N20系列属于特细型,先端外径仅2.2mm,但无工作孔道,限制了临床应用。我们希望后期研发技术能在保障气管镜超细先端外径的前提下,增加了工作通道直径,提供优秀清晰的成像,使得超细支气管镜设备的临床实用性大幅度提高,以此解决 4mm 以下直径支气管所在的肺外周"诊断盲区",提高肺外周结节的整体诊断率。

(二) 导航设备在肺外周结节诊断中的作用

结合上篇背景介绍,我们知道肺结节已成为临床常见病多发病之一,而精准评估肺结节性质成为临床当务之急。近年来随着相关技术的蓬勃发展,多款全肺导航系统的面世使可弯曲支气管镜对外周肺结节的取材得以实现。全肺导航系统引导下经支气管镜肺活检(transbronchial lung biopsy,TBLB)具有其独特优势,包括微创操作、直观且诊治一体、几乎无 CT 辐射、借助自然腔道拓扑特征而抗运动干扰强等诸多优点。目前较为成熟的全肺导航系统包括虚拟导航系统和电磁导航系统。虚拟导航支气管镜(virtual brochoscopic navigation,VBN)技术是将患者的高分辨率胸部螺旋 CT 图像以医学数字成像和通信(digital imaging and communication in medicine,DICOM)数据格式导入导航系统中,然后抽取支气管树及血管图像,形成 3D 气管支气管影像及肺血管影像。临床实践中,可通过 VBN 计算出达到外周肺病灶的路径,并与气管镜图像实时匹配,以指导术者准确到达外周病灶。单独依靠 VBN,常很难确认取样工具是否抵达病灶,故一般情况下常需联合 X 线透视、CT 或 R-EBUS 等技术实现外周肺结节(peripheral pulmonary nodules,PPLs)诊断。一篇关于 VBN 对 PLLs 应用系统综述显示,VBN 总体诊断率为 73.8%,对于 ≤2 cm PLLs 诊断率为 67.4%;其并发症发生率和常规支气管镜检查基本相似(1%),远远低于经皮肺穿刺。与 VBN 稍有不同,电磁导航支气管镜(electromagnetic navigational bronchoscopy,ENB)的操作步骤包括术前虚拟路径线规划和术中磁导航两个步骤。在虚拟成像的基础上,配备电磁探头实时引导。操作时患者处于三维磁场中,通过插入支气管镜中的电磁探头实时匹配实际图像与虚拟图像,从而准确地引导电磁探头到达病变部位。ENB 用于 PPLs 诊断率波动于 38.5% to 77.3%。Eberhardt R 等报道了他们随机对照研究结果,ENB 诊断价值低于期望值,R-EBUS,ENB 及 R-EBUS 联合 ENB 诊断率分别为 69%、59% 和 88%。一项多中心前瞻性研究,评估了 581 例经支气管活检(transbronchial biopsy TBB)肺外周结节病例,结果显示,未使用 R-EBUS 和 ENB 情况下诊断率 63.7%,R-EBUS,ENB,ENB 联合 R-EBUS 诊断率分别为 57.0%、38.5% 和 47.1%。

一篇综合各种导航性支气管镜技术包括 GS,VB,ENB,R EBUS 等的 meta 分析显示,导航性支气管镜总体诊断率 70%(46%~86.2%),与结节直径有关,总体上高于常规支气管镜活检,低于 TTNA,但安全性高远远高于 TTNA,主要为气胸(1.5%),仅 0.6% 需置管引流,无严重出血和死亡报道。综合来看,导航支气管镜技术并发症少,对提高诊断率均有不同程度帮助。随着当前设备更新、诊治技术不断进展,其临床地位越来越受重视。根据病灶位置、病灶大小、与气道关系、并发症风险及操作熟练的专家等多种因素,导航气管镜技术在某种层面上可以与 TTNA 等同或互补。

但令人遗憾的是,尽管导航气管镜技术面世已 10 余年,无论单用导航技术还是联合多种现有技术手段包括超声、X 线透视等,其对 PPLs 的总体诊断率仍在 70% 左右波动。至 2015 年,新的全肺导航 lung pro 系统升级带来了新的经支气管镜气道外导航技术(Bronchoscopictransparenchymal nodule access,BTPNA),其对 PPLs 的总体阳性率也只能达到 83%。究其原因,现有主流气管镜的硬件瓶颈及现有计算机成像系统的技术瓶颈为其核心问题。目前市场上几家成熟的全肺导航系统,包括美国 Veran 公司的 The SPiN Thoracic Navigation System 磁导航系统、Broncus 公司 LungPoint 的 VBN System 及美敦力的 Super Dimension 电磁导航系统,尽管在操作流程方面存在一定差异,但其计算机虚拟支气管树成像的核心技术都是类似的,对于 3mm 以下的微小气道重建均欠理想。这使得导航支气管镜技术在肺外周 6~8 级以下的病灶取材阳性率大大下降,使得呼吸介入医师们"全肺可及"的梦想变得遥远。因此,后期若能攻克导航技术的技术成像瓶颈,提高重建精度,使得微小气道成像成为可能,将能进一步提高导航支气管镜技术对肺外周结节的诊断率。

(三) AI-ROSE 在呼吸内镜介入诊断中的作用和前景

对于微小的肺结节来讲,取到的每一块组织都非常珍贵,为了实现术中精准取材,最大程度保障内镜下每一钳的阳性率,呼吸介入病学的专家们创新性的把显微镜搬到了呼吸介入的手术室,便于实时指导取材的准确性,这就是快速现场评价(Rapid on-site evaluation,ROSE)ROSE 技术。ROSE 检查具有很强的时效性,能通过实时反馈提高细针穿刺或活检标本的合格率及诊断率,减少穿刺次数,从而缩短支气管镜检查的操作时间,降低操作相关并发症风险,进而降低患者的整体医疗费用。

随着人工智能技术(Artificial intelligence,AI)走进病理分析领域,病理分析不再局限于传统的定性分析,而是逐渐向定量分析过渡。定量化病理诊断是指以特征学习为基础,从病理切片中提取特定组织结构,形成定量化指标,如有丝分裂数目、肿瘤的实质与间质的比例、黏液湖和癌细胞的比例等,协助病理诊断,其诊断结果更加客观。基于深度学习的病理切片图像的定量分析研究是数字病理分析的大势所趋。例如卷积神经网络(Convolutional Neural Network,ConvNet)是深度学习最常用的网络结构之一。

人工智能技术中的神经网络(Artificial neural network,ANN)一直被探索应用于图像分析和自动诊断的复杂过程。近年研究发现,基于 ConvNet 的深度学习技术适用于图像分析,其在疾病的早期检测和组织分类方面具有重要价值。在医学领域最成功的应用是影像学、病理学和皮肤学的图像分析,其分析速度快,准确度能与临床医学专家媲美。病理图像是多数疾病诊断的金标准,尤其在癌症领域,病理学家通过评估标本的大小、形状、有丝分裂计数、颜色和纹理等属性进行诊断决策。其中细胞病理学诊断在很大程度上依赖于图像,目前基于图像特征的 ANN 在胃肠系统、甲状腺、乳腺、泌尿系统、积液的细胞病理学诊断中均已得到广泛应用。特别是用于宫颈癌检测的 ANN,自动细胞学筛查系统 PAPNET 是目前宫颈癌检测应用最成功的 ANN 模型之一。与常规人工筛查相比，PAPNET 系统的阳性或疑似病例检出率高出 20%，假阴性率降低约 2 倍，人工筛查为假阴性的玻片中有 1/3 被重新归类为异常。ROSE 相关的医学影像属于细胞病理学范畴，目前国内及国际上基于 ROSE 平台开发 ANN 的研究未见报道，因此该医工转化方向具有独特的创新意义。

目前在开展 ROSE 的医院，ROSE 的具体操作者多数是经过相关培训取得资格证书的临床医师，而非专业的病理科医师，对 ROSE 的判读存在一定程度的偏差。因此成为一名合格的 ROSE 人员不仅要具备病理学及细胞学基础，还要掌握肺脏介入各项常规手段，培养周期长，专业性极高。因此国内目前并未广泛开展，其重要限制瓶颈即为专业人才的缺乏。而且由于医师本身具有主观性，不同医师的阅片结果存在差异。同时，对病理玻片行人工镜检，过程费时费力。在病理切片数字化的背景下，人工智能技术走进 ROSE 是大势所趋，可以大力提高诊断效能，节省人力成本，提升整体医疗辅助诊断水平。

二、介入治疗

可降解支架在各种良恶性气道狭窄中的应用及前景

自从 Dumon 设计的硅酮支架面世以来，气道支架(airwaystenting,AS)为快速缓解各种良恶性气道梗阻提供了一种微创及高效的治疗选择，且扩张作用能相对持久。但不可否认的是，气道支架的置入也带来了大量的临床问题。例如最早面世的硅酮支架，最为严重的问题是支架移位、腔内黏液阻塞、细菌定植等问题；自膨胀金属支架的移位率有所下降，但极易刺激肉芽组织增生导致管腔再次闭塞、取出困难、发生支架断裂、继发感染甚至刺激肿瘤生长等，随着放置时间延长会导致更多的问题。

一个理想的气道支架必须具备可靠的支撑性、易于放置或移除、尽量避免刺激肉芽增生、能够模拟气道生理等功能。事实上我们很难找到这样一种支架。近年来有多位学者在改进支架性能和减少并发症方面持续探索。例如药物洗脱支架可能是一种防止肉芽肿和恶性组织形成的新方法。例如在支架中加入抗癌或抗增殖药物例如雷帕霉素或者顺铂。目前已经有一种可生物降解的顺铂洗脱支架面世(局部释放顺铂至少 5 周)，专门用于改善中央气道狭窄，但还在动物试验阶段尚未应用于人体。该类型支架的的潜在缺陷在于可能会增加气道瘘或者食管瘘风险。

生物可降解支架被认为能在一定程度上规避常规支架带来的不良事件。但目前在人体内的应用非常有限，可参考数据少之又少。目前有报道可降解支架用于 6 例肺移植术后的气道吻合术后并发症(Airway complications of bronchial anastomosis,ACBA)及 2 例合并气道支气管软化症(tracheobronchomalacia,TBM)的儿童。初步证实疗效不错，但可降解支架更多适合于暂时性的气道狭窄，或对于良性气道狭窄也许更为适合。报道称 60% 的患者需要再次置入支架，因此可降解支架还需要进一步的研发空间，例如个体化的降解时间和支撑强度，这也是需要医工转化研发的重点方向之一。

参 考 文 献

[1] Wahidi MM,Govert JA,Goudar RK,et al. Evidence for the treatment of patients with pulmonary nodules: When is it lung cancer?: accp evidence-based clinical practice guidelines (2nd edition). Chest,2007,132:94-107.

[2] Welker JA, Alattar M, Gautam S. Repeat needle biopsies combined with clinical observation are safe and accurate in the management of a solitary pulmonary nodule. Cancer, 2005,103:599-607.

[3] Kaneko M,Eguchi K,Ohmatsu H et al. Peripheral lung cancer: screening and detection with low-dose spiral CT versus radiography. Radiology,1996,201: 798-802.

[4] Choi JW,Park CM, Goo JM,et al. C-arm cone-beam CT-guided percutaneous trans-thoracic needle biopsy of small (</= 20 mm) lung nodules: diagnostic accuracy and complications in 161 patients. AJRAm. J. Roentgenol,2012,199: W322-330.

[5] Gould MK,Fletcher J,Iannettoni MD,et al. Evaluation of patients with pulmonary nodules: When is it lung cancer?: accp evidence-based clinical practice guidelines (2nd edition). Chest,2007,132:108-130.

[6] Rivera MP,Mehta AC. Initial diagnosis of lung cancer: Accp evidence-based clinical practice guidelines (2nd edition). Chest,2007,132:131-148.

[7] Shinagawa N,Yamazaki K,Onodera Y,et al. FActors related to diagnostic sensitivity using an ultrathin bronchoscope under ct guidance. Chest,2007,131:549-553.

[8] Ali MS,Trick W, Mba BI, et al. Radial endobronchial ultrasound for the diagnosis ofperipheral pulmonary lesions: a systematic review and meta-analysis. Respirology,2017,22: 443-453.

[9] Steinfort DP,Khor YH,Manser RL,et al. Radial probeendobronchial ultrasound for the diagnosis of peripheral lung cancer: systematic review and meta-analysis. Eur RespirJ, 2011,37:902-910.

[10] Sehgal IS,Dhooria S,Bal A,et al. A retrospective study comparing the ultrathin versusconventional bronchoscope for performing radial endobronchial ultrasound in the evaluation of peripheral pulmonary lesions. Lung India,2019,36:102-107.

[11] Oki M,Saka H,Ando M,et al. Ultrathin bronchoscopy with multimodal devices forperipheral pulmonary lesions. A randomized trial. Am JRespir Crit Care Med, 2015, 192: 468-476.

[12] Toshiyuki Sumia, Takumi Ikedab, Takeyuki Sawaia, et al. Comparison of ultrathin bronchoscopy with conventional bronchoscopy for the diagnosis of peripheral lung lesions without virtual bronchial navigation. Respiratory Investigation,2020,3:2212-5345.

[13] Asano F,Eberhardt R,Herth FJ. Virtual bronchoscopic navi-

gation for peripheral pulmonary lesions. Respiration, 2014, 88:430-440.

[14] Ost DE, Ernst A, Lei X, et al. Diagnostic Yield and Complications of Bronchoscopy for Peripheral Lung Lesions. Results of the AQuIRE Registry. Am J Respir Crit Care Med, 2016, 193:68-77.

[15] Leong S, Shaipanich T, Lam S, et al. Diagnostic bronchoscopy--current and future perspectives. J Thorac Dis, 2013: S498-S510.

[16] Eberhardt R, Anantham D, Ernst A, et al. Multimodality bronchoscopic diagnosis of peripheral lung lesions: a randomized controlled trial. Am J Respir Crit Care Med, 2007, 176: 36 41.

[17] Wang Memoli JS, Nietert PJ, Silvestri GA. MEta-analysis of guided bronchoscopy for the evaluation of the pulmonary nodule. Chest, 2012, 142:385-393.

[18] Felix JF Herth, Ralf Eberhardt, et al. Bronchoscopic transparenchymal nodule access (BTPNA) first in human trial of a novel procedure for sampling solitary pulmonary nodules. Thorax, 2015, 70:326-332.

[19] Majid A, Fernandez-Bussy S, Kent M, et al. External fixation of proximal tracheal airway stents: a modified technique. Ann. Thorac Surg, 2012, 93:167-169.

[20] Saji H, Furukawa K, Tsutsui H, et al. Outcomes of airway stenting for advanced lungcancer with central airway obstruction. Interact. Cardiovasc. Thorac Surg, 2010, 11: 425-428.

[21] Noppen M, Piérard D, Meysman M, et al. Bacterial colonization of central airways after stenting. Am J Respir Crit Care Med, 1999, 160: 672-677.

[22] Lemaire A, Burfeind WR, Toloza E, et al. Outcomes of tracheobronchial stents inpatients with malignant airway disease. Ann Thorac Surg, 2005, 80: 434-437.

[23] Husain SA, Finch D, Ahmed M, et al. Long-termfollow-up of ultraflex metallic stents in benign and malignant central airway obstruction. Ann Thorac Surg, 2007, 83: 1251-1256.

[24] Saad CP, Murthy S, Krizmanich G, et al. Self-expandable metallic airway stents and flexible bronchoscopy: long-term out-comes analysis. Chest, 2003, 124: 1993-1999.

[25] Hohenforst-Schmidt W, Zarogoulidis P, Pitsiou G, et al. Drug eluting stents for malignant airway obstruction: a critical review of the literature. J Cancer, 2016, 7: 377-390.

[26] Chao YK, Liu KS, Wang YC, et al. Biodegradable cisplatin-eluting tracheal stent for malignant airway obstruction: in vivo and in vitro studies. Chest, 2013, 144: 193-199.

[27] Lischke R, Pozniak J, Vondrys D, et al. Novel biodegradable stents in the treatment of bronchial stenosis after lung transplantation. Eur J Cardiothorac Surg, 2011, 40: 619-624.

[28] Zając A, Krysta M, Kiszka A, et al. Biodegradable airway stents: novel treatment of airway obstruction in children. Adv Clin Exp Med, 2019, 28, 961-965.

6 2020 早期肺癌微创介入治疗年度回顾

李 强

肺癌的发病率和病死率居全世界癌症的第一位。2019年全球癌症统计数据表明,当年约有210万新发肺癌病例和180万死亡病例,肺癌死亡人数占癌症总体死亡人数的18.4%。我国每年新发肺癌病例超过70万,死亡人数超过60万,带来了严重的经济社会负担。肺癌患者的预后上很大程度上取决于疾病发现时的临床分期。对于非小细胞肺癌(non-smallcelllungcancer,NSCLC)来说,我国Ⅰ期NSCLC患者5年生存率约为70%,Ⅱ期约50%,Ⅲ期约15%,而Ⅳ期仅为5%左右。因此早期诊断和根治对于改善肺癌患者预后占据至关重要的地位。

根据2020年第六版NCCN指南,早期肺癌被定义为Ⅰ期和Ⅱ期,不伴有淋巴结转移的肺癌。目前对于这一部分患者,临床上的早期筛查及诊断手段主要包括肿瘤标志物、胸部CT等。但目前,临床常用的肿瘤标志物如癌胚抗原(CEA)、神经元特异性烯醇化酶(NSE)、细胞角蛋白19片段(CYFRA21-1)、鳞状上皮细胞抗原(SCC)、胃泌素释放肽前体(Pro-GRP)、糖类抗原125(CA125)等对于早期肺癌诊断的灵敏性和特异性都相对较低,而基于胸部影像的肺癌筛查诊断方式也暴露了假阳性高、电离辐射暴露等问题。因此寻求高效、安全的早期肺癌诊断方式是亟待解决的重大临床问题。

对于已经确诊的早期肺癌患者,手术是目前的首选治疗方式。然而外科手术的实施,前提条件是患者具备足够的心肺功能支持,事实上临床中很多肺癌患者合并了COPD、心功能不全等疾病,这限制了外科手术的开展。目前对于这一部分"无法手术"的患者,立体定向放射治疗(sterotacticbodyradiotherapy,SBRT)已经成为被多部指南推荐作为首选治疗方案。近年来,随着支气管腔内超声、虚拟支气管镜导航和电磁导航及支气管镜机器人等技术的发展,射频消融(radio frequency,RFA)、冷冻和微波等技术的进步,早期肺癌的诊断和介入性根治有了更多的选择。本文将对呼吸介入领域近年来在早期肺癌诊断、治疗的进展进行回顾,以期为致力于早期肺癌介入性根治领域研究的同道提供一些帮助。

一、早期肺癌的诊断技术进展

(一)支气管镜机器人

近年来随着外科手术机器人技术的快速发展,加之人工智能技术的日益成熟,应用于临床的内镜机器人也应运而生。2016年5月,美国的AurisHealth公司对外宣布,该公司研发的ARES(AurisRoboticEndoscopySystem)成功获得美国FDA批准应用于临床。这是一款专门用于肺部疾病诊疗的内镜机器人。在其基础上,该公司又进一步研发了Monarch机器人内镜平台,并于2018年3月通过了FDA的批准。Monarch平台采用熟悉的类似控制器的界面,医师可以使用这种界面将灵活的机器人内镜导航到肺部外周,同时改善伸展范围、视力和控制。Monarch平台通过基于患者自身肺部解剖结构的三维模型的计算机辅助导航将传统的内镜视图结合到肺部,为整个手术过程中的医师提供连续的支气管镜视觉。另外,Monarch系统不需要使用过时的单手界面,让用户通过扭转来操纵内窥镜,而是允许通过一个类似游戏手柄的工具,进行更加人性化的控制。除此之外,Monarch平台还有其他有别于传统内镜的部分,其中包括一个可伸缩的嵌套式内镜,可以更轻松地通过S形弯曲的解剖结构进行导航。

在获得FDA批准之后,很快便在位于加利福尼亚州山景城的ElCamino医院开展了临床研究,在17例入组患者中有15例成功取到了病理标本,这意味着美国第一个支气管镜机器人系统成功实现了临床应用。在2019年完成的后续多中心临床研究中,该手术机器人系统进一步证明了其在外周肺结节诊断方面的独特优势。随着Monarch系统的使用,由于机器人支气管镜能够更深入的进入肺部,并精确地将活检器械引导至最困难的结节,因此该技术提供了在较早阶段诊断肺癌的能力。

(二)荧光成像技术

"荧光"是一种特殊的物理现象,是指某些物体在特定波长光线的照射下可辐射出波长比照射光线长的光,我们就称其为"荧光"。20世纪初,人们就发现人体组织存在荧光现象,并发现肿瘤组织和正常组织的荧光显像不同。人体内的荧光反应物质(荧光载体)有很多种类,包括:色氨酸、胶原、弹力蛋白、紫菜碱、磷酸吡哆醛等。人体组织辐射荧光的波长和强度决定于其中不同荧光载体的含量、入射光的最大吸收和反射值及入射光源自身的特性。当一束442nm的单色光照射在黏膜上时,上皮下的荧光载体被激发,辐射出波长较长的光线。这种荧光是混合光,由波长520nm的绿光和波长630nm的红光组成。其中,绿光较强、红光较弱,显示屏上看到的是绿色图像。在有组织增生和原位癌(carcinoma in situ,CIS)的部位,荧光辐射会减弱,并且以绿光减弱更明显,图像就会偏红色。利用肿瘤组织和正常组织荧光显像的不同,就能分辨普通光线下无法发现的早期肿瘤病灶。

与肉眼可以看见的普通光线不同,支气管黏膜的自发荧光非常微弱,不通过一定的辅助技术,肉眼是无法看到的。目前通常采用的技术分为两大类:①增强照射光的强度和纯度,采用特殊摄像机增加感受荧光的灵敏性;②应用能在肿瘤组织浓聚的光敏药物,增强肿瘤组织的荧光辐射。根据所用技术的不同,可将荧光支气管镜分为两大类:激光成像荧光支气管镜(laser imaging fluorescence endoscopy,LIFE)和自荧光成像支气管镜(autofluorescence imaging bronchoscopy,AFI)。已经有研究证实,这两种类型的荧光支气管镜都可以有效提高中央型早期肺癌诊断的灵敏性和特异性,但由于镜体较粗、可弯曲程度不足,暴露了对于外周肺结节诊断能力较低的缺陷。2019年加拿大团队研发了一种新型的激光成像荧光导管,这种导管可以通过超细支气管镜的操作孔道到达肺外周部位,在实现肺外周结节的早期诊断的同时还能进行激光治疗,这进一步拓宽了荧光支气管镜在早期肺癌诊断和治疗中的应用范围。

二、早期肺癌的介入性根治技术进展

(一)微波消融

微波是一种频率300MHz至300GHz、波长为1mm至1m范围的高频电磁波,通过插入的微波消融(microwave ablation,MWA)针集中能量,周围产生的电磁场从915～2450 MHz,波长为12～25cm,使组织中的电解质离子随微波频率高速振荡,电解质(偶极子)的束缚电荷也随微波频率作相应的位置移动,为克服所在媒质的黏滞性而耗损的微波能量转变为热能,使肿瘤组织中心温度升高,最高温可达100℃以上,周边也可达60℃以上,从而使肿瘤组织凝固坏死,这种类型的热消融对组织传导的依赖较少,产生均匀的消融区域,破坏肿瘤微血管,使肿瘤细胞变性坏死,减少机体的肿瘤负荷,同时刺激机体免疫系统,提高机体免疫功能,起到抑制肿瘤细胞复发、扩散的作用,因此已经被用于经皮治疗各种器官的肿瘤。对于早期肺癌的根治,2014年国内的研究团队所进行的一项单中心临床研究显示:在47例Ⅰ期无法手术的NSCLC患者中,经过CT引导下微波消融治疗后,肿瘤复发的中位时间为45.5个月,术后1、3、5年局部控制率分别为96%、64%和48%,术后1、2、3和5年的总生存率分别为89%、63%、43%和16%,中位生存期和总体生存率(overall survival,OS)中位数分别为47.4个月和33.8个月。≤35 mm的肿瘤与>35mm相比有更好的生存率。这个单中心研究显示CT引导下经皮微波消融治疗早期外周NSCLC患者是安全有效的。该团队随后即在国内进一步开展了多中心的临床研究,结果显示:在中位随访时间27.94个月内,经过CT引导下微波消融治疗患者3年的局部控制率、生存率和OS率分别为98%、100%和96%。CT引导下经皮微波消融主要的并发症包括气胸(48.1%)、咯血(28.8%)、胸腔积液(23.1%)和肺部感染(7.7%)。目前的研究结果显示CT引导下肺外周结节的微波消融治疗是安全有效的。

(二)冷冻消融

经皮冷冻消融治疗(percutaneous cryotherapy,PCT)主要是指在CT引导下将冷冻探针插入肿瘤组织,通过氩氦刀冷冻系统进行消融。PCT治疗早期周围型肺癌的临床报道目前相对较少,但总体疗效比较理想。Yamauchi等研究了22例Ⅰ期NSCLC患者共34个肿瘤25次PCT治疗的临床结果显示,在12～68个月的观察期内,只有1例肿瘤出现了局部进展(3%)。治疗后患者总的2年和3年生存率分别为88%和68%,中位OS为68个月,无病生存期(46±6)个月。治疗相关的并发症主要为气胸(28%,1次需要胸腔闭式引流),胸腔积液(31%),无并发症相关死亡。国内近期完成的一项经皮冷冻消融治疗肺磨玻璃结节的前瞻性多中心临床研究显示,14名入组患者在经过冷冻消融治疗后,磨玻璃结节在24个月的随访之后均完全吸收,3名患者在治疗后出现了气胸,5%的患者出现了肺功能下降但1个月后基本恢复正常。目前证据显示,经皮冷冻消融治疗早期肺癌的疗效明显、确切且安全。

(三)射频消融

射频消融(radiofrequency ablation,RFA)治疗恶性肿瘤是90年代初兴起的一项新技术。射频发生器产生近400～500kHz的高频电流通过消融电极插入肿瘤,组织中的导电离子和极化分子在射频交变电流作用下快速反复振荡。但由于各种导电离子的体积、质量及所带有的电荷量不同,它们的振动速度也就不同,因此会剧烈摩擦,产生大量热量。由于消融电极周围的电流密度极高,因此电极周围就会形成一个局部高温区,当温度达到60℃以上时,组织中的蛋白质会变性,肿瘤细胞不可逆转性坏死。同时,在凝固坏死区外,还有43～60℃的亚疗区,在此区域内的肿瘤细胞被杀灭,凝固性坏死和组织的碳化会增加组织阻抗,减少电流流动,从而保护周围正常肺组织。由于肺是含气组织,因此在RFA过程中,肺组织电阻高、热传导能力差,因此合理的穿刺点及足够的热量决定消融体积。同时热消融技术仅限于肿瘤局部控制,因此对有任何区域淋巴结转移的病例不适用。目前美国胸科医师学会指南将经皮穿刺消融作为Ⅰ期NSCLC患者的一种治疗方案。来自美国外科医师学院肿瘤组的前瞻性试验Z4033的结果显示,经皮RFA治疗NSCLC,术后1年的OS率为86.3%,2年的OS率为69.8%。在同一研究中,肿瘤<20mm且一般状态评分为0分或1分的患者在2年时分别获得了83%和78%的存活率。鉴于这些结果,美国胸科医师学会在最近对<30 mm肿瘤的治疗推荐中包括了RFA。经皮RFA治疗中,气胸是最常见的并发症,其中10%～50%的患者需要胸腔闭式引流。延迟性气胸很少见,这通常认为是支气管胸膜瘘发生的征兆。同时,采用多极RFA也增加了肺部并发症的风险。Kashima等研究发现,在所纳入的420例患者中每次RFA治疗后的并发症包括:无菌性胸膜炎(23%)、肺炎(18%)、肺脓肿(16%)、需要胸膜粘连术的气胸(16%)和支气管胸膜瘘(0.4%)。出现这些并发症的主要危险因素是肺气肿和既往放疗史,因此合适病例的选择和从技术上消融针通过较长路径的肺组织能

减少并发症发生。

（四）激光消融

多年来，支气管镜下激光治疗一直是治疗中央性气道狭窄及气道肿瘤病变的重要手段。随着气管镜达到远端病变的能力的提高，肺周围性病变的激光治疗也逐渐被研究者所重视。目前的主要策略是通过传输光纤将激光传输到肺外周病灶区域进行消融，然而在更狭小的气道中精准的消融病灶是困难的，因此研究者们在激光传输光纤末端设计了不同形状发射头以达到精准消融的目的。Casal等发表了他们命名为支气管镜激光间质热疗的一项动物研究提示了该种治疗方式的可行性，同时正在进行一项关于早期NSCLC和转移灶切除后消融的支气管镜激光间质热疗临床实验也正在进行当中。

（五）支气管镜热蒸汽消融

支气管镜热蒸汽消融目前主要应用于肺气肿患者肺减容术，即在目标肺减容肺段近端经支气管内输入高温水蒸气，水蒸气经支气管传送到远端肺组织，触发气道和肺实质发生纤维化修复为特征的炎症反应，通过此种纤维化修复牵拉及远端肺组织发生肺不张而达到肺减容的目的。在周围型肺癌研究方面，研究者们也试图用更高温度的热能完全灌注远端肺实质，因此引起的炎症、肺不张及缺血坏死达到消融肿瘤的目的。我们看到这种技术相对于其他技术的潜在优势是肿瘤不一定需要直接进入，能判断准确肿瘤所在的亚段气道就足够了，因此推测经支气管镜下热蒸汽消融周围型肺癌理论可行。有研究者在健康猪肺上通过该技术做了动物实验，需要330cal及以上的治疗能量水平才能在75%～88%的消融中实现均匀坏死，但是肺内侧支旁路通气问题削弱了疗效，增加了并发症，这需要进一步研究。目前已经有两项注册的临床研究在澳大利亚及意大利两家机构正在进行当中。

三、SBRT与介入消融技术在早期肺癌根治中的应用

SBRT是瑞典神经外科医师LarsLeksell基于颅内立体定向手术技术在20世纪50年代提出的概念。在20世纪80年代，基于线性加速器的立体定向手术技术平台被开发和使用，由瑞典和日本科学家首次报道体定向放疗在颅外肿瘤治疗中具有良好的安全性和可行性。在此基础上德国小组开始研究SBRT在无法手术的肺和肝脏肿瘤中的应用并取得了初步成果，2000年以后，这一技术得到迅速推广。SBRT综合多种技术手段来实现精准的放疗，尤其是对于那些受呼吸运动影响的肺内小病变效果明显，这些技术包括：四维CT（三维CT的基础上联合动态时间维度扫描来精确实时监测肿瘤动度）、多野适形、调强光束、弧形照射、容积图像引导等技术，这种治疗模式需要尽可能缩小照射的边界，既提高了局部治疗的精确性，又可以减少对正常脏器的损伤，达到精准治疗。目前SBRT已经被多个国际学会明确为无法手术的NSCLC的标准治疗方式。

近年来随着介入性消融技术的发展，呼吸介入领域研究者开始关注消融技术与SBRT在治疗早期肺癌方面的疗效对比及分别的适用人群。19年的一项研究纳入了15,792名NSCLC患者，其中14,651（93%）名接受了SBRT治疗，另外1141（7%）名患者接受了经皮消融治疗。结果显示SBRT在总体OS方面优于经皮消融治疗，但对于直径<2cm的肿瘤二者无明显差异。另外一篇文章探讨了SBRT和经皮热消融治疗的优劣对比。作者指出经皮热消融可能能够降低SBRT带来的与高放射剂量相关的放射性肺炎等不良反应，同时还能保持良好的治疗有效率。同时也有研究者指出经皮消融治疗可以作为SBRT治疗失败后的补救治疗措施。

四、总结与展望

随着人口老龄化的进程及肺癌筛查技术的进步，早期周围型肺癌的检出率逐年增加，伴随而来的是早期肺癌中很大一部分患者可能无法行外科手术。因此探索早期周围型肺癌的非手术治疗方法成为焦点。基于目前影像学定位技术及支气管镜导航技术的发展，CT引导下的经皮消融技术及经支气管镜消融成为手术替代治疗方法。目前SBRT技术治疗早期非手术周围型肺癌为多家共识所推荐，多家单中心正在进行的RFA、MWA和PCT的局部疗效果也获得了良好的结果。另外，目前多个经支气管镜热蒸汽消融、支气管镜激光间质热疗治疗技术目前多个临床试验正在进行。这些非外科手术技术具有多方面优点，包括对心肺功能及机体基础状况要求低、创伤小、手术时间短、费用低、术后恢复快、并发症发生率低、可重复性好及对肺内多原发肿瘤有更大优势等。虽然上述技术取得了良好的效果，临床上也证实可行，但都局限于单中心及临床医师经验报道，缺乏技术上的统一性及标准管理流程，今后需要开展大规模、多中心、随机对照研究，来制定指南或专家共识以指导临床应用。随着肿瘤免疫学研究的深入，继发于冷、热消融后机体的抗肿瘤反应会极大促进以上技术的进步。另外，支气管镜机器人的研发成功，联合人工智能导航技术使内镜医师更容易到观察肺外周病灶，未来通过支气管镜机器人治疗早期周围型肺癌前景可期。考虑到将部分癌症视为慢性疾病的观点，未来的策略应该将消融联合药物治疗作为常规治疗手段。经支气管镜治疗早期周围型肺癌的低创伤性、低风险性和可重复性是最大优点，值得进一步研究探索。

参 考 文 献

[1] Ferlay J, Colombet M, Soerjomataram I, et al. Estimating the global cancer incidence and mortality in 2018: GLOBOCAN sources and methods. Int J Cancer, 2019, 144（8）: 1941-1953.

[2] Ettinger DS, Wood DE, Aggarwal C, et al. NCCN Guidelines Insights: Non-Small Cell Lung Cancer, Version 1. 2020. J Natl Compr Canc Netw, 2019, 17(12): 1464-1472.

[3] Koike T, Koike T, Sato S, et al. Lobectomy and limited resection in small-sized peripheral non-small cell lung cancer. J Thorac Dis, 2016, 8(11): 3265-3274.

[4] Maconachie R, Mercer T, Navani N, et al. Lung cancer: diagnosis and management: summary of updated NICE guidance. BMJ, 2019, 364(l1049).

[5] Rojas-Solano JR, Ugalde-Gamboa L, Machuzak M. Robotic Bronchoscopy for Diagnosis of Suspected Lung Cancer: A Feasibility Study. J Bronchology Interv Pulmonol, 2018, 25(3): 168-175.

[6] Chen AC, Pastis NJ, Jr., Mahajan AK, et al. Robotic Bronchoscopy for Peripheral Pulmonary Lesions: A Multicenter Pilot and Feasibility Study (BENEFIT). Chest, 2020.

[7] Kinoshita T, Effat A, Gregor A, et al. A Novel Laser Fiberscope for Simultaneous Imaging and Phototherapy of Peripheral Lung Cancer. Chest, 2019, 156(3): 571-578.

[8] Yang X, Ye X, Zheng A, et al. Percutaneous microwave ablation of stage I medically inoperable non-small cell lung cancer: clinical evaluation of 47 cases. J Surg Oncol, 2014, 110(6): 758-763.

[9] Yang X, Ye X, Lin Z, et al. Computed tomography-guided percutaneous microwave ablation for treatment of peripheral ground-glass opacity-Lung adenocarcinoma: A pilot study. J Cancer Res Ther, 2018, 14(4): 764-771.

[10] Yamauchi Y, Izumi Y, Hashimoto K, et al. Percutaneous cryoablation for the treatment of medically inoperable stage I non-small cell lung cancer. PLoS One, 2012, 7(3): e33223.

[11] Liu S, Zhu X, Qin Z, et al. Computed tomography-guided percutaneous cryoablation for lung ground-glass opacity: A pilot study. J Cancer Res Ther, 2019, 15(2): 370-374.

[12] Howington JA, Blum MG, Chang AC, et al. Treatment of stage I and II non-small cell lung cancer: Diagnosis and management of lung cancer, 3rd ed: American College of Chest Physicians evidence-based clinical practice guidelines. Chest, 2013, 143(5 Suppl): e278S-e313S.

[13] Dupuy DE, Fernando HC, Hillman S, et al. Radiofrequency ablation of stage IA non-small cell lung cancer in medically inoperable patients: Results from the American College of Surgeons Oncology Group Z4033 (Alliance) trial. Cancer, 2015, 121(19): 3491-3498.

[14] Anderson EM, Lees WR, Gillams AR. Early indicators of treatment success after percutaneous radiofrequency of pulmonary tumors. Cardiovasc Intervent Radiol, 2009, 32(3): 478-483.

[15] Kashima M, Yamakado K, Takaki H, et al. Complications after 1000 lung radiofrequency ablation sessions in 420 patients: a single center's experiences. AJR Am J Roentgenol, 2011, 197(4): 576-580.

[16] Casal RF, Walsh G, Mcarthur M, et al. Bronchoscopic Laser Interstitial Thermal Therapy: An Experimental Study in Normal Porcine Lung Parenchyma. J Bronchology Interv Pulmonol, 2018, 25(4): 322-329.

[17] Sabath BF, Casal RF. Bronchoscopic ablation of peripheral lung tumors. J Thorac Dis, 2019, 11(6): 2628-2638.

[18] Gompelmann D, Shah PL, Valipour A, et al. Bronchoscopic Thermal Vapor Ablation: Best Practice Recommendations from an Expert Panel on Endoscopic Lung Volume Reduction. Respiration, 2018, 95(6): 392-400.

[19] Harris K, Puchalski J, Sterman D. Recent Advances in Bronchoscopic Treatment of Peripheral Lung Cancers. Chest, 2017, 151(3): 674-685.

[20] Leksell L. Sterotaxic radiosurgery in trigeminal neuralgia. Acta Chir Scand, 1971, 137(4): 311-314.

[21] Uematsu M, Shioda A, Tahara K, et al. Focal, high dose, and fractionated modified stereotactic radiation therapy for lung carcinoma patients: a preliminary experience. Cancer, 1998, 82(6): 1062-1070.

[22] Uzel EK, Figen M, Uzel O. Radiotherapy in Lung Cancer: Current and Future Role. Sisli Etfal Hastan Tip Bul, 2019, 53(4): 353-360.

[23] Ager BJ, Wells SM, Gruhl JD, et al. Stereotactic body radiotherapy versus percutaneous local tumor ablation for early-stage non-small cell lung cancer. Lung Cancer, 2019, 138: 6-12.

7 慢性血栓栓塞性肺动脉高压的介入诊疗

周 玮

肺动脉高压(PH)是一种罕见疾病,可由多种病因导致。慢性血栓栓塞性肺动脉高压(Chronic Thromboembolic Pulmonary hypertension,CTEPH)是毛细血管前肺高压的一种形式,其原因是肺血栓栓塞的不完全溶解及肺血管床内形成慢性、纤维化、血流受限的血栓。属罕见病范畴。在肺高压分类中属第4类。一般指急性肺栓塞患者经过正规抗凝治疗3个月右心导管下平均肺动脉压力(mPAP)≥25mmHg,肺小动脉楔压(PAWP)≤15mmHg即可诊断。

肺通气灌注显像(V/Q)是评估疑似CTEPH的肺动脉高压患者的初步筛查试验。V/Q扫描对灌注异常的检测高度敏感(96%～97.4%),提示CTEPH发生的可能性。正常的V/Q扫描将CTEPH诊断排除在外,其阴性预测值接近100%。低特异性限制了其诊断CTEPH的效用,任何异常灌注扫描都需要进行其他的影像学最终确定诊断。如CT肺血管造影、磁共振成像和(或)导管下肺血管造影。CT肺血管造影在评估怀疑为CTEPH的患者中起着至关重要的作用。CT肺动脉造影可显示各种异常,如肺动脉内再通或有血栓栓塞物质,支气管动脉旁侧应。CT肺血管造影的额外好处是评估潜在的实质肺实质和纵隔疾病、检测出V/Q肺扫描中可能出现灌注缺陷的其他肺血管疾病,如肺动脉肉瘤、肺静脉闭塞病或纤维化性纵隔炎,帮助它们与CTEPH区分。CT肺血管造影的缺点是在段和段以下血管中检测CTEPH的敏感度较低。

目前,CTEPH首选的治疗方法仍然是肺动脉内膜剥脱术(PTE),一旦确诊为CTEPH,患者将接受PTE手术治疗。如果认为无法手术,或PTE手术后持续出现症状性肺动脉高压,或存在不可接受的风险-收益比,则考虑采用靶向治疗和(或)球囊成形术(BPA)。患者经常接受联合药物治疗和BPA,以获得最佳的血流动力学和临床结果。手术可以减轻症状,减缓肺动脉高压的疾病进展。PTE手术5年和10年生存率分别为82%和75%,住院死亡率为2.2%,常见并发症为心律失常、心包或胸腔积液、肺不张、伤口感染和谵妄。严重的再灌注肺水肿(RPE)在PTE患者的发生率9.6%。(数据来源:加州大学圣地亚哥分校的研究小组报告)。

BPA手术约20年前被作为一种治疗不可手术的CTEPH患者的替代疗法,但是由于主要并发症的频繁,该方法被放弃。在近5年里,这一手术经过了不断改进,获得了越来越多的阳性结果和来自世界各地不同中心的安全数据。2015年欧洲心脏病学会/欧洲呼吸学会肺动脉高压诊断和治疗指南建议:那些技术上不能手术,或者对PTE的风险-效益比率不佳的CTEPH患者使用BPA,(推荐类别IIb,证据水平:C。目前报道的手术死亡率为3%(1.3%～24%),残留肺动脉高压:11%～35%再灌注肺水肿:5.5%～19.3%。

BPA的手术适应证为:①症状性、无法手术的CTEPH;②持续/复发性CTEPH;③作为快速恶化的CTEPH患者在PTE之前稳定的过渡治疗选择;④可与PTE结合,用于治疗一个肺的手术可及性病变和对侧肺的不可手术疾病。

研究证明,BPA短期疗效包括心肺血流动力学、肺灌注、运动耐受性、世界卫生组织功能等级和6分钟步行距离改善;血流动力学的改善(mPAP和PVR)与治疗血管的数量成正比;生活质量的改善和症状的缓解与肺动脉高压的降低程度不成比例。目前来自日本7个中心的数据显示,2004-2016年,308例CTEPH患者接受BPa,共1408次手术,3年生存率94.5%,mPAP降低44%(43.2～24.3mmHg)。

加州大学圣地亚哥分校使用该技术治疗38例患者(183次手术),严重并发症0%,手术相关的轻度咯血6.6%。完成1年随访的20例患者中,mPAP降低26%(39.1～28.8mmHg)。

CTEPH是一种诊断不足的疾病,外科PTE仍然是首选的治疗方法。确定手术的可操作性是很有挑战性的,而且手术专家有限。经皮介入治疗不可手术的CTEPH结果越来越令人兴奋,来自世界各地多个中心的数据显示BPa治疗CTEPH的临床可行性。里奥西瓜特仍然是唯一被批准的靶向药物治疗方法,也是治疗PTE后不可手术或持续性肺动脉高压的重要辅助手段。

8 经支气管肺活检和消融治疗进展

孙加源

随着低剂量CT筛查应用普及,肺结节发现率增加,降低了肺癌死亡率,但其有较高假阳性率。因此,术前明确肺外周病变(PPL)的性质具有重要意义。经支气管肺活检(TBLB)作为诊断PPL的主要方式之一,相比经胸壁针吸活检(TTNA)经自然腔道进行,气胸、出血发生率明显减低。在导航系统引导下细镜支气管镜联合径向支气管内超声(EBUS)、引导鞘管(GS)进行的 TBLB 已成为经支气管方式诊断PPL的标准术式。随着支气管镜技术的发展,出现了外径3mm的超细支气管镜,并显示了其相比细支气管镜的诊断优势。支气管征对TBLB诊断率有很大影响,对于无支气管征的PPL,其诊断率较低,而支气管镜经肺实质结节取样术(BTPNA)的出现使得这部分PPL的诊断率有了很大程度改观。

手术切除仍然是目前早期周围型非小细胞肺癌(NSCLC)根治方法,但许多高龄或合并症较多的患者无法耐受手术切除。对于这类患者,消融治疗是推荐的,目前常用的热消融治疗,如射频消融(RFA)、微波消融(MWA),多数经胸壁方式进行,其气胸、出血发生率与TTNA相同。正是由于经支气管方式的独特优势,近些年一些学者在经支气管消融治疗周围型肺癌方面也进行了积极探索。

本文就周围型肺癌通过经支气管方式诊断和消融治疗进展做一总结。

一、超细支气管镜在肺外周病变中的诊断价值

超细支气管镜(UTB)与目前使用的细支气管镜(TB)(外径4mm,工作通道2.0mm)相比,可以到达更远端支气管,从而使普通支气管镜下不能直视的部分PPL变成UTB下可以直视的管腔内病变,联合导航支气管镜可以更加准确到达PPL所在远端支气管,进而提高TBLB诊断率。最早出现的UTB外径2.8mm,工作通道1.2mm,不能联合EBUS使用,限制了其在PPL中的诊断价值。新出现的外径3mm的UTB,其工作通道为1.7mm,可以通过直径1.4mm的高频超声探头使用,具有更大优势。

日本学者Oki等早在2010年就已开始对外径3mm UTB的诊断价值进行了研究,在4个中心前瞻性入组肺结节直径≤3cm且怀疑为肺癌的患者,随机分配到UTB组和TB-GS组,两组均联合使用虚拟导航(VBN)、EBUS和X线透视,UTB组由于工作通道小无法使用GS,TB组联合GS。研究共入组310例患者,最终305例纳入分析,其中UTB组150例,TB-GS组155例。结果显示,UTB相比TB可以到达更远端支气管(中位数 5级 vs 4级,$P<0.001$),且显著提高肺结节的诊断率(74% vs 59%),两组并发症发生率无差异(3% vs 5%,$P=0.595$)。

在上述研究中TB-GS组使用的是1.5mm的小活检钳,而TB工作通道2.0mm可以不联合GS,从而可以使用1.8或1.9mm的标准活检钳或经支气管针吸活检(TBNA)进行取样。已有研究证明,使用TBNA或标准活检钳可以提高TBLB诊断率,该团队又进行了一项多中心随机对照研究,研究人群与上述研究相同,随机分配到UTB和TB组,不同的是在本研究中TB组使用1.95mm GS联合1.5mm活检钳和(或)1.8/1.9mm活检钳而不使用GS,且当肺结节EBUS影像不可见或者临近时,可以使用21G TBNA针进行取样。本研究共入组360例患者,最终356例纳入分析(肺结节中位直径19mm)。结果显示UTB组诊断率明显高于TB组(70.1% vs 58.7%,$P=0.027$)。UTB组操作时间明显缩短(中位 24.8min vs 26.8min $P=0.008$),并发症发生率分别为2.8%和4.5%($P=0.574$)。

以上两项多中心研究证实了UTB相比TB对肺结节具有更高诊断率,但两项研究均在X线透视辅助下进行,其在无X线透视辅助下对肺结节的诊断价值尚需进一步探讨。

二、支气管镜经肺实质结节取样术在肺外周病变中的诊断价值

BTPNA技术是通过在LungPro导航系统引导下经肺实质建立隧道,从而实现病变的抵达。Herth等开展的一项单中心可行性研究,对12例进行BTPNA获取样本的受试者术后立刻接受了肺叶切除术或全肺切除术,其中10例获取样本,活检检出率为100%;另外2例患者因支气管镜无法充分明确地可以创建通道至肺结节,因此未能获取标本;该研究中没有因建立隧道导致的不良事件报道。后续该团队又对6例拟接受支气管镜活检的患者进行BTPNA获取样本,活检检出率为83%。在其上市后的临床研究中,有包含中国在内的全球共10家中心、共106例受试者接受了经BTPNA技术取样活检。入组的结节平均大小为2.41cm,中位数为2.1cm,经BTPNA技术实现取样的

活检检出率为84.8%,无支气管征结节的活检检出率为80%,2cm以下结节的活检检出率为80.6%,2cm以上结节活检检出率达87%,严重并发症发生率为0.8%。

上述研究证明了BTPNA技术对PPL诊断的可行性、安全性和有效性,为无支气管征PPL的诊断提供了新的方法。

三、经支气管消融治疗周围型肺癌进展

Tsushima等最早报道了经支气管RFA的动物研究,比较两种不同RFA导管消融对正常羊肺的安全性和可行性。该团队研发了3种规格的经支气管冷循环射频消融针,并对3种消融针的周围型NSCLC消融效果进行了临床研究,明确了不同消融针的消融范围。该团队后续又报道了经支气管冷循环RFA的临床研究,该研究入组20例患者,包括23个肿瘤,局部控制率达到82.6%,中位PFS 35个月,5年生存率61.5%,仅3个患者发生了消融相关的急性发热、胸痛反应,未见其他严重并发症。Ferguson等的会议摘要报道了在3头猪上进行的经支气管MWA动物实验,证明了其可行性和安全性。

我们中心自2015年开始开展电磁导航引导下经支气管RFA,初期对3例患者(2例IA肺癌,1例肺转移瘤),截至文章发表时,其中2例患者术后均随访1年。我们中心在经支气管MWA方面也做了一些探索,在2016年4月首先进行了电磁导航引导下无水冷MWA治疗周围型肺癌。后续联合国内厂家研发了用于消融恶性肺部磨玻璃病变的柔性水冷微波消融针,并通过动物实验完成相关性能测试,研究发现经支气管微波消融后24h,尽管支气管粘膜上皮会有凋亡损伤,但支气管软骨并未破坏,且这种损伤在1个月内会逐渐重构和修复,在理论上证明了经支气管微波消融PPL的可行性和安全性。该研究被德国和美国权威呼吸介入专家关注,发表述评肯定了本研究对开展经支气管微波消融具有重要理论价值。截至到目前,仅有1篇会议摘要报道了3例肺部转移瘤的患者接受经支气管MWA治疗,其在原发性周围型肺癌中的疗效尚无数据,我们中心目前正在进行经支气管水冷MWA治疗早期不可手术周围型肺癌的临床研究,并于2018年6月施行了国内首例电磁导航支气管镜联合CBCT引导下经支气管MWA。此外,我们还研发了经支气管用柔性冷冻消融针用于肺部肿瘤消融治疗,其工作直径2.33mm,离体动物实验证实消融针头端降温可至−150℃以下,经过两个低温循环,冰球范围≥30mm,证实了经支气管低温冷冻消融的可行性。

目前经支气管消融治疗周围型肺癌这一新兴领域还处于探索阶段,需要不断积累经验、开展大样本随机对照多中心研究提供更多循证依据。

四、小结和展望

支气管镜技术是肺癌诊疗的有效手段,与经胸壁方式具有同等重要的价值,并且二者可相互补充,在肺癌诊治过程和全程管理中起着不可或缺的作用。随着支气管镜新技术的不断涌现,将会有效指导肺外周病变的诊治,在不能手术和多原发早期肺癌诊治领域具有潜在的应用前景。

参 考 文 献

[1] Aberle DR, Adams AM, Berg CD, et al. Reduced lung-cancer mortality with low-dose computed tomographic screening. N Engl J Med, 2011, 365: 395-409.

[2] Howington JA, Blum MG, Chang AC, et al. Treatment of stage I and II non-small cell lung cancer: Diagnosis and management of lung cancer, 3rd ed: American College of Chest Physicians evidence-based clinical practice guidelines. Chest, 2013, 143: e278S-e313S.

[3] Scott WJ, Howington J, Feigenberg S, et al. Treatment of non-small cell lung cancer stage I and stage II: ACCP evidence-based clinical practice guidelines (2nd edition). Chest, 2007, 132: 234s-242s.

[4] National Comprehensive Cancer Network. NCCN clinical practice guidelines in oncology. Non-small cell lung cancer. Available from URL: https://www.nccn.org/professionals/physician_gls/default.aspx#nscl. Accessed February 29, 2020.

[5] Oki M, Saka H, Ando M, et al. Ultrathin Bronchoscopy with Multimodal Devices for Peripheral Pulmonary Lesions. A Randomized Trial. Am J Respir Crit Care Med, 2015, 192: 468-476.

[6] Chao TY, Chien MT, Lie CH, et al. Endobronchial ultrasonography-guided transbronchial needle aspiration increases the diagnostic yield of peripheral pulmonary lesions: a randomized trial. Chest, 2009, 136: 229-236.

[7] Kunimasa K, Tachihara M, Tamura D, et al. Diagnostic utility of additional conventional techniques after endobronchial ultrasonography guidance during transbronchial biopsy. Respirology, 2016, 21: 1100-1105.

[8] Herth FJ, Eberhardt R, Sterman D, et al. Bronchoscopic transparenchymal nodule access (BTPNA): first in human trial of a novel procedure for sampling solitary pulmonary nodules. Thorax, 2015, 70: 326-332.

[9] Harzheim D, Sterman D, Shah PL, et al. Bronchoscopic Transparenchymal Nodule Access: Feasibility and Safety in an Endoscopic Unit. Respiration, 2016, 91: 302-306.

[10] Sun J, Vichani A, Criner GJ, et al. Late Breaking Abstract-Safety and Performance of Total Lung Access to Peripheral Nodules in prospective, multi-center study, 2019, 54: OA1614.

[11] Tsushima K, Koizumi T, Tanabe T, et al. Bronchoscopy-guided radiofrequency ablation as a potential novel therapeutic tool. Eur Respir J, 2007, 29: 1193-1200.

[12] Tanabe T, Koizumi T, Tsushima K, et al. Comparative study of three different catheters for CT imaging-bronchoscopy-guided radiofrequency ablation as a potential and novel inter-

ventional therapy for lung cancer. Chest, 2010, 137: 890-897.
[13] Koizumi T, Tsushima K, Tanabe T, et al. Bronchoscopy-Guided Cooled Radiofrequency Ablation as a Novel Intervention Therapy for Peripheral Lung Cancer. Respiration, 2015, 90: 47-55.
[14] Ferguson J, Egressy K, Schefelker R, et al. Bronchoscopically-Guided Microwave Ablation in the Lung. Chest, 2013, 144.
[15] Xie F, Zheng X, Xiao B, et al. Navigation Bronchoscopy-Guided Radiofrequency Ablation for Nonsurgical Peripheral Pulmonary Tumors. Respiration, 2017, 94: 293-298.
[16] Yuan HB, Wang XY, Sun JY, et al. Flexible bronchoscopy-guided microwave ablation in peripheral porcine lung: a new minimally-invasive ablation. Translational Lung Cancer Research, 2019, 8: 787-796.
[17] Pritchett MA, Schirmer CC, Laeseke P. Melting the tip of the iceberg: bronchoscopic-guided transbronchial microwave ablation, 2020.
[18] Hohenforst-Schmidt W, Zarogoulidis P. Time to get started with endobronchial microwave ablation-chances, pitfalls and limits for interventional pulmonologists. Translational lung cancer research, 2020, 9: 163-167.
[19] Zheng X, Yang C, Zhang X, et al. The Cryoablation for Peripheral Pulmonary Lesions Using a Novel Flexible Bronchoscopic Cryoprobe in the ex vivo Pig Lung and Liver. Respiration, 2019, 97: 457-462.

9 从呼吸介入发展谈临床创新

陈成水　金旭如

一、呼吸介入取材技术促进弥漫性肺病变诊治的进步

呼吸介入的发展一定是伴随着临床疾病诊疗给临床医师提出的新问题，在不断创新中走向进步的。回到20年前，伴随着我院当时大量开展的肾移植工作，呼吸科医师接触到一批肾移植术后弥漫性肺炎的病患。该类患者疾病进展迅速，病情危重，却病因不明。疾病的明确诊断首先要通过有效手段获取具有代表性的病变标本，患者的血液标本、痰液标本通过常规检验均无法为我们提供有价值的诊断信息，于是我们想到了呼吸介入取材技术，通过支气管镜到达患者肺部病变部位取材进行相应的检验，为诊断提供最直接的病变部位的标本，理论上应该是最有价值的信息。而在弥漫性肺部渗出、呼吸衰竭的状态下，如何谨慎地通过支气管镜肺泡灌洗、肺活检，获取患者病变部位的肺泡灌洗液、肺组织，并且处理好气胸、呼吸衰竭等并发症，在当时缺乏成熟经验的情况下，都需要临床医师的大胆创新，严谨诊疗。而获取标本后的检验过程更是一个创新的过程，肺泡灌洗液的常规涂片染色、病原菌培养等均未能获取有价值的诊断信息，那么病变肺组织的病理切片中能否找到病原踪迹？HE染色、PS染色、抗酸染色等常规光镜下病理检查未能发现有价值的诊断信息，那么我们能否创新性的利用电镜，来观察病变组织及细胞的更细微结构，去寻找病原的蛛丝马迹？结合大量的文献查阅，我们终于在电镜下找到我们以往不认识的存在于病变组织细胞内外的耶氏肺孢子菌的包囊和滋养体，再回头看病理切片HE染色，甚至肺泡灌洗液沉渣涂片革兰染色，便都找到了耶氏肺孢子菌的可疑病原体。这些临床检验的经验，使得今天，我们无须电镜检查，通过普通病例切片及肺泡灌洗液，进行针对性银染，便可确诊耶氏肺孢子菌病。20年前，我院创新性应用电镜检查结合呼吸介入取材技术诊断耶氏肺孢子菌病的过程，同时助推了弥漫性肺部病变支气管镜介入取材技术的成熟与发展。以我们20年前呼吸介入诊断中的创新性经历，已可见呼吸系统疾病的诊断过程中标本及取材技术的重要性，而经支气管镜介入取材技术的创新和进步，也引领了呼吸介入诊疗技术的起步与发展，促进了呼吸学科的发展。

二、肺癌诊断的临床需求促进了呼吸介入穿刺技术和导航技术的发展

经支气管针吸活检术（TBNA）发明之前，纵隔淋巴结病变的诊断只能通过创伤性大、费用高的纵隔镜来实现。早在20世纪40年代，阿根廷Schieppati便首次开展硬镜下隆突下淋巴结穿刺术。20世纪80年代，美国约翰霍普金斯大学的Ko-Pen Wang教授使用纤维支气管镜操作TBNA并改进穿刺针及穿刺方法，使得TBNA技术得到推广，在此过程中，Ko-Pen Wang教授不断改进TBNA的相关技术与穿刺针等操作器材，如建立王氏淋巴结穿刺图谱，推出王氏TBNA针，设计制作穿刺针固定器等，在不断的创新实践中让TBNA技术走向成熟。但TBNA毕竟是盲检，是否可以在TBNA基础上加用超声成像，将TBNA的盲穿，变成超声影像引导下的直视下活检取材？早期的创新探索是将超声波探头经支气管镜工作孔道送至靶目标附近，探查肿大的淋巴结或肿物，确定确定病灶、异常淋巴结位置及其周围血管的关系后，拔出超声波探头，送入穿刺针对选定的穿刺目标抽吸活检。尽管这种支气管内超声（endobronchial ultrasound，EBUS）探查后的TBNA提高了传统TBNA的取材成功率，但并非实时TBNA，活检效率的提高仍有空间。于是临床医学家与医疗器材工程学家们从1992年开始，研发一体化的搭载电子凸阵扫描超声探头的超声支气管镜（convex probe EBUS，CP-EBUS），2002年开始奥林巴斯公司和日本千叶大学胸外科安福和弘医师共同专注于适合于临床应用的CP-EBUS的研发和改进，时至今日，形成了配合通用型超声内镜图像处理装置使用，带操作孔道，配合多种规格穿刺针的新一代超声光纤电子支气管镜，这种创新与改进，使得临床医师能够更加安全、高效、方便的进行EBUS-TBNA操作。为了能够更加精准地取材，研发团队又在超声图像中应用了一种可以测量组织硬度的新技术：弹性图（图11-9-1）。一般认为恶性肿瘤组织的硬度要大大高于良性病灶组织或正常组织，因此在超声弹性图上呈现蓝色图像，有助于选择最佳的靶活检区域。

除了超声引导下经支气管活检取材，临床医师们更早以前就开始透视引导下、CT引导下的经支气管活检取材，并且至今仍有在临床应用。为了精准定位，临床医学家与医学工程学家不断开发新技术应用于支气管镜诊疗过程中，包括基于CT图像的非实时的虚拟导航支气管

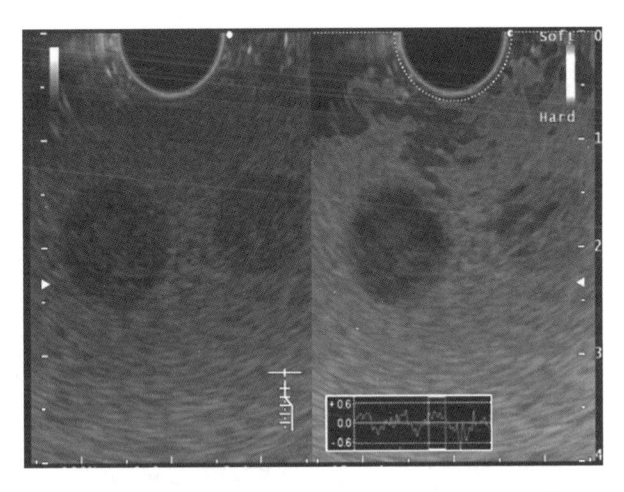

图 11-9-1 超声弹性成像,硬度较高的病灶部位显示蓝色

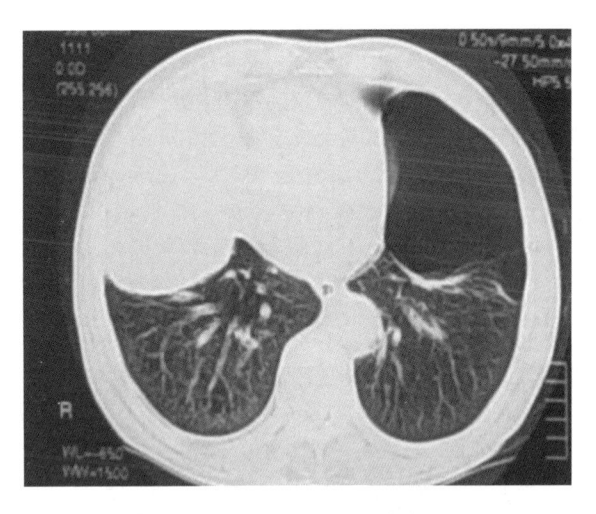

图 11-9-2 治疗后 3 个月腔内液平面

定位系统,实时图像引导导航系统,电磁导航引导系统等。由此可见,从使用纵膈镜进行纵膈淋巴结取材,被经支气管镜 TBNA 抽吸取样所替代,再改良为超声下经支气管穿刺抽吸取样(EBUS-TBNA)并结合超声弹性成像等技术,如今开发出各种经气道导航技术,其发展历程其实就是呼吸介入技术发展的一个缩影,是不断创新改进的成果。

三、临床问题是呼吸介入技术创新的源动力

1. 临床上,呼吸内科医师常常会遇到重度肺气肿,巨型肺大疱的患者,由于患者肺功能极差,不能耐受外科手术,而内科药物治疗无法改善患者呼吸费力症状。于是我们创新性为患者实施微创介入的经皮肺大疱穿刺封闭术:C 形臂机定位下经皮穿刺,大疱腔内留置引流管,肺大疱腔内注入纤维蛋白胶,胸腔内留置气胸引流管。术后 7d 患者进行穿刺封闭术的右侧肺大疱内出现液平面,治疗 3 个月后肺大疱内被液体充满(图 11-9-2);治疗 6 个月后肺大疱明显缩小(图 11-9-3);治疗 12 个月后患者右侧肺大疱疾病消失(图 11-9-4)。而术后 3 个月、12 个月的各项肺功能指标也明显好转(表 11-9-1)。

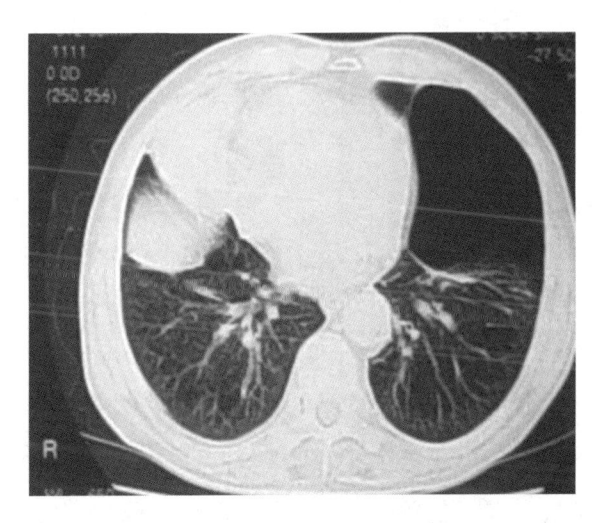

图 11-9-3 治疗后 6 个月体积缩小

表 11-9-1 肺大疱穿刺封闭术术前、术后 3 个月、12 个月肺功能对比

	术前基础值	术后 3 个月	术后 12 个月
FEV1	0.97L	1.10L	1.30L
	%pred38	%pred42%	%pred58%
FVC	2.08L	2.18L	2.93L
	%pred 65.1	%pred 68.1	%pred 88.6
FEV1/FVC	46.74	50.45	48.91
6MW	140m	200m	350m

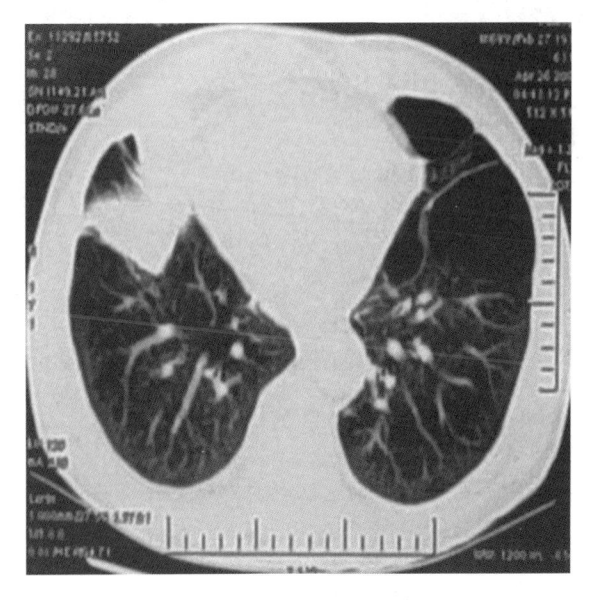

图 11-9-4 治疗后 12 个月明显缩小

在施行经皮肺大疱穿刺封闭术的过程中,我们发现部分患者经皮肺穿刺置管不成功,借助胸腔镜我们发现部分患者肺大疱疱壁坚韧增厚,导致穿刺置管困难,无法施行穿刺封闭术。为解决这一临床问题,我们开始尝试胸腔镜下肺大疱消融术治疗无法耐受外科手术的巨型肺大疱患者。一例两侧多发肺大疱,本次合并右侧气胸(图 11-9-5)入住我科,因肺功能差,无法耐受手术,给予内科胸腔镜下肺大疱消融术。术中可见脏层胸膜表面肺大疱(图 11-9-6),消融后肺大疱萎陷(图 11-9-7)。

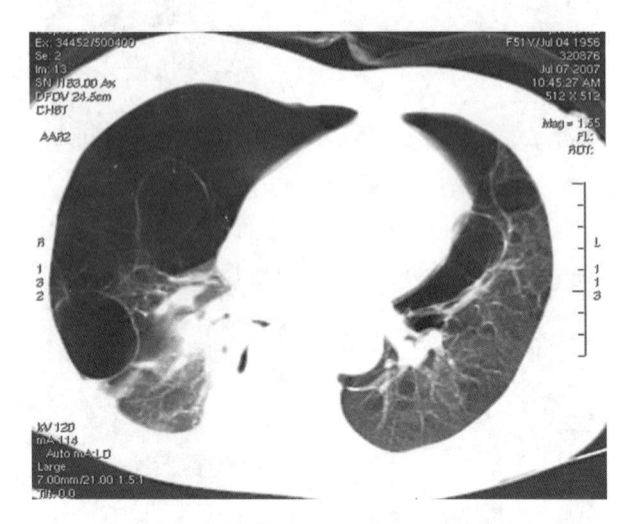

图 11-9-5 术前右侧气胸、两侧肺大疱

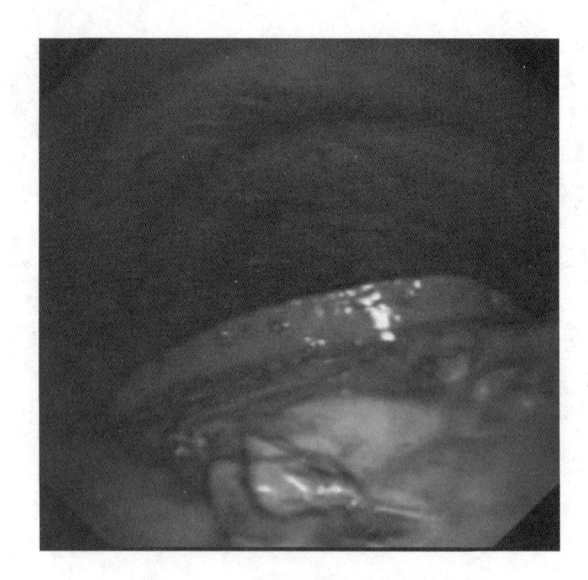

图 11-9-7 胸腔镜肺大疱消融术后

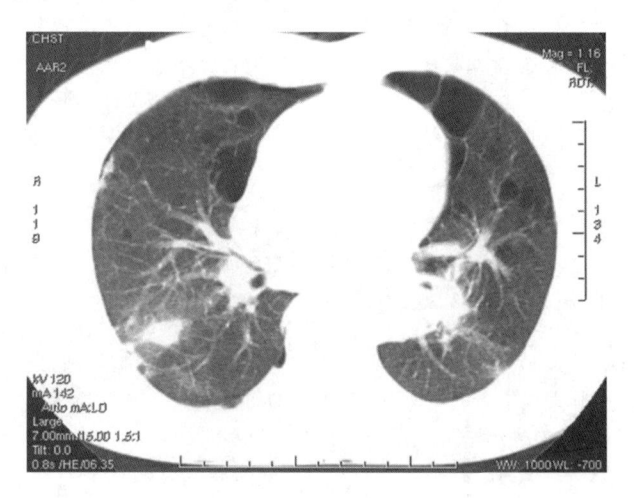

图 11-9-8 胸部 CT:胸腔镜大疱消融术后 3d

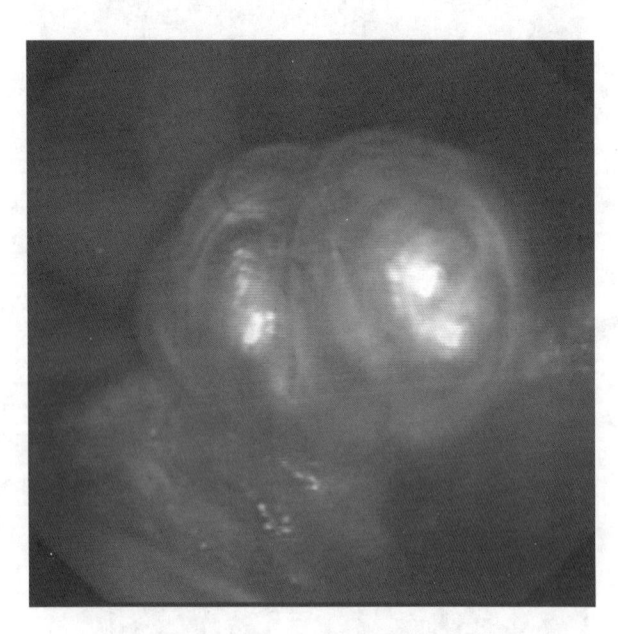

图 11-9-6 胸腔镜下肺大疱

3 d 后,患者气胸、肺大疱均消失(图 11-9-8),肺功能得到明显的提升(表 11-9-2)。

实践证明,对于不能耐受的巨型肺大疱患者,经皮肺大泡穿刺封闭术和胸腔镜下肺大疱消融术都是相对安全、有效的介入微创治疗方法。

表 11-9-2 胸腔镜肺大泡消融术前、术后 1 个月肺功能变化

肺功能	术前	术后 1 个月
FEV1	40.7%	42.2%
FVC	57.6%	61%
FEV1/FVC	54.71	52.99
RV/TLC	55.6	54.4
DLCO	47.9%	37.3%
6 min 步行距离	335m	586m

2. 气道支架的置入是十分普遍的治疗良、恶性气道狭窄的手段。但实践过程中开通气道似乎十分容易,维持气道通畅却不那么容易,其中的原因之一:支架边缘刺激正常气管壁黏膜产生肉芽从而堵塞支架。此种情况在气管、左右主支气管 Y 形支架置入时的左主支气管远端更为常见。分析原因可以发现,由于 Y 形硅酮支架夹角固定,而人体左主支气管与气管中线夹角相对较大,导致 Y 形支架置入后左支与左主支气管形成夹角(图 11-9-9),支架远端

边缘与支气管壁形成切迹,从而刺激管壁黏膜增生肉芽(图11-9-10)。于是,利用硅酮支架可裁剪,可拼接的特点,应运而生了各种创新DIY。针对Y形支架夹角固定的问题,我们将两个直通支架用连接片缝合的方法拼接在一起,制成左右支夹角活动的V形支架(图11-9-11),置入后支架最大程度上与患者的左、右主支气管角度适型吻合,从而避免了支架边缘对支气管壁的切割作用,很大程度上减少了刺激肉芽生成的副作用。同样是临床中遇到的问题启发思考,针对气管直筒硅酮支架容易移位的难题,我们创新了穿刺法固定支架内垫片的方法,来固定气管上段直筒支架(图11-9-12)。

得益于呼吸介入实践中不断遇到的问题,和积极的创新性探索,我们进一步拓宽思路,利用工程学和医学生物材料学的进步,开始探索3D打印技术在气道支架中的应用(图11-9-13)。相信更多的创新会在呼吸介入实践得到实现。

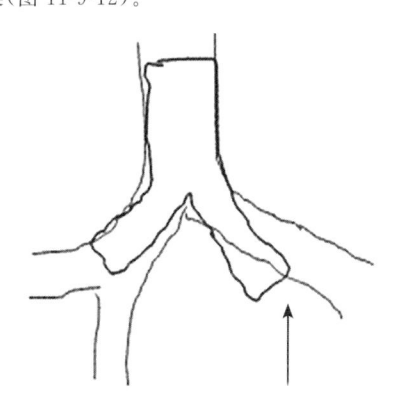

图11-9-9 支架末端与气道纵径成角

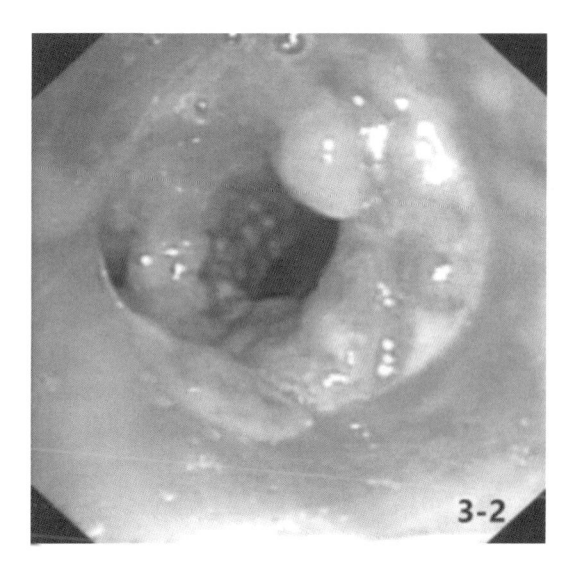

图11-9-10 支气管壁黏膜增生肉芽

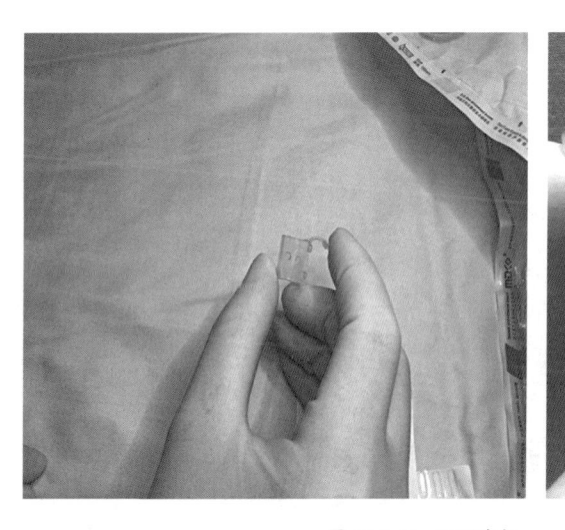

图11-9-11 V形支架

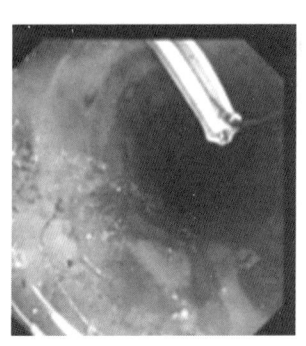

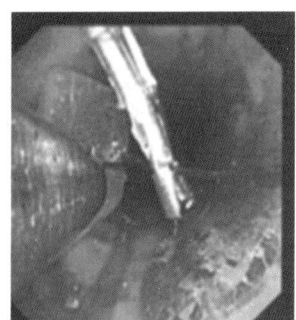

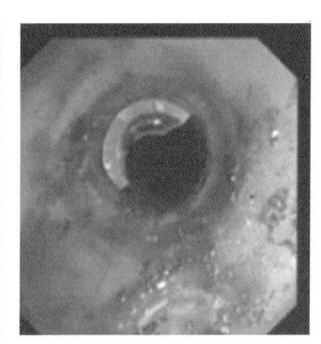

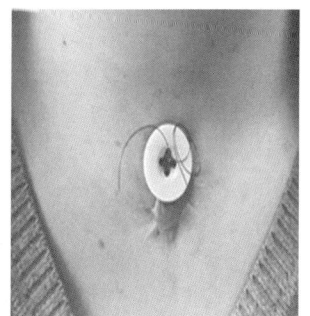

图11-9-12 直筒支架

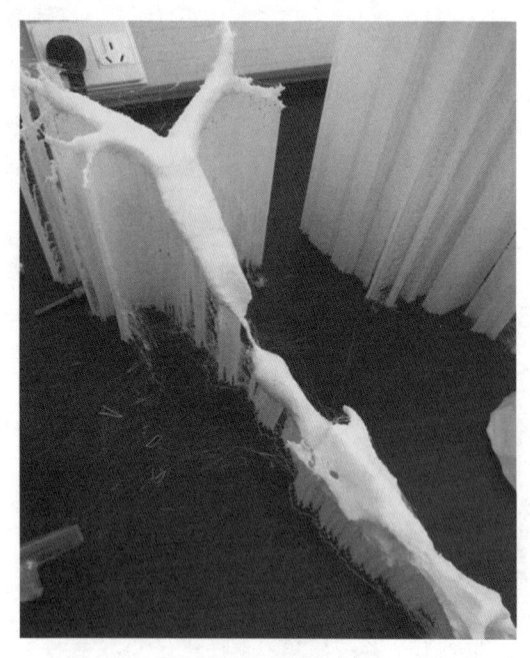

图 11-9-13　3D 打印技术在气道支架中的应用

3. 临床上我们常常还会遇到的更加危急、更加凶险的病症：大咯血，死亡率可高达 60%，常常让临床医师措手不及，救治过程没有绝对有效的手段和必胜的信心。在大咯血的救治过程中最关键的措施就是防止咯血窒息，挽救生命。而现有的手段中：内科药物疗效差；支气管动脉栓塞需要术前术中患者相对稳定状态，且术前需完善 CT 支气管动脉造影明确血管分布来提高支气管动脉栓塞成功率，这些措施都需要患者相对稳定的状态和时间来完成；外科手术切除，由于术前出血部位定位不充分，容易造成手术部位的误判，且术中气道安全也得不到彻底的保障。而气道内介入球囊封堵出血部位支气管，避免窒息大气道，便成为以上这些治疗手段成功实施的前提和关键。但当前气道内介入球囊封堵技术难度大、操作复杂，疗效不稳定，费用高，以至于难以推广。针对现行经气管镜气道球囊封堵术需导丝引导，需做导丝交换，球囊容易移位，球囊容易漏气的缺点，我们对封堵球囊做了创新性设计（图 11-9-14）：增加球囊导管的整体韧性，增强推送性能，从而实现自导引；其次球囊前端加长导丝来防止球囊移位；球囊导管后端设计可拆卸注射接口，导管经支气管镜置入气道后可直接留置，撤出气管镜，从而避免了导丝交换的步骤，操作简单；球囊导管末端单项活瓣设计防止漏气。功能设计的创新还需要产品的技术创新来实现，其中包含了材料的创新：硬度渐变管材的创新，实现了导管力传递性的提升和推送性能的增强；还包括工艺的创新：多段渐变管材连焊接工艺的创新，保证了密闭性与力学性能。该新型气道球囊导管现已申请专利，进入产品改进的最后阶段，有望在近期投入生产，投入临床应用，最终使经气管镜气道球囊封堵术成为临床上操作简便，快捷，疗效稳定，费用低廉的治疗大咯血的常用呼吸介入治疗技术，惠及更多了患者。

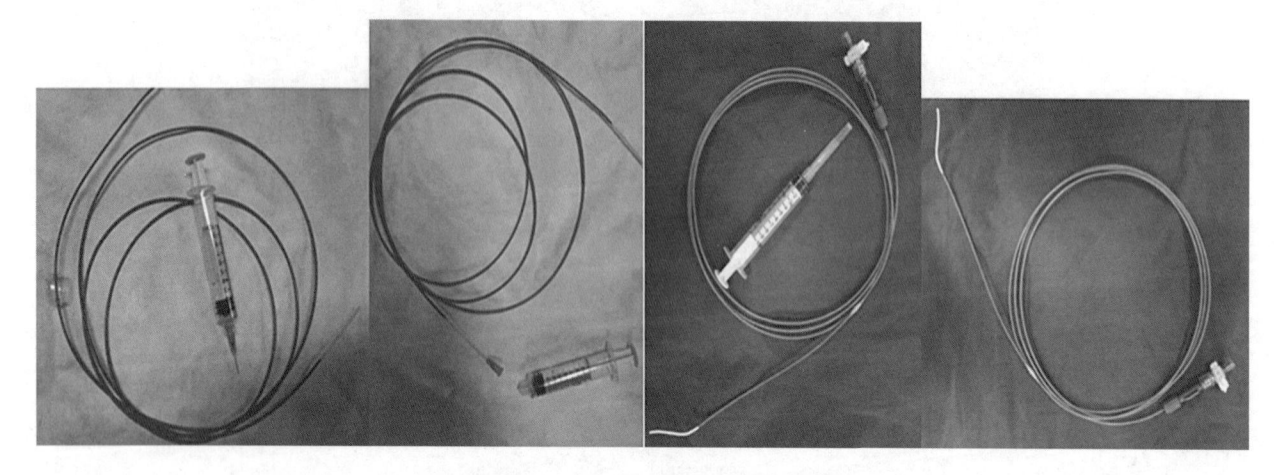

图 11-9-14　新型气道球囊导管试样图

4. 临床上在恶性气道狭窄患者的呼吸介入治疗过程中，我们常常为气道肿瘤组织清除后短时间增生再狭窄，即使狭窄段置入支架，肿瘤组织也会在短时间内增殖长入金属裸支架的网孔，造成再狭窄。于是我们创新设计可携带粒子的金属气道支架，用于恶性气道狭窄的气道开通和维持。所有的创新一开始都是基于基本理念：放射性粒子附着在金属支架上，支架置入恶性气道狭窄段，在开通气道的同时利用放射性粒子的照射作用抑制恶性肿瘤生长，甚至使肿瘤组织萎缩，从而维持气道通畅。但是具体实施的时候，会在各个细节上遇到诸多困难。比如，如何将粒子附着在金属支架上？金属支架上的粒子需多少量？如何分布？才能达到所需的放射剂量又不至于损伤正常组织黏膜引发并发症？根据不同的肿瘤累及面，粒子分布该做怎样的调整？附着了粒子后支架体积增大，该如何推送至狭窄气道局部？等等这些问题都是创新探索中需要我们一一去解决的新问题。这个过程中，跨学科协作起到了重要的作用，与国内放射性粒子应用专家团队共同探讨研究，根据放射性粒子剂量分布，设计出硅胶管捆绑金属支架，粒子 W 形平行分布置入的模式（图 11-9-15）。

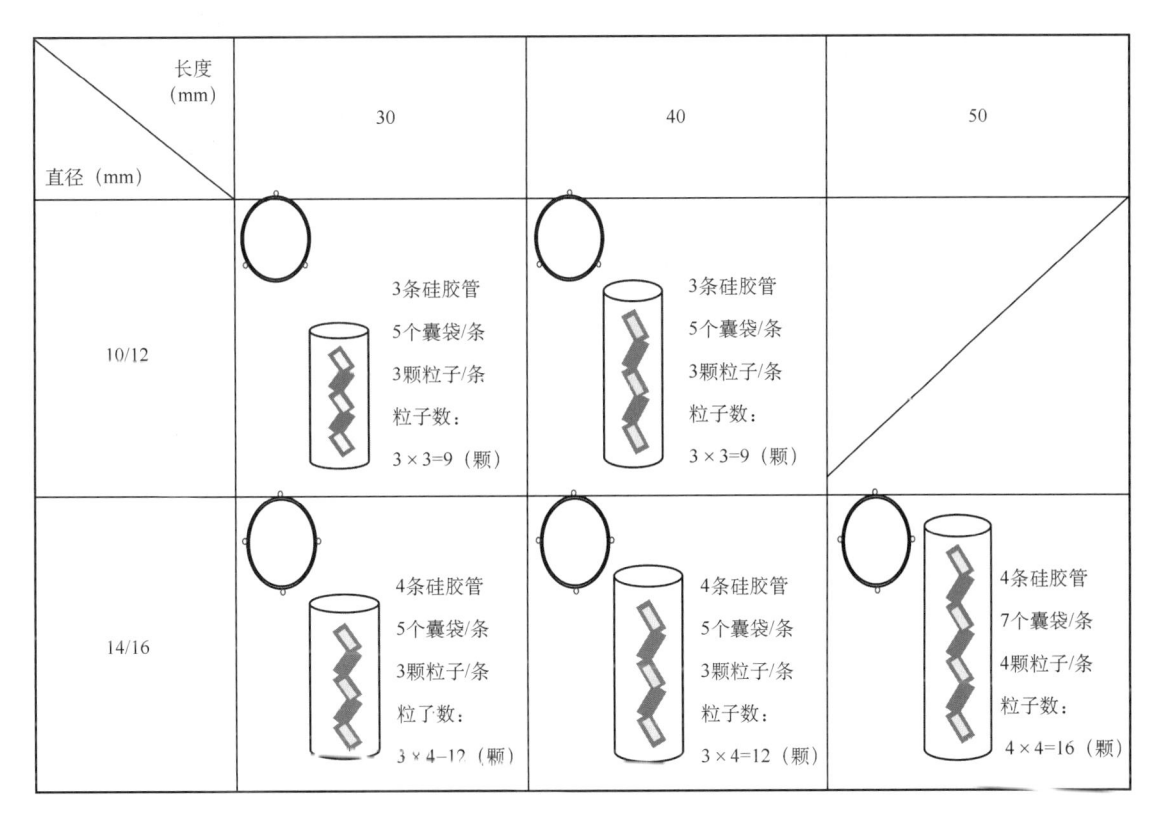

长度(mm) 直径(mm)	30	40	50
10/12	3条硅胶管 5个囊袋/条 3颗粒子/条 粒子数： 3×3=9（颗）	3条硅胶管 5个囊袋/条 3颗粒子/条 粒子数： 3×3=9（颗）	
14/16	4条硅胶管 5个囊袋/条 3颗粒子/条 粒子数： 3×4=12（颗）	4条硅胶管 5个囊袋/条 3颗粒子/条 粒子数： 3×4=12（颗）	4条硅胶管 7个囊袋/条 4颗粒子/条 粒子数： 4×4=16（颗）

图 11-9-15　支架选择及粒子

一例肺恶性肿瘤累及左、右主支气管导致左、右主气管狭窄的患者，在支气管镜介入治疗下左、右主支气管分别置入了带粒子金属支架。术后患者短期内在行支气管镜检查，发现金属支架腔内可见多量白色坏死物，给予支气管镜下清理后官腔通畅。之后患者未接受其他抗肿瘤治疗（无法耐受）。3个月后复查，患者左右主支气管腔内金属支架在位，官腔通畅。该例带粒子支架置入达到了预期的治疗效果和目的（图 11-9-16）。

此外，我们还在肺器官模型、功能支气管镜等方面进行着创新探索。可以说面对层出不穷的临床问题，我们的创新点无处不在，尤其在呼吸介入诊治技术领域，可以说近年来呼吸介入技术飞速发展，正是基于临床医学家与医学工程学家们的创新性实践。

创新有多种方式，包括模仿他人的引进吸收、基于启发的跟踪创新及自主创造的引领创新。创新可以发生在技术方法领域，设备材料领域。创新需要充分的时间去思考，需要知识产权的保障去激发，需要名誉、利益的保障去激励。创新还需要研究、转化和生产的平台，让创新型的临床人才去发现问题提出解决方案、让创新型的工程人才去解决问题、最终通过生产人员来实现创新。归根结底，对临床医师来说，只有保持一颗在临床工作中一旦发现问题，一定要解决问题的初心，保持耐心，坚定信心，才能实现创新。

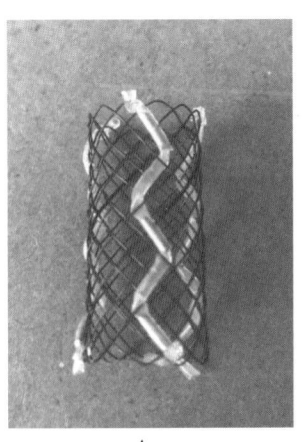

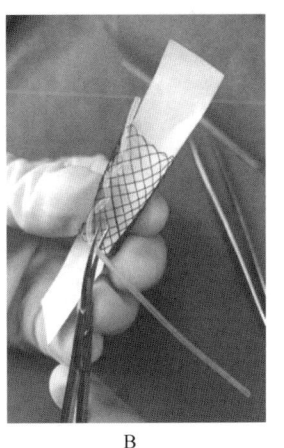

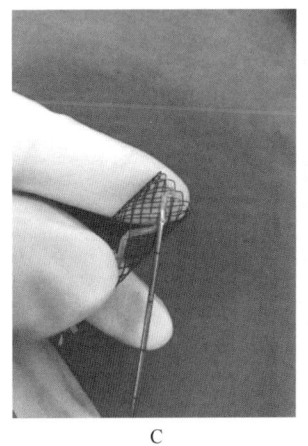

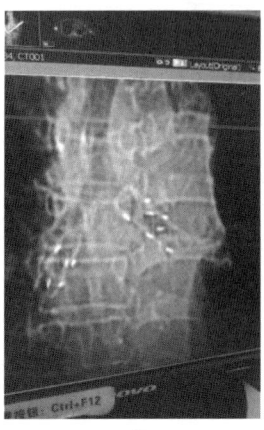

A　　　　B　　　　C　　　　D

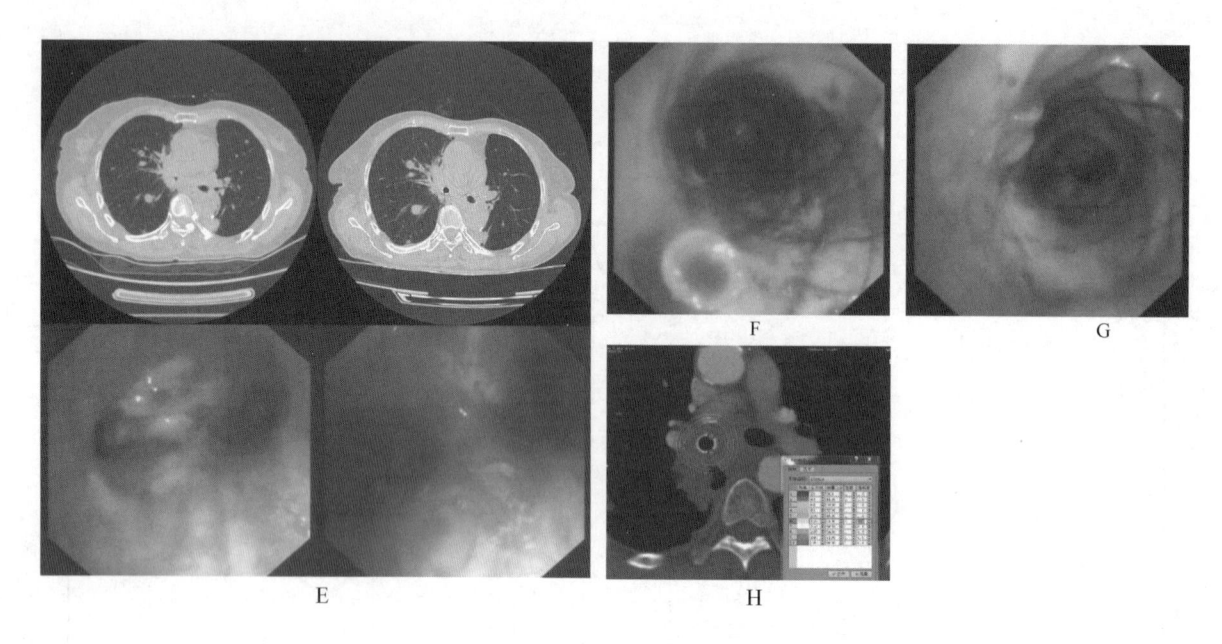

图 11-9-16 带粒子支架

参 考 文 献

[1] Na Zhu, Dingyu Zhang, Wenling Wang. A Novel Cornavirus from Patients with Pneumomia in China, 2019, THE NEJM, 2020.

[2] Qun Li, Xuhua Guan, Peng Wu. Early Transmission Dynamics in Wuhan, China, of Novel Coronavirus-Infected Pneumonia. THE NEJM, 2020.

[3] Herth FJ, Becker HD, Ernst A. Ultrasound-Guided Transbronchial Needle Aspiration: an Experience In 242 Patients. Chest, 2003, 123: 604-607.

[4] Herth FJ, Becker HD, Ernst A. Conventional vs Endobronchial Ultrasound-Guided Transbronchial Needle Aspiration: a Randomized Trial. Chest, 2004, 125: 322-325.

[5] Ono R, Suemasu K, Matsunaga T. Bronchoscopic Ultrasonography in The Diagnosis of Lung Cancer. Jpn J Clin Oncol, 1993, 23: 34-40.

10 人工智能-快速现场评估场景的研发及应用

张 新

组织活检是诸多呼吸系统疾病诊断和鉴别诊断的关键。其中支气管镜活检应用最广泛，其次是经皮肺穿刺活检。但这些活检并不能保证很高的阳性率，尽管应用多种导航技术，支气管镜对肺外周病灶活检的阳性率只有60%～80%，TBNA也经常存在取样不足的问题，而当病理报告显示阴性结果时，患者不得不接受再次活检，既增加了患者痛苦，又耗费医疗资源。现场快速病理评估技术(Rapid On-site Evaluation，简称ROSE)可以在5～10 min快速反馈活检初步病理结果，有提高活检阳性率、减少重复活检次数、优化标本后续检测流程等作用，是气管镜活检操作重要的辅助手段。ROSE技术也可用于其它各种诊断性介入操作，如肺穿刺、胰腺穿刺等。

ROSE技术的开展离不开病理医师的现场支持，然而受限于我国病理师生资源严重不足，注册病理医生仅1万多人，缺口高达4万～9万人，因此ROSE技术的临床应用推广受到极大限制。一些呼吸科医师经短期培训从事ROSE判断工作，但毕竟难以达到病理专业医师的水准。

近几年人工智能(artificial intelligence，AI)技术在国内外得到快速发展，通过深度学习，对细胞病理图像识别的准确性逐步靠拢临床应用的需求。将人工智能图像识别技术应用于组织活检的快速现场评估场景(AI-ROSE)，很有可能解决到现场病理医师不足的问题，而且通过大量数据的训练，人工智能判断的准确性和速度有可能超过低年资病理医师。为此，我们提出了开发AI-ROSE机器的构想，并与上海杏脉信息科技有限公司开展合作开发研究，目前已开发出染色的病理涂片显微扫描、良恶性AI判断、恶性区域自动定位的AI-ROSE一体机，即将开展前瞻性临床验证工作。

AI-ROSE研发内容包括细胞病理的数字化、病理类型的标注、类似显微镜视野小图的AI识别、对整张病理扫描片的AI识别、AI识别的扩展和泛化性研究等。AI识别包括良恶性的判断、病理亚型的判断、标本量是否足够的判断等，其核心在于良、恶性细胞病理的准确判断。

我们首先选择了约300例支气管镜活检时制作印片行ROSE人工判断的病例，包括EBUS-TBNA、TBB、TBLB等多种活检方式，参照组织病理诊断结果，标记扫描小图近万张。这些图片按良、恶性二分类进行深度学习，通过不断优化算法，最终在测试集中达到AI诊断AUC98%。扩大病例，将恶性病例细分为鳞癌、腺癌、小细胞癌、NSCLC-NOS、其他恶性肿瘤等亚型，AI判断等AUC也达95%以上。通过优化算法，基于病例的AI判断准确性也得到了提高，对162例独立测试集病例的对照研究显示，高年资脱落细胞病理医师、低年资病理医师、AI-ROSE判断的准确性分别为95%、91%、88%，AI-ROSE与低年资医师的准确性无显著性差异，而且该组医师有大比例不确定性诊断报告，包括将恶性报告为见异形细胞、恶性可能等，AI-ROSE的判断却非常明确。使用不同的扫描仪和扫描参数测试，本研究结果基本能够重复，反映了该AI算法有良好的泛化性。当然，扫描与AI识别整合在一起形成一体机，则更有利于控制扫描条件，提高判断的稳定性，也增加了临床应用的便利性。

AI研究涉及的医学场景已不少，但落地困难是一个问题：一般病理影像AI识别的准确性达到90%～95%并不很难，但达到99%以上就非常困难，而病理诊断要求99%以上准确性毫不为过，故而AI病理诊断还有很长的路要走。AI-ROSE这一应用场景落实到临床和商业应用有一个独特可行性优点，ROSE只是反馈给操作医师标本量是否足够、初步诊断的辅助技术，文献报道病理医师ROSE病理诊断与最终组织诊断的一致率经常在80%～90%，因此AI-ROSE被临床实践所接受的难度并不高，易于落地应用。而且，AI-ROSE并不排斥临床医师的判断，它快速显示恶性区域、显示AI判断恶性的概率，这都有可能辅助临床医师提高判断的准确性。通过增加病例数量，相信AI-ROSE判断多种良恶性病理亚型的能力将不断提高。

总之，本研发工作显示AI-ROSE有潜力成为不依赖于现场病理医师、有临床应用价值的AI设备，其判断准确性不亚于低年资病理医师，其临床应用有利于ROSE技术的更广泛开展，提高活检工作质量。

11 肺结节工作室建设与运行

郭述良

根据 2018 年世界肿瘤筛查,肺癌为发生率及死亡率最高的恶性肿瘤。肺癌恶性程度高,预后差。早期肺癌患者 5 年术后生存率可高达 90% 以上,而我国,约 75% 的肺癌患者在诊断时已属晚期,5 年生存率仅为 15.6%;我国肺癌防治经济负担现状严峻,据统计,2015 年我国肺癌医疗总费用高达 243.1 亿元,约为卫生总费用的 0.6%。早诊、早治率低为其重要原因。而早期肺癌通常表现为无症状性肺结节,在多项大型肺癌检查试验中,肺结节的检出高达 50.9%,根据美国国家肺部筛查试验研究(National Lung Screening Trial Research Team, NLST)的数据,经过 3 轮的低剂量 CT 筛查后,肺癌高危人群总体死亡率降低了 20%。然而,由于特异性较低,其假阳性率高达 96.4%。而传统肿瘤标志物对早期肺癌的敏感性及特异性不足。同时目前研究较热门的如外周血循环异常细胞、甲基化、外周循环肿瘤细胞检测等液态活检对肺结节的辅助定性能力有限,而且价格较高,亦不能满足肺结节患者的实际需要,因此,很多肺结节患者反复多次科室就诊,病例资料散乱,诊疗流程复杂,缺乏个体化诊治意见,以致过度诊治或误诊漏诊。因此,怎样跟踪和整合患者就诊信息,掌握肺结节的发展演变规律,做到对肺结节的早诊早治,是提高早期肺癌诊治的关键。

随着大数据时代的到来,利用科技化、信息化的技术对患者进行精细化管理已成为未来医学发展的热潮。根据健康中国 2030 计划,对于肺癌实施慢性病综合防控战略,强化早筛早诊早治、分级诊疗医联体建设、信息化智能化管理及健康知识宣教,以提高肺癌的早期精准诊治。基于目前我国肺癌诊治严峻的形势及在国家政府的统筹下,2019 年重庆医科大学附属第一医院重庆市肺结节管理工作室作为首批重庆市中青年医学高端后备人才工作室成立,开启了肺结节全程管理新模式。

重庆市肺结节管理工作室是以人工智能影像早筛为基础,4D 呼吸介入(经气道、经胸、经肺血管、经食管)微创技术为特色,多学科或远程专家 MDT 会诊,患者全程智能跟踪管理的肺结节精准诊治一体化中心。本中心与国际、国内先进水平接轨,通过对肺结节患者全程数据规范化管理,为患者提供个体化健康知识、智能随访、大数据跟踪,实现肺结节早诊早治与精准诊治。

一、肺结节工作室的建设

(一)平台建设

1. 肺结节全程管理数据库平台　纳入肺结节患者人口统计学资料、临床信息、影像、实验室、病理检查、诊断/治疗/随访信息、疗效评价、不良事件、经济负担、生命周期等全程资料,并建立部分患者标本库、样本库,记录 MDT 会诊意见及标记临床或者科研关注患者。

2. 肺结节人工智能分析平台　将人工智能(AI)纳入肺结节全程管理过程,通过 AI 自动化分析初步对肺结节进行良、恶性及病理预判,辅助肺结节临床决策。

3. 肺结节多学科会诊平台　工作室与放射科、核医学科、肿瘤科、胸外科、病理科、分子中心、表观遗传学中心等科室组成的 MDT 团队,建立了一个"1+X"工作室院内合作平台,以分子基础支撑临床,全面协作,对疑难病例患者提出个体化诊治方案。

4. 肺结节远程会诊平台　实现了与其他医院的双向会诊,通过线上病例分享及交流,解决了肺结节患者远程就诊问题,也有利于带动并提高区域医院对肺结节的诊治能力(图 11-11-1)。

5. 国际/国内合作平台　作为西部地区第一家中国肺癌联盟肺结节诊疗分中心,牵头及带动了西部多家医院建立了肺结节管理工作室,并建立了长期学术合作关系,并与世界著名呼吸介入诊疗中心——德国海德堡大学胸科医院建立战略合作平台,与国际接轨。

(二)团队建设

由重庆市卫生健康委员会主管,组建了一支 12 个多学科诊疗、管理、研究和教学培训专家团队。

1. 科内团队　由郭述良科主任牵头,以气道、经胸、经肺血管、经食管组成的 4D 呼吸介入微创技术全面覆盖,实现现代、可视、多方位辅助肺部疾病诊治。

(1)经气道:普通气管镜、超声气管镜、导航气管镜、支气管冷冻肺活检等;

(2)经胸:CT 引导下经皮穿刺肺活检;

(3)经肺血管:肺血管介入;

(4)经食管:食管超声。

2. 院内团队　呼吸科、放射科、核医学科、肿瘤科、胸外科、病理科、分子中心、表观遗传学中心等科室组成的 MDT 团队,从分子基础到临床全面解剖肺结节。

3. 国内团队 与复旦大学附属中山医院呼吸内科主任白春学教授合作,成立了中国肺癌防治联盟重医医院肺结节诊治分中心。

4. 国际团队 为德国海德堡大学胸科医院签署战略合作医院。

(三)管理机制建设:系列流程及制度,确保规范运行(图11-11-2)

内部人员管理制度:博士7人,硕士1人,每月集中学习并汇报科研进展情况,确切落实并负责如下工作:肺结节注册登记管理及随访;肺结节人工智能分析;肺结节多学科会诊;肺结节远程会诊;肺结节科研与教学;临床信息数据库及组织标本库建设。

二、科学技术

(一)信息化、智能化云服务

包括:以人群精准分类模型为基础以智能引擎为驱动实现患者诊后个性化管理;自动跟踪随访任务执行;患者诊后不失联,全方位提升患者服务感知;实现复诊管理闭环。

(二)科技合作——医工合作、医企合作

1. 与信息技术有限公司合作开发(肺结节全程管理数据库),一体化全程追踪并记录患者肺结节演变,诊治流程及后期随访等。

2. 肺结节人工智能分析系统、MDT远程会诊软件:辅助临床决策,协助提高早期肺癌早诊、早治率,并为患者就诊提供便捷。

三、医学核心实力

传统经支气管活检术(TBLB)诊断价值与病灶大小有关,价值有限,诊断效能低下。

对于恶性病变,诊断率20%~84%;对于良性病变,诊断率35%~56%;对于直径<2cm外周结节,诊断率14%~31%。

(一)建立了现代、可视、微创、快速的肺结节精准活检诊断技术

1. 导航+径向超声引导下的肺结节精准活检技术

(1)导航支气管镜:分为电磁导航支气管镜(ENB)和虚拟导航支气管镜:为近年来最先进的支气管技术,根据术前完成的胸部CT进行术中路线设定,根据导航引导的支气管进入病变部位取材,使传统气管镜无法检查到的周围肺组织病变的检测成为现实,进一步提高了对周围肺结节的诊断效力。

(2)超声支气管镜:支气管内超声引导下肺活检术(EBUS-TBLB)在常规支气管镜基础上能在术中实时进行支气管超声检测,使病灶清晰可见。对肺结节的诊断能力高于常规支气管镜。

(3)超细支气管镜+径向超声+C形臂机:可以到达更远端病灶,进一步提高对周围性病变诊断的阳性率。

ROSE:快速现场评价,逐渐覆盖至我科所有内镜检查及其他活检方式。

优势:确保活检质量;肺癌、结核等的快速诊断;减少活检次数、时间、并发症;并指导标本合理分流。

2. 在国内率先建立了肺结节的经支气管冷冻肺活检技术-大样本取样技术。

经支气管冷冻肺活检(transbronchial cryobiopsy,TB-CB)是将冷冻探头经支气管伸入远端小支气管,利用冷冻探头在冷冻过程中的黏附性,将探头周围的肺组织暴力撕裂,获得组织学标本的一项技术。

优势:TBCB具有创伤小、标本大且质量高、并发症少。

3. CT引导下疑难高风险肺小结节经皮穿刺活检术,在国内呼吸界居一流水平,西部领先。

CT引导下经皮穿刺活检:术中通过CT对病灶定位,确定穿刺点、穿刺深度、角度,精准取材,对外周性肺结节的诊断具有较高的效能。实现了对肺结节的精准取样和快速诊断。

(二)快捷精准微创诊疗一体化平台肺结节

射频消融:射频消融(radiofrequency ablation,RFA)是应用消融电极,在超声、CT引导下经皮穿刺,或者在手术过程中、胸腔镜下,使射频电极进入实体肿瘤组织,然后在消融电极针前端伸展出9个锚形细电极丝,插入到肿瘤组织中,通过射频输出,使病变区组织细胞离子震荡摩擦产生热量,局部温度达90℃以上,通过加热的温度来杀灭肿瘤组织病变组织发生凝固性坏死,最终形成液化灶或纤维化组织,同时实时调节监控温度,从而达到局部消除肿瘤组织的目的。

适应证包括:

1. 肺原发癌

(1)高龄、心肺功能差,不能耐受外科手术的早期肺癌;

(2)拒绝外科手术的早期肺癌;

(3)早期肺癌外科或SBRT后孤立转移多原发癌;

(4)多原发癌,≤3个,最大直径≤3cm,没有证据表明淋巴结或远处转移;

(5)全身治疗后局部复发的单个病灶;

(6)单肺单病灶。

2. 肺转移癌

(1)转移至肺部的原发癌具有相对良好的生物学特征;

(2)原发癌控制较好,单侧肺部转移数目≤3个,最大直径≤3cm,或单个转移<5cm,没有其他脏器转移。

实施流程:AI恶性概率分析→CT引导穿刺活检→ROSE现场快速诊断→现场经皮经胸射频/微波消融。

建立肺结节的Hook-wire定位技术帮助胸外科和病理科术中和术后精准、快速找到肺结节。

四、制定了肺结节精准处置流程（图11-11-1）

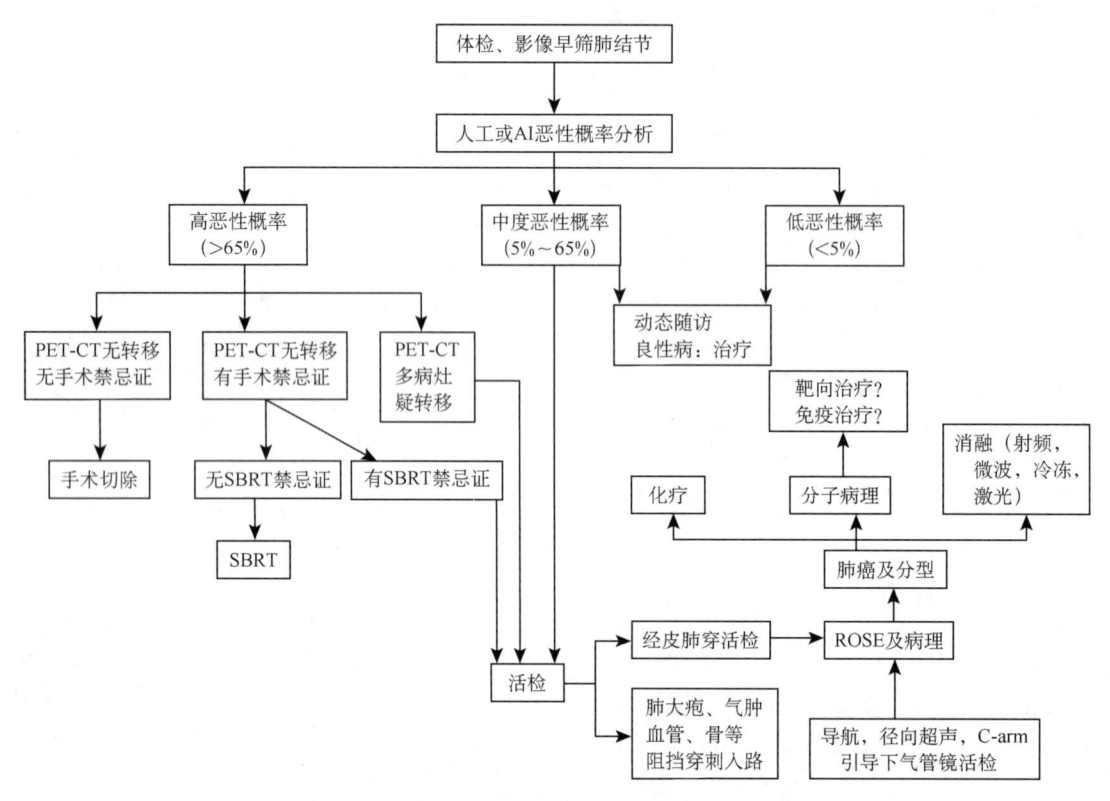

图11-11-1 肺结节精准处置流程图

五、肺结节就诊绿色通道

1. 患者持肺结节专病门诊＋普通门诊就诊卡→肺结节工作室（登记，影像学阅片，AI分析，知识宣教，并给与下一步诊治方案）。

2. 患者复诊CT后→肺结节工作室。

肺结节就诊绿色通道大大提升了肺结节患者就诊的便捷性。

参 考 文 献

[1] Freddie Bray, BSc, MSc, et al. Global Cancer Statistics 2018: GLOBOCAN Estimates of Incidence and Mortality Worldwide for 36 Cancers in 185 Countries. CA: Cancer J Clin, 2018, 68: 394-424.

[2] MMurakami S, Ito H, Tsubokawa N, et al. Prognostic value of the new IASLC/ATS/ERS classification of clinical stage IA lung adenocarcinoma. Lung Cancer, 2015, 90(2): 199-204.

[3] 中华医学会呼吸病学分会肺癌学组 中国肺癌防治联盟专家组.肺部结节诊治中国专家共识.中华结核和呼吸杂志，2015, 38(4): 249-255.

[4] 蔡玥, 严宝湖, 周恭伟. 2011-2015年中国肺癌直接经济负担及次均费用分析. 中国卫生统计, 2018.

[5] Field JK, Duffy SW, Baldwin DR, et al. UK Lung Cancer RCT Pilot Screening Trial: baseline findings from the screening arm provide evidence for the potential implementation of lung cancer screening. Thorax, 2016, 71: 161-170.

[6] van Klaveren RJ, Oudkerk M, Prokop M, et al. Management of lung nodules detected by volume CT scanning. N Engl J Med, 2009, 361: 2221-2229.

[7] Denise R, Aberle, et al. National Lung Screening Trial Research Team. Reduced Lung-Cancer Mortality with Low-Dose Computed Tomographic Screening. N Engl J Med, 2011, 365: 395-409.

[8] Libby, Daniel M, et al. Managing the small pulmonary nodule discovered by CT. Chest, 2004, 125(4): 1522-1529.

[9] Walid A, Baaklini, Mauricio A, et al. Diagnostic yield of fiberoptic bronchoscopy in evaluating solitary pulmonary nodules. Chest, 2000, 117(4): 1049-1054.

[10] Ye, et al. Guidelines for thermal ablation of primary and metastatic lung tumors. Journal of Cancer Research and Therapeutics, 2018.

[11] Expert consensus workshop report: Guidelines for thermal ablation of primary and metastatic lung tumors Journal of Cancer Research and Therapeutics, 2018.

12 活瓣肺减容的患者选择和并发症的处理

李 明 王昌惠

自本世纪初以来,内科肺减容技术得以迅速发展并不断完善,一方面得益于手术的疗效,另一方面,更重要的是,手术的安全性相较外科肺减容术(LVRS)大大提高。

在内科肺减容术广泛运用之前,重度肺气肿患者多采用外科手术治疗。NETT 研究是针对外科肺减容最经典的研究,共纳入 1218 名晚期肺气肿患者,比较外科肺减容手术和单纯内科治疗的疗效。研究发现以非上叶病变为主和高运动能力的患者不能从手术中获益,反而有死亡风险增大的可能,这一类患者没有体现出比内科治疗更多的获益。随后的研究也进一步明确了外科肺减容术的局限性:①手术创伤大,术后并发症多,如术后漏气等并发症发生率高,占术后患者的 40%~50%;②手术费用高,住院时间长;③肺功能恢复是以短期死亡率升高为代价的;④手术的远期疗效尚不肯定。因此当内科肺减容技术表现出良好的疗效和并不严重的并发症后,人们开始不断开展临床研究来完善内科肺减容的技术和适应证。

下面要着重讨论常见的内科肺减容技术患者的选择和并发症及其处理。支气管镜介入医师一方面要有过硬的操作技术,另外一方面要掌握内科肺减容技术的并发症及其处理。这有利于我们选择合适的患者,更好的理解手术原理和操作。因此对于内科肺减容术的并发症需要深入理解,充分认识,全面评估,合理应对。

一、活瓣肺减容患者的选择

目前应用最广的支气管内活瓣是由 Emphasys 公司(Emphasys Redwood City,CA,USA)生产的,其第一代为 Emphasys EBV,是硅酮镍钛合金的圆柱形结构,内有一硅酮鸭嘴样单向活瓣。后 Emphasys EBV 外形改为近端大,远端小的多边形柱状结构,中心为鸭嘴样单向活瓣,称为 Zephyr EBV。Zephyr EBV 在欧洲已经批准临床应用于治疗严重肺气肿,我国也已于 2010 年获得批准,目前在国内多家医院应用于临床治疗。

此外,Spiration IBV 活瓣(Olympus,Inc,Japan)也较为常见,其近端是被覆薄膜的镍钛记忆合金伞形结构,中心有金属杆便于活检钳取出,远端有 5 个带钩尖的固定锚可将活瓣固定在支气管壁上,避免活瓣移位。吸气时伞形结构撑开阻塞气流进入远端气道,呼气时气流自伞形结构与气道壁之间的缝隙排出,并可排出远端气道分泌物。

新近研发的 Miyazawa 活瓣(Novatech,France)为硅酮单向活瓣,远端为一环形结构,利于活瓣的放置和调整位置,近端是一单向活瓣,可呼气时排出气道远端气体,活瓣侧面设计了多个小凸起以利于活瓣固定在气道内,整个活瓣没有金属材料,避免了对气道的损伤。尚需要更多数据和研究评价 Miyazawa EBV 的疗效和安全性。

合理的患者选择往往对最终疗效起着至关重要的影响。除肺功能的要求外,大多数学者认为不均质肺气肿及完整的叶间裂是肺减容术成败及临床疗效的关键。美国和欧洲的研究数据支持活瓣减容成功的两个共同的评价条件是:靶肺叶被 EBV 完全封闭,确保没有气体从临近部位通向终末气道;完全的叶间裂,也就是靶肺叶和相邻肺叶间没有旁路通气。高分辨 CT 能较为准确的评估叶间裂的完整性,然而若有怀疑应行 Chartis 检测进一步明确。

与传统外科减容术类似,以肺上叶病变为主的非均质性小叶中心性肺气肿患者和低运动能力的肺气肿患者能从手术中获益。但近年来的资料提示以下几点值得注意:残气量和侧支通气量是最重要的纳入标准,也有学者认为无论是均质或非均质性肺气肿患者,只要够耐受的治疗过程和任何潜在的并发症,都可考虑活瓣肺减容治疗。

根据国内外的临床病例报道和循证医学研究,支气管内单向活瓣肺减容术疗的适应证为:

1. 诊断为重度或极重度 COPD 的患者,经过戒烟、规范内科药物治疗 3 个月后,运动耐力仍然明显下降者。

2. 年龄<80 岁。

3. FEV1 15%~45% 预计值,TLC>100% 预计值,RV>150% 预计值。

4. 胸部 CT 为显著的非均质性肺气肿,且叶间裂完整(无旁路通气)。

5. 静息状态下呼吸室内空气时,血气分析 $PaCO_2$<50 mmHg(1 mmHg = 0.133 kPa),PaO_2>45 mmHg。

6. 康复治疗后 6MWT≥140 m。

7. 戒烟 4 个月以上。

另外结合我们的实践经验,以下几点需引起大家的重视:患者的叶间裂需完整;如有陈旧结核,纤维条索等,容易发生气胸;目前对部分内容仍有争议,如目前认为均质型也可获益,故已不再强调必须为非均质型。

以下情况应视为禁忌证。

1. 绝对禁忌证

(1)置入心脏起搏器、除颤器等其他电子设备的患者。

(2)急性心肌梗死 6 周以内。

(3)严重心肺疾病无法进行支气管镜操作患者。

(4)麻醉药物过敏,无法实施支气管镜者。

(5)无法纠正的出凝血功能障碍者。

(6)已完成 BT 治疗的患者。

(7)康复治疗后 6MWT<140 m。

(8)一氧化碳弥散量(DLCO)≤20% 预计值。

(9)需呼吸机辅助呼吸,或静息状态下需持续吸氧(吸氧浓度≥6L/min)以维持 SaO_2 >90% 者。

(10)巨大肺大疱。

(11)$α_1$-抗胰蛋白酶缺乏症。

(12)曾进行开胸手术者。

(13)痰多、各种感染活动期。

2. 相对禁忌证

(1)因其他疾患未停用抗凝药物或抗血小板药物者;

(2)哮喘未能控制导致肺功能损害严重者;

(3)既往有致死性哮喘发作者;

(4)未控制的其他合并症。

为保证患者治疗安全性和有效性,在术前还需进行全面的评估。

(1)症状、用药规范及依从性。

(2)呼吸困难程度、肺功能状况、BODE、6min 步行距离。肺功能是评估手术风险和安全性的重要检查。但重度降低的 FEV1 并非绝对禁忌证。

(3)合并症及手术风险评估:合并疾病如糖尿病、冠心病等,是评估手术风险的重要因素,必要时评估心功能水平(如超声心动图检查或心肌酶、血清脑钠肽等),并应做好相应的围术期处理预案。

(4)HRCT:主要是判断肺部是否存在其他疾病和结构性异常,以及判断非均质性肺气肿的程度,叶间裂的完整性,帮助选择靶肺叶。

(5)判断非均质性肺气肿需要进行定量 CT,计算各肺叶肺气肿百分数。应选择肺气肿百分数最高,与同侧相邻肺叶肺气肿百分数差值最大的肺叶作为目标肺叶。目标肺叶与同侧相邻肺叶间的叶间裂完整性需做高分辨 CT,并从横轴面、矢状面和冠状面判断叶间裂完整性,即在至少 1 个薄层 CT 扫描轴位层面上显示 90% 以上的叶间裂,可认为叶间裂完整。如果多个肺叶符合上述严重肺气肿标准,应做肺灌注扫描,选择相对低灌注肺叶为治疗目标肺叶。目前多不推荐单独仅做右中叶肺减容,因为相对其他肺叶,右中叶容积小,即使完全阻塞气道出现肺不张,邻近肺叶复张对整体肺功能影响较小,难以显著改善患者的运动耐力和生活质量。

(6)术前对患者行充分告知和宣教,术前按常规支气管镜检查完善相关血常规、凝血、乙肝、梅毒、HIV、心电图等检查,测量生命体征,做好术前评估;术前向患者及其家属讲解 BLVR 的手术必要性和手术风险,做好心理护理,减少紧张恐惧心理;均签署经支气管镜单向活瓣减容术知情同意书。

(7)常规气管镜检查术前准备和术中心电生命征监测,根据情况可选用局部麻醉结合镇静和镇痛、静脉全身麻醉等方式。患者接受了纤维支气管镜检查、靶气道直径测量,选择相应直径大小的活瓣置入。

尽管在术前进行了仔细的选择和全面的评估,患者仍有可能出现一些并发症,如何处理并发症,也是治疗成功的关键。

二、支气管活瓣肺减容术的并发症及处理

支气管活瓣肺减容引起的并发症主要包括肺炎、COPD 急性加重、气胸、活瓣移位等。2014 年 IBV Valve trial 入选 142 例治疗组和 135 例对照组。研究中没有发生活瓣移位、咳瓣或严重的器械相关性肺炎。没有发生严重的与器械有关的不良事件。与对照组(n = 5 或 3.7%)相比,治疗组中 SAE 明显增加(n = 20,14.1%)。对 SAE 的分析显示,没有一种类型的事件导致两组差异。共发生 28 次 SAE(治疗组 20 例,对照组 5 例),其中 19 次为非手术或器械相关。6 次 SAE 是程序相关的,3 次被认为是设备相关的。3 个设备相关事件是与完全闭塞治疗相关的气胸。在 5 例治疗患者中发生的 6 次与程序有关的 SAE,包括 2 次 COPD 加重,2 次呼吸衰竭,1 例次死亡,1 次支气管痉挛。在所有不良事件(包括中度和轻度事件)中,57% 的治疗组和 48% 的对照组发生在手术后的前 4 周内。

(一)肺炎

1. 发生率 VENT 研究报道活瓣肺减容术后 90d 肺炎的发生率,治疗组为 4.7%,对照组为 2.0%。其中活瓣靶叶肺炎发生率 1.9%,非靶叶肺炎的发生率为 2.8%,与对照组 2.0% 相仿。

2. 原因 活瓣靶叶肺炎的发生与活瓣植入及气管镜在局部操作相关。而非靶叶肺炎的发生可能与手术操作相关,也可能与本身患者肺功能较差、呼吸道粘膜功能减退、容易继发细菌感染相关。

3. 临床表现 Snell 等在 2003 年首次报道支气管活瓣(EBV)肺减容用于肺气肿患者的队列研究。在 30 d 的研究期内没有发现重大的危及生命的并发症。第 37 天 1 例患者发生肺炎,需要使用抗生素并住院 10 d。2014 年 IBV Valve trial 中,活瓣治疗位置仅有 3 例(2.1%)发生肺炎,无严重肺炎发生。在非活瓣位置共有 26 例肺炎发生,前 4 周发生 6 例(23%)。发生严重肺炎 3 次,其中对照组 2 次。

4. 治疗 活瓣肺减容术后肺炎的治疗多为手术或者活瓣相关肺炎,抗感染治疗应着重覆盖 G^- 杆菌,同时加强化痰治疗。雾化吸入糖皮质激素和支气管扩张剂对肺炎的吸收消散也有一定的帮助。

5. 预防 ①选择患者病情稳定和一般情况相对较好的时机进行手术。②术前术后应该加强雾化治疗。③术中应减少肌松药物的使用。④手术操作时间应尽可能不超过 1h。⑤对于预计可能出现肺炎的患者,术前可考虑预防性使用抗生素。

(二)COPD 急性加重(AECOPD)

1. 发生率 2014 年 IBV Valve trial 中,最常见的不良事件是慢性阻塞性肺疾病(COPD)急性加重。与对照组相比,0~4 周时,治疗组(44 例)在支气管镜检查后 COPD 急

性加重发生率更高。而第5~24周,治疗组与对照组比较,COPD急性加重没有差异(治疗组51例,对照组41例,$P=0.45$)。

Snell等在2003年还报道手术后第11天,1例患者出现感染诱发COPD加重,另1例患者在第21天出现感染诱发COPD加重。1例患者出现少量、无症状的气胸,经简单的吸氧治疗好转。在随后的243 d的随访中,发现另外两例因感染诱发COPD急性加重。未出现咳嗽增加、活瓣移位和呼吸衰竭等并发症。这一研究促进了活瓣肺减容技术的临床运用。

在VENT等RCT研究中统计COPD急性加重的发生率,手术组19.7%,对照组20.5%,两组没有统计学差异。

2. 原因 活瓣肺减容术后出现AECOPD,一方面与手术及麻醉应激相关,另一方面与活瓣植入后诱发的感染或者痰液引流不畅或者活瓣移位等有关。

3. 临床表现 术后AECOPD多表现为咳嗽、咳痰、气促等症状加重,如果合并感染可能出现发热甚至合并肺炎等表现。

4. 治疗 与一般的AECOPD治疗相同,治疗原则也是解痉平喘等,首选雾化吸入治疗,必要时给予静脉激素等。如果考虑细菌感染诱发,抗生素须覆盖G-杆菌。

5. 预防 ①术前术后应该加强雾化治疗。②术中应减少肌松药物的使用。③手术操作时间应尽可能不超过1h。④术后继续按照标准治疗方案治疗并坚持戒烟。

(三)气胸

1. 发生率 活瓣肺减容术后出现气胸的概率并不低,2013年单中心回顾性分析显示,活瓣肺减容气胸发生率最高可以达到23%。

自VENT研究之后,活瓣肺减容所致气胸的发生率有所上升。这可能与更加严格的患者筛选有关,因为较低的旁路通气提高了成功率,但同时也提高了气胸的发生率。

Gompelmann等纳入VENT研究的欧洲和美国亚组数据及多中心Chartis数据进行研究,共421例肺气肿患者接受EBV肺减容手术。其中26例出现气胸,发生率为6.2%。除去1例患者因活检导致气胸,真正由于EBV手术导致的气胸患者为25例,发生率为5.9%。分析气胸的位置发现,EBV放置在左下叶的情况下,气胸发生率为10.3%,其次为EBV放置在上叶(8.7%)。因此,靶叶为左肺的EBV肺减容治疗后,气胸的风险似乎较高。EBV放置后气胸发作的中位时间为2 d(0~272 d)。气胸的中位持续时间为11 d(2~73 d)。

25例患者中有17例(68%)长时间漏气7 d以上。

2. 原因 作为单向阀,活瓣设计目的,就是放置在高度膨胀而没有旁路通气的靶叶中。其目的是为了诱导靶叶的减少和改善呼吸力学,从而改善临床症状。Brown等研究表明,靶叶体积的减少部分被重新分配到同侧肺叶,只有一小部分重新分布到对侧肺。这一结果解释了为什么这些患者的总肺活量的净减少即使是在靶叶的大幅度萎缩的情况下也是适度的。在EBV治疗后,气胸的发生通常包括未治疗的同侧叶和(或)由于单向阀存在而无法再扩张的已破裂的靶叶。手术后靶叶容积减少,同侧未治疗肺在胸腔内扩张以占据新创造的空间。在某些情况下,肺的一侧的体积会迅速变化(这可能与张力变化有关),在某些情况下会撕裂已经受损的肺组织。靶叶的缩小,容积转换引起未处理的同侧叶张力改变,可能是气胸的主要危险因素,然而这一假说尚未得到正式的检验。目前在同侧非治疗的叶中肺大疱的破裂被认为是气胸最常见的原因。

另一种机制可能是由于患者本身的胸膜粘连而导致的肺叶移位和破裂。以上几种机制导致的气胸,可能引起支气管胸膜瘘。如果不进行胸管引流治疗,可能导致气胸的进一步进展。当然气胸多数情况下并不合并支气管胸膜瘘,在这种情况下,急性肺叶塌陷导致周围的负压突然增加,从周围组织和血液中产生的气体进入围绕着塌陷裂口周围的胸膜空间,而相邻叶的内部胸膜与胸膜壁层之间的密封保持完整,此时仅仅引起气胸,而不会导致支气管胸膜瘘。在这种情况下胸膜腔内的空气会随着时间的推移而自行消退,此时不需要胸管引流。最后,从理论上讲,气胸也的机制也可能是靶肺叶体积急性减少引起的气压性创伤反应,此时靶肺叶的支气管被活瓣阻塞,因此不会形成支气管胸膜瘘。这些患者的气胸量比较少,而且可以采取密切观察的策略。

3. 临床表现 少量气胸患者仅出现胸闷,气胸明显时可出现气促加重,不能平卧,血氧饱和度下降,严重者甚至血压下降。

4. 治疗 对于气胸的处理,有时需要胸导管引流,必要时支气管镜检查或视频辅助胸腔镜检查。此外,张力性气胸是一种危及生命的状况。因此,气胸的患者应留院观察48~72h。

如果气胸量少可先行观察,无须处理。如果量较大,并引起患者明显的气促和低氧血症,可先移除部分活瓣,观察气胸进展,必要时可移除全部活瓣,行胸腔闭式引流。如果是严重甚至张力性气胸,需要立即置入粗管闭式引流(慎用橡皮管或猪尾巴管等细管),病情稳定时移除活瓣,然后加强营养支持,促进破裂的肺愈合。手术并非严重气胸的首选处理方式,因为风险太大,患者有极大可能无法耐受手术或者因为术后并发症死亡。事实上针对支气管活瓣肺减容术后出现气胸的处理,已经达成共识,具体可见图11-12-1。

在VENT研究的25例患者中,21例(84%)气胸在观察或胸腔引流后解除。1例患者(4%)接受了胸腔引流,随后在同侧肺未治疗的肺叶植入2个附加活瓣进行治疗。在漏气解决之后,移除后植入的附加活瓣。在另1例患者(4%)中,胸腔引流治疗后漏气未解除,因此需要开胸手术。在1例(4%)患者中,胸腔引流、移除活瓣和胸腔镜手术均未能解决气胸,最终需要开胸手术来封堵漏气。1例患者(4%)由于气胸和并发肺炎在瓣膜植入后12 d重新住院,给予胸腔引流和抗生素治疗。在随后的过程中,发生呼吸衰竭,进一步需要机械通气和移除活瓣。经过长时间的重症监护后,取出胸管并脱机。然而,随着时间的推移,患者一般状况持续恶化,在瓣膜治疗后85 d死亡。

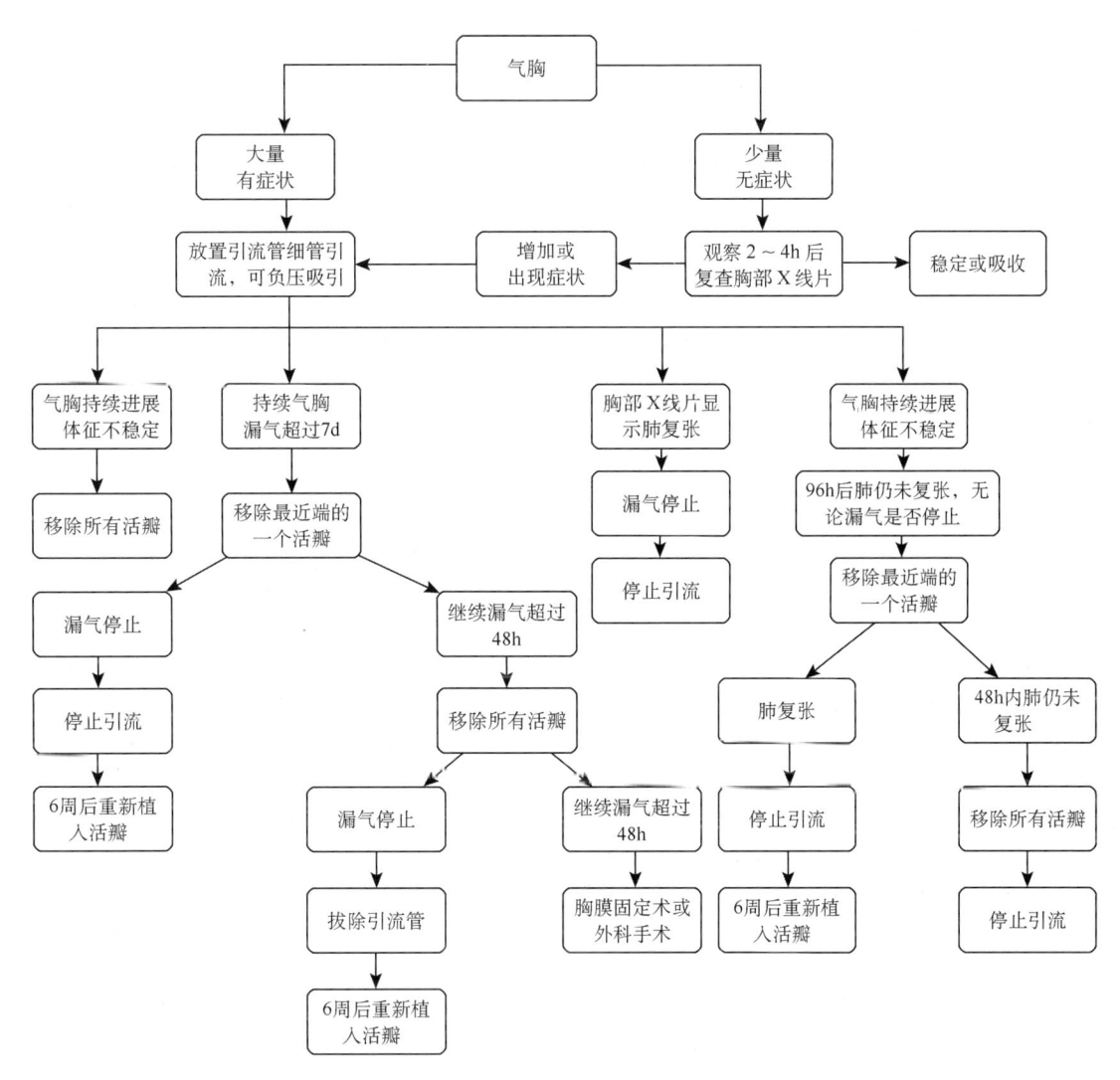

图 11-12-1 支气管活瓣肺减容术后气胸处理流程

由于治疗患者多数叶间裂完整和无旁路通气,支气管活瓣肺减容术后出现气胸可能提示患者的获益更明显。25 例发生气胸的患者中有 17 例(68%)叶间裂完整,旁路通气(CV)较少。7 例患者叶间裂不完整,剩余 1 名患者无法评估叶间裂完整性。参考总患者人数,获得以下数据:经 EBV 治疗后,叶间裂完整的患者中 10.6% 发生气胸,而叶间裂不完整的患者仅 3% 发生气胸。

20 名气胸受试者接受高分辨率 CT(HRCT)评估靶叶容积缩小百分比(TLVR)。结果表明气胸患者达到高 TLVR。在 VENT 研究欧洲亚组中,6 个月的随访后发现气胸患者平均 TLVR 高达 60%±38%。在多中心 Chartis 试验中,在 1 个月的随访中发现气胸患者平均 TLVR 为 75%±30%。总之,三项研究中 EBV 治疗后出现气胸的患者平均 TLVR 为 65%±36%。

对于叶间裂完整的 17 例患者,3 例患者无法进行 TLVR 评估。其余 14 例患者平均 TLVR 为 58.4%。7 例不完全裂隙患者中有 5 例平均 TLVR 为 41.3%。在 25 例患者中,20 例中 180 d 平均 FEV1 变化为 15%±15%,平均残气量(RV)变化为-10%±14%。因此,肺功能参数的改善,特别是呼气肺体积的减少似乎与高 TLVR 有关。在 19 名患者中,6-MWD 略有增加(平均 6 MWD 增加 2 m±50 m)。评估了 12 例患者的 SGRQ,改善了-7 分±12 分。在气胸患者中,45% 的患者在 6 个月时 FEV1 升高了 15%,58% 的患者 SGRQ 改善了 4 分。在发生气胸的患者中,18% 的患者在 6-MWD 中经历了≥15% 的改善。

因此虽然气胸是 EBV 肺减容手术的并发症,但在 FEV1 和健康相关生活质量方面似乎并不会对临床结果产生负面影响,患者反而可以获得较高的 TLVR。

(四)肺不张

1. **发生率** 肺不张的发生率一般取决于靶叶是否存在旁路通气及活瓣放置是否合适。因此各个研究报道肺不张发生率从 0%~56.5%。

2. **原因** 支气管活瓣肺减容后出现肺不张,提示靶叶没有旁路通气,并且活瓣位置良好,导致靶叶被活瓣完全阻塞引起肺不张。肺不张可能提示肺减容达到良好的疗效,甚至可能提示患者获得更好的预后。

3. **临床表现** 活瓣阻塞所致肺不张患者一般没有明显的临床症状,多数在复查 X 线胸片或 CT 等影像时发现。

如果是痰液阻塞或者感染所致肺不张,可能会出现发热、咳嗽、咳痰等症状。

4. 治疗　EBV 肺减容的数据提示术后肺不张的患者生存期更长。Hopkinson 等研究 EBV 治疗患者 19 例(其中肺不张 5 例),随访 6 年发现肺不张患者的生存率更高,无一人死亡,而无肺不张患者死亡 8 人。这一数据与两组患者的基线肺功能、生活质量、活动耐量、急性加重率和影像表现无关。二者唯一有差别的在于肺不张患者组的 BMI 更高(平均 28.4 kg/m^2)。

因此不论是手术即刻或者是延迟出现的肺不张患者,均无需过度紧张。密切观察患者的生命体征,排除过多分泌物或感染所致的阻塞后,无须特殊干预,随访即可。

对于活瓣移位的问题,一方面应该在不同的位置选择合适大小的 EBV 或 IBV 活瓣,规范操作。另一方面术后适当的镇咳治疗也是必需的。当然最重要的是术后 1 月左右,如果疗效不符合预期,可以考虑复查肺 CT 或气管镜观察活瓣位置。如果活瓣出现明显向外的移位,可考虑调整或更换活瓣(尤其是 EBV 活瓣);如果活瓣向内移位,需要判断是否有漏气,可表面注入生理盐水,观察气泡产生情况,气泡较多时需考虑更换活瓣(尤其是 IBV 活瓣)。

(五)活瓣移位

1. 发生率　活瓣植入后多数情况下都会发生一定的移位。影响肺减容疗效的移位发生率可以达到 10%。

2. 原因　IBV 活瓣因为尾部装有倒钩,活瓣可能向支气管远端移位,因此如果活瓣大小不适合近端支气管或者放置时尾部没有与远端支气管壁接触,活瓣可能进一步发生移位;EBV 主要靠周边支撑力来固定,因此更多的是向外移位,因此活瓣大小不合适近端支气管或者活瓣尾部没有支撑在合适的远端支气管分叉处,那么活瓣也可能进一步发生移位。除了活瓣本身结构的原因,术后患者剧烈咳嗽,不适当的运动,都可能导致活瓣的移位。

3. 临床表现　轻度移位不影响肺减容效果,通常无明显的临床表现。如果发生明显的移位,活瓣与支气管壁出现间隙,肺减容的效果不明显,或者患者自觉症状改善后再次回复到手术前,此时应该考虑活瓣移位可能。

4. 治疗　轻度的移位通常是无须处理的,并不会影响疗效。但是如果术前检测靶叶无旁路通气,术后 1 个月患者肺功能或者活动耐量等无改善,此时可考虑行 CT 检查,观察活瓣的位置(也有活瓣肺减容指南建议术后 1 个月如果无肺不张出现,均应行 CT 扫描观察活瓣位置),如发现活瓣与支气管间有空隙,应考虑气管镜调整或更换活瓣。

5. 预防　①针对不同的靶叶和支气管选择合适的活瓣(包括合适的大小和类型)。②进一步规范手术操作,EBV 选择合适的释放位置和 IBV 释放时选择合适的深度和角度。③术后适当镇咳治疗,适度活动。

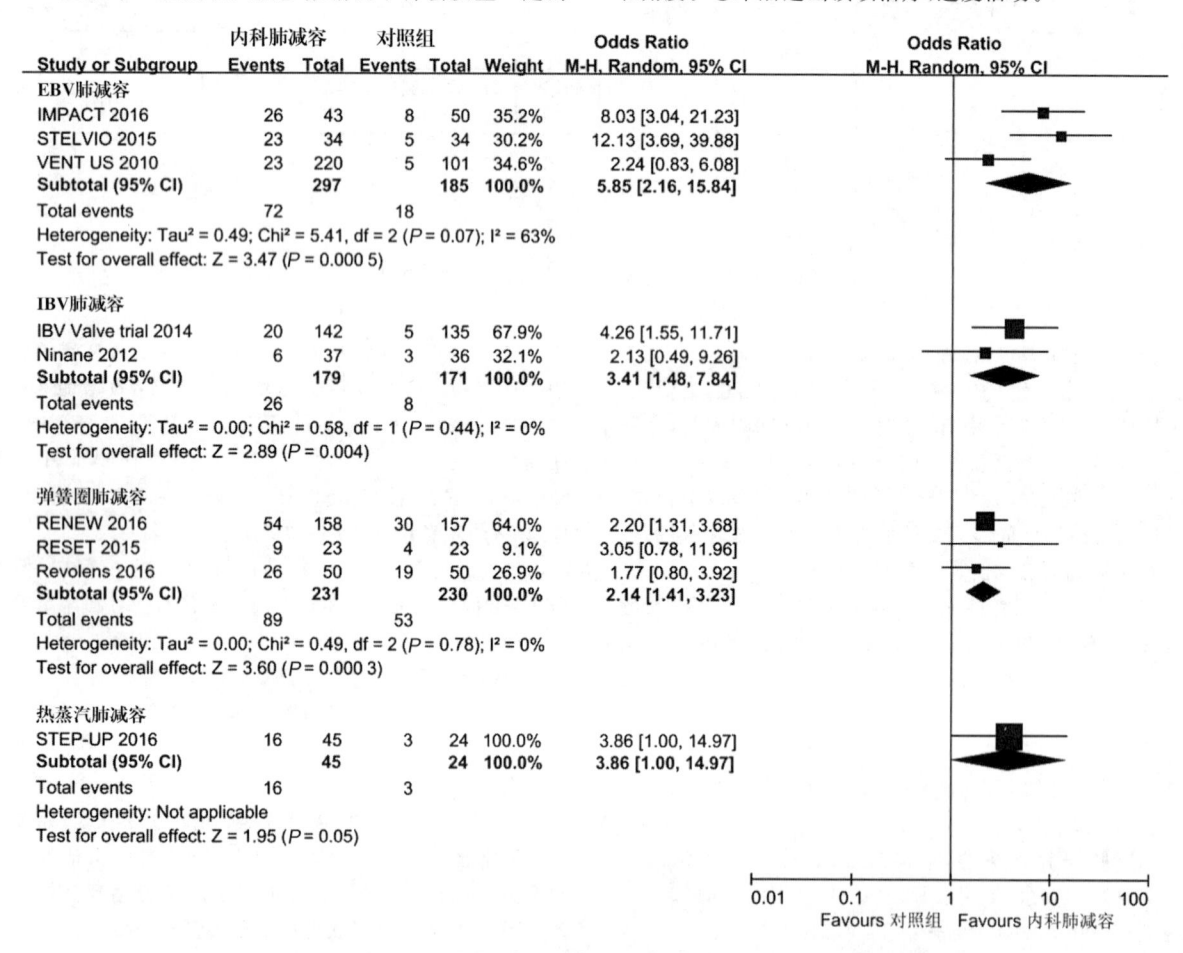

图 11-12-2　RCT 研究中,主要的内科肺减容术治疗组和对照组总体并发症的森林图

(六)死亡

1. 发生率　术后90 d死亡率,BeLieVeR为8%,IMPACT研究为0。术后12个月死亡率,VENT研究欧洲亚组为5.4%,VENT研究美国亚组为2.7%。但是所有的RCT研究治疗组和对照组的死亡率均无统计学差异。

2. 原因　①术后AECOPD,进展为呼吸衰竭导致死亡。②其他严重并发症,如胃肠道出血和多脏器功能衰竭等。

3. 临床表现　2010年,VENT研究在新英格兰杂志发表。术后90d内,EBV治疗组两例患者(0.9%)死亡,对照组在此期间没有死亡;治疗组17例出现急性加重需要住院,对照组为1例;治疗组12例出现咯血,对照组没有。一年后,两组的死亡率相当(治疗组为2.7%,对照组为2.9%),而治疗组的COPD急性加重(9.3%),咯血(6.1%),活瓣移位(4.7%)和气胸(4.2%)等并发症发生率较高。因此总体来说活瓣肺减容手术严重不良反应发生率与对照组类似,其可能导致的各项非致死性不良反应都在可接受的范围内。

2012年Ninane等报道IBV活瓣肺减容术,治疗组1人死亡,而对照组没有死亡。

2014年IBV Valve trial中死亡患者治疗组6例,对照组1例,没有器械相关性死亡。3例死因为心血管病(对照组1例为第26天死亡、治疗组2例为第95、165天死亡)。1例死亡(第82天)与COPD加重相关,进展为呼吸衰竭。1例死于胃肠道出血(第59天),另1例死于肝硬化和多器官功能衰竭(第190天)。

参 考 文 献

[1] Cetti EJ,Moore AJ,Geddes DM. Collateral ventilation. Thorax,2006,61:371-373.

[2] Gierada DS,Yusen BD,Villanuenval A,et al. Patients selection for lung volume reduction surgery:an objective model based on prior clinical decisions and quantitative CT analysis. Chest,2000,117:991-998.

[3] DJ Slebos,PL Shah,FJF Herth,et al. Endobronchial Valves for Endoscopic Lung Volume Reduction:Best Practice Recommendations from Expert Panel on Endoscopic Lung Volume Reduction Respiration,2017,93(2):138.

[4] Felix J. F. Herth,Dirk-Jan Slebos,et al. Endoscopic Lung Volume Reduction:AnExpert Panel Recommendation-Update2019. Respiration,2019,5:1-10.

[5] Come CE,Kramer MR,Dransfield MT,et al. A randomised trial of lungsealant versus medical therapy for advanced emphysema. Eur Res J,2015,46(3):651-662.

[6] Davey C,Zoumot Z,Jordan S,et al. Bronchoscopic lung volume reduction with endobronchial valves for patients with heterogeneous emphysema and intact interlobar fissures (the BeLieVeRHIFi study):a randomised controlled trial. Lancet,2015,386(9998):1066-1073.

[7] Eberhardt R,Gompelmann D,Schuhmann M,et al. Complete unilateral vs partialbilateral endoscopic lung volume reduction in patientswith bilateral lung emphysema. Chest,2012,142(4):900-908.

[8] Wood DE,Nader DA,Springmeyer SC,et al. The IBV Valve trial:a multicenter,randomized,double-blind trial of endobronchial therapy for severe emphysema. JBronchology & Interventional Pulmonology,2014,21(4):288-297.

[9] Valipour A,Slebos DJ,Herth F,et al. Endobronchial valve therapy inpatients with homogeneous emphysema:results from the IMPACT study. Am J Res CritCare Med,2016,194(9):1073-1082.

[10] Ninane V,Geltner C,Bezzi M,et al. Multicentre European study for the treatmentof advanced emphysema with bronchial valves. Eur Res J,2012,39(6):1319-1325.

13 再生医学在气道疾病中的应用

宋新宇　李时悦

气道疾病严重威胁着人类的健康,不可逆的气道损伤使这类疾病存在持续加重的特点。再生医学作为一门新兴的学科,为治疗气道疾病带来了新的思路。通过再生修复损伤细胞、调节损伤局部微环境和替代损伤组织等方式,从而重建气道的结构和功能。以间充质基质细胞、基底细胞和组织工程气管为代表的再生医学治疗工具,目前在慢性阻塞性肺疾病、闭塞性细支气管炎、支气管扩张、支气管瘘和气管狭窄等疾病治疗方面均取得了一定进展,初步证实了再生医学方案的安全性。目前,再生医学逐步应用于更多的疾病,气道疾病的临床研究也将把再生医学的应用推向新的高度。

气道是呼吸系统导气部的重要部分,按解剖位置和组织学特点分为近端气道和远端气道。气管和(左右)主支气管进入肺逐渐延伸为叶支气管、段支气管、小支气管、细支气管和终末细支气管。气管和主支气管作为近端气道,是连接喉部和肺的管状结构,对于维持通气功能有着重要的作用。以气管为例,其内侧覆盖有假复层纤毛柱状上皮,含有纤毛细胞、杯状细胞等,与局部驻留免疫细胞构成了气道的第一道屏障;另一方面,气管的C形软骨环、软骨间韧带及气管膜部平滑肌共同构成了气管独特的半刚性、半弹性结构。而远端的气道管腔变窄,假复层纤毛柱状上皮逐渐变为单层柱状上皮,纤毛细胞减少;同时,支撑的软骨环逐渐消失,以更大弹性的肌性管道替代软骨管道,以适应肺的呼吸作用。

作为与外界交通的重要结构,气道极易受到空气中病原体、有毒有害气体、颗粒和变应原等物质的刺激。气道的损伤既包括以上物质对气道结构的直接损伤,也有局部驻留的免疫细胞对其进行免疫应答后引起局部微环境紊乱和上皮复旧异常,从而出现气道损伤的疾病表现。近端气道的结构在人体内具有唯一性,尤其是气管C形软骨环,使得气管在呼吸产生的气流影响下仍维持管径不变。而发生于近端气道的疾病也多与管径缩窄以及气管结构破坏有关。这类疾病多为局部病灶,但往往损伤创面大,常规的治疗不能满足解剖重建的要求。而远端气道分布广泛,管腔窄,与呼吸性细支气管相连,更易使有害物质沉积,形成局部反复刺激,从而导致持续的炎症反应。常规的内科治疗以抗炎为主,对于复杂的免疫微环境紊乱和已经损伤严重的气道没有保护和修复作用。正是由于气道疾病病灶的解剖位置、结构和功能的特殊性,传统的治疗不能满足其功能的重建,需要运用再生医学的手段进行治疗。

再生医学(regenerative medicine)是通过生命科学、药学、材料科学和工程学等多学科交叉的手段,来创建活的功能组织的过程,用于修复或替换那些由于衰老、疾病、创伤或先天因素而失去功能的组织或器官功能。从20世纪90年代再生医学开始兴起,在许多难治性疾病中取得了突破性的进展,当中最具有代表性的就是异体造血干细胞移植治疗恶性血液系统疾病。结合气道疾病的特殊性,医学界也利用再生医学的手段对许多疾病进行了大量基础和临床研究。其主要方法包括细胞或细胞产品治疗和组织工程材料置换治疗。本文基于已经完成临床研究介绍目前再生医学在气道疾病治疗中的应用。

一、用于治疗气道疾病的再生医学工具

(一)间充质基质细胞

间充质基质细胞(Mesenchymal stromal cells,MSC)是一种可以向多种中胚层谱系分化的干细胞。20世纪60年代,有学者在体外对骨髓进行培养时发现了一群可以贴壁并形成集落生长的纤维样细胞,移植到小鼠体内分化成为成骨细胞。这群细胞除了维持骨骼的动态更新外,还通过旁分泌对造血微环境提供支持。后来证明这群细胞还可以向骨、软骨、脂肪和肌肉等方向分化。因此,也有学者称之为"间充质干细胞(Mesenchymal stem cells)"。这类细胞除了在骨髓中存在,在体内的外周血、脂肪组织、脐带、羊水、胎盘、牙髓、脾、肺、肾和表皮等组织器官的间质中也有分布,其在不同的组织微环境中发挥着不同的作用。国际细胞与基因治疗协会(International Society for Cell and Gene Therapy,ISCT)对MSC的定义如下:人源MSC须表达CD105(SH2)、CD73(SH3/4)和CD90,同时不表达CD45、CD34、CD14、CD11b、CD79a、CD19和HLA-DR,并且能在体外向成骨细胞、成软骨细胞和脂肪细胞分化。但是,不同的培养条件、供者和组织来源都会影响MSC的功能及表型。

MSC具有较强的自我更新能力。并且,因其低表达MHC Ⅰ,不表达MHC Ⅱ,不会引起T细胞活化,具有低免疫原性,异体来源MSC不会引起免疫排斥反应。自我更新能力、多向分化潜能及低免疫原性使MSC成为备受关注的干细胞。除此之外,MSC通过旁分泌细胞因子及免疫调节蛋白,对免疫细胞进行广泛的调控,具有强大的免疫

调节作用,使免疫微环境整体趋于相对稳定;也可分泌生长因子促进血管生成及内源性的干细胞再生及修复。自2004年使用MSC治疗第一例移植物抗宿主病(GVHD)以来,医学界利用MSC进行了大量自身免疫性疾病相关的治疗。目前,在GVHD、系统性红斑狼疮、克罗恩病、急性心肌梗死等疾病的治疗方面都取得了进展。

气道炎症损伤是远端气道疾病最常见的病理生理改变。外界的有害刺激和机体的自身免疫相关因素,均可以在小气道表现为不同程度炎症改变,进而引起气道损伤。但不同的刺激引起的细胞因子谱不尽相同,常规的类固醇激素仅是无选择性的抑制炎症反应。而MSC强大而广泛的对免疫微环境的调控可以更有效地完成对局部炎症的控制,同时通过旁分泌生长因子促进内源性细胞的再生。MSC向软骨的多向分化能力,也有对气道支撑结构重建的潜力。另外,肺血管血容量大,肺毛细血管网发达,具有高容量低阻力的特点,MSC经静脉给药后可以更长时间驻留在肺毛细血管中。因此,MSC在气道疾病的治疗当中有着巨大的应用潜力。

(二)基底细胞

基底细胞(basal cell,BC)分布于气管支气管树假复层纤毛柱状上皮的基底膜附近,是气道内的一种多能干细胞。在人的气道中,BC分布于整个气道直至细支气管;相反,在啮齿类动物中,BC仅局限于大气道内,散在分布于纤毛细胞、分泌细胞和神经内分泌细胞之间。在细胞表型方面,基底细胞主要通过特异性转录因子TP63、角质蛋白KRT5和KRT14及神经生长因子受体NFGR的表达来鉴定。基底细胞对整个气道内稳态和损伤后修复发挥着重要作用。为研究BC对气道上皮损伤的修复作用,一项对小鼠萘气道损伤模型的谱系追踪研究表明,BC既能自我更新,又可分化产生纤毛细胞和分泌细胞。另有报道,在流感病毒感染的小鼠模型中,感染的肺部在接受p63/krt5双阳性细胞移植后,这些细胞可分化为Ⅰ型和Ⅱ型肺细胞及细支气管分泌细胞,而p63/krt5细胞的缺失会导致修复过程的失败,从而对小鼠气道和肺造成结构和功能上的影响。Meyer等在体外培养人BCs的研究表明人支气管基底细胞在体外培养条件下能分化成气管上皮。此外,只需经气管镜刷检,研究者便能获取组织并在体外进行基底细胞的分离、扩增,在特定的培养环境中,这些细胞可在短期内大量扩增并维持其多向分化的能力,目前已形成相对稳定的工艺制备支气管基底细胞。

一般情况下,气道损伤后将会启动基底细胞修复,但在某些疾病过程中会引起基底细胞数量和群体的改变及微环境的变化。广泛的研究表明许多气道疾病,如闭塞性细支气管炎、支气管扩张和慢性阻塞性肺疾病(COPD)等疾病均提示与基底细胞的损伤、耗竭甚至变异有关。由于基底细胞具有多向分化气道上皮细胞的能力,并易于提取和扩增,结合呼吸介入技术,可以准确地将扩增后的基底细胞呈递送到损伤的气道处,来完成对损伤气道的修复。目前,我们开展了多项评估安全性和有效性的临床研究,其中部分已经取得了较好的结果。

(三)组织工程气管

组织工程气管主要指通过组织工程学构建的具有组织相容性并可充分血管化的三维结构气管,主要用于长段气管损伤的修补。其主要分为合成材料气管和同种异体脱细胞气管。合成材料气管在3D打印技术的支持下具有极高的可塑性,可针对患者具体情况个性化定制;而脱细胞气管则是通过手术或酶解将同种异体气管内表面的黏膜结构去除,避免了强免疫原性的上皮细胞引起免疫排斥作用的同时,保留了气管的机械结构,而随着对于MSC和BCs认识的加深,解决了困扰气管移植研究多年的移植段血管化及再上皮化问题,MSC更是拥有分化形成软骨组织的潜力。目前,呼吸学界在通过组织工程气管解决复杂气管病变的过程中取得了较好的短期结果,但在长期随访过程中仍暴露其存在的多项问题。

二、再生医学在气道疾病中的应用

(一)慢性阻塞性肺疾病(COPD)

COPD是一种持续不可逆气流受限为特征的小气道疾病,其主要的病理生理特点为反复存在的炎症导致小气道损伤及肺气肿。目前完成较多的是研究是利用MSC治疗COPD。大量体外细胞实验和COPD动物模型验证了MSC治疗的有效性,证明了MSC以旁分泌或直接细胞接触的方式,通过产生VEGF、HGF及EGF等细胞因子,抑制血管内皮细胞和气道上皮细胞的凋亡,促进毛细血管内皮修复及小气道结构修复;此外,通过IL-8、IL-1β和TGF-β等细胞因子促进肺泡巨噬细胞细胞从M1向M2极化,升高抗炎/抑炎因子的比例,恢复正常的蛋白酶及蛋白酶抑制剂的比例,从而改善气道的免疫微环境,抑制气道内的炎症反应。此外,随着对MSC的作用机制研究加深,科学界也对使用MSC外泌体进行了临床前研究,也有研究使用了GM-CSF等细胞因子或低氧培养环境对MSC进行预处理,这些研究取得了较好的疗效。在前期临床研究的基础之上,近些年也完成了5项MSC治疗COPD的临床研究。

2009年一项骨髓来源MSC治疗急性心肌梗死的随机、双盲、安慰剂对照的临床试验当中,MSC治疗组的患者FEV_1占预测值比例(FEV_1%)比安慰剂组明显升高,引起呼吸学界的注意。2011年巴西完成了第一例COPD细胞治疗的临床研究(NCT01110252)。这项研究所使用的并不是MSC,而是通过粒细胞集落刺激因子(G-CSF)刺激自体产生骨髓单个核细胞(BMMC),体外处理后经静脉回输$1×10^8$个BMMC完成治疗。该研究纳入4例患者,为单臂、开放标签设计。所有患者在注射MSC1个月后FEV_1%占预测值比例有所改善,但之后又出现下降。有2例患者分别在治疗后第12个月和第27个月死于院内感染,另外2例患者的FVC均较治疗前有所升高。随访持续3年,患者生存质量明显好转,患者在治疗过程中未出现与MSC有关的不良事件。虽然病例数量少,但是初步证明了MSC治疗的安全性。

2012年美国完成了一项多中心面向GOLD(COPD全球倡议)分级Ⅱ和Ⅲ级的中到重度COPD患者的Ⅰ期临床研究(NCT00683722)。该研究设计为双盲、随机分组,设置安慰剂对照,共有62例患者纳入研究。MSC治疗组患者前 4 个月每个月接受 1 次静脉输注 MSC 治疗,每次细胞用量为 1×10^8 个骨髓来源 MSC。2 年的随访结果表明,COPD 患者没有发生与 MSC 相关的不良反应,但是在肺功能、生存质量指标及 COPD 的加重频次方面两组患者没有差异。MSC 治疗后第 1 个月血清 C 反应蛋白(CRP)水平明显的下降,反映出 MSC 在抗炎方面的作用。这项研究有力地证明了 MSC 在治疗 COPD 的安全性。

2015 年荷兰完成了一项面向重度肺气肿和 $FEV_1\% < 40\%$ 的 COPD 患者的 I 期临床研究(NCT01306513)。该研究设计为单臂、开放标签,共有 10 例患者纳入研究,主要方案是,在外科肺减容术(LVRS)间隔给予 2 次自体 MSC 治疗,使用 MSC 数量为 $(1\sim2)\times10^6$ 个骨髓来源 MSC/kg 体重。患者在接受第一次 LVRS 时完成自体骨髓来源 MSC 的提取,扩增 6~10 周后通过静脉回输体内。第 1 次输注完成后 1 周完成第 2 次 MSC 输注。再经过 3 周接受第 2 次 LVRS 治疗。研究结果显示,所有患者没有发生与 MSC 相关的不良事件,经过 MSC 治疗后的肺未发生纤维化,而且经过 MSC 干预后的肺泡间质的内皮细胞的标记物 CD31 升高了 3 倍。这项临床研究证明,MSC 参与治疗重度 COPD 是安全的,但是研究者认为患者的体重增加和肺功能的改善是因为 LVRS 的原因。

2017 年巴西完成了一项面向 GOLD 分级 III 和 IV 级 COPD 患者的 I 期临床研究(NCT01872624)。该研究为单盲、随机分组,设置安慰剂对照,共有 10 例患者纳入研究。患者在接受支气管单向活瓣(EBV)置入后,EBV 联合 MSC 组同时经气道注入 10^8 个异体骨髓来源 MSC,单纯 EBV 组经气道注射等体积生理盐水。术后 90 d 内经 4 次随访,结果显示所有患者没有发生与 MSC 相关的不良反应,在 2 项生存质量评价(BODE 和 mMRC 评分)方面,EBV+MSC 组优于 EBV 组,并且 EBV+MSC 患者在第 30 天和第 90 天随访时血清 CRP 水平较单纯 EBV 组患者 CRP 水平降低。但是 6 min 步行试验(6MWT)及基础代谢率(BMI)两组之间没有差异,肺功能和胸部影像两组之间没有差异。这项研究同样证实了 MSC 治疗的安全性,CRP 的下降也反映了 MSC 在降低全身炎症反应的作用。

2020 年越南完成了首例利用脐带来源 MSC 治疗 COPD 的临床研究(ISRCTN70443938)。该研究为单臂设计,治疗使用的细胞为脐带来源 MSC,共有 20 例患者完成了这项研究。每个患者的体重以 1.5×10^6 个脐带来源 MSC/kg 的标准计算用量,经静脉输注完成治疗。治疗完成后 6 个月随访结果显示,患者在随访期内没有发生与 MSC 治疗相关的不良事件发生,相比较于治疗前,患者的 MMRC 评分、CAT 评分及加重次数均减少,但是 $FEV_1\%$、CRP 和 6MWT 较前无明显改善。这项研究证明了脐带来源 MSC 治疗 COPD 的安全性。

目前国内已开展了人自体支气管基底层细胞移植治疗重度慢性阻塞性肺气肿的实验性医学研究,目前已取得初步进展 COPD 目前治疗使用的 MSC 以骨髓来源和脐带来源为主,未完成的研究当中较多项目使用的是脂肪来源的 MSC。已经完成的研究均初步证明了 MSC 治疗 COPD 中的安全性,在患者生存质量和抗炎效果方面也取得了较好的结果,但是肺功能、影像学等方面的改善还需要继续完成更多的研究来论证。

(二)闭塞性细支气管炎

闭塞性细支气管炎(bronchiolitisobliterans,BO)是一种小气道阻塞性疾病,以远端及终末细支气管纤维化狭窄或阻塞为特征,引起持续气流受限、进行性呼吸困难。它是骨髓、肺和心肺移植的常见并发症,也见于某些肺部感染、药物不良反应、毒性气体吸入和自身免疫性疾病。当 BO 发生在肺移植后或造血干细胞移植后则被称为闭塞性细支气管炎综合征(BOS),是肺移植和造血干细胞移植后最常见的非感染性并发症之一。当前对 BO 的治疗主要是基于类固醇免疫抑制剂疗法,除了疗效差外,不良反应明显,从而增加了 BO 的死亡风险。在细胞治疗方面,目前研究较多是使用 MSC 治疗 BO。小鼠气管移植 BOS 模型的研究表明,骨髓来源的 MSCs 可调节免疫微环境,通过 MSCs 来源的 PGE2 促进巨噬细胞释放 IL-10,抑制 IL-6 和 TNF-α 的产生,从而减少炎症反应阻止 BO 进展。此外,更多的研究表明,不同来源的 MSC 对治疗小鼠气管移植模型中 BO 的发生具有保护作用,可通过调节免疫细胞功能、减少气道炎症细胞的浸润来缓解 BO。

在一项针对肺移植患者的单中心临床研究中,Keller 等向 9 例肺移植患者并发中度 BO 的患者静脉输注异体来源的骨髓来源 MSC,输注后未发生不良反应,表明其是安全且耐受性良好,但在疗效方面,细胞治疗后 1 d、7 d 和 30 d 的结果与治疗前结果相比,肺功能、气体交换能力和生化检测指标没有明显改善。但是观察过程中所有患者均未出现与 MSC 相关的不良反应。

南方医科大学南方医院 2019 年完成了一项 MSC 治疗异基因造血干细胞移植后对基础标准治疗无效 BOS 的一项多中心前瞻性队列研究。项目共纳入了 81 名患者,为开发标签设计,分为 MSC 联合基础治疗(类固醇激素和阿奇霉素)组及基础治疗组。所使用的的细胞为异体骨髓来源 MSC,根据每个患者的体重以 1.5×10^6 个 MSC/kg 体重计算细胞用量,每周经静脉输注,共进行 4 次治疗。3 个月后评估治疗效果,MSC 联合基础治疗组 $FEV_1\%$ 下降速率较基础治疗组明显减慢,同时组内患者分泌 IL-10 的 $CD5^+$ B 细胞数量明显减少。MSC 联合治疗组(71%)比基础治疗组(44%)的治疗反应率有所提高。这两组患者在感染和白血病复发率上没有差异,同时也没有发生与 MSC 治疗相关的不良反应。因此,MSC 治疗对于 BO 的具有较好的安全性,但在疗效方面,未发现 MSC 治疗可逆转 BO 的自然病史,机体的内环境、移植后患者体内复杂的免疫状态和免疫抑制药物的使用可能影响了 MSC 对 BO 逆转的潜在作用。目前的临床研究由于患者的异质性及纳入研究的病例数较少,仍需进一步更多临床研究进行验证疗效。

(三)支气管扩张症

支气管扩张症(bronchiectasis)是由多种原因引起气道管腔扩张伴有管壁纤维性增厚,这种气道变形和持续扩张由于管壁支撑结构被破坏后受到外周肺组织瘢痕牵拉所导致的,支气管壁上皮增生伴鳞状化生。该病病程迁延,并有反复感染,主要方法为对症治疗或手术切除病损,亟需探索新的治疗方法。2018年,上海肺科医院带领的团队报道了首个基底细胞移植治疗支气管扩张症患者的研究。该研究纳入了2例确诊为非囊性纤维化支气管扩张症的患者,经支气管镜将自体 SOX9⁺ 基底细胞分别注入不同的肺叶中。细胞移植治疗后患者呼吸困难、咳嗽等症状改善,运动耐力提高,肺功能检测指标如 FEV_1、FVC 和 DL-CO/VA 均有显著恢复,1位患者 CT 提示支气管扩张部位局部修复,整个随访期间未出现相关不良事件。随后,该研究团队开展进一步的研究,纳入7例非囊性纤维化支气管扩张症患者,细胞治疗后患者 FEV_1 较前有改善,患者胸部 CT 扫描未观察到支气管扩张进展,随访期间表现出良好的安全性和积极的治疗效果。目前针对干细胞治疗支气管扩张症的研究均为初步的探索性研究,纳入的患者数量相对较少,基底细胞治疗的安全性和有效性仍需更多的临床试验进行验证。

(四)支气管胸膜瘘

气管瘘同样是气管完整结构受损所导致的一类疾病,根据瘘管形成后所连通腔隙可分为气管食管瘘、支气管胸膜瘘等,多由于外伤、恶性肿瘤或手术等引起,也见于先天发育不良。这类疾病临床处理复杂,瘘口易反复感染,难以治疗。2007年报道了首例使用自体脂肪来源 MSC 成功治疗气管纵隔瘘的病例。患者因气管肿瘤出现气管纵隔瘘,大小约 10mm。使用纤维蛋白胶混合 9.8×10^6 个自体脂肪来源 MSC,经支气管镜递送于瘘口处封堵。瘘口经治疗被封堵,并出现上皮化。2年随访未出现其他并发症。

而后,Petrella 等利用山羊模型完成 MSC 治疗支气管胸膜瘘,证实 MSC 治疗比常规治疗对瘘口的愈合更有效果,MSC 通过旁分泌以及间质细胞分化使得瘘口外围成纤维细胞增殖以及纤维基质沉积从而阻塞瘘口;MSC 的抗炎作用也对于所构建的急性瘘口模型有所帮助。在此基础之上,该课题组首次在人体上使用骨髓来源 MSC 治疗支气管胸膜瘘。患者在接受右全肺切除术后发生右主支气管胸膜瘘,抽取患者骨髓提取自体骨髓来源 MSC,经支气管镜下将 10^7 MSC 注射于右主支气管残端瘘口处,60 d 后复查显示瘘口完全封闭。支气管镜活检发现瘘口形成了纤维固有层,表面覆盖鳞状上皮。之后,也有研究采用自体脂肪来源 MSC 治疗了3例支气管胸膜瘘口的患者,均取得成功。福建医科大学附属第二医院进行了我国首例脐带来源 MSC 治疗支气管胸膜瘘的工作,2×10^7 个 MSC 是用气管镜递送到大小为 5mm 的瘘口,同时静脉输注 2×10^7 个 MSC,2年随访无瘘口复发。

因此,MSC 在治疗气管瘘方面具有一定的优势,在控制复发率、并发症等方面优于常规疗法。但目前还需要更多的病例来进行安全性和疗效,同时需要更多的基础研究明确相关的治疗机制。

(五)气管/支气管狭窄

良、恶性气管/支气管狭窄是最常见的近端气道疾病,缩窄的管腔严重影响患者的正常呼吸,严重者可导致患者死亡。对于长段气管损伤的患者,手术切除过长的气管直接吻合会导致吻合口张力过高,而气管移植受限于移植物来源不足。目前主要的气管重建技术是同种异体气管移植或是通过肋软骨加强前臂桡侧皮瓣等自体组织移植。组织工程气管利用同种异体气管,结合体外脱细胞技术或合成材料气管技术,得以完成定制个性化气管支架的工作,并在临床初步得到应用。

脱细胞技术是通过手术剥离或温和的酶将同种异体气管表面高度免疫原性的黏膜组织去除,保留软骨结构,从而得到生物相容性高的脱细胞气管支架。2012 年,Elliott 等报道了脱细胞气管支架治疗一名先天气管狭窄的患者。脱细胞支架利用骨髓来源 MSC 将其包裹,然后通过加入 TGF-β 诱导分化为软骨细胞。自体上皮细胞利用补片植入到腔内,局部利用促红细胞生成素(EPO)的方式促进血管化。2年的随访显示气管移植段逐渐上皮化,支架置入使塌陷的气管保持稳定。患者身高增长,但移植段并未出现异常,并能恢复正常生活。

合成材料方面,Omori 等报道了首例合成材料气管修补案例,在聚丙烯网状管的基础上覆盖胶原海绵,在移植前将自体血液注入,共4名患者接受了此类合成材料的移植,并进行了 8~34 个月的随访,发现经过在置入后 2~22 个月的时间内,移植段上皮化情况良好。Zopf 等通过 3D 打印技术构建了可生物吸收的聚己内酯夹板用于支气管塌陷的治疗,在1年的随访期内管腔无明显狭窄。

就现有研究报道而言,组织工程气管短期内疗效显著,可以完成气道解剖重建。但需要气管介入治疗长期的支持,表明这项技术仍处于早期,对于气管机械特性、血管化、黏膜覆盖等要素已初步认识,但如血管化不足、感染、软骨细胞再生不足、再上皮化不足以及脱细胞工艺本身可能对气管结构造成的影响都需要进一步研究。MSC 和气管上皮细胞的参与虽然可以形成具有一定功能的结构,但这些"种子"细胞多大程度的参与了修复仍不清楚。

气道疾病的防治一直是呼吸学界的重大课题,因其结构和功能的特殊性,目前的治疗方案仍然不能较好的解决这一难题。干细胞治疗和组织工程材料的气管支架目前成为气道疾病治疗的两大方案。MSC 对应是解决气道的炎症损伤,BC 面向的是气道的再生修复,气管支架是为了完成大气道的重建。此外,基础研究中,包括全肺支架、肺来源的 MSC 的研发继续为临床提供着新的思路。这当中有好的结果,也有失败的案例,带给我们诸多思考。

需要利用新技术完成更深层次的机制研究指导未来的治疗方向。越来越多的基础研究发现,气道上皮细胞和微环境在反复的复旧过程中会出现偏移,从而走向疾病的表型,而这个过程是复杂的,单一的修复结构或微环境均不能使之恢复正常。炎症一直被认为是 COPD 中最核心的发病机制,但近期的一项研究表明,在 COPD 患者中,有3种变异的干细胞发生异常分化,导致气道内黏液分泌增多和气道上皮鳞状化生。这也可以为 MSC 治疗 COPD 不能改善肺功能做出一定解释,即 MSC 缓解了现存的炎症反应,但是对于这类已经异常的干细胞是没有作用的,因此气道损伤仍然存在。而这也进一步提示,在 MSC 治疗的基础之上,利用结合分子技术沉默这部分干细胞再使用 BC 重建气道上皮或许可以成为一个备选方案。另外,这种围绕再生医学的基础研究也可以为挑选合适的临床适应证提供更有力的理论依据。

需要围绕患者继续深入研究,患者的异质性和再生医学产品的一致性需要我们着重关注。所有的技术开发都是以患者为出发点,根据目前已经完成的临床研究,在进一步追加随访时间的和更大样本的患者参与研究的同时,也应把研究对象具体到每一个患者,即在已经完成的研究的患者身上寻找突破点,明确治疗成功和失败患者的原因。不仅可以对未来设计更有针对性的干细胞或产品,也可以根据疗效为适合或不适合再生医学手段干预的患者进行进一步分群,更精准地选择患者。如何利用相对宏观的临床指标选择患者是临床医师和科学家们需要进一步讨论的重点。

总体而言,再生医学为气道疾病的治疗提供了新的思路,在安全性上取得了一定程度的验证,是非常有前景的新的治疗方法,但再生医学治疗气道疾病仍然有很长的路要走。

参 考 文 献

[1] Rackley CR, Stripp BR. Building and maintaining the epithelium of the lung. The Journal of clinical investigation, 2012, 122(8): 2724-2730.

[2] Lane SW, Williams DA, Watt FM. Modulating the stem cell niche for tissue regeneration. Nature biotechnology, 2014, 32(8): 795-803.

[3] Friedenstein AJ, Petrakova KV, Kurolesova AI, et al. Heterotopic transplants of bone marrow. Transplantation, 1968, 6(2): 230-247.

[4] Ding L, Morrison SJ. Haematopoietic stem cells and early lymphoid progenitors occupy distinct bone marrow niches. Nature, 2013, 495(7440): 231-235.

[5] Crisan M, Yap S, Casteilla L, et al. A perivascular origin for mesenchymal stem cells in multiple human organs. Cell stem cell, 2008, 3(3): 301-313.

[6] Murray IR, West CC, Hardy WR, J, et al. Natural history of mesenchymal stem cells, from vessel walls to culture vessels. Cellular and Molecular Life Sciences, 2014, 71(8): 1353-1374.

[7] Dominici M, Le Blanc K, Mueller I, et al. Minimal criteria for defining multipotent mesenchymal stromal cells. The International Society for Cellular Therapy position statement Cytotherapy, 2006, 8(4): 315-317.

[8] Yin JQ, Zhu J, Ankrum JA. Manufacturing of primed mesenchymal stromal cells for therapy. Nature biomedical engineering, 2019, 3(2): 90-104.

[9] Le Blanc K, Tammik C, Rosendahl K, et al. HLA expression and immunologic propertiesof differentiated and undifferentiated mesenchymal stem cells. Experimental hematology, 2003, 31(10): 890-896.

[10] Le Blanc K, Rasmusson I, Sundberg B, et al. Treatment of severe acute graft-versus-host disease with third party haploidentical mesenchymal stem cells. The Lancet, 2004, 363(9419): 1439-1441.

[11] Cole BB, Smith RW, Jenkins KM, et al. Tracheal basal cells: a facultative progenitor cell pool. The American journal of pathology, 2010, 177(1): 362-376.

[12] Hong KU, Reynolds SD, Watkins S, et al. In vivo differentiation potential of tracheal basal cells: evidence for multipotent and unipotent subpopulations. American Journal of Physiology-Lung Cellular and Molecular Physiology, 2004, 286(4): L643-L649.

[13] Zuo W, Zhang T, Wu DZA, et al. p63+ Krt5+ distal airway stem cells are essential for lung regeneration. Nature, 2015, 517(7536): 616-620.

[14] Imai-Matsushima A, Martin-Sancho L, Karlas A, et al. Long-term culture of distal airway epithelial cells allows differentiation towards alveolar epithelial cells suited for influenza virus studies. EBioMedicine, 2018, 33: 230-241.

[15] Butler CR, Hynds RE, Gowers KH, et al. Rapid expansion of human epithelial stem cells suitable for airway tissue engineering. American journal of respiratory and critical care medicine, 2016, 194(2): 156-168.

[16] Van Niel G, d'Angelo G, Raposo G. Shedding light on the cell biology of extracellular vesicles. Nature reviews Molecular cell biology, 2018, 19(4): 213.

[17] Hare JM, Traverse JH, Henry TD, et al. A randomized, double-blind, placebo-controlled, dose-escalation study of intravenous adult human mesenchymal stem cells (prochymal) after acute myocardial infarction. Journal of the American College of Cardiology, 2009, 54(24): 2277-2286.

[18] Ribeiro-Paes JT, Bilaqui A, Greco OT, et al. Unicentric study of cell therapy in chronic obstructive pulmonary disease/pulmonary emphysema. International journal of chronic obstructive pulmonary disease, 2011, 6: 63.

[19] Weiss DJ, Casaburi R, Flannery R, et al. A placebo-controlled, randomized trial of mesenchymal stem cells in COPD. Chest, 2013, 143(6): 1590-1598.

[20] Stolk J, Broekman W, Mauad T, et al. A phase I study for intravenous autologous mesenchymal stromal cell administration to patients with severe emphysema. QJM: An International Journal of Medicine, 2016, 109(5): 331-336.

[21] de Oliveira HG, Cruz FF, Antunes MA, et al. Combined bone marrow-derived mesenchymal stromal cell therapy and one-way endobronchial valve placement in patients with pulmonary emphysema: A phase I clinical trial. Stem cells translational medicine, 2017, 6(3): 962-969.

[22] Bich PLT, Thi HN, Chau HDN, et al. Allogeneic umbilical cord-derived mesenchymal stem cell transplantation for treating chronic obstructive pulmonary disease: a pilot clinical study. Stem Cell Research & Therapy, 2020, 11(1): 1-14.

[23] Barker AF, Bergeron A, Rom WN, et al. Obliterative bronchiolitis. New England Journal of Medicine, 2014, 370(19): 1820-1828.

[24] Guo Z, Zhou X, Li J, Meng Q, et al. Mesenchymal stem cells reprogram host macrophages to attenuate obliterative bronchiolitis in murine orthotopic tracheal transplantation. International immunopharmacology, 2013, 15(4): 726-734.

[25] Keller CA, Gonwa TA, Hodge DO, et al. Feasibility, safety, and tolerance of mesenchymal stem cell therapy for obstructive chronic lung allograft dysfunction. Stem cells translational medicine, 2018, 7(2): 161-167.

[26] Chen S, Zhao K, Lin R, et al. The efficacy of mesenchymal stem cells in bronchiolitis obliterans syndrome after allogeneic HSCT: A multicenter prospective cohort study. EBioMedicine, 2019, 49: 213-222.

[27] Lesan A, Lamle AE. Short review on the diagnosis and treatment of bronchiectasis. Medicine and pharmacy reports, 2019, 92(2): 111.

[28] Ma Q, Ma Y, Dai X, et al. Regeneration of functional alveoli by adult human SOX9+ airway basal cell transplantation. Protein & cell, 2018, 9(3): 267-282.

[29] Sun F, Cheng L, Guo H, et al. Application of autologous SOX9+ airway basal cells in patients with bronchiectasis. The Clinical Respiratory Journal, 2020.

[30] Álvarez PD-A, García-Arranz M, Georgiev-Hristov T, et al. A new bronchoscopic treatment of tracheomediastinal fistula using autologous adipose-derived stem cells. Thorax, 2008, 63(4): 374-376.

[31] Petrella F, Toffalorio F, Brizzola S, et al. Stem cell transplantation effectively occludes bronchopleural fistula in an animal model. The Annals of thoracic surgery, 2014, 97(2): 480-483.

[32] Petrella F, Spaggiari L, Acocella F, et al. Airway fistula closure after stem-cell infusion. The New England Journal of Medicine, 2015, 372(1): 96-97.

[33] Álvarez PJD-A, Bellido-Reyes YA, Sánchez-Girón JG, et al. Novel bronchoscopic treatment for bronchopleural fistula using adipose-derived stromal cells. Cytotherapy, 2016, 18(1): 36-40.

[34] Aho JM, Dietz AB, Radel DJ, et al. Closure of a Recurrent Bronchopleural Fistula Using a Matrix Seeded With Patient-Derived Mesenchymal Stem Cells. Stem cells translational medicine, 2016, 5(10): 1375-1379.

[35] Zeng Y, Gao H-Z, Zhang X-B, et al. Closure of bronchopleural fistula with mesenchymal stem cells: case report and brief literature review. Respiration, 2019, 97(3): 273-276.

[36] Elliott MJ, De Coppi P, Speggiorin S, et al. Stem-cell-based, tissue engineered tracheal replacement in a child: a 2-year follow-up study. The Lancet, 2012, 380(9846): 994-1000.

[37] Omori K, Tada Y, Suzuki T, et al. Clinical application of in situ tissue engineering using a scaffolding technique for reconstruction of the larynx and trachea. Annals of Otology, Rhinology & Laryngology, 2008, 117(9): 673-678.

[38] Omori K, Nakamura T, Kanemaru S, et al. Regenerative medicine of the trachea: the first human case. Annals of Otology, Rhinology & Laryngology, 2005, 114(6): 429-433.

[39] Hornung A, Kumpf M, Baden W, et al. Realistic 3D-printed tracheobronchial tree model from a 1-year-old girl for pediatric bronchoscopy training. Respiration, 2017, 93(4): 293-295.

[40] Rao W, Wang S, Duleba M, et al. Regenerative Metaplastic Clones in COPD Lung Drive Inflammation and Fibrosis. Cell, 2020.

致知力行　继往开来　相聚2020世界支气管和介入呼吸病学大会

王广发

介入呼吸病学学组自2011年成立以来,在中华医学会领导及钟南山院士、王辰院士的关心、指导下,在呼吸学分会历任主委的领导下,在学会常委、委员的支持下,以推动我国呼吸内镜和介入呼吸病学事业健康发展为己任,以团结、包容、进取、创新的理念引导我国介入呼吸病学队伍建设,将规范、普及、提高作为学科发展的目标。倡导和崇尚民主、和谐、向上的学术氛围。目前我国基本完成了对国外技术的跟踪和全面接轨,技术规范程度大幅度提高,没有发生行业性的技术滥用,在业界对介入呼吸病学技术获得了广泛的认知和普及,并且实现了部分技术的自主创新。

遍及全国、数量众多的学术研讨会、技术培训班、动手培训项目,极大提高了我国推广呼吸内镜技术普及程度,推动了我国呼吸内镜技术的规范、普及、提高。推动了我国介入呼吸病学技术的快速发展,通过引进、吸收和自我创新,迅速填补了我国介入呼吸病学与国际水平的巨大差距,引进及创立了我国介入呼吸病学领域的众多新技术、新疗法,建立、培养、塑造了我国介入呼吸病学的优秀团队,并实现了从追踪到超越的转变,使我国站到了世界介入呼吸病学领域的前列。

过去10年,我国完成了众多介入呼吸病学技术的引进、消化和吸收,并将血管介入技术和经胸壁的介入技术纳入我国介入呼吸病学的技术范畴。在钟南山院士的直接领导下,介入学组高质量地完成了IBV肺减容的临床研究,获得了国际学术界的高度评价。硬质镜技术在我国的受到重视并获得了普及,使我国难治性中心气道狭窄的治疗治疗水平居于世界前列。内科胸腔镜技术向呼吸内科的回归,气道内超声及各类导航技术日益普及,慢性气道炎症性疾病的介入治疗也如雨后春笋,迅速在我国得到推广。使我国的介入呼吸病学技术获得了均衡、全面的发展。在良性中心气道狭窄的治疗上取得了共识,提高了水平。结合我国疑难病多、困难气道患者多的特点,完成了许多具有世界级难度的高质量创新手术。此外介入学组成员追踪技术前沿,完成了许多具有中国特色的技术创新,大大提升了我国在国际介入呼吸病学界的地位和影响力。

为规范介入呼吸病学技术,介入呼吸病学学组在过去10年致力于介入呼吸病学技术的规范化。注重中西部的技术推广及促进京津冀协同发展,技术培训和普及特别关注了新疆、内蒙、甘肃、河北等地区。完成了2019版成人诊断性可弯曲支气管镜检查术应用指南、经支气管镜冷冻活检专家共识、良性中心气道狭窄专家共识、支气管镜诊疗操作相关大出血的预防和救治专家共识、难治性气胸专家共识、活瓣肺减容专家共识、气道肿瘤光动力治疗专家共识等技术文件。2020年新冠疫情全球流行,介入学组在全球发布了首个2019新型冠状病毒感染疫情防控期间开展支气管镜诊疗指引,受到了国际学界的关注和高度评价,为新冠疫情的控制做出了贡献。在国家卫健委的领导下,以介入呼吸病学学组为骨干的专家组制定了我国呼吸内镜诊疗技术管理规范、四级呼吸内镜诊疗技术培训基地遴选标准等行业标准,并撰写了国家级的培训教材,为推动我国介入呼吸病学事业的快速、健康发展做出了突出贡献。

通过加强与国外介入呼吸病学术界的交往,通过请进来,走出去,积极开展国际间的交流合作。积极参加国际学术会议,向世界展示国际介入呼吸病学的面貌和水平。在连续两届世界支气管和介入呼吸病学大会上,我国的参会人数、投稿量均排在参会国家或地区的首位,我国的专家也多次站到国际介入呼吸病学顶尖学术讲台上作报告。随着我国介入呼吸病学技术水平的提高,获得了国际介入呼吸病学界的认可,2014年王广发教授代表中华医学会呼吸病学会,到日本京都召开的WABIP董事会进行申办陈述,以24票对1票的绝对优势成功获得了2020年世界支气管和介入呼吸病学大会的主办权,极大提升了我国在国际学界的地位。通过与国家卫生健康委国际交流中心合作,2019年开展了对外交流参访活动,即向国外学习先进的技术和管理经验,也向国外介绍中国介入呼吸病学的技术水平及经验。

一场新冠疫情席卷全球,改变了世界,也改变了我们。原定于2020年4月16—19日在上海召开的第二十一届世界支气管和介入呼吸病学大会(WCBIP,World Congress of Bronchology and Interventional Pulmonology)暨第八届中华医学会介入呼吸病学学术会议因疫情的缘故而未能按时召开。对于会期的延误,我们深表遗憾。经与WABIP

的商定，将WCBIP2020延迟至2020年11月19~22日召开，又应医学会的要求，会议将主要以虚拟会议的形势召开。这些或多或少带给我们些许遗憾。然而学术不分线上、线下，既然是国际会议，我们将一如既往地向世界展示我国介入呼吸病学的面貌和风采。对此我们进行了精心的准备。此次会议的主题是"New Land, New Scope"。"New Land"寓意为支气管和介入呼吸病学是现代呼吸病学的新领域，这一领域的最新进展是现代呼吸病学领域最为活跃的前沿之一。"New Land"也意味着WCBIP是首次在中国这样的发展中国家举办，这些国家和地区对WABIP而言是一片新的希望原野。"New Scope"代表新的内镜，意味着更多新的介入呼吸病学技术在WCBIP2020展现并会令人瞩目。"New Scope"也将意味着中国、印度等发展中国家，进入WABIP的新视野，并在这一组织内扮演越来越重要的角色。WCBIP2020也将展现介入呼吸病学领域的崭新风景，也将因众多发展中国家和地区的参与而为WABIP带来多彩、光明的明天。

此次会议收到来自34个国家和地区的稿件600余篇，是WCBIP有史以来稿件最多的一次。我国的稿件数量占到了2/3，也创造了我国参加WCBIP依赖的奇迹。相信通过与国外的交流，让世界了解我国介入呼吸病学的发展，同时也让我们看到当今世界介入呼吸病学的最新进展。大会共收到300余个学术专题的建议，从中筛选出近100多个专题，包含300多个讲题。讲者来自全球，既有叱咤介入学界的老将，又有朝气蓬勃的新秀，既有发达国家的专家，也有发展中国家的学者。其内容既有中心气道相关疾病的治疗，又有慢性气道疾病的治疗和最新肺癌微创治疗技术的进展。既有肺癌的各类诊断技术，又由冷冻肺活检等间质病相关诊断技术。既有最新的技术发明，也有规范化的技术操作。我们还将有血管介入及经胸壁的介入纳入此次会议的内容。另外，我们还将有新冠肺炎的相关研究进展。可以说，这次会议的学术内容将会琳琅满目、精彩纷呈。这次的会议企业也积极踊跃参加，卫星会、冠名专题会、企业研讨会等会议设置，将给企业展示其最新技术和产品的机会。技术操作录像展示、病例讨论将为介入呼吸病学实战提供重要的借鉴。

攀枝一树艳东风，日在珊瑚顶上红。春到岭南花不少，众芳丛里识英雄。中国的介入呼吸病学已有了长足的发展。WCIBP2020提高了一个契机，让中国的介入呼吸病学界向世界展示自己的进步与自信。我国的介入呼吸患者以自己的执着、奉献与追求，成就了我国介入呼吸病学的辉煌与荣耀。然而，前有古人，后更会有来者，相信中华医学会呼吸病学会介入呼吸病学学组的后继者们将传承优秀的学科文化，创造中国介入呼吸病学的明天，将我国介入呼吸病学事业带上新的高峰。让我们一起致知力行，继往开来，相聚WCBIP2020！